NURSING PRACTICE AND HEALTH CARE

A FOUNDATION TEXT

Third Edition

EDITED BY

Sue Hinchliff
MSc, BA, RGN, RNT
Head of Continuing Professional Development,
Royal College of Nursing of the United Kingdom

Sue Norman
RGN, NDN Cert, RNT, BEd(Hons)
Chief Executive/Registrar, United Kingdom Central
Council for Nursing, Midwifery and Health Visiting,
London

Jane Schober
MN, RGN, RCNT, DipN, DipNEd, RNT
Principal Lecturer (Nursing), De Montfort
University, Leicester

A member of the Hodder Headline Group
LONDON • SYDNEY • AUCKLAND
Co-published in the United States of America
by Oxford University Press Inc., New York

First published in Great Britain in 1989 by
Arnold, a member of the Hodder Headline Group,
338 Euston Road, London NW1 3BH

http://www.arnoldpublishers.com

Co-published in the United States of America by
Oxford University Press Inc.,
198 Madison Avenue, New York, NY 10016
Oxford is a registered trademark of Oxford University Press

Second Edition 1993
Reprinted 1994

Whilst the advice and information in this book are believed to be true and
accurate at the date of going to press, neither the editors nor the publisher
can accept any legal responsibility or liability for any errors or omissions
that may be made.

British Library Cataloguing in Publication Data
A catalogue record for this book is available from the British Library

ISBN 0 340 69230 8

Commissioning Editor: Clare Parker
Project Editor: Catherine Barnes
Production Editor: Julie Delf
Production Controller: Rose James
Cover Design: Julie Martin

Typeset in 9.5/12pt Palatino by
J&L Composition Ltd, Filey, North Yorkshire
Printed by The Alden Group, Oxford

CONTENTS

LIST OF CONTRIBUTORS   VI
FOREWORD   IX
PREFACE TO THIRD EDITION   X
ACKNOWLEDGEMENTS   XII

CHAPTER 1   NURSING TODAY AND TOMORROW   1
Jane Salvage

CHAPTER 2   THE PHILOSOPHY OF HEALTH   17
Alan Cribb

CHAPTER 3   THE SOCIAL CONTEXT OF HEALTH   35
Paul Watt and Barbara J. Harrison

CHAPTER 4   PROMOTING HEALTH   71
Sally Kendall

CHAPTER 5   PRIMARY HEALTH CARE   103
Margaret Edwards

CHAPTER 6   HOMEOSTASIS AND NATURE–NURTURE INTERACTIONS: A FRAMEWORK FOR INTEGRATING THE LIFE SCIENCES   122
John Clancy and Andrew J. McVicar

CHAPTER 7   COMMUNICATING FOR HEALTH   149
Paul Barber

CHAPTER 8   THE NATURE OF STRESS AND ITS IMPLICATIONS FOR NURSING PRACTICE   166
Elisabeth Clark and Susan E. Montague

CHAPTER 9   THE PATIENT AS A CONSUMER OF HEALTH CARE   205
Judith Chamberlain-Webber

CHAPTER 10   **MANAGING HEALTH CARE DELIVERY**   **230**
Tom Keighley

CHAPTER 11   **NURSING: ISSUES FOR EFFECTIVE PRACTICE**   **251**
Jane E. Schober

CHAPTER 12   **SPIRITUALITY**   **274**
David J. Stoter

CHAPTER 13   **ETHICS, MORALITY AND NURSING**   **291**
Verena Tschudin

CHAPTER 14   **DEVELOPING THE 'PERSON' OF THE PROFESSIONAL CARER**   **309**
Paul Barber

CHAPTER 15   **EXPERIENCING AND MANAGING PAIN: THE PATIENT–NURSE PARTNERSHIP**   **337**
Eloise C.J. Carr

CHAPTER 16   **PROVIDING A SAFE ENVIRONMENT – THE MANAGEMENT AND PREVENTION OF INFECTION**   **363**
Jennie Wilson

CHAPTER 17   **WOMEN'S HEALTH**   **396**
Mary Hamilton and Judy Reece

CHAPTER 18   **MATERNITY CARE**   **421**
Maureen D. Raynor

CHAPTER 19   **FAMILY-CENTRED CARE**   **457**
Norma Whittaker

CHAPTER 20   **NURSING'S CONTRIBUTION TO THE HEALTH CARE OF CHILDREN AND ADOLESCENTS: SOME PRINCIPLES FOR PRACTICE**   **478**
Chris Caldwell and Katy Lee

CHAPTER 21   **MENTAL HEALTH NURSING**   **515**
Stephen Firn, David L. Parker and Gregory Philip Rooney

CHAPTER 22   **CARE OF THE PERSON WITH A LEARNING DISABILITY**   **540**

David Sines

CHAPTER 23   **FIRST LINE CARE**   **565**

Marion Richardson

CHAPTER 24   **PRINCIPLES OF ADULT NURSING**   **590**

Nick Salter and Ruth Beretta

CHAPTER 25   **CARE OF ADULTS IN HOSPITAL**   **611**

Sharon L. Edwards and Kim Manley

CHAPTER 26   **CARE OF THE OLDER PERSON**   **662**

Hazel Heath

CHAPTER 27   **CARING FOR THE DYING PATIENT – PRINCIPLES OF PALLIATIVE CARE**   **692**

Penny Smith

GLOSSARY   **713**
INDEX   **727**

LIST OF CONTRIBUTORS

Paul Barber PhD, MSc, BA, RNT, RNMS, RMN, SRN
Director, School of Postgraduate Educational Studies, University of Surrey, Guildford

Ruth Beretta RGN, DipN, RNT, BSc(Hons), MA
Senior Lecturer, Department of Nursing and Midwifery, Faculty of Health and Community Studies, De Montfort University, Charles Frears Campus, Leicester

Chris Caldwell RSCN, RGN, BSc, PGDipEd, MSc
Lecturer, Royal College of Nursing Institute and Practice Development Facilitator, Guy's and St Thomas's NHS Hospital Trust, London

Eloise C.J. Carr BSc(Hons), RGN, PGCEA, RNT, MSc
Senior Lecturer, Institute of Health & Community Studies, Bournemouth University, Royal London House, Bournemouth, Dorset

Judith Chamberlain-Webber BSc(Hons) RGN
Clinical Editor, *Nursing Standard*, London

John Clancy BSc(Hon), PGCEA
Lecturer in Physiology Applied to Health, University of East Anglia, School of Health (Nursing and Midwifery), Norwich

Elisabeth Clark BA(Hons), PhD
Head of Distance Learning, Royal College of Nursing Institute, Royal College of Nursing, London

Alan Cribb PhD
Deputy Director, Centre for Public Policy Research, Kings College London, Cornwall House, London

Margaret Edwards BA(Hons), MSc, PGCE, RGN, RM, RHV, DNCert
Lecturer in Nursing, Department of Nursing Studies, Kings College London, Cornwall House, London

Sharon L. Edwards RGN, DipN(Lond), MSc, PGCEA
Senior Lecturer, University of Hertfordshire, Department of Nursing and Paramedic Sciences, Hillside House, Hatfield Campus, Hertfordshire

Stephen Firn RMN, MSc, BSc
Director of Nursing and Quality, Oxleas NHS Trust, Pinewood House, Bexley Hospital, Bexley, Kent

Mary Hamilton RGN, RM, MTO, BA, MSc
Principal Lecturer in Midwifery, Faculty of Health and Community Studies, Charles Frears Campus, Leicester

Barbara J. Harrison BA, MA
Professor of Sociology and Head of Department, University of East London, Dagenham, Essex

Hazel Heath MSc, BA(Hons), DipN(Lond), CertEd, FETC, ITEC, RGN, RCNT, RNT
Chair, Royal College of Nursing Forum for Nurses working with Older People and Independent Nurse Advisor, Loughton, Essex

Tom Keighley
Director of International Development, School of Health Care Studies, University of Leeds, Blenheim Terrace, Leeds

Sally Kendall PhD, BSc(Hons), RGN, RHV
Professor of Primary Health Care Nursing, Centre for Research in Primary Care, Newland Park Campus, Buckinghamshire Chilterns University College, Chalfont St Giles, Buckinghamshire

Katy Lee BSc, RGN, HV
Primary Health Care Nurse (Children), Chertsey, Surrey

Andrew J. McVicar BSc, PhD
Principal Lecturer, School of Health Care Practice, Anglia Polytechnic University, Chelmsford, Essex

Kim Manley MN(Wales), BA, RGN, DipN(Lond), RCNT, PGCEA
Course Director MSc in Nursing, Royal College of Nursing Institute, London

Susan E. Montague
Principal Lecturer/Scheme Tutor, Adult Nursing & Health Sciences, University of Hertfordshire, Hatfield Campus, Hatfield, Hertfordshire

David L. Parker RMN, RGN, BN, MA, CertEd
Principal Lecturer, Mental Health Nursing Specialism Leader, School of Health, University of Greenwich, London

Maureen D. Raynor RMN, RN, RM, ADM, PGCEA, MA
Midwife Teacher, Division of Midwifery, University of Nottingham, Faculty of Medicine and Health Sciences, Nottingham

Judy Reece MA, BA(Hons), RMN, RGN
Senior Lecturer in Nursing, Department of Nursing and Midwifery, Faculty of Health and Community Studies, De Montfort University, Scraptoft Campus, Leicester

Marion Richardson BD(Hons), RGN, RCNT, DipN(Lond), CertEd, RNT
Senior Lecturer, Department of Post-Registration Nursing, University of Hertfordshire, Hatfield, Hertfordshire

Gregory Philip Rooney BA(Hons), ENB 650, RMN, RNT
Lecturer/Practitioner, Oxleas NHS Trust and University of Greenwich, London

Nick Salter BSc(Hons), DipN(Lond), CertEd (Adults), RGN, RNT
Senior Lecturer and Subject Leader, Department of Nursing and Midwifery, Faculty of Health and Community Studies, De Montfort University, Scraptoft Campus, Leicester

Jane Salvage BA, MSc, RGN, HonLLD
Editor-in-chief, *Nursing Times*, London

Jane E. Schober MN, RGN, RCNT, DipN, DipNEd, RNT
Principal Lecturer, Department of Nursing and Midwifery, Faculty of Health and Community Studies, De Montfort University, Scraptoft Campus, Leicester

David Sines PhD, BSc(Hons), RMN, RNMH, PGCTHE, FRCN, RNT
Professor of Community Health Nursing and Head of School of Health Sciences, University of Ulster, Newtownabbey, County Antrim, Northern Ireland

Penny Smith RGN, RM, HV
Director of Home Care, St Christopher's Community Palliative Care Services, London

Reverend David J. Stoter AKC, JP
Manager of the Chaplaincy and Bereavement Centre, Queen's Medical Centre University Hospital Trust, Nottingham

Verena Tschudin BSc(Hons), MA, RGN, RM, DipCouns
Senior Lecturer, University of East London, London

Paul Watt BA(Hons), MSc, MPhil, CertEd
Senior Lecturer, Department of Sociology, University of East London, Essex

Norma Whittaker BA(Hons), MA, RGN, RNT, DipN, DipHS, PGD, CertEd, CMB part 1 Cert
Senior Lecturer in Nursing Studies, Department of Nursing and Midwifery, Faculty of Health and Community Studies, De Montfort University, Charles Frears Campus, Leicester

Jennie Wilson BSc(Hons), RGN
Senior Nurse, Nosocomial Infection Surveillance Unit, Central Public Health Laboratory, London

FOREWORD

The increasing complexity of nursing work requires the proper and intellectual study of the subjects which come together to provide the intelligence which makes nursing so particular and special.

There is little doubt that over the next decade nursing will continue to change and develop and respond to the requirements of new technologies and demands of practice. Nurses who are prepared through diploma and undergraduate degree programmes must be flexible, well-grounded in their subject and aware of the latest thinking in their profession. The right kind of preparation for practice must offer a blend of theoretical, clinical and reflective experiences, and the way in which these interact is important. General textbooks offering a blend of academic subjects which inform practice and help in the understanding of practice are vital to the development of students, who face a bewildering array of new experiences.

The chapters which are to be found within this text offer a comprehensive and thorough briefing, not only on the subjects which contribute to the practice of nursing, but also on those which form and assist in the planning and management of care and indeed the particular requirements of mental health, the care of children, family-centred care, maternal health and learning disability. A book such as this is difficult to write and it can be hard to balance the relevant subjects; however, what the reader will quite clearly find in this third edition is that the expert subject contributors and the editors have managed to do this with considerable skill.

Two previous editions of this highly successful text book have proved to be one of the more popular core text books for nurses working towards first level registration. The content is aimed quite deliberately at the common foundation programmes and adult branch of students undertaking the Diploma of Higher Education for Nursing. There is much within this book which is useful to students undertaking other courses, most particularly registration diplomas and degrees, and to those who have returned to nursing after a break from the profession.

Tony Butterworth
January 1998

PREFACE TO THIRD EDITION

The third edition of this foundation text reflects the numerous changes – both overt and more subtle – that have taken place in nursing over the 5 years since we prepared the second edition. Change in professional practice is most often evolutionary, and less often sudden, and so it is always a salutary experience to use the work on a new edition to contemplate the directions in which practice has advanced.

In order to help the reader to focus on change within nursing practice and wider health care policy issues we have commissioned a new start to the text, by asking Jane Salvage to move from the present to the future in her thought-provoking chapter on Nursing Today and Tomorrow.

There are two other completely new chapters. One is on Spirituality, by the Reverend David Stoter, who is well versed in the needs of health care professionals in relation to offering support, both to patients and clients and also to each other. The role of nurses in meeting the spiritual needs of those for whom they care has received less attention than it deserves, and by offering David Stoter's insights to the reader we hope to go some way towards rectifying this omission.

The other new chapter, Family-centred Care, gives a pointer to the growing acceptance of the importance and role of the family and significant others in the health of those whom we nurse.

When we were planning this edition we decided that it was not the place of a foundation text for nursing practice, such as this, to expound on the sciences that underpin care, such as psychology, physiology, pathology and sociology, and so chapters in earlier editions that related to these areas have been omitted. We have, however, retained and revised the chapters where such disciplines underpin and impinge on health issues, such as Chapter 6 on Homeostasis and Nature–Nurture Interactions and Chapter 3 on The Social Context of Health.

All the chapters that appeared in the second edition have been radically revised, and we are pleased to welcome a number of new authors to our team, who have contributed their own understandings and perceptions of the issues discussed. We are also grateful to the authors who continue to support this popular text and for their commitment to their subjects, which is reflected here.

We do not envisage that the reader would begin at the beginning of a text such as this and read through to the end, but rather that he or she would dip in and out of it as their studies and practice require. However, if the chapters are read sequentially, some apparent repetitions will be noticeable, such as several references, for example, to inequalities in health. When topics like this are revisited in different chapters it is because we feel that such reiterations are valid, important and offer fresh and differing insights to each chapter in which they appear.

The reader who is familiar with the preceding editions would not only be able to trace something of the progress in, say, primary health care or consumerism in health care – an interesting study in itself – but would also be able to make some deductions about changes in textbook design over the decade since the first edition was published.

This new edition offers a number of devices and features within the text, which, we hope, will make it easier to study, such as:

- Boxed introductions at the start of each chapter, to signpost it for the reader
- Boxed summaries at the end of sections of each chapter to help to recapitulate
- A conclusion section at each chapter end to summarise the arguments
- Chapters firmly grounded in practice to facilitate application
- The inclusion of vignettes or practice scenarios where they can illuminate the text
- Emphasis placed, where appropriate, on equal opportunities and a multi-cultural perspective

- Use of a terminal glossary for words that are not explained in the text, glossary inclusions being emboldened where they first appear
- Annotated further reading, selected to take the reader on in his or her thinking.

Finally, a new design and colour have been used within the text to make it more attractive and to highlight the features referred to above.

We hope that you will find this text both valuable and enjoyable as you use it to guide you through your studies and practice in nursing. As editors we have gained immense satisfaction from seeing the book develop through three editions alongside advances in nursing practice, education and research.

Readers should note that the views expressed are those of the individual authors and not necessarily those of the editors.

Sue Hinchliff
Sue Norman
Jane Schober

London, 1998

ACKNOWLEDGEMENTS

To reach the third edition of a learning text in a complex and rapidly changing field, such as nursing practice and health care, is a major achievement. It is the contributors who have created this success and we would like to thank warmly all those who have committed their time and expertise in writing for this text, of which we can all be proud.

CHAPTER ONE

NURSING TODAY *and* TOMORROW

Jane Salvage

- Map of this chapter
- A European overview
- Health for All
- Health care reform
- New roles and new professionalism in the UK
- An education revolution
- Looking to the future
- Conclusion

This chapter takes a panoramic view of nursing today. Starting with an overview of the political, social and health status of Europe, it locates nursing in the UK in a wider global context. WHO's Health for All movement and its emphasis on primary health care are advocated as a helpful policy framework for nursing, although a brief analysis of European health care reform suggests that these approaches are not high on the political agenda. Moving on to assess the role and influence of nursing on health care reform in Europe and the UK, the chapter reaches pessimistic conclusions. However, it points to many interesting developments that demonstrate how nursing is responding to change and being shaped by it. Special attention is paid to changes in the nursing role. Changes at the 'top' and 'bottom' of the profession, also linked with changing patterns of care delivery and a revolution in nursing education, are seen to have potentially far-reaching effects on health care and nursing.

The chapter ends with a plea for a new type of professionalism that looks beyond territorial boundaries and tunes in to the real needs of society and individuals. The weaving together by nurses and patients, in partnership, of the physical, social, emotional and spiritual domains of human life in order to create patterns of care and relationships that are truly holistic and healing is a ripe area for development.

In looking at the future, it is useful to begin by looking at the present – and the past. We need to look at the past both to learn from it and to move on from it. Our attempts to forge a better future are often tragically constrained by the baggage of the past – as current events remind us, whether close to home in Northern Ireland or in countries further afield ravaged by war. In the early 1990s, for example, euphoria over the collapse of the Berlin Wall and the totalitarian systems of Eastern Europe and the former Soviet Union rapidly turned to disillusionment, even despair, and people's intentions to live in peace and harmony evaporated almost overnight. In 1997 the UK experienced a less dramatic but nevertheless marked change of mood, from the stagnation of the last years of Conservative government to a new spirit of optimism and willingness to tackle our most intractable problems (such as the troubles in Northern Ireland) following the election of a new Labour government.

Many nurses, when they look into the future, find their mood swings confusingly between optimism and disillusionment. As the millennium approaches, speculation mounts on the future of the nursing professions and of the health care system itself. The pace of change is so rapid and the current situation so full of variety and apparently contradictory trends that it is possible to produce evidence to sustain many conflicting prophecies. This chapter develops its own speculations by looking first at the present and at some of the most striking features of the current nursing and health care scenario. It is offered not as an authoritative statement, but as a personal reflection; its ideas are drawn from experience, reading and discussion rather than a systematic literature review. The key point of concern is not the nursing profession itself, but the health needs of society and the individual people it serves – alongside a belief that a healthy profession is an important vehicle for achieving better health for all, and that the need for good nursing is universal and timeless, whatever the current configuration of lay and professional care.

MAP OF THIS CHAPTER

This chapter is written primarily for a UK readership, but any consideration of the future of British nursing cannot ignore the wider European context. Controversy continues to rage about what our relationship with continental Europe should be, and even about the definition of Europe itself. The term is often used as a synonym for the European Union (EU), currently comprising 15 member states including the UK and likely to expand further in the next few years. The EU's directives and regulations, as agreed by all member states, have a direct and indirect influence on nursing in many ways; for example, the directives on harmonisation of qualifications aim to maintain standards while enabling workforce mobility between countries, thus having an impact on nursing education in all 15 countries. A wider definition of Europe is adopted by other bodies such as the

World Health Organization (WHO), whose European Region comprises 50 member states, including the 15 successor republics of the former Soviet Union, and thus extends territorially from Greenland in the west (a dependency of Denmark) to Vladivostok in Russia's far east, and to the Mediterranean and the central Asian republics in the south.

However defined, there is no doubt that Europe will continue to be a major influence, with implications for nursing. This chapter therefore begins with an overview of the current state of Europe and its key health issues. Health care reform and the role of nursing are considered from the perspective of the WHO's goal for Health for All and its emphasis on primary health care as the means to achieve it. Current trends in UK health care and nursing are considered, paying special attention to the question of changing roles. Finally, some questions are offered for debate about the future of nursing: what strengths can the profession build on to ensure that it equips itself to meet future needs, and what areas of neglect should be addressed?

A EUROPEAN OVERVIEW

When the Cold War ended, Europe once again became whole. After the Second World War the map of Europe had been redrawn and its borders and systems remained fairly stable for 40 years, until those unprecedented changes began in the countries of Central and Eastern Europe and the former Soviet Union in the late 1980s. As the Iron Curtain lifted, countries about which those in the West knew very little took their place on the international stage once more, and we realised that our conception of 'Europe' as essentially the European Union was inadequate. Nevertheless the EU has expanded despite considerable opposition within many member states, and plays an ever greater part in national affairs. It continues to struggle with the issue of extending membership to Eastern Europe, while trying to comprehend and respond to the changes in the east which have had such a major and as yet unmeasurable impact on the rest of the continent.

Eastern Europe paid a heavy price for its gains in freedom and democracy – severe political, economic and cultural problems, which eroded the fabric of society and drove millions of ordinary people into poverty and sickness, and into migration. Years later, many of those countries are still volatile and armed conflict has taken a terrible toll in the former Yugoslavia, the Caucasus, the Russian Federation and elsewhere. The social cost of the changes continues to be enormous and it is impossible to predict where it will all lead – but we know that health and social problems do not respect national frontiers despite attempts to erect walls around the EU's Fortress Europe.

One indicator of the dramatic changes is the sudden appearance of newly independent countries and new nation states. In 1988 WHO had 32 member states in Europe, and by the 1990s it had 50 (for historical and political reasons the WHO European Region includes all 15 former USSR republics, Israel and Turkey as well as Central/Eastern Europe and the EU). When I joined WHO in 1991 it lacked not only contacts and relationships with many of those Eastern European countries, but knew little about them. Even the countries themselves lacked information, for a variety of reasons; government chief nurses, for example, might not know the true extent of common health problems or the size of their nursing workforce.

WHO's European nursing and midwifery unit spent 4 years in the early 1990s collecting data and feeding them into 46 Country Nursing and Midwifery Profiles, later summarised as a description and analysis of the current situation in Europe (Salvage and Heijnen, 1997). For the first time, nurses and others can take a comprehensive look at the real picture of nursing and midwifery across Europe, make comparisons and map trends. Now that this baseline has been established, further analysis and trend-spotting can be undertaken and it should become easier and more accurate. This information is used in this chapter to encourage understanding of British nursing in a European context. What emerges time and again is the universal nature of the issues affecting nursing, and the common and often timeless nature of the challenges it faces both in improving the quality of care and in winning recognition of its contribution to health. The vast majority of problems that are assumed to be specific to local situations turn out to be common themes elsewhere, suggesting that long-term solutions lie less in tinkering with systems than in more radical social change, for example in the position of women.

THE SOCIOPOLITICAL CONTEXT

Data on nursing and midwifery should be interpreted in the light of the overall social, political and health context of the region. Here are some of the key facts. The population of Europe (defined here as the member states of the WHO European Region) is around 842 million and expected to rise slowly. Fertility rates have fallen, marriage is becoming less frequent and divorce is increasing. The population continues to age, with a notable increase in people aged 60–79; the economically active population is also ageing. These statistics indicate complex interlocking factors stemming from sweeping social, political and cultural changes throughout the region. Traditional family and community structures are breaking down, migration to escape war and poverty is soaring, isolation and insecurity are much more marked, and stress – manifested in the growing abuse of drugs and alcohol – is high. All this and more takes its toll on people's mental and physical health (WHO, 1994).

Within nearly every country, East and West, there is a widening health gap between rich and poor; the UK is no exception, as the Black Report documented long ago (Townsend et al., 1988). While the rich minority in every country are more healthy and live longer, the larger number on low incomes are sicker and die younger. There is also a widening health gap between East and West, with people's health generally improving in the West and deteriorating in the East. In health services, there is a wide quality of care gap between West and East, caused partly by the crisis now engulfing the health care systems of eastern countries, but also partly attributable to their historical neglect of nursing and midwifery.

The WHO data show huge variation in nursing and midwifery across the region. Interestingly, as the 1995 WHO Global Expert Committee on Nursing observed, there is no direct correlation between the socio-economic condition of a country and the scope of nursing practice. In other words, the expectation that rich countries have a more powerful and effective nursing profession than poor ones is not always fulfilled. Regardless of their development status, the effective delivery of nursing services is impeded in many countries by a variety of factors. These include the following, which may sound familiar:

- The exclusion of nurses from policy making and decision making at all levels of the health care system
- Shortages of appropriately trained nurses relative to needs
- Insufficient financial support
- Undervaluing of nursing, and concomitant subordination to medicine
- Continuing gender discrimination – nursing everywhere is women's work and shares the characteristics of other female-dominated occupations, i.e. low pay, low status, poor working conditions, few prospects for promotion and poor education.

Starting points and initial conditions differ widely between countries, and so do the ways they tackle the issues, but it is possible to distinguish some emerging trends. On the positive side, there is a growing awareness throughout the European region of the need to examine the role of nursing. Attitudes towards the position of nursing in society and its role in health care are slowly changing, and the perception of nursing as a low-status occupation requiring minimal training, and the associated undervaluation of humanistic, psychosocial care, is beginning to alter, though the process is very slow and uneven. This is especially marked in the former Communist countries, where the Soviet model of health care, with its almost complete neglect of nursing, gradually superseded existing national nursing traditions. In Romania, for example, all nursing schools were closed in 1978 and were only reopened in 1991 following the overthrow of the Ceausescu regime. In the UK itself, it has taken decades of painstaking effort to secure greater autonomy for nursing, and even today the real nature of modern nursing work is barely understood outside the profession.

Meanwhile nurses, like all other health care providers, are under increasing pressure to prove they are good value for money, which has spurred greater efforts to measure the outcomes of nursing interventions (particularly in the UK and northern Europe). Both trends have promoted a growing interest in nursing education and research. Key issues include curriculum review and reorientation to primary health care; new programme development, especially in higher education; training of nurse educators and researchers; provision of high quality educational materials; continuing profes-

Table 1.1: The Health for All nurse

Nursing's mission
To help individual people, families and groups to determine and achieve their physical, mental and social potential, and to do so in the context of the environment in which they live and work.

The nurse's functions
- Promotion and maintenance of health
- Prevention of ill health
- Care during illness, rehabilitation and dying

Adapted by the author from the 1988 Vienna Declaration on Nursing (Salvage, 1993).

sional development; and closer links between education, services and research departments.

This complex picture of social, political and economic change must form the backdrop to any consideration of the future of nursing. It significantly influenced WHO programmes. The 1993 WHO publication *Nursing in Action* described visions, goals and policy guidelines that had mostly been developed during the 1980s and earlier through consensus processes involving thousands of nurses from many countries (Salvage, 1993). Its forward-thinking view of the nurse's role in helping to achieve the goals of Health for All, summarised by the author in Table 1.1, looks familiar to UK nurses but for many countries it is revolutionary. Yet the First WHO European Conference on Nursing, which laid down the framework for the future of nursing, took place in Vienna in 1988 when the epochal changes had barely begun. This provoked some hard questions as the new Europe of the 1990s took shape. Was the Vienna Declaration and subsequent WHO (and other international) guidance relevant only to Western Europe? Those visions, goals and guidelines must constantly be reviewed to ensure they are still useful. How relevant will they be in the next century?

HEALTH FOR ALL

One of the most exciting moments in my WHO career was waking up somewhere in central Asia, dazed and jetlagged, and drawing back the curtain of my 16th-floor hotel window to find a breathtaking panorama of the snow-capped Tien

Shan (Celestial Mountains) with a huge, modern building directly beneath. I was in the capital of the newly independent ex-Soviet state of Kazakhstan, a new WHO European Region member state, looking down on the Palace of Lenin, venue of the famous 1978 WHO international conference at which the Alma-Ata Declaration was agreed. Like many people, I had hardly realised that Alma-Ata was a place although I had studied the declaration, a remarkably radical statement that both captured and stimulated a new approach to health care, shifting the emphasis firmly to promoting health and preventing ill health through healthy public policy and primary health care.

By 1984 WHO's European parliament, the Regional Committee for Europe, had used the declaration as the basis of a policy framework setting out the improvements in health expected by the year 2000 and describing strategies for achieving them through healthier lifestyles, improvements in the environment, and provision of high quality health services. These strategies, it was proposed, could be implemented using a target approach: 38 Health for All targets and related indicators. The targets were intended to support the formulation of health and health care policies and their implementation in member states, and the indicators would enable comparisons between countries and the monitoring of trends.

The endorsement of this framework by all member states was very encouraging and health policy development took a big step forward. In England, it led to the *Health of the Nation* strategy which, while focusing more on an individualistic, 'lifestyles' approach to health gain than on the wider policy measures also required, was nevertheless a step in the right direction. As yet, however, there has been no real progress towards the primary target of health for all – equity. Closing the health divide by improving the health of particular population groups, at least to the level of the differences that existed at the beginning of the 1970s, is today's major challenge, in the UK and everywhere else. In the UK, important new steps are being taken to tackle it, beginning with a government review and updating of the aforementioned Black report on inequalities in health.

PRIMARY HEALTH CARE

The Alma-Ata declaration had stated that primary health care, in its fullest sense, was the route to health for all. It urged governments 'to give high priority to the full utilisation of human resources by defining the technical role, supportive skills, and attitudes required for each category of health worker according to the functions that need to be carried out to ensure effective primary health care'. This implies that nursing should be a key component of primary health care, and therefore an essential vehicle for health for all.

Today virtually all the countries of Western Europe have adopted policy goals that propose to shift health care delivery towards primary health care and closer to the community, workplace and home, with less dependence on institutional care. The primary health care approach is certainly better understood by health professionals today, but as Robinson and Elkan point out (in Salvage and Heijnen, 1997), 'there is still a need to educate policy-makers and the public at large that nursing's most effective contributions to the overall health of the population are based in the community'. Despite the rhetoric, progress in reality has been uneven and slow. Most European countries still support the hospital sector at the expense of the community, too often reinforced in poorer countries by the policies of major aid agencies and bilateral government projects. The strings attached to their loans and grants often reinforce market forces at the expense of equity and social justice; privatisation at the expense of socialised health care; and medical power at the expense of multidisciplinary work and patient power.

Many Western countries state that the development or maintenance of community nursing is a priority – with a trend towards establishing home visiting services to support ageing populations. As WHO notes, these services are well established in countries such as Scandinavia and the Netherlands, but relatively underdeveloped in others such as France, the Mediterranean and the Republic of Ireland. WHO data also show that there are relatively few nurses working in the community in the countries of Central and Eastern Europe and the former USSR, owing to poor status, pay and working conditions and a lack of relevant basic and continuing education (Salvage and Heijnen, 1997). Those countries are now beginning to redevelop primary health care services and to reassess medical and nursing roles, with promising moves to create better policy, improve training, and foster more autonomy and accountability – although results as yet are few.

COMMUNITY NURSING IN THE UK

Is community nursing in the UK in a better state of health than its European counterparts? The picture is mixed. The predicted shift of care from hospital to the community has been virtually imperceptible despite repeated rhetorical statements from government ministers about their commitment to a 'primary care-led NHS'. There are many reasons for this, including the push to reduce hospital waiting lists, the unexplained increase in emergency admissions, and the growth of the elderly population. Above all, however, it appears that the present system militates against such a shift because of the huge fixed costs of any hospital. These combine with tight budgets to guarantee that in most cases money simply cannot be released from the acute sector to fund a shift of services into the community.

At the same time, there are counteracting pressures to concentrate acute services in larger, more centralised sites. The result is that, contrary to some expectations, the great majority of NHS nurses remain hospital-based. Indeed, their role in hospitals is set to expand significantly in some areas, whereas in some community nursing services nurses have been made redundant, with cuts in school nursing causing particular concern. Yet all may not be lost. Some nurses argue that the rhetoric of a primary care-led NHS, combined with the increasingly influential role of the general practitioner in purchasing health, opens up new opportunities for nurses as direct employees of GPs or contracted workers. The number of practice nurses has risen dramatically in a few years to an estimated 20 000, despite accusations that they carry out similar functions to existing community nursing roles but with less training, and that they are a throwback to the days of doctors' handmaidens. Certainly, there now seems to be less pressure to dilute the skill mix in GP-based teams, as GPs appreciate the value of qualified nurses, and district nurses and health visitors are increasingly likely to be attached to GP practices (see Chapter 5).

Community nurses must take the initiative and show why and how they are so well placed to promote community health and demonstrate their success in securing more equitable, effective, needs-led primary care. The overall policy context is broadly more supportive of values which are important to all disciplines of community nursing. There is a greater emphasis on public health, with recognition of the importance of the collective approach; recognition of the importance of partnership and user involvement; and renewed interest in multidisciplinary working. These values have long been at the heart of community nursing, but are now much more overt in policy documents. However, policy makers are still unclear about the distinction between 'primary health care', which they too often equate with the personal medical services provided by general medical practitioners, and 'public health' with its roots in the broader vision of Alma-Ata and Health for All. Alternatively, it could be argued that they understand the distinction well enough but are unwilling to upset the powerful GP lobby.

HEALTH CARE REFORM

Primary health care in the UK and in most other countries is often described by policy makers as a key aspect of health care reform, which is a major issue nearly everywhere. In the countries of Central and Eastern Europe and the former USSR there is much debate about how far the Soviet model of health care, which dominated all those countries to a greater or lesser extent, can or should be adapted to new needs. Formidable problems are emerging from the efforts to impose rapid change – often too quickly and with incomplete understanding of the policy options, not to mention poor resources. Their concerns about how to find the right balance between public and private health care provision are echoed in Western Europe, where many if not most countries, faced with apparently endless needs and resources that cannot keep pace, are experimenting with different approaches to the structuring and financing of health care systems and the rationing of services.

The frequent reference to primary health care in this context is encouraging but seems to be rooted more in rhetoric than reality. Primary health care is difficult to organise and deliver and its successes are not easily measured in league tables and statistical indicators. It remains the poor relation of acute hospitals, who are not going to give up their lion's share of resources and prestige without a fight. In many Western countries the locus of power has shifted from hospital consultants to executive managers, whereas in the east, where the GP role barely exists, hospital doctors are still in the driving seat and regard health care reform as a synonym for privatisation, which they see as the route to improving their own income and status. Either way, west or east, nursing remains marginal and nurses are seen not as active partners in reform discussions but as subordinate workers who carry out others' orders, whether managers or doctors.

In the UK, a radical Conservative government drove health care reform forward on free market principles from the early 1990s, imposing many major changes on the health service. Yet, although many of the changes were ideologically driven, others that were regarded as part of the reform package actually arose from other motivations and other sources. Indeed, it is difficult to generalise about 'reform' for that reason. In any case, as one commentator put it, 'you never start from the Year Zero in the NHS'. Change is much more difficult than it might seem on paper because of entrenched attitudes and structures, especially in a huge 50-year-old organisation like the NHS, and lasting changes are likely to be incremental and gradual despite government attempts to force the pace. Nevertheless, it is increasingly acknowledged that health care in Europe as a whole is in a state of 'permanent transition'; although the change of UK government in 1997 signalled to many that more extreme commercialising measures would end and some changes would be reversed, or at least softened, but there will be no return to the supposedly golden days of the early NHS when most care was free at the point of delivery.

A NEW PATCHWORK OF NURSING SERVICES

One trend unlikely to be reversed in the UK is the growth of the independent health sector, which now accounts for £7.2 billion of annual spending, compared to £35.4 billion spent on the NHS (Cole,

1997) – a 1:5 ratio. Health care in the UK has always been a mixed economy but the range of providers is greater than ever and likely to grow further, with the non-profit sectors providing more services. Nurses are increasingly likely to be employed outside the NHS, whether by nursing homes, social services, charities or independent nursing agencies.

The 1:5 non-NHS:NHS expenditure ratio given above is closely matched in nursing numbers, with the independent sector in England employing 48 000 nurses compared to 238 000 in the NHS. (It is a very different story with unqualified staff, the independent sector employing 77 000 compared to just 107 000 in the NHS.) Of those 48 000 qualified nurses, 8000 were working in private hospitals in 1994 and 40 000 were in nursing and residential homes (all figures taken by Cole, 1997, from official sources where available). Private acute hospital numbers have probably reached their peak, but the nursing home sector is bound to increase significantly, fuelled by a combination of the increase in the elderly population, gradual withdrawal of the NHS from long-term care provision and new arrangements for insurance-based care. The independent sector will continue to provide a further employment option for many disillusioned NHS nurses, and may come to account for a larger and larger share of the nursing workforce. It also offers promising opportunities for innovation, as entrepreneurial nurses may find more freedom to develop nurse-led initiatives and creative new services there than in the more hidebound NHS structures – and to sell their services to individual or corporate purchasers.

FORGOTTEN RECIPES FOR SUCCESS

The major resource of every health care system, NHS and independent, is the people who work in it, yet discussion of health care reform still focuses obsessively on funding and structures. In the long run the achievements of any service will be influenced primarily not by the choice of structure or funding mechanism, important as these are, but by how well it develops, motivates and deploys its staff. The quality of the contribution of each person, from the top manager to the floor cleaner, is central to success or failure. Major reform of nursing and midwifery should therefore be an important aspect of health care transition, but it rarely is.

Although it does not grab the headlines like other measures such as the commercialisation of medicine or the emergency supply of drugs, such reform could arguably have a greater long-term impact.

Nurses and midwives, as the largest single group of health professionals in Europe, are fundamental to health care and exert great influence – even if indirectly. If the reform agenda fails to inspire them, its long-term success must be doubtful or even impossible. Around five million people work in the nursing services of the 50 WHO European member states, promoting health, preventing disease and providing care. Even the World Bank (1993), bastion of the free market, has identified nursing and midwifery personnel as the most cost-effective resource for delivering high quality public health and clinical packages. These factors link nursing's fortunes much more closely to the reform of health care systems than is usually recognised.

This presents a major challenge to every country's health services. Plans for health care reform are unlikely to succeed in isolation and in the absence of concurrent plans for the best use of human resources for health. To put the case at its most extreme, no system can work properly if its best staff have left or are demoralised and demotivated. A comprehensive national health care plan must include these issues as part of its strategy, and tackle them at the same time.

Good management is crucial to success here. People with management capabilities must be identified and trained in order to create a core of managers with modern management skills – a combination of leadership and administrative expertise. Few people, whatever their background, can automatically be good managers without extra training and in-service development. They may be doctors, nurses, other health professionals, experienced managers from other sectors, or specially recruited general management trainees. The management style of the organisation is also critical: evidence suggests that the most successful organisations are those that motivate their staff, reward them for good work, and involve them in decision making. Good management therefore includes paying attention to organisation development and to creating incentives for all staff.

One aspect of organisation development which is of special relevance when considering health care reform is the management of change. Professional and management training needs to accept change as the norm, and to give people the capacities to respond effectively in terms of the structures in which they work, the patterns of their work, the tools they use and their responses to new evidence. Organisations and individuals unable to be flexible and sensitive to change or to handle its impact on people and institutions will fail to thrive in the Europe of the future.

VALUE FOR MONEY?

The experiments prompted by health care reform and a more mixed economy of health, with not only nursing homes but other providers such as voluntary agencies playing a bigger role in health and social care, have already led to some interesting innovations. Yet, as argued above, the reformers' overriding concern with finance, and the associated structural issues, tends to focus on the historically dominant acute hospitals and medical profession, and is detrimental to nursing and midwifery, which are marginalised. Like the UK, many countries are aware of the need to tackle such issues as staff recruitment and retention, education and quality of care, but they are not generally high on the political agenda.

Ironically, though, nurses' salary costs lie at the heart of health service economics. When NHS Trusts have to balance their books substantial cuts to their workforce are inevitable, and tend to fall most heavily on the largest group of staff. Indeed, the NHS reforms and associated events have instilled a sense of Darwinian struggle for survival in those occupations which cannot easily prove their value in mathematical formulae (even medicine, traditionally exempt from such scrutiny, has started to feel the economists' hot breath on its neck). Nursing is having to justify its position as never before.

Having to prove your professional worth seems insulting to people who struggle daily in difficult circumstances to provide high quality care for little financial reward. Yet it cannot be denied that a surprisingly large proportion of the work of health care professionals – doctors, nurses, physiotherapists and others – is ineffective and even harmful. This rather shocking statement is supported by evidence from many countries, including the USA and the UK, and is probably true of most countries. Even where clear evidence exists, staff continue to use dangerous or outdated interventions, which injure patients and waste money. Perhaps it needs the brutal goad of economics to galvanise a critical mass in the professions into evidence-based practice, stimulating them to scrutinise their work to ensure that it is appropriate and effective. However, the pioneering work done by nurses on audit- and research-based practice, long before the medical profession took the issues on board, is yet another unsung story of nursing innovation.

Relevant tools include quality assurance systems, clinical audit, clinical research, strategies for research implementation, and continuing professional development. The principles underlying these interventions are relevant to any health care system and the tools can be adapted according to its stage of development. The importance of peer and patient review of the effectiveness of health care interventions also points to a new type of professionalism that emphasises working in partnership with patients and populations – and is linked to another key theme, power-sharing.

NEW ROLES AND NEW PROFESSIONALISM IN THE UK

The nursing professions have always inhabited a rather uncomfortable social space somewhere between the 'true' (i.e. male-dominated, powerful, elitist) professions such as medicine and law, proletarian occupations such as domestic work and health care assistants, and unpaid 'women's work' in the family home. This has often been regarded as a weakness, and nurse reformers have sought greater power by mimicking the institutions and culture of the true professions. Now, however, it can be seen more clearly that nursing's proletarian nature may be a source of strength and equips it much better for the future than traditional upper-middle-class occupations, whose patrician style is increasingly at odds with ordinary people's expectations and desires. As Celia Davies has brilliantly argued, 'we need a new professionalism to fit the changed circumstances in which we find ourselves at the end of the 20th century' (Davies, 1996a). She calls for reflective practice rather than mastery of knowledge; empowered patients and colleagues joining in interdependent decision processes, rather than unilateral decision making; engagement rather than detachment; and specificity of practitioners' strengths rather than interchangeability of practitioners (Davies, 1996b).

It can be argued that nursing is already moving in this direction and that some of its greatest achievements, including the small but significant caring acts which affect thousands of lives every day, spring precisely from the values and practices Davies advocates. The 'new nursing', with its emphasis on nurses' therapeutic relationships with patients, may in part represent a bid for more professional power but it has also stimulated important changes in care delivery, which give patients more power and more choice, and pays more regard to their individual needs and wishes (Salvage, 1992).

Throughout Europe, consumer demands for greater involvement and control in public services such as health care are also reflected at the macro level. Decentralisation is a strong theme of health care reform and indeed of societies in general, promising greater decision making power at local level. In the UK a good example is the trend towards devolution of greater independence to Scotland and Wales, which will also affect health services. If decentralisation is to have any beneficial effect, it means devolving authority and responsibility down to the 'lowest' possible levels. People must be given the authority to make decisions on the issues that lie within their competence, whether they are clinical, administrative or support staff. In return for giving them this authority and expecting them to be responsible and accountable for what they do, the organisation must offer them proper training and support, and respect the integrity of their decisions.

Power-sharing is not simply a matter for health service staff. Power must also be shared with the users of services. Participative care is essential for effectiveness and efficiency, not just a luxury for consumer-oriented societies. It means involving citizens directly in every stage of health care, from service planning to evaluation. It means offering them genuine choices based on full information, and evolving new styles of professional behaviour based on doing things with patients rather than to them. After all, people should really be considered not as consumers of health services but as producers of their own health. Ultimately, the major human resource of any health care system is its citizens.

CHANGING BOUNDARIES

This panoramic sweep of health, health care and nursing issues in Europe has at many points touched on the question of the nurse's role. Professions like to regard their roles as timeless, wrapped round with self-justifying rhetoric about how indispensable they are, or how they are the only ones who can provide a certain service or uphold certain values. Yet the nursing profession is a relatively new social institution, even though nursing care is as old as humanity itself. Recently, much anguished debate in UK nursing circles has focused on trying to distinguish between what aspects, attributes or values of organised nursing are indeed timeless, and what can or must change as society and its needs and demands change. This is a crucially important debate, but the pressure-cooker atmosphere in which it is conducted does not encourage calm, reasoned reflection; managerial and financial pressures have tended to force nursing into a corner, provoking the fear and uncertainty that lead to territorial defensiveness and introversion rather than a balanced consideration of fitness for purpose. In other words, the debate often starts at the wrong end – with nurses and what they do rather than with patients and what they need.

In a more logical world, many questions about role would be solved by adopting that focus on the client. Proper workforce planning would be an essential component of an effective health care strategy – not as a head-counting, number-crunching pseudo-science, but as a cool consideration of how best to ensure that the profile of the health care labour force was designed to meet people's needs for health care, and of the appropriate steps necessary to match the supply of staff to the demand. This is a complex exercise involving at least the elements shown in Table 1.2.

In real life these logical steps are hard to follow, dogged as they are at every turn by tradition, custom and practice, and vested interests. Yet the costs of ignoring them are huge. The lack of such an approach means that NHS staff will continue to be passive or resistant vessels for whatever change the decision makers want to impose, rather than active partners in the process. A recent report predicts that 'the greatest change within the acute sector will not be in the nature of hospitals, nor in the use of their sites, but in their staff'. It

Table 1.2: Some elements of successful workforce planning

- Identification of health care needs.
- Decisions about how the service aims to meet those needs.
- Clarification of the role and functions of each group of staff, including doctors, nurses, other therapists, auxiliary staff and other support workers.
- Clarification of the contribution to be made by patients, clients, families and lay carers.
- Review of educational initiatives to ensure staff, patients and carers are properly prepared for their roles.
- Planning the best mix of grades and skills in the health care team, based on the agreed role and function as well as experience of each member.
- Determining the number of staff needed in each grade, and regulating labour supply (recruitment and training) accordingly.
- Offering incentives (pay, better working conditions, development opportunities and so on) to attract and retain high quality staff.

suggests that reshaping the acute sector will require about a quarter of the total health care workforce to change their jobs over the next few years (cited in Cole, 1997). Such massive change will cause yet more chaos unless a radical new approach is taken to workforce planning and staff participation.

SKILL MIX ISSUES

Policy and managerial interest in changing roles in nursing in the UK too often focus on how to reduce costs – stirring up more fear in the profession and driving it back into its corner. Any discussion of more cost-effective staff training or deployment immediately falls foul of this defensiveness – with some justification, since deskilling and dilution of skill and/or grade mix has been too many nurses' experience. A typical example of how such attempts to open the debate can backfire was a report from the University of Manchester Health Services Management Unit (HSMU) which aimed to answer the key question: 'If we were designing the workforce today for tomorrow's health service, what would it look like?' (HSMU, 1996).

To most nurses' dismay it proposed a new generic health worker – whose core would be nursing – together with a big increase in support workers to meet the changing needs of the service. It was immediately construed as an attack on nursing (though few read the report) and as further evidence of the lack of respect and understanding of nursing skills. Interestingly, similarly radical ideas were put forward earlier in the 1990s but few have been translated into action; despite the continuing talk of multiskilling and generic health workers as well as generic nurses, there is little evidence of any widespread enthusiasm for the first two ideas. More positively, the changing political climate has spawned new pilot projects that attempt to bring staff organisations and managers together in joint initiatives looking at workforce planning and career structures.

Rumours of nursing's death may in fact have been greatly exaggerated, and the latest official workforce figures bear this out (Cole, 1997). The number of qualified nurses in the NHS fell by only 2.2% between 1989 and 1994, and the 1994 figure was only 1.3% lower than the previous year. During the same period, the number of qualified nurses in the independent sector rose by nearly 20 000, and the number of practice nurses doubled from 4600 to over 9000. In other words, the number of practising nurses across all sectors has risen by around 19 500 in England alone since 1989. The overall picture is clear: there has not been a massive increase in unqualified staff at the expense of trained nurses; in fact, the global picture is of healthy increases in both the qualified and the unqualified workforce. Even within the NHS, the reduction in qualified staff is smaller than most predicted, as is the increase in unqualified staff. It would appear that skill mix exercises have not had the Draconian impact many feared.

Why should this be? Part of the answer is that acute, labour-intensive services have not been cut back as fast as predicted. Beds may have gone, but more patients are being treated and this high throughput requires high numbers of skilled nurses. There have also been openings for nurses to take over aspects of junior doctors' roles in hospitals, and to join the ever-expanding GP practices. Over and above that, nurses remain the core of the health service workforce. Nursing is not subject to competitive tender, and it is essential in keeping the daily work of most services going. So it is difficult for managers to get to grips with radical overhaul in this area, even if they wanted to. Maybe the message that good, efficient care needs to be delivered by qualified nurses is beginning to get through.

The other factor that has altered recently is supply and demand. In the mid-1990s health authorities could pick and choose their nurses; now it is rapidly becoming a seller's market. Although the number of qualified and unqualified nursing staff has risen, the number of learners fell by 30%, which could lead to a shortfall of trained nurses at just the time when their services are in high demand. As a result managers may be forced to dilute their skill mix whether they like it or not. By the time nursing students are coming through in sufficient numbers again, the long-term damage may already have been done.

MINI-DOCTOR OR MAXI-NURSE?

The question of the nurse's role has always preoccupied the profession, partly as an expression of its insecurity and partly as a reflection of the difficulty of putting into words many of the most important values and attributes of nursing at its best. Besides, roles rarely remain unchanged for long, and the division of labour within health care has always been contentious. Alongside the efforts – real and imagined – at 'giving away' aspects of the nursing role to support workers or others in generic roles, there is a parallel readjustment of boundaries under way at the top of the practitioner scale.

Both hospital and community nursing seem to be travelling simultaneously down two different and almost contradictory paths. One focuses on taking on aspects of the doctor's role, typically including delegated medical tasks – sometimes because the doctor recognises the nurse's superior expertise, but more often because the task is routine, unpopular or time-consuming, or is easily delegated. Sometimes nurses take on medical tasks in unpopular locations, with unpopular client groups or at unsocial times such as nights and weekends. Others take on tasks that doctors do not do well, or that they see as trivial, such as giving health advice.

Where it gets confusing is that alternatively, and sometimes in the very same posts, nurses are developing genuinely innovative roles, often with underserved groups such as homeless people or sex workers; meeting care needs of people with specific conditions such as diabetes or asthma; or responding to new developments that create new needs, such as genetic counselling. Some of this work is extremely creative and research is beginning to demonstrate its value to patients. It is seen as becoming not a mini-doctor but a maxi-nurse, expanding the nurse's true nursing role.

Therefore it can be argued that there are two major areas of change, at the top and the bottom of nursing. At the most advanced and expert end of the practice spectrum, nurses are taking on ever more adventurous, unorthodox and innovative roles. The nurse practitioner in primary health care is a widely debated example but there are countless others, where the nurse uses and expands nursing expertise as a complement to the work of other professionals. Clinical specialist nurses in medically defined specialties, mental health nurses in advanced therapeutic roles, theatre nurses performing surgery, community nurses coordinating packages of care for elderly or chronically ill people all demonstrate a huge variety of skills and knowledge being attuned to patients' needs. Perhaps it does not really matter whether they are mini-doctors or maxi-nurses if patients are getting better care.

KEY INFLUENCES ON ROLE CHANGE

Such developments are made possible not only by the dynamism and intellect of individual practitioners, but by the willingness of professional colleagues to assimilate these changes and the impact on their own practice; the willingness of managers to help professionals reconfigure their services; and the willingness of patients to accept new types of service and professionals stepping beyond their traditional boundaries.

Other less altruistic factors may be equally important in shaping new roles: the long-overdue decision to reduce the number of hours worked by junior hospital doctors was implemented not by employing more doctors to make up the shortfall, but by making nurses take on some of the doctors' responsibilities. Some have done so happily, some reluctantly; some with extra training, some without. Largely unwittingly, this has opened doors that would otherwise have remained shut in most nurses' faces. Some critics see this as further exploitation of nurses and dilution of the nurse's

caring role; others see it as a gift, an unprecedented chance to revolutionise nursing practice and status.

Either way, it may with hindsight prove to be one of the biggest levers for change in late twentieth century nursing. There are exciting options on offer for those nurses who can put their case persuasively. Yet nursing has been tying itself up in knots: ever sensitive to real or imagined slights from the doctors, some bridle at the idea of being duped into doing their dirty work, even if the individual nurse finds it interesting and rewarding. In the prevailing professional paradigm, those who enjoy being medical technicians, such as nurses who have trained to perform minor operations or procedures such as endoscopy, have their authenticity challenged, as though by liking this work they are less caring or are betraying the real values of the profession.

As humans so often do when confronted with uncertainty, some sectors of nursing opinion have reacted by attempting to exert tight control over these developments – for example, by urging the regulatory body to open new registers for 'advanced' or 'expert' practitioners, with specific role descriptions and prescribed clinical and educational experience as a prerequisite for taking on these roles. While it is essential that the public is protected from inadequately prepared practitioners overstepping the limits of their competence, such moves seem to be more concerned with internal professional demarcations, rewards and jealousies than with the needs of patients.

At the other end of the spectrum, as discussed, fears are widespread that qualified nurses will be replaced by cheaper options such as health care assistants or auxiliary workers. There is nothing new in this: much if not most direct, hands-on care in institutions has always been given by unqualified staff, and the profession has continually fought to retain control of these workers and to replace them, wherever possible, with registered nurses. The evidence of the effectiveness of an all-registered nursing workforce is not extensive enough to persuade managers to invest the initial greater cost, even if the staff were available. What perhaps is more noteworthy is the growing professionalisation of the health care assistant; although numbers have not boomed as some predicted, nevertheless the growth in this group of workers is big enough to provoke the Royal College of Nursing into wondering whether they should be admitted into membership. The close approximation between NVQ level 3 in health care and pre-registration nursing education begs the question of what accreditation of prior learning or experience should be offered to those health care assistants who wish to proceed to nursing and raises tricky issues about the entry gate to the profession.

Taken together, these two trends at both ends of the profession illustrate the fluidity and complexity of nursing's professional status. As university-educated, high-flying practitioners move into semi-medical or more autonomous nursing roles, the top of the profession shifts 'upwards' (how soon before these practitioners demand comparable pay and conditions with doctors?). Meanwhile, with the cessation of enrolled nurse training, the gap at the 'bottom' is filled by health care assistants with NVQ training, by experiments with generic workers or multiskilling, and, as always, by nursing auxiliaries and other support workers: these are the people giving much, if not most, hands-on care in formal settings, casting doubt on the extent of the influence of the much-vaunted changes in care delivery methods and philosophies.

All these developments have different, even contradictory implications. In analysing them we should remember the many reasons underlying role change. Historical, class and gender factors influence the division of labour in health care more strongly than ideals: such factors include government policy decisions that have nothing to do with health; the state of the labour market; the demands/desires of the dominant profession; the demands/desires of the subordinate profession; the attitudes of the employer; the attitudes and aptitudes of the individual nurse; legal constraints; trade union pressure, including restrictive practices; and working conditions, especially for women with children/dependants. The needs of the population or the individual user are probably the least influential factor.

For whatever reason, the role of the nurse will continue to evolve. She/he will be more accountable for her/his actions and more the judge of her/his own competence; the recent UKCC guidelines for professional practice (UKCC, 1996) provide a somewhat daunting reminder of the legal and policy constraints that hedge in professional practice. The changes are undoubtedly taking some nurses into areas beyond 'traditional' nursing. They may also lead to some practitioners feeling a stronger identity with non-nurses in the same clinical field than with nurses in other clinical fields, which could have far-reaching implications for the professional identity and unity of nursing.

Meanwhile, provider institutions will continue to enjoy considerable independence in how they interpret and implement government guidance, with ever greater fragmentation of the service; a number of apparently contradictory trends could therefore coexist. For instance, skill mix exercises may well reduce the qualified workforce sharply in some areas but have no impact elsewhere; multi-skilling will be pursued by some trusts but not others; pay may vary from one part of the country to another; and some organisations will pursue a very traditional model of nursing whereas others will push the concept to its limits. It will be more and more difficult to make sustainable generalisations.

AN EDUCATION REVOLUTION

A further factor fuelling these changes is the extraordinary flowering of nursing education. The last decade saw dramatic reshaping of pre-registration programmes under the banner of Project 2000, which, despite inevitable teething problems, is beginning to produce a new generation of nurses whose education has laid the foundations of life-long learning, and who want to remain in clinical practice. Educated to diploma or degree level in higher education settings, they are confident, articulate and not content to be medical hand-maidens and will continue their professional and personal development in a variety of courses and self-directed learning experiences. Not to be outdone by the new generation of nurses, thousands of more mature nurses are taking post-registration courses and first and higher degrees, often in their own time and at their own expense. Nurses are one of the groups who study Open University courses most enthusiastically and epitomise the virtues of the democratisation of further and higher education. Few other occupational groups can surely match the educational commitment of nurses, though sometimes it springs from fear of losing your job (nurse teachers, for example) or of being left behind in the promotion race (nurse managers).

Offering both stick and carrot, the UKCC, nursing's regulatory body, took the bold step of introducing a requirement that each nurse, midwife and health visitor on the register should prove his/her entitlement to practise by providing evidence of professional updating (UKCC, 1994). The requirements of its PREP scheme for post-registration education and practice are modest enough but the move itself is revolutionary and far-reaching. It reinforces the lifelong learning commitment in a focused way and obliges employers and educators to consider how they can meet the continuing education needs of qualified staff.

This flowering of nursing education and continuing professional development has begun to raise the academic credibility and currency of nursing as well as the educational level of individual nurses. New nursing departments and research units have opened in universities, new professorial chairs have been created, and growing numbers of nurses are publishing research studies in books and scholarly journals. Fears that Project 2000 graduates would be lacking in practice skills do not appear to have been justified, despite heated and often ill-informed debate; far from being motivated only to achieve promotion into management, these graduates seem strongly committed to remaining in practice roles in the early stages of their careers.

Nevertheless, serious problems remain. The relationship of academic study to practice, and whether Project 2000 graduates are sufficiently well equipped to meet health care needs, especially in such a rapidly changing environment, are still unclear. Research into education outcomes and fitness for purpose is highly complex and as yet underdeveloped, and its findings do not necessarily point clearly to what changes should be made. Further anxieties focus on whether health service structures and attitudes are flexible enough to accommodate these new professionals; the erosion of nursing management and clinical leadership posts, although to some extent offset by new clinical specialist posts, has reduced the opportunities open to motivated and dynamic practitioners. Meanwhile, the morale of those expected to supervise and teach pre-registration students and junior practitioners is low; many who do not have academic qualifications, and lack the confidence, time or desire to acquire them, describe a feeling of being 'sidelined' by the profession, with little respect paid to their years of experience and intuitive skills.

Finally, the goal of Project 2000 was to ensure that nursing was relevant to health needs in the year 2000 and that milestone is nearly on us: will a Project 2020 soon be needed?

LOOKING TO THE FUTURE

All these issues provide endless fuel for controversy in professional nursing circles. They seem important, but nurses sometimes lose sight of the real question: what difference does all this make to patients? Does what people want from their nurses remain fundamentally unchanged, and if so, are we focusing on the right things?

The report of the so-called Heathrow debate of 1993, when the four UK government chief nurses brought together a small expert group to consider the challenges for nursing and midwifery in the twenty-first century, argued the existence of something it called 'the nursing constant', a key subset of characteristics that represented the 'fundamental attributes of a nurse' (Department of Health, 1994). 'The work of the nurse, whatever the setting, draws upon a tradition of caring, based around both skills and values,' it said. This work includes:

- A coordinating function
- A teaching function, for carers, patients and professionals
- Developing and maintaining programmes of care
- Technical expertise, exercised personally or through others
- Concern for the ill, but also for those currently well
- A special responsibility for the frail and vulnerable.

It is hard to dispute these functions, which have been extensively explored in recent years; but consider the viewpoint of other health professionals. Is there any reason why a doctor could not sign up to such a description? If, as seems very probable, there is still more that unites the health professions than divides them, a new inclusive agenda for the future, which concerns itself not so much with drawing lines between different professional territories, but with how the professions' combined skills can best meet patients' needs, could be drawn up.

REACTING AGAINST MATERIALISM

The 'nursing constant' alluded to above runs deeper than the rather functional list of values, attributes and roles listed at Heathrow. Every skilled nurse knows that the subtle processes of healing, of living with disability and of dying a good death have strong psychological, emotional and even spiritual dimensions, although they can be difficult to put into words. This is an area where nursing can really come into its own in future.

More and more people, reacting against the gross materialism and greed of the late twentieth century, are looking for a spiritual dimension in their lives; seeking healing and meaning in making deeper connections with others, in work and personal life. For a minority this may mean involvement in organised religion, but for most it takes more diffuse forms. In nursing, this spiritual revival glows in the explosion of interest in complementary therapies. From aromatherapy to massage, the ancient healing arts are putting nurses back in touch with values and experiences that are in danger of being destroyed by rapid patient throughputs, cash crises and staff shortages. Indeed, in combination with the deceptively simple acts of 'basic' nursing care, they give nurses the chance to practise the interpersonal and technical skills that attracted them to nursing in the first place.

Nursing's achievements, in complementary therapies and in more mainstream domains, epitomise the type of skills, knowledge and attitudes that could be heavily in demand come the millennium. In fact they are heavily in demand now, but society and individuals are still too frightened to acknowledge openly the depth of their need. As the pendulum swings back to humanitarian values, nursing will be increasingly appreciated – not patronisingly, but a true appreciation, at last, of the fact that people's physical, intellectual, emotional and spiritual faculties are intertwined, and that caring for another person means paying attention to all those dimensions and their interaction.

Nursing can lead itself and others in that humane direction, but only if nurses can get in touch with their own power and believe in their own potential. This requires what has been dubbed the 'remoralisation' of nursing, in both its meanings: raising morale but also reinforcing the moral roots of the profession. This will not be a restrictive Victorian morality, but a reaffirmation of the key values shared by many in every health care occupation and by many service users and carers. It could form the basis of alliances across professional, gender, race, class and cultural divides, in projects and ways of working that not only tolerate but also celebrate differences while developing shared visions and goals.

BEYOND ORTHODOX POLITICS

In their necessary efforts to make the world sit up and take notice of them, nurses have emphasised their uniqueness. Healthy self-esteem is essential, but this focus on uniqueness has sometimes been a mask for insecurity. It is time to adopt a different strategy, not least because nurses do not have a monopoly on caring, and such statements alienate potential allies among patients, carers, support workers and other professionals. As argued above, we need a revitalised form of professionalism that empowers patients and involves all colleagues in an interdependent decision making process that sees responsibility as collective as well as individual.

This does not mean nurses can give up the more orthodox forms of political activity where they have made such great strides. Strong professional organisations, trade unions and networks are still vital to fight for nurses' rights, influence decision making and court public opinion. Better pay, working conditions and child care, better staffing levels, improved education, adequate research funds, a functioning clinical career structure and representation of nurses at the highest levels of management and policy making are all important aims to be fought for relentlessly.

Not much headway will be made, however, unless nursing in the next century works on the issues raised by the new professionalism, such as how to develop specific practitioner strengths without retreating into tribalism, and how to share decision making with clients and communities. In doing so nurses should remember that they may sometimes feel weak but are actually, in many ways, strong. Nursing is the biggest health profession (and the oldest); health services would collapse without it, it enjoys enormous public support and most of the time it provides excellent service.

CONCLUSION

This chapter has taken a panoramic view of nursing today. Starting with an overview of the current political, social and health status of Europe, it has attempted to locate nursing in the UK in a wider global context. WHO's Health for All movement and its emphasis on primary health care have been advocated as a helpful policy framework for nursing. However, despite lip-service to it, a brief analysis of European health care reform shows that Health for All and primary health care are not high on the agenda.

Moving on to assess the role and influence of nursing on health care reform in Europe and the UK, this chapter reaches pessimistic conclusions. However, it points to many interesting developments that demonstrate how nursing is responding to change – and being shaped by it, willingly or not. Special attention is paid to the prevailing preoccupation with changes in the nursing role, which is not a new phenomenon but has special and current interest. Changes at the 'top' and 'bottom' of the profession, also linked with changing patterns of care delivery and a revolution in nursing education, are seen to have potentially far-reaching effects on health care and nursing.

Finally, this chapter ends with a plea for a new type of professionalism that looks beyond territorial boundaries and tunes in to the real needs of society and individuals. One area seen as ripe for development is the weaving together by nurses and patients, in partnership, of the physical, social, emotional and spiritual domains of human life in order to create patterns of care and relationships that are truly holistic and healing.

Peering into the crystal ball may not reveal a clear future, but it shows us that nursing will always be needed, and that its dearest values may

be about to make a big comeback. Our troubled world badly needs them.

REFERENCES

Cole, A. (1997). The state we're in. *Nursing Times*, 93(4), 24–7.

Davies, C. (1996a). Cloaked in a tattered illusion. *Nursing Times*, 92(45), 44–6.

Davies, C. (1996b). A new vision of professionalism. *Nursing Times*, 92(46), 54–6.

Department of Health (1994). *The Challenges for Nursing and Midwifery in the 21st Century. The Heathrow Debate, May 1993.* Department of Health, London.

HSMU (1996). *The Future Health Care Workforce.* HSMU, University of Manchester, Manchester.

Salvage, J. (1992). The new nursing: empowering patients or empowering nurses? In *Policy Issues in Nursing*, Robinson, J., Gray, A. and Elkan, R. (eds). Open University Press, Buckingham.

Salvage, J. (ed.) (1993). *Nursing in Action: Strengthening Nursing and Midwifery to Support Health for All.* World Health Organization Regional Publications, European Series No. 48. WHO, Copenhagen.

Salvage, J. and Heijnen, S. (eds) (1997). *Nursing in Europe: A Resource for Better Health.* World Health Organization Regional Publications, European Series No. 74. WHO, Copenhagen.

Townsend, P., Davidson, N. and Whitehead, M. (1988). *Inequalities in Health: The Black Report and The Health Divide.* Penguin, Harmondsworth.

UKCC (1994). *Post Registration Education and Practice.* UKCC, London.

UKCC (1996). *Guidelines for Professional Practice.* UKCC, London.

WHO (1994). *Health in Europe.* WHO Regional Publications, European Series No. 56. WHO, Copenhagen.

WHO (1995). *Report of the Global Expert Committee on Nursing.* WHO, Geneva.

World Bank (1993). *Investing in Health.* World Development Report. Oxford University Press, New York.

CHAPTER TWO

THE PHILOSOPHY *of* HEALTH

A l a n   C r i b b

■ Introduction
■ Healthy things
■ Conceptions of health – negative, positive, broad and narrow
■ Holism
■ What is well-being?
■ The subjective perspective
■ Social well-being
■ What is health?
■ Assessing ill health and quality of life
■ Conclusion

The main aim of this chapter is to ask fundamental questions about the meaning of health and the ways in which our ideas about health affect health care and health policy. It considers the advantages and disadvantages of using different ideas about health, including, for example, 'broad' versus 'narrow', or 'positive' versus 'negative' ideas. The importance of these issues for measuring health is set out. The chapter presents the arguments but the reader is invited to come to his/her own conclusions about key questions:

■ Is health something objective or a matter of subjective judgement?
■ Is health absence of disease, or well-being, or something in between the two?

INTRODUCTION

This chapter is about two things. It is about the idea of health and it is about the process of trying to understand this idea. Ideas shape everything we do. Our personal ideas about what matters shape our individual lives; and social ideas shape the institutions and cultures in which we live and work. This certainly applies in the world of health care where most people spend their lives working in settings in which ideas are built into the system. Their objectives, the shape of their day and their every task are defined by other people's (e.g. policy makers', manager's) ideas about what matters. One thing we can do, to lessen this domination, is to spend some time reflecting on these

ideas, where they come from, and how far they make sense to us.

Vast quantities of time, energy and resources are spent in the name of ideas like 'health' and 'well-being'. Yet, if we were to ask what these ideas mean, most of us would probably look blank; furthermore we might be accused of fussing. 'Never mind what they *mean*, let's go on and do some work!' I have a lot of sympathy with this attitude but I do not believe it can be left at that. We still have to decide what sort of work health workers should do. How far, for example, should health workers spend time 'just talking' to people, or getting involved in community projects? Or are these things on the margins of health care? One way of approaching questions like this, and I stress only one way, is to ask about the meaning of health. What is it that health workers are trying to bring about: what is health?

The obvious problem is that different people have different ideas about what health is. Different groups of professionals, and different individuals inside and outside health care, all tend to disagree. It has become customary in situations like this to ask for a definition. Unfortunately, this is to misunderstand the situation in two important respects. First, definitions only work within a framework of agreement. If a number of people get together and agree to define the word 'paper' in a certain way, this may prove to be useful, providing they do not expect others automatically to change the way they use the word. (As part of a scientific community this can work well, and these are called **stipulative definitions**.) Second, the whole business of definition does not work well with words that refer to some abstract social concepts like 'equality', 'happiness' or 'health'. These concepts, which are closely tied in with people's emotions and values, have the characteristic of having a number of conflicting meanings. They are inherently debatable or, to use the technical expression of philosophy, *essentially contestable* (Gallie, 1964). That is, we cannot reduce their meaning to a single definition without taking sides in an important debate. Any stipulative definition would not only be ignored by others, but would be attacked for missing 'the real meaning' of the concept.

Thus in what follows I will not be looking for the definition of health but rather exploring its meanings.

Box 2.1

In this chapter I will only really consider three kinds of definition in depth:

- Health as absence of disease
- Health as well-being
- Health as personal capacity or resources for living.

I will normally use the word **conception** rather than the word definition. This is a word philosophers use to stand for the different meanings of a complex concept. It is a broader term than definition, and, unlike the latter, it makes no claim to be definitive in the sense of universal or final. It is possible for the same person to operate with several different conceptions of health, although they

may have a preferred one. Indeed, I shall argue that this would be to their advantage.

However, this chapter is not simply going to be a catalogue of the meanings of health. It is also about the process of clarifying these meanings and it raises a host of surrounding questions such as: 'How should we think about health, what attitudes, what types of knowledge are required?' 'What are the implications of thinking about health for health care policy and practice?'

Key Points

- Exploring the meanings of health is one way of shedding light on the nature of health care and the work of health professionals.
- It is not possible to have an agreed definition of health; rather there are different conceptions of health each of which 'tells a different story'.

HEALTHY THINGS

Let us begin with a question which looks superficially the same as 'What is health?' but is in fact different: What do we mean by the word 'healthy'?

Many things are said to be 'healthy'. A run round the park, wholesome food, a glowing complexion, our pets or plants. Aristotle distinguished between the different senses of the word and also explained that all these senses are related:

'Everything which is healthy is related to health, one thing in the sense that it preserves health, another in the sense that it produces it, another in the sense that it is a symptom of health, another because it is capable of it.'

(Aristotle, 1941, page 732)

Some things preserve or produce health, and some things are symptoms of health. But this does not tell us what health is. Aristotle's other category takes us a little further by indicating that only some sorts of things are capable of having health. Thus pets, plants and people can literally be healthy whereas rocks, watches and tables cannot be. We can think of ways in which watches, for example, might be described as healthy in a metaphorical sense, but we normally reserve the word 'health' for living things. Health and life are inextricably linked.

If we think of biological characteristics of life – movement, reproduction, exchange with the environment, and growth – we see immediately that there are many things that can affect the quality of life. A rock does not share any of these characteristics, does not perform any complicated functions, does not have a biological identity, does not have any potential to realise and consequently cannot fail to realise potential.

Watches, and other designed objects, only have some of these characteristics. Objects can be good *for a task*, a rock may make a good doorstop, a table may be well or badly designed to do its job, but these things cannot simply *be* well. Living things can also perform tasks but in addition to this their life systems can work well (or badly), i.e. they are 'beings' which can *be* well or healthy. This gives us an idea of what it is to have health. But someone might object that this is too limited an idea. The account so far equates health with good biological functioning, but – the objector might say – for humans functioning and growth are not merely biological; they involve the functioning and growth of personality, of projects, of goals and of autonomy.

If we are to seek to understand the 'good functioning' of a person, we need to consider more than biology; likewise, the causes and effects of 'good personal functioning' or 'well-being' will be much broader than the causes and effects of good biological functioning. The causes or determinants of good biological functioning are broad-ranging and include our genetic make-up, behaviours, relationships, and physical and social environment. But the range of causes relevant to our functioning successfully as a person is almost unlimited. Certainly, factors such as architecture, music, religion, as well as politics and economics (and all the others relating to biological health) seem potentially relevant. This is what lies behind the debate about narrow versus broad conceptions of health (which should not be confused with the debate about so-called 'negative' versus 'positive' conceptions of health, see below).

Health can be used to refer to a relatively narrow range of characteristics – roughly all those characteristics which humans share with plants and other animals. Alternatively, it can be used to refer to a very wide range of characteristics such that we talk about things like a healthy personality or even a healthy attitude to life. Some people

will only feel comfortable with the narrow usage and see the broader one as a kind of metaphorical extension of it. Others will take the broader usage to be equally valid.

> **Box 2.2**
>
> The examples with which we began all relate to the narrow conception of health. A run round the park preserves or produces health. The person who runs can possess health, and a glowing complexion can be a sign of health. We could call these three ways to be healthy:
>
> - 'Health causing'
> - 'Health possessing'
> - 'Health enjoying'.

Many attempts to understand what it is to be healthy fail because they do not distinguish these different senses. It is worth noting that a person can be healthy in all three ways. If the parts of their life systems (e.g. their kidneys) are working well, these are healthy ('health causing' to the person); the person can function well as a whole (possess health), and thereby experience a high quality of life (be 'health enjoying').

> **Key Points**
>
> - Only living things can possess health although many other things are related to health (e.g. by causing or undermining health).
> - Health refers to something like 'the good functioning and development' of living things; but the good functioning of people involves a lot more than biology.

CONCEPTIONS OF HEALTH – NEGATIVE, POSITIVE, BROAD AND NARROW

A negative conception of something is a picture of what it is not. To paint a negative picture of poverty we might talk about the characteristics of wealth. Wealth allows people choices, it enables them to live in comfort, it gives them some sense of security about the future. To be poor is not to have any wealth, it is not to be able to enjoy any of these benefits. Similarly, there is a tradition in theology that talks about God in negative terms. He is not made of matter, He is not petty or selfish. Again, political activists sometimes talk about an ideal future society in negative terms. There will be no oppression, no prejudice and no discrimination. In some cases it is because of the lack of an appropriate language in which to couch a positive description that a negative one is used. Sometimes it is because a state of affairs is largely understood as the absence of something, as poverty is the absence of money, that a negative description seems appropriate. Some people define health this way:

'As a physician, I am content to define health as the absence of disease.'

(Scadding, 1988)

This is a negative, and also a narrow, conception of health. It suggests that a living creature is healthy to the extent that it does not suffer from diseases or disability. It is a very clear and useful definition, and we should not be put off it completely just because it is fashionable (in some circles) to dismiss it.

It is possible to demonstrate its usefulness by making a simple analogy. Imagine someone employed to test and report the quality of jigsaw puzzles. He/she has to put each one together and jot down any comments. It is not difficult to imagine him/her ending up with two piles of boxes. In one pile every box would have 'fine' or 'OK' marked on it, but the other pile would contain a range of labels – 'missing pieces', 'broken pieces', 'mis-shapen pieces', 'the wrong pieces', and so on. On the face of it there is not much to be said about the good quality puzzles but much more to be said about the puzzles that fall short in some way. There are countless ways that a person can fall short of being 'fine'. The whole of medicine depends on the careful cataloguing and description of types of disease and disability. To define health as the absence of disease is to put the emphasis on the traditional role of medicine, i.e. the prevention, cure or alleviation of diseases. It also serves to rule out speculation about 'health' as some kind of mysterious substance or process. Just as darkness is not a special kind of stuff, but only the absence of light, health is just another word for being disease-free.

We can imagine negative but broader conceptions of health although they are not employed as commonly. There are many ways in which people can fall short of being 'fine' that do not amount to diseases. People can be ignorant, or confused, or frightened, or alienated, or exhausted, and so on, and we might wish to conceive of health as the absence of these 'disabling states'. Are the narrow or the broader negative conceptions enough?

Let us take the narrow negative one first. Surely health is not exactly like darkness in being only an absence of something? A brick wall is disease-free but it is not thereby healthy. Health, thought of as good biological functioning, can be catalogued and described in the same way as diseases. Indeed, the two processes of description are inseparable. Just as it would be impossible to recognise a poor jigsaw puzzle without having a picture of what a good jigsaw puzzle should be, it is impossible to understand disease without at the same time having an understanding of a healthy organism. They are two sides of the same coin. So when health is seen as the absence of disease a normal background state of affairs is presupposed. This background norm can be summarised as 'biological fitness and efficient functioning'. It is a positive conception of health, a conception which aims to inform us about what health is, not simply what it is not.

It is, however, much more problematic to articulate a broad positive conception of health. Having noted that there are many ways in which a person can fall short of being 'fine', can we say what it is to be fine, to be functioning well, not just biologically, but as a person? Does it not follow from the above arguments that here, too, we must have some picture of a normal or satisfactory state of affairs if we are prepared to identify certain states as falling short of it? This is what is often referred to as 'positive health' or 'personal and social health' and distinguished from a so-called medical model of health which equates health with freedom from disease. Another way in which this point is made is to talk about the merits of a holistic approach, or a holistic conception of health. There is a danger here of confusing two distinct points. It is possible to advocate a holistic approach without necessarily wishing to *define* health in a very broad way. In the next section we will look at a holistic approach, and in the following one at a 'holistic definition', i.e. a broad positive conception of health which equates health with well-being.

Key Points

- A narrow negative conception of health is one which defines health as the absence of 'bad functioning' understood narrowly, e.g. health is the absence of disease.
- A broad negative conception of health is one which defines health as the absence of 'bad functioning' understood broadly, e.g. health is having 'nothing wrong with you' – not being distressed, confused, sick, and so on.
- A narrow positive conception of health is one which equates health with some relatively narrow set of good attributes, e.g. health is biological fitness and efficient functioning.
- A broad positive conception of health is one which equates health with a relatively open-ended set of good attributes, e.g. health is being happy, well-balanced, fulfilled, and so on.

HOLISM

Holism means paying regard to the whole. At one level this means we should not treat the different physical systems of the body as if they were really separate because in fact they make up an interconnected whole. It also means that we should not treat individuals as if they were separate from their immediate or total environment. For some practical purposes we can behave as if these separations were possible but unless we appreciate the artificiality of these distinctions we will never understand health.

At another level to pay regard to the whole means recognising that persons are part of a range of systems, not all of which are physical. It is now commonplace to hear about psychosocial factors in health and disease. These relate to the psychological and social components in the lives of people. Those who advocate holism are usually drawing our attention to the importance of these components. If we wish to look after people, it would be absurd not to have a concern for their states of mind, their relationships or their social circumstances. Yet a large part of what is intended in the critique of 'the medical model' is to say that this is precisely what can happen if we become narrowly focused on the need to diagnose and treat disease.

The narrow focus can come about in a number of different ways. It is sensible for health workers to focus on diseases; this is often the major preoccupation of all parties. The patient's life may be threatened, he/she may be in pain or substantially incapacitated. A high priority has to be attached to addressing these issues. It is not surprising that individual health workers get into the habit of giving these issues priority and then sometimes do so when it is inappropriate. But it is too simple to see this only as a product of individual habit formation; it is normally a product of systems or policies of care. Take, for example, the case of screening for breast cancer. Here an elaborate system has been developed to enable the early detection and treatment of breast cancer. This is an expensive, and an administratively and technically sophisticated, task. It would be a waste of a good deal of human resources if it failed in its chief objective of early detection, and this must be the priority of the service. Yet, by its very nature, its clients are well women who have social and psychological needs other than those relating to breast cancer, and for whom an invitation to screening may be experienced as an additional burden, and a source of disquiet or alarm. A holistic service would attempt to give a certain priority to meeting these concerns as well as the clinical ones, and fortunately these issues were considered in the planning of the UK Breast Screening Programme (Gray and Austoker, 1989), but it is easy in this case to see that the service is essentially a disease-centred one. The same is true of most other systems and policies of the health service, leading to the much repeated complaint that it is really a 'disease service'.

We have added psychological and social components to biological ones. But this still treats people as complicated objects made up of interacting systems; it does not seem to treat them as themselves.

Box 2.3: Reflection

Imagine someone who studied health sciences and systems coming up to you and saying: 'I understand what makes you tick.' What would he/she have to know about? He/she would presumably know something about biochemistry, anatomy and physiology. He/she would have to know something about psychology, sociology and other human sciences. Perhaps he/she has gone further and has interviewed your family, friends, teachers and so on. He/she now claims to be an expert on you. How would that claim make you feel? Despite the attention, it would make most people feel strangely disregarded. Not only because someone had gone behind their back but also because they had been treated merely as an object of investigation, not as a full person. After all, you would expect to be consulted about who you are; you probably feel as if you are the expert about yourself.

Here we are touching on a very deep problem about the scientific study of humans. To see someone as conforming to scientific generalisations is to some extent to 'reduce' their behaviour to these generalisations. **Reductionism** is the opposite of holism. There are times when it is useful and even necessary, but it can also lead to a dangerous partial-sightedness. The so-called medical model is criticised when it reduces people to bearers of disease. But merely adding on psychological and social models does not get rid of reductionism. It is still possible to reduce a person to 'an introvert' or 'a single, white, middle-aged male', etc. Individuals are individuals, and we have our own sense of who and what we are; we are subjects as well as objects. Whatever we may say when we are being 'intellectual', we do not feel in our bones that our life and behaviour can be entirely explained by the generalisations of science; we feel that we are at least partly authors of our own life, and expect to be treated as such.

Thus a holistic stance entails bringing more and more into our gaze. Ultimately, it means we have to encounter the person with whom we are dealing. As we enlarge our perspective, something new comes into focus. We move from a cold consideration of arrangements of matter to a meeting with a person, an equal who looks back at us with his/her own interests and concerns in mind.

Hence systems of care can fail to be holistic if they neglect properly to consider the psychological and social needs of people. But they can also fail to be holistic if they neglect to meet properly the individual concerns and needs as felt by, and voiced by, those who are receiving care. No system of care can claim to be holistic if it leaves the individual person (on his or her own terms) out of the picture.

It is because of the merits of a holistic approach that some people advocate the use of a holistic, or very broad, conception of health. The most

famous of such conceptions is offered in the World Health Organization Constitution:

'Health is a state of complete physical, mental and social well-being and not merely the absence of disease and infirmity.'

(WHO, 1947)

If we put aside the word 'complete', which would entail that nobody could ever qualify as healthy, this is another very useful, although rather imprecise, definition. It offers a broad and positive conception of health. It equates health with well-being and it makes clear that this involves a good deal more than physical well-being or good biological functioning. But it does not make clear exactly what this 'more' is.

Hopefully, everyone is agreed that when we are dealing with people we should have regard to their whole well-being and not just their physical health. However, it does not follow from this belief that we must operate with a holistic conception of health. Some people may prefer to restrict the use of the word 'health' to the narrower conceptions and use other words, like well-being or welfare, to stand for the broader ones. There are advantages and disadvantages to both approaches. Using a broad conception of health makes it more difficult to fall into the trap of reducing people to mere bodies, but it can mean that health professionals lose sight of the limits to their responsibility and expertise in an effort to look after 'the whole person'. On the other hand, using a narrow conception keeps the focus on definite objectives, but this tends to be at the expense of reductionism.

Key Points

- A holistic approach to health care sees people as complex wholes who need to be understood both in their social context and from their own personal standpoint.
- It is possible to take a holistic approach to health care without subscribing to a holistic, or broad, conception of health.

WHAT IS WELL-BEING?

What is well-being? This is a question that has been asked in many different forms through the centuries, and it is a question that each of us asks in our own way whenever we make major decisions in our life. What is a good life, a happy life, a full life? What is it to be fulfilled, to flourish, to make the most of things? I will not pretend to answer it here but rather to point to certain aspects of its scope and complexity. It is a very demanding question but at the same time it is a question that anyone who claims to care for people must confront.

A fashionable answer would be to say that a person's well-being is whatever he or she chooses it to be. You may value some things, I may value others. It is a matter of opinion, or subjective judgement. This is the kind of thing a child might say to his/her parents: 'You have your ideas about what's good for me, I have mine.' In many ways the view that it is all subjective seems plausible, yet it cannot be entirely right. The expression 'one man's meat is another man's poison' is used to sum up this stance, but we also know that in most cases this expression is not *literally* true. In broad terms, it is possible to say what substances are poisonous to human beings, and these things are normally poisonous to all human beings. We would regard somebody who said that he/she could choose what was a poison as being stupid, as trying to ignore objective facts.

So it looks as if the answer to 'what is well-being' is partly subjective and partly objective. This is one reason for using a fairly narrow and biological conception of health. Here it is possible to generalise about what is good and bad. Humans have a definite physical constitution, which has to be respected. At the other extreme there are many areas, such as our choice of wallpaper, where it seems clear we are dealing with subjective judgements about what suits us. This suggests we can divide the answer to the question about well-being into two parts – a part to do with facts and a part to do with values. It could be said that whether or not we identify our well-being with our family or money, etc., is a matter of values but that there are certain things, such as food and shelter, which are simply good as a matter of fact. The further we move away from the biological facts of life, the further we get into the realm of personal beliefs and values. Perhaps the best example of this is religious belief. Some Christians, for example, believe that no-one can be fully well unless he/she has come to accept the 'Good News' of Christianity, and this remains so no matter how physically healthy

he/she is, or how well he/she may feel. (Note that it may be essential to understand this if you knew you were caring for such a person.)

But this distinction between factual judgements and value judgements is too simple-minded, as a closer look at examples shows. The Christian and the atheist are not merely agreeing to differ over personal values: they are disagreeing about what the facts are. The former is claiming that it is objectively the case that human welfare will be improved by recognising the existence of God, the latter is claiming that there is no God. It is difficult to imagine a more important disagreement. For our purposes this disagreement also indicates something important. It indicates the sheer scope of the question about well-being, and that it is possible to subscribe to very broad conceptions of well-being as being of general, and not merely personal, applicability. Many people, and perhaps all of us to some extent, feel that we can make judgements about what would improve someone else's well-being that extend beyond the remit of biological science. Indeed, there is a long tradition, rooted in classical philosophy, of debating the nature of the good life. Plato debated the relative merits of a life based on the pursuit of pleasure, the pursuit of status or the pursuit of knowledge (Plato, 1982). These debates have recently been revived both in mainstream philosophy and in health care analysis (Moore, 1994). And those who participate in such debates look to them for insights of general applicability.

Box 2.4: Reflection

It is worth stopping to take stock. We have identified two sorts of questions about well-being. Some questions appear to be open to a generalisable answer, others appear to be a matter of personal judgement. Not only is there considerable disagreement about the answers to some of these questions, but there is also disagreement about which of two categories they fall into. Whether or not we can live well without air clearly falls into the first category. Whether we enjoy drinking coffee or tea clearly falls into the second category. Whether or not it can be good to have many sexual partners, or take 'hard drugs', or have an abortion do not obviously fit into either category. People would not only disagree about the answers (even given a specific instance) but would disagree about whether or not these questions are entirely a matter for personal judgement.

Many of the issues that health workers have to cope with fall into the 'in-between' category where both factual evidence and value judgements are relevant. Hence it is necessary both to look at what evidence there is about how, in general, these issues affect well-being, and also to be self-conscious about our own values and the values of those for whom we are caring.

Thus we return to the importance of recognising people as subjects and not merely as objects. Because there is so much scope for disagreement about well-being, we often place a strong emphasis on the judgements people make about their own well-being. Some of the time this is because they are the judge, the experts, about what seems to suit them. This is the case if we are getting them to choose the least bad side-effects of different therapies. But some of the time it is because we are treating their views (with which we may disagree) about a debatable subject, like bringing up their children, with respect. It is not because any view, or any choice, about well-being is as good as any other.

So we can see that the idea of well-being is very unclear. Not only does it encompass all aspects of life, but its meaning is subject to the most profound disagreements about the nature of the world, about human nature, and about what makes up a good or full life. However, perhaps it is possible to say something helpful about well-being. First, it does appear to have a subjective element – being well is surely connected in some way with believing or feeling that one is well. Second, we can say that at least some 'objective' social and environmental conditions, such as the existence of food and shelter, are necessary for the existence of well-being. These are the subjects for the following two sections.

Key Points

- Well-being is a very broad-ranging and unclear idea yet it is necessary to think about it if we want to care for other people.
- There is considerable disagreement about how far well-being is something we can generalise about and how far it is a matter of subjective judgement.

THE SUBJECTIVE PERSPECTIVE

There is another starting point from which to begin thinking about health: our own subjective perspective. It follows from what has already been said about holism and well-being. Let us start from an experience that is fairly common: a time during which we feel we are becoming unwell. It would be helpful to think about what goes through our minds at such a time. We might worry about our immediate commitments: perhaps there is something that has to be done for work; perhaps we are looking forward to going out. We might look around for explanations: perhaps we are overtired; perhaps we are imagining it; perhaps it is something we ate. We might start to look into the future: 'Should I buy in some provisions, will I miss next week's trip?' Maybe we know exactly what it is; it is a condition we live with permanently which affects what we can and cannot do; perhaps it is getting gradually worse and the whole future looks bleak and uncertain.

Thought experiments like this highlight a couple of key things about the nature of health and well-being. First, there is a gap between how we feel and other people's assessment of how healthy we are. We may feel unwell and yet hesitate to talk to anyone else about it, least of all a health professional, for fear of not being taken seriously. Conversely, we may feel fine and happy but other people may see signs that make them concerned about our health. Second, feeling unhealthy, in however broad or narrow a sense, is never experienced as only physical symptoms. It is always experienced as a threat to, and a disturbance in, our life patterns, and sometimes as a threat to our life itself. Health is about changes in biography, not just biology.

For these reasons the distinction between broad and narrow conceptions of health seems less appropriate to the subjective perspective. Clearly, there are very 'broad' phenomena, such as anxiety about the future of the world, and very 'narrow' phenomena, such as a headache. But on the whole feelings of 'dis-ease', broad or narrow, are actually experienced as affecting life as a whole. Disease and well-being cannot be easily separated.

Also, for these reasons, social scientists who are interested in studying experiences of health and illness have to use very different methods and conceptions from those working in the clinical and biological sciences. For a start, they tend to talk about 'illness' rather than 'disease'. The latter refers to a clinically defined pathological abnormality, whereas the former refers to a person's subjective experience of ill health (Taylor and Field, 1993). We are the authorities about whether or not we are ill in this sense, but we may not know whether we have a disease. It is possible to feel ill without having a disease, and to have a disease without feeling ill. It should be clear that if we see health as the 'absence of illness' we would have a much broader, but rather less definite conception of health than if we define it as 'the absence of disease'. Again it seems to me that what really matters here is not whether or not we operate with a broad or narrow definition of health but how we treat people. People who feel ill are manifestly in need of respect and care whether or not a pathological abnormality is detectable.

Another respect in which the sociological perspective differs from the perspective of clinical science is the context in which ill health is seen. Whilst studying disease you are interested in things such as micro-organisms, the physical environment and DNA. Whilst studying illness, which may be the consequence of disease, you must look at things such as personal and working relationships, cultural beliefs, and social and economic structures. This is the shift from biology through biography to sociology. For the experience of illness is not only shaped by an individual's own decisions and beliefs; all experiences and beliefs are shaped by the social world in which we live. We have to live with the language, the values and the constraints that are more or less given to us; and we experience ill health through this framework. This means that people of different cultures, or subcultures, might be expected to have rather different ways of making sense of experiences of health and illness. Norms and attitudes to the body, to personal space, to professional–client relationships, to gender expectations, to death, and to what is serious and so forth can vary between cultures. An awareness of this fact has to be balanced against the danger of 'labelling' people according to stereotypical beliefs about other cultures.

Box 2.5

It is crucial that those who participate in health care are aware of both the personal and social significance of ill health. Without this awareness they may totally miss the mark about what actually matters to people. This is why communication between health professionals and so-called 'lay people' or patients is so important. It is not about a mere 'transfer of information' so that the professional can check hypotheses about signs and symptoms. It is to find out how the patient feels, how he/she makes sense of what is happening to him/her, what his/her hopes and fears are, and what he/she thinks should and should not be done. It is to try to see the world from the patient's perspective.

Even with the very best will in the world, communication between professionals and 'clients' may be limited. It is important to understand that people tend to have a public version and a private version of their concerns (Cornwell, 1984). The latter may only be shared with trusted friends or family members or with others who 'speak the same language'. The formal situation of an encounter with health professionals normally entails the presentation of the public face. On occasions, a 'transfer of information' approach may be enough, e.g. when prescribing reading glasses. On other occasions (e.g. counselling someone who is going blind), a patient-centred approach is essential. Most situations in health care involve a mixture of these demands, and a skilful communicator will know how to move between them, and not to get stuck in one mode.

Cross-cultural communication is particularly important and challenging. Here, where there is the greatest need for person-centred communication, there is the greatest danger of resorting to a 'transfer of information' stance in inappropriate circumstances. There may be barriers to both spoken and body language, and institutional or personal racism, as well as divergence of cultural beliefs and norms. There are no easy answers to these challenges, but there is always scope for positive action to increase access, uptake and satisfaction with services – but this will usually involve changing services.

This introduces another factor which underlines the value of the subjective perspective: the question of power. Enabling people to communicate, and treating what they say with respect, is enabling them to participate in care. Illness is often experienced as a loss of control over our affairs. It is possible to see health care as an attempt to restore control. Yet most health care settings are made up in such a way that they make non-professionals feel relatively powerless, thereby compounding the problem. Some of this is inevitable. An unfamiliar environment, bad memories or associations, and lack of technical expertise all lead to feelings of powerlessness. And patients normally lack real knowledge and power which others have, particularly knowledge and power connected to the management of disease. Yet there is a lot that can be done, through dialogue, to give patients greater control over their care. This power-sharing need not be confined to one-to-one interactions but can be built into the way institutions work, the ways in which the health care agenda is drawn up, and the way in which resources are allocated. As well as important differences there are a lot of commonalities between the perspectives of individual patients. Taken together, and taken seriously, they would make for a different health service.

Key Points

- One important aspect of exploring the meaning of health is to try and understand the meaning of health from the personal and subjective standpoint.
- The meanings that make up individuals' experience of health and illness require us to bring together biographical and sociological (as well as biological) frames of reference.
- Unless we attend properly to individuals' own points of view, we fail to respect them. Furthermore, we will not be able to communicate with them, care for them or empower them effectively.

SOCIAL WELL-BEING

The famous World Health Organization (WHO) definition of health refers to 'social well-being' as part of health. Sometimes this is taken to refer to an aspect of personal well-being, i.e. that aspect of an individual's welfare that stems from the quantity and quality of social relationships and social support that he/she enjoys. But it is also possible to interpret it in a wider sense as the well-being of society. If so, is there more to a healthy society than the health of the individuals who make it up?

Even if we operate with a narrow conception of health, these are important questions. Aristotle's distinctions are helpful here. Society itself cannot possess health, only individuals can do that, but it can be healthy in the sense of 'health causing'. This is the reason so much emphasis has come to be placed on health promotion. As well as aiming to develop personal skills, health promotion seeks to 'Build Healthy Public Policy; Create Supportive Environments; Strengthen Community Action; and Reorient Health Services' (WHO, 1986a) – in other words to help bring about a healthy social and physical environment. The following two chapters deal, in depth, with the social context of health and health promotion, respectively, but it is worth introducing some issues about the relationship between individual and social well-being here.

One way into these issues is by looking at what has become the accepted technical usage of the terms 'impairment', 'disability' and 'handicap' (WHO, 1980). These terms are often fudged together in ordinary usage, but for the purposes of scientific classification and communication the WHO have produced three useful stipulative definitions. In brief, an impairment is a physical or psychological abnormality that may, or may not, lead to a disability. A disability is a loss of function experienced by the impaired person which in turn may, or may not, lead to a handicap. And a handicap is some social disadvantage suffered by a person because of his/her disability. Thus it is possible to have an impairment (such as slight damage to one ear) that does not cause any significant disability (such as loss of hearing) or handicap. It is equally possible to have a disability (such as short-sightedness) that does not cause any significant handicap. Note that as we move from impairment to handicap we are moving from a medical, through a functional, to a social conception of health.

Leaving aside the exact technical specification of these three terms, the distinctions between them are most useful. It is plain that if we want to reduce handicap, we must address social factors. Someone who cannot walk has, by definition, a substantial disability, but he/she only has a substantial handicap if the world in which he/she lives makes it impossible for him/her to enjoy equal opportunities. Just as we turn to physical remedies for disability, we need social action to address handicap. Often the cause of handicap is

the attitudes of others either individually or collectively embodied in institutions, policies or
actions. These points do not only apply to those
with recognised disabilities: they apply equally to
anyone who is put at a social disadvantage. Some
people are handicapped by physical disabilities,
others by gender, race, social class or other factors.

The existence of discrimination and inequalities
takes us on to social well-being in the broader
sense, and to politics. It is well known that there are
inequalities in patterns of disease and death, as
well as in access to health care and health promotion. These inequalities are intimately tied in with
more general inequalities such as those in material
living and working conditions (Townsend et al.,
1990). It is very tempting for those interested in
maximising health to assume that everything possible should be done to reduce all such inequalities.
Unfortunately, this is too simplistic. If we take
health to refer to something narrow, such as the
absence of disease, then there are other social
goods that we may also value (such as personal liberty and market competition), which might be
undermined in the pursuit of equal health. However, if we see greater equality as part of what we
mean by social well-being or 'a healthy society',
then this is fine providing that we accept that it is
also a political judgement about the nature of a
good society. There is always a danger of trying to
smuggle in our moral or political values disguised
as neutral-sounding references to health.

What is undoubtedly the case is that expectation and quality of life are related to divisions of
wealth, status and power. For many this is a forceful political argument. Even those who are quite
happy to see inequalities in houses, cars and holidays often find it difficult to accept that one person should live for longer than another for reasons
of wealth. This is because in most people's minds
health is seen as a basic need, or even a basic entitlement. It is felt to be a minimum requirement of
life, and it is uncomfortable to admit that our
social or economic arrangements do not distribute
this basic good equitably. These feelings and
judgements are not only important politically;
they also indicate something about what health
means to many people.

Key Points

- The physical and social environment, including
  social attitudes, is a crucial determinant of health.

This is the insight at the heart of health promotion.
- It is difficult to separate out our 'health-related'
  values from our moral and political values but it is
  useful to be self-conscious about the overlaps
  between them.

WHAT IS HEALTH?

Thus far we have explored some of the issues
around narrow and broad conceptions of health.
We have noted that it is possible to have negative
and positive versions of these conceptions, and
that it is possible to assess our state of health from
an internal subjective perspective or from an
external perspective. The only two definitions we
have looked at, health as absence of disease and
health as well-being, seem to be at two extreme
poles. The former is a narrow negative conception
and the latter a broad positive conception. The former would entail health assessment being made
from an external, 'objective', perspective, the latter
has a subjective as well as an objective dimension
(see also Chapter 4).

Box 2.6: Reflection

There are two main routes that could be taken from
this point and they are both worthy of serious attention. On the one hand, it could be said that there is
no need to look for a definitive conception of health.
Individuals might have preferred definitions or conceptions; they may choose to use rather different
conceptions in different circumstances. All that matters is that they are self-conscious about their use of
the word 'health', and that they are willing and able to
make clear how they are using it. On the other hand,
it could be said that we do need to look for some
more definitive conception. That there must be some
compromise between, or common denominator lying
beneath, the variety of conceptions. This way, by identifying the 'true' definition of health, we will not only
clarify things further, but we will also provide a conception which everyone can come to share. It is
worth spending some time pursuing this goal, even if
some people see whatever emerges as just one more
conception.

The search for a compromise seems sensible, as freedom from disease seems too narrow and well-being too broad. Also a compromise seems quite possible if we return to the idea with which we began, of health as 'good functioning' whether that be the good functioning of the body or of the person as a whole. The problem is that the general formula of 'good personal functioning' is useful at an abstract level but the minute we try to specify it further we get tangled in a web of value debates. There is a mass of moral, political and religious disagreements about what it is to function well as a person.

However, there is a way forward. Some authors have argued that there are certain basic elements in common between all conceptions of well-being. So although we may not be able to agree about the full meaning of well-being, we should be able to agree about a core meaning, that part which relates to essentials or basic needs (Plant *et al.*, 1980; Doyal and Gough, 1996). The argument is that whatever conception of the good life we have there are certain requirements that need to be fulfilled in order for us to attain it. *Physical survival* is one of these requirements, and we saw in the section on well-being that conditions like food and shelter can be seen as 'objective' parts of well-being. But, it is argued, another such requirement is *autonomy* or self-determination (i.e. the capacity of an individual to make and carry out choices on his or her own behalf). For how could we say that someone was functioning well as a person, let alone that he/she was trying to meet his/her own conception of well-being, if he/she lacked any measure of autonomy? In turn, we can see that there are conditions, such as physical functioning, education, and some level of social and economic opportunity, that are necessary conditions for autonomy.

These arguments, therefore, make space for a conception of health between the two extreme poles. Health could be seen as the state of having one's basic needs satisfied, or more positively as having the necessary resources to live one's life as one chooses. This is the kind of conception that the WHO have moved towards in recent years.

'Health is, therefore, seen as a resource for everyday life, not the objective of living; it is a positive concept emphasizing social and personal resources, as well as physical capacities.'
(WHO, 1986b)

This is also the frame of reference that informs David Seedhouse's (1986) influential work on the meaning of health. His conception of health is a carefully articulated version of 'the resources for living' or what he calls 'the foundations for achievement' approach:

'A person's optimum state of health is equivalent to the state of the set of conditions which fulfil or enable a person to work to fulfil his or her realistic chosen and biological potentials.'
(Seedhouse, 1986, page 61)

Although this is not offered as a final definition, but as a way of delimiting the meaning of health, it is certainly very useful and thought provoking. Anyone who is interested in this subject would do well to read the whole of the book from which this quotation is taken. But the essence of the conception is clear. Health is seen as the foundations or conditions necessary to live one's own life to the full. These conditions will include such things as physical fitness, food and shelter but also things like education, self-confidence and access to opportunities. Although most of these necessary conditions will be the same for all people, some of them will vary according to the circumstances and the particular life goals individuals have. Finally, as with any sensible conception, there are degrees of health depending on how many of the foundation conditions are realised. This final conception of health sees health as 'personal and social resources', where 'resources' is understood in the broadest, and not merely monetary, sense.

This conception of health overlaps with a famous sociological definition of health as 'the state of optimum capacity of an individual for the effective role and tasks for which he has been socialised' (Parsons, 1981). It emphasises the idea of health as the capacity to function well. However, there is also a crucial difference. According to Seedhouse, the yardstick for 'good functioning' depends partly on the choice of the individual concerned, and not on the norms or expectations prevailing in society at the time.

Perhaps we have arrived at the ultimate destination. It is up to you to decide. Here we have a relatively clear conception of health that is neither too narrow nor too broad. One clear advantage of this sort of conception over both the narrow and broad conceptions is the way they relate to mental health. According to the disease-freedom model, mental health only exists as the absence of patho-logical abnormality. This seems wrong for two reasons. First, there is the highly controversial reduction of mental ill health to physical pathol-ogy; mental illness seems better described in behavioural rather than physical language. Sec-ond, it seems that there is much more to the posi-tive conception of mental health than the absence of mental illness, however the latter is under-stood. But the broad conception of complete men-tal well-being seems far too vague and all-encompassing. We would probably regard anyone who thought he/she had complete mental well-being as mad! Ideas such as 'self-realisation' seem to demand too much. The conception of health as necessary resources for a full life sug-gests a compromise picture of mental health. To have mental health would require a certain level of autonomy, and in turn this would depend upon conditions such as understanding one's environ-ment, self-confidence, and a relatively supportive (as opposed to oppressive) social environment. All these resources are necessary for adequate-to-good mental functioning. They are practical and positive considerations, more than just the absence of something, and less than perfection.

From this example we can see the practical implications of the 'resources conception'. It draws attention to those conditions that either enable, or block, the realisation of potential. Thus health workers can put their own energies into providing those resources that are most needed. They need not be completely preoccupied with diseases (although these can be important blocks to potential); neither need they be overwhelmed by the endless range of things that affect well-being.

It would be tidy to end this section here. But a concern for truth does not always coincide with tidiness. Indeed, when Seedhouse identifies work for health as the provision of 'foundations for achievement' he writes:

> 'The common factor is, on the face of it, blindingly simple, but on analysis the idea soon becomes plagued with difficulties.'
> (Seedhouse, 1986, page 63)

I will give a brief indication of two possible diffi-culties, the first arguably trivial but the second rather more important.

The first difficulty is this: how can food, shelter, clean air, or employment be part of a person's

health when they are 'outside' the person. They are clearly 'health causing', and therefore have implications for health work, but it seems to be odd to see them as part of someone's health. I would prefer to see health as referring to an indi-vidual's physical and mental resources, that is, to personal resources, rather than to both personal and social resources (whilst noting that the former are dependent upon the latter). What do you think?

The second difficulty is more complicated and more challenging. Is the idea of basic resources or foundations really neutral between all the various conceptions of well-being? It can be argued that it is not, that this conception of health actually rests upon a particular conception of well-being, in which personal well-being is closely identified with the exercise of autonomy or choice. Accord-ing to this conception of health someone whose foundations are in place is in effect healthy, and there is no reason, nor right, for health workers to interfere in his/her life. This applies even if he/she uses his/her autonomy to choose to smoke, or over-eat, or even to commit suicide. So long as he/she is autonomous, he/she is healthy. Many people who have more definite views about health and well-being will find this implication difficult to accept. Once again you must decide what you think.

Key Points

- There is a 'compromise' between the extremes of 'absence of disease' and 'well-being' which views health as 'resources for living'.
- This 'resources' conception meets a number of the limitations of the other two conceptions and it is a plausible candidate for being 'definitive', but it faces difficulties of its own.

ASSESSING ILL HEALTH AND QUALITY OF LIFE

One of the reasons for trying to clarify the mean-ing of health is so that we can assess the health of individuals and populations. This is an essential dimension of health care. It should be clear by now that we cannot ask how healthy someone is without specifying a conception of health. So many apparent complications and paradoxes come about because this is ignored. Someone who is diseased may be healthy in the sense that he/she does not feel ill, and/or in the sense that he/she has the resources to function well, and/or in the sense that he/she is enjoying considerable personal well-being. It is possible to generate countless examples in which people can be judged to be unhealthy (according to some conceptions) *and* healthy (according to others). Even within a conception of health, individuals can be both healthy and unhealthy, just as a glass can be both half full and half empty, because health is always a matter of degree.

It seems, therefore, that it is important to understand the contestable meaning of health, and to be able to appreciate the move between the various conceptions discussed previously. But from another point of view all of this seems most unhelpful. Suppose you were given a health care budget to manage. There would be two questions you would feel obliged to answer: 'On what, and on whom, should we spend this money?' and 'Having spent money, are we doing as much good as possible?' These questions give rise to many complexities which it is not possible to explore here; however, we can see that these questions could be raised by asking about the health of populations before or after care. Imagine how you would feel faced with the reply: 'We cannot tell you what the health of this population is; there are a countless number of answers, it all depends what you mean.' This may well be true but it will not do as an answer. It is necessary to fasten upon some indicators of whether or not health care or health care policies are improving health. This is becoming increasingly important with the growth of evidence-based practice which requires us to state the effectiveness of our interventions in explicit (and demonstrable) terms. Here we face a practical challenge which opens up all the above theoretical discussions. Should our indicators be negative or positive, broad or narrow, subjective or objective? This question has to be tackled at policy level and at the level of practice.

We cannot avoid making some very general policy decisions about the purposes and priorities of health care. These decisions are either 'made' implicitly by what happens to be provided, or they can be made explicitly. One way of doing so explicitly is by advocating a particular conception of health. Thus if we accept that health care is, in broad terms, the promotion of personal autonomy,

we would look to increase some indicators of autonomy. Or we could say that health is, in broad terms, absence of medically defined pathology, and aim for lower indications of disease. However, although a decision about the purposes and priorities of health care is inevitable, it does not follow that this decision is the same as deciding upon a conception of health.

Box 2.7

It is worth emphasising this. Take an individual who is a car mechanic. She may believe that it is part of her job to keep owners informed, reassured and satisfied. But no-one would think that all this is part of the *meaning* of 'car maintenance'. Similarly, it is perfectly possible to subscribe to a narrow conception of health but also to believe that health care should aim to meet other aspects of well-being.

What matters, what is essential, is that the overall purposes or ends of health care are decided upon. Only then, when we have decided what we will count as a benefit, can we assess the costs and benefits of various patterns of provision. So although what we are assessing can be summarised in broad terms as 'ill health' or 'quality of life', in practice we will use a wide range of concepts like 'needs' or 'satisfaction' in the process of assessment.

These general questions of policy or philosophy are notoriously difficult, and in some ways things are easier at the level of practice. Any particular practitioner can focus on his or her own medium- and short-term objectives and ask how far these are being met. This is what makes evidence-based practice possible. Up to a point appropriate indicators will be suggested by the objectives. If the objective of a particular intervention is pain relief, then assessment will depend upon subjective reporting of pain; if it is to increase mobility, it will be possible to use more generalisable measures, and so on. This does not tell us how to combine such assessments into more holistic indicators. Nor can these limited indicators be used to justify forms of care, for it is always necessary to ask the general policy question: 'Why should we be doing this at all?' But these sorts of narrow indicators do offer a start in the process of assessing ill health or quality of life. Also it would be foolish in the extreme to rely on a very general conception of health to assess the outcome of specific interventions. Such a conception would form a valuable part of an overall evaluation, but we will also want to know whether the intervention meets its specific objectives.

There are two particularly influential approaches to the assessment of ill health that roughly correspond to the two questions raised above. In order to assess the health of populations so as to determine what kind of health care to offer, it is necessary to employ some form of **needs assessment**. In order to assess any improvement in the health of individuals or groups who have received care, it is possible to use a **quality of life measurement scale**.

As we have seen, the concept of need is intimately connected with the conception of health as personal resources. (The negative version of the 'resources conception' would be that health equals the absence of basic needs.) It is therefore sensible to use the concept of need in order to identify what to provide, but many people would see it as too broad. They would want to distinguish between general needs and health needs where the latter means the ability to benefit from actual or potential health care (Stevens and Gabbay, 1991). Once again the scope of needs assessment depends on whether we use broad or narrow, subjective or objective indicators. However it is interpreted, it depends on systematic social and epidemiological research. In order to assess the needs of a local population researchers will look at some combination of death and disease (mortality and morbidity) statistics, use of services, expressed needs or demands of patients, and subjective concerns of some sample of the population as a whole.

Most forms of needs assessment (and quality of life instruments) involve *measurement*. This makes a special demand on those who practise it. Measures taken at different times and places have to be comparable. That is, they have to be *reliable*. They also have to be accurate, or *valid*, indicators of whatever they set out to measure. For these purposes a vague conception is not good enough: it is necessary to use a stipulative technical definition (sometimes called an **operational definition**). For example, and to oversimplify, we could choose to define someone's need for health care as 'the number of visits made to clinics or hospitals'. Even this would provide some kind of indication of need, and it would enable us to provide comparable and reliable measures. However, we can

see that there would be a considerable gap between this measure and our normal conception of health need. The more sophisticated the measure, the narrower this gap would become, but there would always be some gap. The challenge is to find practical and reliable measures which are as valid as possible. Above all, it is vital not to confuse a measure of needs or ill health with the full meaning of these concepts.

All of this applies equally to quality of life measures. Quality of life is a good shorthand phrase for the overall aim of health care; it is the effect of possessing health. Health care can only be properly evaluated if improvements in quality of life as well as quantity of life are taken into account. To this end a number of quality of life scales or measures have been developed and checked for their **reliability** and **validity** (Bowling, 1997). These are ways of estimating the overall quality of life of individuals according to combinations of narrow indicators. Some of these indicators, or criteria, are dependent upon professional observations, but most are decided by the subjective reporting of the patient. In this way, diverse criteria such as mobility, or depression, or social support can be translated into an overall score or picture of quality of life. Many of these scales are very sophisticated and holistic in ambition. However, it should be clear how difficult it is fully to capture quality of life even with the most sophisticated measure. As with needs assessment the only option is to choose an approach which best fits the purpose to which the measurement is going to be put.

Elsewhere I have argued that it is possible to see the elements of quality of life on a map which, roughly speaking, moves from the public to the personal (Cribb, 1985). At one extreme are the most public and generalisable determinants of quality of life, what might be called 'quality of lifestyle'. These relate to people's capacities and restrictions in their work, social and home life. These elements are the most easily quantified and compared, but they are too blunt to provide good assessment of quality of life as a whole. At the other extreme is what could be called 'sense of life'. This relates to the individual's subjective perspective on his/her life, its meaning and value. Experiences of health and illness are enmeshed in a web of fears, beliefs and commitments from the most mundane to the most profound. It would be impossible to understand, or assess, an individual's quality of life without taking this into account. But it does not lend itself to measurement. In between these extremes are less specific elements of outlook or subjective well-being, what might loosely be called 'mental health'. Here both measurement scales and more subjective forms of assessment are possible, and can be combined.

From this we can see that the process of measurement, which is essential if proper assessments and comparisons are to be done, pushes us towards a more generalisable, 'scientific' or reductionist stance. Thus there is a constant danger that we will forget the importance of the person-centred or subjective perspective.

Key Points

- Assessing health care needs and the effectiveness of health care interventions depends upon some understanding of the nature of health.
- Practical decisions need to be made in order to produce suitable indicators of need or quality of life for particular purposes. But these decisions do not resolve the philosophical issues; they merely suspend them.
- There is an inevitable tendency for measures of health to favour narrower and more generalisable conceptions of health.

CONCLUSION

Thinking about the meaning of health takes us in many different directions, and raises many questions and uncertainties. These complexities stem from the fact that thinking about health is thinking about the basic nature of life, of people, and of the world in which they live. We cannot neatly separate health issues from non-health issues. Neither can we completely separate factual questions about health from value questions.

For practical purposes we sometimes have to divide the world into supposed health domains (e.g. the local 'health' centre) and non-health domains (e.g. the local tax office). But it only takes a moment to see that this separation is false. There is no domain of activity that is not connected with health in the sense that it does not affect people's state of health, or their experience of health and illness. In order to avoid getting entangled in value debates about health, we might decide to employ a narrow, 'scientific' conception or defini-

tion of health. We might choose to see health as the absence of disease, and thereby leave all the complications, abstractions and disagreements behind whilst we get on with clinical science and practice. I hope that what has been said above is enough to show why this 'trick' will not work.

Many value questions arise regardless of how we define health. First, there are questions about the distribution of health, the targeting of health care and the rectification of inequalities. The answers to these questions cannot be found in clinical science but only through moral and political reflection and analysis. Second, there are questions about *how* to behave towards people, and how to take their perspective, and their values and objectives into account. Once again there are no universal scientific solutions. Finally, there are questions about the general well-being of people, about what is in their overall interests. These arise whether or not individuals are well enough to express their own views or preferences. Focusing on diseases does not make these larger concerns disappear.

There is yet another reason why the resort to scientific language does not avoid the need for value judgements. An important complication, which has not been discussed above, can be indicated briefly here in order to make clear that this chapter is the beginning rather than the end of the debate. That is, even apparently scientific classifications or descriptions of ill health are not entirely free from value judgement. The ideas of physical impairment or disease depend upon an idea of a range of normality. But the definition of this range of normality is arguably determined in part by cultural and value judgements (Kennedy, 1983; Scadding, 1988).

None of this is to say that the conception of health as the absence of disease is not useful. I have tried to show that there are advantages and disadvantages with this narrow conception, as with the broader conceptions of 'personal capacity or resources' and 'well-being'. It is merely to emphasise that we cannot solve the problem of health care by fastening upon a definition of health. Some of the time it is helpful to use a conception of health that concentrates on specific measurable objectives; some of the time it is helpful to be reminded of the infinite variety of elements that can contribute to life's quality; and it is always helpful to remember that health care involves enabling individuals to function well as people and not just as biological organisms.

Thinking about the meaning of health is necessary if we are to decide what kinds of knowledge, attitudes, and values should be built into health care; but it is only a start.

Summary

Thinking about the meaning of health is one way of being reflective about the purposes and processes of health care and health policy. There are advantages and disadvantages of working with both narrow and broad conceptions of health. A narrow conception lends itself to measurement and generalisation but may fail to capture important aspects of well-being. A broad conception reminds us of the complex and rich range of ways in which peoples' lives can go well or badly but makes generalisation difficult. There is a 'compromise' conception which sees health as resources for living but this, too, is open to objections. Whichever conception of health we use (and perhaps we should move between different ones) it is necessary to have regard to those aspects of health which are relatively objective (which apply to people in general) and those which are more subjective. In order to do this we need to combine biological, biographical and sociological perspectives and to respect the individual person's own voice.

REFERENCES

Aristotle (1941). *The Basic Works of Aristotle*. Random House, New York.

Bowling, A. (1997). *Measuring Health*. Open University Press, Buckingham.

Cornwell, J. (1984). *Hard-earned Lives*. Tavistock Publications, London.

Cribb, A. (1985). Quality of life. *Journal of Medical Ethics*, 2(3), 142–5.

Doyal, L. and Gough, I. (1996). *A Theory of Human Needs*. Macmillan, London.

Gallie, W.B. (1964). *Philosophy and Historical Understanding*. Chatto and Windus, London.

Gray, J.A.M. and Austoker, J. (1989). *Draft Guidelines on Improving Acceptability*. Screening Publications, Oxford.

Kennedy, I. (1983). *The Unmasking of Medicine*. Granada, St Albans.

Moore, A. (1994). Well-being: a philosophical basis for health services. *Health Care Analysis*, 2(3), 207–17.

Parsons, T. (1981). Definitions of health and illness in the light of American values and social structure. In *Concepts of Health and Disease*, Caplan, A.L., Englehardt, H.T. and McCartney, J.J. (eds). Addison-Wesley, New York.

Plant, R., Lesser, H. and Taylor-Gooby, P. (1980). *Political Philosophy and Social Welfare*. Routledge and Kegan Paul, London.

Plato (1982). *Philebus*. Penguin Classics, Harmondsworth.

Scadding, J.G. (1988). Health and disease: what can medicine do for philosophy? *Journal of Medical Ethics*, 14(3), 118–24.

Seedhouse, D. (1986). *Health: The Foundations for Achievement*. John Wiley & Sons, Chichester.

Stevens, A. and Gabbay, J. (1991). Needs assessment needs assessment. *Health Trends*, 23(1), 20–3.

Taylor, S. and Field, D. (1993). *Sociology of Health and Health Care*. Blackwell Science, Oxford.

Townsend, P., Davidson, N. and Whitehead, M. (1990). *Inequalities in Health*. Penguin, Harmondsworth.

WHO (1947). *World Health Organization: Constitution*. WHO, Geneva.

WHO (1980). *International Classification of Impairments, Disabilities, and Handicaps*. WHO, Geneva.

WHO (1986a). *The Ottawa Charter of Health Promotion*. WHO, Geneva.

WHO (1986b). A discussion document on the concept and principles of health promotion. *Health Promotion*, 1(1), 73–6.

FURTHER READING

Bowling, A. (1997). *Measuring Health*. Open University Press, Milton Keynes.

A guide to the methods of, and challenges of, 'operationalising' and measuring health.

Plato (1982). *Philebus*. Penguin Classics, Harmondsworth.

A discussion of well-being and the role of pleasure within it, which will also serve as an introduction to the classical debate about these questions.

Seale, C. and Davey, B. (eds) (1996). *Experiencing and Explaining Disease*. Open University Press, Buckingham.

A reader that illustrates the importance of including the subjective perspective in our understanding of health and illness.

Seedhouse, D. (1986). *Health: The Foundations for Achievement*. John Wiley & Sons, Chichester.

An influential and accessible argument about conceptions of health and their practical importance.

CHAPTER THREE

THE SOCIAL CONTEXT *of* HEALTH

Paul Watt and Barbara J. Harrison

- Sociological approaches to social inequality
- Defining and measuring health
- Class and health inequalities
- Gender and health inequalities
- 'Race', ethnicity and health inequalities
- Health care and social divisions
- Tackling health inequalities
- Conclusion

The aim of this chapter is to provide a sociological analysis of the social context in which health and health care occur. It provides a brief introduction to a number of sociological theories and their treatment of social inequality. The chapter concentrates upon the ways in which three aspects of social inequality, namely class, gender and 'race', affect both people's health and the process of health care itself, and hence give rise to health inequalities. Suggestions are made regarding the ways in which these health inequalities can be reduced at a number of policy levels.

SOCIOLOGICAL APPROACHES TO SOCIAL INEQUALITY

The previous chapter has explored the various ways in which health has been defined. In this chapter we will be considering how people's health is affected by their social circumstances. We emphasise the way in which individuals share common life experiences and problems with others and how these experiences follow certain social patterns. In so doing, we are developing what the American sociologist C. Wright Mills called 'the sociological imagination', in understanding the connections between an individual's private troubles and what Mills refers to as 'the public issues of social structure' (1970, page 14). Sociology is concerned with describing, under-

standing and explaining the regularities and recurring patterns of social life, including those concerned with inequality, or what sociologists call 'stratification': 'we can virtually define the core of sociology as an inquiry into the origins, characteristics and consequences of social inequality defined in terms of power, status and class' (Turner, 1986, page 30). The rest of this chapter will deal with the question of how three aspects of social inequality, namely class, gender and 'race', affect people's health.

Within sociology there is a range of theoretical perspectives that refer to the different ways in which sociologists look at social reality, in terms of how they understand and explain social phenomena, including stratification (see Abbott and Wallace, 1996; Giddens, 1997). In broad terms, sociological perspectives can be divided into two:

- Macro-perspectives, which are concerned with understanding and explaining large-scale social processes, usually in relation to entire societies, for example, a nation state
- Micro-perspectives, which are concerned with small-scale social interaction involving a few people and these are the areas of sociology which are closest to psychology, especially social psychology.

In this chapter, we will be concerned mainly with the macro-perspectives since it is these which have had most to say about social stratification. The main theoretical perspectives are summarised below.

MARXISM

Marxism derives from the work of Karl Marx, the nineteenth century German social theorist and revolutionary. Marx concentrated on the form of stratification which is called social class (Edgell, 1993). Marx argued that, under capitalism, industry and commerce or, as Marx terms it, 'the means of production', is owned by a relatively small group of people called the 'bourgeoisie' or capitalist class. According to Marx, this class only gains profits from its ownership of factories, offices and banks because it exploits a much larger class, the 'proletariat' or working class, which, because it does not own the means of production, is compelled to sell its labour to the capitalist class in exchange for wages. The relationship between these two classes is an antagonistic one in Marxist theory and results in class conflict, and ultimately revolution. In terms of health, Marxists argue that ill health largely arises from the social inequality that exists as a result of the class-based nature of capitalist society, not only in terms of the effects of work on people's health, for example industrial accidents, but also in terms of the health-damaging impact of products that are sold by capitalist firms solely for profits, notably cigarettes (Doyal, 1979). Although the influence of Marxism within sociology has declined in recent years, it is still nevertheless arguable that Marxism provides a powerful analysis of the dynamics of social inequality within contemporary capitalist society (Gubbay, 1997).

WEBERIAN SOCIOLOGY

Unlike Marxism, Weberian sociology does not prioritise class over other forms of stratification, for example, inequality based upon racial or religious differences. Instead, its founder, Max Weber, argued that there are three main types of stratification which arise out of differences in power within a society (Saunders, 1990):

- Class
- Status
- Party.

For the purposes of this analysis, we will ignore the latter and concentrate on classes and status groups. Classes, for Weber, are phenomena that arise out of the distribution of property and occupational skills (including qualifications) in a market society, so that using Weber's analysis one can identify several classes in modern society. One notable attempt to apply Weberian theory to class analysis has been the study of **social mobility** by Goldthorpe in which he uses a complex array of seven class positions based upon occupations and their rewards in terms of income, job security, exercise of authority, etc. (Goldthorpe, 1980; Erikson and Goldthorpe, 1993).

Status groups arise out of the possession of what Weber calls 'social honour' or prestige. Examples of such status groups can be seen in the caste system in India or the racial division between 'whites', 'blacks' and 'coloureds' which used to exist under the apartheid regime in South Africa. Such status groups are not classes because their position does not depend upon economic factors, but instead on possession of some socially significant marker which distinguishes that group from others, for example, skin colour or other physical characteristics. This aspect of stratification is discussed later in the chapter.

FEMINISM

Feminists have been responsible for highlighting two issues that have provoked important insights into the social context of health. The first is that a distinction is made between the categories of sex and gender. 'Sex' refers to the biological differences between men and women, whilst 'gender' is the social construction of masculine and feminine behaviour, that is, the socially acceptable behaviour expected of the two sexes in different societies. Feminism has pointed out how men and women are socialised into their respective gender roles and how these roles are irreducible to biological differences between the sexes (Abbott and Wallace, 1996). The second issue feminism has raised is that gender is more than the playing of roles; instead, it is argued that gender relations are based upon inequality of power between men and women and that this power takes the form of patriarchy or 'the generalised power of men over women' (Ramazanoglu, 1989, page 15). We will discuss the relevance of patriarchy for health when we look at gender in more detail later in the chapter. It is important to note that there are different types of feminist analysis, including Marxist feminism, radical feminism and black feminism (see Abbott and Wallace, 1996).

FUNCTIONALISM

In contrast to the previous theories, functionalism assumes a consensus model of society characterised by order and stability; this order is based upon agreement over the values held by the members of society. Functionalism asks the question, 'what is the function of the component parts of the society in relation to the maintenance of order in the social system as a whole?' It uses an organic analogy: in a body, each particular organ plays a vital role in the maintenance of the whole body, and in a similar way each part of society fulfils a particular function for the whole society. An example is the system of stratification itself. Functionalists argue that stratification is both universal, in that it exists in all known societies, and necessary, in that it plays a vital role in ensuring that the most talented people in a society are enticed into the most important positions; this is done since those positions receive more rewards, in terms of income and prestige, than less important positions (Saunders, 1990).

SYMBOLIC INTERACTIONISM

A micro-level perspective which has been very influential in the sociology of health is symbolic interactionism. This theoretical approach is also concerned with issues of power and inequality, but it is concerned to see how power operates at the level of face-to-face interaction. According to this perspective, people interact with others on the basis of symbols and language, which are modified in the process of interaction itself. Using mental illness as an example, symbolic interactionists are not concerned with the social structural causes of mental illness, which Marxists argue are related to class inequality, but instead with the social processes by which certain people's behaviour comes to be interpreted as mental illness, in other words, power at the micro-level. Interactionists regard mental illness as a form of **deviance**, that is, behaviour which breaks the social rules. Interactionists are concerned to show how certain behaviour comes to be seen by others as deviant and, importantly, what is the role of those people, in this example psychiatrists, who 'label' others as deviant. The emphasis on the labelling of deviance by people in authority is termed **labelling theory** and has been usefully applied in relation to the mental health of women and minority ethnic groups, as we will see in later sections. An excellent example of an interactionist account of life inside a mental hospital is *Asylums* by Erving Goffman (1968).

POSTMODERNISM

The newest theory in sociology, and certainly one that is extremely influential, is that of postmodernism. This approach to inequality tends to take the line that structural notions of inequality, as for example in the Marxist theory of class, are antiquated in that they are based upon a view of society rooted in notions of social production, employment and work. Postmodernists, on the other hand, argue that production is no longer the fulcrum of contemporary Western societies, but that instead consumption and consumerism are more important. As such, the emphasis is less on inequality, but instead on notions of difference; rather than seeing society as being divided into unequal groupings (classes or racialised groups), postmodernism stresses the manifold varieties of ways in which people construct their identities, for example, around sexual preferences, belief systems, consumer tastes, ethnicity, age groups, etc.

(Bradley, 1996). For many postmodernists, issues of power and inequality recede into the background in the face of the complexity of lifestyle groupings in Western societies (Crook *et al.*, 1992).

POVERTY RESEARCH AND EMPIRICISM

The tradition of research on poverty goes back to the early twentieth century studies of Booth (1905) in London and Rowntree (1902) in York. Both men were concerned to gather the 'facts' about poverty in these cities so as to provide the evidence to assist in the alleviation of social conditions for the worst-off via social reform. In the sense that the studies were concerned with using social surveys to collect data on the extent of poverty, these studies can be regarded as 'empiricist' because they were not testing out any kind of theoretical hypothesis, but were merely concerned to gather the 'facts' about incomes, living conditions, etc. Strictly speaking, this research on poverty does not constitute a theoretical perspective in sociology at all, since it neglects social theory. However, it is important to include it here since it has played a very important role in terms of both measuring the extent of inequality and understanding the linkages between inequality and health. Modern exemplars of the poverty research tradition include Townsend (1979) and Hills (1995).

There are usually two ways in which poverty is defined:

- Absolute poverty: people are classified as poor if they have insufficient resources to acquire the basic essentials for a healthy life; that is, food, clothing and shelter. The poverty line, then, is the point at which people's resources fall below a level adequate to maintain their physical efficiency. The absolute definition of poverty is meant to be cross-cultural and trans-historical, but problems of making comparisons over time have led most contemporary poverty researchers to use a second definition of poverty, that is, a relative one.
- Relative poverty: in this, poverty is relative to the general standards of living that exist in a society at a particular point in time. As those general living standards change historically, so should our conceptions of poverty. Relative poverty involves lacking the resources to participate fully in the life of the society:

'Individuals, families and groups in the population can be said to be in poverty when they lack the resources to obtain the type of diets, participate in the activities and have the living conditions and amenities which are customary, or at least widely encouraged or approved, in the societies to which they belong. Their resources are so seriously below those commanded by the average individual or family that they are, in effect, excluded from ordinary living patterns, customs and activities.'

(Townsend, 1979, page 31)

For some contemporary writers on health, it is relative poverty, rather than absolute poverty, which provides the key to explaining inequalities in health (Wilkinson, 1996), and we will discuss this research below.

Key Points

- Sociology is centrally concerned with the issue of social inequality, or 'stratification'.
- Within sociology there are a number of sociological theories or 'perspectives'.
- Each perspective emphasises different aspects of social inequality and offers differing explanations for this inequality.
- This chapter looks at three aspects of inequality: class, gender, and 'race'.

DEFINING AND MEASURING HEALTH

The previous chapter was concerned with identifying the various concepts of health that have been used in the past and currently. In the sociological literature on health, various measures of health are used, including the following:

- Mortality rates: these measure the number of deaths in a given population; for example, the infant mortality rate is the number of deaths of children less than 1 year old per thousand live births.
- Morbidity rates: these measure the amount of illness or disease in a population, for example, the number of people in a given population who have been diagnosed by their general practitioner as having chickenpox. The General Household Survey, a national survey carried out annually by the Office for National Statis-

tics (previously the Office of Population Censuses and Surveys [OPCS]) includes a measure of morbidity based upon people's own assessment of whether they have a 'longstanding illness' (OPCS, 1996).

Whichever measure of health is used, sociologists have drawn attention to the fact that such measures are social constructions themselves: in other words, they are the creations of researchers, employed in particular organisations, who have specific objectives in mind. We will be commenting on the limitations of various measures of health throughout this chapter.

CLASS AND HEALTH INEQUALITIES

CLASS AND INEQUALITY IN BRITISH SOCIETY

The class-based nature of British society has often been remarked upon, and until relatively recently British sociology was itself said by lay people to be 'class-obsessed'. Sociologists have been able to establish links between class, as measured by occupation, and a whole range of social phenomena, including educational achievement and voting behaviour, as well as health (Abercrombie and Warde, 1994). The most commonly used measure of class in relation to health is not actually derived from either Marx or Weber, but is the Registrar General's (RG) social class schema based upon the government's classification of occupations (Table 3.1) which has been in existence since 1911 when it was first used to measure inequalities in infant mortality rates. As Edgell (1993) argues, the schema relies on a shared notion of occupational status hierarchy, and as such could be located within a functionalist theoretical framework. Feminists have criticised both the RG and Goldthorpe class schemas because they allocate married women a class position based upon the occupation of their husband (Abbott and Wallace, 1996). The debate is highly complex, but as we will see below, it does relate to issues of gender and health.

The concept of social class has come under increasing criticism in the last few years for what some sociologists, notably postmodernists, claim is its lack of applicability to an increasingly plu-

Table 3.1: The Registrar General's social class schema

Class I	Professional occupations (e.g. doctor, solicitor)
Class II	Managerial and technical occupations (e.g. nurse, manager)
Class IIIN	Skilled non-manual occupations (e.g. secretary, clerk)
Class IIIM	Skilled manual occupations (e.g. ambulance staff, electrician)
Class IV	Partly skilled occupations (e.g. hospital porter, bus conductor)
Class V	Unskilled occupations (e.g. cleaner, labourer)

Adapted from OPCS, 1991.

ralistic and culturally diverse society in which consumerism and lifestyle loom far more importantly than social class (Crook *et al.*, 1992). Although many Marxist and Weberian sociologists refute such claims about the 'death of class' (Goldthorpe and Marshall, 1992; Edgell, 1993; Watt, 1996), it is nevertheless recognised that class, by itself, cannot adequately account for all of the divisions in society, and that importance needs to be given to other forms of inequality, notably gender, 'race' and age, as well as class (Bradley, 1996).

If there is some dispute as to the relevance of class as a concept, what is far less in dispute is that British society has become far more unequal in terms of the distribution of income and wealth during the last 20 years, which has resulted in the growth of poverty and deprivation (Hills, 1995). In Britain there is not an 'official' poverty line, but one frequently used measure is the number of people living on or below the **income support** (previously supplementary benefit) level. This rose from 14% of the population in 1979 to 24% of the population in 1992, or 13 680 000 million people (Oppenheim and Harker, 1996). There is considerable dispute as to whether the income support/supplementary benefit level is an accurate indicator of poverty, with some poverty researchers using 150% of this level as being an indication of poverty.

EVIDENCE ON CLASS AND HEALTH INEQUALITIES

The links between class and ill health were documented during the nineteenth century by a range of social reformers, as well as revolutionaries such as Marx. They all addressed the appalling living and working conditions of the working class during the early phase of industrial capitalism, which led either directly or indirectly to illness, disease and premature death. A series of state welfare reforms were introduced this century to combat the poverty and ill health of the working class, including the creation of the National Health Service in 1948 by the Labour government. Given that the NHS provided health care free at the point of delivery, it was commonly assumed that the links between ill health and class would be broken. In addition, the **full employment** which Britain had during the 1950s and 1960s and the gradual improvement in living standards should have also meant that the relationship between class and ill health would become a thing of the past.

Unfortunately, this was not in fact the case. The Black Report on health inequalities gathered data on class and health for the period of the early 1970s and was published in 1980. The Report used the Registrar General's (RG) social class schema and it showed that wide class variations in mortality rates existed for all age groups, so that the mortality rate increased as one moved down the RG class scale from class I (professional) to V (unskilled manual). The Report also found that rather than such class inequalities diminishing in size, they had in fact increased for the period 1930–72. So the Report confounded expectations that, after 20 years of the NHS, class inequalities would have diminished. The newly elected Conservative government in 1979, under Mrs Thatcher, responded very coolly to the Report's findings, especially the suggestion that the government should embark on a comprehensive anti-poverty campaign if the class differentials were to be reduced. A second report on health inequalities, called *The Health Divide*, was published in 1987 by Margaret Whitehead. This report found that all of the major diseases follow class gradients, with the lower social classes being far more likely to have such diseases at every stage of life, the exception being malignant melanoma – skin cancer, usually caused by too many holidays in the sun! *The Health Divide* also found that mortality differentials had in fact widened since the Black Report (both reports can be found in *Inequalities in Health* by Townsend et al., 1988a).

The most recent evidence, shown in Table 3.2 below, is based upon data for males and compares death rates at three times: 1970–72, 1979–83 and 1991–93 (Drever et al., 1996). This table clearly shows that there has been a widening of health inequalities since the early 1970s, so that the **standardised mortality ratio** (SMR) in 1991–93 is almost three times higher in class 5 compared to class 1, despite the overall reduction in mortality rates over the period. Figure 3.1 shows that significant class differences in longstanding illness continue to exist in both women and men.

Although the Conservative government had a generally dismissive view of the research on health inequalities during the 1980s, there has been more recent government interest in the topic, as seen in

Table 3.2: SMRs by social class for males aged 20–64, England and Wales, 1970–93

Social Class	SMRs (standardised mortality ratios)*		
	1970–72†	1979–80, 1982–83	1991–93
I	77	66	66
II	81	74	72
IIIN	99	93	100
IIIM	106	103	117
IV	114	114	116
V	137	159	189
England and Wales	100	100	100

* A standardised mortality ratio (SMR) is a measure of death rates. The average for males aged 20–64 in each time period is 100. SMRs below 100 indicate lower than average mortality, and SMRs higher than 100 indicate higher than average mortality.

† 1970–72 used age groups 15–64.

Adapted from Drever et al., 1996, page 19.

the Department of Health (DoH) report *Variations in Health: What Can the Department of Health and the NHS Do?* (DoH, 1995). However, whether this shift in government interest is genuine or not is highly debatable (Wainwright, 1996).

EXPLANATIONS OF HEALTH INEQUALITIES

The Black Report offered four possible explanations for the health inequalities which it found and *The Health Divide* replicated these explanations. We will briefly consider these in turn, plus a fifth omitted from the Black Report list, namely social support:

- The artefact explanation
- Theories of natural and social selection
- Cultural/behavioural explanations
- Materialist/structuralist explanations
- Social support.

The artefact explanation

This explanation suggests that the method of measuring social class using the RG schema artificially inflates the size and importance of mortality differentials in the following ways:

- There are substantial differences in SMRs within each social class, which means that the

SMR for each class is only a crude average (Jones and Cameron, 1984).

- There are problems with utilising the RG social class schema to measure changes in health inequalities over time, given that the size of the classes has changed considerably; for example, between 1931 and 1981 classes I and II have increased in size whilst classes IV and V have shrunk (Carr-Hill, 1987).

It would seem, then, that the RG schema is probably not the best measure of class for determining the nature of the relationship between class and health. However, this does not mean the relationship found in the Black Report is artificial. There is evidence that the use of the RG scale as a measure of socio-economic inequality actually *underestimates* the impact of such inequality on health. The *Whitehall Study* of 17 000 male civil servants (Marmot, 1986) found that the mortality gradient is actually much steeper than the Black Report found for social classes, since the mortality rate of the lowest grade of civil servant is three times higher than that of the highest grade. Such results would suggest that the RG schema is simply not finely tuned enough to pick up all the impact of socio-economic inequality on health.

Further evidence that the class-based inequalities are not artefactual comes from a recent study by Bartley *et al.* (1996). They compared mortality rates for a sample of men aged 15/16–64 using two measures of social class: the Registrar General's

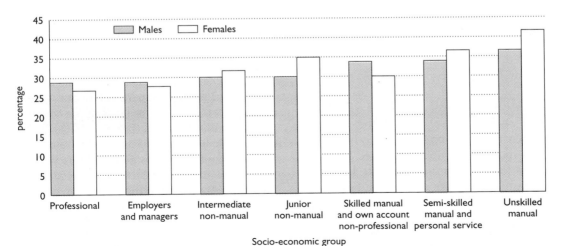

Figure 3.1: Prevalence of reported longstanding illness by sex and socio-economic group of head of household: Great Britain, 1994
(Source: *Living in Britain: Results from the 1994 General Household Survey*, the Office of National Statistics, Crown Copyright, 1996)

and that originally devised by the Weberian sociologist Goldthorpe (Erikson and Goldthorpe, 1993). The findings were that similar class-based mortality differentials were found using the two schemas. This gave credence to the view that differences in mortality between social classes are not the result of the schema used to measure class, but are real differences.

Theories of natural and social selection

This explanation accepts that social class inequalities in health exist, but argues that the inequalities are caused by a process of health selection. This means that people with poorer health are more likely to move down the class scale (they experience downward social mobility) and so concentrate in the lowest classes; for example, illness in childhood can result in absence from school which in turn leads to educational failure and an unskilled job. This works in reverse for people in good health who would tend to travel up the class scale. *The Health Divide* did find some evidence to support the health selection explanation of health inequalities, although Blane *et al.* (1993) argue that in itself this explanation has only a minor effect on the overall class gradient in health.

Cultural/behavioural explanations

According to these explanations, health inequalities arise because working-class people, particularly those in semi- and unskilled occupations, have adopted more health-damaging behaviour than have middle-class people and are also less likely to utilise preventive health services, including antenatal care and vaccinations. We will examine use of such services later in the chapter. Attention here is focused on four aspects of behaviour which most epidemiologists agree have an independent impact on health: cigarette smoking, food and nutrition, exercise in leisure time, and alcohol consumption. All except the last, drinking alcohol, follow clear class gradients in that manual workers are more likely to smoke, eat more fatty foods and less fruit and fibre, and take less exercise. The position is reversed for alcohol consumption, especially for women: those women living in households headed by a professional are

more likely than women in semi-skilled and unskilled households to drink more than the recommended sensible level and are also less likely to be non-drinkers (OPCS, 1996). Apart from alcohol consumption, therefore, working-class people seem to lead less healthy lifestyles than the middle classes and it is this which is said to cause their poorer health.

To say that working-class people lead a less healthy lifestyle does not in itself explain why this might be the case. There are two different theoretical interpretations of the evidence:

- Individualistic: this suggests that the unhealthy lifestyles of manual workers stem from their actions as individuals; in other words, the lower classes have in some sense chosen to lead such unhealthy lifestyles by their choosing to smoke, eat fatty foods, etc. This view of human behaviour is individualistic since it locates the source of behaviour in the 'free' choice of individuals. It is a view which historically is associated with conservatism (Turner, 1986) and what has come to be known as the **'New Right'**. Edwina Currie, a junior Health Minister in the 1980s, described the links between ill health and poverty: 'the problem very often for many people is just ignorance ... and failing to realise they do have some control over their own lives' (Townsend *et al.*, 1988a, page 12). As Smith and Nicolson (1991) argue, this emphasis, by politicians and other people in authority, on the ignorance of working-class people in relation to health goes back to the late nineteenth century. Such individualistic explanations for the unhealthy lifestyles of the working class are often criticised by sociologists, largely because they tend to ignore the social basis of human behaviour, although they still remain the basis of much contemporary health education (Beattie, 1991).
- Cultural: this emphasises how individuals share common beliefs and customs with each other; in other words, they share a common **culture**. According to this approach, behaviour such as smoking and drinking alcohol are not isolated aspects of working-class life, but they derive their meanings from within working-class culture as a whole. For example, smoking has a cultural acceptability amongst manual workers since it is seen as a form of leisure activity, as witnessed in pubs in working-class

areas and in factory canteens. During the last 20 years, smoking has become a form of despised activity amongst middle-class people so that there is greater group pressure to give up the habit amongst professionals and managers compared with manual workers (Hart, 1985).

The cultural explanation for health inequalities is not one which has gone unchallenged. One problem with it is that it can abstract 'culture' from the rest of the lives of the working class, chiefly in relation to material factors such as the income people have or the kind of houses they live in. For example, in relation to smoking, Graham (1987), in a study of young mothers on low incomes, has shown how smoking offers them very positive benefits in allowing them to cope in situations of little money but constant demands from children. Smoking means that these mothers can gain some form of psychological release from emotionally challenging situations they cannot physically escape. Blaxter (1990) has pointed out that behavioural factors, such as smoking and drinking, actually have a greater influence on the health of the middle class compared with those in poor material circumstances. It would seem, then, that less healthy lifestyles cannot in themselves account for all the health inequalities which the Black Report found and this is certainly the conclusion drawn by this report and *The Health Divide*. Marxists argue that the emphasis on the purchasing habits of the population neglects the way in which the production of health damaging products, such as cigarettes, is based upon what is profitable in capitalist society and not what is healthy (Doyal, 1979).

Materialist/structuralist explanations

These types of explanations focus on the role of social structural factors in causing health inequalities, that is, the working and living conditions which arise out of people occupying a position in the class structure. The Black Report states that such materialist explanations are the most important and further evidence supports this claim (Blane, 1985). In short, the argument is that health is affected primarily by people's working environment and their material resources, or rather lack of such resources, such as income and access to good quality housing. Since manual workers and their families are more likely to live in poor quality

housing and have low incomes, it is little wonder that their health will be worse than those people in higher class positions. In other words, the major problems underlying health inequalities are those associated with poverty and deprivation.

One methodological issue to bear in mind is that although poverty is more likely to affect manual workers and their families, by no means all manual workers are poor. Wilkinson (1989) has pointed to wide income differentials within each class as measured by the RG scale, so that class position is only an approximate measure of deprivation and poverty. Gender and racism, as well as occupational class, also determine who is poor or not, as we will see later on in this chapter.

Some research has tried to separate measures of material deprivation from social class in order to see if it really is the material factors which play the largest part in explaining health inequalities. Townsend *et al*. (1988b) did exactly this by looking at the health of people living in 678 wards in the north of England. They constructed a health index and a deprivation index based on the following four factors:

- Unemployment level
- Non-ownership of a car
- Non-ownership of a house
- Overcrowding.

They found that variations in health tended to correspond closely with variations in material deprivation and certainly closer than with occupational class. This suggests that class inequalities in health are probably more a result of material deprivation, which is linked to class but not adequately measured by class schemas such as that of the RG (Wilkinson, 1989).

Let us see, in more detail, how material factors associated with deprivation can affect health:

UNEMPLOYMENT

The following statement from the *British Medical Journal* starkly illustrates the impact of unemployment on health:

> 'the evidence that unemployment kills – particularly the middle aged – now verges on the irrefutable.'
>
> (Smith, 1991, page 606)

Mass unemployment returned to Britain during the 1980s, reaching a post-war peak of over 3 million officially unemployed in 1986, a condition which most people thought had disappeared for good since the Depression of the 1930s. Unemployment declined during the late 1980s, but increased again during the recession of the early 1990s. In December 1996, it had fallen to under 1.9 million, or 6.7% (ONS, 1997a).

Surveys have shown that there is a higher incidence of mortality and morbidity amongst those who are unemployed compared with similar people who are in employment (Benzeval *et al.*, 1995). Whilst there is evidence of the effects of unemployment on mortality and morbidity, there is some debate as to which aspects of unemployment have the most effect. Hakim (1982) suggests that two processes could be at work. One is the impact of economic instability and financial insecurity upon levels of stress; Moser *et al.* (1986) found that deaths due to suicide and lung cancer were much higher amongst the unemployed and both of these are linked to stress and stress-related activity. The second process is the poverty associated with unemployment, particularly long-term unemployment (Oppenheim and Harker, 1996).

INCOME

The Black Report concluded that low income was one of the main reasons for the health inequalities which it found. Those people on low incomes are restricted in the kinds and even quantities of food which they can buy:

> 'women who have to count every penny have less opportunity than women who are relatively comfortably off to concern themselves with issues of goodness; they are constrained to buy what they can afford to ensure that their families eat properly.'
>
> (Charles and Kerr, 1988, page 169)

Given the links between diet and health, income would seem to play a major role in explaining the relationship between class and health. Income is also important in relation to other areas of social life which also impact upon health, for example, the capacity to heat one's home as well as opportunities for socialising (Kempson, 1996).

HOUSING

In the 1930s great attention was paid to the condition of slum housing in British cities and the effects of overcrowding and insanitary conditions on health. Considerable slum clearance took place in

the 1930s and the large-scale building of council houses in the 1950s and 1960s was thought to have broken the links between working-class health and housing. However, the Black Report and *The Health Divide* both pointed to research which showed that such optimism was premature. Both reports made the general finding that mortality rates for all classes were highest in council and private rented dwellings compared with owner-occupied housing. Since the working class are more likely to live in council housing, this must explain some of the class differential in health. Byrne *et al.* (1986) also found that there were significant differences in health *within* the council housing sector, with those people living in 'difficult to let' estates reporting the worst health. Studies have noted the effects of damp and mould on health, particularly in relation to respiratory symptoms amongst children, as well as other ill effects of poor quality housing, including infestation, accidents and psychological stress (Best, 1995).

Homelessness is another housing-related factor which affects the health of many people today. The number of households accepted as homeless by local authorities has increased from 53 000 in 1978 to 150 500 in 1994, whilst nearly 48 000 households were living in temporary accommodation, including bed and breakfast, in 1994 (Lund, 1996). How does homelessness affect health? For those sleeping rough, the effects on health are only too obvious:

> 'once on the streets it is hard to keep healthy. The shelter, warmth, and privacy often taken for granted do not exist; good food may be hard to find or expensive; it is almost impossible to keep clean; "minor" illnesses are hard to cure.'
>
> (Lowry, 1991, page 87)

A recent report from the homelessness charity Crisis found that the average life expectancy for those living on the streets of London actually dropped to 42 in 1995, down from 47, 4 years previously, with common causes of death including heart disease, pneumonia and suicide (*The Guardian*, 2 December 1996, p. 7).

A survey of the health needs and problems of homeless families living in temporary accommodation was carried out by the housing charity Shelter (Miller, 1990). Many of the respondents were seriously concerned about their children's health and development, since most accommodation lacked a place for children to play in. Cooking facilities were often negligible which meant families lived on expensive, poor quality take-away food. Given this catalogue of material and social deprivation, it is unsurprising that nearly half the respondents had health problems they believed were caused by their accommodation, including depression and physical illnesses such as asthma.

WORK

Work itself, meaning here paid work, can be a cause of ill health and even death. In the nineteenth and early twentieth centuries, poor health and deaths in industrial work were a regular feature of working-class life. Increased government intervention in health and safety at work, including the 1974 Health and Safety at Work Act, did lead to a reduction in industrial injury rates, although the level of injuries in manufacturing industry rose considerably during the early 1980s (Tombs, 1990). Chemicals, fumes, dusts and other toxic substances can cause industrial diseases, including direct poisoning, allergies, congenital abnormalities or various forms of cancer (Doyal, 1979). Both industrial diseases and accidents are more likely to affect manual workers and this partially explains the class inequalities in health, particularly for men. Office workers also suffer from specific industrial hazards, such as **repetitive strain injury** which can occur in the wrists of data processor operators and telephonists, amongst others (Ewan *et al.*, 1991). The level of control over their job experienced by workers could also be a factor in determining the higher mortality rates amongst junior as opposed to senior office workers (Marmot, 1986). Work environments, the pace and organisation of work can all impinge on morbidity.

Social support

A fifth possible explanation for health inequalities is the amount and quality of social support people receive. The importance of social support in health and illness has been recognised ever since Durkheim's classic study *Suicide*, originally published in 1897, which linked suicide levels to the extent of social integration. For example, he found that single, widowed and divorced people are more prone to suicide because they have fewer social ties (Durkheim, 1952). More recently, in a survey of social support ties amongst pregnant women in England, Oakley and Rajan (1991) found that working-class women were no more likely to be closely involved with their relatives than middle-class women and that the latter had more support from both their friends and male partners than the former. Although this study is necessarily limited to a particular social group, it is suggestive that the class differences in health may be due to differences in the levels of social support between the classes. The *Whitehall Study* of civil servants (Marmot, 1986) also found evidence for an association between social support and mortality rates.

One of the most important recent analyses of health inequalities is that by Wilkinson (1996). In this he draws upon international data to show that in developed industrialised societies the countries with the best health are not those that are the richest, but those that are the most egalitarian, defined as those that have the least unequal income distribution. Average life expectancy is 2 or 3 years longer in countries such as Sweden and Japan, which have smaller income differences, compared with Britain or the USA. In fact, although the USA is the richest country in the world, death rates in Harlem, New York City, are higher at most ages than those that exist in Bangladesh, one of the poorest countries in the world. Wilkinson (1996) argues that the reason for this state of affairs lies in the idea that more egalitarian societies are characterised by higher degrees of social cohesion, or social support. Lack of social support and cohesion is fostered by higher levels of relative poverty, and results in greater levels of psychosocial stress, which in turn leads to illness and premature death. In other words, it is not absolute poverty that is crucial, but relative poverty and its impact on the social fabric.

The issue of social support is also an important issue in relation to assumptions about family and kin obligations and inequalities in both the availability and 'cost' of informal care, and access to a variety of community health and social services. There are, as we show later, gender, 'race' and ethnic dimensions to this kind of social support.

Key Points

■ Class inequalities in health have widened since the 1970s.

■ A number of explanations have been put forward for such health inequalities.

- The most important explanation appears to be the materialist one, which emphasises deprivation and inequalities in material resources, including income and access to good quality housing.
- Levels of social support and cultural variations in lifestyles also seem to play some role in explaining health inequalities.

GENDER AND HEALTH INEQUALITIES

GENDER

As we saw earlier, gender refers to the socially constructed relations between the sexes. Feminists have drawn attention to the manner in which gender acts as a form of stratification which exists not only in the so-called private sphere of the family, but also in the public world of industry, commerce and politics (Abbott and Wallace, 1996). The nuclear family is structured along gender lines, with the vast bulk of domestic labour, in the form of housework and child care, being carried out by women. In terms of employment, it is clear that paid work is stratified by gender with women doing different kinds of jobs from men and frequently being employed in low-paid and low-status occupations. Feminists have demonstrated that most areas of social life are structured by gender, including health and health care which are examined here.

EVIDENCE ON GENDER AND HEALTH INEQUALITIES

The broad conclusion on gender differences in health is that, on average, women live longer than men, but that they suffer more ill health than men. In 1994 men in the UK could expect to live to over 74 years of age compared with a life expectancy for women of over 79 years (ONS, 1997b). Excess male mortality exists in every age group from birth upwards. Amongst young people, the main cause of the gap between the sexes is the greater incidence of accidents and violence. *The Health Divide* found evidence that the sex differences in mortality for certain causes of death may be nar-

rowing in more recent years, for example in relation to deaths due to lung cancer in which the male:female ratio declined from 9:1 in 1960 to 4:1 in the late 1970s.

Does class make a difference to the mortality differences between men and women? As the Black Report showed, the death rates for men aged between 15 and 64 are nearly twice that of women in every occupational class, so the relationship between sex and mortality is not specific to any one class. However, there are class differences in the mortality rates of women as there are for men. Given the limitations of the RG class schema as applied to women, where women were traditionally grouped into classes on the basis of their husband's occupations, including on death certification, researchers have devised other measures for assessing inequality in women's mortality. One study utilised a composite measure of women's class position based upon:

- Their own employment
- Their **housing tenure**
- Whether they had use of a car.

This study found that for women 'high mortality is associated with working in manual occupations, living in rented housing, and with no car in the household' (Pugh and Moser, 1990, page 110).

What of differences in morbidity rates? Women on average have higher rates of both acute and chronic illness. Evidence from the 1994 General Household Survey (GHS) shows that on three measures of self-reported morbidity (restricted activity, longstanding illness and limited longstanding illness) there is both an upward trend in reported morbidity since the early 1970s and an excess of women in all (OPCS, 1996). In addition, the 1994 GHS data show that women have more days of acute sickness than men, and a small excess in hospital admissions. However, *The Health Divide* found that age affects this relationship, with boys and young men more likely to have higher rates of serious illness than girls and young women, whilst women are more likely to record higher levels of illness than men from middle age. There are also differences between men and women in the prevalence of particular complaints, which also vary by age. For example, women report more musculoskeletal problems and genito-urinary complaints (a category which encompasses reproductive disorders), whereas men report more respiratory disorders. Differences between men and women in reported morbidity for mental illness are also significant, showing an excess of morbidity in women (Graham, 1993).

Arber (1990) found that morbidity is also affected by the social class of the woman, so generally higher-class women report less long standing illness than lower class women. But she also found that marital status also seems to affect a woman's health, with married women having better health than single women, whilst divorced, separated and widowed women have the worst health of all. What is interesting from Arber's work is that for married women, social class measured by their own occupation showed a different pattern of morbidity. Women who were employers or managers had poorer health than other women in non-manual occupations and men in the same class (see Figure 3.2). This demonstrates the importance of developing new analyses of women's health in relation to their own circumstances and suggests that occupational status may have a different significance for women.

EXPLANATIONS OF HEALTH INEQUALITIES

The Health Divide suggests that the four explanations for class inequalities (artefact, natural selection, cultural/behavioural, materialist/structuralist) are also potential explanations for gender inequalities in health. We will examine each of these in turn, and in addition we will consider a fifth possible explanation which focuses on patriarchy.

The artefact explanation

The emphasis here is that the relationship between gender and health is actually an artificial one created by the measures of health used. Morbidity rates based upon use of the health services, for example, number of visits to a GP, may not be an accurate indicator of women's own ill health, but may arise because women are more likely to visit the GP on behalf of others, notably children (Abbott and Wallace, 1996). *The Health Divide* suggests that it could be that women are more likely to report illness than men, either to the health service or to an interviewer asking questions about health. This explanation suggests that the gender **role** into which women are socialised means that it is more acceptable for women to admit to illness and hence not to carry out their normal role obligations. Women's greater reporting of ill health may then reflect gender differences in the acceptability of going to seek medical assistance or in simply admitting to ill health, with men conform-

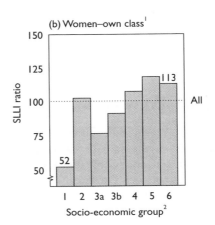

Figure 3.2: Standardised limiting longstanding illness ratios by class for women (20–59) (age-standardised)
Notes: [1] Women with husbands are classified by their husband's occupation; women of other marital statuses are attributed to their own (current or last) occupational class. [2] Socio-economic group: 1, higher professional; 2, employers and managers; 3a, lower professional; 3b, supervisory and junior non-manual; 4, skilled manual and own account; 5, semi-skilled manual and personal services; 6, unskilled manual
(Source: Arber, 1990, page 83. Analysis based on General Household Survey 1981–82)

ing to cultural stereotypes of masculinity and under-reporting illness.

Other research has suggested that consultation rates are deficient because 'women are more likely than men to suffer in silence' (Abbott and Wallace, 1996, page 168). This is because women have the major family responsibilities of domestic work, child care and care for other relatives, and therefore tend to treat their symptoms as normal and find ways of living with them to perform everyday duties. Popay (1992) strongly suggests it is difficult to argue that women who combine the roles of housewife and mother with those of paid work have as much time to report as full-time housewives or employed men. Here, then, we can see a more feminist interpretation of the gender differences in morbidity rates which suggests that such rates actually underestimate the extent of such differences. Brown and Harris (1978) found a large **illness iceberg** of unreported depression amongst a sample of women in London which supports the view of women suffering in silence.

There is a further way of extending this argument, which requires questioning the assumption that there are objectively identifiable categories of illness or symptoms to be acted upon; in other words, subjectively these symptoms will mean different things to people and it is this which affects their behaviour. Popay (1992) has shown that surveys indicate women report an excess of 'tiredness' compared to men, and in her own case studies were more likely to complain of 'severe tiredness'. However, she notes that 'tiredness' is complex; different types of tiredness arise in different social contexts and across the social classes.

Theories of natural selection

This explanation suggests that differentials in health between the sexes are not a product of gender processes at all, but are simply the result of biological differences between the sexes. There are clearly biological explanations for some of the differences in the types of illnesses experienced by men and women, most centring around the differences in the reproductive systems of the two sexes. However, the incidence of illness and mortality associated with women's reproductive systems, including maternal mortality, varies from society to society. The fact that, in all Western societies, women have a greater life expectancy than

men should not be allowed to obscure the fact that in some developing societies this position is reversed. The so-called natural longevity of women has only been so in relatively recent history: it is actually socially variable. In Britain, the fact that women live longer than men partly explains the higher rates of morbidity amongst women, since women are more likely than men to experience those chronic illnesses which are associated with ageing.

Whilst it would be naive to discount the effect of biology on health differences between the sexes, it must also be remembered that feminists have argued that biological explanations for the health of women have frequently been used as a means of controlling women by the male-dominated medical profession. Historically, in medical theories, women's health and social roles were considered to be determined by their reproductive biology but not on the basis of any clinical evidence (Harrison, 1995). Many aspects of women's health, for example, anorexia nervosa or pre-menstrual syndrome, are still explained in biological terms, which may actually serve to ignore or play down the role of social factors in producing illness.

As this short discussion has suggested, it is not a simple matter to disentangle biological from social factors in relation to gender differences in health. One example of where a biological inequality interacts with material and cultural disadvantage is in relation to the transmission of HIV (human immunodeficiency virus), the virus which leads to AIDS (acquired immune deficiency syndrome). Women are at greater risk than men of contracting HIV from a single act of intercourse and each sexual partnership, deriving in part from the 'fluid dynamics of unprotected sex' (Doyal, 1995, page 78). This biological inequality is further exacerbated by gendered inequalities in heterosexual relationships and the structured disadvantages of income.

Cultural/behavioural explanations

This approach, as we have seen in the section on class, focuses on those aspects of 'lifestyle' behaviour that are associated with health: cigarette smoking, excess alcohol consumption, poor diet and lack of exercise. Hart summarises the reason for the higher rates of male mortality, particularly after middle age:

'It is the greater male consumption of socially legitimate drugs, alcohol and cigarettes, which appears to underlie the vulnerability of men' [to an earlier death].

(Hart, 1989, page 133)

As with men, the major causes of death amongst women are circulatory diseases (coronary heart disease and stroke) and cancers. The major 'risk factors' in relation to coronary heart disease are smoking, high blood cholesterol and high blood pressure. Cholesterol levels are linked to the amount of saturated fat in the diet, whilst blood pressure is influenced by several factors, including obesity and heavy drinking. The two most important causes of cancer are smoking and diet, although breast cancer is linked to 'early menarche (age at first period) and first pregnancy delayed until after the age of 35' (Smith and Jacobson, 1988, page 52). There are difficulties, here, as research on causal factors remains contentious (for example, regarding cholesterol, alcohol consumption limits and during pregnancy, as well as the role of genetic predisposition).

Both Foster (1995) and Nettleton (1996) have argued that such controversies over the proliferating research on 'risk' factors has not prevented health promotion campaigns treating them as confirmed, and Foster suspects that this is not unrelated to the vested interests of industry and the state. Furthermore, it could be argued the concept of 'risk' is the new substitute for 'culture' or 'lifestyle' in the way it is used. It is translated on to individuals, and it is 'risky' individuals and 'risk groups' who are identified as the danger and become the target of campaigns and even stigma (see Nettleton, 1996). However, it would seem that lifestyle factors such as smoking and diet play some role in relation to the major 'killer' diseases.

From a feminist perspective, smoking cigarettes, drinking alcohol and taking exercise can only be understood in terms of the fact that such activities are a consequence of the structuring of social life and social relations along gender lines. So leisure itself is strongly associated with gender (Deem, 1986). The 1994 GHS (OPCS, 1996) data show that men are more likely to drink more than the sensible limits (as defined by units). Smoking has also been historically linked to cultural notions of gender. Until the 1950s smoking amongst women was heavily stigmatised; it was seen as

'unfeminine'. However over the 1950s and 1960s this changed, reflecting changes in gender relations and women's sense of their own identities (Hart, 1989). The closing of the gap for male/female rates of death due to lung cancer mentioned earlier could be linked to the narrowing of the gap between male and female cigarette smoking. The major concern here is with the pattern of smoking in young people. In 1994 23% of girls compared with 19% of boys were regular or occasional smokers and there has been an increase in prevalence since 1982 (see Table 3.3; ONS, 1997b). Overall, although the proportion of adults smoking has been declining in both men and women, it is unlikely to meet the Health of the Nation Target of only 20% still smoking by the year 2000.

Of course, this emphasis upon healthy lifestyles focuses solely on health as being a matter of consumption. From a Marxist or socialist feminist perspective, issues of consumption cannot be divorced from issues of production. The increase in female smoking across the century can be linked to the enormous power of the tobacco industry in both advertising cigarettes and in attempting, in various ways, to blunt the effectiveness of anti-smoking campaigns (Jacobson, 1988). Similarly with food:

'When faced with the power of the food manufacturing industry and agribusiness to control the food available in the shops, exhortations to individual women to make their families' diets more healthy without, at the same time, exhorting the food producers not to produce food which is dangerous to health, seem designed to divert attention from those who have the power to change things and increase women's burden of anxiety and guilt.'

(Charles and Kerr, 1988, page 125)

So far we have concentrated on those aspects of health behaviour that are associated with some of the major degenerative and ultimately fatal diseases. We have argued here that to reduce health behaviour to smoking and drinking is in itself a very narrow conceptualisation of a 'healthy lifestyle'. Individuals are 'blamed' for their unhealthy lifestyles rather than understanding that these have a structural and material basis. Graham (1987, 1990, 1993, 1994) has long argued that smoking in women is related to social disadvantage, although not racial disadvantage since smoking among black women is considerably

Table 3.3: Cigarette smoking among children:[1] by gender

England	Percentages		
	1982	**1986**	**1994**
Boys			
Regular smoker	11	7	10
Occasional smoker	7	5	9
Used to smoke	11	10	7
Tried smoking	26	23	21
Never Smoked	45	55	53
All boys	100	100	100
Girls			
Regular smoker	11	12	13
Occasional smoker	9	5	10
Used to smoke	10	10	8
Tried smoking	22	19	17
Never smoked	49	53	52
All girls	100	100	100

[1] Aged 11–15 years.
Source: Smoking Among Secondary School Children Survey, Office for National Statistics *Social Trends* 27, Crown Copyright 1997, page 131.

lower than among white women. It is living conditions that sustain particular kinds of lifestyle. Graham's work has stressed that to understand women's health adequately it is necessary to take into account the fact that it is women who do most of the health work in society, both formally in terms of nursing care (the vast majority of nurses are women), and informally in terms of the caring role which women adopt in the family by caring for children, husbands and other relatives, and often in conditions of poverty. This health work reflects the sexual division of labour in the family. The caring which women perform in the family can itself be detrimental to their health in terms of producing both physical and mental illness, largely due to stress, exhaustion and isolation (Lewis and Meredith, 1988). Gabe and Thorogood (1986) found that among both black and white working-class women, tranquillisers were used as a coping strategy for managing stressful lives. We return to some of these issues in the next section, since they are relevant to the material circumstances of women's lives, which should be taken into consideration when examining the relation between health and gender.

Materialist/structuralist explanations

Here the emphasis is on material inequalities between men and women:

- Despite the 1970 Equal Pay Act, women who were full-time employees in 1995 on average earned only 79% of the hourly average earnings of their male equivalents (CSO, 1996).
- Women are also far more likely than men to be in part-time employment.
- Women represent the majority of both the elderly and lone parents living on income support.

As a result of these inequalities, 'women are at far greater risk of poverty than men; at any given stage in their lives, women are far more likely than men to be poor and their experience of poverty is also likely to be far more acute' (Millar and Glendinning, 1989, page 363).

However, it is not only that women are more represented amongst those groups who are prone to poverty. Glendinning and Millar (1992) point out how resources are not equitably distributed *within* families, so that in low income households men are likely to retain some money for their own personal use whereas the same is not true of women, whilst it is women who are most likely to do without. Even in higher income households that possess large consumer durable items such as cars, these are more likely to be used by men than women (Beurat, 1991). There is not space here to go into the reasons for the gendering of poverty except to say that social policies in terms of benefits and child care provision, as well as the disadvantaged position of women in the labour market, are important factors (Glendinning and Millar, 1992).

One of the consequences of the increase in divorce since the 1960s has been the growth of lone parent families, although this is not the only factor. In 1994, they accounted for 8% of all households in Britain (OPCS, 1996). Approximately nine out of ten lone parent families are headed by women. Lone parent families are far more likely to be in poverty than two parent families, such that over 70% of lone mothers were in receipt of income support by the late 1980s (Millar, 1992). The greater extent of poverty amongst lone parent mothers, compared with fathers, is largely explicable in terms of the fact that lone fathers are more likely to be in full-time employment. The poverty of lone parents, and particularly mothers, cannot be separated from the employment position of women generally and aspects of social policy such as child care policy (Millar, 1992). Popay and Jones (1990), using the GHS, found that lone parents were in poorer health on all measures than parents living in couples. However, there are gender differences within lone parents, with mothers likely to have poorer health than fathers on all measures except that of longstanding illness. Given the lower proportion of lone mothers with child care arrangements and their greater poverty, the parenting demands on lone mothers are likely to be greater than those on lone fathers. Apart from the impact of material circumstances upon health, Popay and Jones (1990) argue that social isolation is an important contributory factor in the poor health of both lone mothers and fathers. It is important to note, as Popay and Jones do, that many lone parents provide positive and enjoyable lives for their children and themselves, but the effort to provide a positive life and maintain the welfare of others can mean that they pay a high price in terms of their future health status.

How does the material deprivation experienced by women affect their health? It affects it directly in terms of the fact that women on low incomes cut down on the amount and the quality of food (Charles and Kerr, 1988; Graham, 1990) that they consume and this has obvious health effects. It also means that women are less likely to make use of preventive health measures, such as screening services or antenatal classes, because they are difficult to get to without access to a car (Beurat, 1991). Payne (1991) also points out that women tend to spend more time at home than men and so the ill health effects of poor quality housing are likely to affect women more than men.

In recent years a number of researchers have been trying to determine the relative effects of domestic labour and paid work on health. For example, Hunt and Annandale (1993) found that paid work was an important factor in contributing to 'malaise', as based on a composite measure of a number of reported difficulties, for example, inability to sleep and feeling run-down. Although paid work affected both men and women, in addition domestic work was an important contributor to women's overall workloads and in itself exerted some influence on their health, whereas the combination of both paid and domestic work led to enhanced 'malaise' for women. These researchers emphasise the importance of treating domestic labour as 'real' work, and that the lack of change in the gendered division of labour continues to impinge negatively on women's health. As Arber (1991) argues, waged work, which is often low paid and part time, and without any change in domestic responsibilities, results in a necessary accommodation to existing inequalities.

Patriarchy

For many feminists, the gender relations and the material inequalities discussed above are manifestations of patriarchal relations between women and men. However, whilst feminists recognise that women are subordinate to men in material ways, for example, due to their occupying low paid and low status jobs, and also in ideological ways, for example, the idea that 'a woman's place is in the home', they also argue that this is not all there is to patriarchy. This system of oppression is also based on more overt forms of social control, chiefly those of violence against women by men. The definition of violence is not clear cut, but feminists have argued that it encompasses a broad range of behaviour including the following: rape, domestic battering, incest, sexual harassment and pornography (Edwards, 1987).

One important aspect of male violence is that the threat of violence can be as intimidating as the actual physical aggression itself. This threat can clearly have profound psychological and even physical effects on women's health. The peculiar feature of violence against women which feminists have pointed to is that, unlike the victims of other kinds of violence, women are somehow held to blame for the damage caused to themselves! It is only recently that recognition of the needs of survivors of violence and sexual abuse has been evident, although sensitive services are still piecemeal. Orr states that nurses should give greater recognition to the problem of violence against women:

> 'battering should be part of the differential diagnosis that nurses make, for the woman may be reluctant to state the problem overtly because of the stigma involved. Women who are victims of any form of male violence may be reluctant to be nursed by male nurses or to be in a mixed ward, but this is one area of patient choice which is not addressed.'
>
> (Orr, 1988, page 129)

This is despite *The Patient's Charter* (DoH, 1991) which provides for it.

This is important because evidence suggests that these forms of violence have increased over recent years. In some cases, as in rape, this may in part be an artefact of reporting behaviour. But recent research suggests that reported domestic violence is still far less than its actual prevalence. Using a household survey in north London, Moody (1996) explored, among other things, women's definitions of domestic violence, their experiences of different types of violence and the impact of these experiences. This showed that:

- 92% of assault involving physical harm was seen as domestic violence
- 80% considered mental cruelty to be so
- 30% had suffered 'composite domestic violence' (that is, more than one kind of action) at some time in their lives from partners or ex-partners

- Over a 12-month period the figures remained relatively high and the violence was often repeated
- Domestic violence results in injury, feelings of fear and insecurity, and being depressed and 'suicidal'
- Prevalence rates indicated that the scale of the problem and, therefore, the potential demand for services, has been underestimated.

Some authors have argued that there are aspects of health care that also perpetrate forms of violence, such as psychiatric incarceration. Kitzinger (1992) has likened much of the medical treatment of women in childbirth to forms of violation, with women often describing aspects of their experience using metaphors from butchery. As with Oakley's (1980) earlier study, such experiences result in poor mental health outcomes for these women. Feminists have also argued forms of patriarchal domination and the exercise of social control are evident in the day-to-day social relations and practice of health care (Foster, 1995).

GENDER AND MENTAL HEALTH

Most of the above discussion on gender and health focuses on the structural determinants of ill health as they differentially affect women and men. Thus we saw how, for example, gender roles and material deprivation could be used to explain the differences in mortality and morbidity rates between the sexes. As regards mental health, women show an excess over men of 'neurotic' psychiatric morbidity, and this remains so in all employment categories (OPCS, 1996). The rates for unemployed and economically inactive women were five times greater than for women working full time, although some social selection effect may operate here, in that illness could be the cause of lack of employment. Several studies have suggested that women's higher susceptibility to neurotic mental illness, such as depression, occurs as a result of the more stressful lives that women lead. This stress can then be explained in terms of the burdens of caring for others, lack of support and material disadvantage. Brown and Harris's (1978) study of women in London demonstrates that such a combination of factors explains the women's chances of becoming depressed, and that having no outside paid work was a factor.

This approach argues that women's greater prevalence of depression is a social product. Miles (1988) found that one important factor as to why women were more likely to develop neurosis than men was that married women receive far less emotional support from their husbands than husbands receive from their wives.

However, as Busfield (1989) argues, this is not the only way in which women's mental illness can be analysed. An alternative approach within feminism looks upon mental illness as a social construct; this approach turns its attention to the definitions of mental health and illness used by GPs and psychiatrists and at how the practice of psychiatry is carried out. In so doing, it draws upon ideas from labelling theory and symbolic interactionism. Labelling theory regards mental illness as a form of 'deviant' or rule-breaking behaviour. Feminists argue that psychiatry itself operates with a sexist conception of mental health whereby women's behaviour is more likely than men's to be considered deviant and is more likely to be defined as 'neurotic'.

Not only are women more likely than men to be labelled as 'mentally ill', but they are also more likely to be given psychotropic drugs. It has been argued that instead of regarding women's problems as arising out of the oppression which they experience in performing the domestic role, psychiatry acts so as to coerce women into accepting that role. Thus, as Penfold and Walker (1984) say, the paradox is that the psychiatry which women turn to for help acts in such a manner as to oppress them further. This feminist critique of psychiatry draws attention to the manner in which the medical profession can 'medicalise' women's problems with living, and in so doing obscure the social origins of such problems by labelling the problems as 'illnesses' which must be treated with drugs. The alternative, stressed by feminist health care practice, dovetails with the emphasis upon **holistic care** in nursing, to consider biography, social context and relationships.

Key Points

- Women tend to live longer than men, but they suffer more ill health.
- As with class, there are a number of explanations for gender inequalities in health.
- A combination of materialist and cultural factors, notably surrounding the domestic division of labour and gender divisions in paid employment, seem to be important in explaining such health inequalities.
- Feminists have argued that patriarchal gender relations, based upon male power over women, are also implicated in various aspects of women's health and in the health care which women receive.

'RACE', ETHNICITY AND HEALTH INEQUALITIES

'RACE', ETHNICITY AND RACISM

This section requires at the outset an examination of what we mean by 'race', ethnicity and racism. Unfortunately, there has been a tendency, including within health research, to conflate or treat these terms as interchangeable, instead of as distinct concepts. This can lead to a certain amount of confusion in trying to understand how the patterning of health, illness and service use might vary across different groups. The onset of ethnic monitoring in the 1980s and its inclusion in the NHS in 1990, followed by an additional question in the 1991 Census, was designed to improve information about ethnic populations. Unfortunately, these new 'measures' continue to use categories which do not reflect the distinction between 'race' and ethnicity. As will be evident, however, not all sociologists agree about such definitions or the relation between them, but it is important to provide a distinction that is useful for understanding health variations. In addition to the discussion that follows, a short definitional summary is provided in the summary box.

'Race' has been commonly used to refer to certain biological differences that are most evident in physical appearance, especially skin colour. This basis for distinguishing between people is regarded as highly dubious, and 'unscientific', accounting for at most 7% of human variation (Bradby, 1995). For some sociologists, the preferred term is ethnicity, whereas others wish to retain a connection between 'race' and racism (Mason, 1994). The contested nature of the concept 'race' is reflected in the use of inverted commas. Ethnicity refers to a group with a common heritage and often destiny, who share a way of life or culture and involves ideas of identity and a sense of belonging (Brah, 1994). In addition, some contemporary analysts, including postmodernist writers, emphasise that ethnicity, like other categories of difference, is unstable and shifting and should not be regarded as a fixed marker of identity. For this reason a number of sociologists have expressed doubt about the validity of the term 'ethnicity' itself as over-stressing a homogeneity of cultural patterns which, in reality, are far more variable and fluid (Ahmad, 1993).

Two issues become apparent if we make this distinction between 'race' and ethnicity. First, there has been an assumption that ethnicity is a property of some groups only, and in particular those who are in a minority. On the contrary, we all have ethnicity. For this reason, it is preferable to use the term minority or majority ethnic groups when we are exploring the variations in social circumstances of different groups in any society. Commonly used categories of minority ethnic groups in this society are Afro-Caribbean or West Indian, African, Indian, Pakistani, Bangladeshi, Chinese, Vietnamese, Arab, Irish, Cypriot, and so on. These broad groupings, however, may also contain further ethnic differentiation, such as between Turkish and Greek Cypriot, or between different Arabic groups. Second, the classification schemes used in the research process use a mixture of terms such as those above (ethnic groups) and white, Black-British (which are not ethnic groups). The problem is that the demands of research for neat, shorthand categories conflicts with the complexity and ambiguity of our social world. These difficulties are also present in the way we communicate, and it is common for the terms black and minority ethnic groups to be used. Donovan (1984) explains the term 'black people', as:

'... a political term, emphasising unity and solidarity among minority groups. The term does not seek to exclude any minority ethnic groups, but in general it tends to refer to people of Asian or Afro-Caribbean descent, who share the common experience of differentiation or racial discrimination in Britain because of the colour of their skin.'
(Donovan, 1984, page 663)

In this section, keeping the above cautions in mind, we will use the terms defined by Donovan above, since much of the work on inequality has concerned these groups. In addition to the difficulties described above, classification schemes have also not always distinguished those who are British-born from migrant groups. This is important because differences in origins, and also experience and circumstances, might differentially affect health. Place of birth is not a good proxy for ethnic group membership. The 1991 Census reveals the number of first generation adults born abroad is diminishing (Raleigh and Balarajan, 1995). Andrews and Jewson (1993) point to a further issue which will assume increasing importance: the number of young people, in particular, whose parents occupy different positions in any ethnic classification.

Before we leave this section two further terms require clarification. Racialised groups are the result when particular groups, including those who constitute ethnic groupings, are constructed in terms of 'race' as a means of delineating collective difference (Mason, 1994). The use of 'white' majority and 'black' minorities is an example of this process and is a product of racism. Racism is the process by which different individuals and groups are negatively constructed and then disadvantaged and excluded by a variety of social practices. Racism is usually divided into two types: personal racism refers to the way in which certain individuals are prejudiced against certain social groups on the basis of some physical characteristic, often, although not exclusively, skin colour. Institutional racism, on the other hand, refers to the way in which one 'racial group' has a position of power over another. Hence in Britain today, institutional racism inheres in the fact that in all the major institutions of society, including government, the legal system, industry and commerce, education and the health service, white people are in dominant positions and black people are in subordinate positions. This is sometimes referred to as systemic racism, and is reflected in values and norms as well as social structures. It is worth noting that this concept of institutional racism has been challenged by Marxists, such as Miles (1989), who argue that racism can only be adequately discussed in relation to class. The relative importance of class and racism in understanding the social position of black people in Britain is a topic of much debate in sociology (Anthias and Yuval-Davies, 1992; Smaje, 1996).

Definitions of 'race' and ethnicity

- 'Race' – used to refer to particular biological markers of differences between people, although actually only refers to small amount of human variation. Often regarded as 'unscientific' and ideological. Some authors stress that as a symbol of difference and as a social relationship, as in racism, it can be retained for analytical purposes.
- Ethnicity – everyone has ethnicity. It refers to real imagined or probable common origins of people.
- Ethnic group – will usually share a way of life and a sense of belonging for members. Ideas of cultural difference are closely tied to ethnicity, but should not be treated as the same.
- Racialisation – is where groups including, but not necessarily coincidental with, ethnic groups are constructed in terms of 'race' for the purposes of defining a collective difference, such as defining Afro-Caribbean, Asian and African people in Britain as 'black'.
- Racism – is a form of exploitation and oppression organised by reference to beliefs about capacities and rights in relation to 'race'. It encompasses the construction of inferiority and social and institutional practices of exclusion and discrimination. Such practices may be personal, and embedded in the organisation and social relations of social institutions. It is also historically specific.

(For further reading on this complex conceptual debate see: Miles, 1989; Anthias and Yuval-Davies, 1992; Brah, 1994; Mason, 1994; Bradby, 1995).

EVIDENCE ON 'RACE', ETHNICITY AND HEALTH INEQUALITIES

Given the clear picture of social disadvantage faced by black people in Britain going back to the 1950s, it is surprising that the study of ethnicity and health had relatively little attention until the 1980s; even the Black Report devotes fewer than two pages to the topic. Both the Black Report and *The Health Divide* concentrated their attention on studies which compared the health of immigrants with that of people born in England and Wales. A recent study by Balarajan (1991) found that deaths due to ischaemic heart disease were much higher in both men and women born in the Indian subcontinent compared with people born in England and Wales, whereas the rates for both men and women born in the Caribbean were much lower than those for the indigenous population. However, Caribbean-born men and women had the highest mortality from cerebrovascular disease. But we have already indicated some of the problems in using such studies to assess the health of minority ethnic groups. Others are discussed here. Similar differentials between minority ethnic groups are shown in relation to a morbidity indicator – limited longstanding illness. When standardised for age, it shows that Bangladeshi and Pakistani groups suffered nearly 60% more than expected given their age structure, whilst Chinese were below what would be expected (see Figure 3.3).

There is considerable evidence regarding the health of ethnic minorities in relation to specific

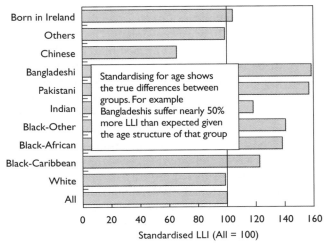

Figure 3.3: Limiting long-term illness: ethnic group: standardised for age
(Source: 1991 Census in *Health Services Journal*, 1993, 103, 30–1)

health conditions. This evidence usually comes from the medical profession and does not necessarily reflect the complete health picture. Furthermore, it has tended to concentrate on those conditions that are 'particular' to certain minority ethnic groups, which has both reflected as well as reinforced a tendency to look for culturally specific explanations and 'culture blaming'. In 1984 Donovan pointed to five main areas of research and research findings:

- Rickets: Asians were more likely to develop rickets than the rest of the population.
- Tuberculosis: higher in all immigrant groups compared with the indigenous population.
- Inherited diseases: **sickle cell anaemia** – an inherited disease which affects Afro-Caribbeans, whilst **thalassaemia** affects a range of groups.
- Mental health: Asian people were less likely to suffer from any form of mental illness than white people, whilst Afro-Caribbeans experienced less depression but had higher rates of schizophrenia compared with the rest of the population.
- Family (usually children's) health: which concentrated on the infant mortality and **perinatal mortality rates**, showing these to be higher amongst Asians with Asian babies having lower birth weights in comparison with white babies, whilst rates of childhood accidents are greater in Afro-Caribbean families.

All these areas remain in the forefront of discussions around the ethnic patterning of health. Further research has demonstrated more variation between minority ethnic groups in the 1990s. For example, although perinatal mortality by country of mother's birth declined amongst all ethnic groups, Figure 3.4 shows that a significant excess among Pakistani and Caribbean-born mothers over UK-born continues. African and Bangladeshi mothers were also at high risk, but those from India and East Africa less so, although still in excess of UK-born mothers (Raleigh and Balarjaran, 1995). There are also variations in cause of infant deaths, indicating that there seems to be no single factor that can be pointed to as an explanation (Andrews and Jewson, 1993), although congenital abnormalities accounted for over half the excess. Important to our discussion about class is that the figures illustrate that, although there is a class gra-

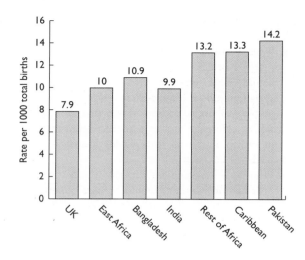

Figure 3.4: Perinatal mortality by mother's country of birth 1989–91 combined England and Wales
(Source: Raleigh and Balarajan, *The Registrar General's Decennial Supplement for England and Wales*, Series DS No. 11, the Office for National Statistics, Crown Copyright, 1995, page 85)

dient within each ethnic group, the excess remains in all social classes (Raleigh and Balajaran, 1995).

Thus Donovan's list does not exhaust the health issues in relation to 'race' and ethnicity and they remain topics which still generate a great deal of heated debate in the sociological and medical literature. In part they have remained so because of the salience of some of these issues for health activists within minority ethnic groups, such as in the case of sickle cell disease, and the inadequacy of knowledge and services to date. Whilst the 1990s have seen other health issues come on to the agenda, particularly aspects of community care, there are many health issues for minority ethnic groups that remain largely invisible to health care professionals. The 1990 NHS and Community Care Act argued that 'good' care was to be sensitive to, and recognise, the 'needs' of minority communities, involving them in planning. However, evidence suggests that access and appropriateness of a variety of community services falls short of such aims. Health patterns and 'needs' for people with mental health problems, disabled and elderly people within minority ethnic groups still require further investigation and response (Ahmad, 1993; Ahmad and Atkin, 1996).

Let us now look at the explanations which have been put forward for these health inequalities and differences.

EXPLANATIONS OF HEALTH INEQUALITIES

As with the previous two sections we will attempt to use the explanatory framework devised in the Black Report and we will also include a fifth possible explanation, that of racism.

The artefact explanation

As we have argued above, there are a number of problems regarding the categories which researchers have used to study the 'racial' or ethnic patterning of health. As a consequence it is possible that differences in the data are not 'real' differences between groups, but are due to how people have been classified. The use of broad categories, for example, may obscure significant differences between groups. Studies based upon comparing immigrants with people born in Britain are not really measuring the impact of ethnicity or racism on health at all, since they exclude those ethnic minority members born in this country and they include, in their immigrant category, white people emigrating from countries such as India (Hunt, 1995). This is important given that migration features as an explanation in its own right (Smaje, 1996).

A further kind of artefact explanation lies in the diagnostic practices of practitioners. Here, it is suggested, the values and expectations about both minority ethnic groups and about presented complaints or symptoms lead to certain diagnostic outcomes. Racism can enter into this process. As we suggest later, it has been argued that the higher incidence of schizophrenia in Afro-Caribbean men is in part a consequence of the way doctors interpret symptoms (Knowles, 1991). This can equally lead to an under-representation as might be the case for Asians, men in particular (Watters, 1996a).

Theories of natural selection

To say that there is a biological basis to differences in the health of minority ethnic groups falls back on the now discredited biological theories of 'race'. Nevertheless, there does seem to be a genetic basis to the two inherited diseases mentioned above, that is, sickle cell anaemia and thalassaemia. As Donovan (1984) says, the Sickle Cell Society has called for more training of health workers and for information on the subject to be more widely available, but Hunt (1995) suggests that professional interest in the disease has not been accompanied by the development of preventive screening and access to diagnostic services. Similarly, Ahmad (1995) points to differences here in screening for phenylketonuria, a genetic blood disorder found in the white population. There has been some suggestion that the high rate of perinatal mortality from congenital abnormalities in babies born to mothers born in Pakistan could have a genetic component, although it is acknowledged that causation is complex and not fully understood (Raleigh and Balarajan, 1995). Overall, explanations for the ethnic patterning for health would seem to lie mainly outside of a biological or genetic cause.

Cultural/behavioural explanations

Much of the work on the health of minority ethnic groups has focused on the cultural differences between the minorities and the white majority. Probably the most famous example of this is the higher rates of rickets found amongst the Asian minorities and the consequent Stop Rickets Campaign launched in 1982. Most researchers agree that vitamin D deficiency is the major factor leading to rickets and the causes of this are said to be lack of sunshine and/or dietary deficiencies. As far as Asians in Britain are concerned, most attention was placed on dietary factors, notably the use of foods other than fortified margarine, as well as the eating of foods high in phytic acid, including chappatis (Donovan, 1984; Pacy, 1989). Some researchers offered a change to Western diet and lifestyle as the solution to Asian rickets. In effect, Asian culture itself has been and is seen as a 'problem' which needs to be changed. Such an approach is culturally insensitive and also neglects the evidence that Western diet is thought to be one factor behind circulatory diseases. There are a variety of other approaches to the phenomenon of rickets amongst Asians, including the provision of vitamin D supplements (Pacy, 1989) or more simply the fortification of chappati flour in the same way that margarine itself was fortified (Donovan, 1984).

Apart from rickets, one other health issue affecting the Asian minority groups which has also led to a major health promotion campaign is that of a high perinatal mortality rate amongst Asian babies. The DHSS and the Save the Children Fund sponsored the Asian Mother and Baby Campaign which began in 1984 and was designed to reduce the perinatal mortality rate by helping pregnant Asian women to make more use of antenatal and maternity services. This campaign raises a number of important issues in relation to the provision of health services for minority ethnic groups (Rocheron, 1988). Certainly some commentators regard this campaign as being an improvement on the Stop Rickets Campaign since it is concerned with providing more responsive health services rather than simply with delivering health educational messages (Ahmad, 1989). However, although Raleigh and Balarajan's (1995) data also indicate that the category 'Asian' neglects the now considerable differences among mothers born on the Asian subcontinent, let alone between these and UK-born, this has not prevented cultural differences being 'blamed' as the case of consanguineous marriages in relation to high rates of congenital abnormality in Pakistani babies illustrates.

The difficulty here is that an emphasis on 'special needs', which could lead to more sensitively geared health interventions, has tended to reinforce the rhetoric of cultural specificity in a way that has marginalised those needs. Culture has also rarely been looked at as a positive contributor to either health, or people's ability to deal with their illness. For example, as Ahmad (1995) in his review of American research on families with sickle cell disease (SCD) notes, mothers are involved in constructing their own meaning of the disease, its normality, which enables pain crises to be coped with in particular ways.

As with the debate over the relative importance of cultural and material factors in the explanation of class and gendered health inequalities, a parallel debate exists in relation to ethnicity and health. Several writers in this field (Ahmad, 1989, 1993; Donovan, 1984; Pearson, 1989) have continued to point to how the focus on the lifestyles of minorities deflects from attention to material deprivation and racial discrimination suffered by Asians and Afro-Caribbeans in Britain. Let us turn first to the materialist explanations.

Materialist/structuralist explanations

Despite evidence of a growing number of Asians and Afro-Caribbeans entering the professional and managerial middle classes (Phillips and Sarre, 1995), it is still true to say that in general terms the minority ethnic groups are significantly materially disadvantaged relative to the white population. They are more likely to live in the decaying inner city areas with their problems of multiple deprivation. The 1995 Labour Force Survey (ONS, 1997b) shows that unemployment was:

- 21% amongst black men
- 18% amongst Pakistani and Bangladeshi men
- 8% amongst white men.

It is likely that some of this difference is due to discriminatory practices by employers. Also noteworthy is the fact that many black people live in poor, often overcrowded housing (Brown, 1985) or, as Hyndman (1990) found for Bengalis in one London borough, it was dampness that put health at risk. In addition, they have a disproportionate number of households in the lowest income bracket (ONS, 1997b). Given these factors, many researchers have argued that material deprivation is at the heart of the health issues faced by the ethnic minorities. Donovan (1984) suggests that of the five health issues focused upon by medical researchers, only inherited disease is unconnected to material deprivation.

Racism

Nevertheless, many writers would add that whilst black people living in inner city areas share the same material disadvantages as the poor white working class, they are subject to another form of social disadvantage, namely racism, which can have direct and indirect effects on health. The most obvious form of racism that can affect health is racial harassment, which can include physical assaults, attacks on property, graffiti, arson, verbal abuse, racist phone calls, etc. The Newham Monitoring Project (1995) had 518 cases reported to it in 1994, as well as many more people using their centre; such figures illustrate the harassment black families are subjected to on a daily basis. Attacks and harassment often leave tremendous physical and mental scarring, not just through actual physical assault, but also the anxiety and fear generated by harassment that is verbal as well as physical. As a study in Leeds by the Independent Commission of Enquiry into Racial Harassment (1987) found, many Asian people were afraid to go out, their children needed to be escorted because of fear of harassment, whilst 45% of the sample had changed the way they lived in some way because of potential harassment. Given that nursing is moving towards a more positive holistic view of health in which the health service user is located within their social environment, it is important that nurses are aware of some of the uglier sides of British society.

In addition, institutional racism can have less obvious, but equally important, consequences for the health of black and minority ethnic groups. For example, local authority housing allocations may discriminate against such groups. There is evidence that Caribbean single mothers are more likely to live in worse housing, notably high-rise flats, than white single mothers (Peach and Byron, 1993); this can, in turn, lead to higher levels of stress.

ETHNICITY, RACISM AND MENTAL HEALTH

One of the areas of health need which has generated considerable research in relation to the ethnic minorities has been mental health. The available evidence suggests that, on the whole, Asian people have less reported mental illness than the rest of the population (Ineichen, 1990), whilst Afro-Caribbeans have less depression but more psychosis, especially schizophrenia, and the ethnic group with the highest rate of mental hospital admissions is the Irish (Littlewood and Lipsedge, 1989). In this section we will be concentrating on the question of Afro-Caribbeans and schizophrenia since it highlights a number of sociological issues in relation to mental health.

Whilst it is well established, in the psychiatric literature, that migrants have higher rates of mental illness than the indigenous populations, suggesting that the stress of migration is implicated, what has recently emerged is that second generation Afro-Caribbeans in Britain have higher rates of psychotic illness than their parents. In addition, this results in higher rates of compulsory admission (Cope, 1989). A recent study in London (Bebbington et al., 1994) shows this tendency for compulsory admission continues although overall rates are lower than Cope's data. The rates for detention of Afro-Caribbeans under Section 136 of the Mental Health Act is two and one-half times that for whites (Pilgrim and Rogers, 1993). Clearly, this later finding cannot be explained with reference to the strains of migration. It could be that socio-economic disadvantages, including racial discrimination, contribute towards the high rates of psychosis amongst second generation Afro-Caribbeans; this is an area which requires further research (Cope, 1989).

Another possibility here, as with gender, is in relation to labelling theory where what is considered 'normal' in one group or society may be considered 'bad' or even 'mad' in another. Psychiatric diagnosis involves value judgements in relation to socially constructed standards of acceptable behaviour and there is evidence that white psychiatrists are more likely to apply the label 'schizophrenic' to Afro-Caribbeans (Knowles, 1991). Littlewood and Lipsedge (1989) give several illustrations of the way in which religious beliefs amongst Afro-Caribbeans in Britain can be misunderstood by psychiatrists if they operate within a strictly **medical model** of mental illness. The danger is that psychiatry feeds off and helps to maintain social stereotypes, particularly that of the 'alien' for Afro-Caribbeans:

'Whatever the empirical justification, the frequent diagnosis in black patients of schizophrenia (bizarre, irrational, outside) and the infrequent diagnosis of depression (acceptable, understandable inside) validates the stereotypes.'
(Littlewood and Lipsedge, 1989, page 251)

Labelling, in the form of cultural stereotyping, also seems to operate in relation to southern Asian peoples. For example, the tendency amongst health professionals to characterise South Asians as likely to turn their problems into physical symptoms and to 'waste' physicians' time will directly impinge on the treatment they are likely to receive (Watters, 1996b).

However, writers have challenged this emphasis on cultural differences and misunderstandings, arguing that it does not sufficiently recognise the importance of power between psychiatrist and patient and crucially the issue of racism (Knowles, 1991). In the mental health field there is no reason to suppose there is not a place for what Ahmad (1996) has called a 'sophisticated conception of culture which is well located within its socio-economic, political and historical context' (pages

428–9). As Fenton and Sadiq-Sangster (1996) show, forms of cultural meaning and expression may be crucial in understanding mental distress among South Asian women. Distinct languages are used to 'display' that distress. What is important is that such culturally specific language forms are not seen, as has often been the case, as yet another cultural deficit. Finally, it needs to be stressed that a wider range of mental health problems and the issues they raise for service use requires moving beyond epidemiological patterns of diagnostic groups among black and minority ethnic groups. We return to issues of culture and racism in relation to health care below.

Key Points

- 'Race', 'ethnicity' and 'racism' have different meanings in the sociological literature.
- There is evidence of continuing inequalities between the health of minority ethnic groups and the white majority.
- Material deprivation and racism are argued by many writers to be most important in terms of explaining such health inequalities, but cultural factors are also thought to play some part.

HEALTH CARE AND SOCIAL DIVISIONS

Having looked at how class, gender and 'race' affect people's health, it is important to examine how these three dimensions of inequality affect the delivery and practice of health care in more detail.

CLASS AND HEALTH CARE

The Black Report argues that the NHS can play a role in ameliorating the inequalities which it found, whilst it recognises that the root of the inequalities lies in social conditions which the NHS by itself cannot tackle. What do the Black Report and *The Health Divide* say about the manner in which the NHS is currently organised and used in relation to class inequalities?

As regards use of the health service, the evidence is not altogether consistent. On the one hand, working-class people make more use of GP services than do middle-class people and they also seem to make more use of outpatient departments at hospitals. Against this must be balanced the evidence which suggests that, relative to their health needs, manual workers actually make less use of the health service than do middle-class people (Townsend *et al.*, 1988). It is difficult to be definitive about this because of the problems in measuring health need. The Black Report found that the use of preventive health services, such as family planning and maternity clinics, cancer screening facilities and dental services, did follow clear class gradients with the lower classes making less use of these services than the higher classes.

Benzeval *et al.* (1995) argue that there are three main barriers to access to health care:

- Geographical: research indicates that health care facilities are more likely to be located in affluent areas, and conversely there are fewer health care facilities in deprived areas. For example, a study in Buckinghamshire found that GP and pharmaceutical facilities were lacking in a deprived area, despite the disproportionate number of elderly people, children and people with limiting long-term illness living there (Watt and Stenson, 1996). Removing this barrier involves having more clinics in deprived areas, or having 'outreach' services which take the service to the user, for example, mobile antenatal clinics.
- Financial: despite the NHS being free at the point of delivery, nevertheless there are user-charges on certain health care items, which can put people off seeking treatment. The timing of service availability can also be detrimental to those particularly on low incomes. This indicates the importance of having flexible opening times in order to maximise the numbers of people who can access the service.
- Cultural: there can be cultural mismatch between lower-class patients, particularly those from ethnic minority groups, as we have seen above, and the health care professionals. Some studies have suggested that the working class make less use of preventive health services than the middle class because the two classes hold different cultural beliefs about health, with the former regarding health negatively, as the absence of disease, and the latter regarding

health as a sense of well-being. Blackburn (1991) has challenged this cultural explanation by arguing that mothers in deprived areas do not have negative attitudes towards preventive services, but that they may not attend child health clinics because of the difficulties of travelling to them or because of the manner in which the clinics are organised, including a formal atmosphere.

A further example of some of these issues is in relation to homelessness and health care. One of the main problems regarding people who are homeless is that they tend to be less likely to be registered with a GP than those who are housed and they may well receive little actual health care despite their greater needs. Research on 'rough sleepers' in London has suggested that they would be more likely to use health care services if the latter were both more accessible and delivered in a non-judgemental manner (Shiner, 1995).

Both Townsend *et al*. (1988a) and Benzeval *et al*. (1995) have a number of detailed recommendations as to how service accessibility can be improved for people who are poor and disadvantaged and readers are encouraged to refer to these.

GENDER AND HEALTH CARE

The above section on gender inequalities in health has focused on only some aspects of what is now a substantial feminist critique of the structure and practices of the health care system as a whole in relation to women's health. This critique, which may be found in a number of sources (e.g. Orr, 1988; Doyal, 1995; Foster, 1995; Nettleton, 1996), has changed slightly in emphasis over the last two decades and has focused on several areas:

- The **medicalisation** of women's health, turning social difficulties and 'natural' transitions into medical events.
- The exercise of patriarchal control by the medical profession in its encounters with women patients and in the surveillance of their health and lifestyles.
- The lack of a holistic approach to health in which emotional and social aspects of women's lives are treated seriously; and socio-economic policies which will address wider aspects of gender inequality which 'cause' ill health.

- The subordination of women within the health care division of labour, and a devaluation of their skills and role in health care, and lack of support for those women who bear the main responsibility for informal health care.

In addition, feminists now put considerable stress on recognising the diversity of women's experiences and health needs, and the cross-cutting of gender with other forms of inequality, such as class, 'race' and ethnicity, disability, sexual orientation and age. Much of the work of feminists working through what Doyal (1995) characterises as women's health movements in recognition of their diversity has included specific campaigns to improve access to women-centred health care. Many groups have been organised to provide support and information to women around specific issues, in a context where these are either lacking or doctor- and male-dominated. It was reproductive rights activists who revealed black women were being prescribed the contraceptive Depo-Provera without knowledge of its side-effects, and raised the suspicion that it was also an attempt to control black women's fertility. Other groups have been formed around issues such as the menopause, breast cancer and older women carers. They utilise principles of self-help, mutual support, building self-confidence and empowerment. In nursing too, as Orr (1988) suggests, this approach involves the sharing of knowledge with clients rather than an emphasis on the nurse being the health care 'expert'.

In many ways, **well women clinics** are models of a feminist health care system. However, as Foster (1991) argues, the danger is that well women clinics, as with many other initiatives, depend on short-term funding and are marginalised within the health care system as a whole. She suggests that feminist health care workers need to begin to tackle the difficult challenge of making mainstream health services more women-centred. The point about challenging mainstream, as some feminists would describe them 'male-stream', is well-taken, but we should not forget that activism outside of these has been successful in changing aspects of health care practice. Changes in place of birth and who cares for women in labour are now evident, and certainly unnecessary degradations (such as shaving) and some surgical interventions have decreased. Equally, it can be argued that women are more likely to be involved in making choices about treatment options when diagnosed with breast cancer, even though such choices will be constrained by other factors such as available services.

There is clearly still much to be done. It is crucial that attention is paid to some of those groups of women who remain invisible within discussions of health needs. This is not easy because not only are the majority of doctors and managers men, but the research agenda is also dominated by men. This can be seen in relation to HIV and AIDS, for example, where there are few services directed at women. The experience of black women in the NHS has been neglected, with what attention there has been directed at maternity care and Asian women (see Douglas, 1992). Morris (1995) has equally drawn attention to how, in health care, disabled women are disadvantaged by the neglect of their care needs by non-disabled people. Stereotyping continues to prevent the delivery of appropriate care. These are just some examples, and we could highlight too the neglect of the largest killer of women after middle age, coronary heart disease, where most health promotion for heart disease targets men.

As with other areas of inequalities in relation to health services, there are opportunities within the context of the health service reforms for nurses and other health workers to take advantage of a new emphasis on 'users' to develop new insights into women's experiences of health care. Hillan (1992), for example, has suggested that nurses and midwives who have patient contact could use this to develop aspects of audit, so that it is less of a counting exercise and more of a reflection of women's views. In this way she suggests there is more chance that audit could be used to inform practice and improve the quality of nursing care. Of course, it is also possible that the recent changes in the NHS will exacerbate existing inequalities, including gender: at present it is difficult to assess. In any case, a number of the issues raised as explanations for gendered inequalities in health are not matters for the NHS alone. However, changes as a consequence of challenges to the medical model of health towards a new paradigm have been identified by Nettleton (1996) as emphasising the psychosocial–environmental/ epidemiological and directing attention to prevention and health promotion. Such an ideological

shift, she argues, does not necessarily mean women's needs will be better addressed. In part, this is because neither the material circumstances of women's lives nor their perceived social responsibility for the maintenance of their own and others' health continue not to be addressed at the policy level.

'RACE', ETHNICITY AND HEALTH CARE

There are two models in terms of ethnicity, 'race' and health care. The first is that of 'ethnic sensitivity' and the second is '**anti-racism**' (Stubbs, 1993). The first, underpinned by a multiculturalist philosophy, argues that the main problem in relation to ethnic minorities and the health services is a lack of effective communication arising out of cultural differences between minority patients and the health service which reflects the majority 'white' culture. In particular, attention is drawn to language differences, dietary customs and religious practices. The ethnic sensitivity approach suggests that health service workers need to familiarise themselves with the culture of minority ethnic groups in order that any communication barriers which prevent effective health care are removed. Emphasis is also put on instituting measures to overcome language barriers, such as the use of interpreters for non-English-speaking patients, and also link workers to improve take-up rates for preventive services. This approach focuses on ethnicity and culture, and in different ways was exemplified in the Stop Rickets Campaign and the Asian Mother and Baby Campaign mentioned above. There are parallels between the ethnic sensitivity approach to health care and the concept of transcultural nursing developed by Leininger in the USA (for a summary and critique of transcultural nursing, see Stokes, 1991).

However, this ethnic sensitivity/multicultural approach has been much criticised by sociologists and health workers, for example Culley's (1996) recent critique in relation to health education, especially from those who emphasise the second model of 'race' and health care, i.e. anti-racism. The argument from this model is that institutionalised racism permeates all the major institutions of society and included amongst these is the NHS; hence racism should be the focus of attention rather than 'culture'. Pearson (1989) illustrates racial inequality in the following:

> 'While a walk around many hospitals would reveal a reasonable number of ethnic minority staff, a disproportionate number are in inferior positions. The majority are in low paid, ancillary and manual jobs, working night shifts and at weekends, in the less qualified echelons of nursing or in "twilight" areas, such as geriatrics and psychiatry, in the less prestigious non-teaching hospitals.'
>
> (Pearson, 1989, page 77)

Midwives were shown to take punitive attitudes (in one case refusing pain relief to a woman who had not attended antenatal classes on the grounds 'she had not learned how to breathe'; Bowes and Domokos, 1996), and Bowler (1993) similarly found stereotypes of Asian mothers and an 'us and them' distinction to be prevalent. A consequence of this was also a denial of pain relief. It could be argued that tackling the issue of racism in the NHS and in nursing is essential in making the health service more responsive to the health needs of Britain's black population (McNaught, 1988; Ahmad, 1993).

One further potential problem with the ethnic sensitivity approach to health care is that there is a danger that it provides a checklist of 'cultural differences' which are really no more than stereotypes, for example, the belief that all Asians in Britain live in close-knit, extended families (Ahmad, 1993). Such stereotypes gloss over class, religious and regional variations within the black community in Britain. They equally tend to reinforce a homogeneity that then neglects how differences within black and minority ethnic groups impinge upon health and access to services. Assumptions concerning family type and household composition have led to the invisibility of informal care where this is occurring, and a neglect of all those who may need care in single person households because of a racist belief that 'they will look after their own', and so services are not needed (Walker and Ahmad, 1994). The literature on informal care remains substantially based on studies of the white population (Atkin and Rollings, 1996).

Some researchers, for example Littlewood and Lipsedge (1989), argue that the 'either culture or racism' debate is a sterile one and that both ethnicity and racism need to be incorporated into an analysis of the health and health care of black people. This recognition of the importance of both cultural factors and the systematic disadvantages experienced by black people, as both users and employees of the NHS, is reflected in recent work in relation to nursing (Gerrish et al., 1996). Good communication, is important for all clients of health services, and access to women doctors, interpreters and advocates are all necessary responses to cultural and material disadvantage.

Gender and disability lead further to what Carby (1982) has called 'simultaneous oppression', which creates additional problems in having one's difficulties recognised and accessing appropriate services. In general, services are organised according to white norms, and poverty and material inequalities will create additional barriers to service use. In a context where many people have already experienced personal racism and institutional barriers to access, the process of building up trust between a service and a local black or minority ethnic group community can be a slow and difficult one, and with resource constraints, many NHS Trusts may find it difficult to invest the necessary time and personnel to do so. The temptation returns to use short-term funding, or to divert the problem to the voluntary sector. Ahmad (1995) found the conclusions of a recent report by leading practitioners on haemoglobinopathies 'depressing reading', and noted that although their concern and recommendations were credible, there was little indication of how these would be put into practice. He stresses, too, the importance of initiatives not limited to the NHS but coordinated packages of care, taking in housing, education and social services as well as the voluntary sector, which are especially important in the care of older and mentally ill people. However, in the 'sidelining' of services around 'special needs' there has been a failure to consider how mainstream services, such as primary health care, community care, health education and hospital care, respond to a diversity of health needs.

There are opportunities within the remit of recent changes in the NHS, which now require the planning of services more directly around identified 'needs', to involve 'users', both actual and potential, in that process. To date, there is still some caution necessary in how that involvement is to be brought about and how empowering of consumers it will be. There is still a widespread distrust among health care professionals and managers of services of the legitimacy of 'lay' expertise (see Popay and Williams, 1994). As Walker and Ahmad (1994) have shown, in community care there is, at best, 'tokenistic' consultation with already marginalised groups, and the gulf between need and available resources results in what has been called 'windows of opportunity in rotting frames'. These are problems besetting community care in general, but they impinge much more sharply on those who already experience multiple disadvantage. In a context of racism there is still a view that the problem is with the clients not the services themselves (Ahmad and Atkin, 1996). At the policy level, the Department of Health has funded the SHARE project, designed to facilitate the development of databases and sharing of resources on 'race' and health, and in its own Ethnic Health Unit aims to effect positive change through the purchasing process (Ahmad, 1996). The difficulty is that, as yet, there is little evidence of strategies being in place to do so, nor of new patterns of care which will ensure greater race equality in health care.

Key Points

- Geographical, financial and cultural factors play a role in preventing adequate access to health care from those people in lower social class positions.
- Feminists have pointed both to the gender divisions and sexism inherent in much contemporary health care and also to the importance of recognising the diversity of women's health needs.
- Both 'ethnic sensitivity' and 'anti-racism' provide frameworks for more adequately addressing the health care needs of minority ethnic groups.

TACKLING HEALTH INEQUALITIES

Whitehead (1995) has provided a useful account of the ways in which health inequalities can be tackled. She suggests that there are four main policy levels at which health inequalities can be addressed:

- Strengthening individuals. This includes both interventions with a behavioural focus, such as providing health information to persuade people to change their behaviour (as in health edu-

cation and smoking), as well as interventions with an empowerment focus in which the emphasis is on trying to build up people's self-confidence and skills, for example, stress management or assisting disadvantaged people to claim rights and services to which they are entitled.
- Strengthening communities. Here the emphasis is on how deprived communities can join together for mutual support. Examples include the partnerships which have developed between council tenants and teams of health professionals, including district nurses, health visitors, doctors, social workers and health researchers, concerned with health and housing conditions (Lowry, 1991; Seymour, 1991). The focus has been on how the residents perceive their own health in public, not individualistic, terms; in other words, their health is directly related to the social conditions in which they live. This 'community development' approach to tackling health inequalities involves a change in the **role** of both health professionals and their clients, with the latter becoming active agents in the creation of their own health care instead of being the passive recipients of professional 'expertise'.
- Improving access to essential facilities and services. This includes much of the public health measures concerned with access to adequate housing, sanitation, uncontaminated foods, safer workplaces, welfare and health services.
- Encouraging macro-economic and cultural change. This is the broadest level and involves national and international policies to reduce poverty and inequality both between and within countries, environmental hazards and equal opportunities.

In a critical article on the Whitehead proposals, Wainwright (1996) argues that in the absence of specific proposals to tackle what is probably the most important source of health inequalities, i.e. the structure of social and economic inequality itself, focusing on the rest will have only a minimal impact on health inequalities. In fact, writing from a perspective influenced by Marxism, Wainwright argues that one of the main effects of the 'strengthening individuals' notion is to make poor people accept their social situation rather than challenge those very circumstances which make them poor and unhealthy to begin with. Although

Wainwright illustrates the political difficulties inherent in genuinely tackling health inequalities, the potential drawback is that this approach can result in a sense of hopelessness and fatalism: 'the problems are so immense, what can any one individual do about them?'

Sociology is not a discipline that suggests that analysing 'problems', such as inequalities in health, is a simple matter or which claims to provide easy solutions. Different sociological perspectives provide different views on the possible directions social change should take if the health inequalities illustrated in this chapter are to be diminished, whereas some sociologists are sceptical about whether sociology should make recommendations for social change at all. However, if inequalities are going to be reduced in health and in the provision of health care, it seems clear there will need to be policy developments and structural change across a number of aspects of society. As we have shown, material factors loom large in explaining health inequalities in general and for particular groups, including women, black and ethnic minority groups, older people and lone parents. As we have seen, such material factors structure lifestyle options and consumption. Wilkinson (1996) has demonstrated that the relative size of income differentials now seems to be the most important predictor of a nation's health for all societies, including our own, and therefore income redistribution must be an important priority for governments. As he argues, improvements in health and income inequalities have occurred in different societies, but 'historical experience shows us that political will is crucial' (Wilkinson, 1996, page 223). One thing which is unclear at the time of writing is whether the new Labour government has such political will or not.

In relation to the NHS, this chapter has implicitly challenged the language of consumerism which frequently dominates discussions of the NHS, whereby health service users are described as 'consumers'. As we have attempted to show, describing the population in such terms gives a spurious uniformity to what is in effect a deeply divided society. However, that does not mean that health care professionals cannot utilise the new rhetoric of 'need-led' health provision, and an emphasis on 'user' involvement to ensure that individuals and groups gain more responsive ser-vices. Much will depend on how health purchasers, providers and planners interpret the challenges of the NHS in the 1990s.

Social change, however, is not just about governmental or professional intervention. Many of the sociological perspectives outlined above emphasise that although people are located within structures of inequality, they are also active agents who can themselves, to some extent, modify and change those structures by their actions. Those groups we have singled out as being the most vulnerable to ill health, the working class, women, black people, poor and homeless people, are not just passive victims of their social position, but are actively engaged in shaping their lives and their health. We have indicated throughout this chapter that nurses need to work with their clients so as to allow these disadvantaged groups in particular to shape their own health care agenda rather than having one imposed upon them by experts, no matter how well meaning. As Marx said, 'the educator must himself be educated' (Bottomore and Rubel, 1963, pages 82–3). In other words, those who are without power and social advantage can teach nurses about the circumstances of their lives and what they think their health needs are. Holistic care is not simply about seeing people in their social environment. It is also, ideally, about trying to shift the power balance towards those people who have least power in this society, so that they can truly fulfil their human potential and take genuine control of their lives; in other words, lead healthy lives.

Key Points

Health inequalities can be tackled by addressing the issue at four policy levels:

- Strengthening individuals
- Strengthening communities
- Improving access to services and facilities connected with health
- Encouraging macro-level social and economic change, notably the reduction of inequality.

CONCLUSION

This chapter has provided a sociological account of the social context of health in which nurses will be operating, focusing on the manifold ways in which class, gender and 'race' affect people's health and also the manner in which health care itself is delivered. Hopefully, the chapter has contributed towards providing the sociological evidence and theories which will stimulate debate amongst both trainee and qualified nurses as to the significance of health inequalities and on the best ways in which these can be tackled in future.

Summary

We have seen in this chapter how British society continues to be structured by deep processes of social inequality. Class, gender and 'race' all operate as important determinants of people's life chances, not least in relation to their experiences of health and health care. Health inequalities in terms of illness and mortality rates exist in relation to class, gender and 'race': those people at the lower end of the class structure have worst health than those at the top end; women tend to live longer than men but have worse health; black people face additional health disadvantages resulting both from their poorer economic position and racism. The delivery of health care itself in the NHS is affected in numerous ways by social inequality and difference. There is a wide-ranging set of policies designed to deal with health inequalities, although more needs to be done at all levels of government and the NHS if such policies are to be genuinely effective.

ACKNOWLEDGEMENTS

The authors would like to thank Anne Chappell for her very helpful comments on an earlier draft of this chapter.

REFERENCES

Abbott, P. and Wallace, C. (1996). *An Introduction to Sociology: Feminist Perspectives*, 2nd edn. Routledge, London.

Abercrombie, N. and Warde, A. (1994). *Contemporary British Society*, 2nd edn. Polity Press, Cambridge.

Ahmad, W.I.U. (1989). Policies, pills and political wills: a critique of policies to improve the health status of ethnic minorities. *Lancet*, 1, 148–50.

Ahmad, W.I.U. (ed.) (1993). *'Race' and Health in Contemporary Britain*. Open University Press, Buckingham.

Ahmad, W. (1995). 'Race' and health: a review article. *Sociology of Health and Illness*, 17(3), 418–23.

Ahmad, W.I.U. (1996). Family obligations and social change among Asian communities. In *'Race' and Community Care*, Ahmad, W.I.U. and Atkin, K. (eds). Open University Press, Buckingham.

Ahmad, W.I.U. and Atkin, K. (eds) (1996). *'Race' and Community Care*. Open University Press, Buckingham.

Andrews, A. and Jewson, N. (1993). Ethnicity and infant deaths: the implications of recent statistical evidence for materialist explanations. *Sociology of Health and Illness*, 15(2), 137–56.

Anthias, F. and Yuval-Davis, N. (1992). *Racialised Boundaries: Race, Nation, Colour, Class and Anti-racist Struggle*. Routledge, London.

Arber, S. (1990). Revealing women's health. In *Women's Health Counts*, Roberts, H. (ed.). Routledge, London.

Arber, S. (1991). Class, paid employment and family roles: making sense of structural disadvantage. *Social Science and Medicine*, 32, 425–36.

Atkin, K and Rollings, J. (1996). Family care-giving among Asian and Afro-Caribbean communities, In *'Race' and Community Care*, Ahmad, W.I.U. and Atkin, K. (eds.). Open University Press, Buckingham.

Balarajan, R. (1991). Ethnic differences in mortality from ischaemic heart disease and cerebrovascular disease in England and Wales. *British Medical Journal*, 302, 560–4.

Bartley, M., Carpenter, L., Dunnell, K. and Fitzpatrick, R. (1996). Measuring inequalities in health: an analysis of mortality patterns using two social classifications. *Sociology of Health and Illness*, 18(4), 455–75.

Beattie, A. (1991). Knowledge and control in health promotion: a test case for social policy and social theory. In *The Sociology of the Health Service*, Gabe, J., Calnan M. and Bury, M. (eds.). Routledge, London.

Bebbington, P., Feeney, S., Flannigan, C., Glover, G., Lewis, S., and Wing, J. (1994). Inner London Collaborative Audit of Admissions in two health districts II: ethnicity and the use of the Mental Health Act, *British Journal of Psychiatry*, 165, 743–9.

Benzeval, M., Judge, K. and Whitehead, M. (eds). (1995). *Tackling Inequalities in Health: An Agenda for Action*. King's Fund, London.

Best, R. (1995). The housing dimension. In *Tackling Inequalities in Health: An Agenda for Action*, Benzeval,

M., Judge, K. and Whitehead, M. (eds). King's Fund, London.

Beurat, K. (1991). Women and transport. In *Women's Issues in Social Policy*, Maclean, M. and Groves, D. (eds). Routledge, London.

Blackburn, C. (1991). *Poverty and Health*. Open University Press, Milton Keynes.

Blane, D. (1985). An assessment of the Black Report's explanations of health inequalities. *Sociology of Health and Illness* 7(3), 423–45.

Blane, D., Davey Smith, G. and Bartley, M. (1993). Social selection: what does it contribute to social class differences in health? *Sociology of Health and Illness*, 15(1), 1–15.

Blaxter, M. (1990). *Health and Lifestyles*. Tavistock/Routledge, London and New York.

Booth, C. (1905). *Life and Labour of the People of London*. Macmillan, London.

Bottomore, T.B. and Rubel, M. (1963). *Karl Marx: Selected Writings in Sociology and Social Philosophy*. Penguin Books, Harmondsworth.

Bowes, A., and Domokos, T.M. (1996). Pakistani women and maternity care: raising muted voices. *Sociology of Health and Illness*, 18(1), 45–65.

Bowler, I. (1993). 'They're not the same as us': midwives' stereotypes of South Asian maternity patients. *Sociology of Health and Illness*, 15(2), 157–78.

Bradby, H. (1995). Ethnicity: not a black and white issue. *Sociology of Health and Illness*, 17(3), 405–17.

Bradley, H. (1996). *Fractured Identities*. Polity Press, Cambridge.

Brah, A. (1994). Time place and others: discourses of race, nation and ethnicity. *Sociology*, 28(3), 805–13.

Brown, C. (1985). B*lack and White Britain: The 3rd PSI Survey*. Gower Publishing, Aldershot.

Brown, G.W. and Harris, T. (1978). *Social Origins of Depression*. Tavistock Publications, London.

Busfield, J. (1989). Sexism and psychiatry. *Sociology*, 23(3), 343–64.

Byrne, D., Harrisson, S.P., Keithley, J. and McCarthy, P. (1986). *Housing and Health*. Gower Publishing, Aldershot.

Carby, H. (1982). Black feminism and the boundaries of sisterhood. In *The Empire Strikes Back: Race and Racism in 70s Britain*, CCCS (eds.). Hutchison, London.

Carr-Hill, R. (1987). The inequalities in health debate: a critical review of the issues. *Journal of Social Policy*, 16(4), 509–42.

Charles, N. and Kerr, M. (1988). *Women, Food and Families*. Manchester University Press, Manchester.

Cope, R. (1989). The compulsory detention of Afro-Caribbeans under the Mental Health Act. *New Community*, 15(3), 343–56.

Crook, S., Pakulski, J. and Waters, M. (1992). *Postmodernization*. Sage Publications, London.

CSO (Central Statistical Office) (1996). Women in the labour market: results from the Spring 1995 LFS. *Labour Market Trends*, 104(3), 91–100.

Culley, L (1996). A critique of multiculturalism in health care: the challenge for health education. *Journal of Advanced Nursing*, 23(3), 564–70.

Deem, R. (1986). *All Work and No Play? The Sociology of Women and Leisure*. Open University Press, Milton Keynes.

DoH (1991). *The Patient's Charter*. HMSO, London.

DoH (1995). *Variations in Health. What Can the Department of Health and the NHS Do?* DoH, London.

Donovan, J. (1984). Ethnicity and health: a research review. *Social Science and Medicine*, 19(7), 663–70.

Douglas, J. (1992). Black women's health matters: putting black women on the research agenda. In *Women's Health Matters*, Roberts, H. (ed.). Routledge, London.

Doyal, L. (1979). *The Political Economy of Health*. Pluto Press, London.

Doyal, L. (1995). *What Makes Women Sick? Gender and the Political Economy of Health*. Macmillan, London.

Drever, F., Whitehead, M. and Roden, M. (1996). Current patterns and trends in male mortality by social class (based on occupation). *Population Trends*, 86, 15–20.

Durkheim, E. (1952). *Suicide*. Routledge & Kegan Paul, London.

Edgell, S. (1993). *Class*. Routledge, London.

Edwards, A. (1987). Male violence in feminist theory: an analysis of the changing conceptions of sex/gender violence and male dominance. In *Women, Violence and Social Control*, Hanmer, J. and Maynard, M. (eds.). Macmillan Press, Basingstoke.

Erikson, R. and Goldthorpe, J.H. (1993). *The Constant Flux*. Oxford University Press, Oxford.

Ewan, C., Lowy, E. and Reid, J. (1991). 'Falling out of culture': the effects of repetition strain injury on sufferers' roles and identity. *Sociology of Health and Illness*, 13(2), 168–92.

Fenton, S. and Sadiq-Sangster, A. (1996). Culture, relativism and mental distress; South Asian women in Britain. *Sociology of Health and Illness*, 18(1), 66–85.

Foster, P. (1991). Well women clinics. In *Women's Issues in Social Policy*, Maclean, M. and Groves, D. (eds). Routledge, London.

Foster, P. (1995). *Women and the Health Care Industry*. Open University Press, Buckingham.

Gabe, J. and Thorogood, N. (1986). Tranquillisers as a resource, In *Tranquillisers; Social, Psychological and Clinical Perspectives*, Gabe, J. and Williams, P. (eds). Tavistock, London.

Gerrish, K., Husband, C., and Mackenzie, J. (1996). *Nursing for a Multi-ethnic Society*. Open University Press, Buckingham.

Giddens, A. (1997). *Sociology*, 3rd edn. Polity Press, Cambridge.

Glendinning, C. and Millar, J. (eds) (1992). *Women and Poverty in Britain: the 1990s*. Harvester Wheatsheaf, Hemel Hempstead.

Goffman, E. (1968) *Asylums*. Penguin Books, Harmondsworth.

Goldthorpe, G. and Marshall, G. (1992). The promising future of class analysis: a response to recent critiques. *Sociology*, 26(3), 381–400.

Goldthorpe, J.H. (1980). *Social Mobility and Class Structure in Modern Britain*. Oxford University Press, Oxford.

Graham, H. (1987). Women's smoking and family health. *Social Science and Medicine*, 25(1), 47–56.

Graham, H. (1990). Behaving well: women's health behaviour in context. In *Women's Health Counts*, Roberts, H. (ed.). Routledge, London.

Graham, H. (1993). *Health and Hardship in Women's Lives*. Harvester Wheatsheaf, Hemel Hempstead.

Graham, H. (1994). *When Life's a Drag: Women, Smoking and Disadvantage*. HMSO, London.

Gubbay, J. (1997). A Marxist critique of Weberian class analyses. *Sociology*, 31(1), 73–89.

Hakim, C. (1982). The social consequences of high unemployment. *Journal of Social Policy*, 11(4), 433–67.

Harrison, B. (1995). Women's health. In *Women's History, Britain: 1850–1945*, Purvis J. (ed.). University College Press, London.

Hart, N. (1985). *The Sociology of Health and Medicine*. Causeway Books, Ormskirk.

Hart, N. (1989). Sex, gender and survival. In *Health Inequalities in European Countries*, Fox, J. (ed.). Gower Publishing, Aldershot.

Health Services Journal (1993). Data briefing, *Health Services Journal*, 103, 30–1.

Hillan, R. (1992). Research and audit: women's views of caesarian section. In *Women's Health Matters*, Roberts, H. (ed.). Routledge, London.

Hills, J. (1995). *Joseph Rowntree Inquiry into Income and Wealth*, Volume 2. Joseph Rowntree Foundation, York.

Hunt, K. and Annandale, E. (1993). Just the job? Is the relationship between health and domestic and paid work gender specific? *Sociology of Health and Illness*, 15(5), 632–64.

Hunt, S. (1995). The 'race' and health inequalities debate. *Sociology Review*, 28–32.

Hyndman, S.J. (1990). Housing dampness and health amongst British Bengalis in East London. *Social Science and Medicine*, 30(1), 131–41.

Independent Commission of Enquiry into Racial Harassment (1987). Racial Harassment in Leeds 1985–1986. Leeds Community Relations Council, Leeds.

Ineichen, B. (1990). The mental health of Asians in Britain. *British Medical Journal*, 300, 1669–70.

Jacobson, B. (1988). *Beating the Ladykillers: Women and Smoking*. Victor Gollancz, London.

Jones, I.G. and Cameron, D. (1984). Social class analysis: an embarrassment to epidemiology. *Community Medicine*, 6, 37–46.

Kempson, E. (1996). *Life on a Low Income*. Joseph Rowntree Foundation, York..

Kitzinger, S. (1992). Birth and violence against women: generating hypotheses from women's accounts of unhappiness after childbirth. In *Women's Health Counts*, Roberts, H. (ed.). Routledge, London.

Knowles, C. (1991). Afro-Caribbeans and schizophrenia: how does psychiatry deal with issues of race, culture and ethnicity? *Journal of Social Policy*, 20(2), 173–90.

Lewis, J. and Meredith, B. (1988). *Daughters Who Care*. Routledge, London.

Littlewood R. and Lipsedge M. (1989). *Aliens and Alienists: Ethnic Minorities and Psychiatry*, 2nd edn. Unwin Hyman, London.

Lowry, S. (1991). *Housing and Health*. London: British Medical Journal.

Lund, B. (1996). *Housing Problems and Housing Policy*. Longman, Harlow.

McNaught, A. (1988). *Race and Health Policy*. Croom Helm, London.

Marmot, M.G. (1986). Social inequalities in mortality: the social environment. In *Class and Health*, Wilkinson, R.G. (ed.). Tavistock Publications, London.

Mason, D. (1994). On the dangers of disconnecting race and racism. *Sociology*, 28(4), 845–58.

Miles, A. (1988). *Women and Mental Illness*. Wheatsheaf Books, Brighton.

Miles, R. (1989). *Racism*. Routledge, London.

Millar, J. (1992). Lone mothers and poverty. In *Women and Poverty in Britain: the 1990s*, Glendinning, C. and Millar, J. (eds.). Harvester Wheatsheaf, Hemel Hempstead.

Millar, J. and Glendinning, C. (1989). Gender and poverty. *Journal of Social Policy*, 18(3), 363–81.

Miller, K. (1990). *Wasting Money, Wasting Lives: The Scandal of Temporary Homes*. Shelter, London.

Mills, C.W. (1970). *The Sociological Imagination*. Penguin Books, Harmondsworth.

Moody, J. (1996). Researching domestic violence: The North London Domestic Violence Survey. In *Gender Relations in Public and Private*, Morris, L. and Lyon, E.S. (eds.). Macmillan, London.

Morris, J. (1995). Creating space for absent voices: disabled women's experiences of receiving assistance with their daily living activities. *Feminist Review*, 51, 68–94.

Moser, K.A., Fox, A.J. and Jones D.R. (1986). Unemployment and mortality in the OPCS Longitudinal Study. In *Class and Health*, Wilkinson, R.G. (ed.). Tavistock Publications, London.

Nettleton, S. (1996). Women and the new paradigm of health and medicine. *Critical Social Policy*, 16(3), 33–53.

Newham Monitoring Project (1995). *Fifteen Years of Resistance: Annual Report for 1994/95*. Newham Monitoring Project, London.

Oakley, A. (1980). *Women Confined: Towards a Sociology of Childbirth*. Martin Robertson, Oxford.

Oakley, A. and Rajan, L. (1991). Social class and social support: the same or different? *Sociology*, 25(1), 31–59.

ONS (Office for National Statistics) (1997a). Labour market data. *Labour Market Trends*, 105(2), S1–S84.

ONS (1997b) *Social Trends 27*. The Stationery Office, London.

OPCS (Office of Population Censuses and Surveys). (1991). *Standard Occupational Classification*, Volume 3. HMSO, London.

OPCS (1996). *Living in Britain: Results from the 1994 General Household Survey*. HMSO, London.

Oppenheim, C. and Harker, L. (1996). *Poverty: The Facts*. 3rd edn. Child Poverty Action Group, London.

Orr, J. (1988). Women's health: a nursing perspective. In *Political Issues in Nursing: Past, Present and Future*, Volume 3, White, R. (ed.). John Wiley & Sons, Chichester.

Pacy, P.C. (1989) Nutritional patterns and deficiencies. In *Ethnic Factors in Health and Disease*, Cruickshank, J. and Beevers, D. (eds). Wright, London.

Payne, S. (1991). *Women, Health and Poverty*. Harvester Wheatsheaf, Hemel Hempstead.

Peach, C. and Byron, M. (1993). Caribbean tenants in council housing: 'race', class and gender. *New Community*, 19(3), 407–23.

Pearson, M. (1989). Sociology of race and health. In *Ethnic Factors in Health and Disease*, Cruickshank, J. and Beevers, D. (eds.). Wright, London.

Penfold, P.S. and Walker, G.A. (1984). *Women and the Psychiatric Paradox*. Open University Press, Milton Keynes.

Phillips, D. and Sarre, P. (1995). Black middle-class formation in contemporary Britain. In *Social Change and the Middle Classes*, Butler, T. and Savage, M. (eds). UCL Press, London.

Pilgrim, D and Rogers, A. (1993). *A Sociology of Mental Health and Illness*. Open University Press, Buckingham.

Popay, J. (1992). 'My health is all right, but I'm just tired all the time': women's experience of ill health. In *Women's Health Matters*, Roberts, H. (ed.). Routledge, London.

Popay, J. and Jones, G. (1990). Patterns of health and illness amongst lone parents. *Journal of Social Policy*, 19(4), 499–534.

Popay, J and Williams, G. (eds.) (1994). *Researching the People's Health*. Routledge, London.

Pugh, H. and Moser, K. (1990). Measuring women's mortality differences. In *Women's Health Counts*, Roberts, H. (ed.). Routledge, London.

Raleigh, V.S. and Balarajan, R. (1995). The health of infants and children among ethnic minorities. In *The Registrar General's Decennial Supplement for England and Wales, Series DS No. 11*, Botting, B. (ed.). HMSO, London.

Ramazanoglu, C. (1989). *Feminism and the Contradictions of Oppression*. Routledge, London.

Rocheron, Y. (1988). The Asian Mother and Baby Campaign: the construction of ethnic minorities' health needs. *Critical Social Policy*, 8(1), 4–23.

Rowntree Seebohm, B. (1902). *Poverty: A Study in Town Life*. Nelson, London.

Saunders, P. (1990). *Social Class and Stratification*. Routledge, London.

Seymour, J. (1991). Whose health is it anyway? *Nursing Times*, 87(15), 16–18.

Shiner, M. (1995). Adding insult to injury: homelessness and health service use. *Sociology of Health and Illness*, 17(4), 525–49.

Smaje, C. (1996). The ethnic patterning of health: new directions for theory and research. *Sociology of Health and Illness*, 18(1), 139–71.

Smith, A. and Jacobson, B. (1988). *The Nation's Health*. King's Fund, London.

Smith, D. and Nicolson, M. (1991). *Health and Ignorance – Past and Present*. Paper given at British Sociological Association Annual Conference, University of Manchester, March 25–28.

Smith, R. (1991). Unemployment: here we go again. *British Medical Journal*, 302, 606–7.

Stokes, G. (1991). A transcultural nurse is about. *Senior Nurse*, 11(1), 40–2.

Stubbs, P. (1993). 'Ethnically sensitive' or 'anti-racist'? Models for health research and service delivery. In *'Race' and Health in Contemporary Britain*, Ahmad, W.I.U. (ed.). Open University Press, Buckingham.

Tombs, S. (1990). Industrial injuries in British manufacturing industry. *Sociological Review*, 38(2), 324–43.

Townsend, P. (1979). *Poverty in the United Kingdom*. Penguin Books, Harmondsworth.

Townsend, P., Davidson, N. and Whitehead, M. (1988a). *Inequalities in Health: The Black Report and The Health Divide*. Penguin Books, Harmondsworth.

Townsend, P., Phillimore, P. and Beattie, A. (1988b). *Health and Deprivation: Inequality and the North*. Routledge, London.

Turner, B.S. (1986). *Equality*. Ellis Horwood and Tavistock Publications, Chichester and London.

Wainwright, D. (1996). The political transformation of the health inequalities debate. *Critical Social Policy*, 16, 67–82.

Walker, J. and Ahmad, W.I.U. (1994). Windows of opportunity in rotting frames: care providers perspectives of community care and black communities. *Critical Social Policy*, 40, 46–70.

Watt, P. (1996). Social stratification and housing mobility. *Sociology*, 30(3), 533–50.

Watt, P. and Stenson, K. (1996). Poverty amidst plenty: hard times in the South East of England. *Poverty*, 95, 13–15.

Watters, C. (1996a). Representation and realities: black people, community care and mental health. In *'Race' and Community Care*, Ahmad, W.I.Q. and Atkin, K. (eds). Open University Press, Buckingham.

Watters, C. (1996b). Representations of Asians' mental health in British psychiatry. In *The Social Construction of Social Policy: Methodologies, Racism, Citizenship and the Environment*, Samson, C., and South N. (eds). Macmillan, London.

Whitehead, M. (1995). Tackling inequalities: a review of policy initiatives. In *Tackling Inequalities in Health: An Agenda for Action*, Benzeval, M., Judge, K. and Whitehead, M. (eds). King's Fund, London.

Wilkinson, R.G. (1989). Class mortality differentials, income distribution and trends in poverty 1921–81. *Journal of Social Policy*, 18(3), 307–35.

Wilkinson, R.G. (1996). *Unhealthy Societies*. Routledge, London.

FURTHER READING

Ahmad, W.I.U. (ed.) (1993). *'Race' and Health in Contemporary Britain*. Open University Press, Buckingham.

This is a very useful collection of readings on 'race' and health.

Benzeval, M., Judge, K. and Whitehead, M. (eds.). (1995). *Tackling Inequalities in Health: An Agenda for Action*. King's Fund, London.

This is an excellent summary of policy initiatives in relation to tackling health inequalities.

Giddens, A. (1997). *Sociology*, 3rd edn. Polity Press, Cambridge.

This is one of the most comprehensive and informative introductions to the discipline of sociology.

Nettleton, S. (1995). *The Sociology of Health and Illness*. Polity Press, Cambridge.

This is a very good introduction to the sociology of health and illness.

Townsend, P., Davidson, N. and Whitehead, M. (1988) *Inequalities in Health: The Black Report and The Health Divide*. Penguin Books, Harmondsworth.

This provides an important discussion of the evidence on health inequalities.

Wilkinson, R.G. (1996) *Unhealthy Societies*. Routledge, London.

This is a highly acclaimed analysis of health inequalities in an international context.

CHAPTER FOUR

PROMOTING HEALTH

Sally Kendall

- Introduction
- Nursing and health promotion
- The challenge of promoting health
- The preventive approach
- The self-empowerment approach
- The radical approach
- Conclusion

The aim of this chapter is to examine ways of promoting and maintaining health which the nurse may apply in clinical practice. To meet this aim, the chapter includes consideration of the relationship between nursing and the promotion of health and the challenge of promoting health. The use of a range of health promotion models, including illness prevention, self-empowerment and radical models, are critically discussed and their application illustrated using examples including **immunisation**, screening, diet, exercise, alcohol consumption and mental health. The importance of promoting human potential through the nurse working in partnership with the patient is a theme throughout this chapter.

INTRODUCTION

The previous chapter has explored in some depth the broad and varied concepts that people may hold about health and some of the possible influences on those conceptions. This chapter will be looking at how we, as nurses, can use our ideas about health and our skills (both in practical nursing and communication) to both promote and maintain health. First, the relationship between nursing and health will be explored. This will be followed by a series of examples of how health can potentially be promoted.

It is not the intention here to define health. You will by now be aware that health is an area of enormous subjectivity and as such is difficult to label or measure in such a way that it can be universally understood. However, it may be useful when thinking about health to refer to David Seedhouse's idea that:

'All theories of health and all approaches designed to increase health are intended to advise against, to prevent the creation of, or to remove, obstacles to the achievement of human potential. These obstacles may be biological, environmental, societal, familial or personal.'

(Seedhouse, 1986, page 53)

Although we may each differ in our understanding of what constitutes human potential, it is at least a phrase unburdened by values related to sickness or wellness. Thus, it is possible to begin to understand how individuals may exist at any point along the wellness–sickness continuum and still be in a position to achieve potential. For example, a young woman disabled by multiple sclerosis may have come to terms with her illness and found a new and satisfying relationship with her family. Another woman of the same age might be physically fit, but find it difficult to handle stress, leading to difficulties in personal relationships and health behaviours, such as smoking. Is it possible to say who is the healthier of these two women? Seen in terms of human potential we can see that they each have obstacles to overcome and each has managed to do so with different degrees of success.

The obstacles to achieving human potential, and the ways in which we as nurses may enable those in our care to overcome them, will form the main focus of this chapter.

NURSING AND HEALTH PROMOTION

Before addressing the nurse's role in health promotion, it is useful to consider what is meant by the term, as there is some debate about the difference between health promotion and health education. In 1984 the World Health Organization (WHO, 1984a) produced some principles of health promotion which are summarised below:

- Health promotion involves the population as a whole in the context of everyday life, rather than focusing on people at risk of specific diseases
- Health promotion is directed towards action on the determinants or causes of health
- Health promotion combines diverse, but complementary, methods or approaches
- Health promotion aims particularly at effective and concrete public participation
- While health promotion is not a medical service, health professionals – particularly in primary health care – have an important role in nurturing and enabling health promotion.

This involves action which:

- Enhances equal access to health
- Develops an environment conducive to health
- Strengthens social networks and support
- Promotes positive health behaviour and appropriate coping strategies
- Increases knowledge and disseminates information.

These principles suggest that health promotion is an activity that nurses, among others, may engage in. Some of these actions will be addressed

later in the chapter. However, Baric (1985) has argued that health promotion is not so much a specific activity as a 'movement towards the achievement of health as a basic right for all'. Whilst he acknowledges that the health care professions have an important part to play in this movement, he suggests that other professions, such as economists and policy makers, should, equally, be part of promoting health for all. One could also argue that if public participation in health is to be realised, then lay people should also form a part of that movement. Baric's discussion concludes that, by defining health promotion as an activity rather than a movement, significant participants may be excluded or marginalised as professionals take on specific activities as part of their perceived role. On the other hand, Baric sees health education as a more active process concerned with raising individual competence and knowledge about health and illness, about the body and its functions, about prevention and coping and with raising awareness about social, political and environmental factors that influence health. Health education should ensure that people are competent and knowledgeable whilst health promotion should facilitate their active involvement in the decision-making process.

Not all authors agree on the difference between health promotion and health education. Tones (1986) has suggested that health promotion is often perceived to be about promoting positive health and well-being rather than just preventing disease. He warns that this could lead to people being promised an idealistic state of health which is unobtainable and also that it can lead to a form of 'healthism'. By this, he means that some elite individuals may manage to achieve a state of health which encompasses physical fitness, freedom from disease, coping skills, satisfactory social relationships, etc., leaving the majority who cannot achieve this feeling that they have failed in some way, whereas they may be constrained by their social and environmental context from achieving positive well-being. Williams (1984) has also cautioned against the over-enthusiastic use of the term 'health promotion' as this may be misinterpreted as a coercive 'sales' strategy to persuade people to 'buy' a health product which they may neither want nor need. Both Williams (1984) and Tones (1986) seem to agree that health education is an activity which promotes health-related learning. As Tones suggests, it may 'produce changes in belief or attitude and facilitate the acquisition of skills; or it may generate changes in behaviour or lifestyle'. Others see health education as a part of health promotion (French and Adams, 1986; Gott and O'Brien, 1990) and that the processes involved depend on the concept of health adopted and the approach to health promotion will evolve from this.

Clearly, there is no easy definition of health promotion, but for the purposes of this chapter health promotion is perceived to be the broader activities which enable people to achieve human potential, of which health education is a part.

Florence Nightingale not only introduced education and training for nurses but also possessed an analytical and forward-thinking mind. Although nursing, as we know it, was only in its infancy under Miss Nightingale's influence, she was already planning for the future direction of nursing in relation to individual and societal change. In 1891 she wrote in one of her letters:

'I look forward to the day when there are no nurses of the sick, only nurses of the well.'
(Nightingale, 1891)

Just over 50 years later Aneurin Bevan had a similar vision when he created the National Health Service. Florence Nightingale saw health in terms of prevention and eradication of disease because of the conditions she observed around her. She saw the main obstacles as bad hygiene, poor nutrition and poverty. It was her aim that nurses in both hospitals and the community should help people to overcome these obstacles. She gave papers at conferences in which she stressed the role of the nurse as a health educator, particularly in the home:

'Health nursing is to keep or put the constitution of the healthy child or human being in such a state as to have no disease.'
(Nightingale, 1893)

Are we any nearer nurses being truly active in health promotion and education than we were over 100 years ago? Is it appropriate that nurses should take on this role? In answer to the first question, there is evidence to show that nurses are engaging in health promotion, but often at a limited level. There are, of course, particular areas of nursing, such as health visiting, school nursing and practice nursing, which do have health education within their brief. Often, however, it is viewed as an area of special interest which is introduced as an 'extra' if time allows, rather than as a continuous thread running throughout their work. Studies in the 1980s undertaken by the Health Education Council suggest that the underlying cause for this lay with the educational preparation of nurses. In 1980 they found that less than one-half of all schools of nursing in England and Wales had a working definition of health education. A later study in 1982 found that nurse tutors were themselves inadequately educated to prepare learner nurses for this role. Other studies have suggested possible inadequacies in nursing which may have contributed to nurses abdicating a health education role. Syred (1981) has argued that nurse education lacks a framework for health education. By this she means that nurses are not taught the necessary concepts or guidelines in order to function as health teachers. However, whilst Syred urges nurses to incorporate the Health Belief Model (Becker and Maiman, 1975) into their care planning, she does not present any empirical evidence on which to base her convictions.

Traditionally, nurses have been taught to nurse the sick within a medical framework, or model, which embodies the principles of diagnosis, treatment and cure. There is no analogous framework for health within nursing, probably because, until the advent of Project 2000, nursing had been unable to unleash itself from the medical model. A study by Lask and colleagues (1994), carried out on behalf of the English National Board, found that whilst some colleges of nursing are beginning to adopt a philosophy of health into the nursing curriculum, there are still a significant number which have not made the conceptual switch from 'sick nursing' to 'health nursing'. It is clearly difficult for a student nurse to internalise and practise as a health promoter if the philosophy has not been part of her socialisation into nursing.

Other studies (Faulkner and Ward, 1983; Macleod Clark et al., 1990) have highlighted interpersonal skills as the factor most lacking in nurses' ability to become health educators. The ability to ask questions sensitively and to listen and respond to the client's needs are undeniably important assets to the health educator. However, as Gott and O'Brien (1990) point out, it is not only communication skills which are relevant to health promotion activities. It is also the ability to understand health behaviour and the contextual nature of this, as well as appreciating the meaning of health promotion.

More recently, a study conducted by Latter (1994) indicates the way in which the organisation of nursing care can influence the direction of nursing practice. In her study of health promotion in an acute hospital setting, Latter found that many nurses felt powerless to practise health promotion due to the pressures of the organisation and the need to get the work done taking priority over the 'hidden' work of health promotion. Latter found that nurses working on a ward where primary nursing was the care delivery system in place, were more likely to perceive themselves as health promoters and were more able to plan this activity as part of patient care. She explains this as being the product of a more patient-centred and autonomous way of working as advocated by the 'new nursing' philosophy (Salvage, 1992). Team working and task-centred working did not have the same 'empowering' effect on the nurses to enable them to practise health promotion. This study therefore begs the question, can health promotion only be practised effectively in settings where primary nursing is in place? In the NHS, decision makers and planners have to look at workforce issues within a business plan which enables the provider unit to reach health targets cost-effectively. For many providers, primary nursing is seen as labour intensive and not cost-effective and it is therefore unrealistic in the late 1990s to expect primary nursing to become the *modus operandi* of nursing. However, many of the principles are transferable into other modes of organisation of care and these include the emphasis on the individual patient with the attendant need to communicate effectively to work in partnership with the patient.

Turning to the second question, how appropriate is it for nursing to move in this direction? The WHO views health promotion as an important activity for all health professionals. At a world conference in 1977 a statement was made which has become known as the 'Declaration of Alma-Ata'. It reads:

'The main social target of governments and the World Health Organization in the coming decades should be the attainment by all citizens of the world by the year 2000 of a level of health that will permit them to lead a socially and eco-nomically productive life. Primary health care is the key to attaining this target.'

(WHO, 1978)

Primary health care includes all health professionals working at the interface between the individual or community and the health care system in operation. Nurses are a very important part of primary health care, working in partnership with their medical and paramedical colleagues. Increasingly, nurses will be expected to practise in primary care and community settings as the NHS moves towards a primary care-led service (DoH, 1996). Whilst a minority of people will continue to be cared for in hospital, the changing emphasis and the changing roles of doctors and nurses which have resulted from a series of policy changes through the 1980s and 1990s, means that nurses have now got to be prepared and competent to carry out a range of skills often without the direct supervision of medical staff or senior nurses.

The WHO set targets (WHO, 1985) related to many aspects of health to be achieved on an international level by the year 2000. For example, one target is that all member nations will have a smoking population of not more than 20%. Other targets are related to environment, lifestyles and research, etc. Some of these targets were adopted by the Department of Health in England (DoH, 1992a) in the Health of the Nation strategy. These targets are summarised in Table 4.1.

The targets proposed by the Department of Health for England were also largely accepted by other countries within the UK, with some local differences and priorities for health taken into consideration. The targets obviously are intended as a strategic way forward for the whole of the health service and nurses are recognised as a part of that strategy in order to achieve the projected health gains. However, bureaucratic decrees are not in themselves reason enough for nurses to accept this challenging role. Indeed, Gott and O'Brien (1990) have suggested that health promotion policies frequently seem to misinterpret or ignore preceding documents, making it difficult for nurses to develop their own policy. An example of this is the Green Paper which preceded the Health of the Nation White Paper *Promoting Better Health* (DoH, 1988) which claims that doctors are in the best position to promote health. It largely ignored the potential role of nurses except as handers-out of leaflets and adopts a 'victim-blaming'

Table 4.1: *The Health of the Nation* targets (DoH, 1992a)

Coronary heart disease (CHD) and strokes
- To reduce death rates for both CHD and stroke in people under 65 by at least 40% by the year 2000
- To reduce the death rate for CHD in people aged 65–74 by at least 30% by the year 2000
- To reduce the death rate for stroke in people aged 65–74 by at least 40% by the year 2000 (baseline 1990)

Cancers
- To reduce the death rate for breast cancer in the population invited for screening by at least 25% by the year 2000 (baseline 1990)
- To reduce the incidence of invasive cervical cancer by at least 20% by the year 2000 (baseline 1986)
- To reduce the death rate for lung cancer under the age of 75 by at least 30% in men and by at least 15% in women by the year 2010 (baseline 1990)
- To halt the year-on-year increase in skin cancer by 2005

Mental illness
- To improve significantly the health and social functioning of mentally ill people
- To reduce the overall suicide rate by at least 15% by the year 2000
- To reduce the suicide rate of severely mentally ill people by at least 33% by the year 2000 (baseline 1990)

HIV/AIDS and sexual health
- To reduce the incidence of gonorrhoea by at least 20% by 1995, as an indicator of HIV/AIDS trends (baseline 1990)
- To reduce by at least 50% the rate of conceptions amongst the under 16s by the year 2000 (baseline 1989)

Accidents
- To reduce the rate for accidents among children aged under 15 by at least 33% by the year 2005
- To reduce the death rate for accidents among young people aged 15–24 by at least 25% by 2005
- To reduce the death rate for accidents among people aged 65 and over by at least 33% by 2005 (baseline 1990)

approach to health promotion which flies in the face of previous documents such as the Cumberlege Report (DHSS, 1986) on neighbourhood nursing and the *Ottawa Charter for Health Promotion* (1986) to which the UK was a signatory. Both these documents acknowledged that nurses had an important role to play and that health promotion should be brought about through public participation and collaboration between different professions and institutions.

In this policy context, it has been difficult for nursing to develop a clear vision of the philosophy, role, educational need and skills required for nurses to be competent health promoters into the next century. There is continual tension between service requirements, professional requirements and patient care. Whilst it would appear that it is appropriate for nurses to promote health, it is not always clear how the profession can rise effectively to the challenge.

Key Points
- Health education is usually accepted as being a part of health promotion.
- Historically, nurses have not played a very active role in health promotion.
- The WHO has established principles for health promotion.
- Nurses, midwives and health visitors have a responsibility to work in a health promoting way.
- The Health of the Nation targets provide a framework for health promotion, but need to be critically evaluated.

THE CHALLENGE OF PROMOTING HEALTH

If it is accepted that it is desirable and appropriate for nurses to be engaged in health promotion, how then can they be prepared to meet the challenge? The major part of this chapter will aim to demonstrate a variety of arenas within which nurses can practise health promotion. Each will be examined in terms of the potential of individuals or communities, the obstacles that work against them achieving these potentials, and the role of the nurse in enabling individuals or communities to overcome these obstacles.

In this context, it is useful to consider how the nurse might practise and not simply what she should do. It is useful at this stage to consider some possible approaches to health promotion. According to Tones (1986), there are three main approaches to health promotion. These can be seen as the traditional approach of health education to preventing illness, the self-empowering approach which enables people to make decisions, and the radical approach which works towards political and social change. Each of these approaches will be considered in more depth and their application to nursing explored.

THE PREVENTIVE APPROACH

Prevention of ill health has traditionally been the aim of preventive medicine and health educationists. In the short term the aim of the preventive approach is to increase people's knowledge about a particular health issue, such as smoking, thereby changing attitudes and behaviour. Ultimately, those using this approach to health promotion hope to achieve changes in **morbidity** and **mortality** statistics, in other words, to reduce the **incidence** and **prevalence** of certain diseases and subsequent deaths from them. This can be illustrated by much of the current work surrounding the human immunodeficiency virus (HIV). Government literature and figures reproduced in newspapers and magazines constantly remind us of the number of people who are HIV positive, the number of deaths from AIDS and the projected numbers for future years if people do not change their sexual and social behaviour. The aim of health educators using a preventive approach is to educate people about the spread of the HIV virus in the hope that this will deter them from engaging in unsafe sex or using intravenous drugs, thereby curbing the increasing numbers of HIV-positive individuals. The educative processes involved may include individual counselling, mass media campaigns, group work, the availability of leaflets and posters, or a combination of these.

In a seminal paper, Caplan (1969) identified three levels of prevention, the preventive approach being appropriate at any one of them. Caplan first suggested his conceptual framework in his discussion of promoting mental health in the community. However, the approach can be applied to a wide range of physical and social conditions as well as mental health:

1 Primary prevention: reducing the risk of members of a community succumbing to a particular disease/obstacle, for example, preventing disease by immunisation.
2 Secondary prevention: activities involved in reducing the duration of an established obstacle, thus reducing its prevalence in the community, for example, screening and early diagnosis of cervical cancer.
3 Tertiary prevention: the prevention of further disability or suffering in those where an obstacle is already established, for example, controlling pain in the person who is terminally ill.

Caplan's framework is not without its critics, primarily because it does appear to maintain the medical model of health care based on disease. It is largely this preventive model which was adopted in the Health of the Nation strategy in the expectation that health targets would be met through the prevention of ill health. However, it is interesting to note that Caplan's original work looked at mental health in the community and by this he was referring to:

'. . . the potential of a person to solve his problems in a reality based way.'

(Caplan, 1969, page vii)

This seems to relate comfortably to Seedhouse's (1986) ideas about health and human potential as discussed earlier and thus Caplan's framework can be seen as a useful tool for approaching health promotion more broadly than the prevention of disease.

The problem with the preventive approach to health promotion is that it takes a very narrow view of health, which is seen purely as the absence of disease. This ignores the more positive view of health proposed by the WHO (1946) and upheld in other documents such as the *Ottawa Charter for Health Promotion* (1986). It also ignores the views of health that lay people themselves may hold. In this sense it can be described as paternalistic, in that the view is taken that health experts know what is best for the good of the people. It assumes, also, that if individuals do not take responsible action to prevent disease, then they are themselves to blame for the consequences. This 'victim-blaming' approach has been criticised for its apparent ignorance of the social and environmental determinants of health and illness as described in a number of reports since the 1980s which have commented on inequalities in health (Townsend and Davidson, 1982, Whitehead, 1988; Benzeval *et al.*, 1995). In this respect it can be seen to be ethically questionable since the very things which the health educator seeks to prevent may, in fact, be caused by the political and economic fabric of society. For example, it could be argued that people turn to drugs in areas of high unemployment as a coping mechanism, thus increasing their risk of drug-related morbidity. But some of the underlying causes of unemployment may be outside the control of the individual so that it is oversimplistic to argue that those who are unemployed should find themselves jobs in order to prevent the uptake of unhealthy coping mechanisms.

The preventive approach may also be seen as economically unsound since, to use Zola's metaphor (cited in McKinlay, 1979), it relies on intensive efforts at fishing people out of the river before they drown rather than concentrating on the factors upstream which are causing them to fall in. In other words, the problems of unemployment and poverty should be addressed at a political level before the blame for health behaviours is laid at the door of the individual.

Having identified some of the limitations of the preventive approach to health promotion, it cannot be ignored that some of the major health battles in Europe and the developing world have been won through primary prevention. This includes the control of infectious diseases such as tuberculosis, diphtheria and smallpox through vaccination programmes that have been largely promoted through the child health clinics and schools.

Traditionally, where nurses have engaged in health-promoting activities it has been at the preventive level and to a large extent this is still the case. For example, the White Paper *Working for Patients* (DoH, 1989a) exhorts general practitioners to be more involved in screening and health assessment, which it suggests can be delegated to the practice nurse. The aim is to increase immunisation uptake and screening procedures for diseases such as cervical cancer and hypertension, thus preventing future disease. Whilst this appears to be an effective measure in which nurses can actively be involved, it appears to be limited by the problems mentioned above. It seems probable that nurses need to consider expanding their role in this area by developing the skills which will enable them to take a more self-empowering approach to health promotion. However, before discussing self-empowerment further, some in-depth examples of the preventive approach will be presented, which can be used to evaluate the method.

PROMOTING IMMUNISATION UPTAKE – AN EXAMPLE OF PRIMARY PREVENTION

Primary prevention involves activities which reduce the risk of members of a community succumbing to a particular disease or obstacle. Some examples include the prevention of communicable disease by immunisation, the prevention of pregnancy by contraception and the prevention of serious injury and death on the roads by seatbelt legislation. It is the secondary obstacles that usually work against people achieving the potential they desire. For example, most people in today's society would find the concept of planned parenthood desirable. However, the human body is regulated by homeostatic mechanisms to produce fertile ova and sperm. It is possible to overcome that primary obstacle to an unwanted pregnancy by using contraception, but experience suggests that the equation isn't that simple. A young woman, for example, may become pregnant in the belief that she was 'safe' the first time she had intercourse without using contraception. The obstacles facing her would be lack of knowledge, possibly pressure from her partner and cultural pressure among peers to engage in unprotected sex. It is in helping people to overcome these secondary obstacles that the nurse can play a major role, using an individualised approach to assess the person's response to the obstacles facing him or her and planning care in partnership to meet these individual needs. For example, a family planning nurse might provide the young woman and her partner with information about fertiliy and contraception, but also explore with them their beliefs and expectations about sex.

The discovery of immunological mechanisms and the development of **vaccines** means that, potentially, humans can protect themselves from any communicable disease of which it has knowledge. Thus, major diseases such as smallpox have been eradicated to an extent which makes immunisation unnecessary on a worldwide basis and other diseases such as diphtheria are well controlled in the Western world. Immunisation policies are developed according to certain criteria such as severity and frequency of the disease. So, for example, in the UK we do not immunise against yellow fever because although it can be severe, it is not very frequent. We do, however, have immunisation policies for infectious diseases such as measles, diphtheria and polio as they are all severe, particularly in childhood, and would be frequent if it were not for the high degree of immunity we now have in the community, known as herd immunity.

To illustrate the issues which are raised when looking at immunisation as a means of primary prevention, whooping cough (*Bordetella pertussis*) immunisation will be used as an example. Whooping cough is a highly communicable bacterial disease which primarily affects the trachea and bronchi. It is typified by paroxysmal coughing which may last for 2–3 months. The disease may be complicated by lung damage, such as collapse or bronchopneumonia, and by cerebral anoxia which can cause brain damage. The majority of complications and deaths occur in infants under 6 months of age. As can be seen from Figure 4.1 a decline in the notifications for whooping cough is closely correlated with a rise in immunisation uptake from 1977 to 1994 (White *et al.*, 1996). It can also be seen that, following a fall-off in the uptake of immunisation in 1974, there were major **epidemics** in 1977–1979 and 1981–1983. This epidemiological evidence collated by White *et al.* (1996) suggests that immunisation against whooping cough contributes significantly to its prevention in the community.

It should be noted, however, that notification of whooping cough (and other infectious diseases) is notoriously poor and it has been suggested that notifications represent the true number by only a third or a quarter (Bedford, 1993). In addition, dramatic declines in mortality from whooping cough (Figure 4.2) have also been apparent from 1953 until 1976. Note, however, that much of the

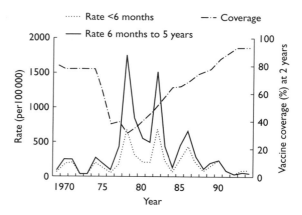

Figure 4.1: Incidence of whooping cough in children by age and vaccine coverage: England and Wales 1969–94 (Source: White *et al.*, 1996, Reproduced with permission of the PHLS Communicable Disease Surveillance Centre © PHLS)

decline in mortality was occurring before 1957 when the vaccine was introduced, suggesting that improved nutritional standards and medical care after the Second World War may also have contributed to this.

The recommended schedule of vaccination is:

First dose – 2 months of age
Second dose – 3 months
Third dose – 4–6 months (DoH, 1992b)

So far, the facts about whooping cough have been presented. With this evidence it would be reasonable to assume that the vaccine is available, parents take it up for their children and whooping cough is well controlled. Unfortunately, it is not as simple as it at first appears. Despite the obvious beneficial effects of immunity against whooping cough, uptake in England has not approached 100%. The real problem with the uptake of whooping cough immunisation is that, although the overall figures have improved, there are still large regional variations. Whilst some may achieve immunisation levels of 80% or 90%, others are in the low 60s. Clearly, control of the disease is impossible whilst there are still large pockets of unprotected children.

As mentioned earlier, there was actually a fall in uptake in 1974 and this can largely be accounted for by the controversy surrounding the safety of the vaccine, when whooping cough vaccine was implicated as the cause of severe brain damage in some children. Some of the effects of this controversy continue today. The most recent

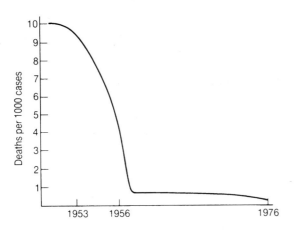

Figure 4.2: UK deaths per 1000 notified cases of whooping cough 1953–76 (DHSS, 1984)

assessment of risk from whooping cough vaccine (DoH, 1992b) suggests that neurological damage occurs so rarely that its frequency cannot be accurately measured. This has to be weighed up against the risks associated with whooping cough itself. The risk of dying from the disease is 1 in 5000 cases (DHSS, 1984). Whilst there is no information available on the long-term morbidity resulting from whooping cough, other factors to consider are the distress for a child with whooping cough and the long-term complications of the disease itself. In addition, parents are put under considerable stress caring for a child with the disease and there are also longer term implications for the community as well as the family, such as caring for the child with disabilities or for the bereaved parents. The implications for promoting immunisation are therefore very powerful. A further potentially forceful pressure on parents to take up immunisation may come as a result of health service legislation, the NHS and Community Care Act (DoH, 1990). As part of the NHS reforms, contracts will be held by general practitioners, which encourage targets in preventive medicine to be met. For example, it is proposed that immunisation rates for each practice population should reach 80%. GPs will not be paid for their immunisation services if the targets are not met. *The Health of the Nation* (DoH, 1992a) strategy recommended a target of 95% uptake for all vaccines by 1995. Thus, there was almost inevitably going to be further pressure on families to take up immunisation, pressure not only from the doctor but possibly also from practice nurses, health visitors and district nurses.

Given the evidence that immunisation against whooping cough is beneficial and that the risks associated with the vaccine are relatively small and are minimised by each individual child's history being considered before immunisation, why is it that the immunisation uptake is not nearer 100%? In other words, what are the secondary obstacles that prevent parents from having their children immunised and how can the nurse help them to overcome them?

Lack of knowledge of the disease and the vaccine

The potential to protect an individual from a communicable disease such as whooping cough may not be achieved through lack of information and fear. People do not always act on knowledge alone, but without accurate information they do not have the foundations on which to base a decision. Perkins (1982) found that parents often had incomplete or distorted knowledge of whooping cough and the effects of the vaccine. Nurses can help parents to reach their decision by assessing the parent's level of knowledge, discussing the arguments for and against immunisation and giving information where appropriate. Alderson *et al.* (1997) found from their qualitative study of professionals' views on consent to immunisation, that doctors and nurses tended to use strategies such as giving detailed information, encouragement, reassurance, listening and overcoming their resistance in cases where parents are undecided. As Perkins (1982) points out, helping the parents to sort out the information involves a partnership between nurse and client. This approach may also involve designing informative notice boards or posters in the clinical area and ensuring that the potential language barriers of those from ethnic groups are addressed.

Restricted access to the vaccine

There could be several reasons for restricted access to the vaccine. There may be geographical difficulties, for example the clinic or surgery may be a long distance from home, involving bus journeys, perhaps with awkward pushchairs and toddlers (e.g. Betts and Betts, 1990). The cost of such a journey might be prohibitive. A study by Spencer and Power (1978) found that child health clinics in deprived areas did not meet the needs of parents in the way that needs were met in areas that were not deprived. Nurses can help by being aware of local immunisation facilities and by supporting parents in relation to their specific needs. In some areas, nurses and health visitors have helped to address this issue through outreach programmes, i.e. taking the vaccine to the child either through home visiting or the use of health buses or drop-in centres.

Inequalities in health

Some research studies have found (Townsend and Davidson, 1982; While, 1985) that there is a lower uptake of immunisation among people from different socio-economic groups. This can be because of social and economic conditions, such as poor housing and unemployment, which may have a generally demoralising effect, leading to apathy and poor motivation. An awareness of these factors and an understanding of the interaction between social factors and health behaviour can enable the nurse to approach parents sensitively in the discussion of immunisation, responding to individual needs as they arise. Blackburn (1991) has argued that research in this area tends to indicate that low income families have the same health goals for their children as more affluent families. Her thesis, based on a review of the surrounding literature and some empirical evidence, is that it is the structural inequalities rather than differences in attitude which lead to a lower uptake of services by lower income parents.

Scenario I

Di Verney is a health visitor working alongside a single-handed GP in Hackney. The practice population is comprised of many elderly people living alone and also many young children. The children are frequently part of a family where there is an absent partner, a step-parent or one or both parents are unemployed. The number of families living on income support is therefore high and the housing is poor, being largely comprised of high-rise flats with little or no safe play areas. There are many signs of vandalism and there is a local drugs problem with dealing openly taking place within the estates. Di has worked hard with the families in the practice to encourage them to take up immunisation for all their children. Some of the parents are keen to protect their children from preventable infectious diseases. Others cannot really see the point of it, but there are parents who do wish to

protect their children but find it difficult or worrying to make the journey to the surgery, which is not based on the estate. What can Di do to improve immunisation uptake, which from her latest audit suggests may be as low as 45%?

Drawing on the preventive approach, Di decides to mount an immunisation campaign in the area. She works closely with the health promotion department to put up posters in the estate shops and to make leaflets available both in the surgery itself and in the estate community centre. She ensures that these are supplied in Punjabi and Urdhu as well as English. Di evaluates this campaign by re-auditing 6 months later. She finds there has been a small but significant increase to 50%. Whilst this is a very positive step, she now has to consider whether a different approach to health promotion would be more effective.

PROMOTING HEALTH SCREENING – AN EXAMPLE OF SECONDARY PREVENTION

We now come to the second part of Caplan's (1969) model of prevention. Secondary prevention can be seen as the activities involved in reducing the duration of an established obstacle. Some examples of secondary prevention are:

- The reduction of mortality from **invasive carcinoma** of the cervix by the early detection of **pre-invasive carcinoma**. This procedure is known as screening
- The reduction of stroke incidence by screening for those with high blood pressure
- Reduction of lung cancer mortality by stopping smoking
- Reduction of antisocial behaviour, accidents and liver disease by stopping alcohol misuse.

Secondary prevention can be loosely broken down into screening procedures and reducing health-damaging behaviours. By routinely examining apparently healthy people, screening aims to detect either those who are likely to develop a particular disease or those in whom the disease is already present but not yet producing symptoms. There are many screening programmes advocated in the UK, among which are included screening for rubella immunity among pregnant women, for phenylketonuria in newborn babies, for the developmental progress of children, and for hypertension. Cervical cancer screening will be used as an example of how screening can be effective, the obstacles that work against people being screened, and the nurse's role. Cervical cancer continues to be a common cause of death among women. In 1987, 1763 women died from the disease (DoH, 1989b). The DoH (1992a) target for invasive carcinoma of the cervix is as follows:

- To reduce the incidence of invasive cervical cancer by at least 20% by the year 2000 (baseline 1986).

Although some risk factors have been identified in its aetiology, for example herpes virus and several sexual partners (Hakama, 1983), there are no proven methods of primary prevention. The only practical way of controlling the disease is therefore early diagnosis by screening. Setting up any screening programme depends on several factors:

- The availability of a safe, repeatable and valid test
- The effect of early treatment on the prognosis of the disease
- The relative costs and benefits of the programme
- The acceptability of the screening programme to the public (Open University, 1985)

In the case of cervical cancer screening, the smear test is available every 5 years to women between 20 and 65 years at family doctors, family planning clinics, well women clinics, and hospital inpatient and outpatient services. It is a safe test involving the removal of cells from the surface of the cervix. The cells are taken from the transformation zone where the columnar epithelium meets the squamous epithelium, with little or no risk to the individual. The test is repeatable and it is valid, i.e. it shows what it is supposed to show. The cost of surgery, radiotherapy and aftercare in the treatment of invasive carcinoma of the cervix is much higher than for the screening procedure and treatment of carcinoma in situ (the pre-invasive stage of the cancer). Of more importance, detection and early treatment of cervical cancer is of demonstrable benefit to the woman concerned. Carcinoma in situ can be treated by laser or surgically (by cone biopsy) which completely removes the altered cells. In almost all cases the woman will go on to lead a normal reproductive life, with no invasive stage of the carcinoma. The screening procedure for cervical cancer is therefore not misleading in its effects on outcomes, i.e.

it does lead to early detection and effective treatment and not just an early diagnosis which could be used to exaggerate survival rates. In other words, women in whom carcinoma in situ has been identified and treated recover; they do not just live longer with the knowledge that they have cancer. Given this seemingly safe and effective screening programme, why is it that up to 2000 women continue to die of cervical cancer every year? The main reason is that many woman are not screened and there are a variety of possible reasons for this.

Fears and beliefs about cancer

One of the obstacles which prevents women taking up the screening service is their fears and beliefs about the nature of cancer. Accepting screening is an acknowledgement of cancer. Despite the fact that many forms of cancer are now curable, many people equate cancer with certain death and prefer to dissociate from it completely. Susan Sontag (1978) has described how it is the metaphorical invasion and destruction of the body by the advancing army of cancer which seems to differentiate it in people's minds from other diseases. Nurses also may find it difficult to discuss cancer, especially in cases where the client is unaware of her diagnosis. Even the discussion of screening can be hard if both nurse and client are trying to avoid the difficult issue of cancer. Being frank about the purpose of cervical screening brings cancer out into the open. It takes a great deal of skill on the part of the nurse if she is to help the client to overcome her fears. A study by King (1987) found that generally older women attributed cervical cancer to a 'germ' or 'smoking' and therefore resisted the test on the grounds that it did not apply to them. She also found that older women tended to resist screening as they felt that it reflected on their morality, as cervical cancer was thought to be a 'dirty' disease resulting from 'promiscuity'. It is now known that cervical cancer is associated with risk factors including smoking, a number of sexual partners, the contraceptive pill and the papilloma virus (McPherson, 1991). Women's beliefs are not therefore without foundation. Nurses can respond to this through accurate and honest information giving, which is tailored to the woman's particular need, and weighing up the costs and benefits of screening for that woman.

FEAR OF THE TEST

King's study also found that resistance to cervical screening among older women was often due to fear of the test itself. It was held to be a painful procedure and many were reluctant to be examined internally, particularly by a male doctor. King concludes that beliefs about the test are the strongest indicators of non-attendance. Nurses can use this research finding by helping women, especially in middle age, to understand the nature of the test and by reinforcing its benefits to all age groups.

Scenario 2

Gill is a practice nurse working with four fund-holding GPs in a large health centre in a Buckinghamshire market town. The practice population is mixed, comprising a proportion of affluent professional families as well as some families from ethnic minority groups and a high proportion of over 60s. Gill and the GPs work to an evidence-based protocol on cervical screening which aims to improve uptake from 80% to 95% over 3 years. The main problem is with the older women. Gill finds they tend to think that cervical screening is no longer a problem for them, or that they are worried about the consequences of such a test. What can Gill do to improve the health of the practice?

In discussion with the GPs, Gill decides to hold a cancer awareness week. She provides posters and leaflets in the health centre and runs a video in the waiting area. She also makes herself available to answer questions for half an hour each day and sets aside a special time in the week for taking smear tests. In addition, Gill arranges for the cytologist from the local hospital to present a 1-hour discussion on cervical cancer during a weekday evening.

Audit 6 months later shows an improvement in uptake in the order of 5%. This is positive, but Gill wonders how else she could approach this problem.

Key Points

- Immunisation and screening have been presented as examples of health promotion using the preventive approach.
- The aim is to prevent disease such as whooping cough and cervical cancer by informing individuals and communities about the possible health risks and the benefits to their health if they accept the services offered.

- Information alone does not always motivate people to take health action. It may be that obstacles, apparently or actually outside their control, are operating and that a different approach to health promotion may be more appropriate.

We will now turn to such an approach which encourages people to develop decision-making skills.

THE SELF-EMPOWERMENT APPROACH

Tones (1986) argues that whilst understanding a health issue may be a precursor to action, it is not sufficient. Thus, health educationists have argued that provision of information should be accompanied by a process of belief and values clarification, which should be followed by development of decision-making skills.

Tones (1991) has defined empowerment as:

'the process whereby an individual – or community of individuals – acquires power, i.e. the capacity to control other people and resources. Self-empowerment focuses on the individual's capacity to control his or her own life'.

The overall aim of the self-empowerment approach is therefore to foster informed choice, which stems ideologically from the concept of autonomy (Harris, 1985). It is important to consider, however, that even in democratic societies people do not always have individual autonomy or a completely free choice about their health. An example in the UK would be the seatbelt legislation. Whilst the law relating to this was brought about within the democratic framework, some would argue that people should remain at liberty to choose whether they wear a seatbelt or not.

A second point in relation to choice is that self-empowerment is about enabling people to make their own decisions even if the decision finally arrived at is not that favoured by the health promoter. It is therefore important to remember that the perceived healthy option is not the only option and to ensure that education for health does not become indoctrination (Campbell, 1990). However, self-empowerment does not simply aim to make people more skilled in their decision making, but to use those skills to empower themselves and others. In this way it is possible that social change can be brought about which would alter the environment in which people seek to become healthy.

Tones *et al.* (1990) suggest that such a process involves addressing issues such as self-esteem and self-efficacy as well as social skills. Self-esteem is important, as individuals who do not perceive themselves favourably may find it more difficult to change or to take health action. Self-efficacy relates to a person's perceptions of his or her own capabilities, which according to Bandura (1977) can be influenced by past experience and through self-mastery by accomplishment of specific actions.

Thus, the self-empowerment approach to health promotion involves much more than preventing disease through the provision of knowledge. The health promoter must be able to provide the information which people need to make an informed choice, but he or she also needs to be able to assess self-esteem and self-efficacy and to appreciate the health beliefs and values of others, as well as to enable people to develop skills in decision making and assertiveness. This clearly requires a great deal of skill and initiative on the part of the health promoter and some nurses may not feel that they are prepared for such a role. For example, ideally, learning how to make decisions should be done in a safe environment (i.e. one where the wrong decision will not result in unfavourable outcomes) and should allow for practice through simulation and role play (Bond and Kendall, 1990). Approaches to learning in the preparation and education of nurses are increasingly looking at adult learning styles which enable students to learn through reflection on experience (e.g. the work of Donald Schon, 1983, is often cited in curriculum development). These approaches to becoming a nurse should, theoretically, enable the practitioner to take a more reflective approach to health promotion practice, which could be seen to be more conducive to the self-empowering approach to health promotion. Currently, there is very scanty evidence which demonstrates the impact of nurse education programmes on the actual practice of nursing and health promotion outcomes.

APPLICATION OF THE SELF-EMPOWERMENT APPROACH TO CORONARY HEART DISEASE (CHD)

Coronary heart disease (CHD) is a major health problem in the UK. Tunstall-Pedoe (1991) cites figures which suggest that besides being the major cause of death for both sexes, it accounted for £500m in treatment costs and £1800m in lost production costs in the mid-1980s. The DoH (1992a) targets for CHD reduction are:

- To reduce death rates for both CHD and stroke in people under 65 by at least 40% by the year 2000
- To reduce the death rate for CHD in people aged 65–74 by at least 30% by the year 2000 (baseline 1990).

One way of reducing the prevalence of this condition and enhancing the quality of people's lives may be through the self-empowerment approach, thus enabling people to make informed decisions about their lifestyle. This may involve considerations of diet, exercise and smoking behaviour.

As Tones *et al.* (1990) suggest, the first stage of self-empowerment may be considered to be information giving in relation to people's beliefs and values. Some background information which may be useful to the nurse is summarised here, followed by discussion of how health may be promoted by enabling people to make informed choices. Smoking is considered as a separate health issue, although it does have significant implications for coronary heart disease.

Background information to CHD

The term coronary heart disease (CHD) includes factors which predispose to acute manifestations such as **atherosclerosis**, and those which precipitate the eventual myocardial infarction, such as plaque rupture, thrombosis and coronary spasm. It is often thought of as a disease of affluence because of its prevalence in the Western world but this is deceptive because it is more likely to be people from the relatively poorer communities who die of it (Townsend and Davidson, 1982). However, it is likely to kill more people from any social group in the UK than any other single cause of death, including cancer. For example, in 1982,

31% of male deaths resulted from CHD compared to 24% from all cancers. For women, the figures were 23% for CHD and 21% for cancer (OPCS, 1982). Currently, England and Wales have the highest rate of death from CHD (about 600 per 100 000) after Finland and Scotland. The lowest rate is in Japan (about 100 per 100 000) (Marmot, 1985). The most recently available figures suggest that in 1987, 81 037 men and 63 824 women died from CHD (DoH, 1989b).

CHD is also responsible for substantial morbidity. The OPCS Report on morbidity (1995) reports on a survey of 60 GP practices in England and Wales, representing 468 042 people at risk from any type of morbidity. In relation to CHD they found that 2% of all people consulted their GP. Prevalence was highest among the 75–84 age group where consultations reached 8%. Clearly, it is a cause of both individual suffering and community concern, since treatment puts a strain on resources in terms of human resources in the health service, hours lost from work due to sickness, expensive surgical procedures, and drugs and rehabilitation. Prevention of CHD could reduce this considerably.

A report of a WHO meeting in 1984 (WHO, 1984b) stated that the debate is now about 'how, not whether CHD could be prevented'. The British Cardiac Society (1987) has recommended that prevention be implemented using both a population approach (i.e. assuming that all members of a community are at risk) as well as a high risk approach (i.e. some members of a community are at higher risk than others and can be identified by screening procedures). One of the conclusions from a seminar held by the National Heart Forum (1995) was, however, that it may be more cost-effective to target those people at highest risk.

The main risk factors which have been identified are raised serum **cholesterol** levels, smoking, hypertension, obesity and alcohol (COMA, 1994). For the purposes of this part of the chapter we will concentrate on serum cholesterol and the role of diet in controlling it.

SERUM CHOLESTEROL, DIETARY FAT AND CHD

Biochemically, cholesterol is an important steroid which forms the basis of many hormones, such as the oestrogens and androgens, and is also an essential component of cell membranes. It is produced endogenously by the liver and and exogenously through the dietary intake of complex lipids including triglycerides (made up of three **fatty acids** which may be saturated and unsaturated) and phospholipids (made up of two fatty acids which are unsaturated).

According to the COMA report (1994) the UK diet provides about 200–300 times more triglycerides than cholesterol. Dietary cholesterol is not therefore as problematic as dietary fat intake. It is the excessive dietary intake of complex lipids which stimulates the liver to produce excess cholesterol exogenously.

Put simply, low density lipoprotein (LDL) cholesterol is that produced by the liver and required for cell maintenance, whilst high density lipoprotein (HDL) cholesterol is the excess cholesterol produced through the dietary fat intake. An imbalance between LDL and HDL cholesterol may cause the abnormal uptake of LDL by the vascular wall, leading to atheroma. Atheromatous plaques in the blood vessels contain a high level of low density lipoprotein (LDL) cholesterol, which appears to be a necessary condition for an atheromatous lesion to occur in the coronary artery wall (COMA, 1994).

Geoffrey Rose, an epidemiologist, sees the role of serum cholesterol in CHD primarily as a population problem (Rose, 1987). In simple terms, he bases this proposal on the fact that among the Japanese (where CHD is not a problem) the mean serum cholesterol is less than 3 mmol/litre. In countries where the mean serum cholesterol level is above 5 mmol/litre, CHD is always a problem. In England, the average serum cholesterol level is 5.7 mmol/litre (Health Survey for England, 1991, cited by White *et al.*, 1993). Bingham (1991) states that a reduction in dietary saturated fats by 10% would reduce the mean serum cholesterol level by 0.4 mmol/litre to 5.4 mmol/litre which could represent a 20% reduction in mortality from CHD. Rose states that by old age, 90% of the UK population have developed a high degree of atherosclerosis and it is therefore everybody's problem. Even among individuals of relatively low risk the commonest cause of death is still CHD.

One way of lowering serum cholesterol levels in the population is through dietary change. Most experts (COMA, 1994) agree that serum cholesterol levels can be controlled by changing the ratio of saturated fatty acids to polyunsaturated fatty acids in the diet. The terms saturated and polyunsaturated refer to the chemical bonding of the fatty acid and its reactivity with oxygen. Thus, polyunsaturates are oxidised much more readily than saturated fatty acids. Saturated fatty acids (SFA) are generally found in animal products, such as meat and dairy produce, whilst polyunsaturated fatty acids (PUFA) are found in vegetable and fish oils, although some are higher in PUFA than others. For example, among the vegetable oils, safflower oil is higher in PUFA than olive oil. There are also exceptions – palm oil is composed mainly of SFA. This demonstrates the importance of accurate food labelling, since foods containing vegetable oils may, on closer inspection, contain a high level of palmitic acid, the main component of palm oil.

The Committee on Medical Aspects of Food Policy (COMA, 1994) made recommendations to the government on how the national diet should change to make appreciable differences to the average serum cholesterol level. COMA made the following recommendations (among others) in relation to dietary fat:

■ That the average contribution of saturated fatty acids to dietary energy be reduced to no more than about 10%

■ A reduction in the average contribution of total fat to dietary energy in the population to about 35%
■ That the average dietary intake of cholesterol should not rise
■ That the dietary energy derived from complex **carbohydrates** should increase to approximately 50%, to replace energy lost through fat reduction.

Bingham (1991) has presented data which represent the necessary changes in dietary fat intake if the DoH targets for CHD are to be achieved:

THE ROLE OF EXERCISE

Exercise can be considered alongside dietary factors, since it is physical activity which determines how much of the energy provided by food is expended. It is the relationship between energy intake and energy expenditure that may determine the degree to which risk factors such as obesity and hypertension are present, although other factors, such as basal metabolism and gender, may also be important. Although the British Cardiac Society (1987) points out that there have been no controlled research studies of the role of exercise

Table 4.2: Possible change in average consumption of foods to achieve government targets for 2005 and dietary recommended values

Food	Present intake (g)	Possible future intake* (g)	Contributions to required alterations in				
			Saturated fatty acids (g)	Non-milk extrinsic sugars (g)	Non-starch poly-saccharides (g)	Starch and other sugars (g)	Proportional change in intake
Wholemeal and other bread	43	110			2.2	50	2.5
White bread	65	85			0.3	10	1.3
Vegetables	135	270			3.0	11	2.0
Fruit	73	110			0.3	4	1.5
Potatoes	132	200			0.8	13	1.5
Biscuits, cakes, puddings	80	40	−2.4	−8			0.5
Whole to semi-skimmed milk	164	164	−2.0				1.0
Saturated to low fat spreads	10	10	−4.0				1.0
Meat to leaner meat	150	150	−3.0				1.0
Chips, crisps and change to lower fat products	62	31	−1.2				0.5
Chocolate	9	5	−0.7	−2			0.5
Sugar, preserves	23	12		−12			0.5
Beverages, soft drinks	100	50		−3			0.5
Total			−13	−25	6.5	88*	

*Includes allowance for the reduction in sources of non-milk extrinsic sugars.

Source: Bingham, 1991. Reproduced with permission of BMJ Publishing.

in primary prevention, there are some studies which appear to demonstrate the protective effect of exercise against CHD. A study by Morris *et al.* (1980) found that British civil servants were less likely to develop CHD if they undertook some vigorous exercise. A study on primates (Kramsch *et al.*, 1981) found that the diameter of the coronary blood vessels was greater in monkeys who were more active and they developed less atherosclerosis than their inactive counterparts fed the same diet. Although this type of evidence is not conclusive, it is widely accepted that exercise may have a protective effect, operating through various mechanisms. These include improved cardiopulmonary function and exercise tolerance, a reduction in platelet aggregation and a possible decrease in blood pressure, as well as weight being more easily controlled (COMA, 1994).

A joint document by the Health Education Authority and the Sports Council (1987) divides fitness into three major areas. Suppleness is the ability to bend, stretch and turn through a range of movements; strength is the ability to exert force for pushing, pulling and lifting; and stamina is the ability to keep going whilst running or walking without getting tired quickly. It is stamina that helps to protect against heart disease and aerobic exercise is recommended to improve stamina. This kind of exercise is usually fairly energetic, keeps the body moving for about 20 minutes at a time and makes the individual fairly breathless. It is known as aerobic exercise because enough oxygen is breathed in to supply working muscles so an oxygen debt is not incurred. Aerobic exercise includes brisk walking, jogging, swimming and cycling, as well as the exercises included in 'aerobic classes'. As with everything else, people's individual needs and abilities will vary and it is important to take account of this when helping clients to plan their exercise.

Self-empowerment and risk factors associated with CHD

Although there have been many reports (Royal College of Physicians/British Cardiac Society, 1976; DHSS, 1981; COMA, 1994) on the dietary aspect of preventing CHD, very few of them address the problem of how the health promoters can encourage the population to change its diet. Even the National Advisory Committee on Nutrition Education (NACNE, 1983), which was led by

a working party from the Health Education Council, fails to give any practical guidelines on how their suggested goals might be achieved. As you will by now be beginning to appreciate, health promotion is not simply a process of giving people information and people changing their behaviour on the basis of that information. Lack of information is only one of the obstacles in the prevention of CHD. We will now turn to those factors which influence whether people change their dietary and exercise behaviour or not and some possible ways in which the nurse can enable them to make the decision to change by using the self-empowerment approach.

INFORMATION GIVING

People need sufficient and accurate information on which to base a decision. The nurse can find out how much the client knows about his/her health by careful assessment and provide clear and accurate information as necessary. This depends on the nurse him or herself being aware of research findings and keeping up to date with new knowledge, or to use another term, to engage in evidence-based practice (EBP). There are various approaches to providing information, which range from the one-to-one interaction, to visual displays, the provision of books and leaflets and group work. Whilst information is important to patient well-being and recovery (Leino-Kelpi *et al.*, 1993), it is probably the style in which it is given and the extent to which this meets patients' preferences which makes the difference to their uptake of the information.

Two recent studies carried out in the primary care setting (Wood *et al.*, 1994; Imperial Cancer Research Fund Study Group, 1995) both highlighted potential problems when nurses carried out health promotion consultations to reduce CHD risk factors. Whilst in both studies the nurses were trained to use a patient-centred approach to the consultation, neither study demonstrated significant reductions in body mass index or cigarette smoking. There were, however, some small changes in cholesterol level and dietary fat intake. These changes were somewhat limited, however, compared to a control group of patients who received no special health promotion intervention. As the nurse consultation was the main component of the interventions, it would appear from these studies that a more empowering approach to health promotion might have yielded more substantial results.

The self-empowerment approach determines that where information is provided, it should not only be accurate but in accordance with the client's needs, values and beliefs. It is therefore imperative that these are established before any information is imparted.

BELIEFS AND VALUES

When trying to empower people to reach healthy decisions in relation to diet and exercise, it is crucial to understand and work with their beliefs and values in relation to food, exercise and the relationship between body, mind and health. For example, an ethnographic study carried out by Davison *et al.* (1991) reports that the people participating in the study carry the notion that heart attacks happen to a particular kind of person, an idea encapsulated by the authors as 'coronary candidacy'. The people who may be identified as coronary candidates included those who evidently display outward signs of recognised risk factors such as obesity, fatty diet and smoking. However, candidates were also identified as those who were worriers, bad-tempered, took excessive exercise or overindulged in activities such as sex and drugs. These indicators of candidacy were used as a retrospective explanation for heart attack, as a predictive indicator and also as a measure of one's own predisposition towards a heart attack. This study provides useful evidence of the

lay explanation for heart attack which may help us to understand the way in which health beliefs influence the uptake of information. The findings from this study would suggest that people may not alter their health behaviour if they do not perceive themselves to be coronary candidates.

The Health Belief Model (Becker and Maiman, 1975) may be a useful tool in aiding the assessment and understanding of people's health behaviours in relation to their health beliefs. This model was originally constructed by Becker and Maiman to try to explain why people do not carry out preventive health action, and some elements of the model (see Figure 4.3) have been shown to be of particular value in explaining health behaviour. For example, Champion (1987) and Stillman (1977) have both demonstrated the particular validity of the variable of perceived barriers to preventive action. These are considered below.

One obstacle which may prevent people from changing their behaviour is their financial situation. Many people believe that eating 'health foods' is more expensive than their usual diet and those in most need of change probably have the lowest income. The Black Report (Townsend and Davidson, 1982, Phillimore *et al.*, 1994) and *The Health Divide* (Whitehead, 1988) both report inequalities in health leading to higher levels of ill health among those who were unemployed and low income groups. Reducing energy intake from saturated fatty acids and increasing the energy

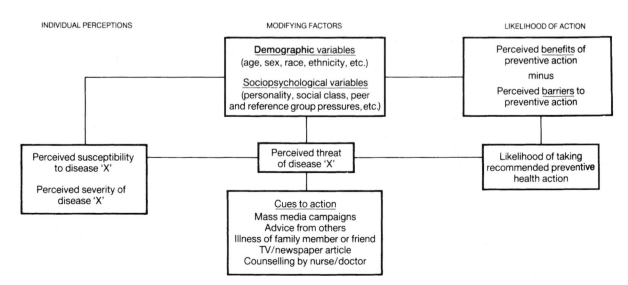

Figure 4.3: The Health Belief Model (Becker and Maiman, 1975)

intake from carbohydrates need not be expensive if carefully planned. For example, oily fish such as mackerel is cheaper than many types of meat, polyunsaturated margarines are cheaper than butter. Wholemeal bread and fresh fruit and vegetables do tend to be more expensive, but they are more satisfying and can be made to go further than the cheaper processed foods. For example, root vegetables are relatively cheap and can fill out a reduced-meat casserole. Simple changes in cooking methods can also reduce fat consumption without affecting the family budget; for example, changing from frying to grilling.

However, there is some evidence to show that people living in the most disadvantaged areas do have to pay more for items such as wholemeal bread. Graham's (1984) research found that large council estates were often built considerable distances from town centres so that shopping involved either expensive journeys by public transport into town or paying higher prices at a local store where healthy alternatives are frequently unavailable. Large supermarkets where foods tends be cheaper are frequently on the outskirts of towns and necessitate the use of a car which many poorer families do not possess. Graham found that women's knowledge in relation to healthy eating was not lacking – they felt prohibited by the factors described and also that they were not doing their best for their families. Therefore, the belief that healthy eating is expensive is not entirely unfounded and it is important to consider these factors when planning for healthy eating with a patient or family. Similarly, exercise can be perceived to be difficult because of expensive equipment, clothing or membership fees. Whilst it can be argued that exercise, such as jogging or walking, is free, women, in particular, may perceive themselves to have problems in carrying out these activities because of the need for child care.

The exploration of attitudes to food and exercise is an aspect of psychology which will not be considered here in detail. An attitude has been defined by Roediger et al. (1984, page 587) as 'a relatively stable tendency to respond consistently to particular people, objects or situations'. This suggests that attitudes can be held towards just about anything, including food, dietary behaviour and exercise, and that although they tend to be stable, they are not fixed. In other words, attitudes are amenable to change and are also open to conflict. Whilst a person may generally behave in accordance with the attitudes held, he may occasionally behave in a way which conflicts with his attitudes. For example, a person may hold favourable attitudes towards reducing saturated fats in his diet, but may also hold favourable attitudes towards cream cakes and chocolate. Therefore, making the decision to change the diet depends very much on how the individual thinks and behaves towards food and his attitude towards health. A fatalistic attitude, for example, would suggest a person who makes comments such as, 'We all have to die sometime so I may as well eat what I like now and enjoy it'. Part of the health promotion process is clarifying people's attitudes in order to enable change, if appropriate.

Attitudes can change but it tends to be a slow process. For example, the general attitude in the UK towards the consumption of polyunsaturated margarines is changing; butter is no longer seen as the only thing to spread on bread! How this change came about is probably due to a number of influences including information from a variety of sources (television, magazines, health personnel, etc.), changes in the availability of foodstuffs in the shops, advertising, and the social pressure to change. A study in Finland (Vartianinen et al., 1987) has shown how a community approach to CHD has changed public attitudes to eating and lowered serum cholesterol levels, especially amongst adolescents. This has involved major changes in the Finnish way of life where dairy produce has traditionally been the staple diet of the population. Finnish nurses have been very active in this project, which has involved changes in school meals, reducing fat content of milk, encouraging retailers to stock less butter and more polyunsaturated margarines and providing farmers with incentives to produce fruit rather than dairy produce. Even if nurses are not taking part in formal research work, it is possible to help to change attitudes towards diet by finding out what the client's beliefs are about diet, exercise and health; using professional skills and knowledge to dispel any false ideas they may hold about dietary fat and its relationship to heart disease. On a wider level, nurses can also be involved in hospital and school food policies and community group work, particularly with women as they do still tend to be the providers of food (Charles and Kerr, 1986).

From the nursing point of view, it is important to take into account cultural attitudes to food before helping a client to plan his or her diet. This implies both finding out from the client what his or her cultural background is and being aware of the dietary preferences of that culture. In a multicultural society, no one could expect you to have a full knowledge of every cultural aspect of diet. Your most reliable source of such information is the client. However, people often need help in clarifying their own beliefs about aspects of their health and this is an important component of the self-empowerment approach, as self-awareness is necessary in facilitating the decision-making process.

DECISION MAKING

Having provided and shared information about diet and exercise, explored and clarified beliefs and attitudes towards behavioural changes in these areas, the final stage of the self-empowerment approach is to facilitate decision making. As a health promoter your aim is to enable decision making, not to challenge the final decision reached. It is therefore important to be aware of your own attitudes towards diet and exercise and to separate those from the client's decision. In order to make effective decisions, people need to have the available options before them, but they also need to have some idea about the potential outcomes of their decision and how this would relate to their own lifestyle and experience. As Tones *et al.* (1990) suggest, there is also an element of psychological control involved with decision making, which may include concepts such as self-esteem and self-efficacy. Whilst it is not possible to explore these concepts in detail here, it is important to recognise that an individual's health behaviour may be regulated by his or her feelings of personal mastery over a particular action, which Bandura (1977) has suggested may be influenced by past experience, observation of others and persuasion. Thus, practice in decision making should be a component of the self-empowerment process, as it may develop or reinforce feelings of personal mastery. Simulation of real-life situations, such as making a choice between walking or catching the bus, role-playing situations which might jeopardise a healthy decision, such as being pressurised to eat high fat foods in a social situation, and rehearsing potential conflict within oneself, can all be useful techniques towards self-empowerment.

It is within such practice situations that self-esteem and self-efficacy can be enhanced, particularly where trust and confidence within a group have been established, as peer support can be very encouraging in making and sustaining a decision. It is not within the scope of this chapter to discuss skills in group work in any detail, but clearly in order to use the self-empowerment approach to health promotion it is a useful attribute to develop such skills, as well as skills in communication and understanding health behaviour. Tones *et al.* (1990) have argued that if the self-empowerment approach can lead to positive changes in self-esteem and self-efficacy then these are positive health-promoting achievements in themselves. In this sense, the self-empowerment approach can be seen not only as an approach to promoting changes in health behaviour, but as a way of directly and positively promoting health.

In summary, there is evidence to show that dietary fat and exercise play an important role in the development of CHD. CHD is thought to be a population problem, i.e. all members of our community are at risk. However, CHD is widely held to be a preventable condition and one of the factors in its aetiology, dietary fat, can be controlled, thus leading to a decrease in the incidence of the disease. Factors which work against people changing their diet in order to reduce serum cholesterol levels and taking regular exercise, are lack of knowledge, existing beliefs and attitudes towards food and exercise, and a need to develop decision-making skills. The nurse has the potential to be influential in helping people to overcome or work around these obstacles by adopting a self-empowerment approach to health promotion.

SMOKING AND HEALTH

There are many behaviours in our society which could be seen as prejudicial to achieving human potential. Among them are misuse of drugs and alcohol, smoking and driving dangerously. Primary prevention of these behaviours begins before they have been started, as in the prevention of smoking among school children. Secondary prevention, however, involves helping people to give up the behaviour before any long-term damage is done. Usually, activities such as drinking and smoking are experienced as enjoyable by the participants and advice to give it up may be seen as an infringement on personal liberty. People are free to make their own choices, but nurses can help them to maintain personal autonomy whilst making the healthy choice and by supporting them in that decision.

As a further illustration of the self-empowerment approach, the use of tobacco will be used to illustrate the obstacles that prevent people from changing their behaviour and the nurse's role in helping them to overcome them.

Background information to smoking

Tobacco smoking is a widespread habit in the UK. The most recent figures suggest that 33% of men and 30% of women smoke (OPCS, 1990). Research which was commenced in 1948 (Doll and Hill, 1952) demonstrated a relationship between smoking and lung cancer and it is now known to be associated with many other debilitating and life-threatening diseases, such as chronic obstructive lung disease and coronary heart disease (Royal College of Physicians, 1983). Smoking is thought to account for up to 18% of deaths from CHD (DoH, 1993b). However, the onset of irreparable disease through smoking is relatively slow. Lung cancer may not be evident for 30 years or more after the commencement of smoking; giving up smoking, even after 20 years, is therefore going to be beneficial. Sandvik *et al.* (1995) found that men who stopped smoking showed lung function performance that mimicked the findings for persistent non-smokers.

This delay in the effects of smoking becoming evident accounts for the observable difference in lung cancer rates between men and women shown in Figure 4.4. This is because women did not take up smoking seriously until after the Second World War – so its effects are only now becoming apparent – whereas men started smoking much earlier. The fact that lung cancer rates for men are declining as cigarette consumption falls is further evidence of the relationship between tobacco and lung cancer. The DoH have set specific targets to reduce smoking rates among young people who continue to smoke at a worrying level (DoH, 1993b).

The relationship between smoking and CHD appears to lie in the way in which smoking affects the balance between serum HDL cholesterol and triglycerides as well as the affect of smoking on increasing the serum fibrinogen level, thus increasing the risk of thrombosis (COMA, 1994). Apart from the long-term consequences, there are

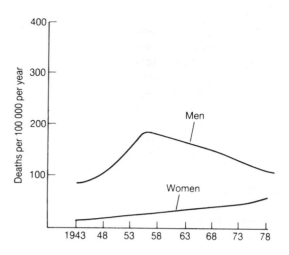

Figure 4.4: Death rates from lung cancer for men and women 1943–78 (Royal College of Physicians, 1983)

immediate benefits of giving up smoking. Ex-smokers report feeling fitter, more energetic, having fewer coughs and colds and having more money available for other things. Given that smoking does have both these long-term and immediate effects on human potential, why don't people give up smoking more readily? There are a number of obstacles to this eventuality which nurses should be aware of and which the self-empowerment approach may help to overcome.

The self-empowerment approach to smoking cessation will be explored by the use of the following scenario.

Scenario 3

Aisha is a primary nurse working on a medical unit. Many of the patients admitted come in with respiratory problems and cardiac problems. Aisha is aware that many of these patients are smokers and that a fair proportion express a wish to give up. Aisha is particularly keen to help a recent patient, Steve, to stop smoking. Steve is 48 and has been admitted for the second time with chest pains. He weighs 95 kg, enjoys eating and drinking with his mates (about 25 units a week) and smokes about 30 cigarettes a day. Whilst Steve is worried about his condition and has expressed a desire to give up smoking, Aisha realises that the need to smoke may be greater than the pressure to give up. Whilst Steve appears to be in control of his life, he is also insecure about his relationships and uses food and smoking as a way of communicating with people. Aisha plans her health promotion with Steve to incorporate a self-empowering approach to stopping smoking.

By exploring Steve's values and beliefs about smoking through a facilitative style using open questions (e.g. What makes you carry on smoking?), Aisha uncovers Steve's belief that he is 'addicted' to nicotine. She is able to draw on the following information to explore this idea with Steve.

HABITUATION/ADDICTION

Many smokers claim they cannot give up because they are addicted. There is still some debate as to whether nicotine is a physically addictive drug, but it is undoubtedly habit-forming and regular smoking maintains the blood level of nicotine. Smokers describe withdrawal effects, such as irritability and depression, when they stop smoking. Pharmacologically, nicotine has paradoxical effects on the body because of its action on both the central and autonomic nervous systems (Ashton and Stepney, 1982). The effects produced, for example, can be both relaxation and a greater ability to concentrate. Such effects appear to habituate the smoker into associating having a cigarette with other activities, such as using the phone, sitting down after a meal or coping with stressful situations. Breaking these rituals can become extremely difficult.

Using the self-empowerment approach to enable Steve to overcome this obstacle is appropriate since it involves not only the information necessary to make a decision, but also clarifying his beliefs and attitudes to smoking and facilitating the decision-making process by enhancing self-esteem and self-efficacy. Aisha started by helping Steve to look more closely at the situations in which he is most likely to smoke and what alternative strategies could be utilised to overcome the need for a cigarette. Thus, Steve says he would find giving up a cigarette during his visit to the pub much more difficult than the two or three he has in the car on the way home from work. Steve thinks he could break the driving and smoking ritual by chewing gum instead. Therefore, Aisha supports the idea that Steve should start with the situation he feels he has most control over. When he has mastered smoking in the car, he can move on to a different situation. It is important that the nurse uses his or her skills in assessment to ensure that decisions reached are, in fact, based on the client's perception of the situation rather than the nurse's own perceptions.

MOTIVATION

Aisha recognised that whilst Steve was motivated to stop smoking, he held conflicting attitudes towards his behaviour and that of others.

Research has shown that the intention of people to stop smoking is closely related to their desire to stop and this in turn is related to their attitude to smoking and health (Mattheson and Marsh, 1983). Attitudes to smoking vary between, 'This is the only thing I have which I enjoy' and 'It's too late to stop now'. Such attitudes may be changed by new knowledge or a new experience (such as the death of someone close from lung cancer or the arrival of a new baby) but information alone is unlikely to change attitudes. Attitudes can change under group pressure, so that although smoking is often commenced and maintained under peer pressure, it can also be peers and social attitudes generally that make people want to stop. Public attitudes towards smoking have changed dramatically over the past 20 years – it is now unacceptable to smoke in many public places such as cinemas and on public transport and even some hospitals. The self-empowerment approach suggests that such attitudes and values should be clarified. As suggested earlier, attitudes are not fixed but people are unlikely to change if they have not thought about their attitude to their own smoking behaviour and that of others. For example, Steve held conflicting attitudes in that he felt positive about his own smoking behaviour but negative towards being in a smoke-filled room. Aisha was able to explore this conflict, thus enabling Steve to understand himself better and his motivations for continuing to smoke or wanting to give up.

COPING WITH EMOTIONS

Smokers frequently use their behaviour as a way of coping with emotions such as stress, anxiety and depression (Maclaine and Macleod Clark, 1991). Dealing with these emotions can be very difficult and may be related to feelings of low self-esteem and lack of personal mastery. Stress may be incurred by the fact that women may take on both domestic responsibilities as well as paid employment and this stress may be partially relieved by smoking.

Aisha was able to explore with Steve the coping strategies that were built in to his smoking behaviour. She found that he was basically a shy person who found it difficult to build lasting relationships. Going to the pub was a way of being with people but he needed the 'prop' of a cigarette in his hand to be able to talk confidently.

By exploring the underlying cause of the stress, Aisha was able to help Steve to identify the first step towards taking alternative stress management measures. However, whilst a nurse may help a client to identify the cause of his stress or anxiety, it is important to be aware of the referral network, such as counselling, if the client needs more than relaxation exercises, for instance. It can be distressing for the client and arguably psychologically damaging if negative emotions are brought to the surface and then left unresolved.

To summarise, Aisha took a self-empowering approach to stopping smoking with Steve by:

- Clarifying his information needs around the idea of smoking as an addictive behaviour
- Exploring his beliefs and attitudes about smoking
- Enabling Steve to consider some situations over which he could have more control and develop mastery
- Enabling Steve to reflect on the alternatives to using smoking as a coping mechanism.

Research has shown that nurses can be effective in helping people to give up smoking (Macleod Clark et al., 1990). This study suggests that the development of communication skills in nursing and health promotion is an important indicator of success. The research has shown that whilst the self-empowerment approach to enabling people to give up smoking does require some counselling skills, even with some fairly basic communication skills nurses can be effective. Exploring the client's perceptions by using open questions and listening skills, for example, were shown to be key indicators of success in enabling people to stop smoking.

Key Points

- The self-empowerment approach to health promotion has been illustrated by addressing two major health issues – CHD and smoking.
- The aim of the self-empowerment approach is to facilitate decision-making skills in the client which will potentially promote a healthy lifestyle.
- For the health promoter, this involves providing information which will enhance informed decision making, clarifying attitudes and beliefs with the client, and facilitating the actual decision-making process.

This may include analysing the client's perceptions of the costs and benefits of behaviour change, as well as considering such factors as self-esteem and self-efficacy.

THE RADICAL APPROACH

Tones et al. (1990) suggest that a third possible approach to health promotion is the radical option. This approach differs from both prevention and self-empowerment in that it attempts to tackle the determinants of health and illness at the social level rather than on an individual level. Whilst the preventive approach, and to a certain extent the self-empowerment approach, are derived ideologically from the concept of responsibility for self, the radical approach acknowledges that the social, environmental and political context, have a major influence on the health of communities. This has been demonstrated by research into inequalities in health, such as The Black Report (Townsend and Davidson, 1982) and upheld by more recent documents (Whitehead, 1988; Benzeval et al., 1995). For example, Whitehead highlights the problem of ill health related to poor nutrition among children and specifically targets the school meals service. Policy changes such as the abolition of price maintenance and national nutritional standards for children have resulted in a haphazard school meals service in which those children who are most needy often fare the worst. This is not an individual problem, but as Lang (1987, cited by Whitehead) puts it:

'Low income is the key link between food, poverty and health. Tackling low income goes entirely beyond the capacity of the local authority and into the realms of benefit policy. Above all, it needs national, not just local action.'

But who is going to instigate such action and do nurses have any role to play here? Arguably, nurses are in a key position to take a radical approach to health promotion. They form a very large body of professionals who ought, through their professional organisations, trades unions and pressure groups, to be able to influence social and health policy. The potential for nurses taking the radical approach will be explored using two health issues as examples – these are alcohol abuse and mental health.

BACKGROUND INFORMATION TO ALCOHOL USE

How much do people drink?

In 1994 the OPCS published the General House-hold Survey (GHS) based on data collected in 1992. One of the topics which they surveyed people about was alcohol consumption. The findings are summarised below:

- In 1992 men aged 16 and over were drinking on average 15.9 units per week, about the equivalent of 8 pints of beer. This was about three times as much as women, who drank, on average, 5.4 units per week.
- Around 27% of men and 11% of women were drinking more than the recommended maximum of 21 and 14 units per week respectively.
- Around 6% of men and 2% of women were drinking more than 50 and 25 units per week respectively. These levels are considered to be dangerous to health.
- There was a small rise from 9% in 1984 to 11% in 1992 of women drinking more than 14 units per week. At the same time, men's intake stayed steady.

The increase in consumption is largely accounted for by the relative price of alcohol in an increasingly prosperous society. For example, in 1950 a bottle of whisky cost the equivalent of 659 minutes of manual work, whilst in 1980 it cost only 153 minutes of manual work (NACNE, 1983). By comparison, the cost of a loaf of bread increased in these terms from the equivalent of 9 minutes of work in 1950 to 10 minutes in 1980. In other words, people are economically in a favourable position to purchase alcohol if they choose to do so.

The Health of the Nation (DoH, 1992a) set the following target for reductions in alcohol consumption:

- To reduce the proportion of men drinking more than 21 units of alcohol per week from 28% in 1990 to 18% by 2005 and the proportion of women drinking more than 14 units of alcohol per week from 11% in 1990 to 7% by 2005.

The Department of Health figures are based on limits for safe drinking which have been established for some time – 14 units per week for women and 21 units per week for men. One unit of alcohol is equivalent to 8 mg ethanol which is the same as drinking one glass of wine, half a pint of beer or one measure of spirits. Whilst these guidelines have been the basis of health education messages regarding alcohol consumption, there has been some debate about the relative risk of drinking alcohol, particularly with regard to a possible protective effect from coronary heart disease. Following the publication of a number of papers which describe this protective effect, the Department of Health set up a working group to review sensible drinking levels. In December 1995 it published a report which suggested that a small increase in these levels would not be hazardous to health and that, indeed 1–2 units per day could be protective against coronary heart disease (DoH, 1995a). The new recommended upper limit was 3–4 units per day for men and 2–3 units per day for women, representing an average increase on the former limits of 0–33% for men and women. This announcement by the Department of Health was qualified by certain caveats – for example, that there are situations in which people should not drink at all, such as before driving, using machinery or electrical equipment and that women who are pregnant should not drink more than 1 or 2 units once or twice a week. The report, nevertheless, had considerable impact on the media, the medical world and the public at large. The medical response was conservative. The BMA and the Royal Colleges of Physicians, Psychiatrists and General Practitioners had already published their own reports on sensible drinking limits during 1995. Both documents reviewed data on the potential protective effects of alcohol on preventing coronary heart disease and both reports concluded that this protective effect in middle-aged men would be offset by other harmful effects of alcohol and that the sensible limits of 21 units per week for men and 14 for women should be retained.

The BMA report concluded thus:

'The current limits of 21 units per week for men and 14 for women, should be maintained but it should not be implied that drinking 21 units for men or 14 for women is the optimum intake for health benefits and reduced risks. The risks of CHD and other alcohol related diseases changes throughout life and for each individual; 1 unit to 21 units for men and 14 units for women, is the recommended low risk range of drinking within which individuals should aim to remain. It should be made clear that whilst there is evidence that drinking up to such levels may provide benefits in terms of reducing the risk of CHD there may be also some risks in terms of other causes of mortality and morbidity including indirect effects. Individuals should be informed that if they drink more than the stated lower risk range of 21 units for men and 14 units for women, they should endeavour to reduce their level of consumption.'

(British Medical Association, 1995, reproduced in *Addiction*, 1996, page 25)

Whilst the final recommendations from the Royal College of Physician's report was identical in its aim to retain the limits of 21 units for men and 14 for women, it did present its conclusions in a slightly different light:

'Whether there is net benefit to the health of individuals from drinking 1–3 units/day (men) or 1–2 units/day (women) will depend on all the other risks related to these levels of alcohol consumption.

For middle-aged men, CHD is the major cause of death. A protective effect of 1–3 units/day may therefore confer an overall advantage.

For younger men the major cause of death is accidents and violent deaths, some sizable proportion of which are alcohol-related. Any increase in consumption in this section of the population could have markedly adverse consequences.

For pre-menopausal women, breast cancer is a more important cause of death than CHD, and there may be a narrow window of benefit before a protective effect against CHD is balanced by a deleterious effect on breast cancer. Recommendations to pre-menopausal women to drink in order to reduce their already low risk of CHD could, therefore, have the consequence of increasing risk of breast cancer.

For all-cause mortality, the risk in men increases from about 3 units/day and in women from 2 units/day. For individuals, then, the window of benefit appears narrow. The evidence reviewed indicates that the current sensible limits of 21 units/week for men and 14 for women should be retained. If an individual has reasons for being a non-drinker, we should not recom-

mend that he or she starts drinking in order to reduce the risk of CHD.'

(Royal Colleges of Physicians, Psychiatrists and General Practitioners, 1995, 29(4), pages 266–71)

The medical advice, therefore, seems reasonably conclusive regarding the concept of sensible drinking for the individual. It perhaps seems odd, then, that the Department of Health was apparently suggesting that increasing the recommended limits for sensible drinking would not only confer no additional health risk but may actually protect against the risk of CHD. Certainly, the medical profession itself found the DoH's advice contentious. For example, in a letter to the BMJ, Griffith Edwards, Emeritus Professor of addiction behaviour, deplored the fact that the public were now faced with confusing advice and that:

'advice from independent medical authorities should be preferred to that of an inter-departmental government body. Civil servants, especially those from the food ministry, are not appropriate arbiters on what doctors say to their patients. That such a group was allowed to advise the public on a matter where there is such strong pressure from commercial interests is deplorable'

(Edwards, 1996, page 1)

Clearly, Edwards is suggesting that the DoH did not present independent evidence and was influenced by membership on the working group which included civil servants from the Ministry of Agriculture, Fisheries and Food, which works closely with the drink industry, which has long lobbied for relaxation in the sensible drinking limits. This is a disturbing possibility.

A further issue raised by both medical reports and taken up by Casswell (1996) in her letter to *Addiction*, is the overall effect on public health of promulgating new low risk limits for alcohol consumption. Whilst there may be some protective effect from CHD for the individual male who is over 40, the overall message could have the effect of increasing the mean (average) alcohol intake for the population, which could increase the overall alcohol-related mortality. Casswell (1996) makes the point that little attention is given to the very small increase in mean consumption that is required to have this effect. She suggests that mass media campaigns on alcohol consumption are not the most effective ways of delivering a public health message because they cannot address individual risk or detail, such as mean consumption. Casswell's evidence suggests that reduction in alcohol-related harm is more likely to be achieved through public policy measures such as taxation, restriction of access to young people and enforcement of drink-driving legislation.

It is the public health and community level of alcohol education that we will concentrate on for the remainder of this section.

Clearly, a great many people drink alcohol regularly, although they may not be alcoholic in the sense that they are dependent on alcohol. They, nevertheless, expose themselves to health risks, such as cirrhosis of the liver, gastrointestinal disturbances, degeneration of the central nervous system, metabolic disorders and an increased susceptibility to infection (Smith, 1981). In addition, there is the risk of accidental death or injury due to the effects of alcohol. The DHSS (1985) estimated that one-third of all drivers and one-quarter of all pedestrians killed on the roads had blood levels of alcohol exceeding the legal limit (80 mg/100 ml). There are also the social consequences to consider – drunkenness contributes to aggressive and abusive behaviour which can be detrimental to the health of families and communities. Women are particularly at risk of violent attacks. Overall the cost of misusing alcohol outweighs the possible benefits and the population as a whole would certainly benefit in health terms from a reduction in alcohol consumption, as indicated in *The Health of the Nation* targets (DoH, 1992a).

There does appear to be evidence that income and social class are associated with alcohol consumption. In a lifestyles survey, Blaxter (1990) found that alcohol consumption was strongly correlated with other 'unhealthy' behaviours, such as smoking and poor diet, particularly among younger men from the manual working groups. Low income was also a strong correlate of alcohol consumption. Power *et al.* (1991) have also found evidence to suggest that young men from the lower social classes are more likely to present with poor health outcomes as a result of alcohol consumption, among other health-related behaviours, than young men from the professional and managerial groups.

The reasons why people become problem drinkers are manifold and it is not appropriate in this chapter to embark on a detailed discus-

sion. Suffice it to say that the research is still unclear because alcohol-related problems such as violence, child abuse and divorce cannot be separated from the underlying cause or other contributing factors. For example, does drink cause divorce or does the trauma of divorce lead to problem drinking? What does appear to be evident is that the harmful effects of alcohol are most likely to occur among communities who are in most need, in terms of income and employment and, by implication, housing, education and health facilities. This would suggest that at least some of the causes of problem drinking lie not within individual control, but rather at a political level. The radical approach to health promotion indicates that by taking political action to change inequalities in health, some of the problems associated with problem drinking could be averted.

NURSING AND THE RADICAL APPROACH TO HEALTH PROMOTION

Traditionally, nurses have not been very active politically. Butterworth (1988) has criticised nurses for their apparent lethargy towards social and national policy issues. The reasons for this seem unclear, but could be rooted in the historical development of nursing as a predominantly female profession with its associated powerlessness in relation to the male-dominated medical profession. This raises many issues about the way nurses perceive themselves and the way they are perceived by the public and professional colleagues. Despite history, some nurses have seen the value of taking collectivist, radical action to put pressure on policy makers. Examples are the radical midwives group, who have campaigned for women to have more choice in childbirth, with some success, as the White Paper *Changing Childbirth* (DoH, 1993a) demonstrated, in as much as the needs of women were very much the focus of the paper. The radical health visitors who support issues such as the new public health movement, which aims to reduce health problems through creating a safer and healthier social environment, have also been active for many years. Now it seems that the DoH and the UKCC are becoming interested in the public health role of nurses as shown by the report from the Standing Nursing and Midwifery Advisory Committee on Public

Health Nursing (DoH, 1995b). It is difficult (though not impossible) for nurses to take a radical approach to health promotion single-handed. One person may be disregarded; a group of people have to be listened to at some level. For this reason, a collectivist approach to a health problem such as the use of alcohol may be most effectively tackled by campaigning and lobbying with other nurses. This could be in association with a professional organisation or trade union, such as the Royal College of Nursing or the Community Practitioners and Health Visitors' Association, or through a local pressure group. In relation to alcohol, the type of campaigns which could be organised include:

- Taxation on all alcoholic drinks to be maintained at the rate of inflation
- Advertising for alcohol to display clear information about alcoholic content and warnings about health risks of drinking
- An annual levy imposed on alcohol advertising which could be used to fund community education programmes
- Clarification and enforcement of the legislation relating to the sale of alcohol to under-18s and to roadside breathalysing
- Lobbying against the promotion of alcoholic drinks which have a particular attraction for young people, e.g. alcoholic lemonade – the so-called 'alcopops'
- Custodial sentences for offences such as dangerous and reckless driving under the influence of alcohol, particularly where the death of a third party is concerned.

The above campaigns could be seen as using the legislative framework to control drinking behaviour. Other, more general, political action which could potentially have a more far-reaching effect on all aspects of health would include lobbying for:

- The right to housing and tackling the problems of homelessness
- Increases in welfare benefits such as child benefit, and the state pension to be raised to a level commensurate with the cost of living
- Provision of state-funded child care for preschool children
- Reduction in unemployment
- Equal distribution of resources for services, such as education and the health service

- Equal opportunities, regardless of gender, race, age or religion.

Nurses form a very large body of people. As individuals, they will have their own political views and will hold their own convictions about health and health promotion. As a profession, they are caring for people who may not have had the education, the wealth or the opportunity to take control of their health and it could be perceived as a professional duty to advocate publicly for those who are disadvantaged or powerless within our society. The next section considers the radical approach to mental health.

Mental health

Mental health is notoriously difficult to define. It can be argued that it means more than just the absence of mental illness, that it refers to a state of well-being, an ability to make rational decisions, a feeling of self-worth. It is encompassed in Seedhouse's (1986) definition of health when he speaks of achieving human potential, but what is the full potential of the human psyche? In many ways mental health is inseparable from physical health if we are referring to a holistic approach to health. Human potential has to be seen in terms of the whole being more than the sum of its parts; the mind and the body are interrelated and the determinants of physical health will, to a great extent, be the same as the determinants of mental health. For example, it has already been noted that poverty makes a significant contribution to ill health. In their seminal study, Brown and Harris (1978) have argued that depression among women is much greater when certain vulnerability factors, such as mother's unemployment, are present and more recently Blaxter (1990) has suggested that income is correlated with poor psychosocial health. These two studies will form the focus of this section as they both suggest ways in which mental health can be promoted through both radical and other measures. *The Health of the Nation* (DoH, 1992a) targets for mental health are:

- To improve significantly the health and social functioning of mentally ill people
- To reduce the overall suicide rate by at least 15% by the year 2000
- To reduce the suicide rate of severely mentally ill people by at least 33% by the year 2000 (baseline 1990).

It is important to note that these targets are more concerned with mental illness than mental health, mainly because it is so difficult to define and measure mental health.

Brown and Harris's (1978) study of depression among women in the community takes a sociological stance. In other words, it looks for causes of depression within the social context of women's lives rather than for a biochemical abnormality within individuals. Brown and Harris interviewed a random sample of women in the community who had not necessarily been clinically labelled as depressed and found that there was a high incidence of women who defined themselves as depressed. Brown and Harris acknowledge that this raises questions of diagnosis, but argue that just because people have not been labelled by the psychiatrist does not mean that they are not experiencing depression.

Having explored a large number of variables which could be related to depression, Brown and Harris put forward a model which proposed some social origins of depression. There is a greater likelihood of major life events, such as a bereavement, leading to depression in the presence of background social factors, such as social class and what they term 'vulnerability factors'; these include unemployment of the woman, three or more children under 15 years, loss of her own mother before the age of 11 and lack of a close and trusting relationship with a partner. Low self-esteem will contribute to an outcome of depression in the presence of these factors. The absence of these vulnerability factors can also be seen as protective against depression, especially where the woman has high self-esteem. But where vulnerability factors lead to low self-esteem and where a life event or difficulty arises (such as death, divorce or separation from children) then depression is likely to occur as a result of a sense of hopelessness about the future and failure to work through grief. Women with high self-esteem are more able to find alternative sources of value and this enables them to resolve their sense of hopelessness.

Brown and Harris's findings appear to indicate that working-class women are much more likely than middle-class women to experience a severe psychiatric disorder in the presence of a life event, which they ascribe to the presence of the vulnerability factors and associated low self-esteem. In other words, working-class women are more likely to be unemployed, without a supportive partner, to have three children under the age of 15 and to have lost their own mother before the age of 11 years. Whilst the authors acknowledge gaps in the research, such as the diagnostic label already mentioned and the difference between depression and the experience of grief, the findings seem to indicate clearly that depression has social origins which could potentially be prevented through political means, such as improving the employment status of women and providing a wider choice of child care facilities, either free or at affordable cost. Brown and Harris do not mention housing as a vulnerability factor. Perhaps there was optimism about housing in the early 1970s when this research was conducted and a municipal housing programme was still in progress. It would be interesting in today's climate to test the model further to see whether housing would feature as a vulnerability factor.

Blaxter's (1990) study was a comprehensive survey of health and lifestyles which was conducted by interviewing a random sample of 9003 people from England, Scotland and Wales. Whilst Blaxter was not attempting to provide a causative model of mental ill health, she was trying to establish some of the major correlates between many aspects of health and people's lifestyles. However, she found very similar relationships between what she terms psychosocial health and income. She found that women on low incomes with no social support were most likely to experience symptoms related to poor psychosocial health, such as depression, worry or sleep disturbances. Overall, it was the young in the 18–39 age group, those who were unemployed, divorced, separated and widowed and single parents of dependent children who were most likely to report high rates of psychosocial malaise.

These findings would appear to support Brown and Harris's thesis that mental ill health has social determinants. Blaxter is particularly concerned with the role that social support plays in the prevention of psychosocial symptoms and its relative protectiveness compared with 'healthy' lifestyles. Perhaps not surprisingly, she found that people with both low social support and 'unhealthy' lifestyles (smoking, drinking, poor diet and lack of fitness) were most likely to experience psychosocial symptoms but either social support or a healthy lifestyle was not protective on its own. A combination of social support and a healthy lifestyle was found to be protective, although only a minority of the sample fulfilled all four lifestyle criteria. Smith and Jacobson (1988) have also explored the concept of social support as a determinant of mental health. Whilst there does appear to be evidence that intimate and trusting relationships can be protective against the negative effects of life events, these authors argue that more research is required into the qualitative nature of social support.

It appears from Blaxter's study that again it is those who are most disadvantaged who are most likely to experience psychosocial symptoms, and whilst the terms of reference and definitions differ from Brown and Harris's earlier study, there do appear to be some similarities. This would suggest that there are some aspects of mental health which can be approached using a radical approach to health promotion, with the emphasis on reducing poverty and unemployment. It seems that the causes of a lack of social support also need to be addressed – is there more divorce among poorer people and if so, is this precipitated by poverty and unemployment? Are the mortality rates higher among those who are poor and is this related to social isolation? We already know that social deprivation is strongly related to ill health (Townsend and Davidson, 1982; Whitehead, 1988, Benzeval *et al.*, 1995); perhaps it is time for nurses to be more pro-active in their response to the research.

Scenario 4

Beth and Mary are community midwives working in Glasgow. They both have a special interest in postnatal depression and have worked closely with their health visiting colleagues both to identify and prevent it. Whilst some parents have found it helpful to have counselling following the identification of postnatal depression, the midwives have conducted their own survey of the community and identified some structural factors which may contribute to a relatively high incidence of postnatal depression. Whilst some of these factors, such as the housing conditions and the employment status of the community, seem insurmountable, the midwives decide to work collectively with both the health visitors and the mothers in the area to gather support for a community drop-in centre. This involves:

- Involvement in local politics – the only available space has been ear-marked for a snooker hall.

- Calculating costs for both short and longer term priorities – e.g. a counsellor in the centre
- Arguing the case for more social support for women with health and social care purchasers
- Presenting convincing evidence to councillors and decision makers
- Campaigning for funds
- Working collaboratively with both professionals and local inhabitants
- Being able to consider the evaluation needs of the project from the outset.

After a great deal of hard work, the drop-in centre finally gets going 12 months later with a small fund from the local authority and some funding from the charity MIND for a limited period. After a further 6 months the midwives carry out a satisfaction questionnaire with the women using the centre and find that they generally find it supportive. However, the midwives are aware that it will take much more time and a very careful evaluation before the real effects of the centre on postnatal depression can be assessed.

Key Points

- The radical approach to health promotion has been addressed by exploring two health issues – alcohol abuse and mental health. This approach sees the determinants of health and illness as being within the social and political arena, rather than within the direct control of the individual.
- It attempts, in this respect, to avoid 'victim-blaming' and to find ways through the democratic processes of lobbying, campaigning, protesting and voting to resolve some of today's major health issues.
- Nurses have not been very prominent in this arena and this may be related to their own position within the health service. However, they do form a very large majority within the health service and there is potential for nurses to influence social policy.

CONCLUSION

In conclusion, this chapter has addressed the promotion of health by looking at the concept of human potential. There are many measures by which human potential can be developed and these have been addressed using three approaches to health promotion. The first approach looked at immunisation and screening within Caplan's (1969) framework of prevention. Nurses have a very significant role to play in helping to prevent ill health by providing people with information which is relevant to their needs and being knowledgeable about the services which are available. The patients and clients in our care have different health needs and individual obstacles to overcome in order to meet those needs. By careful assessment the nurse can identify the patient's needs and use his or her knowledge and skill as a professional to develop and implement a nursing care plan, in partnership with the patient, which will enhance the promotion of human potential.

The second approach, self-empowerment, was illustrated by addressing the issues of diet and smoking. The underlying concept here is that individuals need to develop decision-making skills in order to make healthy choices. It is less paternalistic than the preventive approach, as it assumes that individuals are autonomous beings who wish to make free choices about their lives. It has been argued that nurses can facilitate the decision-making process by providing appropriate information, helping people to clarify their attitudes and beliefs about health and by using more sophisticated skills in communication and group work to enhance decision making. It has been suggested that the levels of skill required to apply this approach in nursing may develop with increasing experience in practice.

Finally, the radical approach was discussed. This approach assumes that health problems are determined by the physical and social environment rather than individual behaviour. It was argued that by changing this environment health problems would be tackled at the 'upstream' level, making it more realistic for people to make healthy choices. For example, social deprivation was seen as an underlying determinant of alcohol abuse and depression among women. As a major workforce, nurses are seen as having a potentially significant role in influencing social policy, but at the moment it appears that nurses are not very pro-active as health campaigners.

Nurses are human beings who also need opportunities to develop their potential and there may be a range of obstacles, both in the work environment and in their personal lives which they need to overcome in order to achieve this. Any of the three approaches discussed may be applied to nurses themselves to promote their own health. In conclusion, you are reminded of Seedhouse's (1986) theory of health when he says:

'Work for health is work which aims to enable and to enhance by providing the foundations for the achievement of potentials.'

(page 74)

Clearly, nursing forms a major part of this work.

Summary

This chapter has considered ways in which nurses can be involved in promoting health. It has been argued that from both policy and care delivery perspectives it is appropriate for nurses to consider the challenge of health promotion. The author has adopted Seedhouse's theory of health as a starting point and also drawn on the principles of health promotion discussed by the World Health Organization. To enable you to develop your arguments and critical thinking about the application of health promotion theory, three approaches to promoting health have been presented. These are the preventive approach, the self-empowerment approach and the radical approach. Each approach offers the practitioner a different way of thinking about health promotion which has been illustrated through use of scenarios.

REFERENCES

Alderson, P., Mayall, B., Barker, S., Henderson, J., and Pratten, B. (1997). Childhood immunisation. Meeting targets yet respecting consent. *European Journal of Public Health*, 7, 95–100.

Ashton, H. and Stepney, R. (1982). *Smoking – Psychology and Pharmacology*. Tavistock Publications, London.

Bandura, A. (1977). Self-efficacy: towards a unifying theory of behaviour change. *Psychological Review*, 84, 191–215.

Baric, L. (1985). The meaning of words: health promotion. *Journal of the Institute of Health Education*, 23, 1.

Becker, M. and Maiman, L. (1975). Sociobehavioural determinants of compliance with health and medical care recommendations. *Medical Care*, 13(1), 10–25.

Bedford, H. (1993). Immunisation: facts and fiction. *Health Visitor*, 66(9), 314–16.

Benzeval, M., Judge, K. and Whitehead, M. (eds) (1995). *Tackling Inequalities in Health: an Agenda for Action.* Kings Fund, London.

Betts, G. and Betts, J. (1990). Establishing a child health clinic in a deprived area. *Health Visitor*, 63(4), 122–4.

Bingham S. (1991). A dietary strategy for England. In *The Health of the Nation: the BMJ View.* BMJ, London.

Blackburn C. (1991). *Poverty and Health – Working with Families.* Open University, Milton Keynes.

Blaxter, M. (1990). *Health and Lifestyles.* Tavistock Routledge, London.

Bond, M. and Kendall, S. (1990). *Improving Your Decision Making.* Distance Learning Centre, South Bank Polytechnic, London.

British Cardiac Society (1987). *Report of the British Cardiac Society Working Group on Coronary Disease Prevention.* British Cardiac Society, London.

British Medical Association (1995) *Guidelines on Sensible Drinking.* BMA, London. Conclusions reproduced in: Commentaries, *Addiction* (1996), 91(1), 25–33.

Brown, G. and Harris, T. (1978). *The Social Origins of Depression: a Study of Psychiatric Disorder in Women.* Tavistock Publications, London.

Butterworth, T. (1988). Political awareness. *Nursing Times.* Community Outlook, December 1988, 20–1.

Campbell, A. (1990). Education or indoctrination? The issue of autonomy in health education. In *Ethics in Health Education*, Doxiadis, S. (ed.). John Wiley & Sons, Chichester.

Caplan, G. (1969). *An Approach to Community Mental Health.* Tavistock Publications, London.

Casswell, S. (1996). Drinking guidelines offer little over and above the much needed health policies. *Addiction*, 91(1), 25–33.

Champion, V. (1987). The relationship of breast self examination to health belief model variables. *Research in Nursing and Health*, 10, 375–82.

Charles, N. and Kerr, M. (1986). Issues of responsibility and control in the feeding of families. In *The Politics of Health Education*, Watt, A. and Rodmell, S. (eds). Routledge and Kegan Paul, London.

COMA (1994). *Nutritional Aspects of Cardiovascular Disease.* HMSO, London.

Davison, C., Davey Smith, G. and Frankel, S. (1991). Lay epidemiology and the prevention paradox: the implications of coronary candidacy for health education. *Sociology of Health and Illness*, 13(1), 1–19.

DHSS (1981). *Report on Avoiding Heart Attacks.* HMSO, London.

DHSS (1984). *Mortality Statistics: Cause, 1983.* HMSO, London.

DHSS (1985). *Drug Mis-use. A Basic Briefing.* HMSO, London.

DHSS (1986). *Neighbourhood Nursing* (Chair: Julia Cumberlege). HMSO, London.

DoH (1988). *Promoting Better Health.* HMSO, London.

DoH (1989a). *Working for Patients.* HMSO, London.

DoH (1989b). *Health and Personal Social Services Statistics for England.* HMSO, London.

DoH (1990). *NHS and Community Care Act.* HMSO, London.

DoH (1992a). *The Health of the Nation.* HMSO, London.

DoH (1992b). *Immunisation Against Infectious Diseases.* HMSO, London.

DoH (1993a). *Changing Childbirth.* HMSO, London.

DoH (1993b). *Key Area Handbook: Coronary Heart Disease and Stroke.* HMSO, London.

DoH (1995a). *Sensible Drinking: the Report of an Interdepartmental Working Group.* HMSO, London.

DoH (1995b). *Making it Happen – Report of the Standing Nursing and Midwifery Advisory Committee (SNMAC).* HMSO, London.

DoH (1996). *Primary Care – the Future.* NHSE, Leeds.

Doll, R. and Hill, A.B. (1952). A study of the aetiology of carcinoma of the lung. *British Medical Journal*, 2, 1271–6.

Edwards, G. (1996) Sensible drinking. *British Medical Journal*, 312, 1.

Faulkner, A. and Ward, L. (1983). Nurses as health educators in relation to smoking. *Nursing Times*, 79(15), Occasional Papers No. 8.

French, J. and Adams, L. (1986). From analysis to synthesis. *Health Education Journal*, 45(2), 71–4.

Gott, M. and O'Brien, M. (1990). The role of the nurse in health promotion. *Health Promotion International*, 5(2), 137–43.

Graham, H. (1984). *Woman, Health and the Family.* Wheatsheaf Publications, Brighton.

Hakama, M. (1983). Cancer of the uterine cervix. In *The Epidemiology of Cancer*, Burke, G. (ed.). Croom Helm, London.

Harris, J. (1985). *The Value of Life*. Routledge and Kegan Paul, London.

Health Education Authority and Sports Council (1987). *Exercise. Why Bother?* HEA, London.

Health Education Council (1980). *Survey of Nursing in England, Wales and Northern Ireland*. HEC, London.

Health Education Council (1982). *Health Education in Nursing – A Workshop*. HEC, London.

Imperial Cancer Research Fund OXCHECK study group (1995). Effectiveness of health checks conducted by nurses in primary care: final results of the OXCHECK study. *British Medical Journal*, 310, 1099–104.

King, J. (1987). Women's attitudes towards cervical smear. *Update*, 34(2), 25.

Kramsch, D., Aspen, A., Abromowitz, B., Kreimendahl, T. and Hood, W. (1981). Reduction of coronary atherosclerosis by moderate conditioning exercise in monkeys on an atherogenic diet. *New England Journal of Medicine*, 305(25), 1483.

Lask, S., Smith, P. and Masterson, A. (1994) *A Curricular Review of the Pre- and Post-registration Education for Nurses, Midwives and Health Visitors in Relation to the Integration of a Philosophy of Health: Developing a Model for Evaluation*. ENB, London.

Latter, S. (1994). Health education and health promotion: perceptions and practices of nurses in acute care settings. Unpublished PhD thesis, Kings College, University of London.

Leino-Kelpi, H., Iire, L., Suminen, T., Vuorenheimo, J. and Valimaki, M. (1993). Client and information: a literature review. *Journal of Clinical Nursing*, 2, 331–40.

McKinlay, J.B. (1979). A case for refocusing upstream: the political economy of illness. In *Patients, Physicians and Illness*, Jaco, E. (ed.). The Free Press, New York.

Maclaine, K. and Macleod Clark, J. (1991). Women's reasons for smoking in pregnancy. *Nursing Times*, 87, 22.

Macleod Clark, J., Haverty, S. and Kendall, S. (1990). Helping people to stop smoking: a study of the nurse's role. *Journal of Advanced Nursing*, 16, 357–63.

McPherson A. (ed.) (1991). *Women's Problems in General Practice*. Oxford University Press, Oxford.

Marmot, M. (1985). Interpretation of trends in coronary heart disease mortality. *Acta Medica Scandinavica*, 701 (Supplement), 58–75.

Mattheson, J. and Marsh, A. (1983). *Attitudes, Behaviour and Smoking*. OPCS, London.

Morris, J., Everitt, M., Pollard, R., Chave, S. and Semmence, A. (1980). Vigorous exercise in leisure time: protection against coronary heart disease. *Lancet*, 2(8257), 1207–10.

National Advisory Committee on Nutrition Education (NACNE) (1983). *Proposals for Nutritional Guidelines for Health Education in Britain*. HEC, London.

National Heart Forum (1995). *Preventing Coronary Heart Disease in Primary Care – the Way Forward*. HMSO, London.

Nightingale, F. (1891). Letter to Mr Frederick Verney on the teaching of health at home. In *Buckinghamshire County Council* (1911). Reproduction of a printed report originally submitted to the Buckingham County Council in the year 1892, containing letters from Miss Nightingale on health visiting in districts, pages 17–19. Requoted from Clark, J. (1973). *A Family Visitor*, page 11. RCN, London.

Nightingale, F. (1893). Sick nursing and health nursing. A paper presented at the Chicago Exhibition. In *Selected Writings of Florence Nightingale*, Seymer, L.R. (ed.). (1954). Macmillan, New York.

OPCS (1982). *Mortality in England and Wales*. OPCS, London.

OPCS (1990). *General Household Survey 1988*. HMSO, London.

OPCS (1994) *The General Household Survey 1992*. HMSO, London.

OPCS (1995) *Morbidity Statistics from General Practice 1991–1992*. HMSO, London.

Open University (1985). *Caring for Health – Dilemmas and Prospects*. Open University Press, Milton Keynes.

Ottawa Charter for Health Promotion, 1986. Drafted by participants in the First International Conference on Health Promotion, November 17–21, 1986, Ottawa, Canada. WHO, Geneva.

Perkins, E. (1982). *Decision Making – The Whooping Cough Dilemma*. Nottingham Practical Papers in Health Education No. 8. University of Nottingham.

Phillimore, P., Beattie, A. and Townsend, P. (1994). Widening inequality of health in northern England, 1981–91. *British Medical Journal*, 308, 1125–39.

Power, C., Manor, O. and Fox, J. (1991). *Health and Class: The Early Years*. Chapman & Hall, London.

Roediger, H.L., Rushton, J.P., Capaldi, E.D. and Paris, S.G. (1984). *Psychology*. Little, Brown, Boston.

Rose, G. (1987). The scale of the problem. Paper given at the first conference of Anticipatory Care Teams, York, October 2–4.

Royal College of Physicians (1983). *Health or Smoking?* Pitman Publishing, London.

Royal College of Physicians and the British Cardiac Society (1976). Prevention of coronary heart disease. *Journal of the Royal College of Physicians*, 10(13), 213–75.

Royal Colleges of Physicians, Psychiatrists and General Practitioners (1995) Working group – summary of Report – Alcohol and the heart in perspective: sensible limits reaffirmed. *Journal of the Royal College of Physicians of London*, 29(4), 266–71.

Salvage J. (1992) The new nursing: empowering patients or empowering nurses? In *Policy Issues in Nursing*, Robinson, J., Gray, A. and Elkan, R. (eds). Open University, Milton Keynes.

Sandvik L., Erikssen, G. and Thaulow, E. (1995). Long term effects of health on physical fitness and lung function: a longitudinal study of 1393 middle-aged Norwegian men for seven years. *British Medical Journal*. 311, 715–18.

Schon, D. (1983). *The Reflective Practitioner: How Professionals Think in Action*. Basic Books, New York.

Seedhouse, D. (1986). *Health – the Foundations for Achievement*. John Wiley & Sons, Chichester.

Smith, A. and Jacobson, B. (1988). *The Nation's Health*. King's Fund, London.

Smith, R. (1981). Alcohol and alcoholism: the relation between consumption and damage. *British Medical Journal*, 283, 895–8.

Sontag, S. (1978). *Illness as Metaphor*. Penguin Books, Harmondsworth.

Spencer, N. and Power, S. (1978). *Nottingham Child Health Survey*. Occasional Paper 14, Leverhulme Health Education Project, Nottingham University.

Stillman, M. (1977). Women's health beliefs about breast cancer self examination. *Nursing Research*, 26(2), 121–7.

Syred, H. (1981). The abdication of health education by hospital nurses. *Journal of Advanced Nursing*, 6(1), 27–33.

Tones, B.K. (1986). Health education and the ideology of health promotion: a review of alternative approaches. *Health Education Research*, 1(1), 3–12.

Tones, B.K., Tilford, S. and Robinson, Y. (1990). *Health Education: Effectiveness and Efficiency*. Chapman & Hall, London.

Tones K. (1991). Health promotion, empowerment and the psychology of control. *Journal of the Institute of Health Education*, 29(1), 17–25.

Townsend, P. and Davidson, N. (eds). (1982). *The Black Report*. Penguin Books, Harmondsworth.

Tunstall-Pedoe, H. (1991). The Dundee coronary risk-disk for management of change in risk factors. *British Medical Journal*, 303, 744–7.

Vartianinen, E., Viri, L., Tossavainen, K., Niskanen, E., Macalister, A. and Puska, P. (1987). Prevention of cardiovascular risk factors in youth (the North Karelia Project 1984–1988). Paper given at the 1st European Conference in Health Education, Madrid, March 25–7.

While, A. (1985). Health visiting and health experiences of infants in three areas. Unpublished PhD thesis, University of London.

White, A., Nicolaas, G., Foster, K., Browne, F. and Carey, S. (1993). *Health Survey for England 1991*. HMSO, London.

White, J.M., Fairley, C.K., Owen, D., Mathews, R.C. and Miller, E. (1996) The effect of accelerated immunisation schedule on pertussis in England and Wales. *Communicable Diseases Report*, 6(6), R86–91.

Whitehead, M. (1988). *The Health Divide*. Pelican Books, London.

WHO (1946). *Constitution*. WHO, Geneva.

WHO (1978). *Report of the International Conference on Primary Care, Alma-Ata, USSR*. WHO, Geneva.

WHO (1984a). *Health Promotion: a Discussion Document on Concepts and Principles*. Regional Office for Europe, Copenhagen.

WHO (1984b). Report of a WHO meeting, October. Quoted in the Report of the British Cardiac Society Working Group in Coronary Disease Prevention, 1987. British Cardiac Society, London.

WHO (1985). *Targets for Health for All. Targets in Support of the European Regional Strategy for Health for All*. Regional Office for Europe, Copenhagen.

Williams, G. (1984). Health promotion – caring concern or slick salesmanship? *Journal of Medical Ethics*, 10, 191–5.

Wood, D.A., Kinmonth, P.L., Pyke, S.D.M and Thomson, S.G on behalf of the Family Heart Study Group (1994). A randomised controlled trial evaluating cardiovascular screening and intervention in general practice: principal results of the British Family Heart Study. *British Medical Journal*, 308, 313–20.

CHAPTER FIVE

PRIMARY HEALTH CARE

Margaret Edwards

- Introduction
- Primary health care – what is it?
- Who delivers primary health care?
- The importance of primary health care
- The goals of primary health care
- Preventive health care and health promotion
- Factors affecting health and individual responsibility
- Primary health care and public health
- The NHS reforms and the New Public Health
- The primary health care team
- Community health profiling and assessment of health needs
- The discipline of community health care nursing
- Challenges and issues for the next millenium
- Conclusion

The aim of this chapter is to explore the importance of primary health care and to examine how the internationally agreed goals can be achieved by the primary health care team within a reorganised NHS. Factors affecting health are explored and the contributions of primary health care professionals to the commissioning process and the 'New Public Health' are discussed. The challenges and issues, and in particular those relating to community health care nursing, are presented.

INTRODUCTION

Primary health care is an elusive and wide-ranging concept. In this chapter an emphasis has been placed on primary health care as it relates to care provision within a recently reorganised National Health Service. This is not to undervalue the international contribution to the debate on the nature and goals of primary health care. It is rather to demonstrate how these can be met within a health care system that is shifting from being acute sector led to one that is primary care led. As general practice is seen as central to the delivery of primary health care, much of the chapter is devoted to those health care professionals who are considered to be the core members of the primary health care team. Inevitably, this means that the valuable contribution of other health care professionals is understated but only for the purposes of this particular exercise. The author wishes to acknowledge the previous work of Elizabeth Raymond in this area and to point out that some of the material presented has been retained from the second edition of the book.

PRIMARY HEALTH CARE – WHAT IS IT?

Defining primary health care can be straightforward or complex depending on whether a biomedical or a broader biopsychosocial perspective is adopted. In Britain and in many Western developed countries primary health care is generally held to be synonymous with primary medical care since health has predominantly been considered a biomedical phenomenon and health care provision has centred largely around services for the sick.

Primary health care in Britain is often defined as those health services which provide the first (*primary*) point of contact for individual members of the public. It is generally thought of as non-institutional, community-based care. This is in contrast to those services (*secondary*) which involve referral to specialist practitioners usually based in or attached to hospitals. In certain countries the public can access specialist services directly, either through visiting independent specialist practitioners or attending polyclinics.

WHO DELIVERS PRIMARY HEALTH CARE?

The organisation of the NHS in the UK has, for the main, centred around a system of general practice where generalist medical practitioners provide continuous care to populations irrespective of gender, disease or organ system. Where specialist attention is required, the general practitioner refers to medical colleagues working within secondary care. Nursing staff, including health visitors, district nurses and practice nurses, have been closely associated with general practice either through a system of 'attachment' serving the same practice population or, as in the case of practice nurses, through direct employment. The Audit Commission (1992) identified a wide range of community health professionals including doctors other than GPs, nurses, midwives and paramedical staff, the majority of whom are employed by Community Trusts (see Table 5.1). Not all the staff listed by the Audit Commission will be found working in every unit.

GENERAL PRACTITIONERS

With the setting up of the National Health Service general practitioners retained the independent status they had previously enjoyed prior to 1946. Since then GPs have contracted with the Health Service, initially with the Family Practitioner Committee and more recently with the new Health Commissions, to deliver core medical services to the patients on their lists. These have been defined as 'reactive services provided to patients who are or believe themselves to be ill, including the reac-

Table 5.1: Community health professionals (excluding general practice staff)

Professions allied to medicine	Doctors and dentists	Nurses
Stoma care	Paediatricians	District health visitors
Occupational therapists	Clinical medical officers	School
Chiropodists	Geriatricians	Community midwives
Speech therapists	Psychiatrists	Community learning disabilities
Physiotherapists	Community dentists	Community psychiatric
Psychologists		Macmillan
Dietitians		Marie Curie
Audiologists		Family planning
Orthoptists		Continence adviser
Health promotion staff		Diabetic liaison
Community pharmacists		Paediatric liaison
		Discharge liaison
		Clinic
		TB
		Nurse practitioner

Source: Audit Commission (1992).

tive management of chronic diseases' (General Medical Services Committee, 1994). General practitioners receive a per capita fee for each patient and additional contracts cover other non-core services such as health promotion and the proactive management of disease.

Although the concept of the primary health care team was first advanced in the early 1920s (Ministry of Health, 1920) it was really only from the late 1960s onwards, following the Report of the Royal Commission on Medical Education (1968), that the attachment of nurses to general practices gained momentum. The Report advocated group practices and argued that GPs needed to delegate a variety of tasks to colleagues in other professions. The Report was unambiguous in its view that the GP would be the leader of any team of health care professionals involved in primary care. Nurses and health visitors were seen as becoming integral members of *medical* practice. Three sets of nurses have been closely aligned with general practitioners: health visitors, district nurses and general practice nurses.

HEALTH VISITING AND DISTRICT NURSES

Prior to 1974 health visitors and district nurses had been employed by local authorities. Both fields of practice started to develop around the middle of the nineteenth century. Health visitors are said to be the descendants of the sanitary visitors who went into the homes of the poor in various parts of the country to teach basic rules of hygiene in response to specific cholera outbreaks. The scheme introduced by the Ladies' Sanitary Reform Association of Manchester and Salford in 1862 is generally regarded as the origin of health visiting. From the beginning, these sanitary visitors were regarded by the Association as health teachers and social counsellors. By the end of the century health visitors were to be found in the employ of the Manchester Public Health Department.

Early in the twentieth century health visiting became associated with the Infant Welfare Movement and practitioners began to take on the image of 'well-baby nurses' involved with the work of the early maternity and child welfare centres. With the passing of the *National Health Service Act* in 1946 it became the duty of all local authorities to provide a health visiting service to every family

with children over the age of 5 years. Although with *The Children Act* (1948) responsibility for child protection passed to social workers, health visitors have continued to have a key role in the prevention, identification and intervention in the event of non-accidental injury to children. Infant and child welfare has remained an important part of health visiting and has tended to occupy the energies of the profession at the expense of a wider public health role.

The middle years of the nineteenth century also saw the birth of district nursing. A number of initiatives providing home nursing to the poor emerged in London at this time but a scheme started in Liverpool by William Rathbone, impressed by the care given to his dying wife by a trained nurse, is generally hailed to be the origin of district nursing. District nursing was only available free of charge to the poor and was provided by a number of voluntary associations in by and large a piecemeal fashion. In 1948 under the *National Health Service Act* (1946) district nursing services were made available to all, regardless of means, and the voluntary agencies acted as agents for local authorities who were the employers of district nurses. The *National Health Service Reorganisation Act* in 1973 saw both health visiting and district nursing brought under the jurisdiction of the NHS area health authorities. It is important to remember that attachment to general practice is a relatively new concept in the development of health visiting and district nursing and this relative newness may account for some of the difficulties that are experienced by these community nurses and general practitioners in fully understanding each other's roles within primary health care teams.

GENERAL PRACTICE NURSING

General practice nurses have a relatively shorter history than health visitors and district nurses but have by definition been closely associated with general practice, having been employed by GPs. Bowling and Stillwell (1988) noted that there were practice nurses as early as 1910. However, official recognition came considerably later (DHSS, 1975). In 1966 the General Practitioner Charter radically altered the way GPs were paid. Among these changes in GPs' terms of service, GPs were allowed a 70% reimbursement to employ a nurse to work in the practice. In the last 20 years the number of practice nurses has grown exponentially from 1500 in 1977 to over 15 183 (9500 whole-time equivalents) in England and Wales in 1993 (Atkin *et al.*, 1994; Smail, J., 1996).

The work of practice nurses has traditionally included wound care, investigative procedures, advising on minor ailments, health education and dietary advice, immunisation, counselling, family planning advice and cervical cytology. For many years practice nursing lay outside mainstream community nursing, having a different employment base. Unlike health visitors and district nurses, practice nurses had little access to appropriate training and gained no professional and academic accreditation (Smail, J., 1996). Practice nursing was not considered to be within the remit of the Cumberlege working group that examined the role and practice of community nursing within the primary health care team (DHSS, 1986a). However, at the present time, community nursing, including general practice nursing, is undergoing a number of changes both in terms of its education and manner of working. Further reference to these will be made later. These changes are occurring in response to new policy directions in relation to the health service as the importance of primary health care within the NHS is recognised.

Key Points

- In the UK, primary health care has been synonymous with primary medical care.
- Primary health care has centred around general practice.
- Health visitors, district nurses and general practice nurses have been most closely associated with general practice.

THE IMPORTANCE OF PRIMARY HEALTH CARE

Studies in the USA and across a number of European countries (Starfield, 1992, 1994) have shown a consistent relationship between the availability of primary care physicians and health levels as assessed by **age-adjusted and standardised overall mortality**, mortality associated with cancer and heart disease, neonatal mortality and life expectancy – even after controlling for the effect of urban rural differences, poverty rates, education and lifestyle, etc. Findings from these studies also suggest that countries where health systems are more oriented towards primary care achieve better health levels, higher satisfaction with health services among their populations and lower costs of services.

With such evidence available it becomes clearer why health care policy in the UK has increasingly focused on primary care as the heart of the health care system within the NHS. A primary care-led NHS centred around general medical practice has been one policy objective (Dorrell, 1996).

The 1991–92 National Morbidity Study found that in Great Britain 78% of the population consulted their GP at least once annually (McCormack *et al.*, 1995). General practice would therefore seem to be a logical fulcrum around which to base primary health care services when first line medical and paramedical care is required. Policy initiatives from the Department of Health (Dorrell, 1996) have tended to view primary health care as care delivered or coordinated by general medical practitioners. This view does, however, pose problems when the internationally agreed goals of primary health care are examined. In 1978, the World Health Organization (WHO), in the Declaration of Alma-Ata, arrived at a definition of primary health care that extended beyond a purely biomedical model.

THE DECLARATION OF ALMA-ATA: AN INTERNATIONAL VIEW OF PRIMARY HEALTH CARE

The Declaration of Alma-Ata takes its name from an international conference held under the auspices of the World Health Organization in the town of the same name in the Soviet Republic of Kazakhstan. Prior to the main conference, the WHO had sponsored a number of national and regional meetings. The main conference was attended by governmental delegations from no fewer than 134 member states together with representatives from 67 United Nations organisations. The immediate outcome of the conference was a declaration setting out, in ten numbered paragraphs, the key concepts of a universal health care system based on primary health care (Smail, S.A., 1996).

The Declaration of Alma-Ata provided a clear statement describing primary care as essential health care which forms the central function and main focus of a country's health system. The Declaration reiterated that primary health care is the first level of contact for individuals, families and the community with the national health system, in the sense that primary health care operates as close as possible to where people live and work. It is further described as the first element of a continuing health care process. The Alma-Ata Declaration is echoed in a UK government discussion document (DHSS 1986b) which described primary health care services as the front line of the health service, as including community health services, and as dealing with over nine-tenths of the contacts the public have with the health service.

The WHO definition of primary health care as 'first contact, continuous, comprehensive and co-ordinated care provided to individuals and populations undifferentiated by age, gender, disease or organ system' is held to be compatible with the current pattern of provision of primary health care services in the UK (Smail, S.A., 1996). Yet even those authors writing from a medical perspective acknowledge that the concept is broader than the customary usage of the term in the UK. The provision of primary medical services forms only one part of an overarching definition of primary health care that has a biopsychosocial basis rather than a purely medical one (see Box 5.1).

and control of locally endemic diseases and injuries; and provision of essential drugs;

4 involves, in addition to the health sector, all related sectors and aspects of national and community development in particular agriculture, animal husbandry, food industry, education, housing, public works, communications, and other sectors; and demands the coordinated efforts of all those sectors;

5 requires and promotes maximum community and individual self-reliance and participation in the planning, organisation, operation, and control of primary health care, making fullest use of local, national and other available resources; and to this end develops through appropriate education the ability of communities to participate;

6 should be sustained by integrated, functional and mutually supportive referral systems, leading to the progressive improvement of comprehensive health care for all, and giving priority to those most in need;

7 relies, at local and referral level, on health workers, including physicians, nurses, midwives, auxiliaries, and community workers as applicable, as well as traditional practitioners as needed, suitably trained socially and technically to work as a health team and to respond to the expressed health needs of the community.

Source: WHO, 1978, extract from the Declaration of Alma-Ata

Box 5.1: Article VII

Primary health care:

1 reflects and evolves from the economic conditions and socio-cultural and political characteristics of the country and its communities and is based on the application of the relevant results of social, biomedical and health-service research and public-health experience;

2 addresses the main health problems in the community, providing promotive, preventive, curative, and rehabilitative services accordingly;

3 includes at least: education concerning prevailing health problems and the methods of preventing and controlling them; promotion of food supply and proper nutrition; an adequate supply of safe water and basic sanitation; maternal and child health care, including family planning; immunisation against the major infectious diseases; prevention

THE GOALS OF PRIMARY HEALTH CARE

The wider overarching remit of primary health care is evident in the goals set by the WHO and embodied in the Alma-Ata declaration. These were stated to be:

- Promotion of health
- Prevention of disease and ill health
- Cure and rehabilitation.

The WHO (1978) outlined the main social target for government as:

'the attainment by all citizens of the world by the year 2000 of a level of health that will permit them to lead a socially and economically productive life. Primary health care is the key to attaining this target. . . .'

(WHO, 1978, Article V, page 3)

In order to achieve the goals outlined at Alma-Ata, primary health care was held to encompass a range of concerns and services. The Declaration included environmental issues such as the provision of adequate water supply and sanitation, prevention and control of locally endemic diseases, and the provision of an adequate food supply. Personal health services listed include maternal and child health care, family planning services, immunisation programmes, a pharmaceutical service, and appropriate treatment of common diseases and injuries. In the Declaration of Alma-Ata, public health services were seen to be as important in meeting the goals of primary health care as are the personal, patient encounter-based services provided by general practitioners, community nurses, pharmacists, dentists, therapists, etc. Until recently, public health measures have not been seen to be part of the work of general practice-based primary health care workers other than health visitors whose origins lie in the nineteenth century public health movements (Cowley, 1996).

Arguably, those goals oriented towards prevention of disease and ill health, cure and rehabilitation have traditionally been accommodated within the primary medical care model and encompass services provided by general practitioners, community nurses and those professions allied to medicine. It is, however, in the area of health promotion that difficulties arise for a system of care that has a predominantly biomedical focus. This is because health is an elusive concept with both objective and subjective dimensions and has to be considered alongside the notion of well-being. As the WHO (1978) recognised, health involves more than just the absence of disease. It is possible to experience well-being in the midst of overwhelming disease and disability (Lindsey, 1996). Conversely, the absence of disease does not guarantee a feeling of well-being. Environmental and social factors contribute as much if not more to well-being than a state of physiological equilibrium alone. Promoting health therefore involves more than preventing ill health though this is clearly an important part of the larger endeavour. The concepts of health promotion and preventive health need to be explored in order to understand how the one fits with the other and how these

internationally agreed goals of primary health care can be achieved by primary health care services.

Key Points

- Highly developed primary care services are associated with increased levels of health and satisfaction with care delivery.
- A large percentage of the population visit their GP at least once a year.
- The WHO definition of primary health care has a biopsychosocial basis rather than a biomedical one.
- Health has to be considered alongside well-being.
- Social and environmental factors contribute to health and well-being.

PREVENTIVE HEALTH CARE AND HEALTH PROMOTION

Preventive health care is often described as operating at three levels, as first outlined by Caplan (1969). According to Caplan, *primary prevention* means the processes involved in reducing the risk that people fall ill. An example of primary prevention is the immunisation programme for children under 5 years. *Secondary prevention* is described as the activities involved in reducing the duration of established cases of a disorder, and thereby reducing the prevalence of the disorder. The emphasis in secondary prevention is on early diagnosis and effective treatment. Screening programmes such as regular child developmental assessments and cervical screening are examples of secondary prevention. In order for a screening programme to be justified, however, the tests used need to be effective in early detection and acceptable to those being tested, and they need to be sensitive and specific enough to avoid **false positives**. Furthermore, there needs to be effective and acceptable treatment available for the conditions detected through the tests. Concern has been expressed, particularly by GPs, about the ethical dimensions of seeking to uncover new cases when resources are not available to treat adequately those who have already been identified as having a particular condition (Mant, 1994).

Caplan describes his third level, *tertiary prevention*, as including rehabilitation services which aim to return sick people as soon as possible to maximum effectiveness. Even where an individual may be suffering from a condition which cannot be cured, it is often possible to reduce the impact of the condition, and minimise or even eliminate side-effects.

General practice and community-based health services have over time operated at each of Caplan's levels of preventive care. Much of the work of health visitors and practice nurses has involved engaging in primary and secondary preventive care whilst district nurses and general practitioners and therapists have concerned themselves with the diagnosis, treatment, care and rehabilitation of ill people. In this way it could be said that the promotion of health has been a long-standing activity within primary health care.

A closer examination of the activities of primary care health professionals would, however, serve to illustrate that for many years since the inception of the NHS promoting health has been conceived in a much narrower way than was outlined in the Declaration of Alma-Ata. Health promotion and health education are often used interchangeably, particularly in general practice. In line with WHO goals, promoting health has increasingly been seen as part of the role of health care workers, including nurses and doctors; yet many of the factors affecting health are seen to lie outside the traditional remit and immediate control of community health care professionals (Mant, 1994).

In the late 1980s, health and preventive health care measures began to gain an increasingly high profile in the UK. The GP contract (Health Departments of Great Britain, 1989), introduced in April 1990, required GP practices to place greater emphasis on health promotion and illness prevention by offering 'health promotion consultations to all patients aged 16–74 years, encouraging women patients to accept screening for breast and cervical cancer and offering an annual home visit to all patients over 75 years, with an opportunity for a health assessment'. By 1993 amendments were made to the contract and the government had introduced a banding system for health promotion in response to criticisms that health promotion clinics could be set up simply to obtain reimbursement rather than because of perceived and identified need (Smail, J., 1996). The banding system represented a more strategic approach to health promotion and payment since practices were required to plan and implement a programme of care for the practice population. Approval for health promotion programmes had to be sought from the Family Services Health Authority (FHSA) (now joined with the District Health Authority to form Health Commissions) and payment only made if programmes were carried out as approved, and every year the practice has to submit an annual report and reapply for health promotion payments to the FHSA.

The GP contract was greeted with much scepticism by general practitioners (Stott *et al.*, 1994) who delegated much of the work required under its terms to a growing army of practice nurses. General practitioners were unhappy that an undue emphasis had been placed on screening and health checks though there was little or no evidence for the effectiveness of many of these activities (Mant and Fowler, 1990). General practitioner objections tended to centre around the fact that health promotion targets and contracts were and have continued to be concerned with the extent of risk identification without consideration of the quality and cost-effectiveness of risk management. Indeed, evidence from the first year of OXCHECK trial (ICRF OXCHECK Study Group, 1994), which studied the effectiveness of health checks conducted by nurses in primary care, led the researchers to believe that the 'real work is not in screening but in providing and sustaining follow-up'.

Health promotion in general practice has been very much about providing health education and risk identification. Health education concerns itself with informing the consumer about prevailing health problems and the methods of preventing and controlling them. In this way health can be said to be promoted. However, as has been pointed out in Chapter 4, health education is only one part of the wider activity of promoting health. This involves not only providing the individual with the information to adjust his or her behaviour but also with the provision of a social, political and economic context in which the person is enabled to change his or her lifestyle. Providing advice and information alone presumes that an individual is free to choose how and where to live.

Key Points

■ The three levels of preventive health care are explored.

- The 1990 GP contract requires practices to be involved with health promotion and screening.
- Health promotion in general practice is often equated with health education and risk identification.
- GPs have been unhappy that there is little evidence for the benefits of some screening procedures.
- Uncovering new cases is not enough: resources for sustained follow-up are required.
- People cannot make health choices if the material circumstances of their lives do not allow them this freedom.

FACTORS AFFECTING HEALTH AND INDIVIDUAL RESPONSIBILITY

For many years now there has been clear evidence (Black, 1980; Whitehead, 1987; Townsend *et al.*, 1988; Wilkinson, 1992) that factors such as poverty, ethnicity and geographical location are important influences on health. None the less, much of health policy in the last 18 years has concerned itself with stressing the duty of individuals to take responsiblity for their own health (Department of Health, 1990) whilst encouraging health care professionals to expend their energies in achieving behaviour and attitude change (Davies, 1996). Attention has been focused on conditions which have variously been described as 'self-induced' or 'diseases of lifestyle'. These descriptions have been applied to conditions such as ischaemic heart disease, lung cancer, alcoholism and addiction, diet-related conditions, and, more recently, AIDS.

Government strategy of the late 1980s and early 1990s demonstrated the belief that behaviour change was the route to improving health. This individualised approach has been said to have sat well with the prevailing ideological disposition to minimise state involvement and maximise personal responsibility in all areas of social welfare (Davies, 1996). This approach to health involves a belief that the role of government, operating through its health care agencies, is to provide information about healthy living in the form of advice. The decision then falls to the individual to make healthy choices. Such a view ignores the fact that the health behaviour of an individual reflects their cultural values and socio-economic

environment (Stott *et al.*, 1994). An analysis of data from 32 countries concerning the distribution of coronary heart disease risk factors including obesity, hypertension and blood cholesterol has revealed that where there is a **high population mean** there is also a long 'high risk' tail (Rose, 1992). Essentially, this means that identified risk factors in a population reflect the nature of that society rather than the behaviour of a few disobedient individuals.

POVERTY, ETHNICITY AND HEALTH

Barker (1992) has described how the poor health record of low income groups is experienced from conception to the grave. A child born into a family where the father is an unskilled worker has twice the risk of being stillborn or of dying in infancy compared with one born into a professional family (Whitehead, 1987). For both men and women the major causes of death are more common for those in social classes 4 and 5. People from ethnic minorities, especially those born in the New Commonwealth, have poorer health and higher mortality rates than the indigenous population (Department of Health, 1995).

In 1980 Douglas Black identified what has become known as the health divide (Black, 1980). Evidence for a widening health divide in the 1990s is to be found even in government publications (Department of Health, 1995).

When the strategic document *The Health of the Nation* (Department of Health, 1992) was published in England outlining the government targets for improving health in key areas (Box 5.2), the word poverty was noted to be conspicuous by its absence (Davies, 1996). Yet poverty has been increasing over the last two decades. The Child Poverty Action Group (1996) has drawn attention to the fact that one in four people (including children) were living in poverty in 1992/93 compared with under one in ten in 1979. Davies (1996) points out that, although unemployed people are at greatest risk of poverty, those in work are not immune. According to Davies (1996) the numbers of those in employment and living in poverty have tripled between 1979 and 1992/93.

Causal relationships are always difficult to establish. Not everyone in similar circumstances succumbs to illness and premature death and the complex relationship between environment,

Box 5.2: Health of the Nation priority areas

- Coronary heart disease
- Cancers
- Mental illness
- HIV/AIDS and sexual health
- Accidents

Key Points

- There is a relationship between poverty, ethnicity and poor health.
- Government policy has focused on behaviour change.
- The strategic document *The Health of the Nation* does not mention poverty.
- Evidence does not suggest that those who are poor are irresponsible.

genetics and lifestyle has not yet been unravelled (Barker, 1992). None the less two phenomena seem to run in tandem. First, there is an ever widening gap between those who are rich and those who are poor (Joseph Rowntree Foundation, 1995) with increased poverty and inequalities in housing, education and health care. Second, the health of those who are poor is measurably inferior to that of those who are better off (Wilkinson, 1992). Explanations from the government of the time for these two phenomena have centred around the inability of those who are poor to manage their affairs in a responsible way and beliefs that with appropriate advice in such areas as choosing a healthy diet health could be improved.

Regarding diet, such beliefs are predicated on the notion that healthy eating is in fact cheaper than the high fat alternatives that prevail in lower socio-economic groups. Research, however, has contradicted the view that it is mismanagement or ignorance that prevents the poor from eating healthily (Charles and Kerr, 1988; Davies, 1996) (see Chapter 4). Paucity of income rather than information has emerged as the main factor preventing the consumption of a healthy diet.

Health promotion interventions aimed solely at providing information on healthy diets are at best an irrelevance and at worst downright insulting to those who do not have the means to alter their food choices. The question then remains as to how health is to be promoted by primary health care professionals when economic and fiscal policy determines the resources available to individuals and governs the choices they make about their health behaviour. The efforts of society as a whole are required if the health of entire populations, not just that of those who are well off, is to be promoted. The issue is whether health care professionals can legitimately move beyond dealing solely with the biomedical problems of individuals and establish a role in contributing to the efforts of society as a whole in improving the public health.

PRIMARY HEALTH CARE AND PUBLIC HEALTH

Many of the improvements in health over the last 150 years are known to be due more to the instigation of wide-ranging public health measures than to advances in medical and nursing care. Closure of the Broad Street pump in 1854, once it was identified as the cause of a cholera epidemic, was more effective in stemming the course of the disease than the efforts of the hard pressed medical officers of the time. Improvements in living conditions have had a greater effect on reductions in infectious disease than the advent of antibiotics. Yet, for patients, both the individual attention provided by health care workers and the public health measures are necessary.

It is increasingly recognised that the well-being of individuals is intimately linked to the health status of the whole community in which they live (Cowley, 1996). Distinctions between traditional individual encounter-based activities of doctors, nurses and others and broader public health measures appear increasingly artifical in the light of the earlier discussions on the influences on health. Acheson in 1988 defined public health as 'the science and art of preventing disease, prolonging life and promoting health through the organised efforts of society'. Using this definition it could be argued that all primary health care activity can be subsumed under the umbrella of public health.

Health professionals working at the individual level have long recognised that the social context has contributed to the ill health of their patients but have not identified a role for themselves in shaping the policies that impinge on health. The reasons for this are several. The education and training of health care practitioners has not until recently prepared them to adopt a public health perspective nor to recognise that their work at the level of the individual is as much part of public health as the laying of drains. The structure and organisation of the National Health Service prior to 1990 did not allow for the needs of entire populations to be considered when planning and operating services. Services provided tended to reflect sectional medical interests and historically determined service delivery rather than being geared to what was required by the population as a whole.

Key Points

- The major improvements in health this century have been due to public health measures.
- The organisation of the NHS has not previously fostered a public health approach to care.

THE NHS REFORMS AND THE NEW PUBLIC HEALTH

In 1990 the NHS underwent a reorganisation that gave prominence to a needs-based approach to health care purchasing (*National Health Service and Community Care Act*, 1990). In one of the government White Papers, *Working for Patients* (Department of Health, 1989), that preceded the *National Health Service and Community Care Act* (1990) the notion of identifying and separating purchasers and providers of health care was promulgated.

The aim of the government was to set up an internal market within the NHS where traditional provider services such as hospitals and community units would need to tailor their services to meet the requirements of designated purchasers. District health authorities and family health services authorities (FHSAs) became purchasers. In 1996 the two authorities merged to form new commissioning agencies.

Commissioning and purchasing are closely related but are not synonymous. According to Goodwin (1995), commissioning is the pro-active approach to developing services in partnership with others concerned, including users. Purchasing describes the technical process of agreeing contracts for services (Goodwin, 1995). Confusion arises because commissioning and purchasing functions are frequently vested in the same authority.

In the past, the range of services on offer in a health district would have been historically determined rather than related to whether the local population actually required the services in the form that they had always been traditionally delivered. For example, across the country district, nursing services would have looked broadly similar irrespective of differences in the population profile and the community's need for district nursing. In terms of acute care, services revolved around the number of historically determined consultant beds for particular specialities. In a health district, monies for diabetic care would have been directed towards maintaining a certain number of hospital beds in spite of the fact that inpatient care may not have been required for the vast majority of diabetic patients, who were then denied more appropriate interventions.

Under the internal market system, existing services would not necessarily continue to be purchased and new services could be commissioned and then purchased from either existing providers or from other groups including social services, private agencies or voluntary organisations. For example, a need for respite care might be identified and the purchasing health authorities would ask for a new service to be set up. The purchasers might ask any of the above-mentioned agencies to set up a service. The commissioned service would then be purchased by the Health Authority. The commissioning of services required carrying out an assessment of population need. The responsibility for identifying these population needs was given to Directors of Public Health. As each of the new commissioning/purchasing authorities came into being they were all required to appoint someone to the role of Director of Public Health.

Initially, the contribution of nursing to public health and the commissioning and purchasing of health care was overlooked (Cowley, 1996). However, in 1993 the Chief Nursing Officer for England asked the Standing Nursing and Midwifery Committee (SNMAC, 1995) to advise and make recommendations to Ministers on developing the role and contribution of nurses, midwives and health visitors to public health. According to SNMAC, public health in nursing, midwifery and health visiting practice was about:

'commissioning health services and providing professional care through organised collaboration in the NHS and society, to protect and promote health and well-being, prolong life and prevent ill health in local communities, groups and populations.'

(SNMAC, 1995, page 5)

The role for nurses midwives and health visitors identified by SNMAC extended beyond the traditional narrower interpretations of public health activity where concerns might have centred, for example, around the prevention and management of infectious diseases. This wider view of public health is sometimes referred to as the 'New Public Health'. The New Public Health is said to have its origins in the report prepared for the Canadian government about the health of the nationals of that country (Lalonde, 1974 in Cowley, 1996). The report demonstrated how all causes of death and disease could be attributed to four discrete and distinct elements:

- Inadequacies in current health care provision
- Lifestyle or behavioural factors
- Issues related to the environment, and
- Biophysical characteristics.

The New Public Health concerns itself with environmental change, personal preventive measures and therapeutic interventions. The concerns of the New Public Health can be seen to mirror closely those of primary health care as defined in the Declaration of Alma-Ata. The reorganisation of the Health Service that occurred in 1990, with its orientation towards needs-based health care purchasing and public health, can be seen as part of the wider movement to shift the emphasis in health care from illness to prevention. In its concern to bring the purchasing decisions nearer to the patient and away from acute care that had previously consumed most of the resources of the NHS, the government gave those general practitioners who wanted it an important role in the purchase of health care.

GENERAL PRACTITIONERS AND FUNDHOLDING

Within the new system general practitioners were given the possibility of being both purchasers and commissioners of care as well as providers of health care under a scheme known as GP fundholding. As general practitioners were perceived to be the lynchpin of a new primary care-led NHS

it seemed logical to transfer much of the purchasing power to those who were thought to be in the best position to identify the needs of the local population through the frequency of their contact.

Within the system of fundholding, GPs were to be given the means to purchase community nursing services and even directly to employ district nurses and health visitors. Many community nurses expressed concern that direct employment by general practitioners would mean a much narrower biomedical focus for their work and actually run counter to meeting the goals of primary health care. The anomaly in the new system, clearer to many away from the policy-making centre, including community nurses, was that general practitioners had little experience or appetite for the public health role and had historically concentrated their energies on providing secondary preventive care to individuals within the narrow confines of the practice population.

Tudor Hart (1988) proposed that there should be a new kind of doctor who would develop a role in caring for the health of the community and, indeed, medical school curricula are increasingly reflecting the need to adopt a public health perspective. Smail, S.A. (1996), however, has described the conflicts in day-to-day practice between adopting a community perspective of care on the one hand and responding to the expressed needs of individual patients on the other. GP fundholding, encouraging as it did a narrow focus on the needs of particular practices, could be said to have been a stumbling block to a population needs-based approach to primary health care. Thus, in spite of the fact that by 1997 GP fundholding had become the predominant model for general practice, the new government outlined plans to replace GP fundholding with GP commissioning where GPs and nurses will take the lead in planning local health services.

Recognition of the potential of nurses to make a significant contribution to commissioning and the New Public Health had come earlier with the previous government. Three White Papers that preceded the *National Health Service (Primary Care) Act* (1997) – *A Service with Ambitions* (Department of Health, 1996a) *Choice and Opportunity: Primary Care – the Future* (Department of Health, 1996b) and *Primary Care – Delivering the Future* (Department of Health, 1996c) – portrayed a willingness, if not always explicit, to recognise the potential role of nurses in primary care. The NHS (Primary

Care) Act provides the opportunity for pilot schemes to be set up for differing ways of delivering medical services. For example, a health authority might be able to employ salaried general practitioners. Possibilities for new approaches to teamwork are thus provided. The emphasis, however, has remained on consolidating the leading role of GPs in primary health care.

Although GPs have increasingly recognised the need to take a more population-based approach to prevention, their requirement to provide medical services to individuals within the practice make it clear that a team-based approach will be necessary to collect the information required to inform purchasing decisions that bring benefits in health for the majority.

Key Points

- The NHS reforms have introduced the process of commissioning for services based on local population need.
- Nurses have an important role to play in the area of commissioning/purchasing and in contributing to the New Public Health.
- Under the system of fundholding, general practitioners have been given the means to commission and purchase health care.
- A team-based approach is required for a comprehensive assessment of local need.
- Fundholding is likely to be replaced by locality purchasing and commissioning.

THE PRIMARY HEALTH CARE TEAM

Nursing in Primary Health Care: New World, New Opportunities (National Health Service Management Executive, 1993) emphasised the importance of teamwork in primary health care. Teams in primary health care have existed for many years though many would argue that the concept has been more easily talked about and aspired to than achieved (Gillow, 1996). Surveys of primary health care teams have identified in varying degrees often low levels of collaboration between GPs and community nurses, and poor teamwork (Primary Care Forum, 1991; Audit Commission 1992). There has been confusion surrounding the membership of primary health care teams

(Southampton Primary Care Development Team, 1993). The Harding Committee (DHSS, 1981) produced a definition of the make-up of the primary health care team as an independent group consisting of GPs, district nurses, midwives, secretaries and receptionists.

This definition does not include the practice manager and general practice nurse who have become an integral part of the primary health care team since the Harding Committee met. The definition also does not include those social workers or community psychiatric nurses who have contact with patients within specific practices. Gillow (1996) has suggested a model for the primary health care team that includes both core and extended membership. Core membership involves a concentration on the defined practice population. Those with core membership are likely to be based within the general practice or close by. According to Gillow, the extended team would comprise those professionals or indeed voluntary agencies who are more likely to be working on a geographical or locality basis and providing a service to several practices.

Many reasons for ineffective teamwork within primary health care have been suggested. These include: separate lines of control, different payment systems, professional barriers and perceived inequalities in status (Audit Commission, 1992). Poulton and West (1993) found evidence of differing priorities from team members. Anecdotally and perhaps evidenced by the concern expressed regarding direct employment, health visitors and general practitioners often have the greatest difficulty with each other within the team. GPs tend to have a better understanding of the work of district nurses whose curative and rehabilitative goals more closely resemble those of the doctors themselves. Firth-Cozens (1992) identified the possession of a common goal as one of the key characteristics of a successful team. If supporting the work of the general practitioner in his or her *medical* work and meeting health promotion targets through health education alone is the aim of team, then conflict is inevitable for those members who have a broader perspective on health and health promotion.

A COMMON GOAL FOR GENERAL PRACTICE

The reorganisation of the NHS has provided a common goal for the primary health care team whether core or extended. Commissioning for health provides an opportunity within general practice for each member of the team to contribute his or her knowledge of the needs of the individuals and groups that are the primary focus of their work. Successful commissioning depends on having a comprehensive picture of need so that the most appropriate type of care can be purchased. For example, a community profile might reveal that there is a high number of emergency out-of-hours GP call-outs and visits to Accident and Emergency departments by parents of young children for minor and self-limiting conditions. An out-of-hours advice centre and minor injuries clinic staffed by members of the primary health care team could be commissioned and purchased to provide a more appropriate and cost-effective service.

The biggest problem encountered by the newly formed purchasing health authorities has been the dearth of information on which to base their decisions. The compilation of general practice profiles is the starting point for the collection of information that will give a locality-wide picture of need.

Key Points

- Primary health care teams can have core and extended membership.
- Teams sometimes have different goals.
- The process of commissioning/purchasing can provide a common goal for the primary health care team.

COMMUNITY HEALTH PROFILING AND ASSESSMENT OF HEALTH NEEDS

A wide range of information exists which can help to identify priority health needs and issues locally (Figure 5.1) although in practice there are many difficulties to overcome if it is all to be put together in a meaningful way to form the health profile of a local community. Health and vital statistics, which have traditionally been regarded as key sources of information, suffer from several limitations. They are inevitably out of date by the time they have been collected and published, so that they therefore do not immediately reflect changes which may be taking place. To date, computerised information systems, intended to speed up the processing of information, often seem to increase the delay, as systems used across the NHS vary and do not 'speak' easily to each other, if at all. Also, in many instances, health statistics relate to populations which contain a number of very different groups, and the larger the population to which they relate, the less likely they are to help clarify local issues.

Caseload analyses comprise one of the most up-to-date sources of information available to primary health care planners. By putting information about caseloads into categories with common characteristics and problems, community nurses may be amongst the first to recognise and identify newly emerging health issues. In addition to information already available from GPs concerning the health problems about which patients consult them, community nurses are likely to be able to shed some light on the dimensions of what has been called the 'symptom iceberg' (Hannay, 1979): in other words, those symptoms which people experience but decide not to report to their GPs, and which reflect unrecognised and unmet health needs.

In recognition of the relationship between social and environmental factors and health, various deprivation indices have been devised, to identify whole populations which are in particular need and vulnerable to poor health. One of these, the Jarman index (Jarman, 1983) was based on caseload information from GPs, who identified various categories of patients who required their services more than the average. Indices such as these can be problematic as they can be skewed by factors including a disproportionate number of elderly people in a population.

Further information about the health of the population can be obtained by using an assessment of the total or global health of the individuals who make up the population. Various global health status indices have been developed and have been described in detail in Bowling (1997).

Compiling a practice profile needs to be seen as everybody's responsibility as each member of

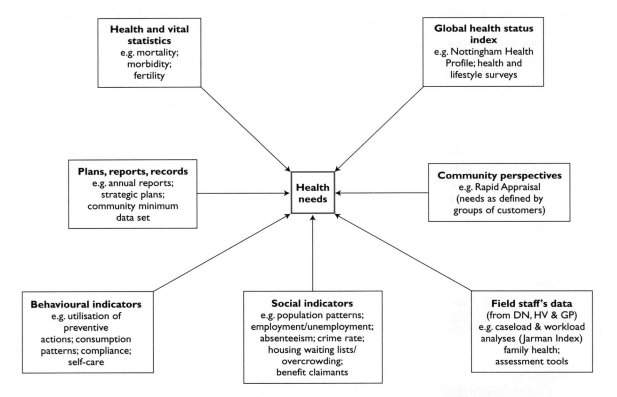

Figure 5.1: Assessment of health needs of local populations – sources of information

the team will have different data to contribute. The district nurse will be acutely aware of the needs and views of housebound elderly people and their carers. Health visitors will have first hand experience of the effects of poor housing on the morale and physical health of their clients. Primary care practitioners are in a position to seek directly the views of the public and to attempt to influence commissioners to reflect expressed needs. Historically, however, it has only been health visitors who have engaged in the active search for health needs and who have undertaken caseload profiles. The new discipline of community health care nursing established as part of the UKCCs Post-registration and Education for Practice (PREP) regulations requires all community nurses to adopt a public health perspective (UKCC, 1994).

Key Points

- There are many sources of information available that contribute to assessment of need.

- Each member of the team can contribute to compiling a practice profile.
- Under PREP all community health care nurses are required to adopt a public health perspective.

THE DISCIPLINE OF COMMUNITY HEALTH CARE NURSING

In 1994 the UKCC detailed the educational preparation required for qualification in community health care nursing. Eight areas of nursing were identified as community specialisms: public health nursing – health visiting; nursing in the home – district nursing; general practice nursing; community mental health nursing; community learning disability nursing; school nursing; community children's nursing; and occupational health nursing. To qualify for one of these specialisms, first level nurses are required to undertake an additional course of study at final year degree level and to achieve discipline specific learning outcomes in both specialist clinical practice and care and programme management. Each of the community specialisms is expected to contribute to strategies that improve the public health, although there is a difference in emphasis for the individual specialities depending on whether the main focus rests with primary, secondary or tertiary prevention.

In creating the discipline of community health care nursing and recognising the specialist nature of community nursing practice the UKCC was acknowledging the complexities of the practice situation for these nurses and was anticipating many of the challenges to be faced by the practice team in meeting the goals of primary health care.

Key Point

■ Under PREP the new discipline of community health care nursing was created.

CHALLENGES AND ISSUES FOR THE NEXT MILLENNIUM

In 1978 the WHO laid down its challenge to world governments for the year 2000. Recent health care policy in the UK has clearly been guided by the WHO goals. The reorganisation of the NHS to reflect the importance of primary health care and the strategic approach to meeting health targets outlined in documents such as *The Health of the Nation* have been on line with international approaches to health care.

There is recognition across both nursing and health visiting and general practice of the need for an intersectoral approach to the promotion of health given the multidimensional nature of health. Health improvement cannot be brought about by the health care sector or any other working alone (Harmond and Crown, 1996). The term **healthy alliances** has been coined to describe projects and initiatives where there is collaborative action between statutory agencies including education, housing, health and social care as well as commerce, industry, voluntary agencies and the community itself. Ashton (1992) has described a number of European and worldwide strategies that describe this approach.

In order to engage in healthy alliances, primary care professionals have to combine an individual-based approach with a public health approach. The individual contact provides primary care professionals with the 'street level' data that are relevant to any wider assessment of need. Where a number of general practices pool the knowledge collected by all the members of the primary health care team a more in-depth picture of local need will be likely to emerge. Community nurses and health visitors in particular have the potential to provide a bridge between primary medical care and public health. The public health role of health visitors and their longer track record in searching for and profiling health needs suggests that they could be the coordinators of commissioning activity within general practice given the calls on GPs to concentrate their efforts on secondary and tertiary prevention.

Although the aim of health for all by the beginning of the new millennium is unlikely to be achieved, the new century will begin with the structures in place to allow for the goals of primary health care to be met. However, having the structures in place does not guarantee that the shift in thinking will occur rapidly. The predominance of the biomedical model of health care has been immense and the shift in emphasis from an acute care driven health service to one in which health care workers perceive health promotion in all its aspects to be their main concern may take many years to occur. Health promotion is now an integral part of pre-registration nurse education. However, the important parts of nursing care are still perceived, not least by students themselves, to be the technical medical tasks, many of which are likely to become redundant as medical science advances. There is also increasing pressure from doctors for nurses to take on many more technical tasks to relieve the strain on medical practitioners (Jarman, 1997).

When the NHS was set up it was thought that the need for acute care would diminish. Demographic pressures, particularly in the form of an ageing population, together with the ability to treat life-threatening diseases more effectively and consumer demand for medical intervention, militate against reductions in the funding of acute care. Threats of hospital closures are met with cries of dismay by the public. Those in need in acute care cannot be abandoned. Yet in their concern to curtail rising health care costs world governments have looked to transferring acute care to primary care locations with the assumption that this is a cheaper option.

Shifting the balance of care without substantially transferring the resources creates a particular tension for primary health care professionals and particularly lay carers whose contribution has traditionally been discounted in the calculations that makes community care a seemingly cheaper option for policy makers. None the less, much acute care is now possible in the home thanks to improvements in housing conditions and the fact that much of the technology previously associated with hospitals has become more portable. Patients often express a preference for home care (Marks, 1991). For many at risk from nosocomial infections hospitals have become dangerous places (see Chapter 16).

Delivering acute care in the home represents a considerable challenge to district nurses and specialist nurses working in the community. Without immediate access to medical advice community nurses have to rely keenly on their knowledge base and need finely honed decision-making skills to decide whether or not medical assistance is required. For many years district nurses and health visitors have provided a gate-keeping service to general practice by discriminating between self-limiting and serious illness and advising accordingly. It is difficult to assess whether general practitioners appreciate the extent to which they have been saved consultations and emergency call-outs by the diagnostic skills of community nurses.

More than any other group of nurses, district nurses are required to be explicit about what constitutes nursing care. The *National Health Service and Community Care Act* (1990) gave social services the lead role in assessing the care needs of elderly and disabled people. District nurses have to be able to determine whether a particular care need represents a deficit in social functioning or whether it is health related. The community care legislation was framed around the premise that health and social care were distinct entities. District nurses have to tread a difficult path around this artificial dichotomy made more contentious by the fact that health care is free but care designated as social in nature may need to be paid for. Community nurses confront the realities of rationing daily. Highly developed analytical skills are required so that equitable and ethical decisions are made.

Recognition of the skills of health visitors and district nurses has been forthcoming in the form of nurse prescribing which is finally likely to be implemented this year. To date nurses at selected pilot sites have been able to prescribe from a nursing formulary. Evaluation of nurse prescribing pilot sites has overall been positive for those involved, including the nurses, general practitioners, practice administrators and patients (Luker *et al.*, 1997). One of the main findings from the evaluation is that the nursing staff involved have been made acutely aware of their responsibilities and accountability when prescribing.

THE SCOPE OF PROFESSIONAL PRACTICE

Expansions in the scope of nursing practice have brought into sharp relief issues of responsibility and accountability. In 1960 Isabel Menzies described how nurses tended to delegate responsibility upwards, looking to medical practitioners and others high up in the hierarchy to take responsibility for nursing actions. Rules were rigorously adhered to. Given the reliance on custom and practice and the whims of ward sisters for nursing care it was perhaps an appropriate form of action to refer to those who had received a more substantial education than that provided by the traditional nurse training. The complexity of health care delivery today makes such a *modus operandi* untenable, particularly where such care is delivered at a distance from medical advice. Changes in nursing education have reflected the need for a higher level of education to underpin sound decision-making skills.

Reflecting the need for nurses to work more autonomously and to extend the traditional boundaries of their role, the UKCC, as the statutory body regulating nursing, midwifery and health visiting in the UK, has established principles that must apply to adjustments to the scope of nursing practice. These principles are laid out in the document *The Scope of Professional Practice* (UKCC, 1992). In this document the onus for ensuring competence is placed primarily with the practitioner who is not restricted professionally in the range of care that he/she may deliver but who is required to ensure that he/she has the necessary expertise and knowledge to deliver that care. The practitioner is also required to recognise the limits of his/her competence, his/her own personal accountability as well as responsibilities for appropriate delegation. Enlargement or adjustment of the scope of personal professional practice 'has to be achieved without compromising or fragmenting existing aspects of professional practice and care ...' (UKCC, 1992, page 6). Adherence to these principles allows nurses to develop innovative approaches to care that are increasingly required across all care sectors. In the community, nurse practitioners have extended the traditional role of general practice nurses whilst district nurses have been able to undertake procedures that have relieved patients of the need for inconvenient and often uncomfortable visits to hospital.

Key Points

- The current framework for the delivery of primary health care presents many challenges and opportunities for practitioners.
- Nurses are likely to take on increasing responsibilities in areas of work previously thought to be the domain of doctors.
- Adherence to the principles for adjusting the scope of professional practice allows nurses to be more flexible in meeting patient need.

CONCLUSION

The reorganisation of the NHS with its emphasis on primary health care can be seen to be in line with the WHO goals. Since 1978, when the Declaration of Alma-Ata was made, the culture of the health service has changed from one in which specialist medical interests dictated the provision of services to one where commissioning is being devolved to those who have the most frequent contact with the greatest number of patients. Since health is a subjective as well as an objective state, needs assessment has the potential to highlight those areas of people's lives that are impeding their well-being and for concerted efforts to be made to improve the public health through the mechanisms of healthy alliances and pressure on the policy makers. Commissioning is in its infancy and many health professionals are yet to appreci-

ate the contribution that they could make to the New Public Health. The demands for curative services are not likely to diminish in the near future and the fruits of prevention and the promotion of health take a long time to ripen. None the less, the first steps have been taken and the opportunities for nurses and health visitors in particular are there to be seized.

Summary

This chapter has outlined the importance of primary health care. It has attempted to describe how the goals of primary health care laid down by the WHO can be met by the primary health care team within a reorganised NHS. An examination of the factors affecting health, including poverty and ethnicity, has illustrated the need for a wider public health approach to the prevention of ill health by all the members of the primary health care team. The potential contribution of nurses to the 'New Public Health' through the process of health needs profiling and the formation of healthy alliances has been emphasised. The chapter ends by highlighting the challenges and opportunities for nurses within the current organisation of the NHS.

REFERENCES

Acheson, D. (1988). *Public Health in England*. HMSO, London.

Ashton, J. (1992). *Healthy Cities*. Open University Press, Milton Keynes.

Atkin, K., Lunt, N., Park, G. and Hirst, M. (1994). *Nurses Count: a National Census of Practice Nurses*. Social Policy Research Unit, University of York, York.

Audit Commission (1992). *Homeward Bound. A New Course for Community Health*. HMSO, London.

Barker, D. (1992). 'Heart Attacks' determined in the womb' cited in *The Observer*, 24 May, 1992.

Black, D. (1980). *Report of the Working Party on Inequalities in Health*, chaired by Sir Douglas Black. DHSS, London.

Bowling, A. and Stillwell, B. (1988). *The Nurse in Family Practice*. Scutari, London.

Bowling, A. (1997). *Measuring Health. A Review of Quality of Life Measurement Scales*, 2nd edn. Open University Press, Milton Keynes.

Caplan, C. (1969). *An Approach to Community Mental Health*. Tavistock Publications, London.

Charles, N. and Kerr, M. (1988). *Women, Food and Families*. Manchester University Press, Manchester.

Child Poverty Action Group (CPAG) (1996). *Poverty: the Facts*. CPAG, London.

Children's Act (1948). HMSO, London. Chapter 43.

Cowley, S. (1996). Health visiting and public health. In *Community Health Nursing. Frameworks for Practice*, Gastrell, P. and Edwards, J. (eds). Baillière Tindall, London, 272–84.

Davies, T. (1996). The politics of 'lifestyle': government policies and the health of the poor. In *Community Health Nursing. Frameworks for Practice*, Gastrell, P. and Edwards, J. (eds). Baillière Tindall, London, 129–41.

Department of Health (1989). *Working for Patients*. Secretaries of State for Health. Cmnd 849. HMSO, London.

Department of Health (1990). *The Health Service. The NHS Reforms and You*. HMSO, London.

Department of Health (1992). *The Health of the Nation: a Strategy for Health in England*. Cmnd 1986. HMSO, London.

Department of Health (1995). *The Health of the Nation. Variations in Health. What can the Department of Health and the NHS do?* Department of Health, London.

Department of Health (1996a). *A Service with Ambitions*. The Stationery Office Ltd, London.

Department of Health (1996b). *Choice and Opportunity: Primary Care – the Future*. The Stationery Office Ltd, London.

Department of Health (1996c). *Primary Care – Delivering the Future*. The Stationery Office Ltd, London.

DHSS (1975). *Nurses Employed Privately by General Medical Practitioners*. HMSO, London.

DHSS (1981). *The Primary Health Care Team Report of a Joint Working Group of the Standing Medical Advisory Committee and the Standing Nursing and Midwifery Advisory Committee*. The Harding Committee. HMSO, London.

DHSS (1986a). *Neighbourhood Nursing: a Focus for Care*. Cumberlege Report. HMSO, London.

DHSS (1986b). *Primary Health Care – an Agenda for Discussion*. Cmnd 9771. HMSO, London.

Dorrell, S. (1996). *Primary Care: the Future*. NHSE, Quarry House, Leeds.

Firth-Cozens, J. (1992). Building teams for effect audit. *Quality in Health Care*, 1, 252–5.

General Medical Services Committee (1994). Core medical services and the classification of general practitioner activity. A discussion paper 9 (mimeo). General Medical Services Committee, BMA House, London.

Gillow, J. (1996). Team building in primary health care teams. In *Community Health Nursing. Frameworks for Practice*, Gastrell, P. and Edwards, J. (eds). Baillière Tindall, London, 207–16.

Goodwin, S. (1995) Commissioning for health. *Health Visitor*, 68 (1), 16–18.

Hannay, D.R. (1979). *The Symptom Iceberg: a Study of Community Health*. Routledge and Kegan Paul, London.

Harmond K., Crown J. (1996). Health for all, healthy cities. In *Community Health Care Nursing. Principles for Practice*, Twinn, S., Roberts, B. and Andrews, S. (eds). Butterworth-Heinneman, Oxford, 44–53.

Health Departments of Great Britain (1989). *General Practice in the National Health Service – the 1990 Contract*. HMSO, London.

ICRF OXCHECK Study Group (1994). Effectiveness of health checks conducted by nurses in primary care – results of OXCHECK study after one year. *British Medical Journal*, 308, 308–12.

Jarman, B. (1983). Identification of underprivileged areas. *British Medical Journal*, 286, 1705–9.

Jarman, B. (1997). Quoted by Walters, A. (1997). News feature. *Nursing Standard*, 11, 376.

Joseph Rowntree Foundation (1995). *Inquiry into Income and Wealth in Britain*. JRF, York.

Lalonde, M. (1974). A New Perspective on the Health of Canadians. Ministers for Supply and Services, Ottawa: Information Canada. Cited in Cowley, S. (1996) Health visiting and public health. In *Community Health Nursing. Frameworks for Practice*, Gastrell, P. and Edwards, J. (eds). Baillière Tindall, London. 272–84.

Lindsey, E. (1996). Health within illness: experiences of chronically ill disabled people. *Journal of Advanced Nursing*, 24, 465–72.

Luker, K.A., Ferguson, B., Austin, L. *et al.* (1997). Evaluating Nurse Prescribing. Unpublished report. Department of Health, London.

Mant, D. (1994). Prevention. *Lancet*, 344, 1343–6.

Mant, D. and Fowler, G. (1990). Urine analysis for glucose and protein: are the requirements of the new contract sensible? *British Medical Journal*, 300, 1053–5.

Marks, L. (1991). *Home and Hospital Care: Redrawing the Boundaries*. King's Fund, London.

McCormack, A., Fleming, D. and Charlton, J. (1995). *Morbidity Statistics from General Practice*. 4th National Study RCGP/OPCS. HMSO, London.

Menzies, I.E.P. (1960). *The Functioning of Social Systems as a Defence against Anxiety: a Report of the Nursing Service of a General Hospital*. Tavistock Publications, London.

Ministry of Health (1920). *Interim Report on the Future Provision of Medical and Allied Services*. By the Consultative Council on Medical and Allied Services (Dawson Committee). Cmnd 693. HMSO, London.

National Health Service Management Executive (1993). *Nursing in Primary Health Care: New World, New Opportunities*. NHSME, London.

National Health Service (Primary Care) Act (1997). The Stationery Office Ltd, London, Chapter 46.

National Health Service Act (1946). HMSO, London, Chapter 81.

National Health Service Reorganisation Act (1973). HMSO, London, Chapter 32.

National Health Service and Community Care Act (1990). HMSO, London, Chapter 19.

Poulton, B. and West, M. (1993). *Measuring the Effect of Teamworking in Primary Care. Audit for Teams in Primary Care – Proceedings of a Conference (July 1993)*. Eli Lilly National Clinical Audit Centre, Department of General Practice, University of Leicester, Leicester.

Primary Care Forum (1991). *A Journey into the Unknown. A Workbook on the Formation of Primary Health Care Teams*. FHSA, Morpeth.

Rose, G. (1992). *The Strategy of Preventive Medicine*. Oxford Medical Publications, Oxford.

Royal Commission on Medical Education 1965–1968 (1968). Report. Cmnd 3569. HMSO, London.

Smail, J. (1996). Shifting the boundaries of practice in practice nursing. In *Community Health Nursing. Frameworks for Practice*, Gastrell, P. and Edwards, J.

(eds). Baillière Tindall, London, 259–71.

Smail, S.A. (1996). Primary care and the general practitioner. In *Community Health Nursing. Frameworks for Practice*, Gastrell, P. and Edwards, J. (eds). Baillière Tindall, London, 28–41.

SNMAC (1995). *Making it Happen: Public Health – the Contribution, Role and Development of Nurses, Midwives and Health Visitors. Report of the Standing Nursing and Advisory Committee*, Chairman Alison Norman. Department of Health, London.

Southampton Primary Care Development Team (1993). *Multidisciplinary Audit by Primary Care Teams Project*, funded by DoH. Southampton Community Health Services Trust, Southampton.

Starfield, B. (1992). *Primary Care: Concept, Evaluation, and Policy*. Oxford University Press, New York.

Starfield, B. (1994). Is primary care essential? *Lancet*, 334, 1129–33.

Stott, N., Kinnersley, P. and Rollnick, S. (1994). The limits to health promotion. *British Medical Journal*, 309, 971–2.

Townsend, P., Davidson, N. and Whitehead, M. (1988). *Inequalities in Health: The Black Report and The Health Divide*. Penguin Books, Harmondsworth.

Tudor Hart, J. (1988). *A New Kind of Doctor*. Merlin Press, London.

UKCC (1992). *The Scope of Professional Practice*. UKCC, London.

UKCC (1994). *The Future of Professional Practice – the Council's Standards for Education and Practice following Registration*. UKCC, London.

Whitehead, M. (1987). *The Health Divide*. Health Education Council, London.

Wilkinson, R.G. (1992). Income distribution and life expectancy. *British Medical Journal*, 304, 165–8.

World Health Organization/United Nations Children's Fund (1978). *Primary Health Care: Report of the International Conference on Primary Health Care, Alma-Ata USSR*. 6–12 September, 1978. WHO, Geneva.

CHAPTER SIX

HOMEOSTASIS *and* NATURE–NURTURE INTERACTIONS: A FRAMEWORK *for* INTEGRATING *the* LIFE SCIENCES

John Clancy and Andrew J. McVicar

- Introduction: what is integrated science?
- Section A: Biological determinants of health
- Section B: The environment and psychophysiological well-being
- Section C: Systems theory and homeostasis – a model for integration
- Chapter summary

The chapter begins by discussing what is meant by the term integrated science.

The rest of the chapter is divided into three sections which explore the concept of homeostasis, the link between homeostasis and nature–nurture interactions and how this linkage provides a framework for integrating the life sciences.

Section A examines the biological determinants of health. Topics explored include reference to and discussion of:

- Homeostasis: the link with health and ill health
- Genes: 'the code of life'.

Section B examines the relationship between the environment and a person's psychophysiological well-being. The following key areas are discussed:

- Nature–nurture interactions in 'physical' and 'mental' health nursing
- Nature–nurture interactions in sensory perceptions.

Section C uses the relationship between systems theory and homeostasis as a model for integrating the life sciences.

INTRODUCTION: WHAT IS INTEGRATED SCIENCE?

The term integrated science is just one of many names given to the area of science which studies the inter-relationship between a person's biological, psychological and sociological make-up. Others include phenomenological, biopsychosocial and the sociopsychophysiological aspects of human beings. 'Biology' usually refers to the anatomical and physiological systems within the body, 'psychology' refers to the study of human behaviour, and 'sociology' concentrates on how societal and cultural norms shape the subjective behaviour of individuals and groups within particular societies and cultures.

The specialists who study these disciplines in isolation – physiologists, psychologists and sociologists – are often referred to as being 'reductionist' because they are studying discrete aspects of human existence in isolation of the others. To avoid such an approach, some specialists study the relationships between two or more of these disciplines. For example, biopsychologists study the correlations between physiological processes and changing patterns of human behaviour, whilst sociopsychologists study how the individual's environment affects psychological processes such as attention, motivation, emotion and memory. Thus, these scientists demonstrate the existence of emergent properties between systems, and so try to explain the complexities of human behaviour as being intrinsically linked to various aspects of the sociological, psychological and the biological make-up of the individual. Integrated science is a relatively new discipline and health care is at the beginning of an exciting era in the development of the knowledge base which focuses on how society shapes the individual's bodily activities.

Nurse education curricula continue to emphasise this 'holistic' nature of health and ill health, since the nursing profession regards approaches such as the 'medical model' as having a reductionist approach. That is, the medical treatment of disorders is viewed as being directed at physiological disturbance; thus, whilst explaining the rationale for therapies, the use of the medical model fails to recognise the broader issues in health and ill health and therefore acts as a barrier to total care.

Holism recognises that the interactions between a person and the environment in which that person lives are significant factors in the shaping of the individual, and are important determinants of well-being (see Chapter 2, page 22, for discussion of the concept of 'well-being'). Consequently, the individual life science subjects provide the knowledge base from which an holistic approach can be developed. However, the applied biological sciences have increasingly become marginalised (Trnobranski, 1993; Jordan, 1994); the current situation is summarised in Figure 6.1(a). If holistic care is the aim, then nurse education must focus the students' knowledge of the biological construct of the individual, and demonstrate how biological functions are influenced by 'psychosocial' interactions (Figure 6.1(b)).

An integrated perspective also encompasses the concept of individualism in relation to the risk factors associated with a patient's illness, since each individual has a unique blend of genes and a unique perceptual view of the environment in which he or she lives (see Figure 6.2). Yet, although the teaching of health from such a perspective may help in the development of a curriculum with a stronger bias towards holistic principles, it may not be able to provide all the answers, since holism, as a concept, incorporates influences which may never be identified (see Figure 6.3).

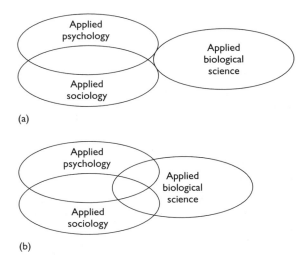

(a)

(b)

Figure 6.1: (a) Today's 'integrated science' approach. Curricula in nursing emphasise psychosocial interactions but marginalise the importance of applied biological studies. (b) Integration of the human life sciences: the first step to holistic curricula

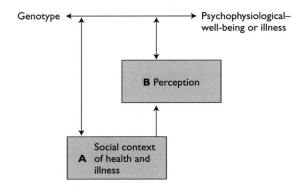

Figure 6.2: Health and illness: an integrated science perspective

A Social context of health and illness (expressed via mortality/morbidity rates):

- Social class differences
- Gender differences
- Ethnicity, racism and health
- Poverty
- Unemployment
- Homelessness.

B Perceptions:

- A behavioural perspective, e.g. classical conditioning, operant conditioning, introspection
- A cognitive perspective, e.g. information processing, motivation, personality, social behaviour

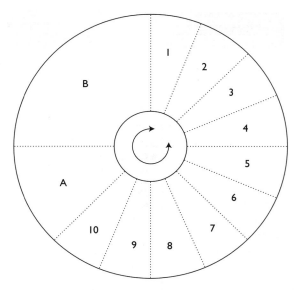

Figure 6.3: Holism: the concept. Interdisciplinary relationships achievable with advancement of knowledge. Segments: 1, primary health care and health promotion; 2, the philosophy and social context of health; 3, spirituality and ethics; 4, individualised care: an integrated science perspective; 5, nursing process, theories and models; 6, care of the child client; 7, care of the adult client; 8, care of the client with a mental health problem; 9, care of the client with a learning disability; 10, care of the midwifery client; A, knowledge which is not known at present but could become available via current research findings; B, knowledge which is not known at present and will never become available. Therefore holism remains a conceptual myth rather than a reality.

On this basis, clinical intervention can be viewed as an attempt to re-establish the health of the patient via working on the subjective elements associated with the illness. Health education advises the patient of the potential risk factors which promote the illness, and levels of pain and distress, in order to minimise their recurrence (see Figure 6.4). The reader is encouraged to preview Chapters 3, 4, 5 and 11 before reading on, so as to increase awareness of issues raised in the remainder of this chapter.

Nursing models provide frameworks for the delivery of holistic care. However, educational curricula do not necessarily support the concept, as identified earlier, and so the integrative nature of the life sciences associated with health and illness needs to be further established so as to improve their application. Although no single theory can apply to all possible situations, this chapter discusses how the concept of homeostasis, and its relationship to systems theory, provides a workable framework for teaching the basis of the concept of health (see Chapter 3, page 38), and so forms a foundation for the application of nursing theory and nursing models (see Chapter 11, page 262) to improve the quality of care.

SECTION A: BIOLOGICAL DETERMINANTS OF HEALTH

Humans are biological organisms. We may have very complex behaviours and cognitive abilities, and we may live in highly sophisticated societies, but nursing should not lose sight of the fact that ultimately our physiological and psychological health depends upon the functioning of biological

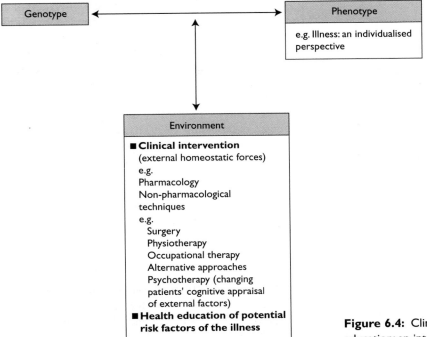

Figure 6.4: Clinical interventions and health education: an integrated science perspective

structures. In the context of this chapter it therefore seems logical first to establish the basis for optimal biological functioning. Two main topics are reviewed:

- The principles of regulation of the internal environment
- The role of genes in cell functions during the lifespan.

HOMEOSTASIS: THE LINK WITH HEALTH AND ILL HEALTH

An introduction to homeostatic control theory

The word 'homeostasis' translates as 'same standing' and is usually taken to indicate constancy or balance. Those students who have entered nursing in recent years having taken courses which have had a significant human biology component are likely to have come across the term, as it is an important concept, especially in physiological studies.

The idea that a constancy of the internal environment is essential to life can be traced to the views of the eminent French physiologist Claude Bernard, in the mid-nineteenth century. The turn of the century produced many important discoveries of how the body is regulated by hormonal and neural mechanisms, and the term 'homeostasis' was finally coined by Cannon in 1932.

Today, the maintenance of the internal environment seems a logical aspect of human function, and homeostatic principles relate to most, if not all, functional parameters (including environmentally induced psychophysiological interactions involved in the subjective perceptions of pain, stress and **circadian rhythms** – Clancy and McVicar, 1992, 1993, 1994a, 1994b). It is erroneous, however, to take the view that homeostasis is simply about constancy.

First, the dynamic nature of control processes dictates that there must be variation – control mechanisms must respond to change and, in promoting responses, will themselves induce variation. Thus, there is a homeostatic *range* within which a parameter is maintained (Figure 6.5). For some parameters, such as body temperature, the range is very narrow. Others, for example blood volume, have a relatively larger homeostatic range. The range reflects the precision with which a parameter is regulated, and individual variation within the population and within each person;

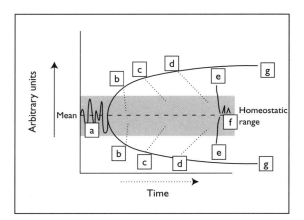

Figure 6.5: Homeostatic control: a, homeostatic dynamism – constantly fluctuating about the mean; b, failure of short-term homeostatic control in restoring homeostasis; c, failure of intermediate-term homeostatic control in restoring homeostasis; d, failure of long-term homeostatic control in restoring homeostasis; e, illness, a homeostatic imbalance; f, patient homeostasis restored by clinical intervention; g, acute or chronic illness not responsive to therapeutic intervention leading to disability or death (Source: Clancy, J. and McVicar, A.J., 1995, *Physiology and Anatomy. A Homeostatic Approach*, with kind permission of Arnold, London)

that is, the range will vary according to each developmental stage of the individual. It also reflects variation in parameter values in relation to sleep–wake activities or circadian patterns.

Second, this level of maintenance could actually be detrimental under some circumstances, as it provides little scope for functional development or change. For example, the maintenance of a constant arterial blood pressure is frequently cited in textbooks as an illustration of a homeostatic process at work. However, it is important that the pressure is increased during exercise, as this helps to increase blood flow through the exercising muscle and so helps to ensure that oxygen supply to the muscle supports the increased demand. The elevation of blood pressure is itself a homeostatic adaptive process, as it acts to provide the appropriate environment for the changing metabolic needs of muscle, and this highlights the most important feature of homeostasis: physiological processes provide an *optimal* environment for bodily function.

Homeostasis, then, is about the provision of an internal environment that is optimal for cell, tissue and organ system function at any moment in time. 'Health' occurs when bodily function is able to provide the appropriate environment. This usually entails an integration of the functioning of physiological systems and its outcome is observed as 'physical' well-being and 'psychological' equilibrium (see Chapter 2, page 22 for discussion of the concept 'well-being'). In order for homeostasis to occur, the body must have a means of detecting change, of assessing the magnitude of the change, and of promoting an appropriate effector response (Figure 6.6; see also Clancy and McVicar, 1996). Feedback processes provide the means of assessing the effectiveness of the reponse.

Homeostasis and ill health

If homeostasis provides a basis for health, then ill health will arise when there is a failure to maintain the control processes involved (Figure 6.5). Imprecise control mechanisms include:

- Receptors which fail to respond adequately to changes in the environment
- Control centres which fail to analyse sensory information, and/or analyse the information incorrectly and send incorrect information to the **effector organs**
- Effector organs which fail to respond to directions from the control centres.

Failure to provide an optimal internal environment will cause further destabilisation, and the integration of psychological and physiological (i.e. psychophysiological) functioning will become impaired. In this way, an environmentally induced change in the activities of one part of the body may have far-reaching consequences for whole body function. Thus, the authors encourage nurses to take a transactional (or interactionist) view regarding the patient's condition (see Chapter 14, p. 320).

All disorders are characterised by a primary disturbance of intracellular homeostasis within tissues somewhere in the body. The disease may be classed according to the primary disorder, such as circulatory, respiratory, endocrine and neuromuscular disease, as a degenerative disorder or tumour of a particular tissue, or as being due to

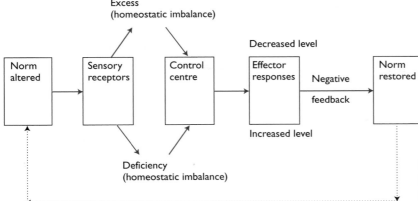

Figure 6.6: Scheme for a homeostatic process (Adapted from McVicar and Clancy, 1998)

immune system dysfunction or infection, but all will have consequences for extracellular homeostasis and hence the functioning of cells and tissues other than those involved in the primary disturbance.

To illustrate this point, we have selected chronic bronchitis, since chronic obstructive airway disease is one of the most common causes of morbidity and disability in the UK. Obstructive airway disease is characterised by difficult expiration. In chronic bronchitis, the obstruction arises because of inflammation of the airways, which leads to excessive secretion by mucus glands, enlargement of bronchial muscle and a thickening of the bronchial walls (Davey *et al.*, 1994). Emptying of the lungs is slowed and there is usually an increased force of muscle contraction during expiration. With more advanced disease there is trapping of air in the lung alveoli.

The decreased ventilation of lung alveoli promotes **hypoxaemia** (if severe, then **cyanosis** will be present) and an increased arterial concentration of carbon dioxide (which leads to respiratory acidosis). Hypoxaemia promotes increased production of red blood cells (polycythaemia), leading to increased blood viscosity. If it is not reversed, hypoxaemia eventually causes **pulmonary hypertension** and **congestive heart failure**.

Chronic bronchitis is caused by the effects of environmental irritants, such as cigarette smoke or other pollutants, or by infection to influence the functions of cells within the airways. Intervention is targeted at reducing the hypoxaemia by increasing airway calibre using bronchodilators, by removing secretions using physical therapy and expectorants, and by oxygen therapy (Clancy and McVicar, 1997). In other words, care is targeted at

restoring blood gas homeostasis by using extrinsic means to support lung function. Note that little can be done to reverse this condition, hence its chronic nature. The environmental cause of the disorder means that a lifestyle change can reduce the risk of developing the condition in the first place, or slow or even halt its progression.

The interaction between cells and extrinsic factors in the aetiology of a disorder, and in caring for people with the disorder, is explored further in later sections of this chapter, since it forms the basis of an integrated, holistic approach to health care.

Homeostatic principles in clinical practice: the nursing process

Clinical intervention in illness and disease is concerned with correcting underlying problems, managing the symptoms, and enabling the patient to come to terms with the 'disorder'. In other words, clinical practice is concerned with restoring, as effectively as possible, the homeostatic status of the patient. By promoting normality, the nurse and health care team are therefore acting as extrinsic homeostatic mechanisms. Homeostatic principles are readily discerned within the stages of the nursing process (see Chapter 11 for further discussion of the nursing process) (compare Figures 6.6 and 6.7). Thus:

1 *Assessment and nursing diagnosis.* The assessment of the health deficit and the needs of the individual correspond to the detection and assessment of change by a homeostatic system. In other words, the nurse is acting as a receptor and monitor mechanism.

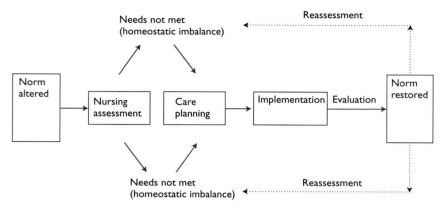

Figure 6.7: Nursing process: a homeostatic mechanism (Adapted from McVicar and Clancy, 1998)

2 *Planning*. The planning stage of the nursing process is analogous to the ways by which homeostatic 'control centres' analyse and determine the responses which the body will need to correct the change.

3 *Implementation*. In the nursing process, implementation refers to putting into action the interventions planned in the previous stage. In a homeostatic perspective this is analogous to the activation of effector organs to produce the appropriate response.

4 *Evaluation*. The effectiveness of care is assessed in this stage, much as feedback processes provide a means of evaluating a psychophysiological response.

5 *Reassessment*. The cyclical nature of the nursing process is emphasised by this stage, in which the patient is reassessed and new care plans considered, if necessary. The dynamism of this process is also observed in homeostatic mechanisms as parameters constantly fluctuate about their means and such changes must, therefore, be constantly reassessed.

GENES: 'THE CODE OF LIFE'

Genes and gene expression

The nucleus of each human cell contains genetic material organised into a set of chromosomes. The chromosomes comprise our genotype (genetic make-up) that encodes the observable and measurable characteristics (the phenotypes) that we inherit from our biological parents. These phenotypic characteristics emerge during embryological development as the genes on the chromosomes express themselves by controlling cell metabolism. It is still uncertain how chromosomes that are identical from cell to cell enable cells to differentiate into a diverse range with specialised functions (i.e. skeletal, digestive, renal, sex cells, etc.), in the different areas of the body, and at a specific time of embryological development (see Figure 6.8).

In 1953 Watson and Crick were awarded the Nobel Prize for discovering that genes are comprised of the chemical deoxyribonucleic acid (DNA). Later research findings demonstrated that the instructions encoded by DNA are transcribed to messenger ribonucleic acid (mRNA) which is then transported out of the nucleus to the cell's ribosomes. In a complex process, other forms of ribonucleic acid then 'translate' the message to synthesise specific proteins, according to the original instructions encoded in DNA, that act to alter cell metabolism (see Figure 6.9, page 130). These changes to metabolism usually involve the production of specialised proteins (and **polypeptides**) called enzymes – biological catalysts which speed up the rate of chemical reaction so that metabolic reactions are compatible with life processes. For this reason the enzymes are referred to as the 'key chemicals of life' since they provide the link between genes and 'physiological' and 'psychological' metabolic activity (see Clancy and McVicar, 1995, for further details). The emphasis in the study of genes is on their role in:

- The maintenance of intracellular homeostasis, or health (see Chapters 2–5)
- Promoting cell specialisation; regulating human development (see later)
- The acquisition of cognitive function
- The subjective perceptions of pain and stress (see Chapters 15 and 8, respectively)

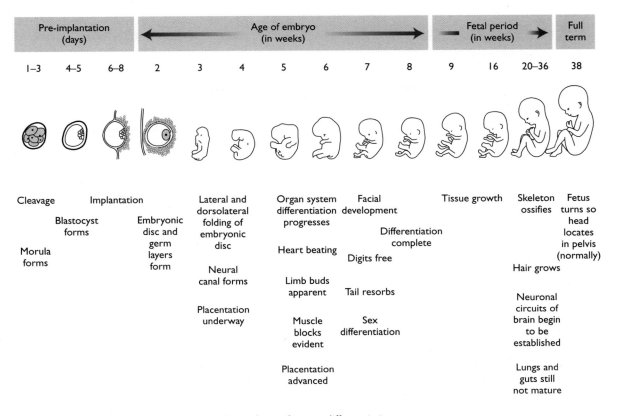

Pre-implantation (days)			Age of embryo (in weeks)							Fetal period (in weeks)		Full term
1–3	4–5	6–8	2	3	4	5	6	7	8	9	16	20–36	38

Cleavage   Implantation   Lateral and   Organ system   Facial   Tissue growth   Skeleton   Fetus

Cleavage

Implantation

Blastocyst forms

Morula forms

Embryonic disc and germ layers form

Lateral and dorsolateral folding of embryonic disc

Neural canal forms

Placentation underway

Organ system differentiation progresses

Heart beating

Limb buds apparent

Muscle blocks evident

Placentation advanced

Facial development

Digits free

Tail resorbs

Sex differentiation

Tissue growth

Differentiation complete

Skeleton ossifies

Hair grows

Neuronal circuits of brain begin to be established

Lungs and guts still not mature

Fetus turns so head locates in pelvis (normally)

Figure 6.8: Embryo/fetal development: chronology of tissue differentiation
(Source: Clancy, J. and McVicar, A.J., 1995, *Physiology and Anatomy. A Homeostatic Approach*, with kind permission of Arnold, London)

■ Illness (see Chapter 2)
■ Clinical interventions (see Chapters 24–27).

However, the question arises as to how it is that gene activity is expressed at the appropriate time?

One way to maintain the steady state of intra-cellular homeostasis, and hence 'psychological' and 'physiological' (i.e. psychophysiological) well-being, is to modulate enzyme production. Various models of how genes are controlled have been put forward. These are mainly based on work with relatively simple organisms, such as bacteria, but they suggest how DNA in all organisms controls enzyme synthesis in response to the presence of substrates (reactants), end-products and/or external regulatory mechanisms. In the context of interactionism, environmental factors can also act as triggers for gene expression, since it is clear that the gene activity necessary for the control of metabolism is environmentally modified.

Gene expression, and its control, has two fundamental roles to play. First, genes are responsible

for enabling the maintence of homeostasis, through controlling intracellular function. Second, genes control human development.

Gene expression: the link with homeostasis and health

As noted earlier, enzymes act as catalysts for chemical reactions (the chemicals involved are referred to as substrates) within the cell, and so promote intracellular homeostasis. Enzyme synthesis may be promoted by the following situations (Figure 6.10):

■ The enzyme concentration is below its homeostatic range, i.e. substrate metabolism is too low. Failure to increase enzyme production will result in deficient substrate utilisation. For example, in hypothyroidism there is a deficiency of thyroid hormone production, which means that the synthesis of enzymes involved in the conversion of glucose into energy is compromised. Cell metabolism is depressed, result-

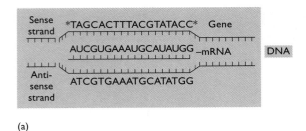

(a)

Codon (triplet)

AUCGUGAAAUGCAUAUGG   Ribosome

(b)

2. Condensation reaction

H₂O

Amino acids

3. Exit

1. Entry

Anti-codons of tRNA   UAGCACUUUACGUAUACC

Codons of mRNA   AUCGUGAAAUGCAUAUGG   Ribosome

Figure 6.9: Protein synthesis. (a) Transcription: messenger RNA synthesis alongside DNA strand in the nucleus. (b) Messenger RNA passes out of the nucleus to become attached to ribosomes. (c) Translation: transfer RNA (tRNA) brings amino acids to the ribosome (Source: Clancy, J. and McVicar, A.J., 1995, *Physiology and Anatomy. A Homeostatic Approach*, with kind permission of Arnold, London)

ing in symptoms such as apathy, slow thought processes and a slowed pulse rate.

■ The substrate is beyond its homeostatic range and so its utilisation must be increased in order to remove the homeostatic imbalance. Failure to do so can have severe consequences. For example, in phenylketonuria there is an inherited deficiency of the enzyme (phenylalanine hydroxylase) required for the conversion of the amino acid phenylalanine into tyrosine, resulting in a build-up of phenylalanine, which inhibits normal brain development in the child.

In health, excess metabolites may be removed in various ways, involving a variety of enzymes:

■ The substance may be stored in a related form. For example, excess intracellular glucose is stored as glycogen via the production of an enzyme, glycogen synthetase.

■ The substance may be converted into another form. For example, **non-essential amino acids** may be transferred (transaminated) into other non-essential amino acids if needed, i.e. if their homeostatic levels are compromised. Alternatively, the excess amino acids may be broken down (deaminated) into energy-producing chemicals (keto acids) and urea. Keto acids are fed into the cellular respiratory pathway and urea is a metabolic 'waste' product and is usually excreted. **Transamination** and **deamination** processes are instigated by the synthesis of enzymes known as transaminases and deaminases, respectively.

■ Toxic substances, for example, alcohol, substances administered as drugs, and those that are circulating hormones are converted to less active forms or are destroyed. A failure to produce the enzymes involved will result in prolonged activities of these substances. This is one of the complications in cirrhosis of the liver, in which liver function is severely disrupted.

It is clear, then, that gene expression is vital to the integrity of metabolic activity in cells. Loss of genes by their deletion or mutation will produce significant alterations to cell metabolism, some of which may be sufficient to induce a disease state.

Most disorders that arise from the inheritance of single defective genes have now been identified; as could be expected, the majority are evident at birth. The most common in the UK is cystic fibrosis in which there is a lack of the protein necessary for the transport of chloride ions across the membrane of mucus-producing cells of the lung and gut (Huether and Andrews, 1994).

Recent years have also provided increasing evidence for genetic involvement in diseases of adulthood. These disorders seem likely to involve mutations in many genes, or altered gene expression (Yarbro, 1992), but the promoting mechanisms are incompletely understood. Some mutations may be inherited, whilst others are accumulated during life.

For example, colorectal cancer tends to occur in middle–late adulthood and its incidence is greatest in countries with high socio-economic standards. Onset of colorectal cancer is related to

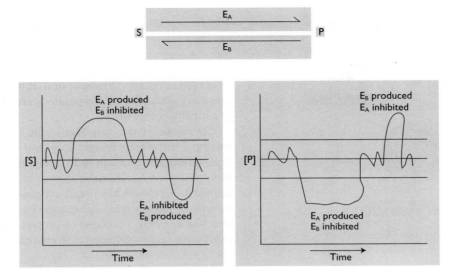

Figure 6.10: Intracellular metabolic homeostasis via enzyme production and inhibition. The reaction goes to the right when there is excess substrate (S) and a deficiency of the product (P). This is controlled by producing and/or activating enzyme A and by stopping production and/or deactivating enzyme B. The reaction goes to the left when there is an excess of P and a deficiency of S. This is controlled by producing and/or activating E_B and by stopping production and/or deactivating E_A. The reaction stops when the homeostatic ranges of both S and P are achieved (Source: Clancy, J. and McVicar, A.J., 1995, *Physiology and Anatomy. A Homeostatic Approach*, with kind permission of Arnold, London)

prolonged contact between the faecal mass and colon mucosa: a diet low in dietary fibre and high in fats increases the risk of developing the cancer because of the accumulation of substances, made by colonic bacteria, that mutate DNA (Henderson *et al.*, 1991). The development of colorectal cancer appears to result from **genetic deletions** from various chromosomes (Department of Health, 1995). Clearly, an individual who inherits some of these deletions will be at increased risk of accumulating the remaining deletions during life, and this helps to explain the occurrence of cancer primarily as a disease of adulthood. Some genes seem to be more crucial in this than others. For example, individuals who inherit one particular altered gene (a **dominant gene** on chromosome 5 [Groden *et al.*, 1991]) exhibit familial adenomatous polyposis coli. These individuals have a high incidence of **polyps** within the colon, and are likely to develop colorectal cancer at an earlier age than those people who do not have the gene.

The reader should note the role of diet (lifestyle) in the advent of this disorder. The aetiology of the cancer is one of gene inheritance (i.e. nature) combined with environmental influences on genes and gene expression (i.e. nurture). The

recognition of environmental modification of genes and/or gene expression will result in further health education programmes, in the not-too-distant future, for the prevention of many common disorders of adulthood including heart disease and insulin-independent diabetes mellitus (Williams, 1994; Department of Health, 1995).

Gene expression: the link with human development

The expression or non-expression of certain genes explains the cell specialisation that occurs during human development. The first stages of cell specialisation occur during the transition of the **morula** into the **blastocyst** and thence into the embryo. That is, all cells appear identical at the morula stage of development, but the blastocyst shows evidence of the first stage of differentiation, since cells specialise into trophoblastic (membrane) or inner mass (embryo) cells (Figure 6.11). The specialisation of the cells of the embryo begins with the transformation of the inner mass into three germ layers: the ectoderm, mesoderm, and endoderm. This differentiation is the second stage of specialisation.

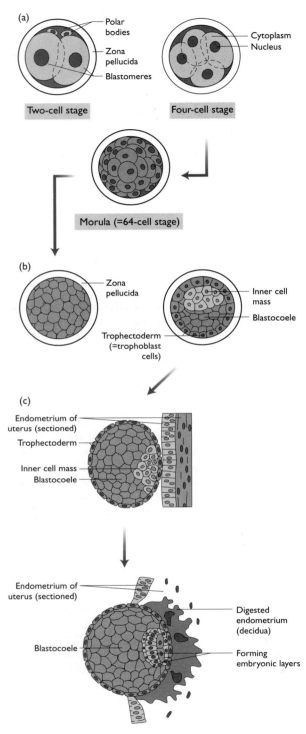

Figure 6.11: Pre-implantation development. (a) Development of the morula from the zygote. (b) The blastocyst (in section). (c) Implantation
(Source: Clancy, J. and McVicar, A.J., 1995, *Physiology and Anatomy. A Homeostatic Approach*, with kind permission of Arnold, London)

The germ layers then differentiate into the cells which constitute the specialised tissues and organs of the embryo. The cells of the body therefore undergo many structural, and hence functional, developments (referred to as the 'principle of complementary structure and function'), and these are enzymatically mediated, and hence are genetically controlled.

Chemicals that interfere with the genes involved in differentiation are collectively referred to as teratogens and can induce severe malformations. They include drugs, dietary factors, environmental chemicals (e.g. pesticides) and infectious agents (e.g. rubella and HIV) (Cefelo and Moos, 1995). The need to protect the embryo from such factors by adequate antenatal and preconceptual care is clear.

Enzyme production is responsible for changing the expression of genes at all of the periods associated with human development – not just embryonic development but also in the development of the neonate, of the infant and child, of the adolescent, and of the adult – and represent a resetting of homeostatic parameters.

Each developmental stage is associated with specific psychophysiological characteristics. Such characteristics involve the functioning, or non-functioning, of cellular enzymes via gene expression and non-expression, respectively. An individual's genes, or genotype, is programmed, and therefore promotes the biophysical and biochemical, anatomical and psychophysiological characteristics (referred to as the phenotypes) of the individual. The expression of genes, however, is modified by environmental cues; hence, the variation in the commencement of each stage accounts for individuality.

For example, the onset of puberty in girls is normally between 12 and 14 years of age, and points to genetic expression occurring during this period (maturity does not occur in the presence of certain chromosomal abnormalities, such as **Turner's syndrome** and **Kleinfelter's syndrome**). Timing of the onset largely depends upon individual exposure to the environmental cues (for example adequate diet) which influence gene expression. The triggers affect higher centres of the brain, mediating the electrochemical impulses involved in the processes of conditioning and socialisation. Such processes influence those genes in the hypothalamus that are responsible for producing and secreting **gonadotropin-**

releasing hormones. Their secretion, and the subsequent action of gonadotropins released by the pituitary gland on the gonads, initiates the onset of puberty/menarche in a defined, controlled way.

It is generally accepted that the stages of development can be initiated prematurely or delayed. For example, premature puberty is common in obese girls and delayed puberty is common in anorexic girls, although there continues to be a debate as to whether or not dietary components are important environmental triggers for gene expression. An integrated science perspective investigates the numerous social, cultural, physical, spiritual and environmental triggers which are responsible for producing obesity and anorexia, and their role in modifying homeostatic processes.

Gene expression and the ageing process

The emphasis on cellular functioning as a basis for health is supported by research which has shed light on the processes of biological ageing. Current theories of the biological basis of ageing focus on the disturbances of metabolism that are observed in cell cultures and in the whole person. Evidence increasingly supports an accumulation of genetic disturbance, and of various chemicals within cells, which ultimately cause cell homeostasis to decline. Such disturbances will also influence the extracellular environment, and this in turn causes the homeostatic ranges of parameters to increase, thus exacerbating age-related changes on tissue functions (Figure 6.12).

Discussion of the various theories of biological ageing can be found in Clancy and McVicar (1995). The most compelling evidence indicates that functional changes during ageing are the consequences of the effects of:

- Cumulative metabolic disturbances arising from damage to mitochondrial DNA by chemicals known as **free radicals** (the 'free radical' theory was first proposed by Harman in 1956)
- Alterations to protein structure during or after synthesis (first proposed as an 'error catastrophe' theory by Orgel in 1963).

The genetic and cellular aspects of ageing imply that its effects on homeostasis are unavoidable. The longevity (i.e. maximum lifespan) of humans is estimated to be of the order of 90–100 years, yet some people live beyond this, whilst the majority do not attain it. This suggests that other factors modify the effects of the ageing process on homeostasis. In fact, the average life expectancy for a person born in the UK 100 years ago was about 50 years, whilst now it is of the order of 75 years. Improvements in diet, public health measures and an increased understanding of disease processes are responsible for much of this change. Research into ageing processes can only increase the understanding of how interactions promote

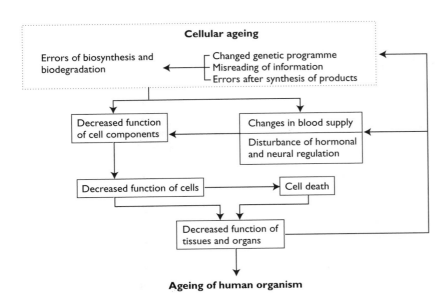

Figure 6.12: Relation between cellular ageing and ageing of the human organism

health and ill health during the lifespan, and so raise average life expectancy still further.

Summary

Homeostasis: the link with health and ill health

- Humans are biological beings. The biological construct of the individual provides the basis for identifying how interactions with the external environment influence the health of the individual.
- The concept of homeostasis helps to explain the importance to health of maintaining an optimal environment within which cells must function. 'Optimal' does not necessarily equate with constancy; it also relates to the control of change observed during daily activities of living, and also during the developmental phases of the lifespan.
- Ill health arises when there is a failure to maintain homeostatic functions, either at tissue or organ levels. The interdependency of tissue functions means that homeostatic disturbances and associated symptoms will also arise secondarily to the primary disorder.
- Health care practices can be related to homeostasis since they provide the extrinsic effectors that act to restore homeostasis.

Genes: the code of life

- Genes regulate the metabolic activities of cells and therefore determine cell functions and hence the environment within and around the cells.
- Genes can exert this control because they contain the chemical codes necessary for the synthesis of enzymes that catalyse metabolic reactions.
- The loss of genes, or interference with gene expression, influences the functioning of cells. The consequences of such loss may be specific to certain tissues of the body, and this illustrates that some genes may be selectively activated depending upon the cell type.
- The capacity for selective activation or deactivation of genes is also responsible for human development.
- Disturbances of homeostasis may arise at any point in the lifespan because of genetic propensity to the condition, coupled with lifestyle/environmental factors that influence genes: this is the basis for an integrated approach to health and ill health.

SECTION B: THE ENVIRONMENT AND PSYCHOPHYSIOLOGICAL WELL-BEING

So far this chapter has emphasised the 'biological' side of health, that is, genes, gene expression and homeostasis. We have also highlighted, however, that these aspects of health are influenced by the lifestyle/culture of the individual. The next sections consider further evidence for an integrated approach to health, and how the impact of our environment promotes individuality.

GENE–ENVIRONMENT (NATURE–NURTURE) INTERACTIONS

'Nature–nurture' discussions figure prominently in holistic approaches to care, particularly when considering those factors which influence the pronounced cognitive and behavioural changes that are observed during the developmental stages of the lifespan, since the genetic and environmental contributions to development are well recognised (e.g. Radford and Hollin, 1991; Bergemann et al., 1993). Such studies frequently attempt to quantify the relative contributions of 'nature' and 'nurture' to human development, and this issue has long been debated.

Unfortunately, the data from behavioural studies tend to emphasise interactions as determinants of mental functions only, and so give the impression that physical health is a separate entity. This dichotomy is encouraged further by the failure of nurse education to integrate biological sciences fully into curricula (Akinsanya, 1987; Jordan, 1994) and by the persistence of nursing (and medicine) to categorise illness as disorders of either mental or physical health. Encouraging health care professionals to discuss the construct of the individual from separate psychosocial and biological viewpoints can only serve to perpetuate the dichotomy.

The exact means by which the environment can influence mental and physical functions are increasingly the subject of research. The following are examples to illustrate some developments in order to demonstrate that the clinical relevance of the 'nature–nurture' question must be considered from a wider perspective, and whenever possible, take into account the integration of the life sciences, if the concept of holistic care is to be furthered.

Nature–nurture interactions in 'mental health' nursing

Psychological and sociological studies have made a considerable impact upon the understanding of the shaping of an individual's behaviour according to societal norms, values and beliefs, yet the continued use of pharmacological therapies, whether as primary or secondary interventions, provides a reminder that the brain is a 'biological' structure and that a lack of 'psychological' equilibrium represents a disturbance of the internal biochemical environment of the brain. Clinical intervention aims to reverse the homeostatic disturbance and this is illustrated by the therapeutic approaches used in the treatment of depression.

Depression is characterised in its extreme by a mood associated with a general feeling of unhappiness and dissatisfaction, and/or a loss of interest and/or pleasure. The majority of studies indicate that the activities of monoamine neurotransmitters (noradrenaline and serotonin in particular) in the brain are reduced in depressive states, resulting in a functional imbalance between certain neural pathways of the brain (Willner, 1985). Clinical intervention entails the use of pharmacotherapy and/or psychotherapy:

■ Pharmacological therapies largely involve the administration of drugs which either inhibit the uptake of neurotransmitter from the synapse, and so prolong its action, or prevent its breakdown by enzymes and so potentiate its release. The efficacy of these drugs in acute care is well established (Morris and Beck, 1974; Wong et al., 1995).

■ Distressing life events and a lack of social support have long been known to act as precipitating factors in the aetiology of depression (Gilbert, 1992), and cognitive–behavioural therapy has been found to be as effective as pharmacological intervention for acute treatment and may even be associated with lower rates of relapse (Swallow and Segal, 1995).

The aim of the above two approaches to care is either artificially to correct the neurochemical imbalance by using drugs, though this does not remove the cause of the disturbance, or to reverse the neurological change which resulted in the imbalance by using psychotherapy. However, comparative studies on the merit of each approach are of little or no value, and an integrated approach should be taken which takes the best of each (Rehm, 1995).

Thus, the cause of depression, and the clinical interventions used to alleviate it, include psychological, biological and sociological factors, disciplines which are predominantly taught separately in nursing and health care curricula. For holistic care the practitioner must consider the integrated life perspective.

Psychiatry utilises the influence of psychosocial interactions in the treatment of disorders of mental health, yet recent studies by geneticists and molecular biologists indicate that (some) behavioural disorders are associated with specific genetic disturbances (see later) and therefore have a primary organic basis. To put these apparently different viewpoints into perspective, it is important first to consider what a genetic basis for behaviour might entail.

Childhood and adolescence are viewed as being the main formative periods of our lives, evidenced by the complexity of psychophysiological development during these periods, though behaviour and personality remain labile throughout life. The formation and maintenance of synaptic connections between appropriate parts of the brain is essential for psychophysiological development and is reflected in the increased complexity and diversity of motor skills and behavioural responses that occur during early childhood. Some of these developments must be genetically determined, since many of the changes are common to all humans (in health and ill health).

The influence of the environment on brain development, and also its influence on adult personality and behaviour, emphasises the plasticity of some neuronal networks. Influencing factors might be 'physical', for example the behavioural actions of steroid hormones released during puberty (e.g. Inoff-Germain et al., 1988). Other influences are social as one's environment and circumstances change through life, and demonstrate how certain synapses can be functionally altered, albeit by a slow process.

So where does this leave the 'nature–nurture debate' in relation to mental health? Our mental faculties have a biological basis, in that sites are identifiable within the brain which have roles in, for example, emotion, aggression, sexual behaviour, perceptions, memories, personality, attitudes, beliefs and values (e.g. Carlson, 1986). The functioning of synapses in neural networks requires the activation of appropriate genes within brain neurones, not only for the existence of the neural components of the brain, but also to promote neuronal growth and to enable a cell to produce the chemicals necessary for synaptic functioning (Figure 6.13). The observable characteristics produced by such genes might be behaviourally or cognitively developed through the individual's subjective perceptions of his or her immediate environment; so there is a genetic basis to all aspects of 'psychological' function (Billings *et al.*, 1992). We prefer, however, to refer to body responses as being psychophysiological in origin, instigated by environmental (social) cues derived through an individual's unique socialisation/conditioning processes.

A genetic basis would help to explain the apparent familial occurrence of many psychological disorders (McGuffin and Thapar, 1992). By implication, gene mutation should be capable of inducing behavioural disturbance by altering neurological structure and functioning. Putative

genes have been identified (McGuffin and Thapar, 1992; Mowry and Levinson, 1993) but the situation is complicated by the likelihood that behavioural traits are characteristics which involve numerous genes, and this increases the complexity of investigation (for example, see Kendler and Diehl, 1993).

Genetic involvement could also help to explain how behavioural disorders are associated with specific neurochemical imbalances, such as those identified earlier in relation to depressive behaviour. Pharmacological therapies target this 'nature' component of behavioural disorders and are an important tool. The increasing recognition of genetic propensity to mental health disorder suggests that the advent of genetic therapies in the not-too-distance future may eventually provide alternative biological means of treatment.

Nevertheless, current pharmacological therapies may not reverse a disorder, and only provide a means of managing it, since they do not recognise the influence of environmental factors on gene expression. Psychotherapy is an alternative that utilises the lability of neural connections to promote appropriate pathways and thus modify behaviour. How such 'environmental' interactions influence the expression of genes and behaviour has not been elucidated. It is clear, however, that

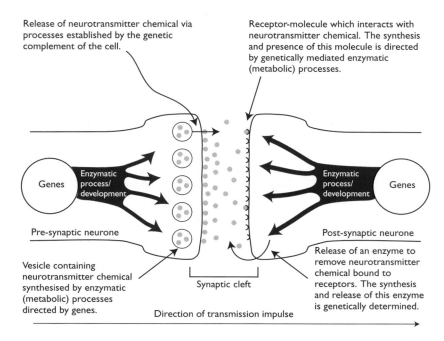

Release of neurotransmitter chemical via processes established by the genetic complement of the cell.

Receptor-molecule which interacts with neurotransmitter chemical. The synthesis and presence of this molecule is directed by genetically mediated enzymatic (metabolic) processes.

Genes

Enzymatic process/ development

Pre-synaptic neurone

Genes

Enzymatic process/ development

Post-synaptic neurone

Vesicle containing neurotransmitter chemical synthesised by enzymatic (metabolic) processes directed by genes.

Synaptic cleft

Release of an enzyme to remove neurotransmitter chemical bound to receptors. The synthesis and release of this enzyme is genetically determined.

Direction of transmission impulse

Figure 6.13: Genes and the functioning of a synapse

to consider only the relative contributions of either genes or environment on mental function is to take too narrow a perspective – much of brain function reflects an interaction of both. (see Figure 6.14).

Nature–nurture interactions' in 'physical health' nursing

The success of some health education programmes to reduce the incidence of physical dis-

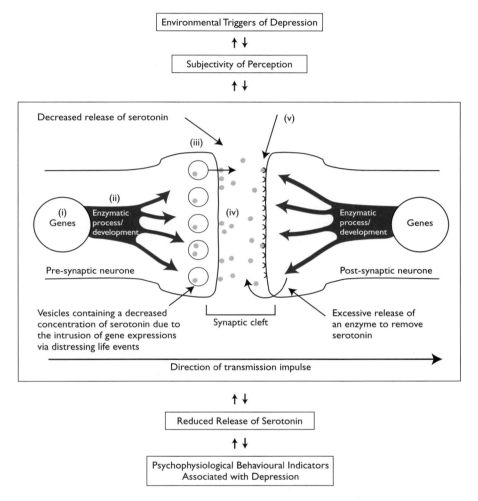

Figure 6.14: Serotonin and depression: aetiology and therapeutic intervention

↓ Aetiology: environmental factors causing a decreased production of serotonin, perhaps via:

(i) inhibiting gene expression for serotonin production, and/or

(ii) inhibiting the enzyme (lock and key inhibition) necessary for the metabolic pathway associated with the production of serotonin, and/or

(iii) inhibiting the release of serotonin via decreasing the permeability of the pre-synaptic membrane, and/or

(iv) synaptic inhibition of serotonin, e.g. enhancing the rate of enzymatic destruction of serotonin therefore inhibiting post-synaptic activation, and/or

(v) post-synaptic inhibition of serotonin via competitive inhibition of serotonin receptor sites.

↑ Therapy: reverses aetiological factors via:

(i) pharmacology approach – tricyclic anti-depressants, e.g. imipramine hydrochloride; serotonin-uptake inhibitor, e.g. Prozac; decrease serotonin breakdown, e.g. monoamine oxidase inhibitors such as Parnate

(ii) cognitive–behavioural approach – decrease distress by altering the patient's perception of capabilities/demands to cope with distressing life events

order indicates that the environment (i.e. lifestyle) has an influence on genetic expression throughout the body. There are numerous examples (Williams, 1994; Department of Health, 1995) but this chapter will focus on two: the occurrence of **atheroma**, and the physical consequences of stress.

ATHEROMA

Atheroma occurs when lipid (mainly cholesterol) accumulates in the walls of blood vessels. Cholesterol is vital to the body, as it is from this lipid that cell membranes and steroid hormones are made. It can be synthesised by the liver from saturated fat or is obtainable direct from our diets, and is transported in the blood, mainly in combination with a protein as a soluble complex called low density **lipoprotein** (Criqui, 1986) sometimes abbreviated as LDLP or LDL. Excess cholesterol removed from tissues is transported in association with a different protein complex – high density lipoprotein (HDLP or HDL). These are biological processes, controlled by genes, and common to us all. Yet there is variation between people in the development of atheroma. This is because atheroma formation is promoted by environmental impacts on cholesterol metabolism:

- Cholesterol is delivered to the tissue to facilitate repair. Excessive or recurrent vessel damage due, for example, to smoking or hypertension will promote its deposition (Ross, 1992).
- The uptake of large amounts of cholesterol or saturated fat from the diet promotes hyperlipidaemia, especially in the form of LDLP, as do the effects of chemicals in tobacco smoke which reduce cholesterol metabolism (Brischetto *et al.*, 1983).
- Normally there is a 2:1 ratio of HDLP:LDLP and this favours the removal of excess cholesterol from tissues. Exercise helps to maintain the ratio, but smoking reduces it and so removes the 'protection' afforded by it (Criqui, 1986).

Consequently, an inappropriate diet, smoking and a lack of exercise are important contributory factors which modify the underlying pathophysiology associated with atheroma (Criqui, 1986; Ross, 1992). Such interactions are major risk factors in the incidence of coronary heart disease in this country. Care is directed at the consequences of atheroma, but also at encouraging individuals to reappraise their lifestyle and so reduce the risk of heart disease.

STRESS

Individuals continually appraise their situations, either consciously or subconsciously, and distress occurs when actual and/or perceived demands placed upon an individual are mismatched with the individual's actual and/or perceived capacity to respond to them (Cox, 1978). The long-term signs of distress are readily discerned and include a diminished attention to detail, forgetfulness, poor work performance, emotional outbursts, sadness, lethargy and apathy (Clancy and McVicar, 1995). These are the so-called psychological indicators of distress and are what most people view as being the consequences of 'stress'. By contrast, stress-related conditions also include cardiovascular disease and gastrointestinal disturbances, and also infectious diseases contracted as a consequence of a depressed immune system. These are the so-called physical aspects of 'stress' and their occurrence, together with psychological indicators, denotes that the impact of **stressors** has exceeded the individual's stress threshold and coping mechanisms, that is, demand capabilities have persistently been mismatched. The position of the threshold is variable between individuals (a factor involved in the subjectivity of stress; Clancy and McVicar, 1993), and within the individual (due to circadian variations; Clancy and McVicar 1994a, b), and therefore influences one's capacity to withstand stressors.

Selye (1976) described the physical responses as a general adaptation syndrome (GAS) dependent upon neural and hormonal activities. He also introduced the concept that our exposure to stressors utilises 'adaptation energy'. The release of hormones in stress responses seems likely to exhibit genetic variation and so, according to the GAS, the amount of 'adaptation energy' that one is born with is likely to be inherited. Its rate of usage, however, depends upon exposure to environmental stressors. In other words, Selye's theory suggests that we inherit a particular capacity to withstand the effects of stressors on psychophysiological well-being, but this capacity varies or is drawn upon according to environmental circumstances and individual perceptions of them. Thus, gene expression is influenced by extrinsic factors and so we have argued that stress should be considered as a sociopsychophysiological phenomenon (Clancy and McVicar, 1993), or in other words, from an integrated science perspective.

Care is targeted at managing the symptoms of stress, at removing the stressor, or at enabling the individual to reappraise the stressor and so remove the capability:demand mismatch.

GENE–ENVIRONMENT (NATURE–NURTURE) INTERACTION IN SENSORY PERCEPTIONS

The previous examples demonstrate how homeostatic disturbance promotes a disease process through a failure to maintain homeostatic equilibrium, primarily caused by a failure of feedback processes. However, it is also the case that our capacity to interpret information regarding the imbalance can also influence our well-being.

The sensing of changes to the parameters of our internal and external environments is central to the whole concept of homeostasis, and hence to health. This requires the presence of specialised receptor cells which are sensitive to specific parameters within the environment. For example, glucose receptors respond to changes in the blood sugar concentration, whilst the eyes detect changes in our visible world.

General principles of receptors and senses

A 'sense' is a faculty by which the body receives information about its internal and external environments. A sense does not necessarily equate with 'sensation' or 'perception', however, as these terms refer to our capacity to be aware consciously of a change in some aspect of our environment; a conscious awareness of a stimulus is frequently not essential. A full discussion of the body's senses can be found in Clancy and McVicar (1995).

The external environment is monitored by the selective sensory receptors of the skin and our 'special sense' organs. Therefore, these receptors provide the link between what constitues the external environment (whether it be physical, social, cultural and/or spiritual) and what will be internalised into mechanisms involved in learning, memories, attention span, motivational processes and perceptions of health, pain and stress, via the conditioning and socialisation processes an individual undergoes throughout life.

The specific type of stimulus detected by a receptor is called its modality, for example touch, pressure, temperature. The properties of receptors are such that many are able to detect individual modalities and their responses only relate to the intensity of stimulation. Some receptors are polymodal and can detect different types of stimuli. Thus, vision involves the detection of light intensity (brightness) and wavelength (colour). The information we receive from such receptors comprises our 'special senses' and is vital in monitoring the world around us.

The complexity of the 'special' senses is such that the receptors are organised into sense organs – the eye, ear, nose, and tongue – which are the vital link for information from our external environment to be internalised into memories, behaviours and conditioning processes. Pain, too, is polymodal and some texts include this as a 'special' sense, although there are no pain sense 'organs' as such. Thus, specific pain centre(s) have not yet been located and the dream of some researchers of finding one pain centre which, if removed, would obliterate pain, has been abandoned (Fordham, 1986).

Receptors are transducers: they convert energy present within the stimulus (for example, heat, light, vision, sound) into electrical energy by altering the electrical properties of the receptor cell membrane. Electrical activity generated by receptors is conducted via sensory neurones to the central nervous system. The impulse eventually arrives in the brain for analysis, coordination and, if appropriate, to convey conscious perception of the stimulus. Interconnections within the brain are highly complex and much is still not understood, but findings from experimental psychology and neurology have shown that they are responsible for psychophysiological well-being (Green, 1995).

Cognitive processes, memories, etc., influence our *interpretation* of sensory information, especially in relation to how stressful our situation is. Stress and pain perception are unquantifiably assessed, since these perceptions are subjectively dependent upon one's genetic capabilities of perceiving these sensations. That is, an individual's genetic ability to produce stress and pain-producing chemicals within the body is cognitively appraised, taking into account the individual's unique environmental experiences of his and her personalised culture, gender, socialisation processes, 'intellectual' development, behavioural patterns, etc.

Of all perceptions, pain is of particular importance to health care. The next section describes the neurophysiology associated with pain perception from an integrated science viewpoint, to illustrate how individuality of our senses, and of our interpretation of those senses, can arise.

Pain: an integrated science perspective

Most people think they know what pain is and yet, from a scientific point of view, it is a state about which relatively little is known. It is difficult for researchers to agree upon a definition and further difficulties arise in developing a suitable theory to account for all the different observations that have been made (Melzak and Wall, 1990). An individual's personality, culture, anxiety level, his or her perception of the painful situation, mood, and social influence, have all been suggested to affect the perception and expression of pain. To understand how pain can be subjective necessitates more discussion than is used in most textbooks when describing this sense.

In order to perceive pain there is usually severe cellular damage or cell death, for example with a **myocardial infarction**, but this is not always the case, for example with **angina pectoris**. Cellular damage results in the release of pain-producing substances, such as histamine, bradykinin-like compounds, serotonin, lactic acid and potassium ions. Prostaglandins are also released and potentiate the effects of other pain-producing substances (Clancy and McVicar, 1998a). The substances combine with binding sites on nociceptors (receptors which respond to harmful stimuli) and are therefore the initiators of the neural transmission associated with the perception of pain following cell damage. In order to evoke a neural impulse, the interaction between pain-producing substances and nociceptors must reach threshold level, i.e. the minimal level of noxious stimulus required to initiate neural transmission. **Depolarisation** (activation) of the nociceptor membrane then occurs and a wave of depolarisation passes along the associated neurones in the form of action potentials (see Clancy and McVicar, 1995, for discussion of action potentials and nerve conduction).

Pain neurones are small diameter, myelinated fibres and smaller unmyelinated fibres, classified as A-delta and C-fibres, respectively (Figure 6.15).

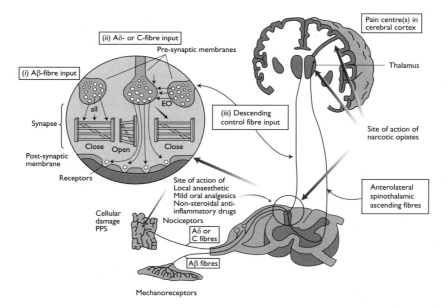

Figure 6.15: The gate control theory of pain perception and management. (i)–(iii), pre-synaptic fibres; P, substance P (excitatory neurotransmitter for transmission of pain impulse); EO, endogenous opiates (neuromodulators of pain perception); INT, inhibitory neurotransmitters; PPS, pain-producing substances.

(Source: Clancy, J. and McVicar, A.J., 1995, *Physiology and Anatomy. A Homeostatic Approach*, with kind permission of Arnold, London)

A-delta fibres comprise the 'fast' pain fibres, whereas C-fibres are 'slow' pain fibres (since faster transmission is associated with thicker fibres and the presence of a myelin sheath) and are involved in sharp, localised pain, and dull, burning, poorly localised pain, respectively (Puntillo, 1988). Nociceptors for fast pain fibres are only located in the skin and mucosal membranes, whereas those for slow pain fibres serve the skin, body tissues and organs, except brain tissue, which therefore is insensitive to painful stimuli.

Melzack and Wall's (1965; cited in Melzack and Wall, 1988) *gate control theory* of pain has become established as the major concept in pain control, and is used here as a basis for linking and integrating what others have labelled the 'sociopsychology' of pain with the 'neurophysiology' associated with pain perception.

THE GATE CONTROL THEORY

The gate control theory proposes that a gating mechanism is present within the dorsal horn of grey matter of the spinal cord, in the layer called the substantia gelatinosa, through which sensory information has to pass before it is relayed to, and perceived in, the brain. It is now generally accepted that there are gating mechanisms at each level of the spinal cord and also at several sites within the brain itself (the thalamus, reticular formation, and areas of the limbic system). The 'gates' are symbolic of junctions, or synapses, between afferent neurones and various ascending and descending tract neurones, and the theory suggests that information can only pass through when the gate is 'open' and not when the gate is 'closed' (Figure 6.15). The opening of the gate is by the release at the synapse of excitatory **neurotransmitter** chemicals. The closing of the gate is brought about by the release of other chemicals, which are inhibitory neurotransmitters and neuromodulators. Clinically, the closing of the gate forms the basis of pain relief (see Chapter 15, page 338; Clancy and McVicar, 1998b).

The gating mechanism depends upon two modifying factors – the balance of activity of afferent neurones that transmit impulses to the gate from sensory receptors, and the control provided by descending neurones from the brain's higher centres.

Balance of activity of sensory neurones The gates receive activity from a variety of receptors,

not just nociceptors. The afferent neurones which provide input to the gates of the spinal cord are:

- The fibres from nociceptors which release substance P, an excitatory neurotransmitter, at the gate. These are the A-delta and C-fibres mentioned above.
- Neurones from other receptors, such as mechanoreceptors (receptors which respond to physical stimuli, such as touch and pressure), that release inhibitory neurotransmitters at the gate. These neurones are classified as A-beta cells and are faster transmitting than those from nociceptors.

If the dominant input to the gate is from the mechanoreceptors, then the gate will close due to the release and action of the inhibitory neurotransmitters. This modifying influence is thought to be the mechanism that relieves pain when the painful area is gently rubbed, massaged or touched, since the mechanoreceptors are stimulated by the contact (Tempest, 1990). According to Melzack and Wall (1988) the application of transcutaneous electrical nerve stimulation, sometimes abbreviated as TENS or TNS, and acupuncture also operate via this method.

By contrast, if the dominant input to the gate is from the pain fibres, the gate may be open and the patient may then perceive pain. Pain perception will still only occur, however, if there is no interference from descending fibres from higher centres within the central nervous system.

Descending control from higher centres The gate control theory proposes that, even if pain fibre input into the central nervous system dominates, the gate may still be closed since higher brain centres (in the brain stem and cerebral cortex) can modify the gating process via neurones that descend to influence neural transmission to or within the brain. These neurones release a variety of opiate chemicals (endorphins, enkephalins and dynorphins) which are the body's own natural 'pain killers'. When released, these neuromodulators may close the gate by inhibiting the release of substance P (see Figure 6.15). Opioid analgesics, such as morphine, act in the same way.

The descending route of pain control forms the psychophysiological basis of distraction and diversion therapies, counselling and the **placebo effect** (Melzack and Wall, 1988) and according to

Whipple (1990) TENS also causes the release of these endogenous opiates.

SUBJECTIVITY OF PAIN

Clearly, there are biological processes involved in the perception of pain, but pain is also a subjective experience, since each individual has a unique range of integrative anatomical, physiological, social, and psychological identities.

Anatomical subjectivity A tremendous variation in human body shapes and sizes exists and it is not surprising, therefore, that the distribution of nociceptors varies between individuals, and hence, in sensitivity to stimuli.

Biochemical and physiological subjectivity Individuals have different production capacities of the biochemicals involved in the transmission of pain, since the person's genotype is responsible for their synthesis. For example, if the genes responsible for the synthesis of pain-producing substances or substance P were mutated or repressed, or the nociceptors become desensitised to them, then it would be possible to experience tissue injury without perceiving pain. Alternatively, people may not report pain, despite tissue damage, if the genes necessary for the production of the inhibitory neurotransmitters and/or endogenous opiates (neuromodulators) are repeatedly expressed, since their high levels would close the gate. Conversely, high levels of pain-producing substances, and consequently substance P, or low levels of inhibitory neurotransmitters and/or endogenous opiates, would lead to pain hypersensitivity. Congenital disorders of pain perception do exist and thus some people are born insensitive to pain, whilst others feel pain without any detectable injury (Melzack and Wall, 1988). Degrees between these two extremes are also likely.

Sociopsychological subjectivity Social factors arising from the development of cultural and spiritual beliefs, and experiences throughout an individual's lifetime, influence the development of the brain and so modify the descending control of the pain gates. Exogenous cues such as hypnosis, distraction, imagery, placebos, conditioning, and biofeedback, can also promote the blocking of transmission of many unwanted stimuli, therefore preventing their perception.

For example, elevated anxiety levels are associated with an increased pain perception (Seers, 1987). The gate control theory would explain this as resulting from depressed endogenous opiate levels, or from increased substance P release; the former is most likely, according to descending control theory. Whichever the case, Sofaer (1983) argued that nursing care should aim to reduce the patient's anxiety before attempting to quantify the pain that he/she is perceiving. Perhaps, then, an appropriate nursing action might be just to empathise, sit and support the patient in pain, since this physical assurance can have analgesic qualities (see Chapter 15, page 354). The health care professional should also be familiar with cultural differences when reducing the patient's anxiety prior to assessing the appropriate care to be implemented.

The importance or meaning of a situation can also affect perception of pain. Thus, when a patient enters hospital (particularly as an emergency) pre-admission pain can seem almost unbearable, whereas post-admission interviews indicate that the pain may have lessened or even disappeared. Although this could be attributed to decreased anxiety, it is also the case that stress and trauma are powerful stimuli for opiate release. Such findings demonstrate how environmental factors, such as the clinical setting, presence of doctors and nurses, and unfamiliar or high technology equipment, may influence gene activity and subsequent opiate release, with the result that pain perception is reduced. This is also a likely explanation for the apparent lack of awareness of injury in instances such as road traffic accidents.

The discussion of the subjectivity of a patient's past experiences, personality typing, social class, and gender in relation to pain are covered in further detail in Chapter 15 and the reader is directed to this chapter for a full description of pain assessment and its management. It is sufficient to note here that pain and nursing are inextricably linked because assessment and management of the pain process is one of the more common roles of the nurse. The measurement of pain, however, is a contentious and controversial issue with debate from two schools of thought. One school believes that pain measurement is necessary and feasible, whilst the alternative view is that pain experiences can never be measured because of its subjective nature (Puntillo, 1988). In addition, there are many pain therapies, and it is hoped that in reading this section the reader will be aware that any pain therapy is only effective if it is adapted to the patient's subjective needs and individualised environment.

Summary

Gene–environment ('nature–nurture') interactions

- Gene–environment interactions can be identified in disorders of both mental and physical health.
- In mental health, genes provide the cellular structures and chemistry necessary for brain functioning. How the cells operate, and interact with other brain cells, is influenced by the social environment, mainly during childhood but also for much of the lifespan.
- The use of pharmacological and psychological therapies in disorders of mental health provides evidence for the nature and nurture components. The term 'psychophysiological well-being' would provide better recognition of this.
- Numerous examples are available to illustrate the role of genes and the environment in physical health, as evidenced by current health education recommendations.

Gene–environment interactions in sensory perceptions

- Sensory receptors provide the means by which the body monitors its internal and external environments. How that information is perceived is affected by socialisation and cultural influences.
- Pain perception provides an example of how sensory perception can be highly subjective.
- The physiology of pain is increasingly explained by reference to the 'gate control theory'. This theory suggests that the neural transmission of information to the brain is influenced by factors within and outside the central nervous system.
- The subjective element in pain assessment and control highlights the genetic and environmental interactions that contribute to this phenomenon.

SECTION C: SYSTEMS THEORY AND HOMEOSTASIS: A MODEL FOR INTEGRATION

The role of nursing care to restore a patient's homeostatic status, and the identification of homeostatic principles within the nursing process, highlight two important aspects in relation to the promotion of homeostasis.

First, psychophysiological parameters are influenced by extrinsic factors (see Chapter 8 for discussion of interactionist theory; see also Figure 6.2). In other words, the external environment acts to induce internal change. Health and homeostasis can only be maintained if the body can respond to such forces.

Second, the factors that promote a change to the internal environment can be influenced by the degree to which they themselves are capable of changing, and to which they act on the individual. In this way, lifestyles can have important implications for health (see Chapter 8 for discussion of life events and daily hassle scales) and clinical therapies can have beneficial (or even adverse) effects. Health education and promotion is aimed at encouraging individuals to adopt a lifestyle which does not compromise homeostatic processes (see Chapter 4). However, what constitutes the ideal lifestyle is transitional, depending upon the most recent influential research data.

The recognition that the body interacts with the external (social, physical, cultural and spiritual) environment is founded within *systems theory*, which views all things, living or not, as components of a wider whole. The theory has been around for many years and Rapaport (1968) provides the following definition of a system:

> 'A whole which functions as a whole by virtue of the interdependence of its parts is called a system.'

Systems can be closed (for example a chemical reaction occurring within a confined and regulated environment, such as a cell's **mitochondria**) or open. Human beings are considered to be 'open' systems as they interact freely with their (physical and social) environment. Pearson *et al.* (1996) noted the properties characteristic of an open system:

- Every order of systems, except the smallest, has a subsystem.
- All but the largest have suprasystems.
- Every system has an arbitrary boundary which distinguishes it from its environment.
- The environment of a system is everything external or internal to its boundary. The envi-

ronment may be immediate or distantly removed.

Systems theory views boundaries as being 'permeable' so that each level interacts with the one below or above it. This interaction between levels means that living systems have a tendency to vary and so move to a greater degree of heterogeneity. The important term here is 'tendency': a system can counteract change provided that certain conditions are met. In other words, a steady state can be maintained, or the change controlled, in spite of continuous interaction with other systems. In order to negate this tendency for heterogeneity, living systems must operate using feedbacks by detecting change and promoting an appropriate response of the appropriate magnitude – in other words by utilising a homeostatic process.

If we view the human body as a system, then sub- and suprasystems can be identified (Figure 6.16). Thus, organs comprise body subsystems, and these, in turn, are composed of further subsystems, that is, tissues and cells. Cells are comprised of organelles, and these consist of chemical molecules and ions. The individual lives within an immediate social suprasystem comprising the family unit/peers/work. These, in turn, have a position within the larger suprasystems that comprise the local and wider communities.

From the nursing point of view, the interactions with the immediate environment are of particular relevance, though the influence of the economic and political climate on that environment is also recognised as a source of illness. This chapter has demonstrated that nursing should view the psychophysiological characteristics of the individual as the net result of the genetic make-up of that individual and environmental influences on gene expression (see Figure 6.2). The application of this, however, requires a definition of 'environment'. If one takes a broad view that it represents the physical, chemical, social, emotional and spiritual circumstances in which the individual lives, then person–environment interactions can be identified in all models of nursing (see Chapter 11, page 262, for a discussion of nursing models). Interactions will include lifestyle influences on the body. Some of these influences, for example, diet, exercise and drug misuse, are well documented and form the basis of health education programmes. Others are only poorly understood, for example, the extrinsic factors (such as stress, see Chapter 8, page 193) involved in the development of many cancers, or in 'modelling' an individual's behaviour. Health education programmes are less apparent in such instances.

One area attracting considerable attention in this interactional view of health is that of psychobiology, or 'mind–body' interactions. The cognitive analysis of situations is an important factor in how we relate to other individuals and situations (Lazarus, 1966), and the factors we use in making that analysis, such as experience and cultural norms, form a boundary between us and our environment, according to systems theory. Links with other functions (i.e. subsystems) of the body come via the voluntary and involuntary nervous systems and the hypothalamic–pituitary endocrine axis, which therefore constitute the systems boundary between the mind and body. Interactions are two-way, however. For example, sex steroid hormones have well documented influences on male and female behaviours, as does pain. The model of holism shown in Figure 6.1(b) then becomes too simplistic. Figure 6.17 is more accurate.

To put this into perspective, interactions between the individual and the external environment act to change the internal environment of that individual. This is the reason, of course, why intrinsic homeostatic processes are so important, since they prevent those changes from becoming destabilising. In preventing or reversing the

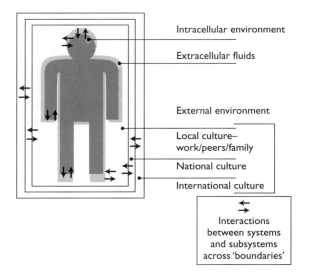

Intracellular environment

Extracellular fluids

External environment

Local culture–work/peers/family

National culture

International culture

Interactions between systems and subsystems across 'boundaries'

Figure 6.16: A simplistic view of systems theory and health (Reproduced from McVicar and Clancy, 1998, with permission)

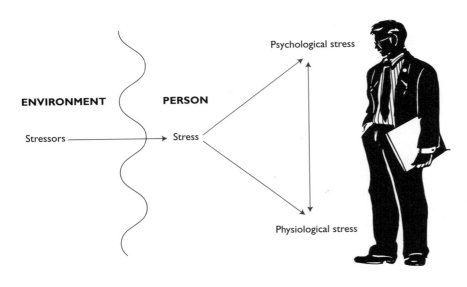

Figure 6.17: An interactional model of holism (Reproduced from McVicar and Clancy, 1998, with permission)

effects of extrinsic influences on the internal environment, nurses are demonstrating homeostasis in action. In fact, we can identify processes analogous to homeostasis at all system levels, even, for example, in government socio-economic policies, directed (we are told) at maintaining and even promoting the well-being of society.

Homeostatic principles, therefore, pervade our lives. The environmental changes that we experience from day to day are stressors which have the potential to induce internal stresses by altering the internal environment.

Whether or not we are able to maintain psychophysiological equilibrium in the face of such stressors is highly subjective for a variety of reasons, including the developmental stage of the individual. Recognising this helps us to appreciate the individualistic nature of health and health care. Systems theory, and homeostasis, therefore, provide a working framework in which to view the health–ill health continuum, and nursing care can be directly related to it.

lifestyle) can be considered as a system or group of systems that interact with the body's internal environments. These latter form the subsystems of the body. Interactions can be viewed as occurring across the 'boundaries' between these systems and subsystems.

- Changes in one system will have implications for those systems with which it forms a boundary. The unique genetic make-up, and the unique upbringing of the individual, determines the stability of the boundaries and this helps to explain where subjectivity arises from.
- Holism can be directly related to systems theory by relating the implications of systems interactions for health. Thus, social practices act to provide some stability in the immediate external environment, whilst homeostatic processes enable us to counteract the effects on the internal environment of any changes that do occur. A failure to do so will alter the state of health and may even precipitate ill health.

Summary

- Interactions can be identified between our external environment and physical and mental functioning. Mind–body interactions are also identifiable and the division of medicine into mental and physical medicine is somewhat artificial.
- Systems theory provides the framework for integrating these life sciences.
- Our environment (culture, peers, family, work,

CHAPTER SUMMARY

The philosophy of holistic care underpins nurse education, but one fundamental point should always be remembered – humans are biological organisms. That is to say, the basic construct of the individual is one of cells, tissues and organs, the functions of which are determined by the genetic make-up of that person. However, genes and gene expression are susceptible to changes in the internal environment and much of our physiological functioning relates to the maintenance of an optimal environment for cellular functions, in other words, to the maintenance of homeostasis. There will, of course, be a genetic basis to those physiological functions, involving the coordinating systems of the body: the endocrine and neural systems. These two systems interact with each other according to our perceptions of the internal and external environments to promote health and development. By their nature, these environments are always changing and our psychophysiological well-being will therefore depend to a large extent on how we perceive change and how we respond to it. Recognising sociocultural influences on neural functions (i.e. neural cells and their interactions), and the effects of diet and environmental interactions to influence the composition of the internal environment, forms the basis of holism and an integrated approach to health care.

People interact with their environment throughout life and it is the interactions between lifestyle and gene expression that are determinants of health and ill health. Academic debate continues regarding the relative role of genes and the environment in developmental processes, health, illness and the subjective perception of pain and stress. That they each have a role is no longer questioned and current thinking argues that it is not enough to consider factors in isolation and ascribe a relative value to their importance in shaping the individual. Whilst it is true that such interactions are poorly understood at present, the continuing identification of genes, and an increased understanding of how they function, are extending the frontiers of medical and health science and seem likely to influence future therapies, approaches to holistic care and health promotion strategies. Nurse educators, practitioners, staff and students should recognise that physical and mental health disorders are not simply physiological, psychological or sociological in origin: physical and mental functioning are strongly interrelated and both are susceptible to extrinsic influences. Although there is a need for health care professionals to understand the principles of each of these sciences, a failure to emphasise their interactions as determinants of health and ill health perpetuates divisions within medicine and acts as a barrier to the aims of holistic care.

ACKNOWLEDGEMENTS

The authors would like to thank our publishers, Arnold (London) for their kind permission to adapt illustrative material produced from our textbook: Clancy, J. and McVicar, A. (1995). *Physiology and Anatomy. A Homeostatic Approach.*

Much appreciation also goes to David Knock, Media Technician, University of East Anglia, for adapting the aforementioned figures and for aid in generating original illustrations.

REFERENCES

Akinsanya, J. (1987). The life sciences in nurse education. In *Nurse Education: Research and Developments*, Davis, B. (ed.). Croom Helm, London.

Bergemann, C.S., Chipuer, H.M., Plomin, R. *et al.* (1993). Genetic and environmental effects on openness, agreeableness, and conscientiousness: an adoption/twin study. *Journal of Personality and Social Psychology*, 61(2), 159–79.

Billings, P.R., Beckwith, J. and Alper, J.S. (1992). The genetic analysis of human behaviour: a new era? *Social Science and Medicine*, 35(3), 227–38.

Brischetto, C.S., Connor, W.E., Connor, S.L. and Matarozzo, J.D. (1983). Plasma lipid and lipoprotein profiles of cigarette smokers from randomly selected families: enhancement of hyperlipidaemia and depression of high density lipoprotein. *American Journal of Cardiology*, 52, 675–9.

Cannon, W.B. (1932). *The Wisdom of the Body.* Norton, New York.

Carlson, N.R. (1986). *Physiology of Behaviour.* Allyn and Bacon Inc., Boston, USA.

Cefalo, R. and Moos, M-K. (1995). *Preconception Health Care. A Practical Guide.* Mosby, London.

Clancy, J. and McVicar, A.J. (1992). The subjectivity of pain. *British Journal of Nursing*, 1(1), 8–12.

Clancy, J. and McVicar, A.J. (1993). Subjectivity of stress. *British Journal of Nursing*, 2(8), 410–17.

Clancy, J. and McVicar, A.J. (1994a). Circadian rhythms I: physiology. *British Journal of Nursing*, 3(13), 657–61.

Clancy, J. and McVicar, A.J. (1994b). Circadian rhythms II: shift work and health. *British Journal of Nursing*, 3(14), 712–17.

Clancy, J. and McVicar, A.J. (1995). *Physiology and Anatomy. A Homeostatic Approach.* Arnold, London.

Clancy, J. and McVicar, A.J. (1996). Homeostasis: the key concept to physiological control. *British Journal of Theatre Nursing*, 6(2), 17–24.

Clancy, J. and McVicar, A.J. (1997). Hypoxia as a failure of respiratory homeostasis. *British Journal of Theatre Nursing*, 6(10), 15–20.

Clancy, J. and McVicar, A.J. (1998a). Homeostasis. The key concept in physiological studies. Neurophysiology of pain. *British Journal of Theatre Nursing* (in press).

Clancy, J. and McVicar, A.J. (1998b). Homeostasis. The key concept in physiological studies. Perioperative pain management. A gate control perspective. *British Journal of Theatre Nursing* (in press).

Cox, T. (1978). *Stress*, 2nd edn. Macmillan, London.

Criqui, M.H. (1986). Epidemiology of atherosclerosis: an updated overview. *American Journal of Cardiology*, 57(5), 18C–23C.

Davey, S.S., McCance, K.L. and Budd, M.C. (1994). Alterations of pulmonary function. In *Pathophysiology. The Biologic Basis for Disease in Adults and Children*, McCance, K.L. and Huether, S.E. (eds), 2nd edn. Mosby Year Book Inc, St Louis, USA.

Department of Health (1995). *The Genetics of Common Diseases. A Second Report to the NHS Central Research and Development Committee on the New Genetics.* Department of Health Publications, London.

Fordham, M. (1986). Neurophysiological pain theories. *Nursing*, 10, 360–4.

Gilbert, P. (1992). *Depression. The Evolution of Powerlessness.* Lawrence Erlbaum Associates, Hove, UK.

Green, S. (1995). *Principles of Biopsychology.* Lawrence Erlbaum Associates, Hove, UK.

Groden, J., Thliveris, A., Samowitz, W. *et al.* (1991). Identification of the familial adenomatous polyposis coli gene. *Cell*, 66, 589–600.

Harman, D. (1956). Ageing: a theory based on free-radical and radiation chemistry. *Journal of Gerontology*, 11, 298–300.

Henderson, B.E., Ross, R.K. and Pike, M.C. (1991). Toward the primary prevention of cancer. *Cancer Science*, 254, 1131–7.

Huether, S.E. and Andrews, M.M. (1994). Alterations of pulmonary function in children. In *Pathophysiology. The Biologic Basis for Disease in Adults and Children*, McCance, K.L. and Huether, S.E. (eds), 2nd edn. Mosby Year Book Inc, St Louis, USA.

Inoff-Germain, G., Arnold, G.S., Nottlemann, E.D. *et al.* (1988). Relations between hormone levels and observational measures of aggressive behaviour of young adolescents in family interactions. *Developmental Psychology*, 24, 129–39.

Jordan, S. (1994). Should nurses be studying bioscience? A discussion paper. *Nurse Education Today*, 14, 417–26.

Kendler, K.S. and Diehl, S.R. (1993). The genetics of schizophrenia: a current genetic–epidemiologic perspective. *Schizophrenia Bulletin*, 19(2), 261–85.

Lazarus, R.S. (1966). *Psychological Stress and Coping Processes.* McGraw-Hill, New York.

McGuffin, P. and Thapar, A. (1992). The genetics of personality disorder. *British Journal of Psychiatry*, 160, 12–23.

McVicar, A.J. and Clancy, J. (1998). Health in the balance. A framework for integrating the life sciences. *British Journal of Nursing* (in press).

Melzack, R. and Wall, P.D. (1988). *The Challenge of Pain.* Penguin, Harmondsworth.

Melzack, R. and Wall, P.D. (1990). *Textbook of Pain.* Churchill Livingstone, Edinburgh.

Morris, J.B. and Beck, A.T. (1974). The efficacy of antidepressant drugs. A review of research 1958–72. *Archives of General Psychiatry*, 30, 667–74.

Mowry, B.J. and Levinson, D.F. (1993). Genetic linkage and schizophrenia: methods, recent findings and future directions. *Australian and New Zealand Journal of Psychiatry*, 27(2), 200–18.

Orgel, L.E. (1963). The maintenance of accuracy of protein synthesis and its relevance to ageing. *Proceedings of the National Academy of Sciences, USA*, 49, 5117–21.

Pearson, A., Vaughan, B. and Fitzgerald, M. (1996). *Nursing Models for Practice.* Butterworth Heinemann, Oxford.

Puntillo, K.A. (1988). The phenomenon of pain and critical care nursing. *Heart and Lung*, 17(3), 262–73.

Radford, J. and Hollin, C. (1991). Intelligence. In *A Textbook of Psychology*, Radford, J. and Govier, E. (eds), 2nd edn. Routledge, London/New York.

Rapaport, A. (1968). In *Modern Systems Research for the Behavioural Scientist*, Buckley, W. (ed.). Aldine, New York.

Rehm, L.P. (1995). Psychotherapies for depression. In *Anxiety and Depression in Adults and Children*, Craig, K.D. and Dobson, K.S. (eds). Century Croft, Norwalk, USA.

Ross, R. (1992). The pathogenesis of atherosclerosis. In *Heart Disease: a Textbook of Cardiovascular Medicine*,

Braumwald, D. (ed.), 4th edn. Saunders, Philadelphia.

Seers, K. (1987). Perceptions of pain. *Nursing Times*, 83, 37–9.

Selye, H. (1976). *Stress in Health and Disease*. Butterworth, London.

Sofaer, B. (1983). Pain relief – the core of nursing practice. *Nursing Times* 79(47), 38–42.

Swallow, S.R. and Segal, Z.V. (1995). Cognitive–behavioural therapy for unipolar depression. In *Anxiety and Depression in Adults and Children*, Craig, K.D. and Dobson, K.S. (eds.). Century Croft, Norwalk, USA.

Tempest, S. (1990). Pain and pain control. 3. Treatment considerations. In *Current Practice in Pharmacy and Therapeutics*, Volume 3, Number 8. Medical Tribune, London.

Trnobranski, P.H. (1993). Biological sciences and the nursing curriculum: a challenge for educationalists. *Journal of Advanced Nursing*, 18, 493–9.

Whipple, B. (1990). Neurophysiology of pain. *Orthopaedic Nursing*, 9(4), 21–32.

Williams, R.R. (1994). Genes and environmental interaction: familial diseases. In *Pathophysiology. The Biologic Basis for Disease in Adults and Children*, McCance, K.L. and Huether, S.E. (eds), 2nd edn. Mosby Year Book Inc, St Louis, USA.

Willner, P. (1985). *Depression. A Psychological Synthesis*. John Wiley & Sons, New York.

Wong, D.T., Bymaster, F.P. and Engelman, E.A. (1995). Prozac, the first serotonin-inhibitor and an antidepressant drug: twenty years since its first publication. *Life Science*, 57(5), 411–41.

Yarbro, J.W. (1992). Oncogenes and tumour-suppressor genes. *Seminars in Oncology Nursing*, 8(1), 30–9.

FURTHER READING

Clancy, J. and McVicar, A.J. (1995). *Physiology and Anatomy. A Homeostatic Approach*. Arnold, London.

This book's special features are that it provides a unique homeostatic approach, which views health as an ongoing process of physiological balance. An integrated science perspective is discussed to key areas of pain, stress, developmental milestones and circadian rhythms.

Clancy, J. and McVicar, A.J. (eds) (1998). *Nursing Care. A Homeostatic Casebook*. Arnold, London.

The editors have specifically developed this book to address the learning needs of nurses who need to apply their knowledge of homeostasis to the nursing care they provide. A wide range of case studies have been taken from the four branches of the Diploma in Nursing (Adult, Child, Mental Health and Learning Disabilities). All of these case studies provide details of symptoms, identify the homeostatic disturbance and show how the clinical intervention and nursing care are aimed at restoring homeostasis.

Cooper, N., Stevenson, C. and Hale, G. (eds) (1996). *Integrating Perspectives on Health*. Open University Press, Buckingham.

This book addresses the issue of the biopsychosocial model of health and is particularly useful for health care professionals who are taught about health and illness in terms of biological, psychological and social factors.

Green, S. (1995). *Principles of Biopsychology*. Lawrence Erlbaum Associates, Hove, UK.

This publication is ideal for students with little background in psychology. It covers the physiological basis of sensations (such as vision), perceptions (such as pain) and motivation (such as hunger) in a simple and comprehensive manner.

Grokr, M.E. and Edith, M. (1989). *Basic Pathophysiology: a Holistic Approach*. Mosby, London.

This book focuses on key concepts such as pain and stress from a holistic viewpoint. It incoporates mind–body interactions in determining health, ill health and restoring the wellness for the patient.

Hall, L.L. (ed.) (1996). *Genetics and Mental Illness: Evolving Issues for Research and Society*. Plenum Press, New York.

This is a collection of essays which focuses on psychiatric genetics. Contributions are from a diverse background in mental health practice.

CHAPTER SEVEN

COMMUNICATING *for* HEALTH

Paul Barber

- Introduction
- Communication: core qualities
- Health: a definition
- Communicating with the self: the role of personal growth
- Developing the self so as to enhance communication
- Becoming a self-creating person: the first duty of a care communicator
- The 'how' of communication: intervention analysis
- Learning from mistakes
- Supervision: care communication by example
- Epilogue

This chapter aims to raise awareness of the dynamics and skills of therapeutic or health-focused communication, with a view to exploring and raising the reader's awareness of:

- How the individual, their attitudes and emotional presence manifest themselves in communication
- Health, what this means and how it informs care communication
- The relationship of personal development to the 'art of communication'
- Intervention analysis, and how we might set about identifying our own communication style
- Professional supervision, and how this can be structured to develop further our ability to demonstrate care through communication.

'I fall far short of achieving real communication – person-to-person – all the time, but moving in this direction makes life for me a warm, exciting, upsetting, troubling, satisfying, enriching, and above all a worthwhile venture.'

(Rogers *et al.*, 1967, page 275)

INTRODUCTION

Periodically within this chapter I offer a critique of professional practice and have set activities entitled 'reflections' to stimulate you into questioning your own clinical practice and professional traditions. Consider for instance, the implications of communication in context of the quote below:

'What is wrong is not the great discoveries of science – information is always better than ignorance, no matter what information or what ignorance. What is wrong is the belief behind the information, the belief that information will change the world. It won't. Information without human understanding is like an answer without a question – meaningless. And human understanding is only possible through the arts. It is the work of art that creates the human perspective in which information turns to truth. . . .'

(Archbishop MacLeish; quoted in BBC radio broadcast, 1991)

This chapter is not about how to communicate. It does not attempt to change you and I doubt if I can teach you anything new. What I am attempting to do is to share with you, to inform you how I view the world and to ask you to consider how my understanding might contribute to your own store of experiential wisdom. This is the essence of good communication, which is educative, challenging of collusion, informative, supportive of self and others, and inviting rather than political. What I communicate is essentially my life experience, bits of me, my values and perceptions created through previous interaction.

What I attempt to communicate in this chapter is a summary of learning gleaned from some 30 years as a care professional. As for the information presented here, I hope you will adopt it for your own use and create something worthwhile from the insights expressed. As I believe we communicate who and what we are in all we do, and because I see the world largely through humanistic spectacles, I emphasise the part personal development plays in communication. Having been bored to death by books that try to reduce communication to a science, I emphasise the 'art' of communication and the role intuition plays in this. In order to provide a framework for self-appraisal, I have also included something on intervention analysis which is less a science than a means of self-assessment and a clarifier of communicative intention, along with occasional activities called 'reflections' so that you can apply insights from this chapter to yourself and to clinical practice. I have also included a little on supervision as an example of how you might further develop your ability to demonstrate care through communication.

Where possible, I offer a critique of nursing practice and its professional traditions:

'Traditions are a splendid thing, but we should create traditions, not live by them.'

(Franz Marc, in Rogers *et al.*, 1967, page 115)

Enquire into yourself and constantly question your own motives, share of yourself, stay curious and respectful of the human condition – and endeavour to communicate this to others, and as long as you have ability to ask for and receive care yourself, I will have little doubt in your skills to communicate care.

COMMUNICATION: CORE QUALITIES

'Knowledge is a function of being. When there is a change in the being of the knower, there is a corresponding change in the nature and amount of knowledge.'

(Aldous Huxley, in Goldberg, 1989, page 135)

Professional development and personal development rest one upon the other. Because care communication is an expression of self, professional helpers need to stay alert to how they, as individuals, offer support to their clients and value the human condition, in short, how they practise the caring arts. In the last analysis the carer's therapeutic use of self underpins care communication. In essence, I believe nursing care is about creating a relationship with the client whereby he/she begins to heal him/herself. For this to happen within the nurse–client relationship, contact, change and communication must be related.

Reflections on the relationship of contact, change and health

- Contact involves the direction of attention, perception, receptivity and empathy towards another. This requires us to let go of our preconceptions and open ourselves up to the enquiry of others. In short, we need to clear and clean the psychological window through which we view the world. Good contact occurs when two people are able to explore each other's reality, see the other and listen to the whole of him/her – while engaging in turn with the whole of him/herself. In the Chinese character that represents 'listening', the heart is also portrayed. When I am fully attuned to another, it is as if I meditate upon him/her while allowing my mind, senses, feelings and intuitions to form an integral 'sense' of him/her. My listening, to be effective, must have heart.

■ Change concerns letting go of the past, exploring the present and risking the future. It involves treating life experimentally and having courage, courage to face up to what does not work in your life and to let old patterns go. As Kierkegaard remarks:

'Life can only be understood backwards; but it must be lived forwards.'

(Kierkegaard, in Rogers *et al.*, 1967, page 167)

For us to live our life in a forward way and to engage the reality of that continuum we call 'health', we must learn to make 'change' a friend, for change is essential to health:

'Health is not an absence of physical or mental dis-ease, nor the experience of continuous physical and mental well-being. It is rather all of these; an ability to move fluidly from one state of being to another. Health is thus an endless flow of changes.'

(Young, 1990)

■ Communication is about sharing and self-understanding. If we have not yet begun to understand ourselves – what of ourselves can we share? Practice is important to communicate efficiently; being aware of those complicated experiences that resonate in our inner world and finding words to express this is essential if communication is to have effect:

'I reject any organized pretence to an objective knowledge of man. I know only what I sweat from my own personal struggle to stay alive. Psychotherapy is not a professional routine. It is a personal venture. The client is "like me". I reject any professional boundary between us. I "make it" as a person or I fail.'

(Richard Johnson, in Rogers *et al.*, 1967, page 67)

■ Good communication, I find, is able to transmit the intimate reality of one person to another, develops a channel along which trust and understanding flow, is relevant to what is happening now, and evokes the creative energy of those involved. Besides being core ingredients of the care relationship, contact, change and communication are the goals of nurse–client interaction and criteria of health.

HEALTH: A DEFINITION

'He [the infant] would laugh at our concern over values, if he could understand it. How could anyone fail to know what he liked or disliked, what was good for him and what was not?'

(Barry Stevens, in Rogers *et al.*, 1967, page 29)

Health, in this chapter, is regarded as a positive quality of well-being, the ability to move in the direction of self-actualisation, to take creative risks and trust in yourself. It is seen to require personal and interpersonal competency. Health is thus an adventure, a state of mind where problems are seen as challenges, symptoms are guides to our lifestyle, and emotions are energies we engage through the act of living. Health is thus the search after our own fullness of being and our ability to relate this to others. In this context, preoccupation with health is not healthy. Health is not a medicated condition nor the building of sanitised defences against the world – this is nearer a fight for survival. Health is an ability to adapt, risk, and to welcome change, rather than a concept to be defined. Health is dynamic; to hold it still long enough for definition is to kill it.

Simply, health is for the joy of it – the creative energy underpinning our ability to grow. Generally, health education has looked at the tasks but missed the processes. The caring professions often echo this, controlling the care environment rather than enriching the individual's potential. Concentration upon disjunction by carers has tended to lead to client care being seen as problematic. It is not by accident that nursing models which emphasise systematic problem solving and task performance have displaced models which attend more centrally to the therapeutic relationship. This is a comment on our professional times and their bias towards a pseudo-scientific rationale.

Reflections upon the nature of health

Personally, I feel much of health education has remained all too mechanical and tended towards:

■ Servicing the body machine
■ Knowing the best foods to feed it
■ Knowing how best to keep it clean
■ Preventing bad habits or curing ill health.

This cognitive, task-orientated approach to health leaves little room for emotional, intuitive or spiritual components of care. The individual's potential for 'personal growth' has all too often played but a little part in modern care practices.

How near is the above definition to the one:

- You operate from?
- Are professionally expected to address?
- Were originally taught?

COMMUNICATING WITH THE SELF: THE ROLE OF PERSONAL GROWTH

'The only dimension of life over which you have limited control is the length. By putting your attention on what you do to extend your life, you can utilize the potential you have for its duration. But be aware that every day you control the depth and width of your experience, your life.'

(Benares, 1985, page 64)

Much of nursing care, though it may be task centred, involves intuitive nurturing and a good deal of self-investment. Because care has more to do with quality than quantity, i.e. what transpires being generally more important than how often it happens, care communication depends more than anything else upon the nature of the nurse–client relationship. Because it is primarily an art, care communication may all too often be professionally labelled as unscientific and as undefinable. When they step out from their role of a 'hands-on' practitioner into the cold light of professional assessment alongside other professionals, many expert nursing practitioners find it difficult to convey what they do.

Traditionally, nurses were not taught the appropriate language to decode interpersonal behaviour – much of which is intuitive – into intellectual terms. The essence of what constitutes care in professional communication has thus tended to be lost.

Although courses leading to registration have recommended an injection of a good deal of science and cognition into care practice in order to remedy role insecurity, the expressive arts of care, which are hard to reference, have tended to remain in the hearts of expert carers. Theories can be taught; attitudes need to be experienced and lived. When a person moves more fluidly between the external universe and the one within him/herself, he/she acquires increased self-understanding and is better equipped to communicate and liberate insight in others.

Personally, I view myself as an evolving organism who, by application of will and consciousness, has the potential to grow in any direction. This potential I see as limited by the choices I allow myself, by what I decide are the fixed boundaries of my behaviour, and by the cultural reality I personally ascribe to. I increase or decrease myself via the tightness of these symbolic boundaries I impose upon myself.

When I start to explore, question and define 'who I am', 'what I do' and 'where I am going', I begin to draw boundaries around myself. The wider I draw these boundaries, the more options I allow myself. The wider I draw my personal boundaries, the richer my potential life experience and personal range.

'Personal growth' can now be seen as an extra, formed from and upon the evolving edge of experience. It is what we gain when we push our boundaries of self a little further out, risk stepping beyond convention – without causing harm to ourselves or others – and when we allow ourselves to experience a little growing pain.

Reflections upon the 'I', my 'culture' and 'personal growth'

Who am I?

- I   My individual self, a continually moving, evolving and changing sense of identity which I invest in my personality, an individually created persona through which I express my consciousness.

What do I do?

- Culture   The medium through which I relate to others, a source of containment and safety, a boundary and provider of language and social reality, the media through which I express myself.

Where am I going?

- Personal growth   The positive dovetailing of myself with my social reality so as to maximise my integration with the whole, my relationship with life, my joyful expression of health, spiritual aspirations and acceptance of universal laws: the seasons, birth, a time to live and a time to die.

DEVELOPING THE SELF SO AS TO ENHANCE COMMUNICATION

'What's to say? I have a feeling that everybody knows everything so far as human interaction goes, and that we only choose to ignore or to forget.'

(Shlien, in Rogers *et al.*, 1967, page 275)

I believe in the last analysis it is the quality of the person, rather than their skills, that elevates professional communication to excellence of care. Such qualities of person do not arise spontaneously from within; they are rather the product of a good deal of uncovering, self-exploration, personal reflection and intrapersonal development. Personal growth and professional development here go hand in hand.

Care communication does not really concern itself with training, nor with moulding or teaching the client what to do nor how to do it. This is nearer propaganda. A truly proficient care communicator would never dream of imposing his/her process upon a client or inducing that client towards imitation of him/herself. Care communication is more to do with unfolding. It is directed towards enabling a client to recover him/herself so that he/she may further self-explore with a view to knowing him/herself better. When we turn to Carl Rogers (1983) for guidance on what we need in order to be more appreciative, self-aware, socially sensitive and valuing of others as communicators of care, he suggests that we need to move away from:

■ Facades, pretence and putting up a front
■ Rigid concepts of 'what ought to be'
■ Meeting the expectations of others for the sake of 'having to please'
■ Pretence and the hiding of feelings.

And that we should seek within to gain greater:

■ Self-direction
■ Positive feelings towards oneself
■ Sensitivity to external events
■ Openness with regard to our inner reactions and feelings.

I have observed that when we acquire these qualities in ourselves, other subtle effects emerge which in turn affect others. We have less need to defend our routines or impose our beliefs, and develop greater tolerance towards the failings of those around us. As we become sensitive to our own inner (intrapersonal) process, we find we can better listen and attend to the inner world of those around us. Good contact and communication with others we find to be nourishing, and in realising this begin to value deep, honest and communicative relationships all the more. At this stage superficial relations are no longer satisfying and we begin to move even further in the direction of sharing our emotions and inner experiences. This is essential for carers; if you are unable to share or honour your own emotional life or experiential depth, how can you value the same in others let alone help them acquire health? Movement in the direction suggested describes 'personal growth' and this, I suggest, is indicative of psychological health.

Over-conformity often blinds us and stills our questioning, suffocating our potential for growth. Almost as a reflex, we may find ourselves – as care professionals – blindly conforming to what appears to be 'the one right way'; nothing kills personal potential or growth as quickly as this. Compulsive behaviour tends towards rigidity, is repetitive and largely unaware. It is the antithesis of growth.

Many of us feel overburdened and clogged up with a host of 'shoulds' and 'musts' picked up in childhood. Professional education all too often adds more to the list. Eventually, if we aren't careful, we spend more time nursing institutional systems rather than our clients.

Changing prevailing patterns of doing things is not easy. Sometimes we come to believe, rather irrationally, that if we step out of line we will be cast out and denied love. This fear of rejection – a relic of the child within us – does much to keep us chained. We forget that by the act of being alive we have the right to be seen, to be heard, to be free, to be loved and respected; these need not be earned.

I know that I experience 'growth' when I step outside the tried and tested, the known parts of me, out beyond my usual personal boundaries, when I risk feeling uncomfortable, embarrassed and shy. Personal growth is comparable to a behavioural spiral which forever strives to conquer more of our experienced reality.

In order for us to 'grow', what is necessary, I would suggest, is an ability to move beyond our present world view, to see things differently and to extend our own personal boundaries. This requires us to forsake the 'known', to step beyond our usual behaviour patterns and engage an unfamiliar world.

Consider, for example, phases of the experiential learning cycle in the model below:

UNCONSCIOUS INCOMPETENCE

At this phase of the learning cycle, we are unaware of what it is we don't know; here ignorance is bliss and we have little incentive to engage in new activity and learning.

During this stage we might say to ourselves: 'I'm fine as I am. Why change things? It would not be me if I were to do things differently.' Often we need to be confronted with our blindness by others, if we are to move beyond this point.

CONSCIOUS INCOMPETENCE

At this stage we become aware of a deficit, a skill we as yet lack and must practise to achieve.

During this stage we recognise that though we attempt to do something we do not yet have the hang of it. Here we may say to ourselves: 'I'm trying but it doesn't feel like me doing it; I still feel very uncomfortable.' We need support and encouragement at this time.

CONSCIOUS COMPETENCE

With practice, our competence grows, we begin to recognise those gains we make and no longer feel deficient.

At this stage our skill grows but we need to concentrate to maintain it. Here we may say to ourselves: 'I can do this now, I can own this skill as my own.' We need to be trusted to monitor ourselves at this time and to make our mistakes without criticism.

UNCONSCIOUS COMPETENCE

In time our skill may become automatic, so much so that we lose awareness of what it is we do.

At this stage, we may say to ourselves: 'I know I can do this but I'm not sure how, it just comes naturally.' At this stage we need help to unpack what it is we do so we may refine the process all over again.

Placing the above in its dynamic whole, it begins to resemble a moving spiral (Figure 7.1).

Letting go of what we know to conquer something new, confronting ourselves with our resistance to learn, risking failure by letting go of the tried and trusted are all part of learning. In this context, shyness and embarrassment are growing pains and part and parcel of the process.

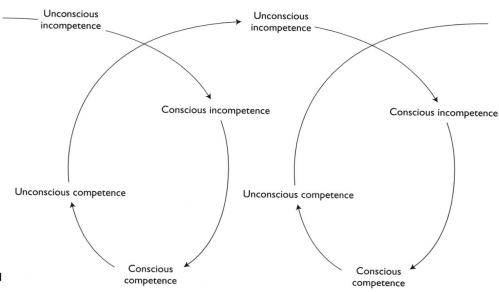

Figure 7.1

Reflection upon the quality of your own professional care

- Who am I as a care giver: how does my role infuse itself with my identity?
- Where have I come from professionally: what am I exploring at this stage of my professional career?
- Where am I going: what is my potential, the direction and purpose I am engaged with, and towards what professional goal does my vision guide me?
- What professionally frustrates me: what are the blocks, constraints and obstacles I see before me?
- How might I better progress: what steps do I need to take, what plans do I need to make, how might I prepare myself?
- Who or what might help me: what resources are available to me, what skills do I need to develop, who might assist me?
- What will it be like when I get there: my imaginative construction of what awaits me, the emotions and energies it elicits, my motivations to continue along my present path?

Consider what you have rediscovered about yourself through the above.

BECOMING A SELF-CREATING PERSON: THE FIRST DUTY OF A CARE COMMUNICATOR

'To become aware of what is happening, I must pay attention with an open mind. I must set aside my personal prejudices or bias.

Prejudiced people only see what fits these prejudices.'

(*I Ching*, 1951, page 345)

The emotional part of ourselves never really grows up. We develop many ways to contain our emotions, to understand and express them, but at root, feelings are ageless. Within us a part has remained unchanged since we were first born. We meet this part of ourselves again when we are infused with emotional energies, such as when we grieve, laugh, experience joy or excitement. A very real part of self care comes from taking time to listen to the child within us, to hear it and meet its needs.

Growth in this context describes the process of self-discovery whereby an individual learns to accept themselves and explores what it is to be a fully functioning human, while moving towards self-actualisation. This latter term requires further consideration.

Maslow (1970) equated the self-actualised person with:

- Being that self which I truly am
- Being all that I have it in me to be.

The self-actualised person was further envisaged as being able to approach life in a fresh and excited way; to view the world through the eyes of a child – with wonder and awe; to be resistant to cultural expectation – though not rebelliously so; to take a philosophical long-term view of his/her life; and as having a good sense of humour. Simply, the self-actualised person appeared to be well integrated within him/herself and able to make direct contact with reality.

Evidence from research into how the self develops (Loevinger, 1976) suggests that individuals some way along the road towards self-actualisation, who are beginning to realise their personal potential and become more integrated, tend to be better able to exhibit the following:

- Tolerance of ambiguity
- Respect for autonomy
- An ability to express feelings
- Flexibility
- Creativity
- Courage to face internal conflicts.

Such persons are well on the way to becoming what Heron (1989) describes as self-creating persons:

'Autonomous behaviour now becomes reflexive. The person becomes self-determining about the emergence of their self-determination. They consciously take in hand methods of personal and interpersonal development which enhance their capacity for voluntary choice, for becoming more intentional within all domains of experience and action.'

(Heron, 1990, page 20)

Perhaps now we are approaching an understanding of what might be called 'super-health' and where our personal potential can lead. Communicating our own 'health' by example, while helping others to uncover and develop their own human potential, is the prime goal of care communication. But how do we communicate the whole of ourselves, keeping our unravelling, receptivity and relationship to the fore while facilitating another towards our vision of health? For this a model is necessary, a conceptual framework with which to gauge where we are and what we do.

Reflections upon what to role model in health communication

Heron (1990) suggests three core intrapersonal processes are ongoing in the self-creating person:

- Unravelling: where the individual activity works on restrictions that emanate from their past, such as childhood traumas and social conditioning, undoing compulsive behaviours and raising to consciousness reflexive conventional habits.
- Receptivity: where the person attempts to become more aware about the exercise of personal choice and power, their intuition, and generally contemplates with enhanced attention what goes on around them.
- Relationship: where attention is focused upon self in relation to others, and the person recognises that personal autonomy only emerges fully in aware relationships with other autonomous persons.

How active are you, generally, in relation to the above?
Where are you strongest and where are you weakest?
In which area should the thrust of your own personal development be directed?

THE 'HOW' OF COMMUNICATION: INTERVENTION ANALYSIS

'I will not let you – or me – make me dishonest, insincere, emotionally tied up or constricted, or artificially nice and social, if I can help it.'

(Gendlin, in Rogers *et al.*, 1967, page 275)

Six Category Intervention Analysis, a device for identifying interpersonal behaviour developed by John Heron (1986), has been taught in the Human Potential Resource Group within Surrey University for three decades, refined in numerous workshops there, and widely applied to nursing (Burnard and Morrison, 1987; Morrison and

Burnard, 1988, 1989; Barber, 1997) and the supervision of carers (Barber, 1991).

Simply, Six Category Intervention Analysis describes six interventions grouped under two subheadings:

- 3 *Authoritative Interventions*: Prescriptive; Informative; Confronting.
- 3 *Facilitative Interventions*: Cathartic; Catalytic; Supportive.

A more thorough overview of these is given in Chapter 14 (Table 14.1) of this book.

In a study by Morrison and Burnard (1989) of 84 general trainees at various points in their 3-year training, findings suggested that students saw themselves most skilled in prescriptive, informative and supportive interventions, and least skilled in confronting, cathartic and catalytic ones. That nurses would benefit from more familiarity with facilitative interventions has been repeatedly suggested in the professional literature (Yura and Walsh, 1978; Marriner, 1979; McFarlane and Castledine, 1982; Barber 1996).

Professional helpers, when they come to act as guardians of their discipline and its formalised systems, have a tendency to behave in a manner reminiscent of critical and/or controlling parents, by using degenerative forms of authority to:

- 'Prescribe' what should happen
- 'Inform' clients of their decision and
- 'Confront' the client when they wish to control his/her behaviour.

Authoritative interventions, when sensitively used and underpinned with support, help to set the scene and define the context in which we relate. Used in an authoritarian rather than an appropriate and supportive person-respecting manner, they feel punitive.

Sometimes, when practitioners take it upon themselves to act as the guardians of a ward or their professional discipline, they overuse authoritative interventions.

Authoritative interventions, when used in a therapeutic way, can set safe boundaries and complement care; when used in the defensive form described in the passage above, they undergo therapeutic degeneration, to manipulate rather than help the client.

Prescriptive or directive interventions are relevant to the delegation of responsibilities and tasks;

they are necessary in climates where a good deal of direction takes place and in times of crisis. They are intended to influence and direct the behaviour of another.

Here, a practitioner may seek to advise, propose or instruct a client to perform certain tasks:

- 'Would you fill in this form for me, please?'; 'You should raise this in the meeting later'; 'Take your medication now, please'.

If overdone, such interventions cause a client to be practitioner-directed rather than self-directed and prevent the growth of self-determination, breed institutionalisation – that is, cause dependence upon systems external to the self, such as the ward and its routines – and undermine initiative and experimentation.

Informative interventions may be used to increase awareness, develop new insight and to transfer specialist knowledge. A practitioner employing these seeks to impart new information. A carer uses this kind of intervention as the primary mode of communication when he/she says:

- 'Your next appointment is for 10 o'clock, Friday next'
- 'Smokers tend to produce less healthy babies more susceptible to disease'
- 'It is common to find your sex drive reduced while taking tranquillisers'.

If overdone, such interventions may blunt self-direction and enquiry, but if left undone a client may feel at the mercy of the clinical environment and a pawn in a medico-professional game.

Confronting interventions help to identify restrictive attitudes and to bring to mind denied aspects of behaviour: for example, when you inform another of the stress he/she generates within you when he/she behaves in a specific way. These interventions challenge the restrictive attitudes, beliefs and behaviours of a client, and bring to attention unseen or avoided awarenesses; in this, they serve a consciousness-raising function. Because these interventions – though informative – are to some degree shock-inducing and communicate uncomfortable truths, they need to be well timed and especially respectful of the client. Examples of such interventions are provided below:

- 'As a drug injector you have a high risk of becoming HIV positive'

- 'You were ill advised not to come sooner; X-rays reveal a growth in your lungs'
- 'You knew what you were saying was false; why did you deceive me?'

If overdone, confronting interventions may give rise to a loss of confidence and security. They can also be perceived as punitive and attacking. If left unsaid, they foster collusion and abet denial, causing a loss of appreciation of differences and personal boundaries, and induce a sense of false security built upon avoidance of the real issues.

We must be alert to the attachment of moral correctness and/or judgemental opinions of right or wrong to authoritative interventions. They should be used in a value-free way to reap the maximum benefit. Tone of voice, posture and presence all play a part here.

Though authoritative interventions are common to professional care, facilitative ones, which honour person-centred care and the authority of the individual client, are a good deal more rare. Cathartic, catalytic and supportive interventions release emotional tensions, liberate awareness and enhance self-esteem.

Cathartic interventions encourage the release of pent-up feelings; they allow for the expressive needs of others. They encourage clients to express painful emotion and discharge bottled-up distress related to, for example, earlier anger or grief. These interventions aim to give the client permission to share and express his/her pent-up emotional energies. It is important that the practitioner pitches the interventions at a level the client is ready for and able to cope with. The nurse or midwife needs to have confidence in his/her own ability to act as an emotional container if he/she is to function successfully in this area. I offer examples of cathartic interventions below:

- 'It's fine to feel sad right now – give yourself permission to feel more'
- 'You look angry – do you have something you want to say to me?'
- 'Follow your body – let it express what it wants to do'.

Cathartic interventions need to be followed by a period of reflection, as catharsis often liberates a good deal of new insight. When pent-up emotions are released, energy is usually freed and new solutions can come rapidly to mind. Heron (1990) makes the point that culturally we are not very well prepared for the exercise of cathartic interventions, emotional control rather than release being the preferred social option in Western society. This I believe is as true of professional preparation, in that emotional energies are pushed underground in clients and carers alike, and emotional release – even in psychiatry – is seemingly viewed with suspicion and a degree of fear.

Catalytic interventions encourage self-reflection and initiate client-centred problem solving. They are used to facilitate independence, self-discovery and self-direction. For example:

- 'How might you change your lifestyle to reduce your present stress?'
- 'In what way can you modify your diet to reduce carbohydrate intake?'
- 'How might you take better care of yourself?'

Catalytic interventions are at heart educational, educating especially the client's ability to manage and change him/herself through self-generated insight. In this, catalytic interventions facilitate client-directed activity and independence and are especially appropriate before discharge from formal care, in the resolution phase of the therapeutic relationship.

Supportive interventions confirm to an individual his/her intrinsic worth and value. They affirm a client's self-image, attitudes and beliefs, actions and creations, and offer unconditional positive regard. They do not collude with a client's rigidities or defences, but rather convey intimate and authentic caring. A carer makes use of such interventions in the following ways:

- 'I feel concerned for you'
- 'I feel very touched by the way you show your appreciation'
- 'I enjoy the communication we share together'.

Sharing yourself with another, honestly saying how you feel, these are part and parcel of supportive interventions; all these undo professional distance, put the person back in the frame and honour the human condition.

Reflection Points

- Imagine three *catalytic* and three *cathartic* interventions you could make to a client who complains of feeling distressed.
- Imagine three *supportive* interventions you might make to a junior member of staff you find in tears after the death of a client he/she nursed.
- A senior colleague demands that you break off from attending to a distressed relative and orders you to help with a new admission. Reflect upon three *confronting* and three *informative* interventions you could make.
- List three *prescriptive* interventions you might make to an insensitive doctor who has just caused undue distress to a newly admitted client.
- Which interventions do you find come easily to you; which are more difficult to construct?
- For each of the six categories of interventions described, list non-verbal ways, such as touch, posture, tone of voice, attitude and manner, in which these interventions might be reinforced/portrayed; e.g. placing a hand gently on a client's shoulder to enable crying (catharsis); staying with a client when he/she is experiencing pain or giving your full attention to a client who is experiencing fear (supportive).

LEARNING FROM MISTAKES

'The only thing that makes life possible is permanent intolerable uncertainty: the joy of not knowing what comes next.'
(Ursula Le Guin, quoted by Hayward and Cohan, 1990)

For every positive and well-timed intervention, there is a series of potentially degenerative ones. Heron (1986) identifies four basic kinds of degenerative response which can affect the six categories described. Such interventions have the characteristics of being:

- Unsolicited
- Manipulative
- Compulsive
- Unskilled.

Unsolicited interventions may occur in relationships where there is no therapeutic contract, that is, where no formal practitioner–client relationship is established. Here a person may take it upon him/herself to inform, confront or advise another inappropriately. This has the likelihood of being intrusive to and disrespectful of the person;

at its most invasive it may be aggressive or stereo-typic. For example, a practitioner may say to a complaining client:

- 'You have no right to complain, this residence has a fine reputation'
- 'You've no one to blame but yourself for your illness'
- 'Don't be silly, you're just down in the dumps, you'll feel better later'.

Manipulative interventions are ones motivated by self-interest and tend to disregard the client's position. These are essentially political and abusive in nature, and involve a good deal of power-play. A more subtle form is when the practitioner manoeuvres the client into saying or doing things that fit the professional belief system in which he/she works, as when a medical rationale is used to explain away discontent:

- 'You're only angry because your hormones are disturbed'
- 'It's normal to be a little depressed and grumpy following childbirth'.

Manipulative interventions are largely deliberate, and have a tendency to be calculated and geared to a specific outcome. Clients are especially susceptible to manipulative interventions:

- When they are newly admitted to a clinical area
- In times of crisis when dependent upon the practitioner and their skills
- When ignorant of the professional and/or clinical rationale employed
- When regressed and disorientated through pain or anxiety.

Students new to the clinical area – who need to feel secure and experience a sense of belonging if they are to learn and survive professionally – are naturally enough prone to be vulnerable to manipulative interventions. As a student myself, I remember receiving manipulative interventions of the following order:

- 'If you don't do things as I want them I'll have you moved'
- 'Don't argue with me, I'm in charge, just do it'.

Compulsive interventions are more a symptom of subconscious distress than a deliberate ploy: for example, when a practitioner unconsciously acts out his/her own stress and frustration to others. Obsessional doing and needless business just for the sake of keeping active so as not to dwell upon internal anxiety and fears are examples of this.

Compulsive behaviours I find commonplace in the helping professions, especially in those areas where routine and set ways of performance are favoured. Interventions such as these include the acts of the compulsive helper, the over-conformist practitioner who fears rejection and obsessionally conforms unquestioningly to routine, the un-assertive nurse or midwife who, through his/her own emotional incompetence, mismanages and/or damages his/her clients. Burn-out can contribute to this. Unexpressed and repressed guilt or shame likewise can drive practitioners on to this self-punishing treadmill.

Interventions here may have the effect of punishing, overlooking and abusing others:

- 'I haven't got time to listen to you now'
- 'You're making far more fuss than is warranted'
- 'You can't be in pain, you had your pain-killers 2 hours ago'.

They may also take the form of colluding with the client:

- 'You're right, what's the point of stopping now when the damage is done'.

Compulsive interventions can only be undone through a practitioner's work upon themselves. Supervision, attendance at assertiveness workshops, becoming a member of a personal growth group or seeking out counselling can all be of help here. Heron observes:

> 'There appears to be one golden rule for all would-be practitioners: never become a helper until you have worked on how angry you feel at your parents' and teachers' mismanagement of you in the interests of making you good.'
> (Heron, 1990, page 147)

Unskilled interventions are simply ones of an incompetent nature. These tend to occur when a practitioner has too few interactive options to mind, is unable to self-assess or evaluate, lacks practice, has received insufficient guidance or supervision, or has had a scarcity of role models to learn from. A general lack of timing, appreciation

	Very common	Common	Infrequent	Rare
Unsolicited				
Manipulative				
Compulsive				
Unskilled				

Which of the above degenerative interventions – if any – do you have a tendency to use?

or sense of occasion characterise such interventions.

All the above examples of degenerative interventions fail to hear or attend to the client, have a defensive or belittling edge, deny the client's reality, and lack the essential ingredient of being at root supportive of the client's worth. Given that degenerative interventions increase stress and illustrate the need for further training and/or quality supervision, their frequency is a valuable guide to the state of health of a ward or care team.

SUPERVISION: CARE COMMUNICATION BY EXAMPLE

'When I feel smashed or trapped or bound or pushed, it is helpful to me to ask myself, "What illusion is fouling me up now?" The illusion is what I think about something. The facts just are. I know this most clearly through reflecting on what happens in emergencies when "there is no time to think".'

(Stevens, in Rogers *et al.*, 1967, page 69)

Hinshelwood (1987) observes that staff individually and as a team take the brunt of desperate demands for relief and reassurance. It is a truism, and a sad indictment of the caring professions and their management, that the staff of caring communities do not experience a sense of being cared for themselves.

Much of communication is symbolic; individuals respond to unique meanings derived from their earlier life events, and negotiate new values via social interaction with others (Blumer, 1969).

For instance, the degree of emotional warmth or distance a client perceives in a nurse may be influenced as much by previous exposure to nurture, gender issues or those personal meanings they attach to dependency and care. What transpires within the nurse–client relationship may similarly affect their attitude to the clinical setting and care service as a whole.

Hidden emotional hurts all too easily arise to complicate practitioner–client communication. Practitioners and clients, though they meet as strangers, are propelled into levels of intimacy rarely found in other relationships. This relationship, where 'intimacy' and 'strangers' combine, demands unconditional trust from clients and their relatives, and puts enormous psychological pressure upon carers to act responsibly, give generously of themselves, and in part play out the role of a perfect nurturing parent. Interestingly, anything less than perfection is rarely tolerated by next of kin or unit managers alike.

Thus, coupled with the managerial stress of the job, professional helpers must also survive those projections – emotional labels – that relatives put their way. To be treated as a 'symbol' and related to as an 'all-knowing' or 'all-giving' provider, to act out the label of the 'perfect parent', is depersonalising, for it reinforces the 'role' rather than the 'person'. The individual within the professional uniform may end up feeling very lonely indeed. It is little wonder carers often report feeling drained, not knowing if they are coming or going, or feel lost even to themselves.

It is a tall order to ask nurses to attend to the hidden agenda attached to communication; it is far better if they are exposed to professional preparation where their interactions are examined, and to clinical supervision of a kind which feeds back to them 'how they are perceived' when they relate.

When carers are left to deal by themselves with the discomforts which emanate from the job, they are ill prepared to learn from their mistakes. Professional guidance, in the form of supervision, seeks to shape uncomfortable and stressful events so as to enhance future skills. Without this, the faults which arise in practice are perpetuated.

Tangled relationships and interpersonal communication in climates where supervision is absent have a tendency to become unnecessarily traumatic.

Nurses, who are thrown together with their clients in situations where anxiety over illness or the prospect of death is to the fore, risk having their own fears evoked. Caring is intimate and can be terrifying, especially when you are there for others (the clients) and there is no-one to support you. Unconscious mental defences naturally arise at such times. Defence mechanisms – coping strategies which give respite from anxiety and protect the self by enabling an individual to deny or distort a stressful event, so as to restrict his or her awareness and emotional involvement with it –

give short-term respite, but in the long term restrict performance and cripple adaptation.

Clarifying and unblocking communication is the salient task of care. It is what carers need to address in client care, and what supervisors must attempt to address with their supervisees. It is therefore useful for carers to acquaint themselves with the more common unconscious defence mechanisms that block or misdirect communication.

In Table 7.1 examples are given of a number of mental defences; these in turn are related to their psychological root and social use (modified from Kroeber, 1963 in Barber, 1991).

I find these mechanisms as common in the staff team as in the client population, and see them as forming a basis for much professional behaviour. Their protracted presence and/or overuse I see as diagnostic of burn-out and the need for clinical supervision. They are also natural enough occur-

Table 7.1: Mental defence mechanisms

Psychological root	In normal coping	As a defence
Impulse restraint or emotional control	→ Appropriate suppression: holding back disruptive impulses, e.g. sexual feelings towards clients	→ REPRESSION: uncomfortable emotions pushed out of awareness; purposeful forgetting
Selective awareness or tuning in to what interests us	→ Concentration: focusing our attention	→ DENIAL: refusal to face up to or recognise undesirable material; arguing black is white
Role modelling or copying the actions of others	→ Socialisation: learning social norms and values	→ IDENTIFICATION: submerging your own identity within another person or group; forever playing 'nurse'
Sensitivity or opening ourselves to others	→ Empathy: identifying similarities between ourselves and others	→ PROJECTION: to project unwanted qualities in oneself on to others; seeing what is really your own anger in another
Impulse diversion or holding on to and releasing emotional energies elsewhere	→ Sublimation: expressing anger harmlessly in sport	→ DISPLACEMENT: to take an emotion from its site of origin and to express it elsewhere; when a senior makes you angry, you then vent your discontent upon a student/client
Time reversal or reliving and/or enacting earlier behaviours	→ Playfulness: letting go of our controls to allow for creative spontaneity	→ REGRESSION: to regress back to an earlier functional and/or emotional level; to be overdependent upon ward routines

rences in professional environments where people spend little time listening to or caring for each other.

Professional carers have a duty to care for themselves, for if they can't receive care themselves they have no business forcing care on others. Nurses who don't care for themselves all too often give out 'dead lifeless care'. Care such as this is damaging and more akin to duty. Though dutiful caring rarely kills anyone, it is, at its core, insensitive and robs the therapeutic relationship of love. Though helping professionals may operate from a basis of care, the culture they have evolved does not, it seems, permit them to show kindness to one another.

Reflection Points

- Which defences, if any, of those described are found in your clinical area?
- Which are you most prone to enact in your professional role?

Professional carers readily become habituated to their clinical world so that they no longer see its faults – indeed, they have a vested interest in not doing so if they are to belong. Accepting everything that their practice throws at them and devoid of quality counselling or supervision, they unconsciously take on high levels of stress and all too easily come to see stress-induced responses – symptoms of burn-out – as relatively normal:

- Inability to concentrate upon the job at hand
- Impulsive acting out of feelings
- Excessive smoking and/or drinking
- Loss of energy
- Preoccupation with work
- Inability to relax
- Absenteeism and sickness
- A chronically disturbed sleeping pattern
- Irritability
- Rapid swings between emotional highs and lows
- Memory disturbances
- The sense that life is a fight rather than something to be enjoyed.

This syndrome of stress may in time become a culture of stress; stressed nurses in turn communicate stress to clients so that before long high levels of anxiety permeate the organisation at all levels. When this occurs, staff can no more recognise stress than a fish can recognise water. Stress now is seen to be a natural feature of the clinical work. Nurses so affected are not without insight; it is rather that they are bereft of the necessary skills to detach themselves from the institutional and professional traditions they live by.

In order to enhance care communication and interpersonal understanding, I suggest a three-pronged approach to supervision, where attention is paid to:

- Unpacking the effects of organisational dynamics, professional collusions and personal defences which breed stress
- Using the unfolding relationship between the supervisor and supervisee as an action guide to what occurs in care communication, the phases of therapeutic engagement, and as a setting where interventions may be practised and new ways of engagement explored
- Developing the potential of the supervised to grow as a person, glean new insight into self, their relationships with others and their professional role.

Essentially, this approach to supervision is experiential, reflective upon the social and personal psychodynamics, and approaches the 'self' and communication expert mentally.

In terms of a definition, we can now say that supervision is the engagement of a relationship where an experienced and hopefully skilled practitioner meets with a less experienced individual to appraise, explore and systematically analyse what makes for good care communication and facilitation, while sharing in a relationship which enacts 'caring for carers'.

Within this relationship, four functions are able to be performed:

1 Education in the necessary knowledge, skills and research-mindedness the job requires; here the nurses explore the skill base they require.
2 Orientation to the clinical area and maintenance of a balance between an 'individual's level of skill' and the 'nature of the work' they are assigned; here, clinical induction occurs and an appropriate mix of personal skill to professional responsibility is established.
3 Support and counsel via the enactment of a therapeutic relationship which nurtures and

Reflection Point

Reviewing symptoms of burn-out described below, tick on the scale provided their frequency within yourself:

	Common	Occasional	Rare	Never
Inability to concentrate				
Impulsively acting from feelings				
Excessive smoking and/or drinking				
Loss of energy				
Preoccupation with work				
Inability to relax				
Absenteeism and sickness				
Disturbed sleep				
Irritability				
Mood swings				
Memory disturbances				
Life more a fight than enjoyment				

Two or more ticks in the common column and you would be wise to slow down, seek counsel or support, and reorganise the balance of your life.

In the light of this exercise, pause to reflect how healthy you consider youself and the culture of your workplace to be.

How does stress in your workplace affect client care?

Reflection Point

What manner of supervision have you received during your professional life? Which of the four functions of supervision described above did it include? Indicate the degree of this on the scale provided:

1 Education in the necessary knowledge, skills and research-mindedness the job requires.

Lots   Some   Little   None

2 Orientation to the clinical area and maintenance of a balance between an 'individual's level of skill' and the 'nature of the work' he/she is assigned.

Lots   Some   Little   None

3 Support and counsel via the enactment of a therapeutic relationship which nurtures and offers care to the supervised.

Lots   Some   Little   None

4 Facilitation of self and interpersonal awareness via experiential exploration and analysis of the developing supervisor–supervisee relationship.

Lots   Some   Little   None

What might you be able to offer if you were to perform as a supervisor within your clinical setting? Relate your answer to the four areas described above.

offers care to the supervised; here, the developmental phases of the therapeutic relationship are engaged, unconditional regard and value for the person of the supervised expressed, and

the formation of a caring relationship experienced by the supervised at first hand.

4 Facilitation of self and interpersonal awareness via experiential exploration, rehearsal and/or

analysis of the developing supervisor/supervisee relationship; here, interactions are analysed, emotional responses explored and new social skills synthesised from experience to inform the supervisee's future clinical practice.

It is not always easy to distinguish between when someone is caring for you or attempting to control you. Carers do not always realise which of these they seek to do themselves.

Supervision needs to untie the social and intrapersonal knots clinical encounters produce, so that new ways of responding and/or ways of being may be liberated and fresh insights emerge for future practice. In this sense, clinical life itself is approached experimentally, what works is retained, and what produces conflict or is deemed to be non-therapeutic is explored in order to illuminate further learning.

EPILOGUE

'The mad are persecuted because so many find it hard to love them. As for madness itself, it is the feeling that we can't love until we have time. Until we love we never have the time.'

(Benares, 1985, page 65)

Summary

In this chapter I have tried to get at the soul of care communication rather than its mechanics, and share some of my thoughts and intuitions as to what this might be. As I glance through the text and reflect on what I have said, I feel a need to make one last statement, one which will somehow integrate the whole. This is it:

Love has to be at the heart of all care communication: love for self – without which we cannot love others – and love for the adventure of life itself – without which there is no such thing as health to self-explore and communicate more fully what it is to be human.

REFERENCES

Barber, P. (1991). *Who Cares for the Carers?* Distance Learning Centre, South Bank Polytechnic, London.

Barber, P. (1997). Caring – the nature of a therapeutic relationship. In *Nursing: A Knowledge Base for Practice*, 2nd edn, Perry, A. and Jolley, M. (eds). Edward Arnold, London.

Benares, C. (1985). *Zen without Zen Masters*. Falcon Press, Phoenix, Arizona.

Blumer, H. (1969). *Symbolic Interactionism: Perspective and Method*. Prentice-Hall, New Jersey.

Burnard, P. and Morrison, P. (1987). Nurses' perceptions of their interpersonal skills. *Nursing Times*, 83(42), 59.

Goldberg, P. (1989). *The Intuitive Edge*. Aquarian Press, Wellingborough.

Hayward, S. and Cohan, M. (1990). *Bag of Jewels*. Intune Books, Australia.

Heron, J. (1986). *Six Category Intervention Analysis*. Human Potential Resource Group, University of Surrey, Guildford.

Heron, J. (1989). *The Facilitator's Handbook*. Kogan Page, London.

Heron, J. (1990). *Helping the Client*. Sage, London.

Hinshelwood, R.D. (1987). *What Happens in Groups*. Free Association Books, London.

I Ching (Wilhelm translation) (1951). Routledge and Kegan Paul, London.

Kroeber, T. (1963). The coping functions of the ego mechanisms. In *The Study of Lives*, White, R. (ed.), Atherton Press, New York.

Loevinger, J. (1976). *Ego Development*. Jossey-Bass, San Francisco.

Marriner, A. (1979). *The Nursing Process*. Mosby, St Louis.

Maslow, A.H. (1970). *Motivation and Personality*. Harper and Row, New York.

McFarlane, J.K. and Castledine, G. (1982). *A Guide to the Practice of Nursing Using the Nursing Process*. Mosby, St Louis.

Morrison, P. and Burnard, P. (1988). Student nurses' interpersonal skills. *Nursing Times*, 84(12), 69.

Morrison, P. and Burnard, P. (1989). Students' and trained nurses' perceptions of their own interpersonal skills: a report and comparison. *Journal of Advanced Nursing*, 14, 321–9.

Rogers, C. (1983). *Freedom to Learn in the Eighties*. Merrill, Columbus, Ohio.

Rogers, C.R., Stevens, B., Gendlin, E.T., Shlien, J.M. and Dusen, W.V. (1967). *Person to Person: The Problem of Being Human*. Condor Books, Souvenir Press, London.

Young, P. (1990). *The Art of Polarity Therapy*. Prism Press, Bridport.

Yura, H. and Walsh, M.B. (1978). *Human Needs and the Nursing Process: Philosophy, Theory, Concept, Process.* Appleton Century Crofts, New York.

FURTHER READING

Barber, P. (1996). The social symbolism of health: the notion of the soul in professional care. In *Insights in Health Care*, Perry, A. (ed.), Chapter 3. Arnold, London.

Useful to those who want to study transpersonal and symbolic aspects of communication further, in a health context.

Barber, P. and Mulligan, J. (1998). The client consultant relationship. In *The Management Consultancy Industry*, Sadler, P. (ed.), Volume 1, Chapter 4. Kogan Page, London.

Though primarily intended for management consultants, the authors relate phases in the consultancy relationship to certain communication styles and relational phases.

Mulligan, J. (ed.) (1988). *Personal Management Handbook.* Kogan Page, London.

Wide-ranging introduction to all aspects of effective communication including: assertion; dealing with difficult people and events; non-verbal communication, etc.

Rowen, J. (1993). *The Transpersonal, Psychotherapy and Counselling.* Routledge, London.

A useful vision of communication as a spiritual experience, as well as counselling in the helping relationship.

CHAPTER EIGHT

THE NATURE *of* STRESS *and*

its IMPLICATIONS *for*

NURSING PRACTICE

Elisabeth Clark and Susan E. Montague

- Introduction
- Sources of stress
- The stress response
- Physiological responses to stress
- Stress and illness
- Conclusion

The subject of **stress** has received considerable media coverage over recent years and has been the focus of much research in a range of settings. The aim of this chapter is to explore the nature of stress and the three main theoretical approaches to studying and understanding stress. Sources of stress in health and illness and their implications for nursing practice are considered. The chapter provides an overview of the nature and function of biological and psychological responses to stress and the relationship between them. The accumulating evidence suggesting how stress might be implicated in the development of ill health is also examined.

INTRODUCTION

Stress is an inextricable part of life. It is, according to the eminent stress physiologist Hans Selye (1976), 'essentially reflected by the rate of all the wear and tear caused by life'.

These introductory remarks beg many questions about the nature, causes and effects of stress. We hope to answer these – and hopefully, to provoke more – within the pages of this chapter.

Despite a huge volume of research and interest in the subject, stress remains a somewhat elusive phenomenon. None the less, the development, in this century, of the concept of stress has contributed significantly to the current understanding

of health and illness. The existence of a relationship between stress and illness has grown to near acceptance in the scientific world (Herbert and Cohen, 1994) and according to Fletcher (1991), few now doubt that psychological factors play an important role in mental health and physical disease.

For all these reasons, we consider it crucial that nurses have a clear understanding of stress, both in everyday life and in relation to ill health. Because of their prolonged day-to-day professional contact with patients and clients, nurses are perhaps the best placed of all members of the health care team to take action to prevent unnecessary stress and to minimise and alleviate prolonged stress. If nurses lack such understanding they may be less able to manage their own lives effectively, to work efficiently, and may unwittingly increase their patients'/clients' experience of stress. The nature of nursing varies widely but is such that the job can and does cause severe stress in its practitioners. It is therefore immensely important for nurses to be sensitive to and to recognise signs of stress in themselves and in their colleagues and to take appropriate steps to alleviate this. It is important to remember here that people are not always able consciously to recognise either the signs of stress in themselves and others, or that they are experiencing stress, or to identify its causes. In other words, they may not be able to articulate their distress clearly. Rather, stress may manifest itself indirectly in high rates of absenteeism from work, turnover and wastage. Despite the high level of interest in occupational stress and its effects, reflected in the ever-increasing literature on the subject, there remains a need in some quarters to challenge the belief that professional workers should be able to cope with difficult situations and that to admit to stress is a sign of failure or weakness.

Understanding stress is, we believe, the key to its prevention and alleviation – and the whole subject assumes even greater importance in circumstances where there are cutbacks in resources, staff shortages and uncertainties created by organisational restructuring and change (Sutherland and Cooper, 1990).

Despite its apparent familiarity and common usage, the term 'stress' is not easy to define and is often used to mean several different things. For instance, it is frequently used to describe subjective feelings experienced when we are under great pressure in our lives, as in 'I'm feeling really stressed at the moment.' It can also be used to refer to those conditions which trigger the negative feelings; for example, 'Things at work are pretty stressful.' If you read a number of books and articles about stress, you will find that various different definitions of the term are used. In trying to make sense of these definitions, it is helpful to understand the main approaches that have been adopted in studying the subject (see Box 8.1) since these influence how stress is defined.

Finally, you will notice that stress is generally thought of and expressed in a negative sense, as illustrated in the above two examples. It is important to realise, however, that stress should not always be construed as negative, unpleasant and potentially harmful. Indeed, as Selye pointed out, positive and pleasurable experiences, such as playing competitive sports and, to quote Selye himself (1976, page 1), 'the ecstasy of fulfilment', contribute to the wear and tear of life. Indeed, in such instances, stress can be considered to be the 'spice of life'. Thus stress can be associated with both positive and negative experience. Selye referred to '**eustress**' and '**distress**' to distinguish between the two. 'Eustress' is the amount of stress necessary for an active, healthy life, whereas when increasing levels of stress become maladaptive (exceeding the person's adaptive capacity to cope) and thus potentially harmful, this is 'distress'. Our focus in this chapter will be on maladaptive stress since it is this which produces most distress and dis-ease.

Box 8.1: Approaches to studying stress

Three main approaches have been used to study stress. One approach views stress as a stimulus – an event or a set of circumstances or conditions which threaten a person's well-being and give rise to a stress reaction. Because of the possible confusion, the term '**stressor**' is sometimes used to describe the stimulus in order to differentiate it from the **stress response**. When someone talks about the 'stress of overwork', they are referring to stress as a stimulus. This idea of stress as a stimulus originated from engineering and the finding that material eventually weakens if unequal pressures are placed upon it. Those working within this tradition aim to identify the particular characteristics of a situation or event that make it stressful.

A second perspective focuses on the set of responses – physiological and/or psychological – that occur when an animal or human is faced with a threatening or demanding situation. This response-based approach has been particularly important in the development of biological concepts of stress. The work of the Canadian physiologist Hans Selye is an example of such an approach to the study of stress. In 1956, Selye published his first major book on the subject, entitled *The Stress of Life* (a second edition was published in 1976). Selye's important ideas about stress are discussed in detail in the section on the physiological responses to stress (page 179).

Both of these approaches, however, fail to take account of the meaning of events. This important realisation provided the basis of a third perspective which is known as the interactionist or **transactional model of stress**. It assumes that stress reflects the relationship (or transaction) between a person and his/her environment. According to this approach, stress should not simply be seen as either a stimulus or a response, but as the product of a person's interpretation of the significance of a threatening event (the stimulus or stressor) and of their resources to cope with it (the stress response).

Demand → Perception → Response

This perspective is derived from the work of Cox and his colleagues at Nottingham University during the 1970s. Cox (1978) describes stress as a 'part of a complex and dynamic system of transaction between the person and his environment' (page 18). He goes on to suggest that 'Stress may be said to arise when there is an imbalance between the perceived demand and the person's perception of his capability to meet that demand' (page 18).

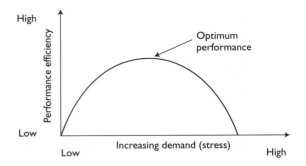

Figure 8.1: The relationship between performance and demand

For the remainder of this chapter, stress will be considered essentially from a transactional viewpoint.

Although we shall be focusing on damaging or harmful stress, it is important to recognise that human beings require some degree of stress in order to function effectively. As already discussed, stress is a necessary part of life and cannot be avoided: it provides the necessary drive and challenge required to maintain life and respond successfully to its changing demands. In particular, as we shall see later in the chapter, we would not be able to alter our level of physical activity or survive injury if these situations did not trigger a stress response. There comes a point, however, when increasing levels of stress become harmful and the demands exceed a person's adaptive capacity and thus their ability to cope, at which point stress becomes dysfunctional. Figure 8.1 shows the relationship between performance and demand. From this you can see the performance is relatively poor at low levels of demand, but improves steadily as the level of demand increases until optimum performance is reached at moderate levels of demand. As demand levels increase further, so performance begins to deteriorate progressively. Welford (1973) claimed that stress occurs whenever the demand departs from moderate levels and this helps to explain why people

working on a monotonous production line often find their work stressful. Low levels of demand can be as stressful as high levels, and produce similar effects on performance.

So when thinking about stress, it is important to acknowledge that it is not simply something negative 'out there' in the environment, but that it depends on an individual's cognitive appraisal of the situation and of the available resources to deal with it. It is not, therefore, possible to identify certain situations as 'stressful' and others as 'not stressful'. Rather, stress must be viewed on a more individualised basis as a function of the interaction between a person and his/her environment. Faced with similar demands, two people may well react quite differently, with one person viewing the situation as a challenge, whilst the other may exhibit symptoms of anxiety and distress. From this it should be apparent that such an approach acknowledges important individual differences and that it fits well within a philosophy of individualised care.

On a methodological note, Cox (1978) points out that the research that is associated with each of the three approaches outlined in Box 8.1 tends to differ in its emphasis. The response model typically treats stress as a dependent variable, describing it in terms of people's responses to threatening stimuli. Meanwhile, researchers who view stress in terms of the characteristics of the stressor (the stimulus) usually treat it as an independent variable, the effects of which can be systematically studied. Finally, those working within the interactionist model usually investigate stress as an intervening variable between stimulus and response.

Key Points

■ Despite a huge amount of interest in the subject of stress, it still remains an elusive concept which is not easy to define.

■ Three main approaches have been used to study stress and influence the way in which stress is investigated in research.

■ Stress is not simply something 'out there'; rather it depends on an individual's appraisal of a particular situation and his/her ability to deal with it. A situation is stressful when the person concerned perceives a mismatch between the demand of a particular situation and that person's ability to cope with it.

■ Physiological and psychological responses in stress represent attempts at dealing with the situation.

SOURCES OF STRESS

If you pause to reflect for a moment on the sources of stress in your life at the present time, you would probably, like me, come up with a fairly long list. My list includes a demanding job of preparing learning materials to tight deadlines and running three distance learning programmes, commuting into London and trying to arrange for renovations to be carried out on the old house in which I am presently living. These and other stressors are likely to be familiar to you.

When thinking about stressors it is important to remember that the majority – with the exception of a disaster (such as a hurricane or flood) or traumatic events (such as a car crash, rape or a life-threatening illness) – should be thought of as *potential* rather than actual sources of stress. Consider the taste for loud music of some young people; whilst this may feature in your own list of stressors now, it may not always have done so. Meanwhile, for some the absence of music might be considered to be a source of stress. Likewise, a parachute jump is likely to be viewed rather differently depending on the individual concerned. Factors such as age, personality and previous experience are likely to affect whether or not a particular stimulus is regarded as stressful by a specific individual.

Returning briefly to disasters and traumatic events, it is important to recognise that they can

have a long-lasting effect on the individual(s) concerned. As a result, certain people go on to develop what has come to be known as **post-traumatic stress disorder (PTSD)**. According to Figley (1986), the main symptoms of PTSD include:

■ A pervading sense of numbness (feeling detached or estranged from other people) and avoidance of thoughts and feelings associated with the traumatic event

■ Re-experiencing phenomena (e.g. nightmares or recurrent intrusive distressing memories of the traumatic event)

■ Symptoms of increased arousal such as being overly alert, difficulty staying asleep, irritability and outbursts of anger.

It is essential for anyone working with individuals suffering from PTSD to have a good working knowledge of bereavement processes since the issue of mortality (one's own and that of other people) often has to be confronted, and terrible, vivid images of death and destruction may be imprinted on people's minds (see Clegg, 1988).

WORK-RELATED STRESS

Your list of stressors may have included a number of work-related sources of stress. Occupational stress appears to occur most frequently in occupations such as nursing, where the physical and psychological demands are high whilst autonomy is relatively low (Lees and Ellis, 1990). Research undertaken in both the UK and the USA has identified some of the sources of stress reported by nurses at differing points in their careers.

In their systematic study of stress in nurse managers, Hingley and Cooper (1986) found that potential stressors could be grouped into nine main categories:

■ Workload
■ Working relationships with more senior colleagues
■ Role conflict and ambiguity
■ Dealing with death and bereavement
■ The conflict between home and work
■ Lack of career prospects
■ Interpersonal relationships with patients/clients, relatives and colleagues

- Lack of resources
- Keeping up with changes.

Looking at this list you will almost certainly agree that these stressors are as relevant in the late-1990s as they were in the 1980s. Indeed, Baglioni and colleagues (1990) identified an almost identical list of stressors in their study of 475 female nurse managers.

Although Hingley and Cooper's study focused on nurse managers, research undertaken with other groups of nurses has identified similar stressors (Marshall, 1980). Perhaps not surprisingly, studies of student nurses have also found that coping with death and dying is frequently listed as a stressor (see, for example, Birch, 1979; Parkes, 1985; Arnold, 1989; Lindop, 1991). Similarly, relationships with colleagues and patients/clients have also been identified (Parkes, 1985; Arnold,

1989; Lees and Ellis, 1990; Lindop, 1991), as has work overload (Parkes, 1985; Lindop, 1991) and coping with changes such as moving wards (Birch, 1979). In addition, lack of confidence and anxieties about carrying out certain clinical procedures (Parkes, 1985; Lees and Ellis, 1990), carrying out tasks in front of others (Kushnir, 1986), and differences between ward-based and theoretical aspects of education (Melia, 1987; Lindop, 1991) are also cited as stressors.

Research by Lees and Ellis (1990) has identified a wide variety of stressors in nursing. As you can see from Table 8.1, no fewer than 26 categories emerged. Fifty-three individuals took part in the study: 20 qualified staff, 20 students and 13 ex-students who had left their training programmes before the end. Several of the stressors, such as dealing with death and dying and conflict with doctors, featured in all three groups, whilst others

Table 8.1: The 26 categories of stressor identified by Lees and Ellis (1990)*

Stressor	Trained	Student	Leaver	Total
Understaffing	75	25	23	43
Dealing with death and dying	25	55	46	41
Conflict with nurses	35	25	46	34
Overwork	25	30	15	25
Conflict with doctors	40	15	8	23
Hours	10	10	39	17
Cardiac arrests	5	30	8	15
Responsibility/accountability	25	5	8	13
Training junior staff	25	0	0	9
Dealing with relatives	15	5	8	9
Lack of resources (beds/equipment)	20	0	0	8
Aggressive patients	10	5	0	6
Study/exams	0	15	0	6
Carrying out certain nursing procedures	5	5	0	4
Feeling inadequate to carry out procedures	0	10	0	4
Seeing patients in distress	0	5	8	4
Staff rough to patients	0	0	15	4
Conflict with 'others' (porters/admin.)	5	0	0	2
Child abuse	5	0	0	2
Dealing with overdose patients	5	0	0	2
Living in nurses home	0	0	8	2
Open visiting	5	0	0	2
Doing the off-duty	5	0	0	2
Disorganisation of workload on the wards	0	0	8	2
Being a new situation for the first time	0	5	0	2
Heat in hospital	0	0	8	2

*For each stressor, the percentage of each group, and of the total group of 53 subjects, citing it as a stressor is given (reproduced with permission from *Journal of Advanced Nursing*)

were found to affect some groups more than others, and some were restricted to one group only. The stressors that affected only one group were specifically associated with that group's role (e.g. only qualified nurses allocate the off-duty roster).

Lees and Ellis also asked respondents to state which incidents and/or situations they found to be the most stressful. For the trained staff, the major stressors were understaffing (75% of the group of trained staff), followed by conflict with doctors (40%). For the student nurses and the student leavers, the main stressor was dealing with death and dying (55% and 46%, respectively).

However, other studies such as Field (1989), Vachon (1987) and Cavanagh and Snape (1993) have reported high levels of exposure to dying patients and to death as a major source of stress for qualified health care staff also.

Some studies have focused on specialist clinical areas and, perhaps not surprisingly, some areas of work have been found to be more stressful than others. For instance, special care baby units (see, for example, Thornton, 1984; Rosenthal et al., 1989; Downey et al., 1995; Oates and Oates, 1995) and critical care settings (e.g. Bailey et al., 1980; Bibbings, 1987; Duggan, 1990; White and Tonkin, 1991; Norrie, 1995) and accident and emergency departments (e.g. Keller, 1990; Hawley, 1992; Sowney, 1996). You will notice that the workload in each of these high dependency areas tends to be unpredictable and involves the use of high technology equipment. A more worrying finding is, however, the lack of support from other nurses which has been cited as a source of stress (Bergh-Braam and de Wolff, 1988; Rentoul, 1989). Do you work in a clinical environment that you consider to be stressful? How do you support colleagues through stressful experiences? If your answer to this latter question highlights a lack of support, you should seriously consider the benefits of introducing support groups and/or clinical supervision to ensure that colleagues receive the support they need to work effectively.

The negative effects of stress may be at least partly responsible for the high attrition rate from pre-registration education programmes. For example, Birch (1979) reported that 66% of the sample of leavers he studied had left because they could not cope with the stress, whilst Beck (1984) found that 20% of students failed to reach their final year at a major teaching hospital because of stress. Other effects include high rates of absenteeism

(Campbell, 1985) and exhaustion (Lindop, 1991). In a further study of over 300 student nurses, Clarke and Ruffin (1992) identified a number of study-related stressors including the use of technical equipment, interpersonal relationships and lack of time for personal/family pursuits.

Since the introduction of the revised form of pre-registration education in the UK in 1989, interest has focused on comparisons between the two forms of preparation and on the levels of stress associated with the revised form (see, for example, Snell, 1995; Power, 1996). In a small-scale study comparing 55 student nurses at the start of their third year and 51 student nurses registered on the Diploma in Higher Education at the start of their Branch programmes, Rhead (1995) found that overall the RGN students were significantly less stressed than the Diploma students. The RGN students found the practical elements of their training to be more stressful than the academic elements, whilst the Diploma students were equally stressed by both the practical and academic elements. Issues concerned with death and patient suffering were a third major source of stress identified by both groups, highlighting the importance of adequately preparing student nurses to cope with death and bereavement.

Evidence suggests, however, that stress among student nurses is widespread and has been reported in a number of countries including Canada (see, for example, Wood and Rubin, 1992; Steen, 1994).

If you are interested in assessing the amount of stress currently in your working life, you might like to complete the Professional Life Stress Scale in Box 8.2. The purpose of this scale is to help you to think about your working life. Fontana (1989) emphasises the importance of treating it as a useful but rough guide to your stress level; it is *not* a precise measurement tool.

Box 8.2: Professional Life Stress Scale

The following instructions are provided by Fontana (1989):

'Complete it [the scale] quickly, and don't think too hard before responding to each question. Your first response is often the most accurate one. As with any stress scale, it isn't difficult to spot what is the "low stress" answer to each question. Don't be tempted to give this answer if it isn't the accurate one. Nothing is at stake. You are as stressed as you are. Your score on the scale doesn't change that, one way or the other. The purpose of the scale is simply to help you clarify some of your thinking about your own life.'

Use the key to assess your results.

1 Two people who know you well are discussing you. Which of the following statements would they be most likely to use?

(a) 'X is very together. Nothing much seems to bother him/her.'

(b) 'X is great. But you have to be careful what you say to him/her at times.'

(c) 'Something always seems to be going wrong with X's life.'

(d) 'I find X very moody and unpredictable.'

(e) 'The less I see of X the better!'

2 Are any of the following common features of your life?

- Feeling you can seldom do anything right
- Feelings of being hounded or trapped or cornered
- Indigestion
- Poor appetite
- Difficulty in getting to sleep at night
- Dizzy spells or palpitations
- Sweating without exertion or high air temperature
- Panic feelings when in crowds or in confined spaces
- Tiredness and lack of energy
- Feelings of hopelessness ('what's the use of anything?')
- Faintness or nausea sensations without any physical cause
- Extreme irritation over small things
- Inability to unwind in the evenings
- Waking regularly at night or early in the mornings
- Difficulty in taking decisions
- Inability to stop thinking about problems or the day's events
- Tearfulness
- Convictions that you just can't cope
- Lack of enthusiasm even for cherished interests
- Reluctance to meet new people and attempt new experiences
- Inability to say 'no' when asked to do something
- Having more responsibility than you can handle.

3 Are you more or less optimistic than you used to be (or about the same)?

4 Do you enjoy watching sport?

5 Can you get up late at weekends if you want to without feeling guilty?

6 Within reasonable professional and personal limits, can you speak your mind to: (a) your boss? (b) your colleagues? (c) members of your family?

7 Who usually seems to be responsible for making the important decisions in your life: (a) yourself? (b) someone else?

8 When criticised by superiors at work, are you usually: (a) very upset? (b) moderately upset? (c) mildly upset?

9 Do you finish the working day feeling satisfied with what you have achieved: (a) often? (b) sometimes? (c) only occasionally?

10 Do you feel most of the time that you have unsettled conflicts with colleagues?

11 Does the amount of work you have to do exceed the amount of time available: (a) habitually? (b) sometimes? (c) only very occasionally?

12 Have you a clear picture of what is expected of you professionally: (a) mostly? (b) sometimes? (c) hardly ever?

13 Would you say that generally you have enough time to spend on yourself?

14 If you want to discuss your problems with someone, can you usually find a sympathetic ear?

15 Are you reasonably on course towards achieving your major objectives in life?

16 Are you bored at work: (a) often? (b) sometimes? (c) very rarely?

17 Do you look forward to going into work: (a) most days? (b) some days? (c) hardly ever?

18 Do you feel adequately valued for your abilities and commitment at work?

19 Do you feel adequately rewarded (in terms of status and promotion) for your abilities and commitment at work?

20 Do you feel your superiors: (a) actively *hinder* you in your work? (b) actively *help you* in your work?

21 If ten years ago you had been able to see yourself professionally as you are now, would you have seen yourself as: (a) exceeding your expectations? (b) fulfilling your expectations? (c) falling short of your expectations?

22 If you had to rate how much you like yourself on a scale from 5 (most like) to 1 (least like), what would your rating be?

Key for Professional Life Stress Scale

1 (a) 0, (b) 1, (c) 2, (d) 3, (e) 4

2 Score 1 for each 'yes' response

3 Score 0 for more optimistic, 1 for about the same, 2 for less optimistic

4 Score 0 for 'yes', 1 for 'no'

5 Score 0 for 'yes', 1 for 'no'

6 Score 0 for each 'yes' response, 1 for each 'no' response

7 Score 0 for 'yourself', 1 for 'someone else'

8 Score 2 for 'very upset', 1 for 'moderately upset', 0 for 'mildly upset'

9 Score 0 for 'often', 1 for 'sometimes', 2 for 'only occasionally'

10 Score 0 for 'no', 1 for 'yes'

11 Score 2 for 'habitually', 1 for 'sometimes', 0 for 'only very occasionally'

12 Score 0 for 'mostly', 1 for 'sometimes', 2 for 'hardly ever'

13 Score 0 for 'yes', 1 for 'no'

14 Score 0 for 'yes', 1 for 'no'

15 Score 0 for 'yes', 1 for 'no'

16 Score 2 for 'often', 1 for 'sometimes', 0 for 'very rarely'

17 Score 0 for 'most days', 1 for 'some days', 2 for 'hardly ever'

18 Score 0 for 'yes', 1 for 'no'

19 Score 0 for 'yes', 1 for 'no'

20 Score 1 for (a), 0 for (b)

21 Score 0 for 'exceeding your expectations', 1 for 'fulfilling your expectations', 2 for 'falling short of your expectations'

22 Score 0 for '5', 1 for '4', and so on down to 4 for '1'

Interpreting your score

Scores on stress scales must be interpreted cautiously. There are so many variables which lie outside the score of these scales but which influence the way in which we perceive and handle our stress that two people with the same scores may experience themselves as under quite different levels of strain. Nevertheless, taken as no more than a guide, these scales can give us some useful information.

0–15 Stress isn't a problem in your life. This doesn't mean you have insufficient stress to keep yourself occupied and fulfilled. The scale is only designed to assess undesirable responses to stress.

16–30 This is a moderate range of stress for a busy professional person. It's nevertheless well worth looking at how it can reasonably be reduced.

31–45 Stress is clearly a problem, and the need for remedial action is apparent. The longer you work under this level of stress, the harder it often is to do something about it. There is a strong case for looking carefully at your professional life.

46–60 At these levels stress is a major problem, and something must be done without delay. You may be nearing the stage of exhaustion in the general adaptation syndrome. The pressure must be eased.

So far we have focused largely on work-related stress, but it is important to acknowledge that stress is not restricted to work and that aspects of our personal lives may also be stressful and affect our work. Many of the changes which occur periodically in our lives, such as moving house or pregnancy, can be a source of stress, since any change – even one that is desired and joyful – requires some form of adjustment. Throughout life, therefore, each of us experiences the need to adapt to new circumstances.

Researchers have spent many years investigating the effects of both positive and negative life events such as moving away from your family home, suffering from a severe illness, marriage, the birth of a child, the death of someone close to you, divorce or promotion at work.

LIFE CHANGES

In 1967, Holmes and Rahe published a scale, derived from clinical experience, which attempted to measure the impact of such life events. This scale, containing 43 items, was developed by examining the case histories of about 5000 individuals and identifying those life events which regularly preceded the onset of illness. They assumed that stress could be induced by a variety of different life events – both positive and negative – which require some kind of adjustment in a person's life. They also assumed that specific stressors could be added up and used to indicate the total amount of stress a person had been under during a specific period of time. So, for instance, if I had experienced 14 of the 43 listed life events over the previous year, then my overall stress score would be 14.

However, implicit in their original scale was a further assumption which Holmes and Rahe were themselves unhappy about: an assumption of equal weighting given to different life events of varying seriousness. Intuitively, a minor traffic offence would seem relatively insignificant when compared with the death of a loved one. They therefore modified the instrument by assigning differential weights to specific life events, using a magnitude estimation procedure. To do this, 394 subjects were informed that the life event of 'marriage' had been assigned an arbitrary value of 50 and they were asked to rate each of the remaining 42 events proportionately as requiring more or less adjustment than marriage. The mean value assigned to each life event was calculated and then divided by ten to give a specific number of life change units (LCU) for each item. Table 8.2 shows the 43 items included in the Social Readjustment Rating Scale (SRRS) which may be used to determine the total amount of life change a person has experienced over a fixed period of time, usually 12 months or 24 months.

When looking at Table 8.2, you might like to reflect on how many of the 43 life events are the concern of a nurse in relation to his or her clients. Let us consider for a moment the likely score of a woman who has just returned to work after maternity leave. Her score will certainly include:

- Pregnancy (40)
- Gain of new family member (39)
- Wife begins or stops work (26)

- Change in sleeping habits (16)

and may also include:

- Change in financial state (38)
- Revision of personal habits (24)
- Change in eating habits (15).

The total number of life change units could, therefore, be as high as 198. The possible addition of other events (such as death of close family member or close friend, sexual difficulties, trouble with in-laws), over which she has little or no control, would increase her score to even higher levels. Thus, knowledge of life events may help you to appreciate the range of stressors which an individual is facing. It should, however, be noted that general life event scales such as the SRRS may not be entirely appropriate for use with specific client groups, such as pregnant women, since they do not include many items relevant to that particular group. As you read about the SRRS several other problems may have occurred to you concerning this approach to measuring stress. If not, pause now to think about any limitations before reading Box 8.3.

Box 8.3: Critique of the Social Readjustment Rating Scale

1. Some items appear ambiguous or vague (e.g. 'change in living conditions').
2. Some items may be more important to certain social groups than others and there may also be cultural differences in the perception/experience of specific events.
3. No consideration is given to the subjective appraisal of potentially stressful situations or events and their meaning for particular individuals as proposed by the transactional model of stress (e.g. a person's reactions to the death of a spouse may depend on a number of factors such as age, length and happiness of the relationship, and dependence on the person who has died).
4. The SRRS is based on Selye's model of stress based on homeostatic readjustments to life changes; it assumes that it is the change itself that is important rather than whether the change is desirable or undesirable (thus an improvement in one's financial affairs is awarded the same score as a deterioration).
5. Individual differences in ability to cope with stressful events are overlooked.

6 Any self-reported measure of life events may be unreliable because it relies on a person's ability to recall the incidence of stressful life events. Thus, the data may reflect a failure to recall accurately and a tendency to be selective. A person's state of mind may influence both what is recollected and how something is recollected (e.g. if a person is feeling unwell, negative events may be over-reported and positive events under-reported).

7 The values assigned to specific items may change over time with changing social situations so one cannot assume that a scale developed in the mid-1970s is equally appropriate in the late-1990s.

Following the publication of SRRS, several more scales have been developed to measure life changes. For example, Dohrenwend and colleagues (1978) produced the Psychiatric Epidemiology Research Interview (PERI) Life Events Scale. They used a large sample drawn from the New York city area stratified for age, gender, marital status, educational level, ethnic group and socioeconomic level. This scale comprises 102 items grouped into 11 topic areas including work, finances, health and family.

An extensive review of the literature on maternal stress by Levin and DeFrank (1988) found stress to be a health risk for both mothers and babies; life change stress was predictive of antenatal complications and of premature labour. As a result, they suggest that those responsible for caring for pregnant women should find out what stressors women are exposed to, offer their support to mothers under stress, and also refer them to appropriate support groups.

In her study of social support during pregnancy, Oakley (1992) found that birth complications were lower in women who had high levels of social support. Meanwhile, a meta-analysis of evidence gathered from 11 randomised controlled trials carried out in different countries including Guatemala, Canada and South Africa found that the continuous presence of a support person throughout labour produced a number of positive outcomes, including a reduced likelihood of medication for pain relief, operative vaginal delivery and an *Apgar score* in the neonate of less than 7 (Hodnett, 1995).

Table 8.2: The Social Readjustment Rating Scale (Holmes and Rahe, 1967)

Rank	Life event	Mean value
1	Death of spouse	100
2	Divorce	73
3	Marital separation	65
4	Jail term	63
5	Death of close family member	63
6	Personal injury or illness	53
7	Marriage	50
8	Fired at work	47
9	Marital reconciliation	45
10	Retirement	45
11	Change in health of family member	44
12	Pregnancy	40
13	Sex difficulties	39
14	Gain of new family member	39
15	Business readjustment	39
16	Change in financial state	38
17	Death of close friend	37
18	Change to different line of work	36
19	Change in number of arguments with spouse	35
20	Mortgage over $10,000*	31
21	Foreclosure of mortgage or loan	30
22	Change in responsibilities at work	29
23	Son or daughter leaving home	29
24	Trouble with in-laws	29
25	Outstanding personal achievement	28
26	Wife begins or stops work	26
27	Begin or end school	26
28	Change in living conditions	25
29	Revision of personal habits	24
30	Trouble with boss	23
31	Change in work hours or conditions	20
32	Change in residence	20
33	Change in schools	20
34	Change in recreation	19
35	Change in church activities	19
36	Change in social activities	18
37	Mortgage or loan less than $10,000*	17
38	Change in sleeping habits	16
39	Change in number of family get-togethers	15
40	Change in eating habits	15
41	Vacation	13
42	Christmas	12
43	Minor violations of the law	11

Interpretation of total score:

- A total score of up to 149 describes no life crisis
- A score between 150 and 199 describes a mild life crisis
- A score between 200 and 299 describes a moderate life crisis
- A score of over 300 describes a major life crisis.

If your score is high, you might like to consider whether it is possible to postpone any events requiring further adjustments in your life over which you may have some control, such as moving house, to prevent your score rising further.

* Please note that in 1967, $10,000 constituted a substantial financial burden. This figure would need to be considerably increased to be equivalent in the late 1990s.

Thus, in addition to calculating a person's overall stress score, it is important to recognise that a number of other factors may influence how someone perceives and reacts to his/her situation. These include personal factors such as individual appraisal of the situation, self-esteem and coping skills, and situational factors such as the amount of support available, the predictability of the stressor and the amount of control that may be exerted over its duration. If, for example, the occurrence of a potentially stressful event can be predicted, this may allow an individual to prepare him/herself. Conversely, uncertainty may make it very difficult to deal with a stressful event. Those who have cared for a person with cancer may already be aware that, for many, it is the uncertainty about whether or not the treatment will be successful that is particularly hard to cope with – the uncertainty of not knowing – rather than the disease itself. Different ways of coping with stress and the issue of control will be considered later.

Moreover, when thinking about a specific patient/client/colleague, it is important to gauge the amount of social support that they have. Any major life event (such as a life-threatening illness, the death of a baby, child or partner, or divorce) is almost certainly more bearable if social and emotional support is available (Schwartzer and Leppin, 1989). Stress may be easier to bear if an opportunity is provided to talk with others who have experienced a similar stressor. To meet this need, a number of national organisations and local groups – such as the Stillbirth and Neonatal Death Association, Cancer Link and the National Association for Staff Support (the latter provides support for health care workers) – provide specialist support.

Wherever possible, health care professionals should encourage individuals who are experiencing stress to seek out some form of social support and make contact with a relevant group or organisation. Four different types of social support have been identified (see Box 8.4). When you have read Box 8.4 pause for a moment to think of at least two patients/clients whom you have recently cared for. For each individual, identify which types of social support might be helpful to him/her and to the family. How might these different kinds of social support be provided?

Box 8.4: Types of social support (Cohen and McKay, 1984)

Emotional support: the expression of concern and care to another so that she/he is comforted and feels a sense of belonging.

Esteem support: giving encouragement and the expression of respect can help to increase a person's sense of worth/self-esteem.

Informational support: involves the provision of information, advice and guidance.

Instrumental support: the provision of practical assistance during periods of stress (e.g. providing transport to and from hospital or respite care for an elderly relative who is being looked after at home to allow the family to go on holiday).

In the light of earlier discussions which have emphasised the importance of the subjective experience of stress, you may be surprised that the SRRS, which uses standardised weightings, has been widely employed in stress research. Certainly, some studies have shown cultural differences and also some age differences. For instance, Ruch and Holmes (1971) found that a group of adolescents rated sexual difficulties as the fifth most stressful item, whilst older adults rated this item thirteenth. Yet even this kind of approach overlooks the issue of individual differences in the perception and subjective experience of potentially stressful events.

Despite reservations concerning the SRRS (see Box 8.3), overall stress scores have been used in a number of prospective studies to predict the likelihood of adverse changes in health of large numbers of subjects (see, for example, Rahe, 1974, 1987; Rahe and Arthur, 1977). Since Rahe was a Captain in the United States Navy, many of the subjects were naval personnel. Small but statistically significant relationships have been reported between the number and intensity of life events and the incidence of illness (as indicated in medical records) whilst living in similar conditions on board ship. Most people, however, appeared to cope with life changes without becoming ill. According to Sarafino (1994), the correlation between individuals' scores on the SRRS and illness is not very strong at only about +0.3. Moreover, correlational data need to be interpreted with care. Any increased susceptibility to illness may not result from the direct effects of the stressful events themselves, but from other associated factors which are difficult to separate from the effects of stress; for instance, a person who has recently been bereaved may not be eating or sleeping properly. Alternatively, poor health may increase the likelihood of experiencing stress-related events such as work difficulties, changes in sleeping habits or marital difficulties; that is to say, early stages of the illness prior to the onset of specific life events may have caused the stressful life events to happen rather than the other way round. Certainly, Hudgens (1974) argued that 29 of the 43 events included in the SRRS are often the symptoms or consequences of illness. Finally, it is also possible that both stress and illness are due to some other, as yet unidentified, variable (such as personality), and that the correlation between the two is spurious.

One further methodological point may also be important. The experience of stress may encourage people to become more aware of their health, take more notice of symptoms they might otherwise ignore, and consult their doctor: the experience of stress may change how people behave in relation to their health. Thus, it would seem reasonable to regard stress associated with life events as a possible predisposing factor in the development of illness. The evidence certainly does not enable us to identify stress unequivocally as a sufficient causal factor.

One further assumption made by Holmes and Rahe has also been challenged; namely, that any change – whether good or bad – requires adjustment and is therefore stressful. However, since an individual's perception of the situation is crucial, one might expect that only undesirable life events are correlated with illness but not desirable events, even though both require some form of adjustment (Suls and Mullen, 1981; Sarason et al., 1985).

THE DAILY HASSLES OF LIFE

If you think back to the SRRS, you will appreciate that the life events included are fairly major, compared with the numerous minor irritations that most of us experience on a daily basis – irritations such as losing one's purse or having an argument with a friend or colleague. In response to this notion, Lazarus and his colleagues developed a scale to assess the daily hassles experienced rather than major life events. According to Lazarus and Folkman (1984, page 376), daily hassles are 'experiences and conditions of daily living that have appraised as salient and harmful ... to the endorser's well-being'. It should be clear from this definition that Lazarus is working within a transactional model of stress where stress is influenced by a person's appraisal of a situation and his/her perceived ability to cope with it. When measuring stress within this conceptual framework, subjective elements such as personal beliefs and appraisal have to be included since the *perception* of stress is more important than the objective event itself. In 1981, Lazarus and colleagues (Kanner et al., 1981) developed the Hassles Scale, comprising 117 items which people may find frustrating or irritating (e.g. losing things, silly practical mistakes). Respondents were required to identify which hassles they had experienced during the previous month and then rate each item on a three-point scale to indicate how severe the hassle had been during that period.

They argued that the impact of hassles may be diminished by 'uplifts' (desirable experiences, such as feeling healthy or relating well with your partner) and developed a 135-item Uplifts Scale. This scale was administered alongside the Hassles Scale and the strength of each uplift was also rated on a three-point scale.

The overall accumulation of daily hassles has been found to be a better predictor of psychological symptoms and health in middle-aged people than major life events (DeLongis et al., 1982). However, the two are almost certainly related. For instance, a major life event such as divorce may create a number of more minor hassles such as sorting out financial arrangements, child care facilities, and so on.

Further research is clearly needed to investigate the obviously complex relationship between major life events, minor frequent irritations and the onset of illness, especially since individual variation has been reported in the way people react. DeLongis et al. (1988) found that whilst most individuals became more anxious as the number of minor hassles in their lives increased, this was not the case for about 30% of people who reported improved levels of coping and more positive mood. This latter group were found to have higher levels of self-esteem and better networks of social/emotional support than those who did not cope as well.

In addition to coping with specific life events and daily hassles, it is also important to be aware that patients and clients may well experience stress in relation to the care they receive.

THE STRESS OF HOSPITALISATION

For those working in a hospital environment which has become totally familiar, it is important not to lose sight of those aspects of the environment and the routine which may be a source of stress for individual patients. There is now considerable evidence that hospitalisation is a stressful experience (see, for example, Franklin, 1974; Ahmadi, 1985; Wilson-Barnett, 1986). A number of studies undertaken in the past 20 or so years have identified specific stressors, measured stress responses and evaluated attempts to alleviate stress (e.g. Langer et al., 1975; Wilson-Barnett and Carrigy, 1978; Johnson, 1983; Wilson-Barnett, 1984; Wilson, 1991; Pattison and Robertson, 1996). It is clearly essential for health care professionals to be aware of potential sources of stress for individual patients so that they may attempt to prevent, or at least reduce, the stress and thereby promote improved physical and psychological well-being in those being cared for.

In this context, it is important to note that many of the physical and behavioural changes associated with stress (such as insomnia, irritability, changes in eating habits) may inappropriately be associated with the primary diagnosis, and other possible causes may be overlooked. Work by Volicer and Volicer (1978) and Wilson-Barnett (1979) and others has shown that the hospital environment is strange and may be associated with unhappy memories. Many patients feel that they lack information or are provided with conflicting information and do not have opportunities to discuss any concerns that they might have. Some resent being made to feel dependent and the loss of control over their own situation and their own bodies. Greater insight into the source(s) of stress for individual patients may be obtained by using the Hospital Stress Rating Scale which was created by Volicer and Bohannon (1975) to assess the degree of stress associated with different aspects of care (see Table 8.3, page 180).

Key Points

- When thinking about stressors it is important to remember that the majority should be regarded as *potential* rather than actual sources of stress.
- Research has identified a variety of potential work-related stressors in nursing. Some clinical areas such as intensive care units and accident and emergency departments have been reported to be more stressful than others.
- Over the years researchers have devoted considerable effort into investigating the impact of both negative and positive life events. The Social Readjustment Rating Scale (SRRS) was published in 1967 to assess the total amount of life change a person has experienced over a fixed period of time. However, there are a number of problems associated with this scale. Rather than assess major life events, other scales have been developed to measure the number and strength of daily hassles and of uplifts experienced.
- A number of factors can influence how an individual perceives and reacts to his/her situation; these include personal factors such as individual appraisal of the situation, self-esteem and coping skills, and situational factors such as the amount of social support available, the predictability of the stressor and the amount of control that may be exerted over its duration.

■ In addition to life events and daily hassles and uplifts, evidence suggests that patients/clients may also experience stress in relation to hospitalisation and the care they receive. It is important, therefore, for all health care professionals to be aware of potential sources of stress in their clinical environment so that they may attempt to prevent or at least reduce the stress experienced and thereby promote improved well-being.

THE STRESS RESPONSE

The stress response has both physiological and psychological components and both these represent attempts at coping with, that is, reducing or removing, the source of stress. The mental and behavioural strategies that make up the psychological component of the stress response (see next section) are called 'coping mechanisms'. These are the responses of the person, which he/she then appraises as being successful or unsuccessful in altering the demand in the desired direction. Such mental and behavioural responses are almost always, if not always, accompanied by a physiological response to the demand. The function of the physiological stress response is to facilitate survival as well as mental and behavioural attempts at coping. As such, the physiological stress response can itself be viewed as a form of coping mechanism.

Physiological coping occurs at an unconscious, reflex level. However, it has been known for many years (Mason, 1971; Frankenhauser, 1975) that the occurrence of these reflexes can be triggered and influenced by the conscious interpretation of events by the cerebral cortex. The conscious interpretation of incoming stimuli from our surroundings, in the form of sight, sound, smell, taste, touch and pain, can trigger physiological reflexes as well as behavioural responses and the experience of emotion (see Figure 8.3, page 182). For example, for a young child, the sight of a syringe may produce all these responses. In an older person, even the conscious interpretation of the likely meaning of an event – perhaps the expression on the face of the nurse in the accident and emergency department who approaches to give news of the condition of a relative – can trigger these physiological and psychological stress responses.

The entire stress response usually leads to physiological, mental and behavioural adjustments which enable a person to cope with demand. If coping is successful that person is likely to learn from the experience and so have an even greater capacity to cope in similar situations in the future. In other words, the stress response has enabled successful adaptation to the demand. However, if coping is ineffective and demand does not abate, the person will continue to experience stress and in time this may lead to structural and functional damage, ill health, exhaustion and, in extreme cases, death.

PHYSIOLOGICAL RESPONSES TO STRESS

HANS SELYE'S THEORY OF STRESS

Biological concepts of stress are grounded in the pioneering and now classical theory of the Canadian physiologist and physician, Hans Selye.

In the 1920s, Selye, then a medical student, reflected on the mechanisms that might underlie what he later called 'the syndrome of just being sick'. This syndrome is composed of a collection of diagnostically unimportant signs and symptoms such as a coated tongue, fatigue, diffuse aches and pains, feeling and looking ill. In other words these features are non-specific and not characteristic of any one disease.

A decade later, Selye was involved in research where rats were injected with extracts of glands of varying degrees of purity in order to identify ovarian hormones and their functions. To his surprise, when he examined the rats' bodies he found the following changes irrespective of the preparation to which the rats had been subjected:

■ Atrophy (wasting) of the thymus and lymph nodes
■ Bleeding ulcers in the stomach and duodenum
■ Enlargement and hyperactivity of the adrenal cortex.

Selye found that this syndrome, which he called the general adaptation syndrome (GAS), was produced by any noxious agent he tried. It seemed to be a pattern of response to the fact of trauma rather than to any specific stimulus or demand –

Table 8.3: Hospital Stress Rating Scale

Factor	Stress scale events	Assigned rank	Mean rank score
1 Unfamiliarity of surroundings	Having strangers sleep in the same room with you	01	13.9
	Having to sleep in a strange bed	03	15.9
	Having strange machines around	05	16.8
	Being awakened in the night by the nurse	06	16.9
	Being aware of unusual smells around you	11	19.4
	Being in a room that is too cold or too hot	16	21.7
	Having to eat cold or tasteless food	21	23.2
	Being cared for by an unfamiliar doctor	23	23.4
2 Loss of independence	Having to eat at different times than you usually do	02	15.4
	Having to wear a hospital gown	04	16.0
	Having to be assisted with bathing	07	17.0
	Not being able to get newspapers, radio or TV when you want them	08	17.7
	Having a roommate who has too many visitors	09	18.1
	Having to stay in bed or the same room all day	10	19.1
	Having to be assisted with a bedpan	13	21.5
	Not having your call light answered	35	27.3
	Being fed through tubes	39	29.2
	Thinking you may lose your sight	49	40.6
3 Separation from spouse	Worrying about your spouse being away from you	20	22.7
	Missing your spouse	38	28.4
4 Financial problems	Thinking about losing income because of your illness	27	25.9
	Not having enough insurance to pay for your hospitalisation	36	27.4
5 Isolation from other people	Having a roommate who is seriously ill or cannot talk with you	12	21.2
	Having a roommate who is unfriendly	14	21.6
	Not having friends visit you	15	21.7
	Not being able to call family or friends on the phone	22	23.3
	Having the staff be in too much of a hurry	26	24.5
	Thinking you might lose your hearing	45	34.5
6 Lack of information	Thinking you might have pain because of surgery or test procedures	19	22.4
	Not knowing when to expect things will be done to you	25	24.2
	Having nurses or doctors talk too fast or use words you can't understand	29	26.4
	Not having your questions answered by the staff	37	27.6
	Not knowing the results or reasons for your treatments	41	31.9
	Not knowing for sure what illnesses you have	43	34.0
	Not being told what your diagnosis is	44	34.1
7 Threat of severe illness	Thinking your appearance might be changed after your hospitalisation	17	22.1
	Being put in the hospital because of an accident	24	26.9
	Knowing you have to have an operation	32	26.9
	Having a sudden hospitalisation you weren't planning to have	34	27.2
	Knowing you have a serious illness	46	34.6
	Thinking you might lose a kidney or some other organ	47	35.6
	Thinking you might have cancer	48	39.2
8 Separation from family	Being in the hospital during holidays or special family occasions	18	22.3
	Not having family visit you	31	26.5
	Being hospitalised far away from home	33	27.1
9 Problems with medications	Having medications cause you discomfort	28	26.0
	Feeling you are getting dependent on medications	30	26.4
	Not getting relief from pain medications	40	31.2
	Not getting pain medication when you need it	42	32.4

and perhaps an experimental replica of the syndrome of 'just being sick'.

Selye found that it was possible to divide the physiological responses associated with the GAS into three quite distinct phases which occur over time (Figure 8.2). He called the initial response the 'alarm reaction'. In this stage, stores of hormone in the adrenal cortex were depleted by increased secretion into the blood. Selye also observed that the blood became more concentrated and that the animal lost weight. No animal could remain in this state for long. It either returned to normal, passed into the next stage of adaptation (or resistance), or died. Progress depended on the intensity and duration of the demand. Selye viewed the alarm stage of the GAS as the expression of a generalised 'call to arms' of the defensive forces of the body.

In the second stage of the GAS, the animal successfully adapted to (or resisted) the effects of the agent (demand) to which it had been exposed. Observed physiological characteristics were quite different from those of the alarm stage. The animal regained weight, blood concentration returned to normal and the adrenal cortex accumulated reserves of hormones.

An animal eventually entered the third phase of the GAS, that of exhaustion, if the effects of the agent continued unabated. Symptoms of exhaustion were essentially similar to those of alarm and the animal died as a result.

Significance of the general adaptation syndrome

Selye called the general adaptation syndrome 'general' because it was produced only by agents

which had a general effect on the body; he called it 'adaptive' because it produced a state of resistance and survival in response to demand. The GAS was a syndrome because its various components were interdependent and coordinated. Selye postulated that the syndrome was produced by 'non-specific stress' and later (1976, page 64) defined stress as 'the state manifested by a specific syndrome which consists of all non-specifically induced changes within a biologic system'. Selye emphasised that the state of stress is manifested only by the appearance of the GAS and defined a 'stressor' as any agent that elicits this syndrome.

By 'non-specifically induced changes', Selye meant those changes that are produced by many agents, as opposed to changes elicited by only one. For example, the characteristic and diagnostic skin rash is a specific effect of infection by the measles virus, whereas a non-specific effect is the inflammatory response which may also be produced by other irritants. It is important to distinguish local inflammation (termed local adaptation syndromes, LAS, by Selye, 1976) from the GAS, which is produced only by agents which have a general effect on the body. Generalised inflammation could therefore activate the GAS.

Selye's very broad concept of stress has been extremely influential and is still used by both biological and human scientists. He was one of the first research workers to claim that inappropriate stress responses can produce physical diseases and named many disorders, including conditions of inflammatory and immunological origin, as being stress-induced 'diseases of adaptation' (Selye, 1946). Research which has developed these early ideas of Selye is discussed in the final section of this chapter.

Selye's description of the specific features of the general adaptation syndrome was, of course, limited by the state of the physiological knowledge and the investigatory techniques available at the time of his original research. Further research, building on that of Selye, has produced more detail of the physiological changes which occur in response to stressors and these are discussed in the next section.

Research has also produced evidence, contrary to Selye's theory, that noxious agents do not always produce the GAS (Mason, 1971). There is also evidence that the response to stress does not always follow the specific pattern described by

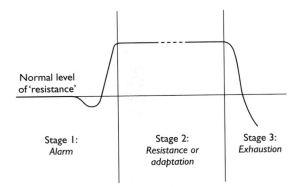

Figure 8.2: The three phases of the general adaptation syndrome (GAS) (Selye, 1976)

Selye. It has been shown (Mason *et al.*, 1976; Terman *et al.*, 1984) that the components of the response can vary with the characteristics of the stressor, between species and between individuals. People exhibit characteristic, possibly familial patterns of response to stress. For example, one person may have gastrointestinal symptoms as the most obvious feature of stress, whilst for another, changes in heart rate, blood pressure and breathing pattern may predominate. Selye's (1976) discussion of 'conditioning factors' goes some way towards making the above evidence compatible with his theory. Conditioning factors may be internal or external to the body and affect the reaction of tissues to stressor agents. External conditioning factors may be concurrent psychological events, for example, whereas internal conditioning factors include inherited characteristics and the effects of past experiences, especially those of coping with that stressor. Despite such discussion, Selye's stress theory is grounded in biology and the body's physiological response to stressors and largely ignores psychological processes or the scope for individual variation in the experience of stress.

PHYSIOLOGICAL CONTROL MECHANISMS IN STRESS

Physiological responses in stress are regulated by the hypothalamus which is a small area of the brain lying, as its name suggests, below the thalamus in the floor of the third ventricle in the brain stem. The hypothalamus controls autonomic nervous activity and hence a number of homeostatic mechanisms, for example, temperature regulation. Through its nervous and vascular connections with the pituitary gland, which lies just below it, the hypothalamus also plays a major role in controlling the secretion of hormones.

The hypothalamus also forms part of the limbic system of the brain. The limbic system is the part of the brain involved in the interpretation of emotion (Ganong, 1995) and has connections with the reticular formation which controls the level of arousal. As well as the hypothalamus having many nervous connections within the limbic system, there are also known pathways between it and the cerebral cortex. These latter pathways are likely to be the ones via which conscious appreci-

ation of events by the cerebral cortex has an effect on physiological function. In other words, the existence of these nerve pathways between the limbic system and the cortex explains how mental events can influence physical response. Stimulation of the limbic system produces the experience of emotions such as anxiety, fear, anger, sorrow and, via the hypothalamus, physiological stress responses. For example, a patient who sees another patient suffer a cardiac arrest may experience both acute anxiety and physiological stress responses. Figure 8.3 summarises the major components in the activation of the stress response. Feedback to the hypothalamus occurs by a number of routes, depending on the nature of the stressor. In stress it may be that the incoming stressor stimuli override normal homeostatic negative feedback mechanisms, thus allowing physiological functioning to take place at levels outside the usual 'normal' range (Toates, 1995).

Acute stress

The physiological changes that occur in the alarm stage of the GAS are short-term responses to cope with acute stress. These responses occur mainly as a result of activation of the sympathetic nervous system, via the hypothalamus, in acute stress and bring about those physiological changes which were first

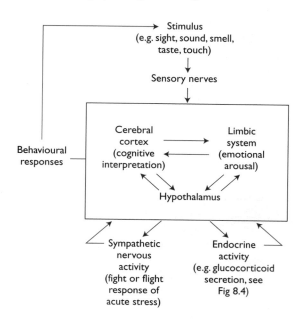

Figure 8.3: The major components in the activation of the stress response

described by Cannon (1929) as the 'fight or flight' response. Sympathetic nervous activity produces reflex responses which are rapid and specific. It also directly stimulates the secretion of the catecholamines adrenaline (epinephrine) and noradrenaline (norepinephrine) from the adrenal medulla. These hormones potentiate and prolong the effects of the sympathetic nervous activity. In humans, adrenaline is the major catecholamine secreted by a factor of about four to one. Although stressor stimuli which increase the secretion of one of these hormones usually increase the secretion of both, this is not always the case. For example, Dimsdale and Moss (1980) have produced evidence to show that heavy physical exercise is associated with a rise in circulating noradrenaline, whereas public speaking has a more marked effect on adrenaline. It has been recognised for many years (Funkenstein, 1955; Frankenhauser, 1975; Asterita, 1985; Toates, 1995) that noradrenaline is associated with the effort and exercise or 'fight' aspect of 'fight or flight' and adrenaline with the responses of fear and helplessness, such as freezing and fleeing. It is likely that the primary behavioural response to threat of primitive man was flight, rather than 'fight'. Nowadays a variety of learnt social and cultural factors may modify such responses.

The second column of Table 8.4 summarises the physiological changes that occur in response to sympathetic nervous activity. A more detailed account of these responses and the physiological mechanisms that produce them can be found in Clarke (1996).

This state of arousal cannot be maintained for long because the physiological changes associated with it disrupt homeostasis and are not compatible, in the long term, with life. If the need for adaptation is very intense and the demand (stressor) not removed, the affected person will become exhausted and die.

Box 8.5: An example of acute physiological stress reflexes in action

The response to a sudden severe haemorrhage
Here, immediate autonomic reflexes function crucially to maintain the blood pressure in order to preserve the blood supply to vital organs such as the heart and brain, so that, despite the blood loss, irreversible ischaemic damage does not occur. Essentially, these reflexes maintain blood pressure by increasing heart rate and force of contraction and by producing vasoconstriction in blood vessels supplying 'non-vital' areas, such as the skin and mucous membranes, gastrointestinal organs, liver, spleen and kidneys. If the response is prolonged these latter organs may suffer ischaemic damage, as a direct result of the acute stress response which has ensured initial survival. For example, acute renal failure is one of the more common complications of severe haemorrhage. Rapid replacement of the blood volume is essential in these circumstances. This reduces the intensity of stressor demand and hence the degree of physiological stress experienced.

If the intensity of the stressor is not so great, for example if the volume of blood loss is not so large or it takes place over a longer period of time, it may be that the short- and longer-term physiological responses can 'cope' with the requirement to adapt to the demand, without additional supportive 'first aid' measures. An excellent, full account of the physiological response to injury of this kind is given by Little (1994).

SIGNS AND SYMPTOMS OF ACUTE STRESS

The majority of the signs and symptoms of acute stress are the direct result of sympathetic nervous arousal. They are summarised in Table 8.4. Symptoms are experienced by the individual concerned and may be communicated to another person, who may be a nurse, whereas physical signs may be directly observed by the nurse. Recognition is the key to prevention and alleviation.

Long-term (chronic) stress

The physiological responses in chronic stress are predominantly the result of increased glucocorticoid secretion from the adrenal cortex, although the secretion of many other hormones is also altered (Toates, 1995). The length of time an individual can remain in the stage of adaptation (resistance) depends on the intensity of the stressor and the adaptive capacity of that individual. If the stressor is not removed, exhaustion will eventually occur when the adrenal cortex can no longer maintain its glucocorticoid secretion. Selye (1976) used the term 'adaptation energy' to describe the energy consumed during stress. He postulated that such energy is determined genetically and is finite, so that when it is used up, exhaustion and

Table 8.4: Physical signs and symptoms which may occur in acute stress

Site	Physiological basis	Physical signs and common clinical measurements	Physical symptoms
Cardiovascular system	Increased cardiac rate and output	Tachycardia Pulse of full volume Raised blood pressure	Pounding heart Palpitations Chest pain Headache
Respiratory system	CNS arousal If the hyperventilation is not in response to physiological need, low pp CO_2 results and leads to vasodilation, fall in blood pressure and, in extreme cases, tetany	Increased rate and depth of ventilation Tetany in extreme cases	Dizziness, faintness, panic (in extreme cases) Tingling in the extremities Muscle spasm (in extreme cases)
Gastrointestinal system	Reduced blood supply to and reduced secretion in gastrointestinal tract		Dry mouth Indigestion/dyspepsia
	Decreased or increased motility of tract	Vomiting Diarrhoea Constipation Anorexia or overeating	Nausea Diarrhoea (often frequent) Constipation Anorexia or overeating
Skin	Contraction of pilomotor muscles Cholinergic sweating Reduced blood supply	Erection of hair Sweating Pallor	Clammy palms
Eye	Contraction of radial muscle	Dilated pupils	Blurred vision
Muscle	CNS arousal	Muscle tension, tremor Muscle spasm in severe cases Lack of coordination	Headache Muscle tension, tremor, twitching Lack of coordination Back pain
General	CNS arousal	Insomnia Restlessness	Insomnia Restlessness Fatigue/weakness
	Increased metabolic rate	Low grade pyrexia	Feeling hot or cold

Reproduced with permission from Boore, J.R.P., Champion, R. and Ferguson, M.C. (eds), 1987, *Nursing the Physically Ill Adult*. Churchill Livingstone, Edinburgh.

death occur. The *stress theory of ageing* has developed from this idea. One important aspect of this theory is the assertion that exposure to stressors accelerates ageing – that is, the greater the 'wear and tear' of life, the faster adaptation energy is consumed. Evidence for the role of stress in the ageing process remains inconclusive. However, the proposition that genetically programmed events may be influenced by life experience of stress is both logical and appealing.

Adrenocorticoid activity in stress

The adrenal cortex is quite distinct, in both structure and function, from the adrenal medulla, despite their close proximity to one another. Unlike the medulla, the secretion of the adrenal cortex is not directly controlled by the nervous system but by the action of other hormones in the blood. Figure 8.4 summarises the negative feedback control of glucocorticoid secretion. Note that,

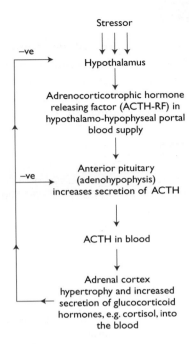

Stressor

−ve

Hypothalamus

Adrenocorticotrophic hormone
releasing factor (ACTH-RF) in
hypothalamo-hypophyseal portal
blood supply

−ve

Anterior pituitary
(adenohypophysis)
increases secretion of ACTH

ACTH in blood

Adrenal cortex
hypertrophy and increased
secretion of glucocorticoid
hormones, e.g. cortisol, into
the blood

Figure 8.4: The control of glucocorticoid secretion

as described earlier, the intensity of the stressor may overcome the negative feedback mechanism.

The physiological effects of cortisol

Cortisol (hydrocortisone) accounts for approximately 95% of the glucocorticoid activity of the adrenal cortex (Asterita, 1985). The main actions of cortisol are on the metabolism of carbohydrates, proteins and fats (Table 8.5). Most changes are catabolic in nature; that is, they break down larger molecules and are sparing of glucose. In most tissues many of these actions are antagonistic to those of insulin and so lead to a rise in blood glucose level. Cortisol is, however, relatively inactive in the heart and brain, so allowing extra glucose to be available to the cells of these organs. In addition to its direct effects, cortisol also has some 'permissive' actions; that is, it must be present to allow some other hormones to affect metabolic reactions. For example, the catecholamines, adrenaline and noradrenaline, require the presence of cortisol in order to influence some metabolic pathways.

Cortisol's anti-inflammatory activity has meant that it and other glucocorticoids can be used therapeutically (steroid therapy) to suppress inflammation in many conditions such as rheumatoid arthritis. However, inflammation is an essential stage in the process of wound healing and if this inflammation is reduced by corticosteroid therapy, wound healing will be delayed. Glucocorticoids are also used for their immunosuppressive effect in reducing rejection in grafting and transplantation. However, high levels of these hormones also reduce white blood cell count and antibody formation, so reducing resistance to infection.

The physiological effects of high plasma levels of cortisol produce Cushing's syndrome. This syndrome can occur pathologically or be due to clinical therapy using the hormones. A fuller account of the physiological effects of cortisol and the mechanisms that produce them can be found in Boore (1996).

According to Hilton (1981), plasma cortisol levels of severely stressed people, for example, postoperative patients and students following oral examination, can be as high as those found in patients with Cushing's disease. Raised cortisol levels are considered by many biologists, including Selye, to be synonymous with stress and it is interesting to consider the possible function in stress of the metabolic changes produced by increased cortisol secretion. This topic is discussed by Asterita (1985) and Toates (1995). In summary, it seems that the role of cortisol is one of:

- Protecting the integrity of the organism against the effect of stressors. It suppresses the less urgent activities of sleep, growth, repair and reproduction, hence making glucose, amino acids and free fatty acids available as an energy source
- Preparing for action, by making available, but conserving the energy source of glucose
- Improving the cells' ability to metabolise anaerobically – possibly crucial in circumstances of maximal survival effort
- Protecting the body from the activity of its natural defences in circumstances where these might get in the way of more urgent metabolic activity. Cortisol acts like a delay switch to turn off several of the body's **defence mechanisms**, for example, inflammation (Munck *et al.*, 1984).

The secretion of other hormones in stress

Although the hypothalamic–pituitary axis and the sympathetic–adrenomedullary axis continue to be the two main areas of research and development in the biological understanding of stress, research evidence suggests that the secretion of nearly every hormone is altered in stress (Asterita, 1985). Mason (1968) pointed out that the stress response produced by the adrenal cortex and medulla are only part of a bigger integrated reaction, which has catabolism and the mobilisation of energy reserves in anticipation of action, as its focus.

The function of physiological responses in stress

The physiological changes of acute stress occur in response to threatening signals and are adaptive insofar as they facilitate effective coping and survival in situations requiring physical activity and in which injury may occur. The stress response

Table 8.5: Physiological effects of glucorticoid (cortisol) secretion in acute and chronic stress

Body function or site	Glucocorticoid effect	Short-term physiological effects	Additional long-term physiological effects
Carbohydrate metabolism	Stimulates hepatic gluconeogenesis	Increased plasma glucose	
	Enhances elevation of blood glucose produced by other hormones, e.g. adrenaline, glucagon		
	Inhibits uptake of glucose by most tissues (not brain) by antagonising peripheral effects of insulin	*Glycosuria (if renal threshold exceeded)	
	Inhibits activity of glycolytic enzyme hexokinase	(Steroid diabetes)	
Protein metabolism	Stimulates breakdown of body protein and depresses protein synthesis	Increased plasma levels of amino acids	*Muscle wasting
		Increased nitrogen content of urine	*Thinning of the skin *Loss of hair
	Stimulates hepatic deamination of amino acids	Negative nitrogen balance	*Depression of the immune response
Lipid metabolism	Promotes lipolysis	Increased plasma levels of fatty acids and cholesterol	*Redistribution of adipose tissue from periphery to head and trunk
		Increased ketone body production and ketonuria	
Calcium metabolism	*Antagonises vitamin D metabolites and so reduces calcium absorption from the gut		*Osteoporosis
	Increases renal excretion of calcium		Kidney stones
Vascular reactivity	Permissive for noradrenaline to induce vasoconstriction	*Prevents stress-induced hypotension	
	Reduces capillary permeability		
Inflammatory response	*Stabilises membranes of cellular lysosomes (inhibiting their rupture) *Suppresses phagocytosis	*Inhibition of inflammation	*Gastric ulceration
	*Reduces multiplication of fibroblasts in connective tissue and hence decreases production of collagen fibres	*Decreased formation of granulation tissue	*Reduced rate of wound healing
	*Inhibits formation and release of histamine and bradykinin	*Reduced allergic response	

Table 8.5: Continued

Body function or site	Glucocorticoid effect	Short-term physiological effects	Additional long-term physiological effects
Immune response	*Reduced immunoglobulin synthesis *Decreased levels of lymphocytes, basophils and eosinophils *Atrophy of lymphoid tissue	*Decreased white blood cell count *Immunosuppression and decreased resistance to infection	
Water and electrolyte balance	Enhances sodium ion and water reabsorption in distal tubules and collecting ducts of renal nephrons Reciprocal potassium and hydrogen ion excretion (mineralocorticoid effect)	Increased extracellular fluid volume	
Blood	*Enhances coagulability *Reduces levels of lymphocytes, basophils and eosinophils *Increases levels of erythrocytes, platelets and neutrophils	*Reduced blood clotting time *Decreased white blood cell count *Haemoconcentration (increased viscosity)	
Central nervous system	*Emotional changes (in excess or deficiency) May facilitate learning and memory (ACTH may independently facilitate learning and memory)	*Emotional changes Increased rate of learning Enhanced learning	

*These physiological effects occur only when high plasma levels of glucocorticoids, similar to those found during steroid therapy, are present.
Reproduced with permission from Boore, J.R.P., Champion, R. and Ferguson, M.C. (eds), 1987, *Nursing the Physically Ill Adult*. Churchill Livingstone, Edinburgh.

varies hardly at all between species and it is likely that such responses developed early in evolution.

Box 8.6: The characteristics of the stress response: a summary

- Central nervous arousal occurs and skeletal muscles tense. The defensive behaviour of freezing and 'playing dead' is a manifestation of extreme muscle tension.
- The pupil of the eye dilates, enlarging the visual field.
- Erection of hair increases the apparent size of the animal (although this response is of little significance in man, it is functional in small furry mammals).
- Nutrients are mobilised in anticipation of a period of fasting and exercise. They are circulated to organs such as the heart and skeletal muscle whose efficient function is crucial to fight and flight.
- Essential organs, such as the brain, heart and muscle are supplied at the expense of those whose function is non-essential in the short term, such as the gastrointestinal tract and kidney.
- Extracellular fluid volume and blood coagulability increase – adaptive responses in case of blood loss.
- Amino acids become available for immediate tissue repair.

It is easy to see that in animal and early human societies, this emergency response to physical threat must often have had survival value. Even today, each time we take exercise or suffer accidental or surgical injury, our ability to produce an acute stress response facilitates survival. As discussed earlier, prompt relief of stress minimises the risk of tissue damage.

Individuals who for some reason are unable to produce an efficient stress response are less able to survive trauma and disease. Loss of adrenomedullary function is not fatal, as sympathetic nervous activity parallels most of the actions of circulating adrenaline and noradrenaline. However, loss of adrenocortical secretion quite rapidly causes death through hypotension, hypoglycaemia and concomitant brain dysfunction.

People suffering from undersecretion of glucocorticoids (Addison's disease) are particularly susceptible to stressors. They may be unable to survive (cope with) quite minor life events, for example, dental extraction, unless they are given artificial hormone cover. People who take glucocorticoids therapeutically and so have artificially high plasma levels of the hormone may also require hormone cover in such situations, because their normal mechanisms of secretion are suppressed.

Today, human stressors are frequently of psychosocial origin and as has been explained in this section, they can also trigger the physiological stress response. If appropriate coping responses do not involve physical exercise and/or injury (as is the case more often than not!) then the physiological stress responses are inappropriate because the resources that are mobilised are not used. In such circumstances sympathetic arousal produces distressing symptoms (see Table 8.4) and in the longer term tissue damage may also occur.

Adrenal reserves of glucocorticoids vary both between individuals and over time for any one person. If a person experiences long-term stress, these reserves are diminished and in very severe cases may become exhausted. This is the parallel of the stage of exhaustion of the general adaptation syndrome. It may also be the physiological reflection of 'burn-out'. Signs and symptoms of impending glucocorticoid exhaustion include feelings of weakness, lightheadedness, extreme fatigue, unease and irritability, gastrointestinal disturbance, low blood pressure, hypoglycaemia and abnormal sensitivity to change in environmental temperature. Clearly the best action is to recognise and help the person to cope with his/her stress before such a situation occurs. If, however, a person experiences these symptoms, rest and relief from stress are imperative. In some circumstances artificial glucocorticoid cover may be necessary.

The similarities between the pharmacological effects of the catecholamines and cortisol and the pathological changes associated with many diseases of civilisation, have led to stress being implicated in the aetiology of these diseases. Although it is known that plasma levels of glucocorticoids as high as those in Cushing's syndrome can induce pathological change, for example, gastric ulceration, the long-term ability of lower plasma levels of these hormones to produce disease, has not yet been elicited.

Evidence for the role of distress in the aetiology of disease is discussed in the last section of this chapter.

Modifying physiological responses in stress

In circumstances where the physiological response to stress is inappropriate, stress can be relieved either by reducing the perceived demand on the individual or by increasing the individual's perceived ability to cope with the demand, for example, by education. Learning a technique such as yoga, transcendental meditation or progressive muscle relaxation can be helpful since successful use of such techniques induces a state that is the opposite of sympathetic arousal (Bailey and Clarke, 1989). Taking exercise is another effective means of stress relief since physical activity utilises the physiological response appropriately. Techniques such as biofeedback systematically train the stressed individual to exercise control over some aspect of his/her stress response.

Tranquillising drugs, alcohol and tobacco relieve stress by temporarily suppressing the person's perception of the demand upon him/her. Their use is associated with other health risks but may be justified in the short term if they help the person to cope until the problem resolves or more effective coping methods are found. These are examples of **emotion-focused coping** (see next section) which is directed at the physiological components of the stress response.

Key Points

■ The stress response has both physiological and psychological components and both of these represent attempts at coping with the source of stress.

■ Physiological coping occurs at an unconscious, reflex level, but can be triggered and influenced by the conscious interpretation of events by the cerebral cortex.

■ Biological concepts of stress are grounded in the pioneering and now classical theory of the Canadian physiologist and physician, Hans Selye, who described the general adaptation syndrome, with its three stages of 'alarm', 'resistance' and 'exhaustion', which was, he proposed, a manifestation of stress.

■ Physiological responses in stress are regulated by the hypothalamus which controls autonomic nervous activity and the secretion of hormones from the pituitary gland.

■ Acute stress, or the alarm reaction, is largely due to the activation of the sympathetic nervous system which brings about those physiological changes which were first described by Cannon (1929) as the 'fight or flight' response.

■ Longer-term stress responses are mainly due to the effects of glucocorticoid (cortisol) secretion from the adrenal cortex, although the secretion of nearly every hormone is altered in stress.

■ Physiological stress responses may be adaptive (appropriate) or maladaptive (inappropriate) in enabling the person to cope with demand, depending on the nature of the stressor which produced them.

■ Stress may be relieved through the use of techniques which modify or utilise the physiological stress responses produced, or which alter the person's perception of the demand upon him/her.

PSYCHOLOGICAL RESPONSES TO STRESS

Despite the limitations of Selye's early research, it stimulated a lasting interest in the subject of stress and much research. This research aimed to discover whether the observation of a characteristic set of physiological reactions to a variety of environmental stressors – the GAS – could be generalised to include the reactions of humans exposed to a range of stressors in their everyday lives. Indeed, Selye's ideas about non-specific responses to stress continued to be influential for a number of years until evidence became available which suggested that some unpleasant conditions did not lead to GAS (Mason, 1971), and that physiological responses may differ according to the nature of the stressor (see, for example, Mason et al., 1976; Terman et al., 1984). Selye's research, therefore, laid the foundations for later studies concerned with the possible influence of psychological processes.

It is now apparent that cognitive and emotional factors intervening between stimulus and response may help to account for observed differences in the endocrine response to stress. Physiological reactions to aversive stimuli appear to be linked to variations in how people perceive the threatening event. This highlights the importance of taking subjective reactions and feelings into account. For instance, Mason et al. (1976) found that humans will produce catecholamines initially when exposed to strong aversive stressors such as heat or noise, but if subjective feelings of competitiveness are minimal, they will not produce the expected increase in cortisol secretion. The absence of cortisol is significant, given the role it is believed to play in inhibiting the immune response. Similar findings have been reported for children admitted to hospital for tonsillectomy (Knight et al., 1979) and for women undergoing breast biopsy for possible malignancy (Katz et al., 1970). Evidence of stress-induced changes in immune activity is now fairly extensive (see, for example, Herbert and Cohen, 1993).

As long as people feel able to meet the demands that are made upon them, they are likely to view stress positively as a challenge. As soon as this situation changes, however, and their ability to cope in relation to the demand decreases, then the all too familiar negative responses to stress occur.

You will almost certainly have experienced a range of feelings associated with the negative experience of 'being under stress'. This may include emotions such as anxiety, fear, guilt, tension, anger, aggression, irritability, depression, tiredness, a feeling of worthlessness, apathy, hopelessness and frustration. Lazarus (1976) refers to these negative emotions which occur as a result of stress as 'stress emotions'. In addition to these negative emotions, stress may impair cognitive ability (Hebb, 1972). You may have experienced this first-hand when you have been unable to concentrate or organise your thoughts logically when sitting an important examination.

According to Lazarus, stress emotions can serve a useful purpose in that they often trigger a variety of behaviours which are attempts to deal with the stressful situation; i.e. most of us are motivated to reduce the unpleasant feelings associated with stress. The way in which we do this has been called 'coping'. We also owe this concept to Lazarus (1966) who suggested that the term 'coping' refers to 'strategies for dealing with threat' (page 151). Cox (1978) suggests that coping is the key to understanding psychological responses to stress.

Lazarus and Folkman (1984) suggest that two rather different kinds of processes may be involved in coping with stress:

- **Problem-focused coping**
- **Emotion-focused coping.**

In the first of these, the individual deals directly with the problem: after evaluating the situation, the individual does something either to change it or avoid it. The alternative process, emotion-focused coping, is a more indirect means of coping, concerned more with reducing anxiety than with dealing with the situation responsible for producing the anxiety.

PROBLEM-FOCUSED COPING

This means of coping involves conscious action and can take several forms. If a potential cause of stress can be anticipated, one may take steps to reduce the harm when it does occur. The provision of information to reduce fear of the unknown is an excellent example of helping to produce this kind of coping. Janis, an American social psychologist, was one of the first people to investigate stress in patients awaiting surgery, and the benefits of giving accurate prior information and reassurance about post-operative discomfort (see Janis, 1971; Langer *et al.*, 1975). The much-cited research of nurse researchers such as Hayward (1975) and Boore (1978) provides further evidence of the benefits of reduced post-operative anxiety levels in patients when they have been given information about what to expect before the operation.

Another example of problem-focused coping is provided by the person who decides to develop new skills (for instance, by attending an assertiveness training course) to deal with colleagues more effectively.

Two further means of problem-focused coping are aggression and escape, which are behavioural responses associated with the physiological acute stress responses of 'fight' and 'flight'. Although each may be effective in the short term, neither allows a person to come to terms with the threat, and each may be responsible for difficulties, such as anxiety, in the longer term. You may either vent your aggression directly on the perceived source of the frustration (for example, in the case of course-related stress, on the college where you are studying) or you may vent your anger on some more readily available target (such as arguing with a friend). For similar reasons, it is not uncommon for patients/clients to become angry with those responsible for caring for them.

Alternatively, the feelings associated with stress may motivate a person to escape from the stressful situation; in this case he or she might decide, if work or studying was the stressor, to leave his/her job or the course. Under normal circumstances, one might argue that escape is more appropriate for physically threatening rather than psychologically threatening events.

EMOTION-FOCUSED COPING

Palliative strategies, such as alcohol, drugs (sedatives and tranquillisers) or relaxation techniques, may be used to moderate the distress frequently associated with a stressful experience by reducing its psychophysiological effects. Psychological mechanisms which distort reality may also be used to moderate distress. When studying the unconscious, Anna Freud (1946) identified a number of psychological ways, known as defence mechanisms, by which a person could deceive himself about the presence of a threat by distorting reality in some way.

Lazarus (1976) suggested that a number of defence mechanisms might be used to reduce the perception of threat, including:

- Denial
- Identification
- Displacement
- Repression
- Reaction formation

- Projection
- Intellectualisation.

You may already be familiar with several of these defence mechanisms. For instance, you may have cared for someone who has a life-threatening disease, but who refuses to accept that he is ill (denial) and thus discounts what he is told about the prognosis. Similarly, intellectualisation may be used by health care professionals to enable them to become emotionally detached from a situation which might otherwise be threatening or intolerable. Professional people may only be able to control their own feelings by not identifying too closely with the suffering of particular patients or clients. Most psychology textbooks will provide a more detailed description of defence mechanisms (see, for example, Chapter 14 in Atkinson *et al.*, 1996).

Although originally used by Freud to describe unconscious mechanisms, Cox (1978) suggests that we may deliberately employ one or other of these defence mechanisms as a means of coping with a stressful situation. Cox also reminds us that such concepts are difficult to evaluate scientifically since they are rather loosely defined (as are many of the concepts deriving from psychoanalytical theory), and they are descriptive rather than predictive. However, he goes on to say:

'Despite this they have, like most psychoanalytic concepts, had some impact on psychological thought and the practice of psychology'.

(page 84)

People probably use both types of coping strategy. Whilst it might appear that problem-focused coping is the more effective approach to adopt, it is important to remember that some problems simply cannot be solved or at least not immediately. For instance, when someone who is close to you dies, you may need some means of emotion-focused coping to reduce the emotional distress in the short term, until you feel ready to face up to the loss and its consequences, and can subsequently seek out more effective methods of coping.

APPRAISAL-FOCUSED COPING

In addition to problem-focused and emotional-focused coping, Moos and Schaefer (1984) identified a third form of coping which they called appraisal-focused coping. As its name suggests,

this type of coping is concerned with attempting to understand the situation and searching for meaning. They suggest this may be achieved through:

- Logical analysis and mental preparation (which is concerned with translating an event that is potentially unmanageable into one that can be managed)
- Cognitive redefinition (involving accepting the reality of the situation and redefining it in ways that are more positive and acceptable)
- Cognitive avoidance and denial (minimising the seriousness of the situation).

According to Moos and Schaefer's theory of coping with the 'crisis' of physical illness (the term crisis is being used here in the Eriksonian view of the life cycle as a series of seven crises), individuals start by appraising their new situation and then employ a range of problem-focused and emotion-focused skills to cope with it. The collective impact of these coping skills can affect the outcome in terms of psychological well-being and may also influence physical well-being (see the next section on stress and illness).

Studies that take account of individual differences, such as coping styles when investigating the benefits of particular forms of social support (e.g. information giving) highlight some important inconsistencies. For instance, Kendall and Epps (1990) found that individuals who preferred to use avoidant coping strategies tended to deny the information given, whilst others actively sought out information in order to prepare an action plan. This may account for some of the differences in research findings you may encounter in your reading. It highlights the importance of focusing on the individual and trying to understand the factors that may be important for that particular person when working with someone who is coping with a stressful situation.

It is now recognised that the success of coping strategies may partly depend on the extent to which people believe that they can control their situation. Seligman's theory of **learned helplessness** originated from a series of studies carried out with dogs (see Box 8.7).

Although this model of learned helplessness in animals is far too simple to explain human behaviour, our ability to cope with stress is likely to be affected by the feeling that we have a certain amount of control over our lives. According to

> **Box 8.7: Seligman's theory of learned helplessness**
>
> Seligman (1975) found that dogs readily learned to escape a mild electric shock by jumping away from the source, and that if a light was switched on briefly before the shock was administered, the dogs learned to avoid the shocks altogether by escaping into the 'safe' area. However, dogs who had previously experienced electric shocks which they had been unable to avoid continued to endure the shocks and sat passively: they did not learn either to escape, or the appropriate avoidance response, even when a new situation allowed them to do so. Moreover, Seligman found that this kind of learned helplessness was very difficult to overcome.

Rotter (1966), people differ in their belief about the degree of control they can exert: some individuals have a greater sense of being in control of their lives than others, which may in its turn affect their coping ability.

If people believe they cannot influence the situation in which they find themselves, then feelings of helplessness are likely to develop and lead to inactivity, as a result of what Lazarus (1976) calls the hopelessness of their situation. In order to help such people, it would be necessary to assist them to re-establish control over their situation by suggesting possible ways of coping. In this context, it is interesting to note the results of a classic study undertaken in a nursing home by Langer and Rodin (1976) in which the residents' perception of control was manipulated by encouraging greater responsibility for certain aspects of their lives (e.g. the movement of furniture, care of a plant, whether or not to attend a film). The reported benefits of perceived control included increased sociability and activity levels of the residents and improved health ratings. These improvements were still evident in an 18-month follow-up study (Rodin and Langer, 1977). Thus, it would appear that even control over relatively minor matters can affect the well-being of elderly people.

MANAGING STRESS

There are numerous strategies, besides alcohol and medication, that may be used to reduce stress, including:

- Giving information
- Relaxation training
- Biofeedback
- Meditation
- Stress inoculation
- Physical exercise
- Assertiveness training
- Counselling
- Sharing the problem with others through support groups.

The list of further reading at the end of this chapter includes a number of useful resources on how to deal more effectively with stress (see, in particular, Burnard, 1991 and Fontana, 1989).

We have already seen that hospitalisation and some clinical procedures are potentially stressful for patients/clients. It is important, therefore, to recognise stressors in the clinical environment and try to reduce stress by altering the way in which a patient/client perceives the environment by providing information and helping individuals to develop appropriate coping strategies. Box 8.8 describes how a fairly simple intervention helped not only male patients who had suffered a myocardial infarction, but also their wives.

> **Box 8.8: In-hospital counselling for male patients and their wives**
>
> The effectiveness of an in-hospital counselling scheme provided by a coronary care nurse has been systematically evaluated by Thompson. Four 30-minute counselling sessions were provided for patients and their wives during the first week in the coronary care unit (CCU), following a first myocardial infarction. The aim of these sessions was to recognise the patients' feelings and reduce fear and uncertainty by giving information about the nature and impact of heart attacks and their management and engender a positive yet realistic outlook. Particular emphasis was placed on the provision of psychological support and the use of positive coping mechanisms and on encouraging involvement in decisions about their care.
>
> Of the 60 patients enrolled on the study, 30 received the counselling sessions (the experimental group) whilst the remaining 30 acted as a comparison group, receiving routine medical and nursing care only. Whilst both groups had similar levels of anxiety and depression at the outset, the experimental group

had significantly lower levels following the counselling sessions. The improvements were still evident 6 months following discharge from hospital (Thompson, 1990; Thompson and Meddis, 1990a, b).

Whilst it may seem obvious that patients and clients need help to cope with stressful experiences, it is also important to acknowledge the consequences of stress for health care professionals. Many learn to cope with the demands of their work, with or without some form of external support, and continue to function effectively. Those who experience difficulties in coping with work-related stressors whilst remaining in the working environment are likely to become exhausted, may suffer burn-out, and may leave the profession or drop out of their education programme. The following comment made by a nurse manager summarises some of the key issues:

'The stereotyped image of the qualified nurse is that she is committed totally to her patients, is skilled, fit and strong, and gives care as opposed to needing it. But of course . . . it just is not true. Nurses need help and support . . . just as much as our students and our patients. Unfortunately this does not seem to be recognised by the public, the organisation, or indeed, the profession itself.'
(Hingley and Cooper, 1986, page 142)

Concern about recruitment, retention and wastage means that gender emphasis needs to be placed on stress management and support groups so that individuals are not left to cope alone. Given our current understanding of stress and its consequences – both for the individual and the organisation – it is important to ensure that no nurse in the future cites lack of support from other nurses as a source of stress as has previously been reported (see, for example, Bergh-Braam and de Wolff, 1998; Rentoul, 1989).

Key Points

- Evidence suggests that cognitive and emotional factors intervening between stimulus and response (i.e. how a person perceives a threatening event) may help to explain observed differences in the endocrine response to stress. It highlights the importance of taking subjective reactions and feelings into account.

- A range of negative emotions is usually associated with the negative experience of 'being under stress', including anxiety, anger, irritability, tiredness, hopelessness and depression.
- Coping skills are the key to dealing with stress. Three types of coping skills may be used: appraisal-focused coping, problem-focused coping and emotion-focused coping.
- The success of coping strategies may be partly determined by the extent to which a person believes he/she can control his/her situation. If a person is feeling helpless, it is important to help him/her to re-establish control over the situation by suggesting possible coping strategies.
- Like patients/clients and student nurses, qualified nurses may also, on occasions, need help and support because of the stressful events they experience; they should not be left to cope alone. Far more emphasis needs to be placed on stress management and on support groups in the workplace, in order to tackle problems associated with staff well-being, morale, sickness rates, recruitment, retention and wastage of staff.

STRESS AND ILLNESS

As long ago as 1932, Cannon suggested that vital body organs could be damaged if the activity of the autonomic nervous system is maintained in a highly aroused state as a result of prolonged exposure to stress. In this section, we shall briefly examine some of the evidence concerning the relationship between physical illness and stress-related factors.

Behavioural medicine has become a recognised interdisciplinary field of study that aims to understand how psychological, physiological and social variables interact to cause illness, and also to identify ways in which health can be promoted. What are your beliefs about a possible relationship between a person's psychological and emotional state and susceptibility to illness? Think for a moment about the following four questions.

Do you believe that:

1 A person is more likely to develop an illness, such as flu, when feeling under pressure?
2 A person's personality can affect the likelihood that he/she will suffer from coronary heart disease?

3 Stress is a causal factor in cancer?

4 Psychiatric illness is associated with changes in immune status?

Whatever your beliefs, it is interesting to note that these and similar assumptions can be traced back to some of the earliest medical thinkers and pre-date the relatively recent growth of interest in this subject (Harvey, 1988).

It is certainly well established that physical illness may be produced in laboratory animals exposed to severe and prolonged environmental stress. Weiss (1972), for example, reported that healthy rats who were able to escape from electric shocks showed fewer gastric lesions than those who were helpless and could not escape. Control rats who received no electric shocks showed no ulceration of the stomach. Similarly, Sklar and Anisman (1979) induced tumours in mice by implanting cancerous tissue and then studied the impact of stress on the rate of growth of these tumours. The tumours of the mice who were exposed to electric shocks grew faster than those of the control mice, and they died sooner.

One cannot simply generalise from animals to humans, and ethical constraints obviously preclude researchers carrying out similar experiments with human subjects. Considerable research has, however, been carried out in relation to people being exposed to respiratory viruses. For example, in a carefully controlled trial undertaken at the (now disbanded) Common Cold Unit run by the Medical Research Council, 394 healthy volunteers were exposed to nasal drops containing one of five respiratory viruses or saline (the control condition). They found a positive correlation between respiratory infection rates and the degree of the subject's psychological stress, even after controlling for other possible contributory factors such as age, gender, season of the year, personality traits, smoking and amount of exercise taken (Cohen et al., 1991). In this type of experimental research, the investigator is able to exert a considerable amount of control over the study and determine which individuals are allocated to specific experimental conditions.

In this field, however, researchers are unable to undertake many highly controlled studies because of ethical and practical constraints. Rather, they are forced to undertake studies which compare the effects of naturally occurring differences in the variable of interest, such as the effects of different levels of stress on the development of illness. So, for instance, a researcher may choose to compare people with high stress/anxiety levels with those with low stress/anxiety levels. Quasi-experimental research does not, however, allow the researcher to identify causal factors. When considering the evidence from such a study, it is necessary to remember that while stress may be identified as a possible contributory factor in the development of illness, illness itself is likely to be a source of stress, thus making it impossible to identify causal relationships unequivocally.

As we shall see, many of the claims that specific illnesses are associated with particular aspects of social behaviour, including stress, have either not been systematically tested or, if they have been tested, the emerging evidence has often been conflicting. One exception to this is the assertion that particular patterns of behaviour predispose people to develop coronary heart disease (CHD).

STRESS AND CHD

Heart disease is a major cause of death in most industrialised countries. Epidemiological data have identified a series of risk factors, including non-modifiable ones, such as family history or a person's gender and other factors that are potentially modifiable, such as smoking behaviour, high systolic blood pressure, raised levels of serum cholesterol (low density lipoprotein in particular), obesity or a sedentary lifestyle. However, even when looked at together, these factors only account for about half the variation of CHD. It would appear that other psychosocial factors also play a role – factors such as levels of anxiety (see Kawachi et al., 1994) and behaviour patterns. The latter possibility has generated a considerable amount of research.

After observing the behaviour of their patients, two American cardiologists identified the major behavioural characteristics of the male who is prone to develop CHD (Friedman and Rosenman, 1959). Their list included:

- Highly competitive behaviour
- Over-commitment to work
- High achieving
- Impatience
- Restlessness
- Hostility

- An exaggerated sense of the urgency of passing time
- The need to do everything in a hurry.

These behaviour characteristics are referred to collectively as the 'type A' pattern of behaviour and have become more common in twentieth century industrialised, urban society. Although this behaviour pattern may resemble a personality type, it is important to remember that the researchers were investigating the relationship between specific behaviours and the incidence of CHD, *not* personality. There is, as yet, no evidence that a particular type of personality is more prone to develop CHD. The 'type B' behaviour pattern, on the other hand, is characterised by more relaxed behaviours.

A double-blind prospective epidemiological study – the Western Collaborative Group Study – confirmed the predictive validity of a type A behaviour pattern. In this study, 3524 American men aged between 35 and 59, who were well at the start, were followed up over 8.5 years. During this time, the drop-out rate was remarkably low and 3154 completed the study. Individuals exhibiting type A behaviour patterns were found to be 2.37 times as likely to develop CHD as were the type B men. Even when traditional risk factors were controlled for, men exhibiting type A behaviours were still about twice as likely to develop CHD. In addition, type A men were five times more likely to suffer a second myocardial infarction than other men with CHD (Rosenman *et al.*, 1975). Similar findings have been reported in other studies (e.g. Steptoe, 1985), including long-term prospective studies (Haynes *et al.*, 1980).

Attempts have been made to explain these findings. It has been suggested that in response to stress, individuals with type A behaviour have higher nonadrenaline levels in the blood and that this may lead to heart lesions and damage to the arteries, and may also increase the extent to which platelets aggregate, making thrombosis formation more likely.

However, the validity of type A behaviour pattern as a risk factor for CHD has been questioned because some studies have failed to find a strong relationship between them (see, for example, Ragland and Brand, 1988a, b). This has led some researchers to suggest that type A behaviour pattern may be too general to be useful and that a specific component of type A behaviour might pro-

vide a better predictor. In particular, hostility has been investigated. A number of studies suggest that hostility is associated with CHD and offers a more valid predictor than type A behaviour (Chesney *et al.*, 1988). The possibility that hostility may be related to some of the established risk factors raises doubt about whether it is appropriate to regard hostility as a strong independent risk factor for CHD. In addition, several studies have failed to find a relationship between hostility and heart disease (e.g. McCranie *et al.*, 1986; Hearn *et al.*, 1989). More recently, anger has been investigated as a specific component of hostility and identified as a potential psychosocial risk factor for heart disease (Mendes de Leon, 1992). It also remains to be seen whether it is possible to modify the behaviours of individuals who have suffered a heart attack, using cognitive and behavioural techniques, in order to decrease the risk of recurrent attacks (Cooper, 1989).

STRESS AND CANCER

Another disease which has received considerable attention is cancer: in particular, the idea that stress may be a causal factor in its aetiology and in the progression of the disease (Sklar and Anisman, 1981). It is clearly important that any empirical evidence is evaluated carefully so that patients are not 'blamed' for their illness. An excellent early review of some of the evidence relating specific aspects of stress to cancer is provided by Temoshok and Heller (1984). They highlight the difficulty of drawing firm conclusions given the diversity of studies that have been carried out. They conclude that the incidence of major life events (such as those measured by the SRRS) appears to be a less important factor than the way in which such events are handled. They also suggest that there is a growing amount of evidence to support the idea that cancers are most frequently found in individuals who do not express their emotions and who react in a hopeless manner to difficult situations.

When reviewing available evidence, it is important to recognise the limitations of research based on retrospective methods which require patients to assess the stress they were under during the one or two years preceding their diagnosis (Blaney, 1985). As for any retrospective data, people's perceptions and memories may become distorted over time, particularly following the diagnosis of cancer. Also, the actual diagnosis probably occurs several years after the disease process has started, so the cancer was probably present before the high levels of stress were reported.

Prospective methods are, therefore, more appropriate to investigate the role of stress in the development of cancer. This involves starting with a healthy group of individuals, assessing them on a range of psychosocial factors and then following up their health status over time. Sklar and Anisman (1981) reported that people who experienced high levels of stress were more likely to develop cancer than those experiencing less stress. Moreover, those already diagnosed with cancer who suffered a relapse within a year also tended to have experienced higher levels of stress and less social support than those who did not have a relapse (see Sabbioni, 1991).

There is also considerable interest in the role that psychological interventions can play in promoting quality of life and alleviating the symptoms of cancer. For example, Simonton and Simonton (1975) used relaxation, mental imagery (focusing on positive outcomes) and exercise programmes to promote a sense of well-being and a good response to treatment with fewer side-effects. In a 15-year follow-up study of women with breast cancer, Temoshok and Fox (1984) showed that poorer outcomes were associated with passive coping styles and with feelings of helplessness (see also Box 8.9).

Box 8.9: A randomised controlled trial to investigate the effectiveness of a cognitive behavioural therapy

Greer and colleagues (1992) investigated the effectiveness of a cognitive behavioural treatment – adjuvant psychological therapy (APT), which focuses on helping patients with cancer to examine the personal meaning of their cancer and how they can cope with it. APT aims to identify an individual's strengths and use these to enhance self-esteem, reduce feelings of helplessness, promote a fighting spirit, challenge any recurring negative thoughts/anxieties, and promote a sense of control. A range of measures was used to assess each participant's psychological state at the start of the study, including the Hospital Anxiety and Depression Scale and the Mental Adjustment to Cancer Scale.

After 8 weeks, patients in the experimental group who had received APT recorded significantly higher scores on fighting spirit compared with those who did not receive the intervention, and significantly lower scores on anxiety, helplessness and psychological symptoms. Improvements of anxiety, psychological symptoms and psychological distress were still evident after 4 months.

At the present time, empirical evidence from both animal and human studies suggesting links between stress and cancer is largely suggestive rather than conclusive. It is important, therefore, not to overstate the case. The effects of stress would appear to be influenced by a number of factors including the source of the stress, when it is experienced and whether or not the stress is chronic. Stress may well play a causal role in the development and progression of cancers by increasing behavioural risk factors, such as heavy smoking, or by reducing the ability of the immune system to fight disease.

STRESS AND THE IMMUNE SYSTEM

Following on from the study of specific diseases, researchers have also been trying to find out how stress may exert its effect. Those working in the rapidly developing field of **psychoneuroimmunology** are trying to uncover ways in which the central nervous system interacts with the functioning of the immune system to affect our susceptibility to disease (Herbert and Cohen, 1993; Evans et al., 1997).

The immune system provides a complex means by which the human body is able to maintain health by protecting itself against disease. An immune response is triggered by invading micro-organisms, such as bacteria or viruses (known as mitogens). There are a number of measures, including the reactivity of T-lymphocytes, the percentages of different types of lymphocyte, and the ratio between different types of cell:

- Helper T-cells which help to generate antibodies
- Cytotoxic and natural killer cells which can destroy tumour cells
- Suppressor cells which can modify the activity of other cells or antibodies.

The effects of a range of stressful events have been studied including marital separation and divorce, bereavement, and caring for a relative with Alzheimer's disease or with dementia. For example, Kiecolt-Glaser *et al.* (1987) studied 34 family care givers of patients with Alzheimer's disease. The care givers were found to be more depressed and to have significantly poorer immune functioning than a comparison group (based on the percentages of total T-lymphocyte and helper T-cells, the ratio of helper to suppressor cells, and the antibody response to a latent herpes virus). In a later study, Kiecolt-Glaser and colleagues (1991) reported that spouses who were caring for a partner suffering from dementia demonstrated suppressed immune system functioning and more days of illness (particularly respiratory illnesses). In a meta-analysis of 38 studies, Herbert and Cohen (1993) found a broad association between chronic stress and suppressed immunity (sometimes referred to as down-regulated immunity).

Immune system activity may also be compromised in people suffering from severe depression. For instance, Stein *et al.* (1985) measured lymphocyte reactivity in a group of severely depressed patients and found it to be significantly lower than that of a carefully matched group of people who were not depressed. The number of T-lymphocytes was also significantly reduced. Similar changes were not, however, found in patients hospitalised for a major physical disorder, patients with schizophrenia, or those suffering from less severe depression.

Current evidence would, therefore, seem to suggest that the activity of the central nervous system and the neuroendocrine system are closely associated with emotional activity. However, the picture is far from clear cut, as Evans and colleagues (1997) remind us. They highlight what they refer to as 'some striking anomalies in the research literature'. The effects of very acute short-term stress on immune function would appear to be very different. Acute stressors such as public speaking, challenging computer games and confrontational role play have been found to result in enhanced immune function, including an increase in the number of natural killer cells (see, for example, Herbert *et al.*, 1994; Delahanty *et al.*, 1996). So there would appear to be important differences between the effects of acute and chronic stress.

Thus, the sheer complexity of the immune system and its relationship with other physiological systems makes it premature to do anything more than speculate about the nature of the relationship between acute and chronic stress and immune responses at the present time (Martin, 1996). This is an area of research that should yield important new findings in the future. If you are interested in this field, you should scan scientific and medical journals such as *New Scientist*, *Nature* and the *British Medical Journal* for the latest published research papers and review articles. For the present time, it remains unclear whether the relationship between stressful life events and the incidence of illness may be due to actual changes in health mediated directly by the immune system, or to lowered capability to cope with disease which is already present. On the other hand, to overlook stress as a possible factor contributing directly to the disease process and its treatment is likely to be an important omission.

A chief concern in the 1990s is the possible relationship between high levels of occupational stress and specific disease. When considering this issue it is important to remember that certain kinds of people may choose stressful jobs in the first place, or even contribute to high levels of stress within their own job: an individual's disposition and temperament is, therefore, a key confounding variable.

Now that we have examined some of the evidence concerning the relationship between stress and illness, we shall return to the four questions set out at the beginning of this section:

- Available evidence suggests that individuals are more likely to develop an illness such as flu when they are feeling under pressure (Question 1).
- Whilst there is evidence that specific behaviour patterns – namely type A behaviours – affect the likelihood that a person will suffer from coronary heart disease, this has not, as yet, been related to personality *per se* (Question 2).
- Question 3 about stress being a causal factor in cancer is not supported by the available data: stress may well be a contributory factor, but correlational data do not enable claims to be made about causal factors.
- Lastly, there is no evidence that psychiatric illness *per se* is associated with changes in immune status (Question 4); people with

severe depression have, however, been found to have fewer T-cells and reduced lymphocyte reactivity.

The answers to these questions highlight the care needed when analysing available evidence and the danger of making unwarranted assertions or generalising the findings too widely. You will notice that at best we can only talk about 'the like-lihood' of something occurring or a high correla-tion between two factors. Individual variation in the experience of stress is certainly evident when one looks at the relationship between stress and health/illness. Although correlational data may enable us to predict the likelihood of a person who exhibits type A behaviours developing CHD, it is important to remember that many people who fall into that category do *not* develop the disease. Moreover, reactions to stressful life events cannot be understood without taking account of factors which mediate their effect, such as degree of antic-ipation and control over the occurrence of an event. Further research is needed to extend our understanding of the highly complex relationship between stress-related factors and the likely onset of specific illnesses.

Key Points

- Whilst there is evidence suggesting a relationship between the incidence of stress and specific types of disease, including coronary heart disease and cancer, the evidence needs to be interpreted with care.
- Correlational data do not allow us to make unequivocal statements about causal relationships. Moreover, data collected within retrospective studies may well be inaccurate since they are largely based on perceptions and memories that may have become distorted with the passage of time.
- Researchers working within the field of psy-choneuroimmunology are investigating the precise mechanisms by which stress may affect our sus-ceptibility to disease.
- An overview of research suggests that there is a broad association between chronic stress and down-regulated immune functioning.
- Whilst current evidence suggests that the activity of the central nervous system and the neuroen-docrine system are closely associated with emo-tional activity, the picture is not clear cut and

there are some important anomalies in the research literature which cannot be overlooked.
- The sheer complexity of the immune system and its relationship with other physiological systems makes it premature to do anything more than speculate about the nature of the relationship between acute and chronic stress and immune responses at the present time.
- This area of research should yield some important new findings in the future and those interested in this field should scan scientific and medical jour-nals for the latest published research papers and review articles.

CONCLUSION

In this chapter we have discussed the nature of and sources of stress and have viewed stress as a phenomenon which is the reflection of an imbal-ance between the demand made upon a person and that person's perceived ability to cope with that demand. Physiological and psychological stress responses, their function in coping and their relevance in relation to health care have been described in some detail and an outline given of some of the evidence for linking stress with ill health, as well as methodological prob-lems associated with such research. It is impor-tant to recognise that the synthesis of research findings on stress given in this chapter represents only an outline of current understanding in what is a major area of on-going research. That stress is an all-pervasive phenomenon in health care is clear. It is equally clear that there is no easy means of tackling the problem. Certainly, the first step is to understand the nature of stress and that it can be, to quote Cox (1978), 'a threat to the quality of life and to physical and psychological well-being'. Next comes the need to develop the skills to recognise stress when it occurs, both in oneself and in others. For most people, dealing successfully with stress is likely to involve quite significant changes in behaviour and lifestyle. One of the major remaining challenges for those involved in health care is to develop creative ways of dealing sensitively and effectively with the inevitable sources of stress associated with their work.

REFERENCES

Ahmadi, K.S. (1985). The experience of being hospitalized: stress, social support and satisfaction. *International Journal of Nursing Studies*, 22(2), 137–48.

Arnold, J. (1989). Experiences and attitudes of learner nurses during their first year of training, Unpublished Report of Manchester School of Management, University of Manchester Institute of Science and Technology.

Asterita, M.F. (1985). *The Physiology of Stress*. Human Sciences Press, New York.

Atkinson, R.L., Atkinson, R.C., Smith, E.E., Bem, D.J. and Nolen-Hoeksema, S. (1996). *Hilgard's Introduction to Psychology*, 12th edn. Harcourt Brace, Fort Worth.

Baglioni, A.J., Cooper, C.L. and Hingley, P. (1990). Job stress, mental health and job satisfaction among senior nurses. *Stress Medicine*, 6, 9–20.

Bailey, J.T., Steffen, S.M. and Grout, J.W. (1980). The stress audit: identifying the stressors of ICU nursing. *Journal of Nursing Education*, 19(6), 15–25.

Bailey, R. and Clarke, M. (1989). *Stress and Coping in Nursing*. Chapman & Hall, London.

Beck, J. (1984). Nurses have needs too II: take time to care for yourselves. *Nursing Times*, 80(41), 31–2.

Bergh-Braam, van der A.H.M. and de Wolff, Ch. J. (1988). Stress among ward sisters. In *Stress and Organizational Problems in Hospitals*, Wallis, D. and de Wolff, Ch.J. (eds). Croom Helm, London.

Bibbings, J. (1987). The stress of working in intensive care: a look at the research. *Nursing: the Add-on Journal of Clinical Nursing*, 3(15), 567–70.

Birch, J. (1979). The anxious learners. *Nursing Mirror*, 148(1), 17–22.

Blaney, P. (1985). Psychological considerations in cancer. In *Behavioral Medicine: The Biopsychosocial Approach*, Schneiderman, N. and Tapp, J. (eds). Lawrence Erlbaum, Hillsdale, New Jersey.

Boore, J.R.P. (1978). *Prescription for Recovery*. RCN, London.

Boore, J.R.P. (1996). Endocrine function: responses to the external environment. In *Physiology for Nursing Practice*, 2nd edn, Hinchliff, S., Montague, S. and Watson, R. (eds). Baillière Tindall, London.

Boore, J.R.P., Champion, R. and Ferguson, M.C. (eds) (1987). *Nursing the Physically Ill Adult*. Churchill Livingstone, Edinburgh.

Burnard, P. (1991). *Coping with Stress in the Health Professions: a Practical Guide*. Chapman & Hall, London.

Callaghan, P. and Morrisey, J. (1993). Social support and health: a review. *Journal of Advanced Nursing*, 18(2), 203–10.

Campbell, C. (1985). Disturbing findings. *Nursing Mirror*, 160(26), 16–19.

Cannon, W.B. (1929). *Bodily Changes in Pain, Hunger, Fear and Rage*, 2nd edn. Appleton Century Crofts, New York.

Cannon, W.B. (1932). *The Wisdom of the Body*. Appleton Century Crofts, New York.

Cavanagh, S.J. and Snape, J. (1993). Nurses under stress. *Senior Nurse*, 13, 40–2.

Chesney, M., Hecker, M. and Black, G. (1988). Coronary-prone components of Type A behaviour in the Western Collaborative Group Study: a new methodology. In *Type A Behaviour Pattern: Research, Theory and Intervention*, Houston B. and Snyder, G. (eds). John Wiley, New York.

Clarke, M. (1996). The autonomic nervous system. In *Physiology for Nursing Practice*, 2nd edn, Hinchliff, S., Montague, S. and Watson, R. (eds). Baillière Tindall, London.

Clarke, V.A. and Ruffin, C.L. (1992). Perceived sources of stress among student nurses. *Contemporary Nurse*, 1, 35–40.

Clegg, F. (1988). Disasters: can psychologists help the survivors? *Psychologist*, 1(4), 134–5.

Cochran, J. and Ganong, L.H. (1989). A comparison of nurses' and patients' perceptions of intensive care unit stressors. *Journal of Advanced Nursing*, 14(2), 1038–43.

Cohen, S. and McKay, G. (1984). Social support, stress and the buffering hypothesis: a theoretical analysis. In *Handbook of Psychology and Health*, Baum, A., Taylor, S. and Singer, J. (eds). Erlbaum, Hillsdale, New Jersey.

Cohen, S., Tyrell, D.A.J. and Smith, A.P. (1991). Psychological stress and susceptibility to the common cold. *New England Journal of Medicine*, 325(9), 606–12.

Cooper, C. (1989). Are Type As prone to heart attacks? *Psychologist*, 2(1), 19.

Cox, T. (1978). *Stress*. Macmillan Press, London.

Delahanty, D.L., Dougall, A.L., Hawken, L. *et al.* (1996). Time course of natural killer cell activity and lymphocyte proliferation in response to two acute stressors in healthy men. *Health Psychology*, 15, 48–55.

DeLongis, A., Coyne, J.C., Dakof, G., Folkman, S. and Lazarus, R.S. (1982). Relationship of daily hassles, uplifts and major life events to health status. *Health Psychology*, 1, 119–36.

DeLongis, A., Folkman, S. and Lazarus, R.S. (1988). The impact of daily stress on health and mood: psychological and social resources as mediators. *Journal of Personality and Social Psychology*, 54, 486–95.

Dohrenwend, B.S., Krasnoff, L., Askenasy, A.R. and Dohrenwend, B.P. (1978). Exemplification of a method for scaling life events: the PERI Life Events Scale. *Journal of Health and Social Behaviour*, 19, 205–229.

Downey, V., Bengiamin, M., Heuer, L. and Juhl, N. (1995). Dying babies and associated stress in NICU nurses. *Neonatal Network*, 14(1), 41–6.

Duggan, N.M. (1990). The stress of working in intensive care: a literature review. *Irish Nursing Forum and Health Services*, 8(5), 22–3, 25–7 and 29.

Evans, P., Clow, A. and Hucklebridge, F. (1997). Stress and the immune system. *Psychologist*, 10(7), 303–7.

Field, D. (1989). *Nursing the Dying*. Routledge, London.

Figley, C. (1986). Trauma and Its Wake, Volume 2. Brunner Mazel, New York.

Fletcher, B. (1991). *Work, Stress, Disease and Life Expectancy*. John Wiley & Sons, Chichester.

Fontana, D. (1989). *Managing Stress*. British Psychological Society/Routledge, London.

Frankenhauser, M. (1975). Experimental approaches to the study of catecholamines and emotion. In *Emotions: their Parameters and Measurement*, Levi, L. (ed.). Raven Press, New York.

Franklin, B.L. (1974). *Patient Anxiety on Admission to Hospital*. RCN, London.

Friedman, M. and Rosenman, R.H. (1959). Association of specific overt behaviour patterns with blood and cardiovascular findings. *Journal of the American Medical Association*, 169, 1286–96.

Freud, A. (1946). *The Ego and the Mechanism of Defence*. International Universities Press, New York.

Funkenstein, D.H. (1955). The physiology of fear and anger. *Scientific American*, 192, 74–80.

Ganong, W.F. (1995). *Review of Medical Physiology*, 13th edn. Large Medical Publications, Los Altos.

Greer, S., Moorey, S., Baruch, J.D. *et al.* (1992). Adjuvant psychological therapy for patients with cancer: a prospective randomised trial. *British Medical Journal*, 304, 675–80.

Harvey, P. (1988). Stress and health. In *Health Psychology: Process and Application*, Broome, A. (ed.). Chapman & Hall, London.

Hawley, M.P. (1992). Sources of stress for emergency nurses in four urban Canadian emergency departments. *Journal of Emergency Nursing*, 18(3), 211–16.

Haynes, S.G., Feinleib, M. and Kannel, W.B. (1980). The relationship of psychosocial factors to coronary heart disease in the Framingham Study Part 3: eight year incidence of coronary heart disease. *American Journal of Epidemiology*, 111(1), 37–58.

Hayward, J. (1975). *Information: a Prescription against Pain*. RCN, London.

Hearn, M.D., Murray, D.M. and Luepker, R.V. (1989). Hostility, coronary heart disease, and total mortality: a 33-year follow-up study of university students. *Journal of Behavioral Medicine*, 12, 105–21.

Hebb, D.O. (1972). *Textbook of Psychology*, 3rd edn. W.B. Saunders, Philadelphia.

Herbert, T.B. and Cohen, S. (1993). Stress and immunity in humans: a meta-analytic review. *Psychosomatic Medicine*, 56, 337–44.

Herbert, T.B. and Cohen, S. (1994). Stress and illness. In *Encyclopedia of Human Behaviour*, Volume 4, Ramachandran, V.S. (ed.). Academic Press, San Diego, California.

Herbert, T.B., Cohen, S., Marsland, A.L. *et al.* (1994). Cardiovascular reactivity and the course of immune response to an acute psychological stressor. *Psychosomatic Medicine*, 56, 337–44.

Hilton, S.M. (1981). The physiology of stress – emotion. In *The Principles and Practice of Human Physiology*, Edholm, O.G. and Weiner, J.S. (eds). Academic Press, London.

Hingley, P. and Cooper, C.L. (1986). *Stress and the Nurse Manager*. John Wiley & Sons, Chichester.

Hodnett, E.D. (1995). Support from caregivers during childbirth. In *Pregnancy and Childbirth Module*, Cochrane Database of Systematic Reviews, Keirse, M., Renfrew, M., Neilson, J. and Crowther, C. (eds). Cochrane Updates on Disk, Update Software, Oxford.

Holmes, T.H. and Rahe, R.H. (1967). The social adjustment rating scale. *Journal of Psychosomatic Research*, 11, 213–18.

Hudgens, R.W. (1974). Personal catastrophe and depression: a consideration of the subject with respect to medically ill adolescents, and a requiem for retrospective life-event studies. In *Stressful Life Events:*

their Nature and Effects, Dohrenwend, B.S. and Dohrenwend, B.P. (eds). John Wiley & Sons, New York.

Janis, I.L. (1971). *Stress and Frustration*. Harcourt Brace Jovanovich, New York.

Johnson, J.E. (1983). Preparing patients to cope with stress while hospitalized. In *Patient Teaching*, Wilson-Barnett, J. (ed.). Churchill Livingstone, Edinburgh.

Kanner, A.D., Coyne, J.C., Schaefer, C. and Lazarus, R.S. (1981). Comparison of two modes of stress measurement: daily hassles and uplifts versus major life events. *Journal of Behavioral Medicine*, 4, 1–39.

Katz, J.L., Weiner, H., Gallagher, T.F. and Hellman, L. (1970). Stress, distress and ego defences: psychoendocrine response to impending tumor biopsy. *Archives of General Psychiatry*, 23, 131–42.

Kawachi, I., Sparrow, D., Vokonas, P. and Weiss, S. (1994). Symptoms of anxiety and risk of coronary heart disease: the Normative Aging Study. *Circulation*, 90, 2225–9.

Keller, K.L. (1990). Sources of stress and satisfaction in the practice of emergency medicine: a comparative study of nurses and physicians. *Journal of Emergency Nursing*, 16(6), 413–14.

Kendall, P.C. and Epps, J. (1990). Medical treatments. In *Stress and Medical Procedures*, Johnston, M. and Wallace, L. (eds). Oxford University Press, Oxford.

Kiecolt-Glaser, J.K., Glaser, R., Shuttleworth, E.C., Dyer, C.S., Ogrocki, P. and Speicher, C.E. (1987). Chronic stress and immunity in family caregivers of Alzheimer's disease victims. *Psychosomatic Medicine*, 49, 523–35.

Kiecolt-Glaser, J.K., Dura, J.R., Speicher, C.E., Trask, O.J. and Glaser, R. (1991). Spousal caregivers of dementia victims: longitudinal changes in immunity and health. *Psychosomatic Medicine*, 53, 345–62.

Knight, R.B., Atkins, A., Eagle, C.J. *et al.* (1979). Psychological stress, ego defences and cortisol production in children hospitalized for elective surgery. *Psychosomatic Medicine*, 41, 40–49.

Kushnir, T. (1986). Stress and social facilitation: the effects of the presence of an instructor on student nurses' behaviour. *Journal of Advanced Nursing*, 11, 13–19.

Langer, E., Janis, I.L. and Wolfer, J.A. (1975). Reduction of psychological stress in surgical patients. *Journal of Experimental Social Psychology*, 11, 155–65.

Langer, E.J. and Rodin, J. (1976). The effects of choice and enhanced personal responsibility for the aged: a field experiment in an institutional setting. *Journal of Personality and Social Psychology*, 34(2), 191–8.

Lazarus, R.S. (1966). *Psychological Stress and the Coping Process*. McGraw-Hill, New York.

Lazarus, R.S. (1976). *Patterns of Adjustment*. McGraw-Hill, New York.

Lazarus, R.S. and Folkman, S. (1984). *Stress, Appraisal and Coping*. Springer, New York.

Lees, S. and Ellis, N. (1990). The design of a stress management programme for nursing personnel. *Journal of Advanced Nursing*, 15, 946–61.

Levin, J.S. and DeFrank, R.S. (1988). Maternal stress and pregnancy outcomes: a review of the psychosocial literature. *Journal of Psychosomatic Obstetrics and Gynaecology*, 9(1), 3–16.

Lindop, E. (1991). Individual stress among nurses in training: why some leave whilst others stay. *Nurse Education Today*, 11(2), 110–20.

McCranie, E., Watkins, L., Brandsma, J. and Sisson, B. (1986). Hostility, coronary heart disease (CHD) incidence, and total mortality: lack of association in a 25-year follow-up study of 478 physicians. *Journal of Behavioral Medicine*, 9, 119–25.

Marshall, J. (1980). Stress among nurses. In *White Collar and Professional Stress*, Cooper, C.L. and Marshall, J. (eds). John Wiley & Sons, Chichester.

Martin, P. (1996). *The Sickening Mind: Brain, Behaviour, Immunity and Disease*. HarperCollins, London.

Mason, J.W. (1968). A review of psychoendocrine research on the pituitary adrenocortical system. *Journal of Advanced Medicine*, 30, 567–607.

Mason, J.W. (1971). A re-evaluation of the concept of 'nonspecificity' in stress theory. *Journal of Psychiatric Research*, 8, 323–33.

Mason, J.W., Maher, J.J., Hartley, L.H., Mougey, G.H., Perlow, H.J. and Jones, L.G. (1976). Selectivity of corticosteroid and catecholamine responses to various natural stimuli. In *Psychopathology of Human Adaptation*, Serban, G. (ed.). Plenum, New York.

Melia, K.M. (1987). *Learning and Working: the Occupational Socialization of Nurses*. Tavistock Publications, London.

Mendes de Leon, C.F. (1992). Anger and impatience/irritability in patients of low socioeconomic status with acute coronary heart disease. *Journal of Behavioral Medicine*, 15, 273–84.

Moos, R.H. and Schaefer, J.A. (1984). The crisis of physical illness: an overview and conceptual approach. In

Coping with Physical Illness: New Perspectives, Volume 2, Moos, R.H. (ed.). Plenum Press, New York.

Norrie, P. (1995). Do intensive care staff suffer more stress than staff in other care environments? A discussion. *Intensive and Critical Care Nursing*, 11(5), 293–7.

Oakley, A. (1992). *Social Support and Motherhood*. Basil Blackwell, Oxford.

Oates, R.K. and Oates, P. (1995). Stress and mental health in neonatal intensive care units. *Archives of Disease in Childhood*, Fetal and Neonatal Edition, 72(2), F107–10.

Parkes, K. (1985). Stressful episodes reported by first year student nurses: a descriptive account. *Social Science and Medicine*, 20(9), 945–53.

Pattison, H.M. and Robertson, C.E. (1996). The effect of ward design on the well-being of post-operative patients. *Journal of Advanced Nursing*, 23(4), 820–6.

Power, P. (1996). High anxiety. *Nursing Times*, 92(5), 58.

Ragland, D.R. and Brand, R.J. (1988a). Coronary heart disease mortality in the Western Collaborative Group Study: follow-up experience of 22 years. *American Journal of Epidemiology*, 127(3), 462–75.

Ragland, D.R. and Brand, R.J. (1988b). Type A behaviour and mortality from coronary heart disease. *New England Journal of Medicine*, 318, 65–9.

Rahe, R.H. (1974). The pathway between subjects, recent life changes and their near-future illness reports: representative results and methodological issues. In *Stressful Life Events, their Nature and Effects*, Dohrenwend, B.S. and Dohrenwend, B.P. (eds). John Wiley & Sons, New York.

Rahe, R.H. (1987). Recent life changes, emotions and behaviours in coronary heart disease. In *Handbook of Psychology and Health*, Volume 5, Baum, A. and Singer, J.A. (eds). Lawrence Erlbaum, Hillsdale, New Jersey.

Rahe, R.H. and Arthur, R.J. (1977). Life-changing patterns surrounding illness experience. In *Stress and Coping*, Monat, A. and Lazarus, R.S. (eds). Columbia University Press, New York.

Rentoul, L.P. (1989). Caring for bereaved relatives: problems and possibilities. Paper presented at the Third Annual Macmillan Conference on Nursing Research and Palliative Care, King's College, London. Cited in Rentoul, L., Thomas, V. and Rentoul, R. (1995). Understanding stress and its implications for healthcare professionals. In *Towards Advanced Nursing Practice: Key Concepts for Health*, Schober, J. and Hinchliff, S. (eds). Arnold, London.

Rhead, M.M. (1995). Stress among student nurses: is it practical or academic? *Journal of Clinical Nursing*, 4(6), 369–76.

Rodin, J. and Langer, E.J. (1977). Long-term effects of a control-relevant intervention with the institutionalized aged. *Journal of Personality and Social Psychology*, 35(12), 897–902.

Rosenman, R.H., Brand, R.J., Jenkins, C.D., Friedman, M., Strauss, R. and Wurm, M. (1975). Coronary heart disease in the Western Collaborative Group Study: final follow-up experience of 8½ years. *Journal of the American Medical Assocation*, 233, 872–7.

Rosenthal, S.L., Schmid, K.D. and Black, M.M. (1989). Stress and coping in a NICU. *Research in Nursing and Health*, 12(4), 257–65.

Rotter, J.B. (1966). Generalized expectancies for internal versus external control of reinforcement. *Psychological Monographs*, 80, 1.

Ruch, L.O. and Holmes, T.H. (1971). Scaling of life change: comparison of direct and indirect methods. *Journal of Psycosomatic Research*, 15, 221–7.

Sabbioni, M.E. (1991). Cancer and stress: a possible role for psychoimmunology in cancer research? In *Cancer and Stress: Psychological, Biological, and Coping Studies*, Watson, C. and Watson, M. (eds). John Wiley & Sons, New York.

Sarafino, E.P. (1994). *Health Psychology: Biopsychosocial Interactions*, 2nd edn. John Wiley & Sons, New York.

Sarason, I.G., Johnson, J.H. and Siegel, J.M. (1978). Assessing the impact of life changes: development of the life experiences survey. *Journal of Consulting and Clinical Psychology*, 46, 932–46.

Sarason, I.G., Sarason, B.R., Potter, E.H. and Antoni, M.H. (1985). Life events, social support, and illness. *Psychosomatic Medicine*, 47, 156–63.

Schwartzer, R. and Leppin, A. (1989). Social support and health: a meta-analysis. *Health Psychology*, 3, 1–15.

Seligman, M.E.P. (1975). *Helplessness: on Depression, Development and Death*. W.H. Freeman, San Francisco.

Selye, H. (1946). The general adaptation syndrome and the diseases of adaptation. *Journal of Clinical Endocrinology*, 6, 117–28.

Selye, H. (1976). *The Stress of Life*, 2nd edn. McGraw-Hill, New York.

Simonton, O.C. and Simonton, S.S. (1975). Belief systems and the management of emotional aspects of malignancy, *Journal of Transpersonal Psychology*, 7, 29–47.

Sklar, L.A. and Anisman, H. (1979). Stress and coping factors influence tumour growth. *Science*, 205, 513–15.

Snell, J. (1995). It's tough at the bottom. *Nursing Times*, 91(43), 55–8.

Sowney, R. (1996). Stress debriefing: reality or myth? *Accident and Emergency Nursing*, 4(1), 38–9.

Steen, L. (1994). So you want to be a nurse? *Canadian Nurse*, 90(10), 55.

Stein, M., Keller, S.E. and Schliefer, S.J. (1985). Stress and immunomodulation: the role of depression and neuroendocrine function. *Journal of Immunology*, 135, 827–33.

Steptoe, A. (1985). Type-A coronary prone behaviour. *British Journal of Hospital Medicine*, 33, 257–60.

Suls, J. and Mullen, B. (1981). Life events, perceived control and illness: the role of uncertainty. *Journal of Human Stress*, 7, 30–4.

Sutherland, V.J. and Cooper, C.L. (1990). *Understanding Stress: a Psychological Perspective for Health Professionals*. Chapman & Hall, London.

Temoshok, L. and Fox, B. (1984). Coping styles and other psychosocial factors related to medical status and to prognosis in patients with cutaneous malignant melanoma. In *Impact of Psychoendocrine Systems in Cancer and Immunity*, Fox, B. and Newberry, B. (eds). C.J. Hogrefe, Toronto.

Temoshok, L. and Heller, B.W. (1984). On comparing apples, oranges and fruit salad: a methodological overview of medical outcome studies in psychosocial oncology. In *Psychosocial Stress and Cancer*, Cooper, C.L. (ed.). John Wiley & Sons, Chichester.

Terman, G.W., Shavit, Y., Lewis, J.W., Cannon, J.T. and Liebeskind, J.C. (1984). Intrinsic mechanisms of pain inhibition: activation by stress. *Science*, 226, 1270–7.

Thompson, D. (1990). *Counselling the Coronary Patient and Partner*. Scutari Press, London.

Thompson, D. and Meddis, R. (1990a). A prospective evaluation of in-hospital counselling for first-time myocardial infarction men. *Journal of Psychosomatic Research*, 34, 237–48.

Thompson, D. and Meddis, R. (1990b). Wives' responses to counselling early after myocardial infarction. *Journal of Psychosomatic Research*, 34, 249–58.

Thornton, S. (1984). Caring for special babies III: stress in the neonatal intensive care unit. *Nursing Times*, 80(5), 35–7.

Vachon, M.L. (1987). *Occupational Stress in the Care of the Critically Ill, the Dying and the Bereaved*. Hemisphere, Washington.

Volicer, B.J. and Bohannon, M.W. (1975). A hospital stress rating scale. *Nursing Research*, 24(5), 352–9.

Volicer, B.J. and Volicer, L. (1978). Cardiovascular changes associated with stress during hospitalisation. *Journal of Psychosomatic Research*, 22, 159–68.

Weiss, J.M. (1972). Psychological factors in stress and disease. *Scientific American*, 226(6), 104–13.

Welford, A.T. (1973). Stress and performance. *Ergonomics*, 16, 567.

White, D. and Tonkin, J. (1991). Registered nurses' stress in intensive care units: an Australian perspective. *Intensive Care Nursing*, 7(1), 45–52.

Wilson, G. (1991). Technology and stress. *Nursing: the Journal of Clinical Practice, Education and Management*, 4(32), 31.

Wilson-Barnett, J. (1979). *Stress in Hospital*. Churchill Livingstone, Edinburgh.

Wilson-Barnett, J. (1984). Interventions to alleviate patients' stress: a review. *Journal of Psychosomatic Research*, 28(1), 63–72.

Wilson-Barnett, J. (1986). Reducing stress in hospital. In *Clinical Nursing Practice: Recent Advances in Nursing 14*, Tierney, A. (ed.). Churchill Livingstone, Edinburgh.

Wilson-Barnett, J. and Carrigy, A. (1978). Factors affecting patients' responses to hospitalisation. *Journal of Advanced Nursing*, 3(3), 221–8.

Wood, V. and Rubin, S. (1992). Rita Kennedy: case analysis for decision-making. *Nurse Education Today*, 12(1), 19–23.

FURTHER READING

Burnard, P. (1991). *Coping with Stress in the Health Professions: a Practical Guide*. Chapman & Hall, London.

Evans, P., Clow, A. and Hucklebridge, F. (1997). Stress and the immune system. *Psychologist*, 10(7), 303–7.

Deals with the relationship between stress and immune system functioning.

Fontana, D. (1989). *Managing Stress*. British Psychological Society/Routledge, London.

Herbert, T.B. and Cohen, S. (1993). Stress and immunity in humans: a meta-analytic review. *Psychosomatic Medicine*, 56, 337–44.

Deals with the relationship between stress and immune system functioning.

Holistic Nursing Practice, July 1991 deals with 'psychosocial nursing and immunocompetence'. See, especially the following papers:

Hillhouse, J. and Adler, C. (1991). Stress, health, and immunity: a review of the literature and implications for the nursing profession. *Holistic Nursing Practice*, 5(4), 22–31.

Houldin, A.D., Lev, E., Prystowsky, M.B., Redei, E. and Lowery, B.J. (1991). Psychoneuroimmunology: a review of literature. *Holistic Nursing Practice*, 5(4), 10–21.

Nguyen, T.V. (1991). Mind, brain, and immunity: a critical review. *Holistic Nursing Practice*, 5(4), 1–9.

Martin, P. (1996). *The Sickening Mind: Brain, Behaviour, Immunity and Disease*. HarperCollins, London.

Messer, D. and Meldrum, C. (eds) (1995). *Psychology for Nurses and Health Care Professionals*. Prentice Hall/Harvester Wheatsheaf, London.

See Chapter 14, Managing stress in health care: issues for staff and patient care; Chapter 15, The consequences of stress; and Chapter 17, Dying and bereavement.

Ogden, J. (1996). *Health Psychology: a Textbook*. Open University Press, Buckingham.

See Chapter 10, Stress and Chapter 13, Psychology throughout the course of illness: the examples of HIV, cancer and coronary heart disease.

Sarafino, E.P. (1994). *Health Psychology: Biopsychosocial Interactions*, 2nd edn. John Wiley & Sons, New York.

In particular, see Chapter 3, Stress – its meaning, impact, and sources; Chapter 4, Stress, biopsychological factors, and illness; Chapter 5, coping with and reducing stress.

Schwartzer, R. and Leppin, A. (1989). Social support and health: a meta-analysis. *Health Psychology*, 3, 1–15.

CHAPTER NINE

THE PATIENT *as a* CONSUMER *of* HEALTH CARE

Judith Chamberlain-Webber

- Health and illness
- The process of becoming a patient
- The experience of becoming a patient
- Towards the patient as a consumer of health care
- Involvement of patients in care
- The nurse's role
- Conclusion

The aim of this chapter is to explore the concept of the patient as a consumer of health care, examining how the person becomes a patient and his/her subsequent role within the health care system. By examining the growth of a consumer ideology within the health service, it describes the changes that have occurred in patients' rights and discusses whether patient choice has really improved as a result. Nurses have been at the forefront of many changes to the status of patients, with initiatives such as patient education, satisfaction surveys and partners in care programmes. How successful these changes have been in improving patient care is explored and some suggestions made for the way forward.

While the language of consumerism is relatively new in the National Health Service (NHS), the concept of the patient as an active 'consumer' rather than a passive 'patient' has gained much ground over the last couple of decades. It is reflected in the new organisation of the health service as a market place, where services which are priced competitively and presented attractively will attract more patients and more resources; where consumer satisfaction surveys are increasingly used, and where quality is monitored and audited.

It is also increasingly reflected in patterns of patient care. Patients are becoming more involved in decisions over their treatment and care, given more information, and allowed to exercise some choice. Increasingly, their individual rights are respected, as are those of consumers of any other service.

HEALTH AND ILLNESS

Concepts of health and illness vary between different societies and different individuals (see also Chapters 1 and 2). As Cribb (1993) pointed out in a previous edition of this book:

'It is possible to generate countless examples in which people can be judged to be unhealthy (according to some conceptions) and healthy (according to others). Even within a conception of health, individuals can be both healthy and unhealthy, just as a glass can be both half full and half empty, because health is always a matter of degree.'

The World Health Organization (WHO, 1978) describes health as 'a state of complete physical, mental and social well-being and not merely the absence of disease or infirmity'. This definition recognises that health is determined not simply by disease but by much wider social, environmental, economic and political considerations. The WHO set targets for health in 1978 in its 'Alma-Ata' declaration, with the slogan 'Health for all by the year 2000', inviting each of its regions to identify appropriate targets for their own areas (WHO, 1978). The European region responded with 38 targets for health, published in 1985 (WHO, 1985).

Health is affected by our lifestyle, for example, tobacco and alcohol intake, physical exercise and stress, and by our environment, through the housing we inhabit and the quality of air that we breathe and the water that we drink. Certain diseases can be linked to particular age or cultural groups; others are more prevalent in particular geographical areas or different socio-economic classes. The link between poverty and ill health has been shown many times, perhaps most notably by Sir Douglas Black in the Black Report of 1980 (Department of Health and Social Security [DHSS], 1980).

When considering patients as consumers of health care, it is important to keep in mind who has responsibility for people's health. How far are we as individuals responsible for the state of our own health, or should the government intervene forcefully in encouraging a more healthy lifestyle? For example, the government can choose simply to educate the public about the dangers of tobacco smoking and alcohol, or it can levy sufficiently high taxes on tobacco and alcohol to act as a powerful deterrent. It can simply warn people that they are more likely to survive a car accident if wearing a seatbelt, or make wearing rear and front seatbelts mandatory.

The government can educate the public on the importance of having children immunised against preventable diseases or it can choose to make immunisation programmes mandatory. It can tackle the link between poverty and ill health by providing better housing and increasing state benefits, or encourage wealth creation by controlling public expenditure and keeping inflation low, arguing that a healthy economy will promote a healthy population.

Over recent years, the government has increasingly concentrated on the prevention of ill health through campaigns, many of which are organised by the Health Education Authority, on areas such as drink-driving, AIDS and HIV, drug abuse and more recently, folic acid intake by pregnant women, early recognition of meningitis, and measles vaccination. The success of these campaigns is often controversial and hard to measure. In the measles vaccination programme in 1994/95, for example, school nurses had difficulty coping with the workload.

HEALTH PROMOTION

In 1989, as part of the NHS reforms (Department of Health [DoH], 1989), it was proposed that the promotion of health should be given a major boost by the government by introducing financial incentives for reaching certain health promotion and screening targets, for example, childhood immunisation rates, cervical screening and, for those over-75, health assessments.

While this certainly encouraged GPs to ensure that patients were being screened, critics pointed to the fact that often it was the well-informed, relatively healthy middle classes who attended, rather than people who were most likely to be at risk, for example, people not registered with a doctor, those with poor diets, people living in poverty, ethnic minorities unable to read English, heavy smokers, etc. Anderson (1983) highlighted that screening could also create an unwarranted belief in the value of such a service and Smail (1990) added that it could create a false sense of security, as a kind of 'life insurance policy'.

The government also set general targets for improving health with the publication of the Green Paper *The Health of the Nation* (DoH, 1991a) and the White Paper of the same name in 1992 (DoH, 1992).

> **The *Health of the Nation* identified three main health challenges:**
>
> - People still die prematurely or suffer ill health from largely preventable conditions.
> - There are significant geographical, ethnic, social and occupational variations in health.
> - There are still marked variations in the quantity and quality of health care in different parts of the country.

The paper thus identified five areas for targeting health improvement and important risk factors. Handbooks have been subsequently published with advice on meeting these targets and the other three countries of the UK have published their own health promotion initiatives (Scottish Office, 1992; Welsh Office, 1994; Northern Ireland Office, 1996). The areas are listed in Box 9.1.

Box 9.1

Health of the Nation targets relate to:
- Heart disease and stroke
- Cancer
- Mental health
- Sexual health
- Accidents.

The risk factors to be targeted are:
- Smoking
- Diet and nutrition
- Blood pressure
- HIV/AIDS.

However, health promotion is not just about illness prevention. The WHO (1978) definition stresses that it is 'the process of *enabling* people to increase control over and thereby improve their health' (my emphasis).

While the Health of the Nation was widely welcomed and long awaited, many were concerned that it over-emphasised individual responsibility and targets as the main focus. As Caraher (1994) wrote: 'Faced with the pressure of meeting targets, issues such as power and control tend to take a back seat.'

Many had already raised criticisms about the potential dangers of health promotion (Crawford, 1977; Grace, 1991). It was suggested that health promotion created a 'victim-blaming' mentality in which people's ill health was their own fault and their responsibility (individualism) rather than that of the government or society. Much health promotion activity centred on teaching or counselling people, which increased the power of the health professional as the teacher and decreased the power of the patient as the learner.

This danger was recognised by Beattie (1990), who developed a model for health promotion in which all discussions with patients are recognised as having elements of power and control which should be shared with the patient.

Table 9.1: Health promotion for the consumer

Ask yourself these questions next time you are involved in a health promotion activity. If you can answer 'yes' to most of these, the activity is probably worthwhile:

- Are clients worked with rather than on?
- Are alternatives presented to clients in terms of lifestyle change/behaviour?
- Are individual needs taken account of?
- Where does the power and control lie in the encounter?
- Are the goals of the health promotion activity negotiated with the client (or are they imposed)?
- Are the health promotion activities evaluated by the clients?
- Are the activities concerned with long-term or short-term outcomes?
- Could the client suggest alternatives to the 'choices' he/she has made?

Based on Caraher (1994).

Clients must have a say in any health promotion activity if it is truly going to empower them to make choices. This may mean that nurses must hand over some of the control and power that they currently possess and help the client to make a choice, rather than tell him/her what to do (Caraher, 1994). Table 9.1 contains some ways to assess whether health promotion is really patient centred.

Key Points

- People can act as consumers of health care before they become patients through health promotion activities.
- The government has increasingly recognised the importance of prevention of illness.
- Nurses must be careful to involve people in making decisions about their health rather than telling them what to do.

THE PROCESS OF BECOMING A PATIENT

Patient care and treatment takes many forms and occurs in many settings. Almost everyone will be a patient at some point in their lives, whether in the primary or secondary health care setting or in NHS or independent health care. Once a health problem is perceived and help sought, the transition begins from person to patient.

Categories of care

The Committee of the Royal Commission on the National Health Service (1979) identified four categories or gradations of care which the individual might need. They are:

- The care which a healthy person will exercise to remain healthy. This includes adopting as healthy a lifestyle as possible, undergoing health checks, such as blood pressure monitoring, breast and cervical screening, bone mass screening for osteoporosis, and ensuring any immunisations and vaccinations required are up to date (as mentioned earlier).
- The self-care which the slightly ill person will exercise, which may involve medication and treatment. People receive information on health from a wide variety of sources including family, friends, newspapers, magazines, TV and radio programmes, including educational programmes, soaps and phone-ins. Most problems are initially – and often completely – self-treated, sometimes with help from a high street chemist. Another important source of help at this level is the many charities and self-help groups, which are often founded because of the lack of advice and support for a particular condition (see the end of this chapter).
- The care provided by a person's family and by health and social services available outside hospital. A huge amount of care takes place informally in the community by family, friends and volunteers with widely varying degrees of support from health and social services. This depends on the degree of illness and disability and dependence, but services that may be available include home help, respite care, community nursing visits and meals on wheels. As people live to greater ages and as the number of people surviving chronic or long-term illnesses increases, this aspect of care will become more and more significant.
- The care which can only be provided in hospital or other residential institutions. This type of care is usually the most significant for a patient, as it is in this setting that the transition from a person to a patient becomes complete. The person is away from home and often family and friends. Much of the status that the person holds in the community is lost as well as the ability to make basic choices about food, clothing and activity. To some extent, patients have to submit to the routine of the institution and the restrictions imposed by the care and treatment they are given.

ALTERNATIVES TO THE NHS

In the initial stages of becoming a patient, the first choice people are faced with is whether to be treated within the NHS or try one of the increasing number of alternative options.

Complementary medicine

Alternative or – as it is more properly called – complementary medicine is becoming an increasingly popular option for patients who wish to choose another form of health care to that available from the NHS.

People turn to complementary medicine for a variety of reasons. They may feel that conventional medicine has failed, having had varied and repeated orthodox treatments which have brought little relief. They may fear the direct or indirect effects of increasingly complex and technologically sophisticated treatments. Patients from different ethnic backgrounds may be accustomed to using different forms of therapy.

These therapies have also traditionally used a more holistic approach to an individual's problem than conventional medicine, often involving extensive questions on diet and lifestyle before any treatments are given. This approach can seem increasingly attractive when GP consultation times are much shorter.

A study by Sharma (1991) showed that all the patients interviewed had consulted conventional practitioners on their condition before turning to alternative practitioners. All said they would continue to consult their GP for any new health problems that occurred.

The medical profession appears to remain largely sceptical and entrenched in its views of complementary medicine. This is mostly because the scientific basis and evidence for the effectiveness of the treatments is still lacking or is of poor quality, much of it being anecdotal. Despite this resistance, complementary therapies are available on the NHS. There are five homeopathic hospitals in the UK and increasing numbers of GP clinics and hospital departments offer these therapies, such as the Outreach Centre in Liverpool and the Gateway Clinic in south London (Stevenson, 1997). The amount of research is also growing and the Research Council for Complementary Medicine holds a database of research, some of which has been conducted by nurses, for example, Dunn (1994) and Corner *et al.* (1995).

Nurses have a responsibility to respect the right of the patient to choose but as interest grows in this area, they should also ensure that they are able to advise patients about the range and effectiveness of therapies now available (Trevelyan, 1995). Many nurses have also recognised the opportunities for extending their practice and emphasising their caring role through providing complementary therapies. As a result, nurse-led therapies such as aromatherapy, massage, reflexology, hypnosis and shiatsu are now available in a range of settings, including hospices, wards and ITU (Stevenson, 1994).

Independent sector health care

Health care provided by commercial companies is a significant alternative to the NHS and there has been rapid growth in the provision of independent sector care over recent years.

In 1994, independent sector hospital and nursing home supply came to 18.9% of the UK total, compared to 15.7% in 1990 and 9.9% in 1986 (Laing, 1996).

Private health companies generally tend to operate in areas of care that are most profitable, for example, routine, non-emergency surgery. Funding mostly comes from insurance schemes, subscribed to either privately or provided as an employment 'perk'. Its attractions are mainly that it offers the patient more control over the timing of treatment and a way of avoiding long hospital waiting lists – hence the predominance of operations such as hip replacement and varicose vein ligation, where NHS waiting lists are long.

Another big growth area has been the provision of long-term care for elderly people. Prior to the changes in the health service, these people were mostly cared for either in local authority residential homes or NHS continuing care units. In 1988, the Griffiths Report stated that the needs of the increasing numbers of elderly people should be met through private sector provision rather than the NHS. Funds were also made available to help those with limited means access private sector provision, resulting in an increase in growth in residential and nursing homes. These changes were crystallised in the Community Care Act 1993 which made local authorities responsible for purchasing care.

> **Key Points**
>
> ■ Patients can choose how they access the NHS, and have the right to choose alternative services to the NHS such as complementary therapies, treatment by friends or paying for care.
>
> ■ The growth in alternative services to the NHS is an indication of the increase in patient choice and therefore consumer power available to patients.

THE EXPERIENCE OF BECOMING A PATIENT

Once a person has decided to seek medical care in whatever form, it is easy for him or her to become subsumed into the identity, routines and regulations of the institution, and for staff to see the person more in terms of his/her physical condition than as an individual.

Patients will automatically be at a disadvantage through lack of medical knowledge. However, if they are in hospital, many other factors come into play, for example, not knowing the ward layout or routines. Having to change into nightwear reduces patients' dignity and sense of personal identity. If they require community care, a lack of knowledge of how the system works may put them at a disadvantage. At the same time, patients may be feeling ill and will almost certainly experience some degree of anxiety. They have to hand over control of their illness and body to someone else who may hold information about them of which they are unaware.

THE TRADITIONAL VIEW OF THE PATIENT'S ROLE

The process of becoming a patient was described as far back as 1951 as assuming the 'sick role'

(Parsons, 1951). Patients are expected to behave in a particular way by the staff and conform to expectations society then has of them.

Patients may have certain rights – being exempt from normal activities and from work, and the right to expect help from health professionals. However, society may also expect obligations from them – to want to get well and to resume normal or near normal activities as soon as possible. In addition, they must do all that is possible to get well, cooperating with those helping them and complying with treatment regimes.

Patients, however, may not always want to behave in this way. A further, debilitating course of chemotherapy, which medical staff say will prolong life but not achieve remission or cure, may be what the family and society expect patients to undergo but the individual may not want this or feel it is in his or her best interests.

Part of the reason why patients adopted the sick role was the belief by society that the doctor knows best and that decisions about health care are best left in the hands of the professionals. As medical care has become more complex and sophisticated, respect for what doctors can achieve has grown and so, as a result, patients have increasingly felt unable to question what a doctor or nurse does. Nursing has been organised traditionally around the completion of nursing tasks rather than the patients, and patients often felt they had to do what the nurse told them.

THE BEGINNING OF CHANGES TO THE PATIENT'S ROLE

Involving patients in care

In the last two decades, the importance of involving patients and giving them information to help them make decisions and feel they have some control has been highlighted. This has made a major contribution to the change in the patient's role.

This fact was recognised as far back as 1983 by the National Consumer Council in its document *Patients' Rights*. It states that patients will:

'get the best from the health service only when they know what is reasonable to expect from it, what their rights and responsibilities are, and when they have the confidence and skill to exercise them. Patients clearly need more and better information about what services are available and how to gain access to them; what choice they have in terms of doctors and services; how they can influence decision-making in the health service; and how they can make a complaint when something goes wrong.'

In a survey of patients who had been in coronary care units, Wallace *et al.* (1985) found huge discrepancies between the information patients wanted and what they received. Ninety per cent wanted information on the cause of their illness and only 40% reported being told about it, whereas 80% wanted information about their medical treatment and only 40% reported being told.

In a study into the problems surgical patients faced after discharge, Vaughan and Taylor (1988) concluded that many people experienced difficulties that could have been removed or alleviated by giving them better information at the time of discharge. Twenty-nine per cent were unsure when they could safely bath or shower and 26% were unsure if their diet was appropriate to aiding recovery. Only one out of a sample of 64 was given any advice on sexual activity following their operation and only two were advised when they could start driving again.

Wilson-Barnett (1979) showed how stress and anxiety are reduced with explanations about hospital procedures, routines and treatment, and Hayward (1975) showed how patients who had received pre-operative information on anaesthesia, operative techniques and post-operative sensations reported less pain and required less analgesia than those who had not been given the same information. Wilson-Barnett (1983) went on to stress the importance of providing patients with the information they need and educating them about their condition as part of total nursing care.

Confirmation of this early work has now been provided by systematic reviews of the literature which has accumulated over the last 30 years. Devine (1992) found that assessing all the studies which have looked at provision of information and support for patients undergoing surgery has shown that beneficial effects can be obtained in reducing patients' pain, distress and recovery time. Similar work on studies of patients with cancer (Devine and Westlake, 1995) has confirmed that providing support reduces patients' pain and anxiety, and improves knowledge.

Nursing philosophy

Nursing itself has also undergone a change in philosophy. The introduction of the nursing process and the development in the 1980s of models of nursing care (Kershaw and Salvage, 1986) redefined the nursing role and emphasised how care should be negotiated between nurse and patient.

Developments such as primary nursing have been instrumental in changing the profession's attitudes to patients (Wright, 1994). The basis of primary nursing is putting the patient first rather than a series of tasks, by one nurse on each shift providing total care for the same group of patients every day. Hegvary (1982) described primary nursing as:

'both a philosophy of care and an organisational design. It is not simply a way of assigning nurses to patients, but rather a view of nursing as a professional, patient-centred practice.'

(Hegvary, 1982, page 2)

The concept of primary nursing requires a change in the nurse–patient relationship to a partnership where the nurse works with the patient, rather than the nurse telling the patient what to do. Wright (1994) summed up primary nurses' roles as:

'They encourage patients to be involved in their own care, to make choices and give information so that the patient can make informed rational decisions. They share their knowledge and skills with the patient. . . . When the patients are unable or unwilling to make their wishes known, the primary nurse uses what knowledge is available of them, coupled with empathy skills, to act as advocate – upholding their wishes when they are unable to do so for themselves, advising in their best interests and being prepared to stand accountable for those decisions.'

(Wright, 1994, page 35)

Another change which has focused nursing towards the importance of the patient has been research into the therapeutic effects of nursing care (Pearson, 1989). Awareness has grown, for example, that communication with patients can have therapeutic effects if the nurse develops a range of skills to become an effective communicator (Schober and Hinchliff, 1995). These skills include empowering the client, using thoughtful silence and open-ended questions, helping the client to see events in context and perspective, and using exploration to help the client to clarify understanding and to describe how he or she is feeling (Murray and Zentner, 1989, pages 52–5).

In the late 1980s, the concept of 'patient-focused hospitals' was developed in the USA, the idea being to make the patient the primary focus of care activities. The idea was introduced into the UK in 1990 when the Department of Health developed three pilot sites which have since been expanded to eight. There are five main features of the approach:

- **Empowerment** of the patient to enable him or her to take control and exercise choice
- Decentralisation of care to each team, delivered in partnership with the patient
- Multidisciplinary working according to the needs of the patient
- Use of care protocols i.e. treatment plans customised for each patient including defined quality standards
- Staff development.

Patient-focused care has been adopted by many hospitals and current findings suggest there are benefits both to staff and patients (National Health Service Executive [NHSE], 1995). However, there has been some concern that managers have adopted the concept with the aim of cutting costs and deskilling nurses (Royal College of Nursing, 1994). Until these issues are resolved, the future of patient-focused care remains unclear.

A recent focus for nursing in the UK has been transcultural nursing, particularly in community nursing. Although the UK has always had people living within its society from many different races and cultures, government immigration policy in the 1950s and 1960s led to the UK becoming indisputably multicultural. There has subsequently been a growing realisation that health care for these people needs to be relevant and meaningful within their culture or they will not benefit from good health care. Dobson (1991) stated:

'As an approach to practice that requires the practitioner to provide nursing care which has meaning for the client in the context of the client's culture, transcultural nursing has become nothing less than a contemporary imperative'

(Dobson, 1991, page 182)

All these changes have strengthened the potential of the nurse's role, redressed the balance in the partnership between patient and nurse, and enhanced the nurse's ability to act as the patient's advocate.

Health service reforms

The real growth of consumer power in the NHS has its roots in the management changes of the early 1980s when, as a result of the Griffiths report (DHSS, 1983), consensus-style management was replaced with executive management. General managers replaced multidisciplinary management teams at unit, district and regional level. On short-term contracts, they were expected to perform as their counterparts in private business – to work to 'targets', to achieve 'efficiency savings' and value for money. Many of these new managers came, as did Roy Griffiths himself, from the private business sector.

These changes, which reflected the much wider alterations in political ideology that occurred in the UK in the 1980s, meant that the NHS was expected to operate more and more as a cost-effective business, providing a quality service with rigorously enforced cash limits. The inevitable consequence of this move to a business philosophy was the adoption of the view that patients should be seen as **consumers** of the service, able to take their custom elsewhere, if services failed to meet their needs.

This also led to an increasing emphasis on making sure services met the demands of the customer. As a result, monitoring and auditing the quality of services became a high priority, with new management posts established in 'customer services' and 'quality assurance', many of them held by nurses.

In 1989, this changing philosophy was embodied in a government White Paper entitled *Working for Patients* (DoH, 1989) which presented the benefits of the changes to the consumer. Money would follow patients, it was argued. Consumer choice would be improved because services would be bought on the basis of which providers offered the best deal – not just the cheapest, but that with the shortest waiting list and the best quality services, detailed in contract specifications, drawn up by the purchaser. Also included in the White Paper were arrangements for auditing the medical services available and for questioning consumers on the quality of the service they received.

Patients were thus encouraged to 'shop around' for health care. In 1990 the process of change reached its zenith with the introduction of the *NHS and Community Care Act* (HMSO, 1990a), in which the NHS was restructured to create an internal market. Health authorities became purchasers of health care, and hospitals and community services became providers. Under the Act, the first wave of hospitals were allowed to become self-governing trusts, funded by the purchasers of their services. Using a similar principle, GPs could choose to become fundholders, buying from provider units the best care available for their patients, in terms of its cost and availability.

The Act also made it easier for patients to change their GP. Opticians were allowed to advertise their services and there were suggestions (since dropped) that dentists and GPs should be allowed to do the same. GPs, however, were required to list the services they offered to help people choose which practice to join.

In 1994, the government made it clear that GPs and community teams were to be at the forefront of future developments with the publication of an executive letter, entitled *Towards a Primary Care-led NHS* (NHSE, 1994). In the document, it states that decisions about purchasing and providing health care should 'be taken as much as possible by GPs working closely with patients through primary health care teams.'

These changes, however, were just the start of a recognition that patients should not simply be passive recipients of care but partners in care.

Key Points

- The patient's role has traditionally been as a passive recipient of care.
- Changes in nursing philosophy over the last few decades such as primary nursing and patient-focused care have played a key part in developing a more patient-centred service.
- The NHS reforms have also led to services becoming targeted at patients' needs rather than the needs of health care staff.

TOWARDS THE PATIENT AS A CONSUMER OF HEALTH CARE

In recent years, there has been an unprecedented increase in the interest and participation of people in their own health care. It is this factor that marks the difference between the patient as recipient and the patient as consumer of health care.

The concept of consumerism carries with it the concept of rights. The consumer is empowered by his or her status; he/she has legal rights, and rights as an individual to choice, self-determination, information and involvement in treatment and care.

It is still a matter of debate, however, as to whether the principles of consumerism can be carried over into a health context. In this section, we will look at the rights that patients have now and whether they are being met and also explore the recent changes in patient choice and information provision.

PATIENT'S RIGHTS AND STANDARDS OF CARE

The patient now has certain rights, both as an individual and in law. As a result of the Patient's Charter (DoH, 1991b), the patient has rights specifically as a user of the NHS.

The charter is not enshrined in any legislation but it can be used as a standard against which care can be measured and a basis for any complaint. It

sets out seven existing rights within the NHS and affirms three new rights (Tables 9.2 and 9.3). It also sets national and local standards which health authorities should adopt (Tables 9.4 and 9.5).

An expanded and updated version was produced in 1995 which introduced several national standards and explained the difference between 'rights' (which all patients will receive all of the time) and 'expectations' (which the NHS aims to achieve).

The patient's rights as an individual may be summarised as follows:

- The right to individualised care. The patient is first and foremost a person and this should be

Table 9.2: A citizen's existing rights within the National Health Service (DoH, 1991b)

> 1 To receive health care on the basis of clinical need, regardless of ability to pay
> 2 To be registered with a GP
> 3 To receive emergency medical care at any time
> 4 To be referred to a consultant, acceptable to the patient, when the GP thinks it necessary and to be referred for a second opinion
> 5 To be given a clear explanation of any treatment proposed, including any risks and alternatives
> 6 To have access to health records and for them to be treated confidentially
> 7 To choose whether or not to take part in medical research or medical student training

Table 9.3: Three new rights (DoH, 1991b)

> 1 To be given detailed information on local health services, including quality standards and maximum waiting time
> 2 To be guaranteed admission for virtually all treatments within two years of being placed on a waiting list
> 3 To have any complaint about NHS services investigated and to receive a full and prompt reply from the chief executive of the health authority or general manager of the hospital. If the patient is still unhappy, the case can be taken to the Health Service Commissioner

Table 9.4: National standards (DoH, 1991b)

> - Respect for privacy, dignity and religious beliefs
> - Arrangements for people with special needs
> - Information to be given to relatives and friends about the progress of treatment, subject to the patients' wishes
> - An emergency ambulance should arrive within 14 minutes in an urban area, or 19 minutes in a rural area
> - Outpatient clinics to give specific appointment times and patients to be seen within 30 minutes of them
> - Operations not to be cancelled on the day of arrival. If an operation is postponed twice, the patient will be admitted within one month
> - A named, qualified nurse, midwife or health visitor to be responsible for nursing or midwifery care
> - A decision should be made about any continuing health or social care needs before discharge

Table 9.5: Local standards (DoH, 1991b)

Health authorities should set and publicise local standards including:

- First outpatient appointments
- Waiting times in Accident and Emergency departments
- Waiting times for being taken home after treatment where transport is required
- Better signposting around the hospital
- Ensuring staff wear name badges

recognised by providing him/her with individualised care. In doing so, nurses must accept that a patient's behaviour is influenced by previous experience, by background and culture, and should avoid making value judgements about lifestyle or behaviours, based on their own values and background.

- The right to holistic care. The patient has a right to have his or her total care needs – physical, psychological and social – taken into account, bearing in mind that they are interrelated.

- Cultural needs. Britain is a multicultural society and this is strongly reflected in the mix of people who seek health care. Patients from different ethnic groups have different lifestyles, family patterns, religious beliefs, dietary habits and attitudes to health and illness which must be understood, respected and, as far as possible, catered for while they are receiving health care.

    Patients from these groups may be more socially disadvantaged than others and many will have problems with language and communication. As a result, they will find it harder to get the information they need to get the best from health care services.

    Health information, particularly in areas where ethnic minority groups are concentrated, must be available in different and relevant languages. Visiting arrangements may need to be more flexible to take account of an extended family structure or religious restrictions on travel on certain days. Hygiene and dietary habits must be respected when planning care and nutritional needs.

- The right to maintain links with home and family. This is especially important for children, for whom the trauma of separation from family can be far worse than that caused by events in

hospital. Since the Platt Report (Ministry of Health, 1959) highlighted the damage that could be caused by such separation, visiting arrangements for children have been completely relaxed in most hospitals.

Open and flexible visiting arrangements are equally important for adults. The involvement of the family in a patient's care should also be encouraged as they may have to take on important aspects of care once the patient goes home.

The effectiveness of the Patient's Charter in improving patients' rights, however, is still an area for debate. McIver and Martin (1996) reported that an information team from the Association of Community Health Councils for England and Wales (ACHCEW) had found that many of the rights specified in the charter were not being met and concluded that the charter had not strengthened the original seven rights.

However, the three new rights had made an impact, possibly by being linked to NHS initiatives, for example, the reduction in waiting times.

The NHS Executive, the body responsible for carrying out government policy, has also attempted to monitor the standards set out. One example of this has been the introduction of league tables which show the performance of individual hospitals against some of the Patient's Charter standards year by year, although they have been criticised for concentrating on 'hard' standards, e.g. number of operations performed, to the detriment of 'soft' standards, e.g. the length of consultation times.

Concern has also been shown over patients' awareness of the charter and therefore its effectiveness in improving consumer power. A poll carried out in 1994 showed that the public had low levels of interest and awareness and considered it was a political initiative closely linked to central government.

McIver and Martin (1996) suggest that if it is truly to increase patients' power, then they should have a greater input into the working of rights and standards and the monitoring of performance, while less independent bodies such as the NHS should decrease their involvement. It remains to be seen whether this will happen.

There are now charters and documents emphasising patients' rights in many specific areas, for example, child health (DoH, 1996), midwifery (DoH, 1993) and mental illness (DoH, 1997).

Child health

The issue of children's rights has received increasing attention over the last 30 years. It is in recent years, however, that the need for children to be able to participate in making decisions about their own welfare has been highlighted by the Children Act (HMSO, 1989).

This change in emphasis has meant that, although family autonomy is paramount, the wishes and feelings of the child are now considered as equally important, particularly in situations which affect them most directly (Atherton, 1994).

Certain rights for children were identified in 1991 by the government (DoH, 1991c) which included a right to privacy, an equal right to information appropriate to their age and understanding, and the right to consent to treatment. Child health nurses, therefore, have to encourage children's participation in care and support their independence, so increasing their autonomy (Akers and Bell, 1994).

Following an Audit Commission report in 1993 which showed a lack of management awareness of the needs of children, the government published the Children's Charter in 1996 which sets out standards for child health services (DoH, 1996). The principles of the Charter, although no different to those of the Platt Report (Central Health Services Council, 1959), were welcomed.

Burr (1996) pointed out that charters appear to have more clout and this provides more ammunition for nurses to persuade managers of the importance of services for children. The key statements from the Charter are in Table 9.6.

The principle of increasing children's autonomy, however, is not as simple as it may seem. The knowledge gap between children/parents and health professionals, and the family's increased vulnerability during illness, makes it easy to exert influence over what decisions are taken (Lowes, 1996). It may also be true that giving more power to the child and parents may be perceived as a threat by nurses and other health professionals. Lowes (1996) concludes that:

> 'Only by nurses becoming more confident of their professional role and more knowledgeable about relevant issues is the child's right to autonomy going to be effectively exercised within contemporary healthcare.'
>
> (Lowes, 1996, page 372)

Midwifery care

Another area of health care that deserves particular mention with regards to patient rights is midwifery.

In 1992, a Select Committee on Health published a report on maternity services (House of

Table 9.6: Some of the recommendations from the Children's Charter (DoH, 1996)

- Parents have a right to information on local child health services
- Children have a right to have access to their health records and to know that everyone working for the NHS has, by law, to keep those records confidential
- In most cases, parents also have access to this information where children are considered too young to make their own decisions
- Parents can expect their health visitor to give them a record of their child's health
- Parents can expect to be told the name of the school nurse and how to contact him/her
- Adolescents can expect to be more and more involved in decisions about their health care and any treatment and prevention measures
- Parents and children can expect to be part of any discussions and decisions about the child's treatment and care, and parents can expect to be kept up to date with their child's progress
- Parents can expect children to have access to an inhaler at school, if necessary
- Parents can expect to have appropriate help and support from the community nursing team when nursing their child at home
- Parents can expect their child to be cared for in a children's ward under the supervision of a consultant paediatrician
- Parents can expect their child to have a named qualified children's nurse responsible for the child's nursing care, whether on an adult or children's ward

Commons, 1992) which was the precursor to the goverment's widely publicised recommendations for midwifery care entitled *Changing Childbirth* (DoH, 1993).

The fundamental principle underpinning all the proposals outlined in the document is that women should be in control of their birth giving. This means they should have choice over, for example, how and where their babies are delivered and they should have continuity of care through the various stages of antenatal and postnatal care. The document sums up this philosophy in the statement: 'The woman and her baby should be at the centre of all planning and provision of maternity care.'

This change towards giving women responsibility for choice over issues to do with the birth of their babies, and stressing that it is their labour rather than that of the various health care professionals involved, represented a dramatic rethinking of the way care should be organised. Midwives, as a result, are expected to take notice of the needs and wants of women in their care and to try and arrange care to fit in with these requests (Flint, 1994). The development of the birthplan was one such way in which women could gain some control over what happens to them during childbirth. Many other schemes are now more widely available partly as a result of the report, for example, **domino** deliveries where the woman is cared for by the same team of midwives throughout, shared care beween GPs and the hospital, and general practice units which are often set up in rural areas to avoid women travelling long distances to hospital.

Research by Too (1996) showed that the birthplan offered only superficial, casual choices. 'Although women were given choices, in practice they were highly constrained. Midwives retained the ultimate sanction on which choices were available to the women.' The midwives felt that women's expectations were too high, and that there were inevitable occasions where the midwife would 'know better'. Too (1996) suggested women, when they receive maternity care, should be entitled to certain rights, which are listed in Table 9.7.

Mental health care

Mental health care and learning disabilities are two areas where patients traditionally have had very few rights or power. The institutions in which these patients were cared for until the 1960s were noted for their dehumanising and controlling effects, caused by the belief that it was in the patients' best interests to be powerless (Goffman, 1968). Attitudes have changed considerably, particularly with the move of patients into the community following the Care in the Community legislation and the power of mental health pressure groups such as MIND. A new Patient's Charter for mental health service users came into effect from April 1st 1997. Patients now have the right to be told about drugs prescribed, possible side-effects and the availability of alternative treatments. The aim of the charter is to help adult mental health patients understand their rights and what standard of service to expect from the NHS.

Table 9.7: The rights of women requiring maternity care (Too, 1996)

- Each woman is a unique individual having inherent dignity, freedom of choice and intelligence
- A woman has the right to be given information in order to make informed choices and decisions
- Midwives need to legitimise the beliefs that women are equal partners in midwifery care by including mutual goal setting and decision making
- In order for an empowerment process to occur, there must be mutual respect, trust and shared responsibility between the woman and the midwife
- Midwives need the self-confidence that stems from appropriate knowledge and expertise. They need self-awareness of their feelings and prejudices
- Midwives must be willing to relinquish control
- Midwives are seen as facilitators and resource persons as opposed to providers of maternity services
- To strengthen their ability to empower, midwives need to be valued and empowered
- Empowerment requires open communication, a nurturing and caring environment, a democratic structure and the support of midwife colleagues or supervisors

Many units have embraced the concept of patients' rights for themselves. For example, Ashworth hospital, which cares for mentally disordered offenders, has introduced its own patients' charter, and encouraged a user-led service to develop, with the introduction of a patient's council where patients can make a contribution to hospital policy and activities (Musker and Byrne, 1997).

LEGAL RIGHTS

The patient has the legal right to decide whether or not to accept treatment – known as informed consent. The onus is on medical staff to explain the implications of treatment and surgery to the patient, and a signed consent form must be obtained for every surgical procedure or invasive investigation that is carried out.

For a person to make appropriate decisions regarding health care and treatment, as much information is required as possible. In practice, as we have discussed, the quality of information given to the patient varies and until recently, patients had no legal right to information concerning their case. Since November 1991, patients have had the legal right to see their medical records, even though doctors will still be able, at their discretion, to withhold certain facts. Doctors will be obliged, however, to make their medical notes more easily understandable (HMSO, 1990b).

The situation becomes more complicated in the case of children or people who are not in a position to make a decision regarding their care. They may be unconscious or they may have some degree of learning difficulty. In such cases, responsibility for informed consent falls upon the parents, guardian or next of kin. If the person acting on the patient's behalf does not agree with the medical staff, however, the case could be decided in court.

Children under the age of 16 years are increasingly being recognised as being able to make a valid contribution to informed consent. The Gillick case in 1987 established the legal principle whereby a doctor could administer treatment, in this case, contraceptive pills, against the wishes of the parent (Dimond, 1995).

However, a child under 16 may not be able to refuse treatment, although the *Children Act* (HMSO, 1989) stresses this is dependent on the level of understanding to be able to make an informed decision. The complexity of this was illustrated in a case involving a 16-year-old girl with anorexia nervosa who refused treatment. The Court overruled her on the basis that 'no minor of whatever age has an absolute right to make decisions on medical treatment, especially when that decision is refusal' (Taylor and Muller, 1995).

There are certain exceptions whereby a patient can be treated without consent, however. They are:

- If a person has a notifiable disease or is carrying an organism capable of causing one
- If a person has been detained under the provisions of the *Mental Health Act* (HMSO, 1983), or the *Mental Health Amendment Act* (HMSO, 1984).

Adult patients, except those in the categories listed above, are free to discharge themselves from hospital, even if medical or nursing staff wish them to stay. They will usually have to sign an undertaking that they are doing so against medical advice and accept personal responsibility for any consequences. In 1997, however, concern was raised over the use of mental health legislation to force women to have Caesarean deliveries (Hewson, 1997). Since 1992, eight cases have occurred, and in seven of them the woman was not legally represented. In two cases, courts ruled that women were temporarily 'incompetent' to decline Caesarean surgery.

PATIENT CHOICE

The choice that patients have in the health care they are given is a key factor in whether they are truly consumers of health care or merely passive recipients. When Roy Griffiths, a Sainsbury's executive, was appointed to chair the 1983 NHS Management Inquiry (DHSS, 1983), jokes and headlines made much of the idea of 'supermarket health care'. But can the philosophy of the supermarket really be transposed on to the health care system? Can people expect to exercise the same degree of choice over their operations as over their oranges? Boxes 9.2 and 9.3 show examples of what being a consumer entails.

Box 9.2: Scenario. Understanding the principles of consumerism (Downie, 1996)

Consumers must have access to the services or goods they require; they must have choice of the goods or services they require; and this will involve competition between suppliers and a fair balance in the market place between supplier and customer; customers must have adequate information on the goods and services they require, and the information must be expressed in clear language; it must be possible for the consumer to obtain redress in the event of poor services or goods; the products or services must be safe and subject to regulation to ensure safety.

Box 9.3: Scenario. An example of consumer autonomy (Downie, 1996)

Suppose that I go into a shoe shop and ask for a pair of strong shoes for walking along country lanes, I try on various pairs which do not appeal to me and then my eye lights on a pair of shiny patent leather shoes and I say I want to buy them. A good salesperson will explain to me that they are not appropriate shoes for my purposes, but if I insist that these are the ones I want the salesperson has no duty to refuse the sale having advised against it. I am here exercising consumer autonomy.

The answer, of course, is no – or, at least, not entirely. First, patients do not necessarily enter the health care system willingly. They do not choose to be ill in the same way that they decide they need more groceries or a pair of shoes. Even independent sector patients, who may be able to choose the timing of an elective operation, have little control over experiencing a road traffic accident or a burst appendix, when they will enter the health care system as an emergency.

As Buchan (1990) pointed out, patients are not always voluntarily making use of the services provided. They may even be uncooperative or even downright hostile; neither can they enter or leave the health care market at will. They are constrained by the availability of services.

Within the NHS, a person has a right, within certain geographical constraints, to choose a GP, or rather apply to be accepted onto a GP's list – the GP can refuse. But at that point, any influence over where and by whom the patient is treated if necessary, effectively ends.

This is not so in the independent sector, of course, or with complementary medicine, which is not publicly funded. Here the only constraints on the patient are price and geographical location. Yet even patients in the independent sector have limited influence over which hospital they are treated in and which medical or nursing staff manage their treatment and care.

During the 1980s, the government sought to introduce greater patient choice into the NHS. Allowing tax relief on private health care insurance for the over-60s offered people greater opportunity to choose to go private. GPs have been required to make public the services they offer, as a way of helping people decide which practice to join. Opticians began to be allowed to advertise their services.

The White Paper *Working for Patients* (DoH, 1989) which heralded the organisational changes in 1990, declared its stated objective was 'to give patients, wherever they live in the UK, better health care and greater choice of the services available'.

The creation of an internal market meant that purchasers (i.e. health authorities and GP fund holders) had the freedom to place their contracts for hernia repairs, hip replacements, etc., with whoever was perceived to be offering the best deal. One of the key tenets of the health service reforms therefore was to improve patient choice, enabling them to change their GP more easily and be treated at a hospital of their choice. How successful the reforms have been in achieving these improvements is open to debate (Paton, 1992).

At the time of the introduction of the reforms, many professional and consumer organisations argued that, far from increasing patient choice, the changes in fact restricted it. Patients were referred for treatment according to local contractual agreements, rather than personal preferences. What limited choice previously existed, they argued – for example, a smaller hospital closer to home in preference to the district general hospital 25 miles away – disappeared, with GPs, in most cases, having to send the patient where the contract was placed.

Likewise, the doctor's freedom to refer a particular patient on professional grounds to a particular consultant went. Patients could no longer be referred elsewhere for treatment if the treatment they required (for example, in vitro fertilisation) was not available in their own heath authority, or be sent to a particular consultant practising in a different part of the country because he or she had some particularly specialised expertise that they needed.

Neuberger (1990) highlighted one of the major flaws in the reasoning behind the internal market as the lack of involvement of the patient in choosing the service. She said:

> 'The problem comes when the purchaser of the services is not the consumer. The purchaser, in this case, is the District Health Authority, in whose interests it clearly is to get services as cheaply and as efficiently as possible. But the consumer who is not paying for services may have other priorities, such as the services being within easy reach of home, or of a particular type.'
> (Neuberger, 1990, page 18)

Current evidence suggests that the early criticisms may have been justified. A survey in 1996 by ACHCEW (Griffiths, 1996) suggests that market forces have failed to deliver significant improvements in quality and patient choice.

The report stated that some patients have become more assertive and aware of their rights. It is not clear, however, that there has been any significant increase in patients' ability to exercise choice about where and how they are treated. In effect, GPs are still often seen as the 'gatekeeper' to the health service for their patients.

This means that though one of the slogans of the NHS reforms – 'the money should follow the patients' – is true, the patient still goes where he/she is sent by the doctor.

One of the key introductions of the NHS reforms to improve patient choice was the system of extra-contractual referrals (ECRs). This meant that if a patient chose to be referred to a hospital that the GP did not have a contract with, money would be made available for the patient to do this. ACHCEW's survey showed that many patients were not aware of the ECR system and that because health authorities varied in their handling of the system, patients' ability to exercise choice depended on where they live.

The report concludes that the system therefore does not effectively guarantee choice for patients in the NHS (Griffiths, 1996).

INFORMATION

A major factor in helping patients to be true consumers of health care is the amount and quality of information to which they have access. We mentioned earlier the traditional lack of communication and information that occurred in the health service which contributed to the lack of power of patients. The importance of giving information was recognised in 1993 by the National Health Service Management Executive (NHSME), as it was then known, as 'the most important factor' in empowering patients.

The population is now generally better informed about health and health care provision than ever before. Documentary programmes show sickness and curing, operative techniques and medical emergencies in unsparing detail. Some programmes chronicle actual events as they occur, while many UK and US hospital soaps, such as *Casualty* and *ER*, cover many aspects of health care in a serious and responsible way.

There are an increasing number of organisations that provide information on medical matters. There has also been a marked increase in the number and power of pressure groups and charities, for example, the National Childbirth Trust, Age Concern, MIND and Mencap. These all provide a great deal of information on a wide range of conditions and the types of treatment and care one can expect to receive.

Many have also set up telephone helplines, for example, the British Association of Cancer United Patients (CancerBACUP), which provide a large amount of advice and support outside the NHS.

Another growing area has been heath care journalism. Many magazines now available in newsagents and bookshops are devoted entirely to health and most women's magazines provide information on health matters and what to expect from the health care system. Women's magazines are often cited in surveys as the favourite source for health information. There are now magazines specifically for men which deal with health-related issues, reflecting a dramatic change from the traditional role of women as the carers of men's health. Although the change is slow, men's health is an area that remains largely neglected (Doyal, 1997).

While information about health is readily available, information about the health service and how to use it is less easy to come by. Some magazines provide both medical information as well as encouraging patients' rights. The best known example is probably *Which?*, which now has a special monthly magazine *Health Which?*. This provides a range of advice from treatment through to how to change your GP if you are unhappy with the service.

Some charities are also more pro-active than others in encouraging patients' rights. The National Childbirth Trust, for example, will frankly advise members on which hospitals are more likely to encourage 'natural' childbirth, or how to arrange for a home birth.

Some of the main champions of patients' rights are the community health councils. These were first introduced in 1974 and there are now 207 in England and Wales. Their job is to review the health services in their districts and recommend any improvements. They have to be consulted by health authorities on any substantial change or variation in service. At a national level, the Association of Community Health Councils for England and Wales (ACHCEW) represents the users of health services and provides a forum for member CHCs. They also advise on and take up patients' complaints, and monitor the number and type of complaints as a measure of public satisfaction. CHCs, however, have no powers to monitor the purchasing decisions made by GP fundholders as opposed to health authorities, and they cannot follow patients from their boundaries if contracts are made with hospitals in different health authorities.

The College of Health, established in 1983, has published several consumer guides to using the health service, on subjects such as alternative medicine, homes for elderly people, obtaining second opinions and hospital waiting lists. Its aims include helping people to make the most effective use of the NHS, improving communication between doctors and patients, and making medical information accessible to lay people. The College also operates a telephone information line giving advice on waiting lists.

The Patients' Association is another organisation which aims to support and advise patients on health service matters. It works to protect and develop the interests, rights and well-being of people who use the health service, and represents patients' interests to many public and government bodies. A list of useful addresses is included at the end of this chapter.

PATIENT COMPLAINTS

For anyone to feel that they really do have rights, it must be possible for them to make a complaint if they feel that their rights have been infringed, and for those complaints to be taken seriously. The NHS Complaints procedures were mostly designed several years before the health service reforms came into place, but the importance of being able to make a complaint was one of the key aspects of the Patient's Charter (DoH, 1991b), as well as the Citizen's Charter for wider public services.

This states that the patient has a right:

'to have any complaint about NHS services – whoever provides them – investigated, and to receive a full and prompt written reply from the chief executive of the [patient's] health authority or general manager of the [patient's] hospital. If [the patient is] still unhappy, [he] will be able to take the case up with the Health Service Commissioner.'

(DoH, 1991b)

A formal complaint is usually made in the first instance to the hospital or community service involved, either verbally or in writing, and it should be immediately reported to the senior manager who is responsible for investigating it. The patient and any staff involved should be kept informed of any steps that are being taken.

Clinical complaints should be referred to the consultant in charge of the case who will discuss how it is to be handled with the senior manager.

Most complaints can be satisfactorily dealt with at local level. Often all the patient will require is an assurance that his/her voice has been heard and that action will be taken. When a complaint is likely to involve litigation, the health authority will seek legal advice and the staff concerned should be made aware of the help that is available to them through their professional association or trade union.

The number of litigation cases has risen in recent years and there is some evidence that fear of litigation can hamper handling of complaints (DoH, 1994).

Cases which appear to involve professional misconduct by a doctor or a nurse will first be examined by the hospital or community services management before a decision is taken as to whether to refer the case to the General Medical Council or, for nursing, to the National Boards in

England, Scotland, Wales and Northern Ireland. They, in turn, decide whether a case should be referred to the Professional Conduct Committee of the United Kingdom Central Council for Nursing, Midwifery and Health Visiting.

The Health Service Ombudsman, formerly known as the Health Service Commissioner, may be involved when a patient feels a case has not been dealt with satisfactorily by the health authority. He/she is appointed by the Crown and is responsible to Parliament, which means he/she is independent of the NHS and the government. Although not entitled to examine clinical cases, he/she can investigate the way clinical complaints are handled. The Health Service Commissioner publishes an annual report.

In 1994, the Department of Health published a report on NHS complaints procedures, compiled by a review committee (DoH, 1994). This was because the procedures had attracted considerable criticism from a number of bodies. For example,

The National Association of Health Authorities and Trusts (NAHAT, 1993) stated:

'The arrangements are seen as being over complex, failing to be user-friendly, taking too long, often over defensive and often failing to give any satisfactory explanation of the conclusion reached.'
(NAHAT, 1993, page 8)

The review committee received evidence showing that complainants could face an uphill struggle in using the complaints procedures, and that patients did not know where to complain because of the fact that nine different procedures were in existence. Those who did manage to complain were frustrated and faced hostile responses. Of those patients who successfully got through to the third stage of clinical complaints, only half were satisfied with the outcome.

The response of the review committee was to publish a set of 67 recommendations to the government to improve the situation, some examples of which are shown in Table 9.8. Since the publi-

Table 9.8: Recommendations to improve NHS complaints procedures (DoH, 1994)

General principles
The following principles should be incorporated into any NHS complaints procedures:

- Responsiveness
- Quality enhancement
- Cost-effectiveness
- Accessibility
- Impartiality
- Simplicity
- Speed
- Confidentiality
- Accountability

- We recommend that every purchaser and provider of NHS services should have simple, readily available written information about how to complain.

- We recommend that complaints procedures empower NHS staff to give a rapid, often oral, response when a complaint is made about a service within their responsibility, and to initiate appropriate action as a result of the information received.

- We recommend that complaints procedures should encourage those handling complaints, including senior staff, to make early personal contact with complainants.

- We recommend that training in complaints handling should be extended to all NHS practitioners and staff who are, or are likely to be, in contact with patients.

- We recommend that all NHS practitioners and staff should be made aware of the support available when a complaint is made against them.

cation of the report, the government has looked at the situation again and a report is expected in February 1997.

Key Points

■ Patients now have many more rights than they used to and they also have more choice about the care they receive within the NHS.

■ Increases in the amount of information available on health and improvements in the patient complaints system have contributed to their enhanced status.

■ There is still clearly much more that could be done to improve patients' choice and involve them in service delivery.

INVOLVEMENT OF PATIENTS IN CARE

The emphasis on involvement of patients in their care has led to many initiatives being set up and various buzzwords and phrases have entered the nursing vocabulary as a result. In this section we shall look at patient empowerment and partners in care, patient surveys and the role of the nurse in empowering patients.

PATIENT EMPOWERMENT

Empowerment is a process in which individuals are enabled to take control of their lives. For patients to have this control they need to have the necessary information and they need to feel that health professionals will listen and respect their views (Elliot and Turrell, 1996).

Patient empowerment could therefore be described as the next step in the process of increasing patients' choice and responsibility for health, started back in the 1980s, which was described earlier. If patients are empowered in this way, they are more likely to have health care that is tailored to their needs and so are more inclined to feel they can help themselves get better.

Patient empowerment, however, has recently become an over-used phrase and, therefore, people can be in danger of forgetting what it really means.

The NHSME (1993) and the Institute of Health Services Management (Fontes and Howland, 1995) both agree that patient empowerment encompasses the following:

■ Equal access to care
■ Getting fair redress for complaints
■ The right to be represented by someone you choose
■ Participating in audit and service development
■ Respecting patient autonomy in health care decisions
■ Maximum availability of information about care and services received.

There are also disadvantages to patient empowerment. Whilst younger patients may be used to living in a consumer society and wish to have choices about their health care, older patients who may be more used to thinking 'doctor knows best', or who may have lower expectations of services available to them, may find it difficult to change to this new way of thinking. In a small survey carried out in a social centre for older people, Cox (1996) found that they had little desire to be involved and empowered in the sense of taking control and influencing events.

Cox suggested this may be because they did not want to have to make decisions, seeing this as an opt-out by hard-pressed health services, and because they did not want to upset an existing good relationship with the staff which empowered them. It might be, therefore, that empowerment is not what everybody wants.

PARTNERS IN CARE

Another step forward in the change from patient to consumer has been the introduction of the concept of partnerships in care between health care staff and patients (Audit Commission, 1993; DoH, 1993). It has been described as the inevitable outcome of consumerism, where the relationship between patient and provider reflects the greater involvement of patients and self-help.

Although there may be much debate about what partnership in care really means, there are key aspects that can be identified, such as relationship, reciprocity, sharing equality, friendship and participation. Concepts such as being empowered, autonomous and patient-centred are also important (Wade, 1995).

Partnership in care can be looked at as a contract that both the nurse and the patient enter into. The nurse brings knowledge, information and skills so that the patient can make informed decisions. The patient, however, keeps overall responsibility for his/her health (Teasdale, 1987). This is similar to the relationship that may exist between a lawyer and a client, for example.

For the partnership to succeed, nurses need to be able to demonstrate unconditional regard, competence, confidence, assertiveness and be genuine and empathetic (O'Donnel, 1993).

It is not always easy for such a partnership to develop. As mentioned earlier, patients may not want to be involved in such a relationship. This may be, for example, because they don't feel able to or don't want to (Teasdale, 1987; Waterworth and Luker, 1990). They may simply want to be looked after (Biley, 1992). Nurses may also find it hard to hand control of the patient's care to the patient.

Closely linked to this idea is another commonly used phrase – patient participation (Brearley, 1990). This can take many forms, for example, involving patients in decision making or encouraging them to perform clinical or daily living skills, or to take an interest in the running of the ward. It is well established in many areas of psychiatric and community care (Saunders, 1995).

What is important, therefore, is that concepts such as partnership in care, patient participation and empowerment are not forced upon patients in the paternalistic style of 'old-fashioned' health care. If patients are really empowered to make choices, their views must be considered and the ability to say no respected.

CONSUMER SURVEYS

As a result of patients being encouraged to be more involved in their care, much attention has been given in recent years to determining patients' views of the care they receive and want. Only in this way can health professionals ensure that they are providing a service which meets the needs of the consumer and which involves them in care provision. The principle was first introduced following the Griffiths NHS Management Inquiry (DHSS, 1983) and was emphasised in the White Paper *Working for Patients* (DoH, 1989). The government also issued guidance on the conduct of consumer surveys and other patient relations activities (Carr-Hill *et al.*, 1989).

Surveys have therefore started to proliferate in a range of settings; for example, Black and Sanderson (1993) looked at the views of patients having day surgery, Bruster *et al.* (1994) surveyed hospital patients, and Walsh (1993) explored opinions in accident and emergency departments.

There are, however, some difficulties with using surveys to find out patients' views, not least of which is that patients tend to give high ratings (French, 1981). Patients also usually record high levels of satisfaction with their nursing care, which may be a reflection of the way questions are asked or the type of question. One attempt to rectify this problem is the development of the Newcastle Satisfaction with Nursing Scales (NSNS) which aims to produce more detailed analysis (McColl *et al.*, 1996). By asking more specific questions, it is hoped that patients' views can be accurately obtained and thus taken into account in planning future services.

Key Points

- Nurses have played a major part in setting up initiatives to empower patients.
- Nurses must ensure that they do not force patients to participate in their care. If patients are truly empowered, they must be allowed to choose what level of involvement they wish to have in their care.

THE NURSE'S ROLE

PROFESSIONAL ACCOUNTABILITY

Patients may, for various reasons, be either unwilling or unable to complain about their care. Nurses, by virtue of their close and continuous contact with patients, are arguably in the best position both to recognise that care falls short of the standards patients have a right to expect, and to complain about it.

According to the Code of Professional Conduct (UKCC, 1992), it is part of the nurse's professional responsibility to do this:

'As a registered nurse, midwife or health visitor, you are personally accountable for your practice, and, in the exercise of your professional accountability, must:

1 Act always in such a way as to promote and safeguard the well-being and interests of patients/clients.
2 Ensure that no action or omission on your part, or within your sphere of responsibility, is detrimental to the interests, conditions or safety of patients and clients.'

(UKCC, 1992, page 2)

This could involve witnessing an infringement of a patient's rights by another colleague. Making such a complaint can be extremely difficult and the staff member may face victimisation from colleagues and management. There can be little doubt that many cases go unreported for this reason.

Nurses who speak out in these situations became known, in the early 1990s, as 'whistle-blowers' and many nurses feared being labelled as such if they complained about standards of patient care (Chapter 13). Perhaps the most well-known speaker against poor standards was Graham Pink, who consistently complained that poor staffing levels at his hospital constituted a danger to patients, but lost his job as a result. Many Trusts introduced 'gagging clauses' in their staff contracts to prevent them from criticising the Trust.

In 1995, Tony Wright MP introduced the Public Interest Disclosure Bill, which is currently being considered by the Commons to protect the rights of individuals who speak out.

PATIENT ADVOCACY

A stage further on from the idea of whistle-blowing is patient **advocacy**, where the nurse in effect is acting on behalf of the patient or in the patient's best interests. In the context of the patient as a consumer of health care, nurses can act as an advocate by, for example, encouraging patients to argue for their rights, or by negotiating the patients' rights on their behalf with a manager. As Beardshaw (1981) said: 'The nurse's role as advocate is a logical extension of the resulting emphasis on patients' rights.'

The UKCC (1996) has outlined the role of the nurse as advocate, stating that:

'Advocacy is concerned with promoting and protecting the interests of patients or clients, many of whom may be vulnerable and incapable of protecting their own interest and who may be without the support of family and friends. You can do this by providing information and making the patient or client feel confident that he or she can make their own decisions.'

There are, however, many ethical, moral and professional difficulties associated with acting as an advocate. For example, arguing that a patient has a right to good care may require the nurse to criticise a colleague who is not giving good care. Nurses, as professionals, are also expected to be accountable to employers and the profession, which makes it difficult for them to act as 'free agents' – a mainstay of an advocate. There may also be a difference between acting in a patient's best interests and safeguarding his or her well-being.

Nurses, however, can and should act as advocates, though they may be placed in situations where they have to choose between their own and the patients' best interests (Gates, 1994).

CONFIDENTIALITY

Nurses may come across large amounts of confidential information in the course of their work and patients expect nurses to act responsibly with any information relating to them personally. If this trust is broken and confidentiality is breached, the nurse may not only break the law but breach a moral code.

The UKCC controls nurses' behaviour in this respect and may revoke registration of a nurse if it is considered that the nurse breached the UKCC's standards (UKCC, 1996) (Table 9.9).

In practice, confidentiality can become very complex and fraught with ethical dilemmas. An example of this is presented in Box 9.4.

Box 9.4: Scenario. An example of breach of confidentiality (adapted from Dimond, 1995)

A woman involved in a serious road accident was admitted to hospital. While on the ward, someone called asking for information on her progress. The nurse taking the call asked who the caller was. The

Table 9.9: Principles of the UKCC position on confidentiality (UKCC, 1996)

- A patient or client has the right to expect that information given in confidence will be used only for the purpose for which it was given and will not be released to others without their permission
- You should recognise each patient's or client's right to have information about themselves kept secure and private
- If it is appropriate to share information gained in the course of your work with other health or social work practitioners, you must make sure that as far as is reasonable, the information will be kept in strict professional confidence and be used only for the purpose for which the information was given
- You are responsible for any decision which you make to release confidential information because you think that this is in the public's best interest
- If you choose to break confidentiality because you believe that this is in the public's best interest, you must have considered the matter carefully enough to justify that decision and
- You should not deliberately break confidentiality other than in exceptional circumstances

answer was 'her husband'. The nurse thus gave the caller full details of the woman's condition. When the nurse told the patient that her husband had called, the patient was angry because she had recently separated from him, had not notified him of where she was now living, and did not want any communication with him because of his violence.

In this case, the nurse should have checked with the patient first, as patients are entitled to withhold information from their relatives and friends.

Woodrow's advice (1996) is:

'As professionals, we have to accept accountability and take responsibility for our own actions. Knowledge and experience may usefully temper our decisions, and our consciences should guide our actions with each case.

Key Points

- The role of the nurse is changing towards one where he/she can act as an advocate for patients.
- Nurses increasingly need to be aware of their accountability to patients and behave professionally when acting in the patients' best interests.

CONCLUSION

The role of patients has changed dramatically over the last few decades and it is clear that the service they receive is more closely aligned to what patients want and need on an individual basis. However, although patients have been given more

choice and power, they are still not able to act entirely as consumers. This is partly because of inherent difficulties in translating a consumer philosophy into a health care service, but also because health care staff are not always able or willing to relinquish their power.

Nurses have come a long way on the road to empowering patients. Changing professional roles or our expectations of ourselves as professionals is not easy (David, 1995). However, nurses still exert considerable power over patients and we need to look more closely at whether we are truly empowering patients and developing open and collaborative relationships (Hewison, 1995).

If patients are allowed to become more involved and have more input into decision making, then they may truly become consumers of health care.

Summary

This chapter has shown how people can act as consumers of health care before they are even ill or become a patient. This is because there is currently a focus on prevention of illness and promotion of health. The government has increasingly recognised its role in encouraging the public to be more health conscious through campaigns and screening programmes. While health promotion activities are generally considered beneficial, nurses must be careful to involve clients in the activities rather than telling them what to do.

Traditionally, the patient has been a passive recipient of care and expected to behave in the way dictated by health care professionals. This situation began to change over the last few decades, as awareness grew of the importance of involving patients in their own care. A concurrent change in nursing philosophy towards a more patient-centred approach and the drastic effects of the health service reforms have all played an important part in setting in progress a change towards a more equal relationship between patients and health care staff.

Patients now have many more rights than they used to and they also have more choice about the care they receive within the NHS. Other changes, for example, to the complaints procedures, have also enhanced their consumer status. However, there are many examples that show patients' rights and patient choice are not always being met and there is clearly plenty of room for involving patients more in the delivery of services.

In their practice, nurses are increasingly becoming aware of the importance of empowering patients to make choices about the health care they need and want. In many cases, nurses are endeavouring to adopt a partnership in care approach with patients. Nurses increasingly need to consider their accountability to patients and behave professionally when acting in the best interests of the patient.

Useful addresses

The Patients Association
8 Guildford Street
London
WC1N 1DT
Tel. 0171 242 3460

College of Health
St Margaret's House
21 Old Ford Road
London
E2 9PL
Tel. 0181 983 1225

National Consumer Council
20 Grosvenor Gardens
London
SW1W 0DH
Tel. 0171 730 3469

United Kingdom Central Council for Nursing, Midwifery and Health Visiting
23 Portland Place
London
W1N 4JT
Tel. 0171 637 7181

Consumer's Association
2 Marylebone Road
London
NW1
Tel. 0171 830 6000

Association of Community Health Councils for England and Wales
30 Drayton Park
London
N5 1PB
Tel. 0171 609 8405

References

Akers, J.A., Bell, S.K. (1994). Should children be used as research subjects? *Nursing Forum*, 29(3), 28–33.

Anderson, R. (1983). Public attitudes to and experience of medical check-ups. *Community Medicine*, 5, 11-20.

Atherton, T. (1994). The rights of the child in healthcare. In *The Child and Family*, Lindsay, B. (ed.). Baillière Tindall, London.

Audit Commission (1993). *Children First*. HMSO, London.

Beardshaw, V. (1981). *Conscientious Objectors at Work: Mental Hospital Nurses: a Case Study*. Social Audit, London.

Beattie, A. (1990). *Teaching and Learning About Health Education: New Directions in Curriculum Development*. Scottish Health Education Board, Edinburgh.

Biley, F.C. (1992). Some determinants that affect patient participation in decision making about nursing care. *Journal of Advanced Nursing*, 17, 414–21.

Black, N. and Sanderson, C. (1993). Day surgery: development of a questionnaire for eliciting patients' experiences. *Quality in Health Care*, 2, 157–61.

Brearley, S. (1990). *Patient Participation: the Literature*. RCN Research Series. Scutari Press, Harrow.

Bruster, S., Jarman, B., Bosanquet, N., Weston, D., Erens, R. and Delbanco, T.L. (1994). National survey of hospital patients. *British Medical Journal*, 309(6968), 1542–6.

Buchan, J. (1990). Caring for the consumer. *Nursing Standard*, 4(18), 46.

Burr, S. (1996). Children's services still inadequate – 37 years on. *Paediatric Nursing*, 8(3), 3.

Caraher, M. (1994). Health promotion: time for an audit. *Nursing Standard*, 8(20), 33–5.

Carr-Hill, I., McIver, S.S. and Dixon, P. (1989). *The NHS and its Customers*. York University Centre for Health Economics, York.

Central Health Services Council (1959). *The Welfare of Children in Hospital* (The Platt Report). HMSO, London.

Corner, J., Cawley, N. and Hildebrand, S. (1995). An evaluation of the use of massage and essential oils on the well-being of cancer patients. *International Journal of Palliative Nursing*, 1(2), 67–73.

Cox, J. (1996). An unwanted concept. *Nursing Standard*, 10(46), 24–5.

Crawford, R. (1977). You are dangerous to your health: the ideology and politics of victim blaming. *International Journal of Health Services*, 7(4), 661–80.

Cribb, A. (1993). The philosophy of health. In *Nursing Practice and Health Care*, Hinchliff, S., Norman, S.E. and Schober, J.E. (eds), 2nd edn. Edward Arnold, London.

David, A. (1995). Power to the parents. *Nursing Times*, 91(9), 26–7.

Devine, E. (1992). Effects of psycho-educational care for adult surgical patients: a meta-analysis of 191 studies. *Patient Education and Counselling*, 9, 129–42.

Devine, E. and Westlake, S. (1995). The effects of psycho-educational care provided to adults with cancer: meta-analysis of 116 studies. *Oncology Nursing Forum*, 9, 1369–81.

DHSS (1980). *Inequalities in Health* (The Black Report). HMSO, London.

DHSS (1983). *NHS Management Inquiry Report* (The Griffiths Report). HMSO, London.

Dimond, B. (1995). *Legal Aspects of Nursing*, 2nd edn. Prentice Hall International, Hemel Hempstead.

Dobson, S.M. (1991). *Transcultural Nursing*. Scutari Press, Harrow.

DoH (1989). *Working for Patients*. HMSO, London.

DoH (1991a). *The Health of the Nation: a Consultative Document for Health in England*. HMSO, London.

DoH (1991b). *The Patient's Charter*. HMSO, London.

DoH (1991c). *Welfare of Children and Young People in Hospital*. London, HMSO.

DoH (1992). *The Health of the Nation*. HMSO, London.

DoH (1993). *Changing Childbirth*. Report of the Expert Maternity Group. HMSO, London.

DoH (1994). *Being Heard*. The Report of a Review Committee on NHS Complaints Procedures. HMSO, London.

DoH (1996). *The Children's Charter*. HMSO, London.

DoH (1997). *The Mental Health Patient's Charter*. HMSO, London.

Downie, R.S. (1996). *A Nurse for All Seasons: Skill Mix, Quality and Education*. Ninth Celebrity Lecture to the NBNI. November 1996.

Doyal, L. (1997). Gendering health: men, women and wellbeing. In *Debates and Dilemmas in Promoting Health*, Sidell, M., Jones, L., Katz, J. and Peberdy, A. (eds). The Open University, Milton Keynes.

Dunn, C. (1994). Sensing an improvement: an experimental study to evaluate the use of aromatherapy, massage and periods of rest in an intensive care unit. *Journal of Advanced Nursing*, 21, 34–40.

Elliot, M. and Turrell, A. (1996). Understanding the conflicts of patient empowerment. *Nursing Standard*, 10(45), 43–7.

Flint, C. (1994). Hailing a new philosophy. *Nursing Standard*, 8(20), 19–20.

Fontes, J. and Howland, G. (1995). *Putting Power into Patients' hands: a Guide for Managers*. IHSM, London.

French, K. (1981). Methodological considerations in hospital patient opinion surveys. *International Journal of Nursing Studies*, 18, 7–32.

Gates, B. (1994). *Advocacy: a Nurses' Guide*. Scutari Press, London.

Goffman, E. (1968). *Asylums*. Penguin, Harmondsworth.

Grace, V.M. (1991). The marketing of empowerment and the construction of the health consumer: a critique of health promotion. *International Journal of Health Services*, 21(2), 292–343.

Griffiths, B. (1996). *How Reformed is the NHS: a Survey of CHCs*. ACHCEW, London.

Griffiths, R. (1988). *Community Care: Agenda for Action*. HMSO, London.

Hayward, J. (1975). *Information: Prescription Against Pain*. RCN, London.

Hegvary, S.T. (1982). *The Change to Primary Nursing*. CV Mosby, London.

Hewison, A. (1995). Nurses' power in interactions with patients. *Journal of Advanced Nursing*, 21(1), 75–82.

Hewson, B. (1997). Whose body is it anyway? *Nursing Standard*, 11(35), 18.

HMSO (1983). *The Mental Health Act*. HMSO, London.

HMSO (1984). *The Mental Health Amendment Act*. HMSO, London.

HMSO (1989). *Children Act 1989*. HMSO, London.

HMSO (1990a). *NHS and Community Care Act 1990*. HMSO, London.

HMSO (1990b). *Access to Health Records Act 1990*. HMSO, London.

House of Commons Select Committee (1992). *Second Report on the Maternity Services* (Winterton Report). HMSO, London.

Kershaw, B. and Salvage, J. (eds) (1986). *Models for Nursing*. John Wiley & Sons, Chichester.

Laing, W. (1996). The independent sector. In *NAHAT 1996/1997 NHS Handbook*. JMH Publishing, London.

Lowes, L. (1996). Paediatric nursing and children's autonomy. *Journal of Clinical Nursing*, 5, 367–72.

McColl, E., Thomas, L. and Bond, S. (1996). A study to determine patient satisfaction with nursing care. *Nursing Standard*, 10(52), 34–8.

McIver, S. and Martin, G. (1996). Unchartered territory. *Health Service Journal*, 106(5521), 25–6.

Ministry of Health (1959). *The Welfare of Children in Hospital* (The Platt Report). HMSO, London.

Murray, R. and Zentner, J. (1989). *Nursing Concepts for Health Promotion*. Prentice-Hall, Hemel Hempstead.

Musker, M. and Byrne, M. (1997). Applying empowerment in mental health practice. *Nursing Standard*, 11(31), 45–7.

NAHAT (1993). *Complaints Do Matter*. Birmingham, NAHAT.

National Consumer Council. (1983). *Patients' Rights: a Guide for NHS Patients and Doctors*. NCC, London.

Neuberger, J. (1990). A consumer's view. In *NHS Reforms: Whatever Happened to Consumer Choice?*, Green, D. (ed.). Institute of Economic Affairs Health and Welfare Unit, London.

NHSE (1994). *Towards a Primary Care-led NHS*. NHSE, Leeds.

NHSE (1995). *Progress with Patient Focused Care in the UK*. Executive Summary. NHSE, Leeds.

NHSME (1993). *Patient Empowerment*. NHSME, Leeds.

Northern Ireland Office (1996). *The Regional Strategy: 1997–2002*. Northern Ireland Office, Belfast.

O'Donnel, M. (1993). How to enable staff to empower patients. *Nursing Standard*, 8(12), 38–9.

Parsons, T. (1951). *The Social System*. Routledge and Kegan Paul, London.

Paton, C. (1992). *Competition and Planning in the NHS. The Danger of Unplanned Markets*. Chapman & Hall, London.

Pearson, A. (1989). Therapeutic nursing – transforming models and theories into action. In *Theories and Models of Nursing*, Akinsanya, J. (ed.). Churchill Livingstone, Edinburgh.

Royal College of Nursing (1994). *Patient Focused Care. Advice Note*. RCN, London.

Royal Commission on the National Health Service (1979). *The Merrison Report*. Cmnd 7615. HMSO, London.

Saunders, P. (1995). Encouraging patients to take part in their own care. *Nursing Times*, 91(9), 42–3.

Schober, J.E. and Hinchliff, S.M. (1995). *Towards Advanced Nursing Practice*. Arnold, London.

Scottish Office (1992). *Scotland's Health: a Challenge to Us All*. Scottish Office, Edinburgh.

Sharma, U. (1991). Using 'alternative' medicine. *Health Visitor*, 64(2), 50–1.

Smail, S. (1990). Health promotion and the new GP contract. *Practice Nurse*, 2(9), 391–2.

Stevenson, C.J. (1994). The psychological effects of aromatherapy foot massage following cardiac surgery. *Complementary Therapies in Medicine*, 2, 27–35.

Stevenson, C.J. (1997). Complementary therapies and their role in nursing care. *Nursing Standard*, 11(24), 49–53.

Taylor, J. and Muller, D. (1995). *Nursing Adolescents: Research and Psychological Perspectives*. Blackwell Science, Oxford.

Teasdale, K. (1987). Partnership with patients. *Professional Nurse*, 2(12), 17–19.

Trevelyan, J. (1995). The new fringe? *Nursing Times*, 91(11), 26–8.

Too, S-K. (1996). Do birthplans empower women? A study of their views. *Nursing Standard*, 10(31), 33–7.

UKCC (1992). *The Code of Professional Conduct*. UKCC, London.

UKCC (1996). *Guidelines for Professional Practice*. UKCC, London.

Vaughan, B. and Taylor, K. (1988). Homeward bound. *Nursing Times*, 84(15), 28–31.

Wade, S. (1995). Partnership in care: a critical review. *Nursing Standard*, 9(48), 29–32.

Wallace, L., Wingett, C., Joshi, M.M. and Spellman, D. (1985). Heart to heart. *Nursing Times*, 81, 45–7.

Walsh, M. (1993). Patients' views of their experience. *Nursing Standard*, 7(27), 30–32.

Waterworth, S. and Luker, K. (1990). Reluctant collaborators: do patients want to be involved in decisions concerning care? *Journal of Advanced Nursing*, 15, 971–6.

Welsh Office (1994). *Caring for the Future*. Welsh Office, Cardiff.

Wilson-Barnett, J. (1979). *Stress in Hospital*. Churchill Livingstone, Edinburgh.

Wilson-Barnett, J. (1983). *Patient Teaching*. Churchill Livingstone, Edinburgh.

Woodrow, P. (1996). Exploring confidentiality in nursing practice. *Nursing Standard*, 10(32), 38–42.

WHO (1978). *Report of the International Conference on Primary Care, Alma-Ata USSR*. WHO, Geneva.

WHO Regional Office for Europe (1985). *Targets for Health for All*, WHO, Copenhagen.

Wright, S.G. (1994). *My Patient, My Nurse: the Practice of Primary Nursing*, 2nd edn. Scutari Press, Harrow.

FURTHER READING

Dimond, B. (1995). *Legal Aspects of Nursing*, 2nd edn. Prentice Hall International, Hemel Hempstead.

This is a good overall guide to many of the concepts surrounding patients' legal rights and includes useful practical examples.

The Health Service Commissioners Annual Report. HMSO, London.

This yearly report looks at cases investigated by the health service ombudsman and provides interesting examples of the type of complaints patients make about the health care they received or did not receive.

Paton, C. (1992). *Competition and Planning in the NHS. The Danger of Unplanned Markets*. Chapman & Hall, London.

This book provides an excellent analysis of the effects of the NHS reforms on patients in both community and hospital settings.

Wright, S.G. (1994). *My Patient, My Nurse: the Practice of Primary Nursing*, 2nd edn. Scutari Press, Harrow.

This book explores the changes in the relationship between nurses and patients which have allowed patients to become equal partners in their care.

CHAPTER TEN

MANAGING HEALTH CARE DELIVERY

Tom Keighley

- Introduction
- The current shape of health services
- Leadership of health services
- The interface between managing care and managing an organisation
- The future of management in health care

This chapter addresses four areas of interest and concern to many nurses in management and leadership positions. The first is the current shape of the health service. Consideration of this extends to the role the independent sector now has, the funding of services and some of the demand issues. The next section addresses leadership styles, their development and how to resource leadership. The third section considers some of the difficult issues that arise at the interface between managing care delivery and managing an organisation. The chapter closes with a more speculative section on the likely future of leadership in health services.

INTRODUCTION

To write about management is to be presented with a choice. Either, the tasks involved and the knowledge and skills required can be described, or, on the assumption that these have already been written about in great detail, one can go on to consider management as a practitioner and as a recipient. To reflect on the process of management in health services it is necessary to appreciate:

- The current shape of those services
- The evolving patterns and styles of management and leadership
- The interface between managing care and managing an organisation
- The possible future scenarios for health care management.

To do this effectively, it is necessary to understand the people involved in these processes, in particular the importance of working with a shared set of beliefs and values, and the relationship between the development of good interpersonal skills and success in achieving change. This chapter addresses these issues primarily from the perspective of the National Health Service but with a clear understanding of the increasing importance of the interface with the independent health care and social care sectors.

THE CURRENT SHAPE OF HEALTH SERVICES

BACKGROUND

This section explains the origins of ths structure and describes the issues that arise as it operates. The shape of the National Health Service (NHS) has taken many hundreds of years to emerge. Central to it is the hospital service, known as the secondary and, in specialist cases, tertiary care provision. The first point of contact with the National Health Service for most people, however, is through the general practitioner (GP) services which offer direct care to patients or can refer them on to hospital-based services. This is known as primary care. The third component of the stucture is made up of the district health authorities. They are responsible for determining the health needs of their community and ensuring that hospital and other community services can meet those needs.

The shape of health services is ever changing. The reasons for change vary continually. Sometimes it is the political ideologies of a particular government that leads to change. In the UK, this is reflected in the various types of legislation determining the nature and extent of health care delivery. Such legislation has been enacted for 400 years, more if local bye-laws are included. On other occasions the motivation is financial. If, for instance, the cost of particular procedures cannot be afforded, those responsible for funding health care reshape service delivery so that they can meet their economic obligations. The USA and some European countries are currently demonstrating this approach. A third motivation for change is dissatisfaction with the quality of health care delivery. Dingwall *et al.* (1988) point to this being a stimulus with a strong historical basis. It was one of the principal reasons for the reform of nursing being actively debated in the pre-Nightingale era. Ironically, it was the need to improve the quality of service delivery and the need to create clear leadership in the NHS, underlined by a reference to Miss Nightingale, that Sir Roy Griffiths (DHSS, 1983) used to legitimate the reforms that his health service review launched. A further major stimulus for change is the cumulative effect of constant experimentation and accumulated wisdom among the many varied health care professionals. This produces an internal imperative for change, driven primarily by a wish to provide ever better care for individual patients and clients.

The health services have a tri-form shape that has only truly emerged since 1985. Although local authorities have long had a responsibility to provide services for elderly people and those in financially straitened circumstances, their remit has extended markedly to include lead responsibility for children, those with mental health problems, and with learning disabilities. In conjunction with this, there has been a most remarkable expansion in the independent health care sector. This has been most marked in the nursing home sector and, currently, approximately a quarter of all nurses in the UK now work outside the NHS. A relationship exists between the expansion of local authority responsibility and the development of the independent sector. The *National Health Service and Community Care Act* (HMSO, 1990) confirmed the responsibilities of local authorities for the care groups identified earlier, based on a full assessment of client need and with the expectation that the independent sector would play a key role in helping to fulfil those obligations. Legislation to change the taxation requirements and the management of personal savings has been enacted to facilitate this.

This distribution of responsibility is an important place to start a consideration of the shape of health care services. It marks the end of an era when the greatest concern had been the closure of large institutions. It signals a political wish to see care provided as locally as possible. This was not without difficulties as it represented not just a shift of many traditional responsibilities from the NHS to other agencies, but a major disruption of the expectations of many people, either about the care that would be available or the careers that might be pursued in the health care professions. Added to this, it has exposed many of the general public to the challenge of living alongside those with a mental illness or a learning disability, perhaps for the first time. The reintegration of people with such problems back into the community reversed the received wisdom of nearly two centuries of health care provision. It is no wonder that the process is not expected to be concluded until at least 2002 or perhaps later, if the problems in generating the finance for the changes persist.

Alongside this on-going process, a major reform of NHS provision has occurred. Announced in 1989 (Secretaries of State for Health, 1989), it introduced three new structures and processes to the NHS:

- A purchasing responsibility for district health authorities
- Hospital and community services reconfigured as providers of health care, to be known as 'Trusts'
- General practitioner services to have a combined purchasing and providing function under the heading of fundholding.

This structure gave new responsibilities to organisations constructed for other purposes. Though not planned for, it meant that there were major cultural and procedural changes to be addressed. The principal challenge faced by all these new organisations was to tie activity to cost. In other words, to relate the delivery of care to the cost of delivering it. While the mechanics of this were emerging in the 1980s, the change in philosophy it represented was enormous. If management of health services is to be understood, each of these new structures needs to be considered both individually and in relation to each other.

DISTRICT HEALTH AUTHORITIES

District health authorities were created to introduce consensus management into the NHS, where all members of the management team considered themselves as equals. Related structures but with slightly different titles and remits were introduced in Scotland, Wales and Northern Ireland. In its time, this was a significant step forward and led to the achievement of a greater degree of ownership of the leadership of health services. It was also the appropriate structure to enable disparate groups of hospitals to be drawn together and resources rationalised, to achieve a more equal spread of those resources across the UK. In the late 1970s, the area health authority tier was abolished and district health authorities inherited many of their functions, in particular, the interface with local authorities.

The change that these organisations faced in the early 1990s was to transform themselves from the direct management of units into structures that could determine the health needs of their local populations and convert that information into contracts of service that could be delivered by the local Trusts. The extent of this change should not be underestimated as the underpinning information to do this was not available, nor were the systems to collect or manage it. To add to the difficulty, the district health authorities were the bodies charged with supporting the units they managed as they made the transition into Trusts. This complex mix of agendas begins to explain why it has taken so long for purchasing to become established in the NHS. It has also generated a completely new debate about the nature and degree of health care rationing that exists in the NHS. This is a debate that will continue ever more rigorously into the future. The concomitant strategies for developing *The Health of the Nation* (DoH, 1991a), and primary care (NHSE, 1994), all point to a political expectation that people will take an increasing responsibility for their own health and health care provision.

This shows a significant change in the way that health services will be provided. Even more importantly, it is a new concept for many people to come to terms with. The notion of cradle to grave health care has been taken by many to mean that one can assume a comprehensive provision of services to meet all needs. So, for example, many elderly people have made no particular provision to meet the costs of their continuing care as they become more dependent. They are, therefore, often outraged that their life-savings are being consumed by the cost of nursing home care when they thought that this would be provided by the NHS. The cost pressures on delivering health care have meant that the funders of health care have had to get people to re-visit that assumption. One way of doing this is to ask people to look at their lifestyles and do those things that will extend the periods that they will enjoy good health. Taking personal responsibility for yourself, either through disease prevention or paying for a proportion of health care services, is a way of responding to the challenges of the future. Most importantly, it requires individuals to be well informed about health and its maintenance, as well as being realistic about how the costs involved can be met.

TRUSTS

Trusts began to emerge from 1991 onwards. These were in three forms:

- Hospital-based services
- Various combinations of community health care services, most often based around mental health and/or learning disability services
- Combinations of the first two, known as integrated Trusts.

The purpose of a Trust was to offer a range of health services that district health authorities or GP fundholders could purchase. Their agendas, therefore, were to develop the range of services on offer and to maximise the number of contracts for which they could compete. This language itself represented such a cultural change that many people felt alienated and marginalised in an organisation that they had entered with a spirit of public, rather than commercial, service. Over time, the smaller, and mainly community-based, Trusts have amalgamated, as responsibility for the care of their clients has been transferred to local authorities, and with it the money. The second major outcome has been the realisation that there is not the need for the number of tertiary care centres that have developed in the larger cities. Most large conurbations are now instigating reviews of the use and distribution of hospital-based services with a view both to reducing the number of beds committed to such work and to achieving a better use of resources. Integrated Trusts, which initially were seen as being a weak option, have emerged as strong players in the system because of the range and flexibility that they represent.

GENERAL PRACTICE

General practice now exists in two forms. The original form emerged with the introduction of the NHS. It consists of doctors working singly or in groups, as independently employed practitioners, fulfilling a contract of service. This contract is now managed through the district health authority. Each practice is a separate and independent business. The purpose of such practices is to offer a full range of primary care services within the constraints of the contract set by the district health authority. Just over half of the GPs in the UK operate in this manner though the proportions vary significantly around the UK. By contrast, GP fundholding is a structural option for all but the smallest of general practices. It allows the GP to take on increasing amounts of service provision and purchasing for the community that they serve. They have, therefore, a dual role, undertaken by separate organisations in the rest of the NHS. They are in the very interesting position of being able to:

- Make their own health needs assessment on behalf of their patients
- Employ a wider range of people to work through their practices
- Negotiate directly with health service providers anywhere to deliver services to their patients
- Develop medical and surgical services to be delivered through their own practices.

This menu of options has only slowly developed but in some parts of the UK it has progressed to such a point that the amalgamation of district health authorities is now being considered, as GP fundholders expand their capabilities. During the implementation of GP fundholding it became apparent that there was the opportunity to unite the two organisations that worked with GPs. In consequence, the family health service authorities, which managed the 'pay and rations' of GPs, were integrated with the district health authorities. This would not have been possible without the increasing independence that GP fundholding achieved. While the move to GP fundholding has not been compulsory, the professional, managerial and financial attractions have meant that it has been widely implemented.

FUNDING HEALTH CARE

These massive changes have inevitably led to health care being a constant on the political agenda. The funding of health care is a government decision. Quarterly reports are generated in the NHS through the year to indicate levels of activity and spending. This information is available to the Chancellor of the Exchequer, when he stands up in the House of Commons to announce the budget for the following year. Health care managers listen carefully to the debate on the budget in the days following the speech, to get the first indications of the sums of money that will be available to them the following year. By April 1 the following year, not only have the district health authorities and GP fundholders received their allocations, the bulk of the contracts have been agreed with Trusts. This is an on-going process. It runs in parallel with the planning and spending rounds of the local authorities and the rest of the public sector. This decision-making process is open to public scrutiny through the parliamentary procedures of question and debate, through the work of such public watchdogs as community health councils and through the public meetings that district health authorities and Trusts run.

The debate about the level of funding for the delivery of health care is a worldwide one. In particular, the developed countries in membership of Organisation for Economic Co-operation and Development (OECD) are all trying to address the challenge of ever-increasing demand for health care and its increasing cost, as set against the availability of funds to pay for it. This is true of all countries, irrespective of the payment system that they use. The underlying challenge is that the combination of increased ability to treat illness along with increased availability of information about treatment, both of which increase public expectation of treatment, are out of step with the money and people to deliver that care and treatment.

Figure 10.1 demonstrates a gradually falling population as fertility rates fall in the OECD countries (EUROSTAT, 1988; OECD, 1988; Nitjkamp *et al.*, 1991). The consequence of this is that not only does the amount of tax available to the Exchequer for the funding of health care and other public sector work fall, but the number of people in the population available to work in humanly intensive services such as health care also diminishes. The rising line shows the increasing lifespan that people will experience over the next half century. This ultimately increases the demand for health care and raises serious questions about the current health care priorities. It points to an increased financial burden being placed on the working population and suggests that it will be necessary in the UK to follow the path of other European countries and put back the age at which pensions and other state support for elderly people becomes available. It is fair to conclude, therefore,

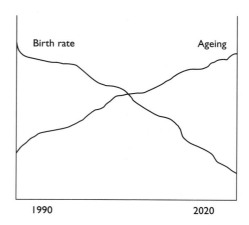

Figure 10.1: Figurative representation of OECD (1988) and EUROSTAT (1988) population data

that the future shape of health care services will continue to change as much as they ever have.

Key Points

This section addresses the overall shape of health care services. It identifies the responsibilities of:

- Local authorities
- The independent sector
- The National Health Service

in the political decision-making framework within which they operate, and places them, briefly, in an international context.

LEADERSHIP OF HEALTH SERVICES

The reforming of health services has led to an unprecedented interest in the nature of such leadership, how it is developed and how it is resourced. This section will review this and, in particular, reflect on:

- Approaches to *quality* in the health services
- the use of *care management systems*
- health service *informatics*.

The overall focus is on practical aspects of leadership.

COMPONENTS OF LEADERSHIP

The challenge facing health service managers was described by Marr (1997) as the need to shift from one end of the leadership style continuum to the other. It requires managers and leaders to come to terms with previously having been developed and promoted through the health service based on their ability to 'control and command', when the new health services require people whose focus is enablement and development of staff. This is a fundamental shift in both thinking and practice. It challenges traditional thinking about hierarchies and chains of command. It requires a transparency of decision making and an ability to relate to staff which has often been advised against in the past. It generates a need to rethink the principles of management. Since the early 1980s a number of authors have been suggesting that management is a separate function from leadership. Yukl (1994), amongst others, suggests that leadership and management are integrated functions. The debate may well prove to be sterile, and whatever the outcome, the challenge is to find ways that enable change to occur. The literature on leadership is more focused in this direction and it is a helpful place to start.

So much of leadership rests on understanding the relationship between:

- Authority
- Accountability
- Responsibility.

These three features have to be considered in all decision-making situations and be agreed, if leadership is to be effective. It is necessary to consider each of these individually.

Authority

Authority is that which legitimates the exercise of power. This is often difficult to understand. People replace a consideration of authority with discussion about qualifications or previous experience or even tradition. In a democratic society, authority is tied to the electoral process, no matter how tenuously. In the NHS it is exercised and delegated in the process of appointing the chairs and non-executive members of the management boards. They have responsibility to appoint the executive members of the board and to hold public meetings. The

chief executives have also been given 'Accountable Officer' status in parliamentary terms which means that they and their officers can be summoned to appear before the committees of the Houses of Parliament to give an account of themselves. This is a major change and underlines the link between the NHS and the political, democratic process of delegating authority.

This form of legitimacy is supported by a framework of civil and criminal law which sets expectations about corporate and personal behaviour in organisations as well as reinforcing the duty to do no avoidable harm. Failure to abide by this legal framework results in court procedures being instigated for reasons as varied as neglect of patients through to embezzlement. In addition to these frameworks, most of the professions involved in health care have codes of professional conduct in order to:

- Make clear to the individual professionals what standards they should adhere to
- Enable members of the public to have unsafe practitioners removed from the registers that allow them to practise.

This provides a comprehensive structure to ensure that the authority delegated to health care professionals and organisations is exercised appropriately.

With this overarching structure in place, it is possible to consider the more routine delegation of authority. One of the problems that occurs in organisations that are going through change is that the exercise of authority becomes obscured. It is by no means unusual to hear people saying nowadays that they do not know who is in charge. The key thing is to be aware of how, and to what extent, authority is being delegated. It is the failure to be clear about this which leads to jobs not being done and people feeling that they are not valued in their roles. Being absolutely clear about the extent of authority being delegated, its duration and in what context it can be exercised, enables people to determine the degree of power it is legitimate for them to use and therefore how they can undertake their role.

Accountability

Aligned to this is the need to be clear about how accountability is to be demonstrated. If, when authority is delegated, it is unclear how individuals are going to be held accountable, they will be unable to determine how they are to be supervised, to what standards they should work and within what timetables they should operate. Accountability can be exercised in a number of different ways. It can take a very harsh form in, a rigid hierarchical system, in which information and commands move in strict lines according to status. This is usually associated with punitive discipline when errors occur and very little creativity among the workforce. By contrast, an increasing number of health service organisations are adopting different forms of matrix management structures in which roles and leadership positions change according to the needs of the organisation. Primary nursing is an example of this in the clinical area. A number of different leadership/management structures exist in organisations and in clinical practice. At one end of the continuum is the classic 'command and control' and, at the other, what looks much more like a project management structure with people coming together to undertake work according to ability and aptitude rather than status. In all of these it is essential to be clear about the degree of delegated authority and the processes by which accountability will be exacted.

Responsibility

To complete this management trinity it is important to consider the nature of responsibility. It takes two major forms, responsibility for self and responsibility for others. In health care services, responsibility for self is often captured in a professional practice code (UKCC, 1992a). These set out the expectations of a profession concerning the sort of behaviour a qualified member of that profession can be expected to exhibit. Wilful failure to adhere to these responsibilities usually results in that profession taking action to exclude the individual from the right to practice. This provides protection for the public and enables a profession to maintain, and continuously improve, standards of professional practice. Increasingly, such codes are associated with minimum criteria for the updating of practice and re-registration for continuing practice. This requires individuals to demonstrate the duration and level of work undertaken to maintain and improve their standard of practice. This can appear to be quite a rigid approach, but regulatory bodies have demonstrated how this can provide a flexible framework for future development in a profession (UKCC, 1992b, 1997). Added to this are the duties of responsible citizenship within the legal and moral framework of the community. Finally, there is the legitimate expectation that, as a health care worker, one will strive to maintain one's health and, when appropriate, keep an employer informed about any significant health problem that might interfere with one's role or function.

Responsibility for others is often a more complex issue. It varies according to position, degrees of authority delegated and the nature of accountability to be exercised. It includes concern for the safety of all in the shared work environment, the need to be explicit with all colleagues about the authority and accountability issues as they affect both yourself and others, and to work only within your levels of knowledge and ability. That final point is an important issue as professionals from all fields can come under pressure to provide service in areas in which they are not adequately prepared. This can occur because of pressure of work and because individual clients have a particular relationship with certain practitioners, and seek help from someone they know and trust rather than a more appropriately prepared person. Being open about such limitations is not a sign of weakness, rather it is a key indicator of mature and caring practice.

In being responsible for others, it is essential to distinguish between the two types of management described previously. Supportive and enabling management ensures equitable and work-related opportunities for development. Paternalistic approaches, using command and control techniques, are often personally intrusive and, most importantly, stifle creativity. It is a very difficult balance to achieve, not least because modern work practices obscure some of the traditional boundaries between employer and employee, or between boss and subordinate. This world of obscured work relationships, as our predecessors would have seen it, is perfectly manageable if there is clarity about authority, accountability and responsibility.

Interpersonal skills

To enable effective and efficient management and leadership, developing good interpersonal skills is essential. Without such skills inappropriate levels of dependency occur, which can act to diminish the ability of individuals and teams to work together (Morton-Cooper, 1997). For many people this is the *art* of management in contrast to the *science* of managing budgets or planning strategy. Acquiring such skills is often what makes management, and leadership roles where they are different, survivable for the individual concerned.

One of the most important of all interpersonal skills is the ability to communicate. This is not simply a facility with words. Much, otherwise good, communication fails to achieve its impact because the fundamentals of effective relating have not been addressed (Watson, 1994; Yukl, 1994). This requires, above all else, a clear understanding of one's own nature and a preparedness to address one's own attitudes, behaviours and knowledge levels about particular issues. This introspection is a critical component of much advocated processes like reflective practice. It is a good example of how good clinical practice is excellent preparation for, and a continuation of, management and leadership in health care. Achieving such a level of self-awareness facilitates all the other components of good communication:

- Clarity of message
- Directness of delivery
- Appropriateness of timing
- Suitability of the environment.

All these features have to be judged according to circumstances, but all the preparation in the world is undermined if the manager/leader has not prepared him/herself. Difficult to define terms like credibility or trustworthiness in managers are used to explain why messages are not comprehended or believed. This always points to lack of personal preparation in management, a deficit which a number of management development programmes are now trying to address. The acquisition of a deep understanding of how to use one's interpersonal skills, and in particular how to use the skills of communication, provides the proper base for the fulfilling of one's responsibilities. In describing the tri-form nature of leadership and management as authority, accountability and responsibility, it should have become very clear that the 'glue' that holds them together is the development and exercise of interpersonal skills. There is no magic in leadership or management,

just the very hard work of constantly clarifying the relevant components of authority, accountability and responsibility and acquiring the interpersonal skills to fulfil them.

Values clarification

A process which can clarify these issues was developed by the RCN Research Society in 1985. It has been used by many organisations since (Figure 10.2).

It provides a framework which enables organisations and individuals to be clear about the six key features of any organisation.

- Stage 1 is to get agreement on the shared beliefs in the organisation. This is important because it is an amalgam of personal philosophies, sociological expectations and psychological frameworks which reflect the mass of beliefs and values that a workforce will contain. The shared set of beliefs is known as an ideology.
- Stage 2 is the identification of key concepts central to determining the purpose of the organisation. This is consciously drawn from Stage 1. For example, if a nursing workforce were to go through this process, concepts like society, person-hood, health or illness might be included, having emerged as important components of the ideology.
- Stage 3 is the most challenging part of the process because value statements about each of the key concepts have to be agreed. These statements must be consciously arrived at, shared by all involved and be sufficiently explicit to gain immediate understanding. These first three stages are central to the successful leadership of the organisation because they clarify the purpose of the organisation and enable the contribution of individual members of the workforce to be elucidated.
- Stage 4 combines the theory and the applied. Using the value statements about each of the key concepts, a framework is determined which relates each of the key concepts into a model which explains their relationships. From this can be deduced the roles and functions required to ensure the delivery of service within the agreed model. This stage, in particular, is heavily influenced by pressures from outside the organisation. These include the financing of the service, the behaviour of the

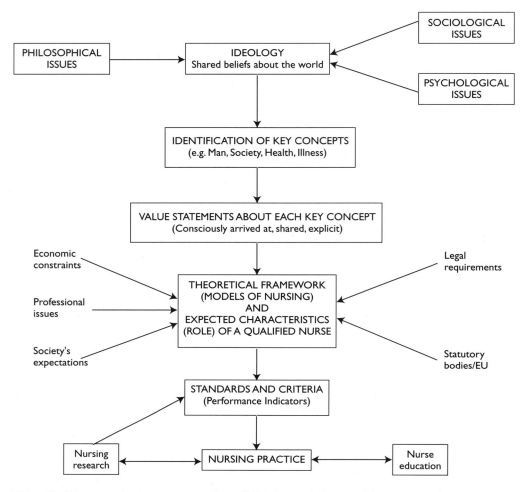

Figure 10.2: Clarifying organisational purpose (from RCN Research Society, Submission to the Judge Commission 1984. Reproduced with permission)

relevant professions, developments in social expectation about the service, new legal requirements or changes in the standards set by regulatory bodies in the UK or European Union.

- Stage 5 is the agreement of standards of, and criteria for, the delivery of care. This is where the effective delegation of authority, which is part of the role determination process, is aligned with the accountability and responsibility processes to enable performance indicators to be determined.
- Stage 6 is the organisation determining a consensus about the work that it does. With a nursing workforce, this is the point at which it can describe what it means by nursing practice. To do this it needs to draw actively on nursing

research and the processes available to educate nurses.

This framework can be used to determine new ways of working and as a tool for investigating or challenging an organisation. For someone new to health care work it provides a series of questions which, if used in this related manner, can offer an explanation of the organisation in which he/she finds him/herself. For colleagues attempting to give an organisation a new direction, or wishing to review the direction they have been pursuing, it offers a framework which can operate cyclically, to give new impetus and direction at crucial times in an organisation's life. This explanation of a particular value's clarification process underlines the centrality of communication in managing and leading an organisation. It also demonstrates that the techniques of good management are often generic.

QUALITY

This is equally true of most approaches to organisational quality initiatives. Much that has been attempted in the NHS has been developed in other management and leadership arenas previously. The government White Paper, *A Service With Ambitions* (Secretary of State for Health, 1996) divided the NHS approaches into two areas:

- Involving users and carers
- Clinical effectiveness and outcomes.

This division of approaches reflects the twin foci of most organisations when considering the quality of their work, responsiveness to customers and product improvement.

Users and carers

Involving users and carers can itself be divided into three areas of work, which are:

- User feedback
- Data collection
- Service planning.

Seeking feedback from users of the health services has developed very significantly in the last decade (Honigsbaum *et al.*, 1997). In the mid-1980s, before the launch of the first quality initiatives, the only feedback from patients was through flowers and cards to clinical staff or through complaints. These usually went to the community health council or occasionally, if to do with medical practice, to the former regional health authorities. Since then, thinking about this has developed in two ways. The first has been to establish systems which elicit systematic feedback from patients about the experience of receiving health care. This was encouraged by the publication of *The Patient's Charter* (DoH, 1991b). This also strengthened the processes that were in place for people to respond directly to organisations about their concerns following treatment.

The second component was to establish systems to involve patients and carers in thinking about current service delivery and how it might be changed in the future. This has taken two forms. Some services have established various types of user groups, which vary in degree of influence from occasional meetings to discuss items selected by the local service managers, through to fully fledged consultative machinery where all management decisions are considered by a user and carer panel before they are placed on a management agenda. This degree of variation demonstrates the extent of the difference it is possible to achieve in involving people in the delivery of local services. The potential that can arise from the fuller involvement of carers and users is great. The information elicited should help in the delivery of current priorities and assist in the determination of future priorities. There should also be a relationship between the work of such groups and both the organisational and clinical audit programmes. The audit reports and the associated discussions help to systematise the work of such groups and integrate their work into the organisation.

Clinical effectiveness and health outcomes

The determination of standards of clinical effectiveness and health outcomes is the reverse of the same quality coin (Unwin *et al.*, 1997). It complements the appropriate involvement of users and carers. The national programme to achieve agreement on health care outcomes has been running throughout the 1990s. The conditions reviewed are dealt with in a comprehensive and scientifically rigorous manner. However, the reports have yet to be vigorously acted upon by the NHS. One barrier has been that the determination of the care outcomes is based mainly on hospital care and excludes complex cases, for example, those conditions that cover a number of medical specialisms. The outcomes measured are, therefore, focused on length of admission or resources consumed. As the bulk of care is delivered in the primary care setting, where a complex mix of conditions is often the norm, an alternative approach might be needed. The future might see the outcomes focus shifting to days lost at school for the child with asthma or the person with Parkinson's disease not reporting problems with their bowels. This would be a good example of how the patient's perspective might be made to fit with the health care professionals' expectations about care delivery.

Current thinking would suggest the need for a small number of national outcomes or indicators developed and agreed by users and the professions and linked to national priorities. These would be added to, and given local meaning through, the contracts set by district health authorities. Such a process could be used to legitimise the standard of service delivery on the agreed outcomes being used as a way of measuring performance. It is acknowledged that achieving this sort of change in the quality of the service requires a different approach to leadership from that which has been the norm in the NHS in the last 10 years (Weightman, 1996; Iles, 1997). Equally, unlike 10 years ago, resources are now available to enable it. They include King's Fund Organisational Audit, ISO 9000, Investors in People, Health Services Accreditation, as well as a wide range of local systems. While rarely being the answer themselves, the attempt to implement them often achieves the degree of culture change required to enable real change in the quality of care to emerge.

Quality remains one of the most nebulous notions in health care. The gap between the client's and the provider's views can seem unbridgeable. Nursing, at least since the time of Nightingale, has taken an active interest in the development of thinking about quality. From a leadership perspective, the debate on quality is important from a number of different perspectives. The first has already been touched on, and that is the relationship between what the client wants and needs from his or her health care experience and how the organisation is led to achieve that. Working with systems that inform the leadership of the organisation what its clients want enables standards of service to be set. In the postwar period in the USA and Canada, a significant volume of research into quality of care occurred. Donabedian (1969) and Phaneuf (1972) did ground-breaking work on nursing audit and the evaluation of nursing care, respectively. In 1971, in the USA, the Joint Commission on Accreditation of Hospitals was established, when it was recognised that audit review alone could not maintain standards of care. This led to a great deal of work on standard-setting systems.

Standards of care

The first modern initiative in this area was the development of the Rush Medicus instrument (Hegyvary and Hausman, 1975). Using the same methodology in the UK, Goldstone and Ball (1984) developed Monitor. The initial version was for use on medical and surgical wards, but versions for mental health, child health, midwifery, and health visiting and caring for older people were subsequently published. In the meantime, the Royal College of Nursing (RCN) had been pursuing its interest in the quality of care, and in 1986, Kitson published a review of the development. The work continued with the creation of the widely used Dynamic Standard Setting System [Dysssy] (RCN, 1990). The significance of the work on standard setting is threefold:

- It reflects the interest of the profession to achieve a degree of uniformity in its practice
- It suggest that patients and employers can expect an equivalence of service given similar conditions applying
- It enables a consistent pricing policy to be created.

All three issues are key to leadership in an organisation because standard setting sets the baseline for discussion about the provision of service. Girvin (1995) stresses that standard setting is not only about achieving agreement about what people do, but is also about enabling people to change in order to do it. This interaction needs to be borne in mind when leading such an initiative.

The development of clinical audit and the use of clinical protocols flows from this. Clinical audit is a multidisciplinary process, described in the 1989 White Paper as:

'The systematic critical analysis of the quality of medical care, including the procedures used for diagnosis and treatment, the use of resources and the resulting outcome and quality of life for the patient.'

(Secretaries of State for Health, 1989)

It is a cyclical process which can be used regularly to review and change processes of care or it can be used as a one-off event to investigate a particular issue. As Sale (1996) points out, it is a complex process requiring clarity of purpose and method. She describes a multi-step process which needs to be followed if useful outcomes are to be achieved. Failure to take such a systematic approach is often the reason why clinical audit cycles fail to be completed.

The development of standard setting and clinical audit has led some organisations to develop clinical protocols. They are usually a combination of elements, including patient tracking systems, anticipated recovery pathways, standard setting and workload measurement. Essentially, organisations try to put them in place to achieve a degree of rationalisation of care across all clients with particular conditions, and to bring a degree of predictability to the associated cost of patient care. It allows clinicians and managers to focus on variations from an expected norm and so facilitates the constant monitoring of care delivery. This has been of interest to the district health authorities who need an ever sharper view about best clinical practice and therefore best spending patterns. Concerns remain about the quasi-legal status of such protocols, especially when someone steps out the agreed protocol because of the individual needs of a patient. However, as Sale (1996) indicates, while the system takes a long time to set up, the principal achievement is that it ensures patients receive greater continuity of care.

Evidence-based care

These developments have been the precursors to the current range of initiatives. They have established frameworks and raised levels of awareness about the need for more systematic approaches to care. This often reflected in the catch phrase 'evidence-based care', i.e. the wish to deliver care that has data to justify it. This is reflective of the wish to continue the move towards determining a rational base for care delivery, something which will consume much time and energy before it is achieved across all aspects of health care delivery.

In considering this a little further, three developments should be noted:

- Pathways of care
- Integrated care management
- Managed care.

It is important to recognise that these are not a hierarchy of development or excellence, rather that different organisations use them either singly or in combination in order to give some degree of assurance to their care delivery. Each of the terms has attracted to itself several slightly different meanings. To demonstrate this, the three headings will be explored in a little detail.

Pathways of care is a title used to include:

- Integrated care pathways
- Anticipated recovery pathways
- Multidisciplinary pathways of care
- Care protocols
- Critical Pathways
- Care Maps® (Johnson, 1997).

Integrated care pathways and multidisciplinary pathways of care share a common focus. They describe care delivery in total rather than separating out the contribution of the doctor, the nurse, the physiotherapist, etc. All health care professionals will be expected to use the one patient record, to report the delivery of care. The benefit to the patient is that a comprehensive record of care is always available and that care is given in a predictable way, determined by the study of many similar and previous cases.

Both of these may well rest on a previous piece of work known as an anticipated recovery pathway. As the title implies, once a diagnosis has been made, within certain degrees of tolerance it is possible to predict, with a high degree of certainty, what the correct course of treatment is and how long it will take to work. This takes much of the myth, mystery and magic out of treatment. As recovery pathways increasingly often indicate the pattern of investigation, the process of diagnosis is also simplified. The predictability of such processes makes it easier to pick up variations from the norm and reduces the likelihood of human error. Care protocols and critical pathways can be as comprehensive as the methods described above. Often, however, they are either unidisciplinary or procedure specific. Their value is that they clarify the actual processes of care being used, get people to come to some agreement about a common approach and then form the basis of audit work to refine what is being achieved. Put crudely, they often clear the ground for the more comprehensive pathway approaches.

The final one on the list is Care Maps®. These are the most comprehensive of approaches which cover the progress of the patient or client, from a multidisciplinary perspective, from the onset of the first sign or symptom through to the achievement of complete recovery, often long after they have left the hospital system. While all the others are used to a certain degree in primary and secondary care settings, this approach offers the best options when attempting to provide seamless care, irrespective of setting.

Achieving clarity of meaning to distinguish between these different approaches is the first and most critical step in developing such pathways. As a tool and an evolving concept, they are an under-researched component of the health service. Their purpose is to:

> 'amalgamate all the anticipated elements of care and treatment of all members of the multi-disciplinary team, for a patient or client of a particular case-type or grouping within an agreed time frame, for the achievement of agreed outcomes. Any deviation from the plan is documented as a 'variance': the analysis of which provides information for the review of current practice.'
>
> (Johnson, 1997, page 16)

This definition captures the essence of pathways and indicates the method of construction and breadth of application. She identifies the benefits as being:

- Improved patient outcomes
- Improved teamwork by care givers
- Improved consistency in care
- Increased patient involvement in care
- Continuous clinical audit
- Clinical and non-clinical resource management
- Continuous standard/guideline monitoring
- Assistance with risk management
- Organisation-wide involvement in a continuous quality improvement process.

Such pathways of care have been developed in a number of acute and non-acute care settings. Integrated care management is often subsumed into any discussion about pathways of care as has already been seen. The important difference is in emphasis. The stress is on multidisciplinary working. Wilson (1992 quoted in Wilson, 1997) defines it as:

> 'a multi-disciplinary process of patient focused care which specifies key events, tests and assessments, occurring in a timely fashion to produce the best prescribed outcomes, within the resources and activities available, for an appropriate episode of care.'
>
> (page 2)

In her subsequent publication, Wilson (1997) places integrated care management in a context of project management, change management and risk assessment. To those new to health care provision it may be difficult to see any difference from a pathways of care approach. The purposes and benefits are very similar. It is a good example of similar approaches being used to slightly different ends in different organisations. Above all, they give organisations the opportunity to develop an approach which is sufficiently different to get the ownership of the staff.

Managed care is a concept which, while not being directly related to pathways of care and integrated care management, completes the picture. It emerged in the late 1980s in the USA, as concerns arose about the cost of health care delivery in disease management began to emerge. It consists of two components:

- Payment for agreed packages of care when patients present with previously agreed conditions
- Agreed approaches to health maintenance by individuals who are part of the scheme.

In the USA, this is usually done through one of the many forms of health insurance available. In the UK, it is reflected in the notion of the managed internal health market (Royce, 1997). The district health authority sets a contract price for so many treatments, to so many patients, at a particular price, and the Trust has to have some certainty that the service can be delivered to a particular standard and within certain predictable costs. The relationship between pathways of care or integrated care management and managed care then becomes obvious. They are the prerequisites for each other.

The interesting thing to note about these developments is that health care professionals put great stress on the need for individualised care and the clinical freedom to make the necessary judgements to meet the individual needs of patients. These three approaches, i.e. pathways of care, integrated care management and managed care, question this autonomy and exercise two fundamental constraints on service delivery, be they publicly or privately funded:

- Cost of service in the light of patient need
- Best practice in centres of excellence are used to set national norms.

This brings a standardisation of care which acts to raise the quality of care while minimising risk and variation in care patterns. The three broad systems generate data in a form which enables judgements to be made about the extent of resource uses on a case-by-case basis, as well as providing a predictive element in the delivery of care. Given that each patient can have his/her own pathway of care laid out once a key point in the investigations has been reached, the role of the health care professional changes from making decisions about the routine, to recognising and responding to variations to the norm. This requires a rather different value set in professional training where the emphasis needs to be on accessing current data on best practice along with information on the management of exceptions to the rule.

For nurses who adopt a notion of holism in their care processes, the implications are clear. In a world driven by the collection of data and the analysis of ever greater data sets, holistic approaches have to be based on interpretation of, and access to, information. While continuing to attempt to meet the physical, psychological, social, emotional and spiritual needs of patients, information, and not just personal assessment and experience, will become the driver. It requires a systematising of the approach to care that can be seen as depersonalising. The added twist in the tail is that as so many more components of health care become information driven, so more patients will gain access to that information. The relationship will become a consultation about shared data rather than care programming determined by the knowledgeable for the ignorant.

INFORMATICS

Informatics in the health service has become the underpinning of these developments in the field of quality. As the technology has developed and with it the facility to use it, so clinical and managerial staff have found a common base from which to discuss service delivery. The Korner Reports of 1982–84 (DHSS, 1982–1984) now seem a distant memory, but they introduced the notion of minimum data sets to the NHS. Those, along with various forms of patient administration systems and finance and staffing management systems, began to provide a structure for the operational manage-

ment information requirements. In 1986, the NHS launched its resource management initiative to improve resource management but also to increase the involvement of clinicians in decision making. Ward, in Morton-Cooper and Bamford (1997), identifies the core information systems to emerge during this period as:

- Patient administration systems
- Case mix management systems
- Clinical information/clinical work stations for medical audit
- Nursing information systems.

Following the publication of *Working For Patients* (Secretaries of State for Health, 1989), there was a need to develop the NHS IT systems. When the strategy was released in 1992 (NHSME, 1992), it had seven elements:

- Hospital information support systems
- Community information systems for providers
- Developing information systems for purchasers
- New NHS patient numbers
- A national thesaurus of coded clinical terms and groupings
- NHS wide networking
- A framework for security and confidentiality.

A novel element in this exercise was to attempt to involve the users of the service. This has not been particularly successful. Overall, however, the NHS has moved forward significantly in its use of information systems. Clinical information systems are still the least satisfactory, often consuming clinicians' time with little feedback to influence their care delivery directly. This continues to be addressed. However, in the fields of personnel, finance, quality management and contract setting, significant progress has been made.

The significance of this for nurses has been the opportunity to become involved in the developments. In particular, nursing-specific systems have been created which have enabled nurses to work with information systems, so enabling them to contribute to the more rigorous thinking about the value of nursing and its place in the health service (Asbridge, 1997). Not only have workload and workforce management systems been developed, but clinically based systems have also evolved. The two major developments, which will have their effect in the next decade, are related. They are the effort to agree nationally and internationally on a set of terms by which nursing practice can be classified, and efforts to get agreement on a framework to enable nursing diagnosis to be recognised and codified. This work will enable a more structured approach to be taken to delivery and evaluation of nursing care.

The implications of this have an impact on the profession, and on the delivery of health care generally. The profession will benefit from having a standardised way of describing and recording its practice. It will lead to clarity about what is and what is not effective. The areas of uncertainty will become clear and be the source of research questions. The subsequent research will add to the quality of nursing care which will be to the patient's benefit. It will strengthen the academic and professional base of nursing practice.

The second set of implications concern the prescribing of care. The adoption of a common nursing language will lead to a rationalising and subsequent systematising of the delivery of nursing care. This will bring nursing care into a position where it will be possible to predict with some accuracy the cost of nursing for patients with particular conditions. It will enable clinical effectiveness and financial efficiency to be assessed simultaneously. Given the wish to develop a fully rational base for nursing care in an era when there is great pressure on resources, this will have its impact on all practising nurses.

Key Points

This section has addressed the changing nature of leadership in the constantly reshaping health services. After describing the relationship between authority, accountability and responsibility, three of the major management tools have been considered:

- Quality systems
- Care management systems
- Health service informatics

all from the perspective of management activity.

THE INTERFACE BETWEEN MANAGING CARE AND MANAGING AN ORGANISATION

This section addresses the nature of clinical management and general or executive styles of management. It includes consideration of career pathways, gender, race and disability issues, as well as how to manage the interface between aspiration and reality when faced with competing, contrasting or conflicting goals.

CLINICAL MANAGEMENT

Clinical management is a term that has emerged since 1974. As part of that reorganisation, doctors and nurses were made members of the district management teams. This meant that clinicians had two management roles:

- Management of the care of patients
- A part in the management of the organisation.

From the late 1980s they took on a third management role:

- Resource management.

This combination of roles has been refined over time. Nurses have, throughout the modern era, played a wide range of roles in organisational management as well as clinical management, but not so with doctors. This lack of interest in this form of management was due to the low regard with which doctors perceived management as a process (Austin and Dopson, 1997). The introduction of the notion of clinical directorates from the early 1990s changed that. It put an emphasis on clinicians (doctors at first, but increasingly nurses) taking responsibility for staff and team management, representation of the directorate at more senior organisational levels, and setting and monitoring standards of service delivery. However, as Fitzgerald (1993) points out, most directors describe their role in change management terms. The increasing contribution that clinical directors are making to negotiating contracts with purchasers confirms this.

The nursing contribution to this development has been twofold:

- Occasionally, and increasingly, as the clinical director, but more regularly as the business manager for the directorate
- Through enhancement of the ward manager role with particular responsibility for advancing clinical practice.

Mares (1996) describes this as care management and describes six core tasks associated with it:

- Deciding the level of assessment
- Assessing need
- Planning care
- Implementing the care plan
- Monitoring
- Reviewing.

This approach helps to distinguish between the contribution to be made to organisational management by nurses and the responsibility to manage themselves and others in the clinical environment.

GENERAL AND EXECUTIVE MANAGEMENT

General and executive management were interchangeable terms in the latter part of the 1980s. During the 1990s a distinction has emerged. General management was introduced into the NHS in 1985 following the Griffiths Report (DHSS, 1983). The intention was to enable the service to move away from a consensus model of governance over to a clearer model of explicit accountability and corporacy. It was an attempt to make the service more businesslike (Ham, 1997). It legitimated the appointment of people with a wide range of managerial experience from outside the NHS. The result was that while the structure of the service did not change, there was a much greater focus on effectiveness, efficiency and variation in service performance.

The executive mode of management emerged with the separation of purchasing and providing in 1989. The creation of boards of non-executive directors, with executive directors directly accountable to them, brought a new sense of purpose to management. While working to objectives had been long established in the NHS, from this point on performance had a financial connotation. In organisational terms, poor performance could result in loss of contracts and with it, loss of associated posts in the organisation. In personal terms, performance was rewarded with enhancements to salary. This approach challenged profoundly the public service ethos that had attracted so many health care professionals into health care. The challenge for senior nurses in Trusts and district health authorities was to continue to operate corporately in these circumstances while still focusing on nursing practice. Asbridge (1997), among others, has pointed to the problem that has emerged of nurses on Trust boards, whose clinical interests and experience do not match that of their equivalent medical colleagues, and who have achieved such elevation because of their general and executive management experience, rather than their ability to lead nursing. This is a challenge for the future. Failure to be professionally competent will undermine the credibility of the Trust nurse position.

It raises question about career pathways for nurses. The traditional career track of staff nurse, sister, senior nurse, nurse director no longer exists. With the passing of this hierarchy has gone the certainty about what constitutes appropriate development. This is compounded by the change in the entry gate to nursing, first to diploma level and increasingly to degree. What is clear is that nursing, as a profession, attracts an enormous range of talent. This is reflected in the range of expert advanced clinical nurses in the profession, the number of nurses in higher education and research, and the number who fill management roles. The difficulty is that the lack of predictability about organisational structure and the traditional UK reticence to invest in staff development (Sisson, 1994) result in uncertainty and lack of motivation to seek development.

Whilst some organisations have attempted to address this and to establish for themselves a reputation as learning organisations (Senge, 1990), the best advice is still that formulated by Kanter (1989). She describes how the more successful organisations use the pressure of change to build in the flexibility to be able to respond to change. Her view is that, even in organisations that are involved in continuous operation, e.g. health services, a project orientation is being introduced. This makes work more measurable and identifies at least notional end-points. To respond to this on an individual basis, Kanter suggests that it is important to maintain one's employability in the widest range of circumstances. This is achieved by constant investment in personal development and is supplemented by a constantly updated portfolio of activity and achievement. It challenges the traditional assumptions about working for one employer for life, and puts the emphasis on skills development and reputation. This is the challenge for nursing, where it is unusual to find such a focus on self, rather than the process for which the individual is responsible.

This raises questions about gender, race and disability in nursing leadership. Nursing is a predominantly female profession and in recent years has become increasingly aware of the inequalities facing women seeking advancement in its own profession (Hutt, 1987) and in the wider health service (DoH, 1992). Burchill and Casey (1996) point out the long history of discrimination and the difficulties arising from trying to tackle it. The disadvantages that nurses experience so often arise from the amount of part-time working they do in their careers, breaks in service for family reasons, lack of flexibility in working hours because of family commitments, as well as straightforward prejudice.

Judi Marshall (1995) describes some of the many difficulties experienced. She recognises that colour and disability simply add to the problem. Despite more than 25 years of legislation in the UK, problems of discrimination remain. Weightman (1996) describes discrimination as occurring at three major points, all associated with the appointment process:

- When short-listing from application forms and CVs
- When testing and interviewing
- When making the final selection.

While proper procedures at this point may keep the process legal, it still permits personal prejudice to have its effect. Employers have a role in ensuring that such prejudice is not exhibited in the workplace.

The positive side of women in management was highlighted by Rosener (1990), who identified women as having an interactive style of management, more suited to transformational management. This is a two-edged sword because there is a danger that women may become associated with jobs that are concerned with caring (Calas and Smircich, 1993), a real trap for nurses in management. Much has been done as a result of the Department of Health (DoH, 1992) strategy to provide women with development opportunities. However, as Marshall (1995) points out, it remains an issue of power, who has it and how it is exercised.

Therefore, the gap between aspiration and reality should be addressed. This gap may occur because of a difference between what an organisation tells its staff and its ability to deliver on that, in which case it has a communication problem. Or it may be due to conflict between the competing/contrasting/conflicting goals of the organisation. Peck (1979) suggests that these are issues of self-management and proposes a fourfold strategy to address them:

- Delaying gratification
- Acceptance of responsibility
- Dedication to reality
- Achieving a balance.

These are the essential components of self-discipline. Iles (1997) points out that these notions were, for centuries, the province of religion. With the decline of theism, they have been increasingly advocated by psychologists as essential to the achievement of mental health. This is especially so when combined with daily reflection on the day's activity and periodic reflection on one's aspirations and the reality of the life to be lived. Together they address the personal side of competing/contrasting/conflicting goals. It also acknowledges the interface between personal goals and organisational expectations. This is likely to be a continuing challenge into the future.

Key Points

This section has addressed a number of the interface issues that arise when managing an organisation. They include:

- Consideration of a number of types of clinical management
- Career pathway issues
- Gender, race and disability
- Competing/contrasting/conflicting goals.

The section concludes with an acknowledgement of the impact that leadership has on people as individuals.

THE FUTURE OF MANAGEMENT IN HEALTH CARE

RESOURCES

The future of health care, and therefore its leadership and management, is all about resources. These are both financial and human. Their availability will depend on political and personal judgements that will be determined by:

- Information systems in the home
- Self-diagnosis and self-treatment in the home
- Changing social expectations about the delivery of health care.

This section will attempt to address these issues and give a sense of the future facing nurses in the next 10–15 years.

The changes in birth rate, life expectancy and their impact on the health care workforce and the ability of the nation to fund health care, were described earlier. This, combined with the increasing cost of health care, as episodes of care become more expensive and an ageing population increases the proportion of society requiring care at any one time, makes it necessary to rethink, fundamentally, what health care is to be delivered, and how. Most worrying of all is the fall in the number of nurses in the workforce (OPCS/HSE, 1995), a trend that is doubly worrying because the number of doctors has risen, indicating significantly increased workloads for nurses. The cyclical nursing workforce shortages indicate the lack of strategic planning that bedevils the health service. It is no consolation to be aware that this problem of lack of resources and lack of strategic planning to address it affects the whole of the developed world (Nitjkamp *et al.*, 1991).

CHOICE

The key to understanding the future of health care is the notion of choice (Honigsbaum *et al.*, 1997). Central to this is the availability of information. Traditionally, access to information has been an issue of control and power. The development of the world wide web and the integration of communication systems means that there is a danger of having almost too much information available. The time is passing when the health care professions can operate on the basis of an otherwise inaccessible knowledge. The development of the Cochrane centres to assess the effectiveness of practice and the work of McMaster University, on the meta-analysis of research findings across the whole of health care, demystifies diagnosis, prescription and treatment. Increasingly, this information will be available in our own homes, and those who wish to make their own decisions about their health care will be equipped to do so.

Honigsbaum and colleagues (1997) have taken their analysis of this across several countries. Much of the work that they report in North America, the Nordic countries, UK and New Zealand is about choices made by health care funders and the interface between available resources and personal choice. Singer (1997) describes different ways in which this is being pursued. Traditionally in the UK, public involvement in decision making has been through representative bodies (e.g. community health councils or specialist interest groups). The more recent development has been through versions of 'health panels' or 'citizen juries' to help formulate a consensus about public expectations (Lenaghan, 1996). However, these are seen as intermediate steps to a fuller system of involvement based on a response by health care professionals to requests for evidence-based care. Once the evidence is in the public domain, as it increasingly is, so the shape and delivery of health care will change.

Combined with this access to information is the increasing availability of self-treatment. This is due almost completely to miniaturisation and simplification of the available technology and modes of therapy delivery. Combined with shortage of resources, this means that people will want to simplify health care delivery and provide as much of their own care as possible. This will result in very different expectations about health care emerging. There will be:

- Increasing demand for evidence-based care
- Higher levels of information available on which individuals will base their health care decisions
- More extensive public debates about the nature of health and illness
- A greater awareness of the ethical issues in health care.

This all suggests greater personal ownership by individuals of their own health care and an increasing wish to control and influence the nature of the environment in which they live.

THE FUTURE OF NURSING LEADERSHIP

The significance of these changes in social expectation for nursing and its leadership is clear. Not only will nursing become better equipped to work with patients in their homes and in hospitals, but they will also develop new working relationships with other health care professionals. There will be significant reprofiling of the workforce which will focus on the essential professions of nursing and medicine. To respond to these challenges, the leadership and management of the profession will need to focus on the agenda described in this chapter to become personally and managerially more competent. The conclusions to draw from this are clear and exciting. The need for nursing will remain and, if anything, expand. The leadership of that nursing workforce will need to be within a development model to respond to all the changes. The individual nurse will need to commit him/herself to life long learning and development, both in his/her professional and private life. The relationship with patients will increasingly be a consultative one rather than interventionist in nature. Finally, among the many other potential outcomes, there will be the opportunity to truly internationalise care delivery. The increasing availabilty of information will enable us to be as knowledgeable as the best practitioners, anywhere in the world. For the leader therefore, it will be a period of facilitation, teaching and creativity as direction and purpose are determined and services delivered. Is there any wonder that so many nurses aspire to lead these services, at every level?

Key Points

This section has provided some well-founded speculation about the future of leadership and management in the health services. It has included reviewing the likely impact of:

- Demographic changes
- Patient/consumer choice
- New roles and relationships.

It concludes in the very firm belief that leadership opportunities will be even greater in the future than they are now.

Summary

This chapter has provided an initial introduction to management and leadership in the UK health services in the late 1990s. It describes the process of change that has led to the current profile of services. The impact of these changes on the nature of leadership is described and the tools that have emerged to underpin it are addressed. Some of the complex interface issues are touched upon and, finally, some thoughts about the future of management and leadership are provided. The chapter is written from the perspective of the human nature of managers and leaders and in the clear recognition that as health services will always change, so will the nature of management and leadership that they require.

REFERENCES

Asbridge, J. (1997). The interview – Jonathan Asbridge. *Nursing Management*, 4(4), 7–9.

Austin, N, and Dopson, S. (1997). *The Clinical Directorate*. Radcliffe Medical Press Ltd, Oxford.

Burchill, F. and Casey, A. (1996). *Human Resource Management – the NHS: a Case Study*. Macmillan Press Ltd, London.

Calas, M. and Smircich, L. (1993). Dangerous liaisons: the 'Feminine in Management' meets 'Globalization'. *Business Horizons*, Mar-Apr, 71–81.

DHSS (1982–1984). Steering Group on Health Services Information, Chairman E. Korner. *Six Reports to the Secretary of State*. HMSO, London.

DHSS (1983). *Recommendations on the Effective Use of Manpower and Related Resources. Report of the NHS Management Inquiry Team* (The Griffiths Report). DHSS, London.

Dingwall, R, Rafferty, A.M. and Webster, C. (1988). *An Introduction To The Social History of Nursing*. Routledge, London.

DoH (1991a). *The Health of the Nation*. HMSO, London.

DoH (1991b). *The Patient's Charter – Raising the Standard*. HMSO, London.

DoH (1992). *Women in the NHS.* HMSO, London.

Donabedian, A. (1969). Medical care appraisal – quality and utilization. In *Guide to Medical Care Administration.* 11. American Public Health Association, New York.

EUROSTAT (1988). *Demographic Statistics (Theme 3: Population and Social Conditions. Series C: Accounts, Surveys and Statistics).* Office for Official Publications of the European Communities, Luxembourg.

Fitzgerald, L. (1993). Clinicians into management: the agenda for change and training. Paper prepared for Professions and Management Conference, University of Stirling, August. Quoted in Austin, N. and Dopson, S. (1997). *The Clinical Directorate.* Radcliffe Medical Press Ltd, Oxford.

Girvin, J. (1995). *Standard Setting.* Macmillan Press Ltd, London.

Goldstone, L and Ball, J. (1984). The quality of nursing services. *Nursing Times.* 29(8), 56–9.

Ham, C. (1997). *Management and Competition.* Radcliffe Medical Press Ltd, Oxford.

Hegyvary, S.T. and Hausman, R.K.D. (1975). Monitoring nursing care quality. *Journal of Nursing Administration,* 15(55), 17–26.

HMSO (1990). *The National Health Service and Community Care Act 1990.* HMSO, London.

Honigsbaum, F., Holmstrom, S. and Calltorp, J. (1997). *Making Choices for Health Care.* Radcliffe Medical Press Ltd, Oxford.

Hutt, R. (1987). *Chief Officer Career Profiles.* Institute of Manpower Studies, University of Sussex, Brighton.

Iles, V. (1997). *Really Managing Health Care.* Open University Press, Buckingham.

Johnson, S. (ed.) (1997). *Pathways of Care.* Blackwell Science, Oxford.

Kanter, R.M. (1989). *When Giants Learn To Dance.* Routledge, London.

Kitson, A. (1986). Indicators of quality in nursing care – an alternative approach. *Journal of Advanced Nursing.* 11(2), 133–44.

Leneghan, J. (1996). *Rationing and Rights in Health Care.* Institute for Public Policy Research, London.

Marr, G. (1997). The leadership challenge in nursing. *Nursing Management,* 3(9), 7–9.

Marshall, J. (1995). *Women Managers Moving On.* Routledge, London.

Morton-Cooper, A. (1997). The politics of healthcare. In *Excellence in Health Care Management,* Morton-Cooper, A. and Bamford, M. (eds). Blackwell Science, Oxford.

NHSE (1994). *Developing NHS Purchasing and GP Fundholding: Towards a Primary Care-led NHS.* NHS Executive, Leeds.

NHSME (1992). *An Information Management and Technology Strategy for the NHS in England.* NHSME, London.

Nitjkamp, P., Pacolet, J., Spinnewyn, H., Vollering, A., Wildero, C. and Winters, S. (eds) (1991). *National Diversity and European Trends in Services for the Elderly.* University of Leuven, Higher Institute of Labour Studies, Leuven.

OECD (1988). *Ageing Populations – the Policy Implications.* OECD, Paris.

OPCS/HSE (1995). *Occupational Health Decennial Supplement.* HMSO, London.

Peck, M.S. (1979). *The Road Less Travelled.* Arrow Books, London.

Phaneuf, M. (1972). *The Nursing Audit.* Appleton-Century-Crofts, Detroit.

RCN (1990). *Quality Patient Care – the Dynamic Standard Setting System.* Scutari, London.

Rosener, J.B. (1990). Ways women lead. *Harvard Business Review,* Nov–Dec, 119–25.

Royce, R. (1997). *Managed Care – Practice and Progress.* Radcliffe Medical Press Ltd, Oxford.

Sale, D. (1996). *Quality Assurance,* 2nd edn. Macmillan Press Ltd, London.

Secretaries of State for Health (1989). *Working for Patients.* HMSO, London.

Secretary of State for Health (1996). *A National Health Service – a Service with Ambitions.* HMSO, London.

Senge, P. (1990). *The Fifth Discipline – the Art and Practice of the Learning Organisation.* Century Business, London.

Singer, R. (ed.) (1997). *GP Commissioning – an inevitable Evolution.* Radcliffe Medical Press Ltd, Oxford.

Sisson, K. (ed.) (1994). *Personnel Management – a Comprehensive Guide to Theory and Practice in Great Britain.* Blackwell Science, Oxford.

UKCC (1992a). *Code of Professional Conduct.* 3rd edn, UKCC, London.

UKCC (1992b). *The Scope of Professional Practice.* UKCC, London.

UKCC (1997). *Scope in Practice.* UKCC, London.

Unwin, N., Carr, S., Leeson, J., with Pless-Mulloli, T. (1997): *An Introductory Study Guide to Public Health and Epidemiology.* Open University Press, Buckingham.

Ward C. (1997). Key concepts in finance and information management. In *Excellence in Health Care Management,* Morton-Cooper, A. and Bamford, M. (eds). Blackwell Science, Oxford.

Watson, T.J. (1994). *In Search of Management: Culture, Chaos and Control in Managerial Work.* Routledge, London.

Weightman, J. (1996). *Managing People in the Health Service.* Institute of Personnel and Development, London.

Wilson, J.H. (1997). *Integrated Care Management.* Butterworth-Heinemann, Oxford.

Yukl, G. (1994). *Leadership in Organisations.* Prentice-Hall, Englewood Cliffs, NJ.

FURTHER READING

Iles, V. (1997). *Really Managing Health Care.* Open University Press, Buckingham.

This book provides readable but in-depth material on the practicalities of management.

Journal of Nursing Management. Blackwell Science, Oxford.

Published six times a year. It provides articles with an academic base.

Morton-Cooper, A. and Bamford, M. (1997). *Excellence in Health Care Management.* Blackwell Science, Oxford.

This text provides a broad-based summary of all aspects of the subject. It has excellent references.

Nursing Management. RCN Publications, London.

Published ten times a year. It provides material on the current nursing leadership agenda.

Sale, D. (1996). *Quality Assurance*, 2nd edn. Macmillan Press Ltd, London.

A good summary of the development of quality assurance and of the current approaches.

Whiteley, S., Ellis, R., Broomfield, S. (1996). *Health and social Care Management – a Guide to Self-development.* Arnold, London.

An excellent summary of management techniques and how to acquire them. It also includes case studies.

CHAPTER ELEVEN

NURSING: ISSUES *for* EFFECTIVE PRACTICE

Jane E. Schober

- Introduction
- Professional requirements for nursing practice
- Understanding nursing
- Individualised care – a practice perspective
- Decision making in nursing practice
- Nursing theory and nursing knowledge
- Care planning for effective practice
- Conclusion

The aim of this chapter is to explore factors which are important to the quality of nursing care with a particular focus on care planning. It is intended that it will contribute to a greater understanding of the influence all nurses have over their own practice, and hence the power and control nurses have over the health of people in need of nursing care. The chapter brings together a number of important issues pertinent to the delivery of nursing care in today's health service.

The nature of individualised patient care and approaches to nursing practice are examined, as are factors influencing the interpretation of nursing activities. Key health care demands for the role of the nurse are also considered. The idea of nursing as a personal service is discussed, as is the influence of attitudes, values and beliefs on nursing.

The chapter goes on to examine the importance of patient participation in care, to discuss the relationship between nursing theory and nursing practice, and to identify frameworks for nursing practice which may be incorporated into care planning.

INTRODUCTION

When you, as a nurse, come to read this chapter, you do so having made decisions to devote time, energy, interest and, perhaps, a career to nursing. Above all you must have commitment to nursing, based on a choice to offer a service to people in various states of health. Whatever you do and say to people in your care depends on the quality of your helping skills and your understanding of their needs. The way you give care is central to the quality of nursing and your influence over this should never be underestimated. Nursing is dynamic and constantly changing in its responsibilities to developments in health care, social needs and professional needs. Illness is an inevitable part of life for the vast majority of people. Your reaction to people who are ill, or who require health care, will be influenced and shaped by your personal qualities, such as your sensitivity, understanding and honesty, as well as the professional attributes, skills, competencies, attitudes and cognitive abilities necessary for effective practice.

Much of the professional responsibility of the nurse is focused on practice and the ultimate well-being of people requiring our services. Nursing is acknowledged as being a practice-based profession. However, for the nurse to practise in ways responsive to the wide-ranging health needs of our society, he/she should be in no doubt about the nature and range of responsibilities which he/she has as a member of the nursing workforce.

Of the developments in nursing in recent years, a number emerge as being particularly significant and relate to the nurse, his/her responsibilities for practice and measures necessary for the promotion and maintenance of standards of care.

PROFESSIONAL REQUIREMENTS FOR NURSING PRACTICE

Whether you are reading this chapter as a pre-registration nursing student or as a registered nurse, you have clearly stated responsibilities for practice. The majority of the professional requirements stem from the Nurses, Midwives and Health Visitors Act (1997) and are encapsulated in the United Kingdom Central Council (UKCC) Code of Professional Conduct for the Nurse, Midwife and Health Visitor (UKCC, 1992a) and the UKCC Guidelines for Professional Practice (UKCC, 1996a).

The standards for education, training and professional conduct are set by the UKCC, which is a statutory organisation charged by Parliament to ensure that the Nurses, Midwives and Health Visitors Act (1997) is implemented appropriately. The purpose of the Act and therefore, professional self-regulation, is to protect the public through professional standards and a professional register. The professional self-regulation facilities, the professional autonomy of nurses, midwives and health visitors in this country, is a privilege not enjoyed in other countries, e.g. in Europe, where often nurses are regulated by the medical profession. The UKCC also sets standards for each of the following:

- Professional conduct for nurses and midwives
- Professional practice
- Professional accountability
- Confidentiality
- Record keeping

- Student nurses and midwives in practice
- Post-registration and practice requirements.

These standards are minimal requirements and it is not unusual for local policies to reflect greater expectations than those required by the statutory body. Contracts of employment and job descriptions, for example, usually serve as clear guidance as to the requirements associated with a role as professional employee, as well as the duties and responsibilities associated with professional registration.

For registered nurses, midwives and health visitors, the legal and professional responsibilities for high standards of practice are clearly stated (UKCC, 1996a). In recent years, additional mandatory requirements for maintaining professional knowledge and competence throughout a registrant's working life have been introduced.

There are four key elements to maintaining registration:

- Completing a notification of practice form at the point of re-registration every 3 years and/or when your area of professional practice changes to one where you will use a different registerable qualification
- A minimum of 5 days *or equivalent* of study activity every 3 years
- Maintaining a personal professional profile containing details of your professional development
- A return to practice programme if you have not practised for a minimum of 750 hours or 100 working days in the 5-year period leading up to the renewal of your registration (from 1 April 2000).'

(UKCC, 1997, page 6)

The purpose is to assure the public that those nurses, midwives and health visitors caring for them are professionally up to date in their knowledge and practice.

THE PERSONAL PROFESSIONAL PROFILE

Since 1995, it has been a requirement for nurses to maintain a profile and usually student nurses and midwives initiate this process during their pre-registration courses.

The profile is:

'a flexible but comprehensive account of your professional development. However, it is more than a record of achievement. It is based on a regular process of reflection and recording that you learn from every day experiences, as well as planned learning activity.'

(UKCC, 1997, page 13)

Guidance is readily available as to how to maintain a profile from local and national nursing organisations as well as there being portfolio documents available on the market (e.g. the English National Board (ENB) portfolio, [ENB, 1991]).

The UKCC (1996b) summarise the benefits of using a profile as follows:

'to help you assess your current standards of practice

■ to develop your analytical skills – these are fundamental to your professional practice and the profiling process will help to sharpen your ability to reflect constructively on and analyse what you do
■ to enable you to review and evaluate past experience and learning in order to plan your continuing education and career development
■ to provide effective up-to-date information for use in application forms and interviews when you apply for jobs or courses
■ to provide evidence of what you have learned from your own experience. This may allow you to obtain credit towards further qualifications from an institution of higher education through schemes such as APEL (accreditation of prior experiential learning) and CATS (credit accumulation and transfer scheme).'

(UKCC, 1996b, page 7)

THE SCOPE OF PROFESSIONAL PRACTICE

In 1992 the UKCC issued guidelines for registered nurses, midwives, and health visitors, designed to support nurses in determining control over their role developments. Six principles were issued (Table 11.1) which encourage nurses to base their decisions for role development, professional education and practice on their evaluation of the needs of patients. This self-determination and professional control had not been widely acknowledged or accepted by nurses prior to this initiative.

Indeed, historically, doctors, for example, had been involved in teaching registered nurses skills and care practices which facilitated nurses' role extension (DHSS, 1977). There had been a natural delegation of clinical responsibilities to nurses as specialised care, technological advances and concern about care coordination developed. Thus, activities, once the domain of medical staff, have been adopted by nurses, e.g. venepuncture, cardiac monitoring and cervical smears, often to the advantage of patient care, though controversies remain over whether nurses who adopt such activities may not fulfil other nursing obligations.

The Scope of Professional Practice is an effective buffer against the risk of the over-delegation of medical tasks to nurses. It encourages nurses to reflect, review and evaluate the activities best undertaken at local level to facilitate the most effective care for patients. It is the responsibility of the nurse to determine whether he/she is sufficiently prepared to undertake new responsibilities in practice. It also encourages the principle of

Table 11.1: The six principles of the Scope of Professional Practice (UKCC, 1992b)

9 'The registered nurse, midwife or health visitor;
9.1 must be satisfied that each aspect of practice is directed to meeting the needs and serving the interests of the patient or client;
9.2 must endeavour always to achieve, maintain and develop knowledge, skill and competence to respond to those needs and interests;
9.3 must honestly acknowledge any limits of personal knowledge and skill and take steps to remedy any relevant deficits in order effectively and appropriately to meet the needs of patients and clients;
9.4 must ensure that any enlargement or adjustment of the scope of personal or professional practice must be achieved without compromising or fragmenting existing aspects of professional practice and care and that the requirements of the Council's Code of Professional Conduct are satisfied throughout the whole area of practice;
9.5 must recognise and honour the personal accountability borne for all aspects of professional practice and
9.6 serving the interests of patients and clients and the wider interests of society, avoid any inappropriate delegation to others which compromises those interests'

multidisciplinary teamworking if decisions for nurses' role development are made with the interests of patients and the organisation of their care in mind.

Nurses, midwives and health visitors are accountable for their practice and have a personal responsibility of saying 'no' to undertaking extended role activities if patient safety is in jeopardy.

Key Points

- Professional and legal requirements for nursing practice are determined by statute and statutory bodies. Additional requirements stem from national and local policies.
- Nurses are accountable for their practice.
- Nurses have responsibilities to maintain their professional registration, their competence to practice and their professional profile.
- Nurses may develop and expand their roles through self-determination while ensuring that interests of patients and standards of practice are maintained.

UNDERSTANDING NURSING

To understand nursing is to appreciate, internalise and be able to offer the optimum response to those needing nursing care. It is the very breadth and detail of nursing responsibilities which make the nature of nursing so complex.

Nursing may be regarded as a bridge between human frailties brought about by changes to health and well-being and the processes which support and heal them, which are enshrined in our ability, as nurses, to care. Nursing is often expressed in terms of caring. Mayeroff (1972) suggested a distinction between caring thoughts and caring actions. Therefore, one may undertake a caring action with or without emotional or intellectual concerns to accompany it.

Reflection Point

As you read the poem here by John J. Bruhn, consider the challenges he raises about the balance between the art and science of nursing. Is it not this need to develop both as a person as well as becoming a skilled, competent practitioner which epitomises the demands of nursing?

The Art of Being Human

What is all this current clamor;
Be more human in our manner
In caring for the sick, the well –
Have we not done so for a spell?

We've expanded science and technology
Found new secrets in biology.
The heart of science; our concern
The art of being human: later learn.

Science helps the sick recover
Secrets of a longer life: discover!
But when the end for each arrives
Science succumbs art survives.

How we live, how healthy we become
Is more art than science for some
The science of wellness less well known
Than the science of sickness with which we've grown.

As health professionals we've much to learn
About health care as a joint concern.
Is it science or art that is most potent?
An endless debate with no rapprochement.

Some special knowledge need I learn
To specialise in this new concern?
Personal growth and awareness required
To become the person you once aspired.

To laugh, to cry, to touch, to feel
Has little scientific appeal.
The art of being human needs reflection
As you prepare to enter your profession

A creed to guide your future direction
Nursing requires skill and affection
A scientist and artist you will be,
And a full measure of satisfaction you will see.
(From Steele and Maraviglia, 1981)

Carper (1978) considered the nature of nursing knowledge and identified four patterns of knowing in relation to nursing:

- Empirical knowledge – this is the science of nursing and includes nursing theories and scientific knowledge, which may be generated from empirical research
- Aesthetic knowledge – this is the art of nursing as expressed and experienced by individual nurses. There is an intuitive element to the

judgements made and it may be seen to be part of expert practice (Hampton, 1994)

- Personal knowledge – this is the insight and understanding individual nurses develop themselves and within the relationships found with patients
- Ethical knowledge – this is the understanding which develops from knowledge, analysis and evaluation of ethical issues, and which has an impact on decision making, values, attitudes and approaches to any nursing and health-related situation.

It can be seen from this insight into aspects of nursing knowledge that the art and science of nursing are clearly expressed.

NURSING AS A PERSONAL SERVICE

When considering nursing, associations are often made with concepts such as vocation and service. Nurturing (from which the word 'nurse' is derived) is a common lay activity, e.g. between parents and their children and between partners, and phrases such as nursing mothers have further associations. In a professional context, nursing goes further, in the sense that the professional nurse carer is charged with responsibilities which stem from statute, codes of professional conduct and employment requirements. There are a range of dimensions to caring which may be summarised as follows:

- The skills, knowledge and practice dimensions
- The emotional perspectives
- The influence of the care environment
- The availability and use of resources.

From the outset, the personal nature of the nurse's work is a key feature. Indeed, the intimate contact between nurses and patients or clients becomes a daily occurrence, not simply in the physical sense (though this, for many requiring care, is the most invasive of all experiences) but also in the social and emotional sense. Elements of oneself, which are usually concealed and the preserve only of family and friends, are made public. Feeling ill, needing an operation and being in pain may be frightening and alienating events and they require professional help. However, these events for health workers are everyday occurrences, they are part of the culture. There is a risk, therefore, of

nurses failing to acknowledge the significance of an individual's health state on his usual functioning.

Henderson (1979) suggests that the nurse who values nursing and its 'personal, individualised and human character' gives 'holistic rather than disease-centred care'. This is not to assume that health care based on a medical model is not individualised, nor that care which focuses on the disease and excludes attention to psychosocial reactions and manifestations is ignoring the individual's unique combination of characteristics and responses. This, at times, will need to be the priority for determining interventions. However, nurses hold a privileged position in the health care service. They hold the key to entering caring relationships at a time when people who are not experiencing optimum health may be at their most vulnerable.

Communication: a key to a personal service

An effective interpersonal relationship between nurse and patient depends largely on communication which is therapeutic and demonstrates respect, concern and care. However, communication problems – and, more specifically, poor information-giving – dominate complaints about the interaction between health care workers and the public (Dimond, 1990).

More than 100 years ago Nightingale (1860) recognised the need for nurses to use social skills, to demonstrate their interest in patients and to avoid impersonal activities. However, despite this clear recommendation, it appears that nurses may have been influenced more by their own expectations of patients.

Stockwell (1972) demonstrated that nurses may be highly selective in their communication with patients. Nurses rewarded patients who knew the nurses' names, who cooperated in their own care and who communicated willingly, by spending more time with them. The 'unpopular patients' in this study were those who complained, were demanding or demonstrated more discomfort than the nurse thought appropriate to the situation. This stereotyped attitude towards patients goes against the ideals of individualised care and the desire to give more time to patients. Menzies (1960) revealed that although nurses perceived the personal fears of patients, they may adopt defensive behaviours, such as avoiding patients' questions, providing negative responses and changing the subject.

One of the most influential statements about nursing is by Virginia Henderson:

'The unique function of the nurse is to assist the individual sick or well in the performance of those activities contributing to health or its recovery (or to a peaceful death) that he would perform un-aided if he had the necessary strength, will, or knowledge. And to do this in such a way as to help him gain independence as rapidly as possible.'

(Henderson, 1969, page 4)

This definition of nursing has been recognised all over the world as capturing the essence of what nurses do. It makes explicit the need to value holistic elements of care through helping, promoting independence and combining artistic and scientific activities. Henderson's definition of the unique function of the nurse skilfully incorporates her interpretation of the 'intrinsic nature of nursing', particularly when considered along with her belief that nursing 'will never be seen as anything less than essential to the human race' (Henderson, 1979).

Care is used here as a specific quality underlying practice, but only refers to activities which are the responsibility of nurses, rather than the value system underlying their execution. The concept of care has far-reaching implications. Griffin (1983) sees care as 'a fundamental concept both in the philosophy of human nature and that of personal relationships with others'. Therefore, in seeking an understanding of care, it is necessary to acknowledge the possible meanings associated with it and relate these to settings associated with the caring professions. Griffin identifies 'interest, concern, guidance, protection and serving' as being on a continuum with 'inclination or liking of a person, attachment or wanting to be near someone'. Therefore, there is more to the concept of care than the skills or actions associated with it. Campbell (1984) views caring as a form of loving characterised particularly by the nature of the companionship between the nurse and patient. He regards companionship as:

a closeness which is not sexually stereotyped; it implies movement and change; it expresses mutuality; and it requires commitment. ... The good companion is someone who shares freely,

but does not impose, allowing others to make their own journey.

It is necessary to consider also that although a nurse may value some, if not all of these aspects of care, he/she may not display them. There may be many reasons for this but there is certainly an interrelationship between the way a nurse values and prioritises these nursing qualities and the way his/her care is practised (Harrison, 1990).

Central to this is a moral aspect of caring. Schrock (1981) examines philosophical aspects of nursing without suggesting specific values for nursing. She suggests that through the analysis of moral concepts the nurse's own beliefs may be explored, so enhancing self-knowledge. She sets forth a selection of concepts here; they include 'telling the truth, respecting physical and emotional privacy, safeguarding adult rights, using but not abusing professional power and preventing incompetent practices'. These examples are essentially patient-centred. Perhaps nurses also need to consider and explore these and other concepts associated with themselves – for example, feelings of fear, embarrassment, revulsion and despair. All these issues imply that the nurse may be influenced by his or her own interests, and so caring activities could be influenced accordingly.

It is suggested that the aspects of care raised by Schrock (1981) – telling the truth and respecting emotional and physical privacy – are concepts which underpin the quality of an interaction between all health care workers and patients. Because in practice, dilemmas may arise from these, it is necessary to find ways of helping staff to clarify them. Values associated with other aspects of care may be more specific in character but are as susceptible to conflict. These include the assessment of pain, maintaining confidentiality and talking about sexual needs. These examples relate to individuals and/or groups of patients, but illustrate issues which should be addressed as part of the preparation of nurses for a particular clinical allocation. This could then be followed up during and after the experience, through the use of specific examples from practice and the analysis of critical incidents.

Personal values and attitudes have a significant effect on problem-solving and decision making; indeed they influence the way needs are identified and prioritised. There is much to be learnt from the exploration of attitudes and values in nursing;

they influence both the developments of nurse–patient relationships and the way care is planned and carried out.

PATIENT PARTICIPATION AND NURSING CARE

The notion of patient participation suggests involving the patient in planning his/her care and is seen as complementary to the concept of individualised care (Brearley, 1990). Patient participation depends on a supportive climate in which problem-orientated, spontaneous, empathic and mutual decision making occurs (McMahon and Pearson, 1991).

Individualised care is the fundamental principle which enables the achievement of this aim, but allowances should be made for those patients who choose not to participate to this extent. In 1987, the Royal College of Nursing (RCN) stated that:

> 'Each patient has a right to be a partner in his own care planning and receive relevant information, support and encouragement from the nurse which will permit him to make informed choices and become involved in his own care.'
>
> (RCN, 1987, page 9)

This could be further determined through the identification and application of appropriate aims for care. The use of a nursing model based on the identified needs of the patient and goals for care which reflect the priorities for intervention from the patient's and nurse's perspective may all encourage patient participation.

INDIVIDUALISED CARE – A PRACTICE PERSPECTIVE

Individualised patient care (IPC) as an aim for nursing practice is established as a nursing policy (DoH, 1991, 1993). In a study by Redfern (1995), nurses identified key characteristics of IPC, examples of which are included here as follows:

- The patient is a unique individual who must be respected
- A one-to-one relationship between the nurse and patient which features elements of continuity of care

- The patient is regarded as a 'potentially active expert' who participates in the care process according to his/her ability and wishes
- Physical, psychosocial, emotional, spiritual and cultural need are addressed without jeopardising patients' privacy
- Nurses may involve the family and friends of patients in assessing and managing care
- Nurses respond to patients' needs and wants as a priority
- Nurses are well informed about patient care and those with the greater knowledge of a patient would contribute to multidisciplinary decision making
- Nurses review and evaluate their practices together.

IPC is demanding, both for the patient and the nurse. Expert judgements are needed to assess continually and evaluate the extent to which the implementation of IPC is appropriate to the person needing care. This is, perhaps, one of the areas which makes nursing so complex. For a commitment to IPC to be rooted in practice, the nurse needs to develop an all-embracing understanding of individuality.

THE NATURE OF INDIVIDUALITY

Carl Rogers (1967) defined the individual as having:

> 'One basic tendency and striving – to actualise, maintain and enhance the experience organism ... The organism woven through struggle and pain towards enhancement and growth.'

The individual (or organism) is a whole being characterised by biological, psychological and intellectual components. These factors influence the internal dynamics of the individual and the way day-to-day situations and stimuli arising from the internal and external environment are processed. Rogers emphasises that nothing is static and everyone faces constantly changing situations. The motivation to grow, develop and enhance oneself is a fundamental drive and it depends on situations or an environment characterised by trust, respect and acceptance. Relationships which bear these characteristics allow those involved to participate and share in decisions and take responsibility for actions. This may be described as a 'healthy' environment. Conversely, an environment which is threatening and stressful, or where people feel undervalued, may result in much of their energy being used to adapt, cope and indeed survive the circumstances they face.

Skilled nurses take into account this range of reactions and respect the fact that each person will react in a way that makes the experience unique to him or her. Skilled nurses also recognise that the needs and wants of those requiring care have marked similarities – this is true of certain physiological responses as well as psychological and emotional responses. Spiritual needs, cultural factors, previous experiences, levels of understanding and ability to communicate and express these needs will shape these responses. However, for the nurse to be aware of this complex interrelationship requires an evolution of skill, insight, intuition and responsiveness which may be seen as characteristic of expert practice (Benner, 1984; Benner and Tanner, 1987).

Table 11.2 summarises factors which limit or facilitate IPC (Redfern, 1995). Here there is evidence of the interrelationship between organisational resources and interpersonal factors for the achievement of IPC. Central to these factors is the need to provide care which facilitates continuity of contact between the same nurse and patients. This is recognised by the work of Bowman and Thompson (1995) who considered that methods of work organisation may be categorised as follows:

- Primary nursing
- Team nursing
- Task nursing.

It is interesting to note that Bowman and Thompson (1995) went on to identify 13 components of nursing work, which reveal key characteristics associated with IPC. These are as follows:

'1 The basis of patient's assessment
2 The assessment and evaluation of the patient
3 The degree of managerial control
4 The accountability for patient care
5 The responsibility for patient care
6 The authority for patient care

Table 11.2: A summary of factors influencing individual patient care

Factors contributing to and facilitating IPC	Factors limiting IPC
Patients' characteristics	**Patients' characteristics**
■ A tendency for partnership in the care process, e.g. longer-stay and younger patients	■ High proportion of high dependency patients demand more nursing time
	■ Rapid patient turnover
	■ Lack of understanding of IPC
Staffing, roles, workload	**Staffing, roles, workload**
■ Adequate staff levels and skill mix are vital	■ Shortage of staff
■ Clerical support is vital	■ Impoverished skill mix
■ Sister's role: support, supervision, encouragement, role model, management of IPC, leadership	■ Workload
■ Support from managers	■ Stress and harassment
Personal qualities of nurses to include	■ Inadequate supervision of students, agency nurses and auxiliaries
■ Belief in IPC	■ Staff turnover
■ Passion for nursing	■ Unforeseen absence
■ Interpersonal skills	■ Lack of clerical support
■ Leadership qualities	■ Lack of support from managers
Ward organisation	**Ward organisation**
■ Ensure continuity of care for patients	■ Task-centred routines
■ Ensure support for students	■ Effects of unforeseen events, uncertainties
■ Involve qualified staff in direct patient care	
The multidisciplinary team	**The multidisciplinary team**
■ Commitment from other professionals to IPC	■ Lack of commitment from other professions to IPC

Adapted from Redfern, 1995.

7　The senior ward nurse's role in decision making

8　The method of communication between professional groups

9　The method of allocating patients to nurses

10　The leadership style operating in the ward

11　Responsibility for communication with relatives

12　The patient's awareness of who has responsibility for care

13　The patient's involvement in care'
(Bowman and Thompson, 1995, page 223)

Bowman *et al.* suggest that assessing care using these items reveals the organisational work method in use and thus how close the working relationship is between nurses and patients.

DECISION MAKING IN NURSING PRACTICE

Actions are inevitably influenced by the attitudes, beliefs and values of individuals who hold them. Decisions for nursing practice need to be informed, systematic and based on sound understanding and interpretation of events, as well as on a thorough knowledge of practice, theory and research.

When the nursing process was introduced into the UK in the 1970s much attention was given to the management and delivery of nursing care. It was implemented as a model of decision making, but great value was placed on the development of nursing records from the assessment, planning, implementation and evaluation framework of a problem-solving approach. Today, there is still great emphasis and value placed on nursing records which reflect these characteristics, without a clear understanding of the distinction between the intellectual thought processes that occur in practice and what needs to be reflected in the written record. As a result, nurses have found themselves overwhelmed by paperwork, often at the expense of interacting with patients. It is widely acknowledged that the effective management of care depends on systematic, holistic care, which promotes shared decision making and the independence of patients and clients. The relationship between IPC and holistic nursing is acknowledged (see also Chapter 24). It is still assumed at national and local level that IPC is the approach to

care to strive for. As an ideal it is commendable but there is evidence that the needs of some patients may not be as all-embracing and as complex as professionals suspect. Indeed, patients often indicate that clear information, accessible, skilled and knowledgeable nurses and freedom from discomfort form the basis of their needs. This is not to simplify the issues. The complexity of need, health and nursing requirements are influenced, for example, by the acuteness of the condition, the dependency and the understanding of the patient and the likely prognosis.

For nursing, effective decision making is central to systematic, patient-orientated care – the nursing process has a contribution to make to this.

THE CONTRIBUTION OF THE NURSING PROCESS TO THE ORGANISATION OF NURSING CARE

The World Health Organization (WHO) definition encapsulates the features of the nursing process by emphasising that many of the characteristics referred to rely on intellectual activities and effective problem-solving and decision making. These contribute to assessing, planning, implementing and evaluating care in a systematic manner.

The WHO (1977) states:

'The nursing process is a term applied to a system of characteristic nursing interventions in the health of individuals, families and/or communities. In detail it involves the use of scientific methods for identifying the health needs of the patient/client/family or community and for using these to select those which can most effectively be met by nursing care; it also includes planning to meet these needs, provide the care and evaluate the results. The nurse in collaboration with other members of the health care team and the individual or groups being served, defines objectives, sets priorities, identifies care to be given and mobilises resources. He/she then provides the nursing services either directly or indirectly. Subsequently, he/she evaluates the outcome. The information feedback from evaluation of outcome should initiate desirable changes in subsequent interventions in similar nursing care situations. In this way, nursing becomes a dynamic process lending itself to adaptation and improvement.'

By implication, any process suggests that there is an identifiable purpose and a system for organising and achieving the purpose. Key features of the process also include inspiration, creativity and productivity. It is the merging of decision-making skills bearing these characteristics with caring activities which is central to the meaning of the nursing process, and thus the effective organisation of care.

By applying this to nursing, it is clear that nurses have the potential for original creative decision making based on the application of sound knowledge and expertise to care situations. There are a number of models of decision making; two are explored here, as they offer some insight to nurses about factors influencing the decision-making process.

THE COMPREHENSIVE RATIONAL MODEL

The nursing process can be likened to the comprehensive rational model of decision making based on the work of Simon (1950). The model contains the following elements:

- Goal-setting
- Identifying ways to achieve goals
- Evaluating each option
- Selecting the optimum solution
- Acting on or implementing the plan
- Review outcome(s).

The similarities with the assessment, planning, implementation and evaluation activities of the nursing process are clear. The model makes a key assumption that the decision maker will take into consideration all possible options and consequences, in the light of a thorough understanding of the situation.

However, in practice this approach will be influenced by time constraints, by habits and routine, and by the current precedent. It is also true that in practice decisions are often taken when the first satisfactory outcome or solution is found. So, when making decisions about care with, or on behalf of, patients, awareness of choices being influenced by what may be the quickest or easiest, rather than the best, solution relies on expert judgement.

THE INCREMENTALIST MODEL

Another model of decision making, the incremental model (Lindblom, 1959), offers a step-by-step approach to decision making. Change is gradual but continuous. The decisions are usually influenced by bargaining processes and a narrower range of options is considered before decisions are reached. By implication those with the greatest power are likely to have the greatest influence. Within the nurse–patient relationship, the nurse holds expert power, as she would usually know more about care and treatment. Thus, the sharing of knowledge is a key way of allowing patients to be part of the decision-making process. This step-by-step approach to decision making may be characteristic of how many decisions are made about care and is more in tune with, for example, short-term goal-setting. It would be useful, also, to consider how a more 'rational' approach would enhance the quality of decision making.

It is important for nurses to consider how their decisions about care are reached and the factors influencing them. This is particularly important in relation to:

- Identifying a philosophy of care for the ward/unit
- The process of assessment, which is the key to effective care planning
- The beliefs and attitudes of members of the care team, which may influence the way care is prioritised – these are usually reflected in the philosophy of care
- How the nurse shares his/her power with the patient in relation to giving information, building relationships and developing a therapeutic partnership for care (see also Chapter 7)
- The way the nurse involves the patient (and his/her family) in the care process, and the appropriateness of this involvement for all concerned
- The motivation and bias of the care team in the light of previous care decisions
- How solutions are reached – whether the nurse is prepared to try alternatives, innovate and initiate as appropriate, or be content with the status quo.

The nursing process should be viewed as a way of making decisions about the care of an individual or a group. However, it does not inform the nurse as to what to assess, what to aim for in care or how to implement care. It is through the development and understanding of frameworks for assessment and care planning that this emerges. Thus, insight into the nursing needs of those requiring care is essential. A means to this end comes from the ability to select and analyse approaches to nursing care which ultimately helps the nurse to plan care to promote the health of the individual. This demands a holistic approach to nursing care where physiological, psychological, social, spiritual and cultural needs are considered. Such approaches to care may be found in a number of nursing models which will be considered later in this chapter and also in innovative approaches to practice which the Burford model identifies (this model is discussed in Chapter 25).

The reference to individuality aims to emphasise some of the implications of approaching nursing as a process of individualised patient care. An adherence to these principles as a means of supporting nursing staff is essential for a healthy, caring climate in which both nurses and patients are trusted, accepted and supported. In many situations this ideal may not be achieved, but striving towards it will provide the motivation for improved practice.

In the context of decision making and problem-solving, the nursing process has a place. However, there is no doubt that moves towards health care practices which focus on effectiveness, efficiency and cost consciousness have influenced health care delivery and thus the organisation of nursing (see Chapter 10). It remains that nurses shape the patients' experiences of health care. This serves as the focus of the next section.

> **Key Point**
>
> Today there exist guidelines in the *Nurses, Midwives and Health Visitors Act* (HMSO, 1997), the Code of Professional Conduct (UKCC, 1992) and from professional organisations (such as the Royal College of Nursing) which advocate that nurses should promote health and prevent illness, be competent in the total planning of care, and use knowledge from the behavioural sciences, physical sciences and nursing research to develop the knowledge, skills and attitudes to provide individualised patient care.

NURSING THEORY AND NURSING KNOWLEDGE

Nursing is essentially a practice discipline, but the quality of this practice depends on attitudes, knowledge and abilities for effective care. The way nurses use knowledge and apply theory will influence their approach to nursing; sound decision making depends on using knowledge expertly (Carper, 1978).

By implication, there appears to be more to the relationship between theory and practice than simply an understanding of what is done and why. In order to discuss the relevance of theory in nursing practice, it is necessary to examine two main relationships – first, the relationship between the knowledge and nursing practice and second, the relationship between the presence of theory, its interpretation, and its relevance to practice. Nurses know how to act, but whether they always have understanding of their actions is debatable. The Oxford English Dictionary defines knowledge as 'theoretical or practical understanding', being 'well informed', and 'familiarity gained by experience'. These definitions imply that knowledge may be acquired *without* theoretical input.

Benner (1984) considered the differences between practical and theoretical knowledge in detail and suggested that those who acquire practical skills may not be able to account theoretically for their actions. She goes on to suggest that knowledge development occurs by extending 'know-how'.

The extension of 'know-how' appears to form a major part of knowledge development in nursing this century. Consider the way nurses in the past have responded to the demands of developments in technology, treatments and patterns of health care; and consider, too, the way that nurses have inherited procedures once carried out by doctors. Historically, rather than research into nursing practice developing, nurses found themselves taking on medical and technical tasks, as medical know-how expanded and developed. Therefore, it may be suggested that the recognition of the relevance of theory was distorted by the preoccupation with watered-down medical know-how.

Today the picture is changing. The growing body of nursing research and knowledge is reflected in nursing texts, nursing journals and in the opportunities for nurses to study nursing and health-related subjects at institutions of higher education. Using theory in practice is regarded as an effective means of introducing change, and research-mindedness as a way of questioning, testing, developing and ultimately generating nursing knowledge.

However, there are two other perspectives which deserve mention of here, namely, knowledge embedded in expertise and the notion that there are complementary areas of practical knowledge. It would be a mistake to assume that just because some practical knowledge may lack theoretical ground, it lacks validity. Benner (1984) suggests that know-how may be acquired through experience, hence leading to expertise, and states that 'adequate description of practical knowledge is essential to the development and extension of nursing theory'.

This conclusion gives clear direction to the way practice may serve the development of knowledge. However, in the UK, it is recognised that the use of nursing research as a means of developing and transmitting knowledge has been very limited – especially before 1980 (Hunt, 1981) – and those who publish research studies have tended to be nurse leaders and lecturers, rather than those working in clinical areas.

In recent years the recognition of the potential of research for the development of nursing has been well recognised through a range of initiatives. These include the contributions of higher education to the research agenda, the development of educational opportunities at degree level for all nurses, national and local research initiatives and the work of key organisations, e.g. the King's Fund.

NURSING THEORY AND NURSING PRACTICE

Chinn and Jacobs (1991) define theory as 'a systematic abstraction of reality that serves some purpose' and which describes, controls and predicts the events that are of concern to the particular discipline. In the light of this, theory of nursing could contribute towards resolving ambiguity by showing what is happening and serving as a predictor of nursing actions.

If theories are able to describe, on the one hand, and predict on the other, there exists a range of potential in terms of their use and development. It is necessary, therefore, to examine the sources and types of theory – particularly since traditionally the use of theory has been limited. Nurses possess a range of personalised theories, demonstrated by the range which exists in some approaches to practice, for example, the prevention and treatment of pressure sores, giving mouth care and offering pre-operative information.

Nurses may view the presence of formal theory with suspicion, particularly as so little practical nursing is carried out by qualified nurses. If theory is unrecorded, not only may it go unquestioned and untested, but it may be generating irregular practices. The importance of theory for practice must be to support practice if its relevance is to be acknowledged. The need, then, is to encourage the development of *inductive* theory, i.e. the development of theory from the study and scrutiny of nursing practice.

This section has examined the relevance of theory to nursing by examining nursing knowledge, the development of theory and the use of theory. There is no doubt that the value placed on the use of theory in practice has been variable, but it remains that nursing theory depends not only on knowledge shared with other disciplines, but also on the nurse's ability to identify with theory and to generate and use it.

The challenge is enormous and, as Fawcett (1993) recognises, practice needs to be validated by research as a means of strengthening the knowledge base of nursing.

NURSING THEORY AND NURSING MODELS

Nursing is a complex activity and may be demonstrated in a wide variety of ways. Models help to make sense of the range of approaches to care by offering a representation of an aspect of reality. Models are essential to the growth of nursing theory and nursing knowledge as they contain the elements of the theory, which may or may not be directly amenable to practice. Models may also contain the ideas and experiences of nurses and it could be said that all nurses have their own model of nursing, which is usually demonstrated through their actions, attitudes and expertise – that is to say, essentially through their practice. These models should be scrutinised and subjected to empirical study.

Nurses who have applied themselves to a greater understanding of nursing through the formulation of a model have usually taken their ideas and their experiences about nursing, health, man and society and sought to explain the interrelationship between them. Specific nursing models (and you will find a small selection summarised in this chapter) assist nurses in their understanding about the nature and complexity of nursing. It is not uncommon to find nursing documentation designed from the features of such work. However, the model itself should not dictate the care for a patient but serve to assist nurses in their decision making and approach to the individual care of patients.

The features of nursing models

Contemporary nursing models have key features in common as a result of this process. These may be summarised as follows:

- Priority is given to the integrity of the individual
- Assessment of the health needs of the individual is the foundation for all decision making and problem-solving activities concerned with care
- Value is placed on the promotion of optimum health for the individual throughout the period of care
- Each model offers a theme or approach to nursing which provides a means of focusing on the needs of the individual – for example, self care, adaptation. Therefore, the model is the guide to the decision-making process.

For clinical nursing practice a model:

'gives direction for the assessment process and provides a systematic approach to patient care. It shows the nurse what to look for and how to provide nursing care.'

(Rambo, 1984, page 5)

In addition, comprehensive assessment establishes an on-going process for the management of patient-centred information; key elements for effective assessment are summarised in Table 11.3.

Choosing a model of nursing

The choice of a nursing model and approach to nursing care may follow one of two general perspectives. The choice may be influenced by the needs of the individual patient and may be chosen following a comprehensive assessment and an understanding of the care priorities. Alternatively, the choice may depend on broader criteria and take into consideration not only the needs of a larger group of patients, but also factors associated with the health care team, the care environment and resources. This is particularly pertinent where the clinical environment is being used for pre-registration or post-registration education.

It is important to emphasise here that care plan design may inhibit or facilitate care. This is particularly so in a clinical learning environment where well-designed records not only allow the features of the model to be made explicit, but also prompt the inexperienced user towards comprehensive assessment and record-keeping.

Table 11.3: Effective assessment: a summary

Effective assessment depends on:

- Prioritising patients' needs to ensure their safety and well-being
- The nurse knowing the general intention of an interaction
- Social skills, which are used to establish a rapport and a relationship which may then develop during the period of care
- Interviewing skills, which are used to gather and give information and to clarify the purpose and intentions of both parties
- Problem-solving and decision-making abilities being applied to the available information
- Observing and using verbal and non-verbal cues
- Learning and listening to what is said and implied – questioning to explore and clarify what is said
- Attending to verbal and non-verbal responses and checking whether they appear to contradict each other
- Using language which is understood and explaining new terms
- Receiving, reflecting on and summarising the points made to check the accuracy of perception and understanding
- Recording what is factual, observable and whenever possible involving the patient with this

Evaluating a model of nursing

Making judgements about the potential value and use of a model of nursing depends on an understanding of the model and a full appreciation of what the model means to those concerned with the delivery of care (see Table 11.4). While the models referred to here are models of nursing, the approaches to care found in each of them have implications for the way health needs are identified, prioritised and how care is planned and delivered. Therefore, it may be said that as a guide for planning nursing care, the choice of model is a reflection of the beliefs and values held by those delivering care and may also be a reflection of the expertise and skills available.

APPROACHES TO NURSING CARE: THE WORK OF KEY NURSE THEORISTS

There are more than 30 theories of nursing and it would be impossible to include them all here. However, this selection is based on their applica-tion to nursing and their use since they were originally published. Despite speculation about their use for care planning, it is noteworthy that these works contribute much to our understanding about the nature and potential of nursing and how nursing may be seen as a response to the needs of those experiencing changes and deficits in their health.

NURSING TO PROMOTE NURSE–PATIENT INTERACTION AND INTERPERSONAL RELATIONSHIPS

These models include the approaches developed by Hildegard E. Peplau (1988) (interpersonal relationships) and Imogen King (1981) (the theory of goal attainment).

The work of Hildegard Peplau: a theory of interpersonal relationships and psychodynamic nursing

Peplau's approach to nursing developed from her work with people who were mentally ill. Her

Table 11.4: Evaluating a model/theory of nursing

The background of the model
Consider the origins of the model, when and where was it devised and how the author developed the model. Answers to these questions will alert the reader to the context of the work and what the original intentions of the model were.

The aims of the model
Examine the aims of the model. These may be expressed as aims of nursing. These will reveal the focus of the model and usually tell the reader whether the approach to nursing extends from the nurse–patient relationship and/or whether nursing aims to respond to states of health. Further understanding of the model will be gained from consideration of any assumptions the author makes about nursing, health, individuals or society.

Definitions and meanings
Identify what the author means by *Health*, *Nursing*, *Man* and *Society*. These concepts will provide an image of the model. They should reveal how the author sees the relationship between a definition of health and how nursing may respond to people with associated health needs in a particular social setting.

Theories associated with the model
Identify any theories or research referred to by the author. This will provide useful insight into how, for example, certain work from the behavioural and social sciences has been applied to nursing through the formulation of the model. It is useful to refer to the original source of these theories for a full appreciation of the work.

Application of the model to clinical practice
Though the author may not offer specific examples of how the model has been used in clinical practice, it should be possible to find examples in the literature of how some models have been applied in both British and American health care settings. (The further reading list at the end of this chapter contains useful examples from British literature.) By considering these examples it is possible to see how models may be interpreted and applied in a variety of ways.

major work was published in the 1950s but readers should not be deterred by its age. The work grew from her insights into how the nurse–patient relationship is, in itself, a therapeutic tool. She states:

'Psychodynamic nursing is being able to understand one's own behaviour to help others identify felt difficulties and to apply principles of human relations to the problems that arise at all levels of experience.'

(Peplau, 1952, page xiii)

THE AIMS OF THE MODEL

The aim of the model is to use the nurse–patient relationship to help patients explore and understand the meaning of their feelings in a way which ultimately offers the opportunity to identify with what is happening and to be involved in care. Peplau describes four phases of the interpersonal relationship:

1 Orientation
2 Identification
3 Exploitation
4 Resolution.

These phases provide a framework for the development of a relationship and should be viewed as overlapping stages made unique by each nurse–patient relationship.

Orientation Orientation occurs at the beginning of the relationship, and is a period during which the nurse and patient can begin to get to know each other. It is a time for the nurse to help the patient recognise his/her needs and for the nurse to be generous with him or herself, to help the patient understand his/her role and explain the nurse's involvement in care.

Identification Feelings are explored to ascertain the nature of the need. The nurse uses positive feedback to support, encourage and help the person gain insight into the nature of his/her behaviour. This is a time for the nurse to promote a trusting relationship and to strengthen bonds which contribute to the person gaining confidence. This phase may be likened to a period of assessment, where needs are explored and identified and goals begin to emerge.

Exploitation This is the time for the nurse to build on the features and qualities of the relation-

ship so far, to help the person take responsibility for identifying further goals.

Resolution New goals replace the old ones and the nurse helps the person prepare for ending the relationship and to be secure away from the support of the relationship with the nurse.

DEFINITIONS AND MEANINGS

Peplau offers the following definitions. Health is defined as:

'a word symbol that implies forward movement of personality and other ongoing human processes in the direction of creative, constructive, productive personal and community living.'

(Peplau, 1988, page 12)

Nursing is defined as a:

'human relationship between an individual who is sick or in need of health services, and a nurse especially educated to recognise and to respond to the need for help.'

(Peplau, 1988, page 9)

Society is not defined, but Peplau encourages the nurse to consider the person in relation to his/her cultural background and environment. This is particularly important when the person is facing changes.

THE NURSE'S ROLE AND THE NURSE–PATIENT RELATIONSHIP

Peplau describes six roles associated with stages of the relationship:

1 Stranger – this is the first role. The nurse and patient meet as strangers. The nurse should aim to extend social skills and establish an atmosphere of acceptance
2 Resource – the nurse offers information. He/she clarifies and encourages patient involvement and patient understanding
3 Teacher – the nurse gives information; he/she guides and facilitates
4 Leader – the nurse leads the process of identification and goal-setting
5 Surrogate – the nurse represents people relevant to the patient, to help him/her to recall feelings and experiences
6 Counsellor – the nurse helps the person reflect, recognise, accept and come to terms with the aspects of experience and feelings.

THEORIES ASSOCIATED WITH THE MODEL

Peplau refers to psychological and psychoanalytical theories and to theories of motivation, personality, psychotherapy and social learning.

Although this work has grown out of caring for people who were mentally ill, Peplau suggests that the principles may be applied to any other setting if an interpersonal relationship exists.

This approach to the formulation and establishment of an interpersonal relationship deserves continued attention and the importance of this work should be valued in all aspects of nursing.

NURSING TO PROMOTE PATIENT ADAPTATION

The key name in the promotion of patient adaptation is that of Callista Roy. Roy's work began in the early 1960s at Mount St Mary's College in California. Her ideas about nursing developed from observation of patients and that they used to adapt to their health states. Much of her early work was with children and she observed their ability to cope with change and adapt to both physical and psychological changes.

THE AIM OF ROY'S MODEL

The focus of the model is the concept of adaptation. Roy sees nursing as a means of promoting adaptation in people requiring health care.

DEFINITIONS AND MEANINGS

Roy's interpretation of health is based on her idea that adaptation is a state of physiological and social integrity. She defines health as 'a state and a process of being and becoming integrated and whole' (Roy, 1989).

Nursing is defined as a theoretical system of knowledge which prescribes a process of analysis and action related to the care of the ill or potentially ill person (Roy, 1984).

Man is defined as a person who is a 'biopsychosocial being in constant interaction with a changing environment' (Roy, 1984).

Rather than a definition of society, Roy defines the environment as 'all the conditions, circumstances and influences surrounding and affecting the development and behaviour of persons or groups' (Roy, 1984).

The concept of adaptation

Roy's study of the meaning of adaptation led her to describe adaptation in relation to nursing and health needs. She suggests that a person responds to different health states according to his level of adaptation. Where a person is unable to adapt unaided to a particular health problem, the nurse intervenes and assesses the nature of the problem. Roy identifies four modes of adaptation which represent her understanding of how people behave and respond (see Table 11.5).

FIRST LEVEL ASSESSMENT

Roy suggests that states of health may affect one or more of these modes (see Table 11.6 for examples). She stresses that each mode is interrelated with the other; for example, a person with a newly formed colostomy may not only need help to cope with the pain following surgery, but also experience feelings of embarrassment about how he or she looks (self concept), anxiety about how he/she is going to cope at home and on return to work (role mastery), and how his/her partner will react when shown the colostomy (interdependence). These four modes form the basis of assessment which is divided into two parts – the first level assessment and the second level assessment.

Each mode is used to guide assessment. The nurse identifies whether the person is adapting or exhibiting problems. Needs or maladaptive behaviours identified from the first level assessment are then assessed more closely to discover more information which will help the nurse to plan care with a greater understanding of the stressors affecting the patient.

Table 11.5: The four modes of adaption identified by Roy (1984)

Mode	Definition
Physiological	Responses to physiological and biological demands
Self-concept	Responses to beliefs and feelings about oneself
Role functions	Responses to role function in relation to one's role set
Interdependence	Responses to relationships with people and other sources of comfort and support

Table 11.6: Roy's first level assessment

		Examples of common adaptation problems
Physiological	**Physiological mode**	
Exercise and rest		Insomnia
Nutrition		Nausea
Elimination		Incontinence
Fluid and electrolytes		Hypovolaemia
Oxygenation and circulation		Dyspnoea
Regulation of temperature, senses and the endocrine system		Pyrexia
Self concept	**Self concept mode**	
Physical self		Loss of libido
Personal self		Guilt, poor self image
Role function	**Role function mode**	
Primary roles		
Secondary roles		Role conflict
Tertiary roles		Role failure
		Role distance
Interdependence	**Interdependence mode**	
Interdependence on others		Loneliness
		Isolation
With others		

SECOND LEVEL ASSESSMENT

The person who is found to be having problems with one or more aspects of his or her health is said to be unable to adapt unaided to certain stimuli in the internal environment (for example, stressors such as infection, immobility, fear and inability to communicate) as well as in the external environment (for example, stressors such as living alone, bacteria and viruses, and lack of information). Each need or problem is explored to reveal the stimuli affecting them. These are classified as follows:

■ Focal – the causative stimulus, the main reason for the problems
■ Contextual – all other stimuli which may influence the focal stimuli
■ Residual – the beliefs, feelings, attitudes relating to the situation as expressed by the person.

The interrelationship between these details illustrates how an understanding of the patient's beliefs would help the nurse plan care specific to the actual problems and, in this situation, the beliefs of the person. It should be noted that not all

focal stimuli have an obvious contextual or residual stimulus. Time spent with the patient and continuous assessment will do much to help and support the patient, allowing more details to emerge.

The use of this model demands that the nurse develops a trusting relationship and is able to maintain his/her contact with the person.

THEORIES ASSOCIATED WITH THE MODEL

Roy refers to the work of Harry Helson (1964) who developed a theory of adaptation. Other work, including that by Hans Selye (1978), is used to refine the concept of adaptation.

Roy's adaptation model offers nurses an approach to care which applies equal attention to physiological, psychological and social aspects of the response to stimuli – whether these be generated from within the person or from the environment. The model also offers useful insights into how knowledge of a patient's adaptation level, coping abilities and associated life experience and beliefs provide a comprehensive base from which to plan care. Thus, goals and interventions are oriented to the promotion of the patient's adaptation level, the nurse acting on his/her behalf as necessary.

This model may be considered where people need help in coming to terms with chronic illness, changes in body image, or are found to be having difficulty coping and adapting.

NURSING TO PROMOTE SELF CARE

The work of Dorothea Orem has been particularly influential in the context of encouraging the patient to be a partner in his/her own care.

Orem's self care model

Orem first published her work about self care nursing in 1971, at a time when consumerism was gaining momentum and the American public appeared to be seeking value for money for their health care as well as looking beyond conventional medically dominated health care services. The concept of self care is explained in detail in Orem's (1995) work and is open to a number of interpretations.

Often 'self caring' appears on British care plans, particularly where people appear to be able to look after themselves. The reality may be that the patient receives little or no care at all. It is important to challenge this notion of 'do-it-yourself care'. This model offers an opportunity to explore the implication of self care nursing, not only for the patient but also for the nurse. Self care nursing is essentially about shifting responsibility for decision making and caring activities appropriately from nurses to patients. It means allowing people to hold on to the control they would normally have over their lives, as they experience the health care and treatment they need.

THE AIM OF THE MODEL

The aim of the model comes from Orem's notion of self care which she sees as:

> 'The practice of activities that individuals initiate and perform on their own behalf in maintaining life, health and well-being.'
>
> (Orem, 1985)

The model provides a means of enabling this to be achieved for people who need interventions, support, teaching and guidance from nurses.

DEFINITIONS AND MEANINGS

Orem suggests that health depends on a person's ability to be self caring, and is therefore a balance between initiating self care and being able to undertake self care activities to meet personal needs. She describes individual needs as 'universal self care requisites' which need to be met in order to maintain health.

The requirements are common to everyone and form the basis of the assessment process. Orem suggests that an individual who is unable to be self caring or be in control of one or more of these areas of need, who needs help or support, is in a state of ill health and requires health care which restores him to a position from which he will once again be as self caring as possible.

Orem also describes 'development self-care requisites' which relate to the experience and maturation of the person. She suggests that people have needs relating to their stage of growth, development and life experiences which should be considered when support is needed for them to be self caring.

The third area of self care requisites relates to the effect of disease, trauma, injury and illness on self care and is called 'health deviation self care requisites'. Included here is the notion that when a person becomes dependent and needs support, he will often demonstrate self care actions when seeking information and help.

These three categories form the basis of the nursing assessment which aims to identify the self care requisites or the actions necessary for the person to be self caring.

CARE PLANNING USING OREM'S MODEL

Nursing is seen as a system in which the promotion of self care is therapeutic for the patient. Care planning depends on the assessment of universal self care requisites, developmental self care requisites, in order to identify the person's self care demands or needs in relation to each requisite, self care ability, self care deficit and potential for self care.

An example of care planning, using Orem's model, based on one need of a young man who incurred facial injuries following a road traffic accident, is given in Table 11.7.

Orem describes three systems or approaches to nursing:

1 Wholly compensatory nursing. The nurse takes responsibility for the total care of a per-

Table 11.7: Care planning based on Orem's model

Universal self care requisites	Self care demands	Self care ability	Self care deficit	Potential for self care
Maintenance of food intake	Well-balanced diet	Unable to tolerate solid food Manages pureed food and prefers to use a straw	Motivation deficit; finds eating a great effort Knowledge deficit relating to the detail of a well-balanced diet	Long-term self care Short-term depends on healing and pain control and return of appetite

son who is unable to carry out any self care activities.

2 Partly compensatory nursing. The nurse undertakes aspects of care that the person is unable to do independently or without help.

3 Supportive-educative nursing. The nurse supports and guides the person to carry out self care which, as yet, he is unable to do without knowledge, skill, practice or assistance.

Care planning, using this model, depends on the nurse adopting one or more of these approaches to care, depending on the needs and skills of the person, his or her willingness to undertake self care activities, and the ability of the nurse to guide, support or compensate for changes that have occurred in a person's ability to be self caring. During a period of care, one or all of the systems may be applied as changes in health and dependency occur.

THEORIES ASSOCIATED WITH THE MODEL

Orem's ideas about nursing and self care have been, by and large, a product of her nursing experiences and her understanding of health care requirements. However, she does refer to other nurse theorists (for example, Imogen King and Virginia Henderson) as well as to sociologists and psychologists.

The self care concept in health care is not attributable to nursing alone. Orem (1984) states:

'The self-care theory component of the general theory of nursing is common to the health professions and to all members of social groups. Physicians as well as paramedical groups help people with aspects of self-care and with development of capabilities to engage in self-care. Persons helped may or may not be in need of nursing or may or may not be under nursing care.'

It is easy to see that the promotion of self care may be closely associated with approaches to health education and prevention of illness, as well as being pertinent to the involvement of people in their health care. These ideas about nursing and self care should encourage nurses to consider the implications of their actions and their relationships with people needing care. To be self-caring, people need information, appropriate support, assistance and help. The nurse also needs to be able to judge with the person whether he or she is willing, able and prepared to participate in this way. There may be patients who are not interested or who are unwilling to undertake self care activities, so offering the opportunity and information for this is vital.

Now is the time for nurses to think more about giving people the choice to participate actively in their own care, and to undertake self care activities as a way of contributing more actively to the maintenance of their own health.

Key Points

- Nursing models, though abstract in nature, have contributed much to the understanding of approaches to nursing care and the development of nursing theory.
- Care based exclusively on a model of nursing may fail to incorporate environmental, contextual, individual and professional influences and may limit the potential and authority of a nurse to develop an individual, systematic and intuitive relationship with patients.
- Nursing theory contributes to our understanding of the complexity of nursing, and the range of needs which may need a nursing response.
- Theories have a fundamental part to play in our thinking, decision making and analysis of care, all of which are essential for effective practice and care planning.

CARE PLANNING FOR EFFECTIVE PRACTICE

A central concern of all nurses is the way care for individual patients is planned and coordinated. Care planning is the process of assessing, planning, implementing coordinating and evaluating care for patients and maintaining appropriate records of the care undertaken.

The Nurses, Midwives and Health Visitors Rules Approval Order (Statutory Instrument, 1989) states a range of requirements for students, before they can register as a nurse. One statement clearly relates to care planning:

> 'the identification of physical, psychological, social and spiritual needs of the patient or client; an awareness of values and concepts of individual care, the ability to its implementation and evaluation; and the demonstration of the application of the principles of a problem-solving approach to the practice of nursing.'
>
> (Statutory Instrument, 1989, page 114)

Earlier in this chapter, factors influencing the ability of nurses to practise and plan care effectively have been highlighted. These include:

- Meeting professional, legal and contractual responsibilities
- Practising nursing competently
- Making effective nursing decisions
- Understanding, applying and evaluating nursing knowledge and theory to care situations
- Developing and maintaining caring, sensitive, interpersonal and interprofessional relationships.

Therefore, the process of care planning and maintaining records of nursing care, whether this is a nursing document or a document incorporating the interventions of the multidisciplinary team, is an expression of the interpretation, analysis and outcomes of nursing interventions which is legally binding.

Other important elements of the care planning process include:

- The standard of record keeping
- The quality of nurse–nurse reporting
- The accessibility of nursing records for the multidisciplinary team.

THE NURSING RECORD

There has been much criticism and concern over the quality of the written nursing record or care plan, particularly since the late 1970s, when the nursing process shaped the design of the nursing record. It is not unusual to see the Health Service Commissioner's (Ombudsman) report cite nursing records as being poor, either because they are scant or because they contain inappropriate information.

Nurses are frustrated by the challenges of record-keeping. Elaborate records are not the answer. Specific factual, accurate and focused care plans are needed.

It is a duty of the nurse to maintain accurate records about the care delivered (UKCC, 1993). The UKCC (1993) states that records should:

> '1 Provide accurate, current, comprehensive and concise information concerning the patient or client and associated observations.
> 2 Provide a record of any problems that arise and the action taken in response to them.
> 3 Provide evidence of care required, interventions by professional practitioners and patient or client responses.
> 4 Include a record of any factors (physical, psychological or social) that appear to affect the patient or client.
> 5 Record the chronology of events and the reasons for any decisions made.
> 6 Support standard setting, quality assessment and audit.
> 7 Provide a baseline record against which improvements or determination may be judged.'
>
> (UKCC, 1993, page 3)

The quality and accuracy of care plans depends on the quality of the assessment process undertaken. Assessment is not simply an activity undertaken during the initial contact with a nurse; it is an on-going process which allows data to be built on and a broad understanding of a patient's circumstances to be developed. It should always be undertaken and supervised by a registered nurse, midwife or health visitor.

The King's Fund (Macguire, 1993) made the following recommendations for nursing records:

> 'whatever the form of record, it should allow for:
>
> - a clear statement of current problems
> - a statement of current capacities

- significant observations
- changes in a patient's condition to be recorded
- changes in instructions to be entered
- entries showing that care has been delivered
- entries evaluating care'

(Macguire, 1993, page 16)

Other standards include:

- All entries should be signed and dated
- All entries by learners/students should be countersigned by a registered nurse
- All entries should be in ink
- Mistakes should be deleted with a line and initialled and Tippex, etc., should not be used
- All records of care for a patient should be kept together
- All records should be legible
- All records should be up to date, i.e. changes should be recorded as soon as possible
- All records should be unambiguous; therefore accurate details, instructions, frequencies and limits should be stated, e.g. 'push fluids' should be replaced by, for example, 'fluid intake: 1500 ml in 24 hours'
- All records should be accessible
- The nursing record is a confidential record and access to it may be restricted. Consent from patients should be gained before those other than paramedics, doctors and nurses have access.

Key Points

- Care plans are the responsibility of all nurses.
- There are standards which must be maintained relating to record-keeping.
- Professional, legal and policy issues influence the quality of care planning processes.

CONCLUSION

This chapter has examined a range of issues which impact on the quality of nursing care and clinical practice. It closes with some thoughts and ideas for you to consider. In an attempt to understand your potential contribution to nursing and health care, it is necessary to consider your place in the much larger scheme of things. Remember, and try to accept, the enormous part you play in the lives of those you care for. You have the power to involve, and be involved with, those who are vulnerable, in need and often fearful and ignorant of what is happening to them and around them. These feelings are true for nurses too; they need to be acknowledged, accepted and worked with, so as to allow greater understanding of the realities of caring. Continue to learn and be receptive to the teaching and skills of others. Use resources like this book, the research undertaken by others and theoretical sources to enhance your own ideas, expertise and practice. Go on learning from those around you – especially the people you care for. They offer the greatest insight into the approach to care they need. The rest is up to you.

REFERENCES

Benner, P. (1984). *From Novice to Expert: Excellence and Power in Clinical Nursing Practice*. Addison-Wesley, New York.

Benner, P. and Tanner, C. (1987). Clinical judgment: how expert nurses use intuition. *American Journal of Nursing*, 87, 23–31.

Bowman, G.S. and Thompson, D.R. (1995). In *Towards Advanced Nursing Practice*, Schober, J.E. and Hinchliff, S.M. (eds). Arnold, London.

Brearly, S. (1990). *Patient Participation. The Literature*. Scutari Press, Harrow.

Campbell, V. (1984). *Moderated Love*. SPCK, London.

Carper, B.A. (1978). Fundamental patterns of knowing in nursing. *Advances in Nursing Science*, 1, 13–23.

Chinn, P.L. and Jacobs, M.K. (1991). *Theory and Nursing: a Systematic Approach*, 3rd edn. Mosby, St Louis.

DHSS (1977). *The Extended Role of the Nurse*. HC(77)22. HMSO, London.

Dimond, B. (1990). *Legal Aspects of Nursing*. Prentice Hall, London.

DoH (1991). *The Patient's Charter*, HMSO, London.

DoH (1993). *A Vision for the Future*. HMSO, London.

ENB (1991). *The Professional Portfolio*. ENB, London.

Fawcett, J. (1993). *Analysis and Evaluation of Conceptual Models of Nursing*, 2nd edn. F.A. Davis, Philadelphia.

Griffin, A.P. (1983). Philosophy and nursing. *Journal of Advanced Nursing*, 5, 261–72.

Hampton, D. (1994). Expertise: the true essence of nursing art. *Advances in Nursing Science*, 17, 15–24.

Harrison, L.C. (1990). Maintaining the ethic of caring in nursing. *Journal of Advanced Nursing*, 15, 125–27.

Helson, H. (1964). *Adaptation Level Theory: an Experimental and Systematic Approach to Behaviour*. Harper and Row, New York.

Henderson, V. (1969). *Basic Principles of Nursing Care. The Nature of Nursing. A Definition and its Implications for Practice, Research and Education*. ICN, Basel.

Henderson, V. (1979). Preserving the essence of nursing in a technological age. *Nursing Times*, 75(20), 12.

HMSO (1997). *Nurses, Midwives and Health Visitors Act (1997)*. HMSO, London.

Hunt, J. (1981). Indications for nursing practice: the use of research findings. *Journal of Advanced Nursing*, 6, 189–94.

King, I.M. (1981). *A Theory for Nursing: Systems, Concepts and Process*. New York, Wiley.

Lindblom, C. (1959). *The Science of Muddling Through*. Open University Press, Milton Keynes.

Macguire, J. (1993). *A Handbook for Nurse to Nurse Reporting*, 3rd edn. King's Fund, London.

McMahon, P. and Pearson, A. (eds) (1991). *Nursing as Therapy*. Chapman & Hall, London.

Mayeroff, M. (1972). *On Caring*. Harper and Row, London.

Menzies, I. (1960). *Social Systems as a Defence against Anxiety*. Tavistock Publications, London.

Nightingale, F. (1860). *Notes on Nursing: What it is and What it is Not*. Dover Publications, New York.

Orem, D.E. (1984). Personal correspondence. In *Nursing Theorists and their Work*, Marriner, A. (ed.), Mosby, St Louis.

Orem, D.E. (1985). *Nursing: Concepts of Practice*, 3rd edn. McGraw-Hill, New York.

Orem, D.E. (1995). *Nursing: Concepts of Practice*, 5th edn. McGraw-Hill, New York.

Peplau, H.E. (1952). *Interpersonal Relations in Nursing*. Putnams, New York.

Peplau, H.E. (1988). *Interpersonal Relations in Nursing*, 2nd edn. Putnams, New York.

Rambo, B.J. (1984). *Adaptation Nursing: Assessment and Intervention*. W.B. Saunders, Philadelphia.

Redfern, S.J. (1995). *The Meaning and Practice of Individualised Patient Care in Nursing. Research Highlights and Implications for Action*. King's College, London.

Rogers, C. (1967). *On Becoming a Person*. Constable, London.

Roy, C. (1984). *Introduction to Nursing: an Adaptation Model*. 2nd edn. Prentice Hall, New Jersey.

Roy, C. (1989). Adaptation models. In *Nursing Theorists and their Work*, Marriner, A. (ed.). Mosby, St Louis.

RCN (1987). *A Position Statement on Nursing*. RCN, London.

Schrock, R. (1981). Philosophical issues. In *Current Issues in Nursing*, Hockey, L. (ed.). Churchill Livingstone, Edinburgh.

Selye, H. (1978). *The Stress of Life*. McGraw-Hill, New York.

Simon, H.A. (1950). *Administrative Behaviour*. Macmillan, New York.

Statutory Instrument (1989). *The Nurses', Midwives' and Health Visitors' Rules Approval Order*. HMSO, London.

Steele, S.M. and Maraviglia, F.L. (1981). *Creativity in Nursing (and other Professions)*. Slack, Thoroughfare, New Jersey.

Stockwell, F. (1972). *The Unpopular Patient*. RCN, London.

UKCC (1992a). *Code of Professional Conduct for the Nurse, Midwife and Health Visitor*, 3rd edn. UKCC, London.

UKCC (1992b). *The Scope of Professional Practice*. UKCC, London.

UKCC (1993). *Standards for Records and Record Keeping*. UKCC, London.

UKCC (1996a). *Guidelines for Professional Practice*. UKCC, London.

UKCC (1996b). Register No. 17. UKCC, London.

UKCC (1997). *PREP and You*. UKCC, London.

WHO (1977). *The Nursing Process*. Report on the First Meeting of a Technical Advisory Group. WHO, Geneva.

FURTHER READING

Benner, P. and Wrubel, J. (1989). *The Primacy of Caring: Stress and Coping in Health and Illness*. Addison-Wesley, New York.

Key aspects of caring for specific client/patient groups are analysed, making this a valuable source of patient-centred details.

Brykczynska, G. (ed.) (1997). *Caring. The Compassion and Wisdom of Nursing.* Arnold, London.

A comprehensive collection of chapters focusing on a range of issues central to nursing care, e.g. ethical and spiritual issues, emotional aspects of caring and patients' experiences of care.

Hugman, R., Peelo, M. and Soothill, K. (1997). *Concepts of Care, Developments in Health and Social Welfare.* Arnold, London.

A four part book which examines a broad range of care issues ranging from theoretical perspectives to contemporary issues relating to the organisation and management of care in practice.

Perry, A. (ed.) (1997). *Nursing. A Knowledge Base for Practice,* 2nd edn. Arnold, London.

A comprehensive collection of chapters written by nurses for nurses, covering a wide range of issues relating to the biological, psychological and sociological aspects of caring.

Schober, J.E. and Hinchliff, S.M. (1995). *Towards Advanced Nursing Practice. Key Concepts for Health Care.* Arnold, London.

A comprehensive text which analyses key concepts associated with the delivery of nursing care, e.g. the individual and strategies for organising care.

CHAPTER TWELVE

SPIRITUALITY

David J. Stoter

- Spirituality, spiritual need and spiritual care
- The nurse in partnership in spiritual care
- The patient in the partnership
- Providing special facilities for spiritual care
- Other issues influencing spiritual care

This chapter aims to explore the concept of spirituality, and ways in which a spiritual basis is an essential component for nursing practice and care. It takes the reader on a journey of personal discovery in developing spiritual awareness, as part of the process of addressing the spiritual needs of patients. A framework for this spiritual component is built up progressively as the reader is invited to reconsider relevant issues including:

- An introduction to the concepts of spirituality, spiritual need and spiritual care, as distinct from religious need and care
- The carer's resources, personal spiritual awareness and needs, skills and experience
- The nurse's role in the caring team, responsibility for spiritual care
- The partnership between patient and nurse – journeying together
- Assessing the patient's spiritual needs and response to illness, loss and recovery, and special situations. Understanding the needs of ethnic and religious groups
- The need for supportive care for the nurse
- The underlying core of spiritual care.

SPIRITUALITY, SPIRITUAL NEED AND SPIRITUAL CARE

THE CONCEPT OF SPIRITUALITY

The concept of spirituality is an elusive one and defies easy definition and this is evident in the range of different approaches expressed by interested writers. It is a concept of particular interest to those who are concerned with the care of individuals, in sickness and in health.

The holistic approach to health care is considered to be important, as it recognises the physical, social, emotional and spiritual aspects of human need. It is, however, the spiritual dimension which is most often misunderstood, and therefore is easily overlooked. Many nurses find it difficult to offer spiritual care appropriate to a patient's needs, partly because there is a lack of guidance and support for them in this aspect of their work. The first step therefore, is to explore the nature of spirituality, spiritual need and to define spiritual care.

THE NATURE OF SPIRITUALITY

The Oxford dictionary is not helpful here, as most definitions tend to perpetuate the traditional associations of spirituality with religion. However it defines 'spiritual' as 'pertaining to the spirit of man', and later refers to spirit as the 'vital principle of man' or 'breath of life'. Taken as a starting point this indicates it is part of the human personality. It both integrates and infiltrates the other three aspects of the personality and is most clearly illustrated in Figure 12.1 below (Stoter, 1995a).

The spiritual dimension can thus be seen as a unifying force, integrating and uniting the other three dimensions of personality. It gives meaning to life as it enables a quest for meaning, and for exploration of the eternal questions about life, reality and the search for identity. It is often expressed through a person's values, beliefs and practices, and in particular it is expressed through relationships. It is therefore vital for nurses to have an understanding of this concept in establishing a good relationship with the patient in the process of nursing care.

Every individual, then, has a spiritual dimension to the personality. Some may be unaware of this capacity, and for some it may be associated with religious rituals, beliefs or behaviours. Not everyone has a religious dimension but everyone has a spiritual dimension, and therefore spiritual need is universal.

THE UNIQUENESS OF THE SPIRITUAL DIMENSION

Spirituality is influenced by the range of life experiences and background a person has, in the same way as the other three dimensions encompass the range of life experiences. It follows that the way in which spirituality is expressed varies with cultural and personal background and beliefs (Labun, 1988).

The nature of influences upon personality is frequently unrecognised in the debate about spirituality and is thus not seen as relevant. It is clear that a person's place of birth can affect religious and cultural practices and outlook and can, therefore, influence his or her spirituality. What is less often recognised is the effect of family background, environmental influences and particularly education and work experience. These areas have a strong relationship with the individual's personal values, self-esteem and approach to major life events.

Family influences are particularly strong, such as the quality of bonding relationships in early years in forming the capacity to love and to be loved. Happy and unhappy events in marriage, and bereavement, for example, are important as is the quality of support given at these times. Clearly, these and many other influences are wide-ranging and vary from one individual to another in their impact on the personality and the way in which they experience and approach life events. It is therefore clear that the nature of a person's spirituality is a unique capacity shaped response in all situations. It is influenced by life experiences, ranging from birth, through the quality of the home environment and family life, to social class and culture. This particular journey through life influences the development of personal attitudes to caring, love, work, life and death and therefore the way the person responds to the needs of others or to life events.

Other writers have echoed this wide-ranging approach to the nature of spirituality. Narayanasamy (1993) says there is no single authoritative definition of spirituality. Some have described it as a 'process' or a 'sacred journey' (Mische, 1982) or 'a belief that relates a person to the world' (Soeken and Carson, 1987). Others describe it as a 'unifying force'. Most writers are agreed that nurses need a thorough understanding of spirituality if they are to offer holistic care. Burkhardt and Nagai-Jacobson (1994) emphasise the need for nurses to have an awareness of their own spirituality, as this is important for expressing spiritual care in practice, and for being attentive to their own personal needs, taking time for themselves to care for their own health and well-being.

SPIRITUAL NEED

It follows from the discussion above that spiritual need is universal, but this need is not always

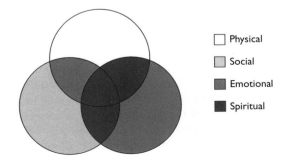

Figure 12.1 The nature of the spiritual dimension

- ☐ Physical
- ☐ Social
- ▦ Emotional
- ■ Spiritual

recognised by individuals. It is important to differentiate between 'human need' and 'human wants' in this context (Stoter, 1995; Farmer, 1996), to establish the understanding and recognition of need in relation to spiritual care.

The fact that spiritual need is so often unrecognised and unexpressed calls for a particular sensitivity on the part of nurses, and requires special skills which are outlined later in this section. The basic spiritual need for each individual is to be accepted and valued for what he or she is. People need to be accepted in terms of previous life experiences, or their values and beliefs – whatever they are, and to be respected and heard on those grounds. This acceptance may involve the carer in sharing the range of emotions the patient experiences, together with areas of confusion and doubt, where the real need is to find a meaning and purpose in the situation and to discuss the way forward or the way to acceptance.

Satisfaction of spiritual need is found in different ways, sometimes within a particular religious faith, through sacraments or worship. It may be through special groups, practices like music, meditation or other therapies or simply through a supportive caring family or relationships. The important issue here is that every individual is unique in needs and expression of these needs. It is also necessary to distinguish between spiritual and religious need, which is just one component of spiritual need.

Understanding the concepts of spirituality and spiritual need is basic to explaining the wider implications of spiritual care, seen as a central component of nursing care.

SPIRITUAL CARE

'Spiritual Care is Anchored in the Ordinary . . . it includes very ordinary things.'
(Report of a Working Party, 1991, page 153)

Spiritual care is not an optional extra to the clearly recognised aspects of health care. It is an integral component of care for all patients, clients, families and staff. It has to be given proper weighting in the assessment of a person's need, and given as much consideration as all other areas of care. It is as important to respond to 'dis-ease' as it is to respond to the disease or malfunction itself.

Spiritual care is a response to basic spiritual need as it arises from the disease or occasion itself, and also from the impact of the symptoms on the individual person. It is also interrelated with other aspects of the person's life, both immediate and past. When someone has experienced bereavement earlier in life, maybe the death of a partner or close friend, if the grief has not been resolved at the time, facing a similar incident may well be a trigger that brings that pain to the surface.

Scenario

Helen, a second year nursing student, a confident, sensible and mature person who took responsibility in her stride, was developing into a competent nurse. A sudden change in her behaviour worried her colleagues as she was showing signs of preoccupation and carelessness. When approached by a colleague she admitted to feeling depressed and puzzled by her own behaviour and readily accepted the offer of discussing this with a counsellor. It emerged that her father had died several years previously and her mother was grief stricken and distracted and Helen had had to shoulder the burden of family responsibility since she left school. The recent death of a patient, for whom she had cared for some time, had brought some of these painful memories to the surface and her unresolved grief meant the pain had to be dealt with. Once the trigger was identified and the grieving process was allowed to take place she soon regained her confidence.

Through this process Helen learned a great deal about the experience of loss, which increased her understanding of the needs of her patients and relatives, and enabled her to stand by others in times of stress and bereavement.

Spiritual care is required to help the person to respond to the effects of treatment given, for example, the provision of care to a person struggling with the impact of radiotherapy. To respond effectively requires an analysis and understanding of what spiritual care really is. The confusion between spiritual and religious care tends to lead to a blurring of definitions and perpetuates difficulties in building a body of knowledge through research in this subject. However, there is evidence of increasing attention in the literature and attempts through exploration to provide more clarity of understanding, particularly for health care providers (Burkardt and Nagai-Jacobson, 1994; Farmer, 1996).

Spiritual care involves responding to the uniqueness of the individual, responding to statements from the very core of the person, whether spoken or unspoken, facilitating the process of search for identity, without a judgemental or dogmatic approach.

Journeying together

Each person involved in the process of giving spiritual care is at a particular point in a personal spiritual journey through life and each individual has a unique way of responding to the exposure to particular events in life. Nothing is ever static, but always changing, and relationships are dynamic and constantly moving. Spiritual care can therefore be described as a response to spiritual needs and the uniqueness of the individual and the particular situation. Spiritual care is focused around the needs of the client or patient, and is offered in the context of a relationship. The patient, not the care giver, defines the territory to be explored (Feifel, 1986), so the carer's approach is through coming alongside the patient and sharing the journey at whatever point the individual has reached. The patient has little choice about the starting point, being caught up in the circumstances of the illness, whereas the carer has the power to choose whether to enter into sharing the journey or not, and has the ability to put parameters in place or to choose to leave that particular journey. The mutual purpose of that journey is to move through a partnership relationship towards recovery or death. It may involve the carer in stepping aside from the place reached in his or her own personal journey for the time being, to walk with the patient at a different pace and in a different direction.

For those of us who are carers in any profession it means starting from where the patient or client is and being willing to allow the itinerary to be set by that patient or client. The process of this journey may well lead to uncharted territory, especially as each time the carer leaves the arena for a while and then returns, the journey is resumed at a different place from where it broke off, and the horizons may have changed. For example, the patient may have had news of a change in treatment or prognosis since last meeting the nurse, or may simply have moved on in his/her thinking.

Religious care

Religious care is often confused with spiritual care, but it is just one aspect of spiritual care in the attempt to meet spiritual needs. Religion can be described as the 'arena' of faith in practice through affiliation with a particular group, church or culture. There are often specific practices or rituals relating to a particular faith; therefore, nurses need to have a sensitivity to cultural and religious differences when planning and delivering care.

Whilst everyone has a spiritual dimension and spiritual needs, recognised or unexpressed, not everyone identifies with a particular religion and some may have stronger identifications than others. Whatever the situation, it is important to recognise the strength of the patient's convictions and the nature of practices to be observed.

> **Key Points**
>
> - The concept and nature of spirituality – there is a wide range of definitions and approaches.
> - The spiritual dimension is unique to each individual, and is influenced by life events and experiences.
> - Spiritual need varies between individuals, hence the importance of a good assessment (see page 282 for an assessment plan) before planning a spiritual care programme.
> - Religious care is only one component of spiritual care.

THE NURSE IN A CARING RELATIONSHIP

The nature of nursing places nurses in a unique position where spiritual care is concerned. Nurses spend more time in close contact with patients than any other professional carer and the nature and quality of nursing care is based very much on the 'partnership' aspect of a relationship with the patient. Partnership implies an aspect of 'being with' or 'staying by' a patient rather than 'doing for' a patient, and being there on equal terms. In this particular situation it is for a limited period and within a particular context, which requires a commitment from the nurse to 'stay with it' (Stoter, 1991; Bayntum-Lees, 1992).

One of the first steps in establishing a relationship of trust with a patient is through offering 'hands-on care' to ensure physical comfort is achieved, and the patient is put at ease. Some very basic considerations may help – for example, ascertaining how the patient wishes to be addressed – not all patients are comfortable with the familiarity of using first names. The skill of helping a person to be comfortable is a powerful tool and its simplicity should not undervalue it as a key to excellence in nursing practice.

Metropolitan Anthony Bloom (1965) talks of the capacity to 'just sit with someone' saying and doing nothing, but 'going so deep in sympathy and compassion that your presence speaks'. This is a presence that puts an emphasis on being rather than doing (Report of a Working Party, 1991).

This relationship is a meeting of two minds – a meeting between equals, where the patient's perspectives and objectives take priority. Sometimes this equation can be reversed, when reinforcing the self-esteem of the carer takes prominence. Any form of proselytising or moral blackmail on the part of the carer is clearly unacceptable and unhelpful.

Spiritual care requires a relationship of trust between the individuals involved. For the carer to come with a 'ready-made package' labelled 'spiritual care' devalues the patient's personal contribution, and denies the opportunity to explore and achieve new learning experiences from the process. Carers need to be prepared to accept the patient's personal agenda and to go in step with the patient's chosen pace if a true partnership is to be developed. A caring relationship requires a 'meeting of equals', and this is a fundamental concept to be observed by nurses involved with spiritual care (Wade, 1995). This idea of 'partnership' is open to a range of misinterpretations among carers. Bayntun-Lees (1992), in a study on nurses, showed how difficult it was for many carers to take this partnership concept into their own belief system, even though they could see it was ideal.

So often there is little attention given to the patient's participation in the caring process. Research in 1989 demonstrated that very often the care plan could underestimate the wishes of the patient in the choice of care or treatment given. (Owen *et al.*, 1989). Bayntun-Lees (1992) comments on the lack of literature available on the partnership relationship, and attempted to rectify this by reviewing the existing literature (see further reading). It is clear that the 'partnership' concept has a wide range of interpretations, in spite of the recognition of its importance as a basis for care, and again shows that nurses still find difficulty in incorporating this concept for attitude change, and in understanding the importance of self-awareness.

Within a reciprocal relationship there is a delicate balance between mutual equality and power or control, and a trusting attitude is important for this relationship to work. Muetzel (1988) pointed out that some patients prefer to have decisions made for them and this too must be respected. Muetzel also presented a useful model of a relationship which described the factors involved in the partnership relationship, and the encounter between nurse and patient. The model shows partnership, intimacy and reciprocity as three major factors involved and these are linked in a triangular relationship and influenced by the atmosphere of the situation, the nature of the personalities and the dynamics of the relationship. (This is expounded more fully in context by Bayntun-Lees, 1992.) Thus the carer's approach to meeting spiritual need requires a wide range of professional skills to be brought into the situation.

The critical review by Wade (1995) examined the research on this subject in detail and supported many of the observations made previously, demonstrating that even though the ideal is now widely accepted in theory, in practice there are many difficulties not yet resolved. For example, successful partnership empowers the patient and this may make the nurse feel threatened by the loss of authority, especially where the patient's views differ from the professional advice. Alternatively, some patients may not wish to be involved in that partnership relationship, and some older people may wish to remain in a dependent relationship. Another constraint occurs when there is pressure to 'get the work done' which allows the carer little time for listening. Wade concludes that 'the partnership in care concept is derived almost solely from the perspective of health care professionals'.

Nurses who are prepared to enter this kind of relationship need very special skills in listening and sensitivity, as discussed later, but also need to be aware of their own vulnerability, in terms of staying with the patient and family in meeting the pain of suffering and loss, which calls for a high level of commitment.

Key Points

- Spiritual care is offered as an integral part of the total care plan for a particular patient.
- It takes place within the context of a relationship, and on a partnership basis.
- The nurse, to be effective, needs a sense of self-acceptance, knowledge and awareness and a willingness to 'journey' with the patient.

THE NURSE IN PARTNERSHIP IN SPIRITUAL CARE

The nurse is clearly a 'major resource' as one of the participants in a relationship where spiritual care is concerned and the patient is the other main resource, and other members of the family and caring team will be involved with either the nurse or the patient from time to time. Each person brings something different into the process, which creates a dynamic and changing scenario.

THE NURSE AS A RESOURCE

The process of offering spiritual care demands a depth of personal awareness, self-development and considerable courage, and can expose the nurse to considerable vulnerability, and at times a feeling of helplessness which may be overwhelming. The nurse, however, brings a range of personal resources into the situation, and each has a unique resource in his/her personal qualities and life experiences, together with professional education and skills to bring to this role. It is often forgotten that professional carers are individuals and therefore influenced by similar life experiences in the same ways as any patient is. Most will have lived as part of a family group within a particular cultural environment where personal values and beliefs have been established. Each personality is shaped by this unique combination of circumstances and this brings a unique resource to the situation. The processes of early bonding and primary socialisation play an important part in the capacity to establish relationships in later life (Storr, 1981). Each person also brings differing degrees of insight, intuition, self-awareness and sensitivity, some of which are inherent in the indi-

vidual and some of which can be enhanced by professional development and the acquisition of skills.

Self-knowledge and acceptance

To be effective in spiritual care a nurse needs to have a sense of self-acceptance and self-knowledge, together with an awareness of the effects of cultural background and personal values and beliefs or attitudes to spiritual care. Clarification of personal perceptions will give confidence to the nurse, and awareness of possible areas where he or she may feel threatened or need clarification. To be effective, the carer needs to be in touch with his or her own feelings and beliefs and secure enough to stand aside from these without imposing them on others, who should be allowed to have their own views. Burkhardt and Nagai-Jacobson (1994) point out that:

'Awareness of one's own spirituality and intentionally caring for one's own spirit are important components in the process of integrating spirituality into clinical practice.'

Reflection Points

A useful developmental exercise for any nurse involved with spiritual care is to consider and write down personal views, values and beliefs on the questions set out here. This can be done individually or within the setting of a support group or with a colleague or friend with whom one can feel comfortable discussing these issues. Views may change as experience and insight is gained:

- Why do people suffer? Is there any value in suffering – if so what is it?
- What is the meaning of life, is there any purpose in it?
- Where do I find a basis for my values and beliefs?
- What are my fundamental beliefs and values?

Some of these questions are fundamental to considerations of ethical issues; knowing or clarifying one's personal views helps to identify the influences that have shaped them and to acknowledge any areas of uncertainty and confusion.

PERSONAL SKILLS

Skills and qualities specific to an individual nurse contribute to effective spiritual care, but in addition there are many valuable skills which can be acquired through practical learning situations and experiences. These include various aspects of:

- Communication skills (these include such things as eye contact, touch and the written word)
- Verbal skills
- Listening skills
- Interpretative skills
- Observation skills
- Reflective skills
- Coping skills.

A good exercise, as a starting point, is for the carer to write down and identify personal individual attributes and resources before reading any further. Often, when a group of professionals is invited to do this exercise, there are blank looks around and a response of stunned silence. Individuals need encouragement to accept that they have valuable gifts and skills to bring to a situation. The tendency is to offer a list in 'textbook' jargon and to overlook really valuable basic life skills.

Reflection Points

This exercise invites you to reflect on, identify and write down your own personal attributes and skills – again they can be considered as a personal exercise or followed through within a group. It is useful to keep the results and repeat the exercise a few months later and observe how the answers have changed.

Reflect on the following:

- Write down a list of your personal attributes and qualities you bring to the situation.
- Identify some of your strengths and weaknesses.
- Think about and identify your special skills, particularly those acquired through professional education.
- Consider the above lists and identify the areas where you would benefit from further tuition or support.
- Recognise and write down the areas where you have particular strengths which could be shared with others.

Communication skills

Communication skills embrace a range of other skills and involve a great deal more than simply talking to a person or passing on information. They are a vital component in establishing the quality of relationship required in spiritual care. Communication is a complex process involving a wide range of interrelated skills, all of which are ultimately involved in the assessment of spiritual need and the delivery of spiritual care.

The three main components to consider in relation to these skills are:

- The source of communication or the person initiating the process and the message
- The message or communication to be shared
- The recipient or person receiving the communication.

The process is not a simple one, as it involves variations in these three elements for it to be received and understood as intended. For example, the initiator and recipient of the message may have very different perceptions and expectations of life and outcomes of illness, which can be coloured by personal hopes and fears, as against the realities of life. Language and culture clearly are strong influences in this situation. An obvious example here is where there are language difficulties. Another example frequently occurs when there is unpleasant news which is completely rejected and unaccepted because the patient is paralysed by fear.

Communication skills include elements of many other skills to a greater or lesser extent. The overall intention is to get the most effective response. They include elements of listening and verbal skills and, in particular, interpretative and coping skills, and involve use of all the senses, all within the context of a good partnership and the ambience of a comfortable and safe setting.

Listening skills

Listening skills can be acquired through teaching and understanding. Listening involves hearing what the patient is expressing not only in words, but all forms of expression. Listening involves hearing what is not being said, for at times what is not being said is more important than what is being said. It means hearing and interpreting the pain expressed through the eyes, through denial or anger or through touch and is an important aspect of assessment. Listening often requires just staying with the patient when there are no answers – perhaps judging when it is appropriate to help him/her to move on, by use of a further simple question or restatement of what has been said.

Verbal skills

Verbal skills, although often perceived to be most important in communication, are at their most effective when combined with the range of other communications described here. Jargon, strong accents or language difficulties may present obvious and basic challenges. These can be especially noticeable where spiritual and religious care are concerned. Jargon may also impede communications between professional carers involved together in spiritual care and interpreters are not always helpful within the caring relationship, where the carer must always be acceptable to the patient.

The use of questions

Questions are an important aspect of verbal skills which require a special kind of skill in spiritual care. Open questions which do not suggest the nature of the answer are helpful here. For example, 'what sort of journey did your visitors have today?' allows a natural opening to talk freely about the family and friends. Probe questions such as 'have you thought any more about the suggestions we looked at last week?' should be used discreetly when a mutual relationship is established with a sense of trust. The patient may need help to carry this further and to accept a plan of action when ready.

Sometimes more searching questions are used as part of a spiritual assessment, relating to the patient's attitude towards life and its meaning or illness. These need to be used with discretion by experienced assessors, once confidence has been gained and within an open relationship. In fact, an experienced nurse may often provide the answers from her own observations without using intrusive questions.

Responding to questions presents considerable difficulty for some, especially when the carer knows there are no answers the patient wants to hear. Simply expressing the question may sometimes be all that is needed. When it is accepted and heard, the patient often feels able to answer it personally, and the carer is then able to stay alongside while the implications are digested. Professional carers need special preparation for skills of

this kind, and this can often be achieved through training in specific skills and the development of self-awareness and self-knowledge, including personal beliefs and values.

Another key area in communication is observation skills using the senses and this will be dealt with in more detail in the section on assessment.

Interpretative skills

Interpretative skills and reflective skills are largely acquired through experience and practice and are very important in terms of assessing spiritual needs.

Example

Lucy was an elderly lady who was meticulous in her dress and personal behaviour and had displayed a stoical approach to her illness and to pain and suffering. She found difficulty in articulating her needs and had an 'old-fashioned' respect, often seen in her generation, for doctors and nurses. When questioned directly she would put on a brave front and say emphatically she was 'very well thank you' and never complained of symptoms.

It was noticed that her denials became increasingly adamant, even though evidence of a progressive tumour was apparent. Understanding and observation of her responses to information led the staff to realise that this emphatic denial hid a deep-seated fear of admitting she was intensely scared of physical mutilation and was suffering from a deep-seated guilt related to her body and fears of retribution for her 'sinful past'.

A careful observation of these signs enabled staff to recognise the nature of her distress and to 'hear' what was *not* being said, and gently to 'give her permission' to share her fears and to accept her condition and to be accepted as she was.

Lucy never learnt to say exactly how she felt, but unspoken messages often passed between them as her carers learnt to meet her on her own territory and to recognise her needs and offer spiritual care in ways acceptable to her. Interpretative skills played a vital part in Lucy's case.

ASSESSMENT SKILLS IN SPIRITUAL CARE

Assessment skills for spiritual needs are important in preparing a care plan and a detailed framework can be found in Stoll (1979), Burkhardt and Nagai-Jacobson (1994) and Stoter (1995a). Any assessment involves the use of a range of skills outlined above, including all the senses which will supply valuable information and need careful recording. This can be done within a framework such as that set out under 'A framework for assessment', below, which may be modified by a particular organisation to suit specific needs.

Sensory skills may have a dual function in that they are often used as part of the healing process for their therapeutic effect as well as for guiding a diagnostic spiritual assessment. They are, for many experienced nurses, part of the armoury of nursing practice skills and include:

- Visual skills – eye contact is an important communication skill, at the same time as it is recording aspects of the patient's condition or response.
- Hearing is similarly an observational and diagnostic skill and an important aspect of listening skills. It is also important to be able to register the quality of silence when there is an absence of or delay in a response. Noticing the quality of voice and speech production may register fear, anxiety or contentment.
- Perceptive skills include use of all the senses to observe the real person and the real need, in addition to what may be spoken, and these skills are also required for a nurse to be aware of her own response.
- Touch, as when registering a patient's condition or response to a situation, is used to convey support and concern. Touch is a key component of therapies, such as reflexology and massage in aromatherapy.
- Observation skills, which include all the above, when combined with perception facilitate the assessment of need.

A framework for assessment

It is clear that there are many basic skills and tools which are useful in an assessment framework, the purpose of which is to give a comprehensive picture of the patient's spiritual need and to allow for questions to emerge.

Several models have emerged for guidance, the best known of which is Stoll's guide for spiritual appraisal, which seeks to explore the situation under four main headings:

- The person's concept of God or deity
- The person's sources of strength and hope
- The significance of religious practices and rituals
- The perceived relationship between the client's beliefs and his/her state of health (Stoll, 1979).

Stoll also outlined specific questions under each of these areas which can be found in a paper by Narayanasamy (1996) and used as a problem-solving approach. Burkhardt and Nagai-Jacobson (1985) also offer a variation on the direct question approach to assessment.

Such models need to be used with caution, however, and more as a guide to the ultimate goal. To approach a sick person with explicit questions of this kind may be too daunting for many, or inappropriate for their religious or ethnic background.

Much of the information required for assessment can be gathered imperceptibly by the use of observation and conversation skills in the process of treatment and thus a picture can be built up gradually without embarrassment or pressure for the patient.

Framework for assessment of spiritual need

A useful framework for assessment of a person's spiritual needs should include observation in the following areas:

- Cultural and environmental background
- Ethnic origin
- General health – including prognosis and treatment
- Mental and emotional well-being
- Relationships within the family and the nature of support from family and friends
- Perception and awareness of his/her condition
- Hopes, fears and expectations
- The person's concept or view of themselves
- The person's support mechanisms or access to external support
- The person's views and beliefs relating to the situation
- Past significant life experiences
- The person's openness and receptivity to help
- Any stated religious beliefs.

Different health care institutions or departments are likely to have different methods of recording on this subject and may develop their own systems, so this assessment may be used as a guide to the kind of observations that are useful. Responses from patients may vary considerably, those who are more articulate being able to formulate well formed responses; but for others the nurse may have to be sensitive to hear what is really being said or implied and precision may be difficult. The goal is to build up a general picture of needs for that individual.

Reflection Points

- Take time to reflect on your particular skills and gifts which you bring to a partnership situation.
- Identify your natural gifts in this situation. Identify the skills you have acquired through experience or training.
- Decide which are strengths and weakness and which of these aspects could be improved.
- How could you make better use of your strengths, and develop the areas where you are less strong?

THE NURSE'S ROLE IN SPIRITUAL CARE

It is clear that nurses have a key role in providing spiritual care. The days when such care was seen as religious care to be passed on to a priest or religious leader are past. The concept of holistic care emphasises the importance of a balance in providing care for all dimensions of the personality. However, in a busy setting where staff carry a heavy workload, the 'doing' aspect of caring takes precedence over 'being' with the patient. Nurses often feel inadequately prepared for this role in spiritual care (Ross, 1994), which calls for a high degree of maturity in a situation which may become threatening (Narayanasamy, 1993).

For this reason, nurses need to understand the concept of spirituality, be aware of their own spiritual needs and be able to recognise spiritual concerns within themselves and their patients and to handle questions about the meaning of life, of purpose, of loss and the importance of belief and value systems. It is very tempting to say to the patient 'I understand how you feel', a particularly unhelpful response as no-one knows how another feels. It is not easy to give permission for the patient to express feelings of terror, fear and anger and to stay with the person entering into that pain – to stay there until he or she comes through to find hope, acceptance or a new way forward in a situation where bland reassurances can only be insincere or trivialise the situation.

Nurses are not alone in providing spiritual care. Everyone who is part of the caring team has a responsibility at some point or another. Sometimes one member of the team may emerge as the right person for a patient at a certain point in time, and that team includes the patient's family and friends, who may be very supportive. Sometimes the patient may prefer not to be too close to family but might prefer a professional carer to share the situation.

The team can also play a supportive role for nurses as well as patients, and the nurse needs to be able to recognise his or her own needs for support and understanding in a situation where patients can be demanding, and to be able to share the situation with others.

Key Points

- There are special skills which contribute to effective spiritual care.
- Communication skills are important and include a range of other skills, such as listening, verbal and interpretative skills.
- Assessment skills also rely on a range of interpretative skills, and an assessment framework provides useful guidance.
- Nurses have a key role as a resource in offering spiritual care, within the professional team.

THE PATIENT IN THE PARTNERSHIP

THE PATIENT'S SPIRITUAL NEED

Patients, like everyone else, have a spiritual dimension, though not every patient is aware of these needs which will be expressed in many different ways. It is important to remember that patients are exposed to a particular experience in becoming a patient, and they are therefore responding to that situation. The experience involves changes in roles and expectations, and it may involve a degree of dependency, which is inherent in an uncertain and unknown situation.

Responses to this situation vary considerably, as some patients express feelings, fears and doubts very openly; others are quiet, or tentative, hiding their innermost doubts and fears. Patients come from a variety of family situations and have lived through many different life experiences which influence the way they respond.

This is where the partnership relationship is particularly important for the nurse seeking to be sensitive to the reality of spiritual need, however it is expressed. The family also needs to be considered, as they too may feel bewildered and scared and this will affect the patient's response. A useful discussion on the 'sick role' can be found in Cox (1982).

THE PATIENT'S RESPONSES IN THE SPIRITUAL CARE PARTNERSHIP

Nurses will be taking in a broad picture of the effect of suffering, pain and other new experiences on patients and noting how such events affect the very core of the being, hopes and expectations of life. They will observe all the effects of suffering in terms of its part in causing 'dis-ease' to the person, rather than just dealing with the disease. There is evidence available which shows there is a relationship between a person's beliefs, values and spiritual awareness and the nature of the recovery to health (Levin, 1994).

We have seen how carers respond in different ways to the need for spiritual care, and in the same way patients respond to life events and illness differently, as a result of differences in personality and life experiences. However, a range of patterns is commonly found in responding to certain situations, such as the way a person responds to grief or trauma. Responses are also determined by the kind of situation faced and the nature and quality of relationships between those involved. The kind of response from a parent losing a child may differ considerably from that of a child losing a parent. The shock of sudden loss or unexpected bad news is likely to manifest itself differently from bereavement that has long been expected. Thus, it follows that the nature of spiritual care given is likely to require different approaches, and the use of different skills from the nurse.

In a partnership the common experience all patients have is that of being a patient. There are various theories and models relating to the nature of the sick role, one well-known example being found in Parsons' (1951) concept of the sick role. This describes the way in which patients have cer-

tain expectations relating to their rights and responsibilities, expectations that treatment and care will be given, and that doctors, nurses and other professionals will offer the necessary treatment – in other words, patients expect to be cared for. Conversely, the patient is expected to behave responsibly, to seek care and, for example, to trust doctors and carry out their advice.

This concept can be fraught with difficulties, especially where patients and their carers have different understandings and perceptions of what is possible or what is reality, or where patients' apparent response to illness is different from how they really feel about it (Friedson, 1975). Nurses also have differences in how they perceive their roles in relation to the patient, for example the partnership concept, where the patient is seen as a member of the caring team and with a right to have a say in the nature of the care given, may be new to some carers (Owen et al., 1989; Bayntun-Lees, 1992).

It is important for carers to be familiar with the range of different responses likely to be encountered in the role of 'being a patient', so that appropriate skills, or other team members, can be introduced into the situation. The important underlying principle is always to 'be with' or 'watch with' the patient – a principle expressed by Dame Cicely Saunders in Hospice Care. There are various other useful theoretical approaches relating to patterns of response, such as Kubler-Ross's description of the process of dying (1969) or bereavement (Parkes, 1975).

Theories and models such as these can be a very useful guide when used as a frame of reference or as an example of what might be expected, but it must be remembered that individuals are unique and may respond differently – dying, for example, is a very personal experience.

Figure 12.2 illustrates the nature of the dynamics involved in the partnership relationship and hence in the wider concept of spiritual care.

THE NATURE OF THE RESPONSE TO SUFFERING

For a nurse to assess spiritual need accurately it is important to recognise the nature of the patient's response to identify the real need. Nurses are well aware of the variations in response to pain, for example, how different patients manifest their dis-

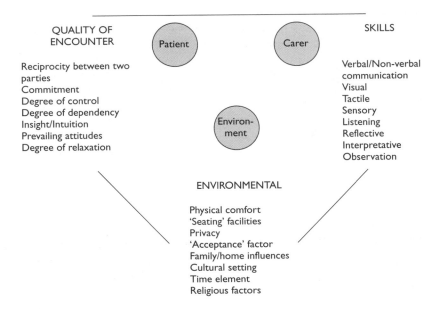

QUALITY OF ENCOUNTER

Reciprocity between two parties
Commitment
Degree of control
Degree of dependency
Insight/Intuition
Prevailing attitudes
Degree of relaxation

SKILLS

Verbal/Non-verbal communication
Visual
Tactile
Sensory
Listening
Reflective
Interpretative
Observation

Patient   Carer

Environ-ment

ENVIRONMENTAL

Physical comfort
'Seating' facilities
Privacy
'Acceptance' factor
Family/home influences
Cultural setting
Time element
Religious factors

Figure 12.2 The dynamics of spiritual care. Factors involved in a partnership relationship in spiritual care

tress. Loss, whether potential, sudden or expected, is a common factor that carers meet and is inherent in most distressing situations encountered by nurses. It may be loss of a partner, child or friend, or there may be physical loss. The process of coming to terms with loss is a very personal one and related to the uniqueness of that person. There is a powerful backward focus on the past and what has been lost and a desperate pain for what can no longer be. With time many patients respond positively, with new determination, and develop fresh perspectives on life, whereas others may find only despair and feelings of mutilation. The carer needs to be able to walk alongside, in step with the patient at a manageable pace. Some examples found in most forms of suffering include:

- Responses to pain and suffering, physical and emotional
- Responses to loss in any of its many forms
- Responses to change in circumstances and life expectations
- Responses to changes in relationships
- Responses to sudden shock or trauma.

The nature of the response, as already indicated, will vary considerably. This is, therefore, a very complex one for nurses who have to be prepared to receive a range of different responses which can include any of the following:

- Anger and violence
- Antagonism – physical and verbal abuse
- Disbelief and refusal to acknowledge reality
- Withdrawal, suppression, despair and possibly depression
- Lack of cooperation
- Paralysis and inability to act, which comes with fear and anxiety
- Acceptance and acknowledgement
- Adaptation and a positive approach.

Any of these can be evident to a greater or lesser degree and some can be very distressing to nurses attempting to meet spiritual need. This is where nurses themselves need acceptance, support and encouragement and due consideration of their vulnerability.

Scenario

An incident was described in the press where a nurse was physically attacked by a patient on a Friday afternoon and went home very scared and shaken. She returned on Monday morning to find herself reassigned to the same patient with no attempt to ask how she felt about this, or to discuss her fears or her own approach. This was clearly a situation demanding more backup from the ward staff and consideration of sensitivity towards the nurse's experience.

So the range of feelings experienced may be expressed in, or through, a wide range of behaviour patterns, many of which are normal and expected. It must be remembered, however, that patients are unique in their personality and experiences and respond to suffering with the whole being, and so no response can be totally anticipated or ignored. For example, an unusual quietness, indifference or lack of response may indicate a person is shattered, stunned or totally repressing the fear.

Other influences may affect the nature and degree of response – nurses will be familiar with the variations in patients' responses to the severity of pain, for example, where patients have different pain thresholds. Alternatively, responses can be influenced by cultural attitudes, if it is expected that grief should be loudly expressed or where a stoical response is considered the norm. All these factors influence the nature and degree of the patient's manifest response to illness and suffering, and clearly this is a complex process, many factors overlapping.

Reflection Points

- Describe ways in which you are most likely to respond to suffering and pain.
- Can you identify any major life events or influences which contributed towards your likely response?

This reflection may be carried out in a group situation or on an individual basis, whichever is most comfortable to you.

One practical way of meeting this kind of spiritual need is through recognition of some of the most specific causes of suffering mentioned above and where particular circumstances can call for a special provision of care. For example, the arrival of a stillborn infant can be anticipated and a special service provided, offering help from staff equipped with special skills and experience. Another example is obvious in the care of patients who know they face a limited lifespan and that long-term incapacity may lie ahead. Certain responses can be anticipated to some extent and special facilities can be built into the caring services to meet these needs.

Key Points

- The patient responds to care within the context of a caring relationship.
- Response varies according to the nature and degree of suffering experienced.
- Response is also influenced by the individual's own personal experiences.
- Some responses are similar in any painful situation, and whilst a pattern in specific situations can often be observed, nurses need to be prepared for a range of variations.

PROVIDING SPECIAL FACILITIES FOR SPIRITUAL CARE

Areas needing special skills or provision of specific spiritual care can thus be found in many situations including:

- Paediatrics, infant deaths and the care of sick children
- Midwifery and obstetrics, including areas like miscarriage and stillbirth, or a malformed baby
- Accident and emergency where sudden trauma calls for special skills
- Major disasters where a well-planned support system, with debriefing and support facilities is needed for staff and victims
- Intensive care, where distressed relatives will need much special care
- Bereavement and loss in its many forms and varieties – the loss of a spouse, child or parent
- Loss of body image and communication
- Long-term illness or disability
- The effects of recovery, rehabilitation and changed circumstances
- Illness in special situations, such as mental health and illness, community care, HIV and AIDS care, alcohol and drug abuse.
- The needs of the family and relatives.

This list is by no means exhaustive but does give a picture of the particular areas where special skills are often required, and increasingly where specialist care is available, through skilled staff and special services.

NEW PERSPECTIVES FOR THE PATIENT

Once diagnoses and treatment are complete, new adjustments to life may well be needed by the patient and family, and this introduces a different phase of spiritual care. For some it may mean the highly personal experience of facing impending death, when questions will be asked and dilemmas ahead will have to be faced. Here the exploration of deeper feelings and fears must be facilitated to allow time and space for the patient to set a personal agenda. Where the nurse responds with openness, the patient is enabled to retain control over the process. It helps if the carer is familiar with and understands the likely expressions of grief, accepting that individuals respond very differently.

It is important to recognise that provision of spiritual care in response to need is a very complex process, meeting, as it does, a complex response to suffering and manifestation of needs in a range of different ways. There are certain principles common to *all* aspects of spiritual care provision, but additional skills are valuable in many areas to meet special situations (a full discussion on these issues can be found in Stoter, 1995a, Chapters 8–15).

Key Points

- Other issues influencing spiritual care include the identification of religious needs and specialist facilities.
- Resources include the family and friends and local community backup and support.
- Resources are found in other team members.
- Staff care is an important component.
- Good spiritual care is an important facet of nursing care.

OTHER ISSUES INFLUENCING SPIRITUAL CARE

MEETING RELIGIOUS NEEDS

Religious need is one of the more obvious elements of spiritual care, especially in the present multi-cultural and multi-faith society. Practical provision is often made for multi-faith needs through the Chaplaincy Department, but nurses will need to have a sound knowledge of cultural and ethnic influences and the practices which affect the care of patients of differing faiths or religions.

Scenario

Most nurses will be aware of differences in dietary needs between different religions, also of requirements for procedures at death. However, it helps to have a more detailed knowledge of customs and rituals. For example, it is important to recognise that Sikhs have very binding food restrictions and prohibitions, and that the dagger is worn as a symbolic representation of readiness for self-defence. The dagger symbol may be worn as a brooch – even in bed or at night – and its removal will cause acute distress for a sick person and his or her family. For Hindus, washing hands and mouth after meals is considered essential, as is a place to be alone for meditation.

These examples are indicative of a wider range of varieties found in a multi-faith society, and often their recognition makes great demands on the nursing staff and provision of practical facilities. This is an area where the acquisition of a knowledge base is an important component of understanding spiritual needs and offering care (Neuberger, 1987).

THE NURSES' ATTITUDES AND APPROACH

The approach to recognising religious needs may be problematic where nurses themselves hold strong convictions. This can present difficulties, for example, if a nurse is asked to enable a patient to practise a ritual unacceptable to the nurse's faith. Enabling does not, however, indicate the carer's agreement with a practice. The only exceptions to this principle are where practices are dangerous to an individual or contrary to law.

Other difficult situations may arise where the issues concerned relate to controversial ethical situations, which pose questions and dilemmas for the patient, family and carer alike. Sometimes several choices are presented, all equally unacceptable, which relate to moral issues. These involve a range of criteria which are available to help in the process towards a painful decision. A knowledge base is always helpful where several choices are involved, but there is often no definite answer which suits everyone and the views, rights and needs of all individuals concerned have to be considered, together with the patient's preferences if known. Where there are no clear cut rules that can be applied, guiding principles have to be observed, such as preserving the patient's dignity and quality of life. The participants will need further care even after decisions are made, especially where feelings of guilt may be involved.

RESOURCES IN SPIRITUAL CARE

Clearly, it is not possible to 'label' spiritual care as the responsibility of one particular person or professional. There are different professionals involved closely with the patient at different stages in treatment. There may well be overlap between roles and this demands recognition of the aims and objectives of care. Nursing staff, it must be repeated, have a major contribution to make, and confidentiality is an aspect which requires trust, understanding and agreement. Confidentiality may present difficulties at times within the staff team, or between staff and family, when a patient raises issues that require consultation. It is helpful for the team to have a recognised agreement on ways to handle any such situations. This also highlights the value of having the patient involved in any discussions on planning care.

The family will be an on-going resource to be considered in many instances, and may need help from one of the many appropriate support groups in existence. There may be a need for continuous counselling or support, extending after the patient has been discharged, and local community services, friends, neighbours and groups can be useful resources.

MAINTAINING THE NURSES' RESOURCES

At various points in this chapter reference has been made to the resources needed and available for staff providing for spiritual care, in what is obviously a complicated process. The first resource is possibly found in colleagues wherever care is delivered, and through other members of the team. But in many of the demanding situations such as those described here a nurse may

have other needs, and provision for these needs should be built into the general staff support system of the organisation, and be made known to each member of staff (for full information on this subject see Stoter, 1997).

Apart from the fact that nurses require informed preparation for spiritual care from their own education department, they need to be able to seek support at the time of need, and appropriate to their own staff development needs. Often this is best given in the work situation by an experienced colleague.

Scenario

Anna was a young nurse in her first year of training, and was approached one day by the staff nurse with:

'Mr Brown in the last bed on the left, has just died, please will you go and prepare him for the mortuary?'

As Anna moved behind the screens, Alison, a third year student nurse nearby, caught sight of her frozen look, as looking at the body, Anna's face drained of colour. Alison followed behind the screen and asked:

'Are you OK – or do you need help?'

Anna replied: 'I know what to do – but I've never seen a dead person before! I'm petrified.'

Alison responded: 'You prepare the trolley and I'll come and *work* with you.'

This she did, chatting in a relaxed way and as procedures were completed she said:

'Come with me into the staff room and we'll have a cup of coffee together and go over what we've just done and how you feel now.'

Anna felt free to explore her panic in a friendly and permissive atmosphere, and so work through her fears and gain confidence, because someone was there on the spot, to listen.

There may be personal issues relating to ethical or moral difficulties, problems of guilt or feelings of inadequacy which arise from the nurse's own experiences or belief. These can be helped through a staff support group, or through reference to a sympathetic counsellor or chaplain, or a friend or colleague externally.

Employers have a responsibility to provide adequate support care, but often this is imposed, *after* the crisis and comes 'too little and too late'.

A good example involving patients, families and staff care can be seen in the ideal approach to a major disaster debriefing and support service, where the system is 'in place' all the time and staff may use the facilities when needed. The need for staff care is often overlooked in long-term patient care, when spiritual demands are often greatest and most demanding for staff and can, if ignored, precipitate post-traumatic stress disorder symptoms (Stoter, 1995b).

Reflection Points

- Identify the sources of staff support in your workplace. These may be a service, e.g. Occupational Health or Chaplaincy Department, or may be a person, e.g. colleague or friend.
- Outline the kind of staff support which could be useful in your own workplace.
- What could you contribute personally to this area of care?

If nurses are to offer high quality spiritual care in hospital or community, attention must be given to their own staff support provision and the caring ethos of the organisation as a whole. Staff who understand their own spiritual needs will offer understanding to patients.

Summary and Conclusion

The breadth of these issues affecting staff care and the quality of patient care reflect the complexity of the nature of spiritual need and that which constitutes spiritual care. A wide range of approaches to this subject and its definitions is prevalent today and further discussion can be found in Farmer (1996). There is a need for yet more clarity and sharpening of perceptions on the subject.

The provision of good spiritual care is clearly an integral part of nursing and health care, from any perspective, and requires a wide range of ingredients and interaction. To be effective it should offer a basis for continuing the journey which does not end once the carer leaves the scene. The successful process grows from the fundamental premise that each patient or client is a human to be respected and accepted as he/she is, with the right to retain and express personal views, beliefs and practices as long as this does not cause offence to others. It requires from the professional the willingness to respect, value and enable these beliefs and practices, even though they may be alien to the professional's own beliefs and practices. This needs the maturity and confidence not to feel compromised by such enabling, and a caring and supportive environment and culture for both patient and professional.

To quote Tschudin:

'... listening with the whole person ... is right at the heart of a helping relationship. By listening we give ourselves to that person at this moment, which is no more and no less than required if we want to help anyone.'

(Tschudin, 1982, page 41)

REFERENCES

Bayntun-Lees, D. (1992). Reviewing the nurse patient partnership. *Nursing Standard*, 6(42), 36–9.

Bloom, A. (1965). Suffering. *Hospital Chaplain's Magazine*, 1(1).

Burkhardt, M. and Nagai-Jacobson, M. (1985). Dealing with the spiritual concerns of clients in the community. *Journal of Community Health Nursing*, 2(4), 191–8.

Burkhardt, M. and Nagai-Jacobson, M. (1994). Reawakening spirit in clinical practice. *Journal of Holistic Nursing*, 12(1), 9–21.

Cox, C. (1982). Sociology. *An Introduction for Nurses, Midwives and Health Visitors*. Butterworth, London, Chapter 8.

Farmer, D. (1996). *Exploring the Spiritual Dimension of Care*, Mark Allen Publishing, Salisbury.

Feifel, H. (1986). In quest of the spiritual component for the terminally ill. Foreword in *Report of the Proceedings at Colloquia at York University*, York.

Friedson, E. (1975). Dilemmas in the doctor/patient relationships. In *A Sociology of Medical Practice*, Cox, C. and Mead, A. (eds). Collins, Macmillan, London.

Kubler-Ross, E. (1969). *On Death and Dying*. Macmillan, New York.

Labun, E. (1988). Spiritual care: an element in nursing planning. *Journal of Advanced Nursing*, 3, 314–20.

Levin, J. (1994). Religion and health: is there an association, is it valid, and is it causal? *Social Science and Medicine*, 38(11), 1475–82.

Mische, P. (1982). Toward a global spirituality. In *Whole Earth Papers*. No. 16. Global Education Associates, East Orange, New Jersey.

Muetzel, P. (1988). Therapeutic nursing. In *Primary Nursing in the Burford & Oxford Nursing Development Units*, Pearson, A. (ed). Croom Helm, London.

Narayanasamy, A. (1993). Nurses' awareness and educational preparation in meeting their patients' spiritual needs. *Nurse Education Today*, 13, 196–201.

Narayanasamy, A. (1996). Spiritual care of chronically ill patients. *British Journal of Nursing*, 5(7), 411–16.

Neuberger, J. (1987). *Caring for Dying People of Different Faiths*. Austen Cornish Publishers, London.

Owen, G.M., Crouch, P. and Wadey, A. (1989). *A Study of the Marie Curie Community Nursing Service*. Marie Curie Memorial Foundation, London.

Parkes, C.M. (1975). *Bereavement Studies of Grief in Adult Life*, 2nd edn. International Universities Press, New York.

Parsons, T. (1951). *The Social System*. Routledge and Kegan Paul, London.

Report of a Working Party (1991). The impact of hospice experience on the Church's ministry of healing. *Mud & Stars*. Sobell Publications, Oxford.

Ross, L. (née Waugh) (1994). Spiritual care: the nurse's role. *Nursing Standard*, 8(29), 33–7.

Soeken, K.L. and Carson, V.J. (1987). Responding to the spiritual needs of the chronically ill. *Nursing Clinics of North America*, 22(3), 603–11.

Stoll, R.I. (1979). Guidelines for spiritual assessment. *American Journal of Nursing*, 9, 1574–7.

Storr, A. (1981). *The Integrity of the Personality*. Penguin Books Ltd, Harmondsworth.

Stoter, D.J. (1991). *Spiritual Care in Palliative Care for People with Cancer*, Penson, J. and Fisher, R. (eds). Arnold, London.

Stoter, D.J. (1995a). *Spiritual Aspects of Health Care*. Mosby, London.

Stoter, D.J. (1995b). *Reflections on Response to Disaster Situations. Hindsight Brings New Perspectives to Preparation*. NASS Occasional paper No. 9. NASS, Woking.

Stoter, D.J. (1997). *Staff Support in Health Care*. Blackwell Science, Oxford.

Tschudin, V. (1982). *Counselling Skills for Nurses*. Baillière Tindall, London.

Wade, S. (1995). Partnership in care: a critical review. *Nursing Standard*, 9(48), 29–32.

Suggestions for further reading

Farmer, D. (1996). *Exploring the Spiritual Dimension of Care*. Mark Allen Publishing, Salisbury.

Kubler-Ross, E. (1969). *On Death and Dying*. Macmillan, New York.

Neuberger, J. (1987). *Caring for Dying People of Different Faiths*. Austen Cornish Publishers, London.

Stoter, D.J. (1995). *Spiritual Aspects of Health Care*. Mosby, London.

Stoter, D.J. (1997). *Staff Support in Health Care*. Blackwell Science, Oxford.

CHAPTER THIRTEEN

ETHICS, MORALITY *and* NURSING

Verena Tschudin

- Beliefs, attitudes and values
- Ethical models
- Rights and responsibilities
- Making ethical decisions
- Some ethical issues concerning patients
- Some ethical issues concerning nurses
- Accountability
- Conclusion

This chapter offers the reader the opportunity to explore principles and theories of ethics and morality. The chapter aims to lead the reader from an exploration of the relationship between personal attributes, attitudes and ways of thinking to making ethical decisions.

The chapter includes discussion of:

- Ways of determining values, attitudes and beliefs, including nursing values
- Ethical models such as deontology, teleology and response ethics, and ethical principles such as the value of life, goodness, justice, truth and individual freedom
- Codes of practice, including the *Code of Professional Conduct* (UKCC, 1992) and *Guidelines for Professional Practice* (UKCC, 1996a)
- Ways of making ethical decisions. Examples relating to nursing are included to illustrate the application of theories and principles
- Ethical issues concerning patients and nurses which include reference to informed consent, confidentiality, trials, conscientious objection and 'whistle-blowing'
- Professional values, including accountability and autonomy, are briefly explored in the latter part of the chapter.

Ethics and morality are concerned with good and right, and being good and doing right. The theoretical study of ethics and morality is therefore *what* and *who* is good and right, who says so, and on what basis. Morality tends to be the domain of the *personal* good and right, and ethics of the *social* good and right. These two aspects necessarily overlap and complement each other.

One way of expressing the personal experience of good and right has traditionally been through the practice of virtue (e.g. prudence, courage, cleanliness, constancy). The more common expression nowadays would be holding certain values (e.g. being creative, having certain experiences, holding particular attitudes). Whichever language or concept a person prefers, what is involved is something chosen and acquired, held as relevant and acted upon. Because of such values or virtues, a person is able to relate to another, at a level which is nurturing and helpful. A person without virtues or values tends to be unstable, shifty, rebellious 'unprincipled' or 'phoney'. It is easy to see that the whole of our society can be described in these terms and that increasing attempts to return to basic morality are made by governments, education, the churches, and many single-issue campaigns, such as changing gun laws.

To be good personally and do right is not enough. Down the ages, philosophers such as Socrates, Kant and Mill have wrestled with the problem of what holds society together, and what *should* hold it together. Is it possible to legislate for morality? For example, a person's sexual morality may lead to illness; does the state then pick up the bill without question? How a child is brought up may be the couple's personal choice, but how does society deal with such problems as parental abuse, neglect, inadequacy and delinquency?

The study of ethics is not only for those with time and opportunity to speculate. It is acutely relevant to those, like nurses, with a 'hands-on' job and often little time to make life and death decisions. The challenge and difficulty of ethics is that it demands reason and reasoning against a setting of human frailty and vulnerability, of feelings and relationships which are stronger than will and mind. It is not in overlooking or avoiding one or other aspect that a decision can be reached or a stance taken; it is through listening, empathy and personal experience of conflict that we come to a decision, a sense of meaning and a capacity to help.

BELIEFS, ATTITUDES AND VALUES

Not only do different societies hold different values; each person holds unique values which differ from other people's and which change through time. To know our own values means that we are more able to live with other people's values, and not expect them to conform to our own.

BELIEF

Belief is the most basic of the values a person holds. It is based more on faith than fact. A person may believe that all people are basically honest; that the earth is good to live on; that the

economy will come right; that the National Health Service (NHS) will survive. There is evidence against all these, but, nevertheless, the belief can survive and drive a person to act according to that basic belief.

ATTITUDES

Out of belief come the attitudes which we hold about ourselves and others. The person who believes that people are basically honest treats all others as honest people and is honest with them. One of that person's attitudes may be to promote honesty. An attitude is not only something of the mind, but something which shows itself in action, particularly in the attitude to those around us. Attitudes are mostly evident in the way we interact with others, creating the 'atmosphere' in places. Examples include respect, dignity, being easy-going; and contempt, being taken for granted and carelessness.

VALUES

Our values are less fixed and more dynamic than either beliefs or attitudes. There is generally an element of motivation or goal in our values. A child's highest value may be to play, an adolescent's, peer relationships. Young adults may be concerned with security in partnership and work. The 'mid-life crisis' is often characterised by drastic changes of values.

Society, background, upbringing and training all shape our values. Our temperament shapes our values, too. An extraverted person will want to be with people, to be at the centre of atttraction, and is happiest in a large ward with plenty going on around. An introverted person gets most energy from being alone, will shun parties, and will be content with solitary occupation. A typical example may be an elderly patient not mixing much with other patients in a ward, perhaps quite content with reading, prescribed antidepressant medication because nurses believed her to be depressed because of her quiet behaviour.

The psychologist C.G. Jung (1964) recognised four different 'functions' by which people orient themselves through experience:

'*Sensation* (i.e. sense perception) tells you that something exists; *thinking* tells you what it is;

feeling tells you whether it is agreeable or not; and *intuition* tells you whence it comes and where it is going.'

(Jung, 1964, page 49)

A person who is more sense-oriented values facts and experiences, is practical and down-to-earth. A person who is attuned to intuition, on the other hand, lives in anticipation, will see possibilities, and functions best with imagination and ingenuity. A thinking type of person prefers to make decisions on the basis of principles and analysis and will therefore often be a good judge, but may come across as cold and calculating. A feeling person will often work in a caring profession, and be working towards harmony, be devoted to people and look for humane and workable solutions. The Myers Briggs Type Indicator (MBTI) – a psychometric questionnaire to determine a person's personality type – is based on these 'functions' (Briggs Myers, 1980).

Keirsey and Bates (1984) recognised another area where temperaments differ – that of judging and perceiving. 'Do I prefer endings and the settling of things or do I prefer to keep options open and fluid?' Given a deadline, a judging person (the word refers more to 'being orderly' than to making judgements) will 'get the show on the road', whereas a perceiving person tends to 'wait and see' what may develop.

This thumbnail sketch of different temperament types will give an idea of the vastness of possible values held by different people. Being of a certain temperament does not mean that a person cannot change; on the contrary, personal growth demands that we become at home in all functions. This is one area where values change and vision is expanded.

Table 13.1: Values

We *have* different values because of our different temperaments:
■ Extravert – Introvert
■ Sensing – Intuiting
■ Thinking – Feeling
■ Judging – Perceiving
We *discover* different values by:
■ Doing a deed (creative values)
■ Experiencing the value (experiential values)
■ Suffering (attitudinal values)

Another way of knowing and learning the values which we hold is through experience. Frankl (1962, page 101) speaks of three types of values:

1 *Creative* values, which we discover through what we do, particularly helping others
2 *Experiential* values are those which we discover through appreciating people, events and artistic and natural beauty
3 *Attitudinal* values are discovered through our reactions to circumstances over which we have no control, such as our own and other people's sufferings (see Table 13.1).

Frankl is specific on two more points: we do not *create* our values, but we *discover* them; and values do not *push* us, but they *pull* us.

NURSING VALUES

The basic personal and temperamental values are expressed through the work or profession someone chooses. Someone with strong person-oriented values is more likely to go into nursing than someone attracted by history and battles, or botany and the outdoor life. The overriding value in nursing must be care: the giving and receiving of caring. All health care worker care, and therefore what is meant by care and caring, needs attention. The practice and the wider significance of the term can vary widely.

The Canadian nurse-philosopher M. Simone Roach (1992) has distilled her thinking on caring into five component parts (Table 13.2). She believes that 'caring is the human mode of being' and that to be truly human is to care. A sick person is restored to health through care; and someone desperately needy is often restored to a sense of well-being by caring for someone yet more unfortunate. This is also an example of how creative, experiential and attitudinal values are discovered.

The component parts of caring all start with the

Table 13.2: The 'Five Cs' of caring

Compassion
Competence
Confidence
Conscience
Commitment

letter C. Compassion is the act of meeting the other where she or he is, and where it hurts. It is a kind of standing alongside, 'being there', not explaining and not identifying but allowing oneself to be touched by one's own vulnerability. This requires listening and hearing what a person is saying, in order to act compassionately, i.e. 'with passion'.

To act compassionately, and correctly, a person has to be competent. A nurse has to be skilled, but more than that. Giving an injection or doing a dressing can be done quite mechanically; doing it in such a way that the patient feels valued as a person is what signifies competence.

That sort of competence instils confidence. Caring is only effective when it is rooted in a relationship which is trusting, respecting and creative. Caring is not arbitrary but is guided by human values. Conscience is the expression of relationships and responsibilities and is the moral awareness of responsibilities to self and others.

None of this would be possible without a commitment to the person, task or cause in question. The nurse has made a commitment to the patient, and the patient or client is now in a relationship with the nurse which is based on a kind of contract, and also on the nurse's compassion, confidence and conscience. Being personally committed is not only ideal for patients and nurses, but sometimes also difficult, especially when, for whatever reasons, optimal care may not be possible, or relationships are abruptly ended due to transfer, duty rotas or changes in the patient's condition.

This highlights and describes what is generally known as an 'ethic of care'. An ethic of care emphasises the human, feeling and relationship aspects and is often seen to constitute the balance to an 'ethic of justice' which is based more on logic and reasoning. An ethic of care is said to be a feminine approach to ethics, while an ethic of justice is a masculine approach, the latter being seen as the medical approach, and the former as that of nursing (Gilligan, 1982). These divisions are disappearing, as both approaches acknowledge the need of the other, and research shows that nurses and doctors, men and women, use both approaches in different situations (Rickard *et al.* 1996), largely occasioned by how close to or far away from the actual person they are (Norberg and Udén, 1995).

Key Points

- Morality and ethics are based on certain values held individually and as a society.
- Beliefs, attitudes and values are held deeply but can (and sometimes must) change.
- Nursing values stem from caring and how this is practised.

ETHICAL MODELS

Many nurses believe that ethics is something difficult, 'bookish', which has little to do with them and their everyday practice. But while they rush to a patient whose intravenous infusion has stopped, another patient calls for a bedpan. Who gets their attention first? An ethical decision will have been made, but on what basis?

With more holistic and patient-centred care, nurses are rightly drawn into case discussions and their views are considered and valued. It is important in all situations to see the issues clearly, to listen carefully to all sides, and to combine reason – rational, theoretical arguments – with emotion – feelings, intuitions and compassion.

Traditionally, two overall models of ethical theory have been described: deontology and teleology. The theories are not meant to be used exclusively, but are more philosophical approaches to help and guide decision making.

DEONTOLOGY

The word *deontology* comes from the Greek *deontos* meaning duty. This theory argues that there are basic duties and obligations which people have. An action is not judged by its consequences, but is either right or wrong depending on whether it agrees with a moral principle or goes against it. Our actions are morally valid if we follow those rules and principles. The main question for deontologists is, 'What *ought* to be done in this situation?'

In the summer of 1996 there were many examples in the press of ethical issues where the public discussion ranged wide:

- A woman who was expecting twins had one fetus aborted because she considered that she could cope with one child, but not with two

- A woman was pregnant with eight fetuses and was unwilling to have them aborted. She had 'sold' her story to a newspaper and was potentially to receive a large sum of money if she could give birth to live babies
- 3000 frozen embryos were destroyed because the law only allowed them to be kept for a certain length of time
- A woman wanted to be inseminated with sperm taken from her husband after he had died unexpectedly. She was refused *in vitro* fertilization (IVF) on the grounds that her husband had not given written consent.

Each of these situations sparked intense discussions in the media. Considered from the point of view of deontology, the people concerned, and those attending them, needed to ask what they *ought* to do, i.e. what their duty was in each case.

TELEOLOGY

Teleology (from the Greek *telos*, end, result) considers an action in view of its consequences. Utilitarianism is a form of teleology which is based on the principle that an action is right if it brings the greatest happiness to the greatest number of people. An action is therefore morally right if its goal is what matters. A historical duty or obligation has no influence in this theory. The main questions are, 'What is the goal?' and 'Is the outcome good?'

Viewed in this light, the various scenarios mentioned above do not depend on duty, but on the outcome of the actions. Thus the woman who had one fetus aborted should presumably be happier at the end because her action (the abortion) meant that she could cope with one child. Similarly, the woman who was expecting eight babies was right not to have them aborted because her goal was to care for them with the money which she was potentially able to receive because of her decision.

The concept of the NHS rests largely on utilitarian principles: to provide health care and treatment for all at the time of need is more desirable than to provide it only for those who can pay, or deserve it.

OTHER APPROACHES

With these two theories largely opposing each other, it is not surprising that other approaches

have been established. *Natural law ethics* is one such theory, taking as its starting point the human rights: the right to life, liberty, happiness, etc. Any interference with bodily functioning is considered a violation of natural law. *Situation ethics* was popular in the 1960s and 1970s. This postulates a person-centred approach rather than principle-centred ethic, and the main thrust is to embrace human creativity, encouraging all that contributes to personal life and freedom (Fletcher, 1967). A further notion, that of *response ethics*, has been put forward by Niebuhr (1963). This approach stresses the meaning of responsibility. The main question posed by this method is not what ought to be done, or what is the goal, but, 'What is happening?' The answer given – the answer made – is based on the responsibility each party has to the other.

This theory rests on the premise that what we have in common is our humanity. In order to stay human (personally) and within humanity (socially) we have to act humanly. How we interpret that humanity colours our actions. Niebuhr stresses that we are creative and responsive human beings, and to remain human we have to be creative and responsive within a framework of freedom and fidelity. Roach's 'Five Cs' of caring fit particularly well into this approach to ethics.

FIVE ETHICAL PRINCIPLES

The above theoretical models are rather abstract. To use them on a day-to-day basis would involve a much deeper knowledge of their intricacies. In order to make these theories accessible, people have established sets of *principles* which need to be considered when making ethical decisions. One such set of principles is outlined by Thiroux (1995) and they are outlined in Table 13.3. These principles are applicable to all walks of life but they can be adapted to suit particular spheres, such as nursing.

The principle of the value of life

Thiroux starts with the principle of the value of life. What we all have in common is life; without human life there would be no 'goodness or badness, justice or injustice, honesty or dishonesty, freedom or lack of it' (Thiroux, 1995). Although we all have life, we each experience it in a way

Table 13.3: Principles of ethics

> The principle of the value of life
> - Human beings should revere life and accept death
>
> The principle of goodness or rightness
> - We should strive to be 'good' human beings and attempt to perform 'right' actions
>
> The principle of justice or fairness
> - Attempts must be made to distribute the benefits from being good and doing right
>
> The principle of truth telling or honesty
> - Meaningful communication – an absolute necessity in any moral system and any moral relationship – depends on truthfulness and honesty
>
> The principle of individual freedom
> - Individuals, with individual differences, must have the freedom to choose their own ways and means of being moral *within the framework of the first four basic principles*

that is unique. This principle is analogous to the notion of 'respect for persons' of other systems (Beauchamp and Childress, 1989). Whenever such terms and concepts are used, one has to ask further, 'What do we mean by life, by respect, by personhood?' It is immediately obvious that there are no black-and-white answers. It also becomes obvious that because of our individuality we all experience these concepts differently and use and apply them differently. When talking with colleagues and patients, we should therefore be wary of assuming that they use the term in the same way as we do. We see this immediately when we look at only one infringement of this principle: abortion.

A person's experience and values will influence his or her view of this subject. One person may see abortion as killing and murder, and wrong without any doubt. Another may argue that a fetus who is not capable of independent life is not a person, or at least not yet. 'Respect for the person' may not only mean that we do not take life, or do not interfere with another's life, but that we do not impose our views on another. Thus we see that this principle of the value of life is the basis not only for decisions about abortion, euthanasia, war, suicide and capital punishment, but also for such concepts as patient advocacy, responsibility and accountability.

By life is not meant 'life at any cost'. In revering life, and the person who has life, we also accept that this life must some day end. With the ever-increasing debate about euthanasia, nurses will be confronted more and more with debates about and requests for euthanasia. On what grounds, then, does a nurse decide what to say and do? We need to have insight and awareness of our own values, feelings and understanding of the facts to be able to argue a case.

The term 'value of life' is used by Thiroux to indicate that 'life' covers more than human life. The traditional term is 'sanctity of life', but this applies only to human life. With increasing awareness of global and planetary life, human life is no longer seen as the pinnacle of existence. In debates about euthanasia, quality of life is more important than quantity, and with xenografts becoming possible, the use of animal life for human purposes is also taking on greater importance.

The principle of goodness or rightness

Morality and ethics are concerned with what is good and right, and what is bad and wrong. But what is good or acceptable when one person holds one set of values and another person holds others? The emphasis which has been put on differing values is reflected in this dilemma. The American Declaration of Independence lists three such 'goods': 'life, liberty and the pursuit of happiness'. Some people may argue that the pursuit of happiness is egoistical, and that a greater good would be the pursuit of truth for knowledge or peace or creativity. 'Good' cannot simply apply to abstract terms. Any good or right that we do is 'good' or 'right' in the context of human experience and in human relationships.

It can be argued that good and right are ideals, and that in daily life there are many times when we fall short of the ideal. This has been recognised particularly in medicine, where it is impossible only ever to do good. For many reasons, treatments and care are often second or third best. In acknowledging this, medicine has established the principle of non-maleficence (i.e. doing no harm). This may seem a negative approach, but it is one that accepts the frailty of human beings and their systems (see 'The principle of justice or fairness', below). Gillon (1986) suggests that:

'we seem to have . . . a perfect duty to all other people not to harm them. On the other hand, we do not have a duty to benefit all other people.'

(Gillon, 1986, page 81)

If goodness and rightness are ideals to strive for, then they can also be seen as calling forth the practice of virtue. Such practice of virtue leads not to smug self-satisfaction, but to creativity, harmony and integration in and between people.

The principle of justice or fairness

Good and right do not only have to be done, but they have to be seen to be done. Where there is harmony and integrity between people, there is also justice. What happens between two people should also happen between societies and nations. By justice is here meant distributive (not retributive) justice. If those with a lot of money would give it to the poor, then the poor would become happy because everybody would then be equal. This is a simple utilitarian argument which has never worked in reality. The basic values of both sides are different, and simply 'giving to the poor' is not respectful of their needs or values. Such paternalistic scenarios are, however, still prevalent, not least in medicine and nursing.

Within health care, the principle of justice or fairness is perhaps the most often quoted principle, as well as the most often violated and idealised. The concept of the NHS is that everybody who needs care or treatment gets it at the time of need. The assumption is that the government, the health authorities, and all with influence on the purse-strings of health care, should ensure that this ideal is upheld. In the present climate of cutbacks, savings and rationalisation, this principle gets quickly distorted or disregarded. It becomes a case of fighting and saving what one can, and priorities are decided not on the basis of who deserves something most, but who can shout loudest. This may sound somewhat stark; however, we see again and again that patients get what they want (or believe they need) by taking their case to the media.

The philosopher Kant (1724–1804) is perhaps best known for his dictum, 'Treat every rational being, including yourself, always as an end and never as a mere means.' This implies respect for all humans; it implies that good and right are done; it implies, above all, that justice is recognised as a basic way of life.

The principle of truth telling or honesty

This principle is probably the most difficult one to maintain or uphold. Human relationships are delicate, and to protect our vulnerability we have built up defences against exposing ourselves to others.

Many patients say that they can cope with bad news or difficult prognoses; what they cannot cope with is uncertainty and deception. Most patients do not need nurses and doctors to tell them the really bad news; they need nurses and doctors who listen to them while they express their feelings, fears and anger, regrets and hopes about what they have come to suspect. Such listening is not easy, because it involves the listener deeply, probably exposing her or his own inadequacies, and fear of saying and doing the wrong thing. This is the underlying reason for the injunction not to 'tell' a particular patient. Patients have been driven to incredible feats in order to find out what their diagnosis and prognosis are.

If one has to give a patient an answer to a particularly difficult question, or to impart unasked-for news, the skill lies in the way the information is given. Respecting the person, valuing him or her as an equal, keeping in mind the good, and trying at least to do no harm – all this helps us to be aware of how such a conversation should be carried out. The challenge is not in how often one has to give bad news, but in how often one has listened, and heard what the person said. We have a truth to give, but more importantly, we have a truth to hear and respect.

The principle of individual freedom

Thiroux (1995) makes the point strongly that individual moral freedom is limited by the other four principles: that there is a necessity to protect and revere life, do good and prevent wrong, treat human beings justly, tell the truth and be honest. In view of the astonishing variety of human values, needs, wants and concerns, this necessity is indeed powerful. We have individual freedom only so long as we do not harm someone in a serious way. A rapist cannot simply apply this principle to himself: the other four principles apply too, and in the light of all these, this 'freedom' of his is not legitimate.

Gillon (1986) makes a distinction between freedom, liberty, licence and doing what one wants to do, and acting autonomously, on the basis of thought or reasoning. A good act may become a virtuous act by the fact of having chosen freely to perform it in a particular way (autonomy as a nursing issue will be examined later).

Bergum (1994) describes one mother's decision for her baby, K'aila, who was dying from biliary atresia.

'He was three months old. The only way to prolong his life would have been to perform a liver transplant. The parents refused the transplant; the doctor reported the situation to the local authorities, and the child welfare department took the parents to court. "In the last week of K'aila's life", says his mother, "we were called on to fight fiercely for him, and at the same time to nurture him tenderly". She says, "I would have been torn for the rest of my life, knowing that I had made a decision which didn't feel right inside. I simply could not bring myself to coerce K'aila to live. By altering his body radically, and then giving him drugs for the rest of his life to prevent his body from defending itself the way it was designed to do, I would be doing violence to him". . . . The court upheld the parents' right to make a decision.'

(Bergum, 1994, page 75)

Bergum stresses the need for participation and collaboration between nurses and patients, trying to understand the meaning an experience has for a patient. This calls for respect for freedom on all sides.

Freedom – liberty, autonomy – is 'built into' the human structure in the same way as life is. And like life, freedom is not absolute: it functions only in relation to other people and other concepts.

These principles are not absolutes, but they can serve as maps on a journey, guiding and directing the decision-making process.

Key Points

- Ethical theories are philosophical guidelines which can direct actions but cannot be used exclusively.
- Ethical principles are not absolutes, but near-absolutes.
- All ethical principles apply in any situation; when one is infringed, they all are eventually.

RIGHTS AND RESPONSIBILITIES

As a society we are more and more conscious of our rights. As citizens we expect to have the right to clean air and water, access to wholesome food, civil and criminal protection, and health care. These rights are on the whole universal.

Other rights, such as freedom of belief, speech and expression, freedom to organise, and freedom from 'state violence' are not nearly as common, certainly not under repressive or totalitarian regimes.

Within these broad rights we hear more subtle rights expressed. In nursing and medicine we hear of the right to receive care, a child's right to love, the right to be heard, the right to refuse treatment, the right to die, as well as the right to live. The rights under *The Patient's Charter* (DoH, 1992, 1995) are clear for all patients, but when delays occur or operations are cancelled the Patient's Charter is of little help to get the situation reversed. The problem may be outside the scope of the personnel immediately involved.

One person's rights are another person's duties or responsibilities. What one person enjoys as a right depends on another person's performance or specific duty. The patient's right to care depends on the nurse's ability and skill, but more still on her or his willingness to perform the task in a humane and caring way. Rights and duties do not go together in a logical relationship, but in a moral one.

In a caring and professional relationship it is expected that the patient's interests must come first. A possibility of conflict arises here when nurses (and other health care personnel) consider that *their* rights are not respected and they might need to consider industrial action. Nurses may argue that because they are not treated adequately, they themselves cannot treat patients adequately. By looking after themselves, they look after their patients. This is an area of rights which needs considerable debate in any given situation.

Another area of debate concerns the rights of patients who attempt suicide, or who request euthanasia. The responsibility of nurses and other health care workers lies in respecting the patient's freedom. A responsible carer does not shrug the shoulders and walk off; rather, she or he hears the words of the request itself, and *in addition*, hears what lies behind them. It is this 'extra', this willingness to respect the whole person and his or her search for meaning, which is part of the special role and responsibility of nurses and carers.

In the present economic climate of health care, where staff shortages are common, time is at a premium. Where time is scarce, good communication is all the more important, because it takes time to hear and say what really matters.

Rights born out of frustration are not, however, 'real' rights. Patients and health care workers claiming the right to a car parking space, being frustrated that an operation has not relieved the pain, or being served a meal on time – all these are often considered as rights. In truth they are demands which correspond more to a want than to a real fundamental human need. All the same, perhaps someone somewhere has not taken seriously his or her responsibility towards a fellow human.

If one is concerned with 'logical' approaches only, then everyone will be out to get as much as they can; everyone will be concerned with their own rights. But the relationship between rights and responsibilities is not logical; rather it is based on morality. We are not born ethical beings, but we become so. We have no intrinsic rights (apart from life and liberty) except those given to us by those who choose to act responsibly. The one who says, 'I have a right to . . .' depends on the one who says, 'I give . . .'. Such giving, caring, sharing of what one has, is what makes a person moral, a 'human being'.

CODES OF PRACTICE

The Code for Nurses, first issued by the International Council of Nurses in 1953 and revised twice, has stood unaltered since 1973. It declares that 'the fundamental responsibility of the nurse is fourfold: to promote health, to prevent illness, to restore health, and to alleviate suffering'. The international flavour of that code is evident in its emphasis on health promotion and the nurse's 'responsibility for initiating and supporting action to meet the health and social needs of the public'.

The publication in 1983 of the first Code of Professional Conduct for Nurses, Midwives and Health Visitors by the United Kingdom Central Council (UKCC) was a significant step forward for these professions in the UK. Many other countries and health care professions have modelled their own codes on that of the UKCC. The Code's third edition has been in use since 1992 (see Table 13.4).

A code of practice (or ethics) is not a legal document, but it gives direction and cohesion to the body for which it has been designed. The UKCC Code of Professional Conduct has become the basis for most major guidance documents (e.g. *The Scope of Professional Practice* [UKCC, 1996b]; *Guidelines for Professional Practice* [UKCC, 1996a]) and is the template against which misconduct is judged.

Such a code has to be wide enough to include many possibilities for action, but also specific enough to enable a nurse to apply it to his or her particular work. Ideally, it should be a distillation of ethical theories and principles, put into a practical framework for action. When an ethical decision has to be made, a nurse should be able to follow the code and decide in which direction it points her or him.

Some of the more obvious areas of ethical concern for a society or profession (such as confidentiality, safety aspects, use and abuse of privilege, refusal of gifts and the use of qualifications for advertising) are expected to be covered in any code of practice. The areas in the UKCC Code which have caused the most concern and debate are the acknowledgement of any limitations of competence (Clause 4), having regard to the environment of care (Clause 11) and having regard to the workload of colleagues (Clause 13). With ever greater pressure on resources of both people and material, these clauses are significant (and called for the publication of *Guidelines for Professional Practice* [UKCC, 1996a]).

Of concern is the frequent reference to 'report to an appropriate person or authority' (Clauses 8, 11, 12, 13). There have been growing numbers of complaints or demands from nurses, usually regarding levels of staffing for safe practice, which have been reported and no action was taken. This has led to cases of 'whistle-blowing' (see below) which have sometimes been dramatic for the nurses concerned.

Safeguarding the interests of patients and clients is and must be the nurse's main duty. How the Code is interpreted in a specific situation is, however, every nurse's own right and duty. Hence

Table 13.4: *Code of Professional Conduct for the Nurse, Midwife and Health Visitor* (UKCC, 1992)

Each registered nurse, midwife and health visitor shall act, at all times, in such a manner as to:

- **safeguard and promote the interests of individual patients and clients;**
- **serve the interests of society;**
- **justify public trust and confidence and**
- **uphold and enhance the good standing and reputation of the professions.**

As a registered nurse, midwife or health visitor, you are personally accountable for your practice and, in the exercise of your professional accountability, must:

1 Act always in such a manner as to promote and safeguard the interests and well-being of patients/clients
2 Ensure that no action or omission on your part or within your sphere of responsibility is detrimental to the interests, condition or safety of patients/clients
3 Maintain and improve your professional knowledge and competence
4 Acknowledge any limitations in your knowledge and competence and decline any duties or responsibilities unless able to perform them in a safe and skilled manner
5 Work in an open and co-operative manner with patients, clients and their families, foster their independance and recognise and respect their involvement in the planning and delivery of care
6 Work in a collaborative and co-operative manner with health care professionals and others involved in providing care, and recognise and respect their particular contributions within the care team
7 Recognise and respect the uniqueness and dignity of each patient and client, and respond to their need for care, irrespective of their ethnic origin, religious beliefs, personal attributes, the nature of their health problems or any other factor
8 Report to an appropriate person or authority, at the earliest possible time, any conscientious objection which may be relevant to your professional practice
9 Avoid any abuse of your privileged relationship with patients and clients and of the privileged access allowed to their person, property, residence or workplace
10 Protect all confidential information concerning patients and clients obtained in the course of professional practice and make disclosures only with consent, where required by the order of a court or where you can justify disclosure in the wider public interest
11 Report to an appropriate person or authority, having regard to the physical, psychological and social effects on patients and clients, any circumstances in the environment of care which could jeopardise standards of practice
12 Report to an appropriate person or authority any circumstances in which safe and appropriate care for patients and clients cannot be provided
13 Report to an appropriate person or authority where it appears that the health or safety of colleagues is at risk, as such circumstances may compromise standards of practice and care
14 Assist professional colleagues, in the context of your own knowledge, experience and sphere of responsibility, to develop their professional competence, and assist others in the care team, including informal carers, to contribute safely and to a degree appropriate to their roles
15 Refuse any gift, favour or hospitality from patients or clients currently in your care which might be interpreted as seeking to exert influence to obtain preferential consideration and
16 Ensure that your registration status is not used in the promotion of commercial products or services, declare any financial or other interests in relevant organisations providing such goods or services and ensure that your professional judgement is not influenced by any commercial considerations

Reprinted with permission of the UKCC.

it is important to be familiar with the Code and to discuss cases and events at ward, departmental and community level, as well as in classrooms and study groups.

Since 1985 the UKCC has published a number of advisory documents. These have been superseded in 1996 by *Guidelines for Professional Practice* which 'has been produced to help to reflect on the many challenges that face us in day-to-day practice'. As such it is achieving its aim and should be consulted widely.

MAKING ETHICAL DECISIONS

It seems that the difference between a problem and a dilemma is that a problem can be solved, but a dilemma is a choice between two or more equally impossible positions. In ethics we are often in such impossible positions. It must be stressed, however, that nurses are rarely in situations where they have to make decisions on behalf of patients; but they are often in positions where they are asked to help patients and clients to make decisions, hence the need to know theories, principles, codes and frameworks for decision making.

Although in many instances, time is of the essence for reaching a decision, it is often not so urgent that good and thorough discussion cannot take place. Then again, this may be difficult because the persons concerned are understandably anxious and perhaps not able to be as objective as might be desired. It is therefore the more important that those, such as nurses, who help a patient to come to a decision, are able to be clear and matter of fact, *and* empathic.

Increasing numbers of patients and clients are concerned with end of life decisions (see Chapter 12). Science and technology have put resources at the disposal of medicine which can prolong life with ever greater success, but often at the cost of the quality of that life. Older people are concerned that they will need more help and be dependent on others who resent caring for them and who do not have the resources for that care because the more spectacular life-saving techniques do not apply to them. The decisions surrounding the beginning and end of life are therefore more likely those which engage the nurses' skills for holistic

and human care. The example given in the following patient study is not untypical.

Patient Study

Mrs Annie James, aged 49, has been getting progressively weaker following a mastectomy 18 months earlier. She has had several episodes in hospital following pathological fractures and also hypercalcaemia. Each time, she was very low but rallied remarkably. This time, though, she seemed not to respond well, and her husband was particularly upset to see her with drips and tubes. They had not talked much about her dying but had concentrated more on living. Mrs James was now not really able to hold a conversation, but her expression had something of a plea which Mr James interpreted as 'I've had enough'. He asked a staff nurse, with whom he had formed a good relationship, if he should ask the doctor that the drip be removed and that his wife be left to die peacefully and without 'heroics'. The staff nurse was not surprised by this question, and she could see how he was in two minds, as his wife had always rallied before. She cannot make the decision for him, but she can help him to come to a decision himself.

MODELS FOR DECISION MAKING

Any decision, even the simplest, goes through a process. Nurses are familiar with the four steps of the nursing process, and in making ethical decisions the process is not very different. The theories, models and principles mentioned above do, however, guide decisions more specifically.

Several nurse authors have devised models for ethical decision making (Brown *et al.*, 1992; Johnstone, 1994; Husted and Husted, 1995) which take these elements into consideration. Johnstone's (1994) model is shown in Table 13.5.

This model is based on process principles. The model used in response ethics (above) is based on moral agency, i.e. it starts with the person and is concerned with the development of the person in the wider social setting. Thiroux's set of ethical principles is also a model for making ethical decisions. These three different types of models complement each other and are indeed all necessary at different stages when making ethical decisions.

Table 13.5: Johnstone's (1994) 'moral decision-making model'

1 Assessing the situation
2 Diagnosing or identifying the moral problem
3 Setting moral goals and planning an appropriate moral course of action
4 Implementing the moral plan of action
5 Evaluating the moral outcomes of the action implemented

In the scenario, the nurse is asked to help Mr James to come to the decision of whether he should ask the doctor to let his wife die peacefully.

What is happening? (Niebuhr's [1963] response ethics, a model of moral agency) must surely be the first question which the nurse needs to ask. This question is so basic that it is, however, often overlooked. Another person's problem causes discomfort, and in order to feel better, we think that we have to give an answer. But the answer is to be given by the person who has the problem, in this case Mr James.

If the nurse asks this question, then he/she has to ask it of Mr James, Mrs James, him/herself, the situation, Mrs James' family, the caring team, the doctor and anyone concerned.

What is happening in terms of illness, prognosis and diagnosis?

What is happening in terms of feelings? fears, hesitation, unspoken and perhaps unfinished business between the couple, memories and expectations of the future now unrealised.

What is happening to Mrs James? What can the caring team contribute?

This question alone can enlighten the situation significantly and bring the people concerned to the point where the decision emerges.

Niebuhr has spoken of a 'pattern of responsibility' which forms when this question is asked. This consists of an initial *response* which is physical, i.e. on being confronted with the challenge, the person experiences perhaps a dry mouth, a fast heartbeat, or an inability to walk. This is caused by memories which are now *interpreted* in the light of the present situation. What happens next is a looking forward, or an *accountability* to the future: 'If I do this . . . that will happen . . .'. If the decision taken is satisfactory, a *social solidarity* will develop in the sense that everybody can benefit. If this is not possible, the interpretation and accountability may need to be examined again.

When the question 'What is happening?' has been asked thoroughly enough, answers will emerge. At this stage the *ethical principles* may have to be addressed and applied. What is the *value of life* of Mrs James, Mr James, the nurse, the doctor and all concerned? What do the people concerned understand their life to mean? How do they react now to life and death? What does each person contribute to life (and death) in the face of Mrs James' suffering? What does each person consider to be *good* or *right* in the present circumstances? What about the issues of *justice*? Should Mrs James receive more care? What care? How would this affect her family? How would this affect the ward where she is? How does such a discussion contribute to the wider issue of care of dying people, and the role which nurses and nursing have in the wider context? If Mr James is unsure about asking the doctor, what is the issue around *truth telling* in this case? What is the issue of truth between Mr and Mrs James as they have not talked about her dying, but only about her living? It may be that here is the nub of the whole problem. But rather than speculate or assume that this is the case, it would be much more worthwhile and empathic to ask Mr James, 'What is happening around the issue of truth or honesty between you?' Finally, as Mrs James seems unable to speak or make a decision, is her *freedom* infringed? Does Mr James feel strongly about his freedom in possibly being responsible for her death at an earlier stage than might be necessary or desired?

Asking these questions and addressing them will never be just an exercise, because the people concerned have been personally involved. Nevertheless, it is possible to see this as perhaps a rather abstract exercise. It is therefore at this stage that the *process model* will come into play, in particular the third question in Johnstone's model: *setting moral goals and planning an appropriate moral course of action.* In Niebuhr's terms, this is his: 'What is the fitting answer?' The emphasis is on the *fitting* or *appropriate,* because no two cases or situations are the same, and when every detail has been considered, the decision is not arbitrary or flighty, but truly a moral or ethical decision.

Thus it can be seen that making ethical decisions is not necessarily difficult, but rather enhancing of the individual; and also, that simply one model is not adequate. The main element in any decision, be this a choice between items in a supermarket or a decision of life and death, is that the person concerned listens to the various elements involved and decides in the most morally fitting way.

Key Points

- The process of making ethical decisions is no different from making many other decisions.
- Nurses are mostly concerned with helping patients and clients to make their own decisions.
- Making ethical decisions demands skills of listening and communicating.

SOME ETHICAL ISSUES CONCERNING PATIENTS

It is often claimed that nurses (and doctors and the public) do not recognise ethical situations when they meet them. It is possible to say that anything which infringes any one of the ethical principles is therefore an ethical situation. Some issues are, however, particularly evident. Those mentioned below are only the most pressing ones.

INFORMED CONSENT

In her book *Whose Body is It?*, Carolyn Faulder (1985) made an early attempt to take the whole notion of consent to pieces. In her view, informed consent consists first of all of *the right to know* and then of *the right to say no*.

In 1990 the Department of Health produced *A Guide to Consent for Examination or Treatment* which states that a patient has the fundamental right to give or withhold consent prior to examination or treatment. The point is made explicitly that:

'the purpose of obtaining a signature on the consent form is not an end in itself. The most important element of a consent procedure is the duty to ensure that patients understand the nature and purpose of the proposed treatment. Where a patient has not been given appropriate information then consent may not always have been obtained despite the signature on the form.'

(DoH, 1990, page 4)

Taplin (1994) describes the results of her research on informed consent and found 'that 15% of the patients interviewed did not even know

what the consent form was for'. Some patients did not know what operation had been performed, some knew partially, and some thought they had one kind of operation when in fact they had another.

It can be difficult to measure consent, and the degree to which it is really informed. In an effort to clarify the meaning of the word 'consent', not only has the adjective 'informed' been used, but also 'true', 'educated' and 'responsible'. This shows the concern underlying this area of care.

It is sometimes argued that it is impossible to give a patient or client *all* the facts needed to make an informed or educated decision, as really only the expert has all the accompanying facts. It can equally be argued that the information *given* will help the patient to decide as the doctor or nurse desires, for if the information which is *withheld* were also given, the patient might decide not to cooperate.

Much consent is implied, such as holding an arm out for a blood test, or opening the mouth for an inspection or treatment. But such consent should not be taken for granted. It is not a signature which counts, but the respect for the other person in the relationship. When consent is not sought, for whatever reason, that person's life is devalued. A paternalistic stance is then taken in which truth telling or honesty is compromised, trust is lost, and individual freedom cannot be exercised. In other words, harm is done and even in a small act, all the ethical principles may have been infringed.

CONFIDENTIALITY

The notion of confidentiality rests on trust. Patients and clients who trust another person with private and personal information about themselves have the right to believe that this information will be used only for the purpose for which it was intended and will not be given to others without permission (UKCC, 1996a).

But what is confidentiality? And what is confidential material? Documents of many kinds are held by vast quantities of health professionals on any one person: the GP, perhaps several hospitals, nurses, physiotherapists, community nurses, family planning clinics and many others. The Data Protection Act 1984 covers typed and computerised material, but not handwritten documents.

Much information passed between patients or clients and nurses is not particularly confidential. When information has to be passed to others for effective care and treatment, it is not only polite but also ethically correct (the principles of the value of life, goodness, rightness, honesty) to tell the patient that this will be done, or at least ask if he or she has any objections to this being done. We often assume that because patients are to be cared for, any treatment is acceptable, but truly ethical care never assumes anything but explicitly asks or tells what may be implied.

According to the UKCC (1996a), disclosure of information happens:

- 'with the consent of the patient or client
- without the consent of the patient or client when the disclosure is required by law or by order of a court and
- without the consent of the patient or client when the disclosure is considered to be necessary in the public interest.

The public interest means the interests of an individual, or groups of individuals or of society as a whole, and would, for example, cover matters such as serious crime, child abuse, drug trafficking or other activities which place others at serious risk.'

(UKCC, 1996a, page 27)

Confidentiality is a complex issue which is easily overlooked and easily breached. If disclosure has to be made, this should only be done after reflection and perhaps talking it over with a trusted person.

INNOVATIVE TREATMENTS

Ethical issues arise mostly at the fringes of care and treatment, when the new is not (yet) integrated. Medicine itself has not made any significant breakthroughs for several decades (since the discovery of penicillin), but technology and science have taken the lead in health care. Innovative treatments such as gene therapies, xenografts, larger and more complex transplants, assisted conception for women beyond the childbearing age, to mention but a few, have all gained in reputation and become acceptable. Again and again it becomes evident later on, however, that patients and clients were not informed well enough about such treatments and their advantages. It is arguable, however, that they could not be

informed, precisely because they were innovative and outcomes could not be known.

The ethical questions surrounding these treatments are not only if they should or should not be done on purely biological grounds, but increasingly on economic grounds also. When such treatments become available, the general expectation rises that everyone should be able to benefit, not only a select few. Can the health service afford such expensive care? Can the treatments be justified when elderly people are not able to get much-needed physiotherapy?

It is impossible to give clear answers to such questions. What is necessary is that nurses discuss these issues, consider their role in them and are prepared to help patients and clients to come to decisions when they are offered or urged to have – or are not offered – innovative treatments. The question of informed consent may here not only involve the truth being given, but what of the truth is not given. This is where the role of nurses as advocates becomes vital.

Key Points

- 'Informed consent' means the process of explaining and discussing with the patient, not simply obtaining a signature.
- Confidentiality is the vital basis for all health care and consent should be obtained before divulging information.
- Giving information without consent must be carefully considered.

SOME ETHICAL ISSUES CONCERNING NURSES

Many of the ethical issues which concern nurses have already been touched upon, and only a few can be mentioned here. For some nurses some issues are not a problem, whereas for others many more issues are real problems. These issues can be seen to relate particularly to rights and responsibilities.

ADVOCACY

Marks-Maran (1993a) states:

'Each of us must begin by clarifying our own values about nursing and the nurse–patient relationship. It is only then that we will be in a position to decide where advocacy fits into our value system. Advocacy, like the Nursing Process, is not just another set of tasks to do for patients. It is a way of being.'

(Marks-Maran, 1993a, page 81)

Advocacy has become something of a slogan among nurses, even though it is far from clear what exactly is meant by the activity. Dictionary definitions see advocacy in legal terms, pleading for another or on behalf of another. In a celebrated article written in 1979, Leah Curtin says that 'the end and purpose of nursing is the welfare of other human beings. This end is not a scientific end, but rather a moral end.' On the other hand, Johnstone (1994) suggests that 'the notion of nurse–patient advocacy is vulnerable to philosophical criticism'. It is unclear precisely what is meant by advocacy in nursing, but nurses have increasingly understood the term to be the most caring aspect of their role.

Different types of advocacy include self-advocacy (when the person is helped to make his or her own case); citizen advocacy (when individuals claim a right as citizens, perhaps appealing to an MP); advocacy partnerships (when groups of people with similar claims join together to make a case which will be stronger than a single or personal one). Nurses may be involved in all types of advocacy. Most likely, nurses will help patients or clients to be self-advocates by giving them information which they may not have had or not have understood fully and then support them in whatever decisions are made. This is essentially what the nurse in the scenario of Mr and Mrs James was asked to do. In many situations nurses will plead with doctors on behalf of patients who are not, or no longer, able to plead for themselves. This normally only happens in severe physical or mental illness. The boundaries of these categories need to be well understood and clearly respected.

The areas in which nurses can, do and should act as advocates on behalf of patients concern:

- The quality of care, corresponding to the principles of the value of life and of goodness or rightness
- The access to care by patients, corresponding to the principle of justice or fairness
- The information regarding care received by patients, corresponding to the principle of truth telling or honesty
- Any alternatives to the proposed care available, corresponding to the principle or individual freedom.

The duty of care demands increasingly a duty to maintain rights and responsibilities. This means also a political awareness. But to exercise one's duty of care in terms of advocacy may require considerable courage. Therefore nurses need to understand 'principles of negotiation, canvassing, and how power is used as a means to influence change' (Albarran, 1995). Advocacy has increasingly been linked to 'whistle-blowing' and how to voice concerns.

VOICING CONCERNS

Witnessing practices which are dubious or unprofessional is disturbing. What can be done about it is rarely clear or without consequences. 'Whistle-blowing' is a form of defence which many nurses have contemplated, some have tried, but few have carried through with success. Unlike in the USA, where 'whistle-blowers' are considered to be heroes, in Britain they tend to be treated with contempt. The health services generally are still in the transition from paternalism and secrecy to equality, egalitarianism and openness. When and where the cultures clash, there will be casualties. Bok (1980) writes about three elements of 'whistle-blowing': dissent, breach of loyalty and accusation. Eby (1994) mentions four ethical concepts which are involved: accountability, loyalty or fidelity, justice and truth.

Perhaps the most common situation within nursing where 'whistle-blowing' is considered or used is when nurses are constantly asked to work with inadequate staff ratios or in unsafe conditions, thereby jeopardising professional practice. Patients and clients cannot, under such circumstances, receive adequate care. If the nurse has made all the normal requests and exhausted appropriate local channels but received no satisfaction, he or she may take the case to the media. By doing this, accusations of breaching confidentiality and loyalty to the employer may follow.

Long before such drastic action may need to be taken, voicing concerns on behalf of the patients and clients is not only right, but is a professional duty and activity. The UKCC Code of Professional Practice (UKCC, 1992) mentions several times (Clauses 8, 11, 12, 13) that in the exercise of professional accountability, nurses must report events and situations which they consider to be contrary to good practice. This cannot be considered 'whistle-blowing' though it may sometimes be called and viewed to be this. When voicing concerns it is important that this is done in the most professional way possible, and some of the points listed by Eby (1994) for those who consider blowing the whistle also apply to less drastic action:

- Talking to families and friends about possible implications from an act of 'whistle-blowing'
- Building up a network of support within the organisation
- Exhaust all the possible 'internal' mechanisms for resolution before going 'outside'
- Make certain that everything is documented. Access to vital documents may be denied as the process develops
- Discuss the situation with either a trade union or professional representative, never attempting action alone.

It must be kept in mind also that what may appear a very clear and simple case seen from the point of view of a particular nurse may, when it is acted upon, take very different routes and uncover aspects which were never envisaged. Nurses have a duty of care and must act in the patient's best interest. Such action demands both compassion and courage, but not martyrdom or heroism.

ACCOUNTABILITY

Accountability is often linked with economy and saving money, but this is too narrow a view of the term.

The UKCC Code of Professional Conduct (UKCC, 1992) states that 'as a registered nurse, midwife or health visitor, you are personally accountable for your practice and, in the exercise of your professional accountability, must . . .'. This stem sentence needs to be seen as introducing each clause separately. In *Guidelines for Professional Practice* (UKCC, 1996a, pages 8–9) accountability is therefore the first topic to be considered. Certain statements are made clearly:

- professional accountability means knowing 'to whom you must answer and how'
- 'no one else can answer for you and it is no defence to say that you were acting on someone else's orders'
- 'professional accountability is fundamentally concerned with weighing up the interests of patients and clients in complex situations, using professional knowledge, judgement and skills to make a decision and enabling you to account for the decision made'.

Accountability arises directly out of responsibility. To say 'I only did what I was told to do' is not good enough. All nurses carry out delegated actions and jobs, but each nurse is responsible for declaring if she or he is skilled to do it; if not, the action must be refused. This is often easier said than done, especially in emergencies. Marks-Maran (1993b) speaks of legal accountability, managerial accountability, professional accountability and moral accountability. In situations when a request for an action has to be refused, all these aspects of accountability come into play.

For any professional to make professional decisions means that there also has to be professional autonomy. Nurses have professional accountability, but if this is denied or interfered with by too many guidelines, policies and directives (e.g. regarding resuscitation, how much care to give, how wounds are to be treated), then professional skill and judgement is no longer possible. The professional responsibility is then to aim to restore this.

PROFESSIONAL AUTONOMY

Nursing has made great strides to establish itself and is largely succeeding in many areas. Key worker systems, clinical pathways, protocols, primary health care, nursing development units and specialist nurses are here to stay. Innovative care is happening, often based on research. Whilst these efforts are laudable, viewed nationally or even globally, they are still only tiny islands in a vast sea of care which is led by other professions. If nursing is to be responsive to the health care needs of the future, then nurses have to be leading in many more areas than they are now. Some examples of how this is possible are described in *Scope in Practice* (UKCC, 1997) where individual initiatives in all branches of nursing, midwifery and health visiting are highlighted. Nursing may have attracted more people who are 'doers' rather than 'leaders', but leaders have always emerged from within the ranks. Leaders have also been suppressed. Nursing alone cannot change the climate, but nurses need to be willing to address the issues of the day. This takes courage. Autonomy can be an exciting and also a frightening prospect. For the sake of patients and nurses, these aspects need to be faced in the future.

Key Points

■ Advocacy is often understood as the most caring element of nursing; this should not be undertaken lightly.

■ Freedom of speech is a fundamental human right; when it is infringed, more extreme measures such as 'whistle-blowing' may become necessary.

■ Accountability and responsibility are the two sides of the coin of professional nursing.

CONCLUSION

An introduction to philosophy was given on the basis of values. Ethics and morality are based on what is good and right. But that may not be enough, and 'excellence' (according to Thiroux, 1995) should be an accompanying factor. Good and right should also exist equally for all: that is, justice must be the outcome. When, because of limited resources, justice cannot be administered with total fairness, some will always receive less than is their due. The question of priorities is therefore acute: will it be the person with cancer, the child, or the elderly man or woman whose life would be transformed with a hip operation? It is not always a question of doing good, but in many circumstances at least avoiding harm needs to be the guiding ideal. This does not only apply to mental or physical illness, but a person's whole life needs to be considered, including the cultural, social, spiritual and psychological aspects. When any aspects are denied, truth seems less than fully present. This leads to justice and advocacy. People have rights to expect and get care, but not at any price. People should not be used as means to ends.

If 'caring is the human mode of being' (Roach, 1992), then caring is what matters most of all. Nurses have always seen caring as their particular hallmark. This caring, characterised by listening and respecting the other and working from within a committed professional relationship, will enhance both the patient or client *and* the nurse. This is an ideal, but ethics is as much about the 'should' and the 'ought' as about the 'is'.

Summary

■ Morality is the personal basis of ethics.

■ Ethics is expressed as behaviour among people.

■ Codes of practice regulate professions and professionals have to abide by them.

■ To make ethical decisions some guidelines are helpful, but essentially all decisions made in daily life are ethical, because they all have consequences which may affect other people.

■ Ethical issues concerning patients also concern nurses, and vice versa.

■ If nursing is to develop, nurses need to contribute to this development. This is not only a professional duty but also an ethical one as patients and clients may otherwise suffer.

REFERENCES

Albarran, J.W. (1995). Should nurses be politically aware? *British Journal of Nursing*, 4(8), 461–5.

Beauchamp, T.L. and Childress, J.F. (1989). *Principles of Biomedical Ethics*, 3rd edn. Oxford University Press, New York.

Bergum, V. (1994). Knowledge for ethical care. *Nursing Ethics*, 1(2), 71–9.

Bok, S. (1980). Whistle-blowing and professional responsibility. *New York University Education Quarterly*, 10, 2–10.

Briggs Myers, I. with Myers, P.B. (1980). *Gifts Differing*. Consulting Psychologists Press Inc., Palo Alto.

Brown, J.M., Kitson, A.L. and McKnight, T.J. (1992). *Challenges in Caring: Explorations in Nursing and Ethics*. Chapman & Hall, London.

Curtin, L. (1979). The nurse as advocate: a philosophical foundation for nursing. *Advances in Nursing Science*, 1(3), 1–10.

DoH (1990). *A Guide to Consent for Examination or Treatment*. Health Publications Unit, Heywood.

DoH (1992). *The Patient's Charter*. HMSO, London.

DoH (1995). *The Patient's Charter and You*. HMSO, London.

Eby, M. (1994). Whistle-blowing. In *Ethics: Conflicts of Interest*, Tschudin, V. (ed.), Chapter 3, 56–84. Scutari, London.

Faulder, C. (1985). *Whose Body is it?* Virago Press, London.

Fletcher, J. (1967). *Moral Responsibility: Situation Ethics at Work*. SCM Press, London.

Frankl, V. (1962). *Man's Search for Meaning*. Pocket Books, New York.

Gilligan, C. (1982). *In a Different Voice*. Harvard University Press, Cambridge, MA.

Gillon, R. (1986). *Philosophical Medical Ethics*. John Wiley & Sons, Chichester.

Husted, G.L. and Husted, J.H. (1995). *Ethical Decision Making in Nursing*, 2nd edn. Mosby, St Louis.

International Council of Nurses (1973). *Code for Nurses*. ICN, Geneva.

Johnstone, M-J. (1994). *Bioethics: a Nursing Perspective*, 2nd edn. W.B. Saunders, Marrickville.

Jung, C.G. (1964). *Man and His Symbols*. Picador, London.

Keirsey, D. and Bates, M. (1984). *Please Understand Me*. Prometheus Nemesis Book Co., Del Mar, CA.

Marks-Maran, D. (1993a). Advocacy. In *Ethics: Nurses and Patients*, Tschudin, V. (ed.), Chapter 3, 65–84. Scutari, London.

Marks-Maran, D. (1993b). Accountability. In *Ethics: Nurses and Patients*, Tschudin, V. (ed.), Chapter 5, 121–34. Scutari, London.

Niebuhr, H.R. (1963). *The Responsible Self*. Harper and Row, New York.

Norberg, A. and Udén, G. (1995). Gender differences in moral reasoning among physicians, registered nurses and enrolled nurses engaged in geriatric and surgical care. *Nursing Ethics*, 2(3), 233–42.

Rickard, M., Kuhse, H. and Singer, P. (1996). Caring and justice: a study of two approaches to health care ethics. *Nursing Ethics*, 3(3), 212–23.

Roach, M.S. (1992). *The Human Act of Caring*, 2nd edn. Canadian Hospital Association, Ottawa.

Taplin, D. (1994). Nursing and informed consent: an empirical study. In *Ethical Issues in Nursing*, Hunt, G. (ed.), Chapter 1, 21–37. Routledge, London.

Thiroux, J. (1995). *Ethics; Theory and Practice*, 5th edn. Glencoe Publishing Co., Encino, CA.

UKCC (1992) *Code of Professional Conduct*, 3rd edn. UKCC, London.

UKCC (1996a). *Guidelines for Professional Practice*. UKCC, London.

UKCC (1996b). *The Scope of Professional Practice*. UKCC, London.

UKCC (1997). *Scope in Practice*. UKCC, London.

FURTHER READING

Chadwick, R. and Tadd, W. (1992). *Ethics and Nursing Practice*. Macmillan, Basingstoke.

This book uses many examples from practice and is accessible for students in its language and its treatment of the subject.

General Medical Council (1995). *Duties of a Doctor*. GMC, London.

This set of attractively produced booklets are 'guidance' for doctors, comprising also a set of principles which doctors must respect. Useful for comparison with the UKCC Code of Professional Conduct.

Hunt, G. (ed.) (1994). *Ethical Issues in Nursing*. Routledge, London.

A very useful collection of essays on most aspects of ethics which nurses will meet in practice.

Kohner, N. (1996). *The Moral Maze of Practice; a Stimulus for Reflection and Discussion*. King's Fund, London.

This slim volume is packed with information, ideally suited to group discussions and as a stimulus for reflection.

Tschudin, V. (1992). *Ethics in Nursing: the Caring Relationship*, 2nd edn. Butterworth-Heinemann, Oxford.

A basic text which gives the reader an overview of ethical terms, theories and principles as used and applied in nursing.

Tschudin, V. (1994). *Deciding Ethically: a Practical Approach to Nursing Challenges*. Baillière Tindall, London.

This text centres around the five principles established by Thiroux. Each principle is addressed specifically in two chapters, based on a case history each.

Tschudin, V. and Marks-Maran, D. (1993). *Ethics: a Primer for Nurses – Workbook (and Workshop Guide)*. Baillière Tindall, London.

The Workbook is designed for individual study of ethics and the Workshop Guide is ideal for teachers and lecturers to take the individual learning further in group settings.

CHAPTER FOURTEEN

DEVELOPING *the* 'PERSON' *of* *the* PROFESSIONAL CARER

Paul Barber

- Surviving: the nurse as an untherapeutic agent
- Harming: the nurse as a persecutor
- Understanding: the personal cost of nursing care
- Facilitating: enabling health to grow
- Reflecting: the nature of nursing care
- Expressing: dynamics of care
- Creating a workable synthesis

This chapter is designed for those who give care and as such is a source of support for the reader. It offers ways of developing further insight into, and understanding of, how we may care for ourselves and others.

The author leads the reader from an analysis of what happens in the real world of caring to an exploration of ways of developing personal insights and understanding of how we may facilitate care for ourselves and for others. Throughout the chapter value is placed on the person, whether the giver or receiver of health care.

The themes of personal and professional growth and development feature throughout the work. The chapter includes reference to and discussion of:

- Ways nurses function, survive and protect themselves from stress
- Factors which may influence care and the nurse–patient relationship
- Processes of understanding and change as they affect the way care is perceived and given
- Ways of 'seeing' and understanding reality. Reference is made to transactional analysis, qualities of care and adaptation which may lead to changes and growth within the individual
- Ways of 'being', of being receptive, open to each other and self-aware
- The interrelationship between thinking, feeling and sensing. This is followed by detailed consideration of styles of facilitation and intervention and their place in health care

The author leaves the reader with a profound message – to know and understand ourselves is the way to the understanding and care of others.

Personal development cannot be separated from professional development; each rests upon the other. Show me how well you share of yourself, understand your own interpersonal processes and are able to communicate this to others, and I'll know how good or bad your nursing care is.

The insights of this chapter have been hard won. As a student nurse I felt devalued and vulnerable, a small cog in the hospital machine. I did not feel listened to by senior colleagues, my questions remained unanswered and my concern with professional 'survival' seemed to displace any aspirations I had towards personal **growth**. Eventually, I 'learnt the ropes' and started to develop the area that gave me the greatest satisfaction, namely, my ability to express myself through 'care'. Strangely enough, though care was said to be at the root of nursing, I saw little demonstrated. As a nurse amongst other nurses I felt uncared for. As a staff nurse I voiced my views with more confidence; I also met much resistance. As a charge nurse the fight was really on and I became aware of the enormous influence brought to bear by the institution on those who dare to suggest change. My resilience owed less to my skills than to my stubbornness. Eventually, I read more, met other dissatisfied carers, and in sharing, started to develop my own conceptual framework. I try to share a little of this in what follows.

Reflection Points

Much of my own growth appears like a letting-go of my defences – rather than the gaining of new skills – as if by unclogging my perceptions I started to appreciate others and care for myself with more honesty. As an educator and therapist I have let go of a lot more. In recent years I have reflected on my earlier journey as a student nurse and begun to value how much my clients and students have taught me. This work is theirs as much as it is mine.

- How have you been changed by your clients?
- What have you got to give to others?
- How good at caring for your self are you?
- Where is your journey as a carer taking you?

SURVIVING: THE NURSE AS AN UNTHERAPEUTIC AGENT

Historically, nursing has rarely been viewed as being a maturing or sensitising influence; it is, in fact, often the reverse (Altschul, 1972; Ashworth, 1980).

Entrants to the profession are observed to commence full of questions, enthusiastic and committed to the ethic of care, but by the time of registration the brighter and more inquisitive amongst their number tend to have left under a cloud of frustration, and those who stayed have done so at a cost, such as a loss of humour, person sensitivity and self-worth (Olsen and Whittaker,

1961). This is sad, for much potential for personal development exists within nursing. All the ingredients are there; nurses face those natural crises of life that further character development, they have responsibility for the care of other individuals, and are required to develop personal and relationship skills within their work. They also have a team available to support and counsel them. This is the potential; it is not the fact, for most nurses are encouraged by their work climate to act contrary to the ideal and divorce themselves from their clients' crises, fear to accept and use their responsibility, are underdeveloped in areas of personal skill, have blunted sensitivities, suffer constant interpersonal stress and are unsupported by colleagues.

Nursing makes incessant demands upon an individual's reserves of counselling and relationship skill, both of which have been largely ignored in **traditional** patterns of basic training (Lamond, 1974).

Nurses work in areas where disease, death, personal loss and the anxieties which arise from these are commonplace; but they are ill prepared to shape 'therapeutically', or to learn interpersonally from, such life crises. Consequently, nurses are more likely to block off their person sensitivity, displace their attention from themselves on to tasks at hand and turn a blind eye to the lessons and wisdom available to them.

Displacement and **denial** are natural defences when individuals are thrown into insecure situations without the necessary skills – and relationship skills were, until comparatively recently, glaringly absent from most training curricula.

In unsafe environments 'survival skills' appear to be more necessary than growth-inducing ones. In nursing, survival mechanisms have all too often triumphed over other features of learning. When you feel insecure and vulnerable you are apt to grip too tightly on to practicalities, focus upon the details of your role and place an inordinate degree of effort in maintaining your professional **status** and personal distance. Everything is viewed as needing a firm outline. There is no time for abstract conceptual reflection. Security is perceived as emanating from tangibles, well-designated roles and maintenance of 'what is' rather than speculation upon 'what might be'. Concerns with 'structure', 'status' and the use of 'power' then come to overshadow relationships.

Undercurrents of **crisis management** and the drawing-up of protective boundaries around nurses frustrate their learning. Anything new is viewed as a threat. In order to learn, individuals must first let go of their prejudices, risk a little uncertainty and appreciate that some discomfort is required as a natural process of 'releasing the old' to 'let in the new'. Discomforts such as these may be equated with 'growing pains', those feelings of unfamiliarity when you leave the tried and tested parts of your life behind a little before the new role you attempt to play becomes you.

'Growing pains' may take us by surprise, producing those fresh awarenesses and confusions that accompany times of transition: when we go for an interview, start a new job or attempt something risky. Simply, they are states of emotional energy we may draw upon to achieve a little extra sensitivity. They are common to the newly qualified staff nurse who first takes charge of a ward.

Too many people view their emotions as 'symptoms' rather than 'energies'. Emotions threaten intellectual clarity; thinking becomes less clear as feelings draw attention to bodily sensations. As most of us have been taught to think – but not to feel – we may see feelings as getting in the way.

Social life is dependent upon a taught reality maintained via right thinking and cultural values.

Professions likewise emphasise an intellectual 'taught reality' which is dependent upon clear thinking. This is no mean thing. Education of the intellect is essential, but we must retain perspective; intellectual cognition is but a feature – not the essence – of an individual. There are other realities open to us associated with feeling, our physical senses, and that ever hard to define perceptive organ we term **intuition**. Nurses need to value all these differing orientations to reality if they are fully to appreciate the situation and sensibilities of their clients.

'Patients' are people who are thrust into strange surroundings while undergoing a crisis of living; intellectual clarity does not come easily to them. An appreciation of emotional and intuitive functioning must be at the fore of care assessment, caring interventions and evaluation. During times of crisis when unruly emotional energies pervade us, we see ourselves as powerless; depression may ensue as our energies reach a low ebb and we become subject to recriminative and self-deprecative thinking. At our most stressed we may regress to childlike states where we are preoccupied with our intuitions and a world of fantasy, and if brought before psychiatrists may – even at this time – be labelled 'psychotic' and in need of care.

To recognise these states in clients is but half the story. Nurses need to be in touch with their own *thinking, sensing, feeling* and *intuitive* processes and have some understanding of how these may be therapeutically shaped to solicit health. This is what holistic models of nursing request of the nurse (Rogers, 1970).

Nurses *must* work towards evolving a sensitivity to the above processes within themselves if they are to develop empathy. The word 'must' is emphasised, for without movement into these areas the nursing profession can never progress. Time after time enquiries have been produced, reports implemented and reorganisations acted upon within our care institutions, but apart from a little tarting up of instrumental activity and the managerial or educational structure, little has really changed. You don't create lasting change from merely placing an old ingredient into a new box. Nursing has been subject to reappraisal and many oddly shaped new wrappings, but its core has been little touched.

The *nursing process* once promised to change all this, not so much in its watered down form of producing ever more records and making the nurse into a ward clerk, but in its more creative mode where the 'process' becomes a socially alert, interpersonal one. Sadly, there is still a dearth of social and personal sensitivity in much of nursing care.

When nurses come to appreciate the full implication of their role as social interactors, perhaps then 'process' changes will be enacted within the profession so that nursing education will be centred and 'growth-orientated', and personnel development will supersede the imposition of systems of control in nursing management. If we perpetuate a failure to 'care for care givers', or to counsel and develop **experientially** the 'humanity' of new entrants to the profession, where will they find a 'role model' of caring? Instrumental nursing activity, devoid of 'care', becomes a nonsense. Doing things to people is not caring.

Nursing can be a nourishing experience for client and carer alike, and solicit personal development in each. This is no pipe dream; we have the necessary knowledge base (Barber, 1990), the skills have been developed (Barber and Dietrich, 1985), and the climate in nursing is constantly subject to change; but first, let us contemplate the costs to the profession when 'care' and 'personal development' are overlooked.

HARMING: THE NURSE AS A PERSECUTOR

Self-worth and personal competence take quite a battering in professional preparation. Before an individual can 'professionally belong' he/she must survive numerous 'rites of passage' – the least of which may be formal examinations – before they become accepted by their colleagues. Dealing with sudden death and handling oneself during crises, counselling relatives, and balancing the conflicting demands of client and institution all relate to this. Proving oneself personally and building emotional competence is all part of the hidden agenda, but you are usually left to your own devices to achieve this.

Facilitating the care of others is a taxing science and an exhausting art. Professions which are empowered to cater for, monitor and/or control the casualties of society take a great deal of stress on to themselves (Edelwich and Brodsky, 1980). Acting as professional parents on society's behalf, nurses receive all the conflict associated with parenting and parenthood. They may be over-invested with responsibility by society and those who employ them, be expected to demonstrate unrealistic levels of expertise even when poorly resourced, and akin to all parents be apportioned undue blame when those they care for deteriorate. In the same way that we distanced ourselves from our parents to acquire adulthood, so our clients may need to reject us to achieve a better sense of their own independence. In this sense the care relationship is often experienced as intrusive and intimate for nurse and client alike, and too close for comfort.

The price of holding an authoritative position and the personal cost of this in terms of intrapersonal disease is nowhere more intense nor better attested than within nursing (Menzies, 1960; Barber, 1996). Indeed, nursing provides us with a lesson as to how the best of intentions may, due to relational stress, end in harm.

Glancing through the nursing journals, one meets glaring examples of insensitive social practice. When I first wrote this account in the late 1980s, I paused to pick an old *Nursing Times* from a pile near my desk, and readily found two examples. In an article entitled 'Facing up to disfigurement', Pamela Holmes (1986) describes the case of a girl in her twenties who needed surgery for two brain tumours:

> 'Her face was badly disfigured and it didn't help that her hair had been shaved off. Anxious about seeing her mother for the first time since this traumatic surgery, the girl approached the ward sister to ask if there was anything that could be done to improve her looks. The sister, who was standing in a group of student nurses, suggested she "put a bucket on her head".'

Later in the same article, a client describes her experience of returning to the ward after facial surgery:

> 'When I was brought back from theatre', she says, 'I didn't have a dressing over my face and all the patients came over to my bed to have a look at what the surgeons had done. It was the most humiliating and degrading thing to have happened.'

Further, in the same journal, another author relates the following:

> 'Some time ago I interviewed a psychiatric nurse who, in a deliberate and measured tone said: "We are looking after people here who are off their rockers, barmy".'

> (Vousden, 1986)

Hopefully times have changed? But I think not. Visiting my mother in hospital in recent years, having a partner who is a nurse, and supervising nurses, I find that professional scapegoating still occurs, especially when a nurse's ego gets bruised or he/she starts to feel trapped and undervalued in his/her work.

Historically, reflecting upon my own clinical experience, while training to be a nurse for those with learning difficulties, I encountered both mental and physical cruelty; it was commonplace to see nurses teasing residents or forcing food quickly down the throats of severely disabled clients so as to have time later to relax and watch the TV. The care of residents was often jokingly referred to as 'farming', and the individuals so 'cared for' as 'animals'.

In my mental nurse training the above picture of alienation was little improved. The staff were very cohesive and powerful and 'care' often masqueraded as rigid regimes of control where staff interests could be presented at the expense of the client group. Staff boundaries were heavily defended and the trappings of nursing status were made much of. For example, keys were dangled from nurses' belts; white coats were worn with pride; badges of office were worn on lapels and **authoritative** professional interventions were the norm.

In general nursing I have found similar non-therapeutic attitudes and behaviours. On the medical wards all patients were forced to sleep, wake and wash at the same time; visiting was restricted; nursing routines were performed – often without purpose – and the patients' feelings and opinions were ridden over roughshod. Before surgery the anxieties of pre-operative patients were ignored and clarifying information routinely withheld. Patients who asked for clarification or argued their case were unpopular; everything seemed to be structured to induce a **learned helplessness** (Seligman, 1975). Both medical and surgical wards perpetuated the unforgivable sin of encouraging their clients to die alone, isolated in side rooms far away from others.

Similar anecdotes to those above come to me still from privately run homes for the elderly. One cannot eradicate nor legislate out negative or shadowy aspects of human nature; such behaviour is part of us all. I guess we must just stay vigilant, on the watch for symptoms of our own arrogance and the potential to over-inflate our ego. Self-absorbed people may have little awareness of their effect on others. Over-identification with a profession can easily inflate an ego and isolate an individual from his/her humanity.

There are many reasons we may cite to excuse the above actions. Indeed, some may have been performed with the very best of intentions. But the fact remains, they are insensitive, unhealthy and run counter to therapeutic care and practice.

But do such insensitive nursing actions still take place in the 1990s? What does your experience as a clinician suggest to you?

With the above in view, and mindful of an earlier concept which stated that stressed people cannot transmit care, reflect upon the following passage which describes the plight of a client whose request to delay a pain-killing injection so that he might better engage with his relative who had travelled some 200 miles to visit brought him in contact with the hard edge of professional politics. This passage also serves to remind us of how rigid we may become and how insulating professional defences can be:

'On what I thought to be my third post-operative day – but was in fact my fifth as I had been unconscious for two days post-operatively – I was approached just before visiting time by the ward sister who told me she was going to give me a pain-killing injection prior to getting me up and sitting me in a chair. As Anna was travelling up from Surrey to visit me, and as the injection cited made me sleepy, I enquired if this could be delayed so that I might remain alert during visiting. This suggestion was not favourably received: I was lectured on how important it was to get up. I agreed, but enquired whether two hours would make such a difference, and repeated my rationale. This did not go down well; I was told I must do as she asked. For whose benefit was this injection being given, I asked. The tempo now increased; we both had the bit between our teeth. I said, with respect, as a client I had a right to be heard; it was important to my own well-being for me to fully contact my kin – they were my lifeline. She objected. Surely, I argued, in these days of nursing process and client-centred care my request was a reasonable enough one to make. She stormed off. My visitors came and went. With their departure I had my injection, was helped out of bed and sat in a chair. While attending to me the sister said nothing. I did not feel forgiven for querying her instructions. A few hours later I heard laughter, the junior nurses and sister were playing, flicking water at one another. When she realised I was watching the sister stopped. I seemed to represent a problem for her, and suspected I had been "hit by a projection". A little after this a doctor was called, and following much furtive glancing the sister came out to tell me I was being transferred out from intensive care. I asked the sister if this meant I was out of danger. She made no answer, but returned to the office where the doctor remained. More furtive glances ensued. I checked myself, surely I was not becoming paranoid; I had earlier been told I would be here for at least a week more. A change of environment felt quite daunting, especially separation from that meaningful contact forged with the night staff. Within the hour porters came to collect me. When a nurse came over to carry the intravenous drips I asked her to relay to the sister and doctor the message that I did not respect their professional cowardice; she looked embarrassed and I doubt if this was relayed.

My move from intensive care felt ill-prepared and emotive. On the positive side, I was aware that I had the resemblance of an emotion forming within me; a potential for anger; confirmation of my ability to experience emotions again.'

(Barber, 1997)

Reflection Points

Are professionals really employed to care for people? And are hospitals designed to provide care? Consider for a moment the ideas floated below:

- Professions are elitist political bodies that protect their own interests.
- Hospitals safeguard society by preventing the ill from clogging up the economy.
- The ill are controlled rather than cared for.
- Hospitals isolate the non-productive from the productive.
- Hospitals are institutions which keep disease out of community sight.
- Community nursing has flowered because it was believed to be the cheapest option.

Which of the above concepts does history favour?

And in terms of nursing and nurses, who or what are they:

- Administering angels?
- Career opportunists?
- Officers of the state?
- Caring or controlling professionals?

UNDERSTANDING: THE PERSONAL COST OF NURSING CARE

In the late 1950s Isabel Menzies Lyth, while conducting a study into low levels of nursing morale, identified ways in which nurses have traditionally structured the social fabric of their clinical environment so as to avoid facing up to, confronting and dealing with intrapersonal and social stress. More recent application of her work (Barber, 1997) suggests her findings have as much meaning today as they did then.

Menzies' study, concerned with the 'nursing service of a general hospital', described the stress that nurses met in the following terms:

'The direct impact on the nurse of physical illness is intensified by her task of meeting and dealing with psychological stress in other people including her own colleagues. It is by no means easy to tolerate such stress even if one is not under similar stress oneself. Quite short conversations with patients or relatives showed that their conscious concept of illness and treatment is a rich intermixture of objective knowledge, logical deduction, and fantasy . . .

'Patients and relatives have very complicated feelings towards the hospital, which are expressed particularly and most directly to nurses, and often puzzle and distress them. Patients and relatives show appreciation, gratitude, affection, respect; a touching relief that the hospital copes; helpfulness and concern for nurses in their difficult task. But patients often resent their dependence; accept grudgingly the discipline imposed by treatment and hospital routine; envy nurses their health and skills; are demanding, possessive and jealous . . .

'Relatives may also be demanding and critical, the more so because they resent the feeling that hospitalisation implies inadequacies in themselves. They envy nurses their skill and jealously resent the nurse's intimate contact with "their" patient . . .

'The hospital, particularly the nurses, must allow the projection into them of such feelings as depression and anxiety, fear of the patient and his illness, disgust at the illness and the necessary nursing tasks. Patients and relatives treat the staff in such a way as to ensure that the nurses experience these feelings instead of, or partly instead of themselves . . .

'Thus to the nurses' own deep and intense anxieties are added those of the other people concerned.'

(Menzies, 1960, page 9)

I make no apology for quoting the above study at length; too few nurses have examined this work or availed themselves of its message. Indeed, many nurses have forgotten to reflect, preferring to act out their stresses through 'doing', rather than confronting and resolving them. Little has changed since Menzies' study. We have modern units, models of nursing at the fore of current practice, but the same old stresses remain, for we have not yet acquired the research awareness and interpersonal skills to deal with the legacy of stress we have inherited via our caring tradition.

Tradition is the more powerful because it is covert and beyond obvious question; what you cannot see you cannot fight.

Traditional power is prescriptive; it allocates power to historically significant agents (such as the hospital institution). This is in direct contrast to the negotiated authority of 'research'.

In such climates questioning is a rarity and 'change' unacceptable. Unanalysed customs are enshrined where tradition is adhered to rigidly, and ward staff subgroups develop a tribal character. Funtionally, traditions provide a sense of permanence and orientate us to an interactive framework, but when oversubscribed they rob us of creative interpretation and interactive space. The values and **collusions** that emanate from traditional practice – nursing's hidden curriculum – are outlined in Menzies' work.

In the same study, Menzies ascribed the following techniques as ploys to alleviate face-to-face anxiety; they were seen as systems of collusive agreements – often unconscious – via which interactive anxieties were dissipated:

1 Splitting up the nurse–patient relationship
2 **Depersonalisation, categorisation** and denial of the significance of the individual
3 Detachment and denial of feelings
4 The attempt to eliminate decisions by **ritual task performance**
5 Reducing the weight of responsibility in decision making by checks and counterchecks
6 Collusive social redistribution of responsibility and irresponsibility
7 Purposeful obscurity in the formal distribution of responsibility
8 The reduction of the impact of responsibility by delegation to superiors
9 Idealisation and underestimation of personal development possibilities
10 Avoidance of change.

It is to be hoped that the above are relics of nursing practice rather than characteristics of its present.

We must redress those defences isolated by Menzies' study if nurses and nursing are to progress – for these are symptoms of a failure to evolve, to face up to the realities of care and to acquire the necessary relationship skills; they are what we must progress from in order to grow as a profession (Barber and Norman, 1987).

Lest you are in danger of too readily believing that Project 2000 and 'the modern nurse' have eradicated the above social dynamics from care, I submit below an extended breakdown of Menzies' categories along with specific examples of the same, gleaned whilst a participant observer/patient within a surgical ward.

Splitting up of the nurse–patient relationship

Here tasks are seen to demand more attention than individuals; patients are treated all the same, personal distinctions are reduced, clinical duties prescribed and listed. Little opportunity is afforded for development of one-to-one relationships; nurse–client relationships are strongly discouraged and professional distance strongly reinforced.

Example

I noted – while a patient in hospital – that nurses were constantly on the lookout for physical jobs to do. This behaviour was strongly reinforced; for example, when a senior member of staff encountered juniors talking to clients, jobs were quickly found for them to do in areas from the individual they had engaged in conversation.

Depersonalisation, categorisation and denial of individual significance

Patients are referred to by their medical condition rather than names. Uniformity of response and client management, attitude and performance is encouraged; individuality and creativity are discouraged.

Example

My own experience testifies to this; I was rarely referred to by my name, but rather identified by my diet, condition, or yet again by my consultant surgeon – 'Dr X's thorax'!

Detachment and denial feelings

Staff are expected to exert strong controls over their feelings; shows of emotion are discouraged and involvement is feared. Staff are disciplined rather than counselled and told what to do rather than listened to or really heard. Clients' feelings are generally ignored and systems of control predominate over systems of care.

Example

Every nurse within the ward appeared to have two forms of presentation or communication style. To colleagues their tone of voice was feelingless and businesslike, and to patients jollying, rather patronising in a playful way, and chiding. When a patient died, no time was set aside for appraisal or mourning. In consequence, nurses plunged themselves into ward tasks with increased energy and were seemingly even more desperate to keep themselves busy.

Decisions reduced and avoided via an adherence to ritual and routine

The anxiety of free choice is replaced with instrumental activity and nursing procedures; decisions are shelved until new policies are formed. Questioning is discouraged and new ways resisted.

Example

To take night sedation at any other than the usual time or to request pain-killers outside of the medicine round produced pronounced tension. Relatively simple requests from patients, such as to delay night sedation or to sleep through breakfast after a sleepless night, were referred by junior staff to seniors, such was the fear of employing one's own initiative.

Responsibility diluted by checks and counterchecks

Individual action is actively discouraged, everything has a tendency to be obsessively recorded. Trust of others – and their skills – is a rarity, fear of failure a constant motivator.

Example

Even aspirin, a common enough drug in the home, was given out in a manner one would expect of a deadly poison. My temperature, pulse and respiration, which I could easily take for myself as a trained nurse, just had to be done for me. Strangely enough, what appeared on my observation chart, the record of my pulse and temperature, was given much more credence than those symptoms I was able to report as an experienced practitioner. Blood pressures recorded by juniors were nearly always checked routinely by senior staff and observations by patients generally given little weight.

Collusive redistribution of responsibility and irresponsibility

Authoritative parts of oneself are displaced on to seniors and irresponsible parts on to juniors; consequently, seniors are seen as parents and juniors as 'childlike'. Personal power is denied and professional autonomy and personal initiative are largely left unused.

Example

It was commonplace to hear juniors being chastised for supposed errors openly in front of their patients. Likewise deviations from routine – for whatever reason – brought quick rebuke. Everything was seemingly directed at keeping the *status quo*.

Responsibility avoided by generalisation and role obscurity

Roles are unspecified, responsibilities blurred and boundaries largely undefined. Ample space is provided for excuses to be found, conflicts ignored and personal responsibilities disowned.

Example

Alongside the need to record things obsessively and to keep the routine operative was another, conflicting thread; here, practitioners would refer everything back to the next level of seniority. This seemed to be in part good sense, to avoid being told off for using initiative, but also appeared to have the flavour of getting back at seniors and acting out passive anger at the system. Seniors in like manner tended to select those individuals who were less compliant or whom they appeared to dislike for the more tedious jobs.

Open disagreements and dislikes were thus avoided, kept under wraps, and punitive power play enacted with the professional veneer well and truly intact.

Delegation to superiors of professional and personal choice

Disclaimed responsibilities are forced upwards to seniors. Staff perform well below their level of competence and skills, and responsibility is shirked.

Example

Largely due to the aforementioned dynamics, seniors were forever overloaded with petty decisions. This in turn reaffirmed what appeared to be a personal need in themselves: to be seen as a 'work hero', a person who gives his/her all and never shirks decisions, an all-giving, all-powerful, indispensable being. Seniors here appeared dangerously close to burn-out.

Idealisation of self and underestimation of the potential to develop

Homage is paid to the belief that 'nurses are born rather than made' and selection of the 'right' people is emphasised over training and professional and/or personal development. Maturity and responsibility are allocated to rank rather than to individual merit.

Example

Personal and professional status within the clinical setting seemed to revolve around rank and rank ordering. This gave immense power to those who knew the routine, the system and other power holders of the hospital. By venerating those who had remained longest in the hospital or one of its specialist areas, routine was safeguarded and change all too successfully resisted.

Avoidance of change

The full consent of everyone is sought before change can take place so progress is as fast as the slowest team member involved. Problem confrontation is avoided; change is avoided for fear of the necessity to restructure existing social defences.

Example

Understandably, in the light of all the above restrictions, change all but failed to permeate the clinical setting. Upon the wall of the nursing office was a chart of various nursing models, individualised Kardex reporting of patients occurred, but I was never interviewed by a nurse in my 2-month stay nor was a care plan produced. Things just went on as they always had done.

Looking at the above social defences, observed in the 1950s and confirmed more recently by my own experiences, I ask myself: do things ever change? When I speak to professional trainees who have reaped the benefit of many years of 'sociology', 'experiential learning' and 'communication studies', they nearly always believe the above to be historical to professional practice. With more thorough reflection and application to their own areas of work, this view changes. Indeed, in line with my own observations (Barber, 1997), they generally report that the above defences are alive and flourishing within their own place of work.

Reflection Points

Reading the 'Rules and Orders for the Government of the Royal Hospital of Bridewell and Bethlem', published 1778, I note the duties of the Matron as: 'to take care the rooms are in every respect in decent order'; 'to let in the women prisoners at all hours of the night should they be brought: and to keep due decorum among them'; 'to take upon her the charge of and be answerable for all the women prisoners'; 'to attend women prisoners when they are burning their straw and cleaning their wards'; 'to take care when the doctor prescribes any medicines'; 'to see that the women's prison be washed once a week and fumigated with tar'. Though this is a historical document over 200 years old, there is something familiar to me. Then, just as now, routines stand in the way of communication and personal care, and individuals are lost within insitutional systems which are supposed to care for them, but which in fact do more by way of managing and controlling them.

- Just what is society seeking to clean away through health care?

- Are more than germs being attacked by sanitation?
- What symbolic rituals are enacted in professional care?
- What do nurses symbolise for others – and what to themselves?

CHANGING: LEARNING TO GROW

'Change' is an interpersonal process, a natural consequence of growth and a requisite of education and personal development. At the last analysis we have no choice but to make 'change' our friend. Nothing is for ever, nothing is permanent, all is in flux. Accepting this fact is the hardest part of change; all too often we have been taught to believe in permanence. We rarely contemplate our own death – that ultimate change awaiting us – or comprehend 'our reality' as a momentary grasping at ever-flowing experience. Everything around us and within us is dynamic. Our pretence to maintain a sense of permanence is understandable; it offers a palliative security. Change implies threat, the letting go of the old known ways. Change is hard work. Successful living requires you to ride upon the crest of the wave of change. To do other than this is to diminish your contact with the world, to retreat into fantasy, to segment yourself, hide from the here-and-now and deny much of your potential; it is also unhealthy.

Health is a state of mind, the ability to make contact with and experience such positive emotions as joy, love and a sense of fulfilment while having the confidence to take risks and live life creatively (Wilson, 1975). Intellectual and physical functions are secondary yardsticks of health to these. Health is an emotionally energised state, and nurses – who concern themselves with the facilitation of health in others – must appreciate both their own and their clients' emotional experience.

Two possible responses to change are illustrated in Figure 14.1. These responses are suggested to be either positive and supportive of healthy outcome, or negative and unhealthy.

Carl Jung suggested there were four major ways of relating to the world: thinking, feeling, sensing and intuition (Jung, 1957).

'Thinking' and 'feeling' are concerned with the way you judge and/or value things. Do you see life from a rational objective standpoint, or are you more inclined towards an inner world view informed by subjective experience and emotion?

'Sensation' and 'intuition', by contrast, are ways of perceiving and gathering information from your environment. Here, you may look out upon the world primarily through your five senses or through intuitive knowing informed by inner certainty.

All these references are important. The science of care is informed by thinking and sensation, the art of expression of care by intuition and feeling.

By self-observation and paying attention to how we use the above dimensions, we may discover a little about how we adapt to change and process the environment.

The art of working through, enjoying and gaining from change is dependent upon our acceptance of it. Acceptance starts the whole process off. Personally, I have found it useful to 'check out' myself when meeting change. To do this I stop, reflect, and explore my 'thoughts', 'senses', 'feelings' and 'intuitions'. I can do this for such diverse issues as a change of job, a quandary of care, the meaning of a recently experienced dream, a life crisis, an essay topic, or indeed, to explore options open to me. I also employ this technique to enable students within my workshops and clients with whom I am working therapeutically to appreciate where they are *now*. For example, if I consider my own immediate reality while writing this tract, the following awarenesses arise:

- *Thoughts*: I'm thinking where best to take this chapter, whether to introduce styles of intervention or continue with the theme of adaptation to change.
- *Sensations*: I'm aware of being warmed by the open fire to my left, cool down my right side, and of my attention being drawn to the flakes of snow falling gently outside the window.
- *Feelings*: I'm feeling low in emotional energy, satisfied with today's work on this chapter, but tired and emotionally flat.
- *Intuitions*: I'm tired and in need of a rest, I will be unable to proceed with clarity unless I take time out from writing for a while.
- *Thoughts*: I'll be more able to continue this work tomorrow; I will try to stop thinking about work until the morning.
- *Sensations*: I'm aware of a sensation of relief at deciding to stop and am aware of my attention drifting away from writing.

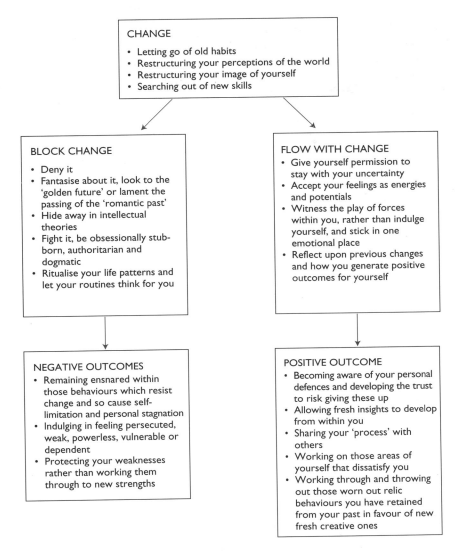

CHANGE

- Letting go of old habits
- Restructuring your perceptions of the world
- Restructuring your image of yourself
- Searching out of new skills

BLOCK CHANGE

- Deny it
- Fantasise about it, look to the 'golden future' or lament the passing of the 'romantic past'
- Hide away in intellectual theories
- Fight it, be obsessionally stubborn, authoritarian and dogmatic
- Ritualise your life patterns and let your routines think for you

FLOW WITH CHANGE

- Give yourself permission to stay with your uncertainty
- Accept your feelings as energies and potentials
- Witness the play of forces within you, rather than indulge yourself, and stick in one emotional place
- Reflect upon previous changes and how you generate positive outcomes for yourself

NEGATIVE OUTCOMES

- Remaining ensnared within those behaviours which resist change and so cause self-limitation and personal stagnation
- Indulging in feeling persecuted, weak, powerless, vulnerable or dependent
- Protecting your weaknesses rather than working them through to new strengths

POSITIVE OUTCOME

- Becoming aware of your personal defences and developing the trust to risk giving these up
- Allowing fresh insights to develop from within you
- Sharing your 'process' with others
- Working on those areas of yourself that dissatisfy you
- Working through and throwing out those worn out relic behaviours you have retained from your past in favour of new fresh creative ones

Figure 14.1: The demands of change on the individual

- *Feelings*: I'm feeling glad to turn away from my work, and am aware of a feeling of excited anticipation in recommencing afresh tomorrow morning.
- *Intuitions*: I'm freer than I suppose, but in fantasy I make myself feel trapped in order to work harder and quicker; that is, I threaten myself into hard work.

My solution seems to stem from my self-awareness; in knowing where I am now and my present state of need, I can relinquish my work until morning. This process is detailed in Figure 14.2 so you may sample it yourself.

Reflection Points

How do you rate yourself in the manner you evaluate and/or constitute your own world view; are you primarily a thinker or feeler? Indicate this on the continuum below:

Thinking _____ Feeling

In which main way do you gather information: via your five senses or intuition?
Indicate this on the continuum below:

Sensing _____ Intuition

How different are you in various settings – at home or work? Or when you lead a team or yet again are a member of it? That is to say, does your rank or status affect how you behave?

It might be interesting for you to examine your nursing notes. What do you portray of yourself in your records; your thoughts or feelings, sensory awareness or intuitions? Personally, I have been surprised by the high ratio of intuitive data I find in professional records which are taken as statements of fact.

Seeing: a transactional view of nursing

Possibly you are starting to ponder just where this discussion is leading. We have identified the lack of relevant preparation in nursing education, the blocks which occur to frustrate personal development, and untherapeutic practices. Change has been addressed – along with those behaviours that enable growth-promoting outcomes – and an awareness exercise has been suggested. But so what?

I have attempted to write this chapter in much the same way as I approach the care of clients. I have introduced my biases and beliefs, provided evidence so that you might understand something of their origin, and shared my own process while directing attention upon 'the present'. What impressions are you left with?

Sometimes we must move slowly if we are to learn. A major fault of the nursing profession is that it spent too much time trying to define 'essences' but failed to appreciate 'existence' and its everyday reality. Many of its theorists would have been better employed exploring how nurses may make better contact with the clinical world in which they work.

Awareness is itself a potent agent of change. Nurses have rarely sought intimate contact with their world – rather distancing themselves from it – with the consequence that little has changed.

Nurses have denied their clients' internal states, paid homage to intellect, but divorced themselves from intuition, feelings and the evidence of their senses. They have forgotten to be 'aware' and 'research-minded'. Nurses have let managerial rituals do much of their thinking for them; likewise the impulse to keep busy in hands and feet has replaced much reflection. Qualitative

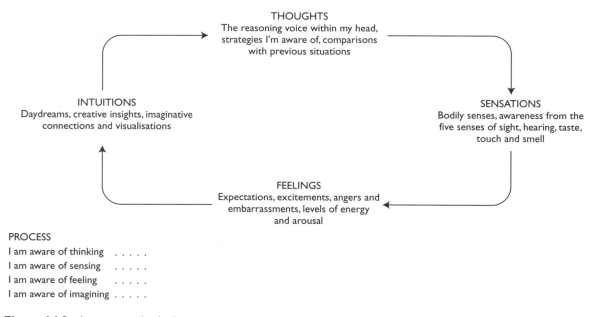

THOUGHTS
The reasoning voice within my head, strategies I'm aware of, comparisons with previous situations

INTUITIONS
Daydreams, creative insights, imaginative connections and visualisations

SENSATIONS
Bodily senses, awareness from the five senses of sight, hearing, taste, touch and smell

FEELINGS
Expectations, excitements, angers and embarrassments, levels of energy and arousal

PROCESS
I am aware of thinking . . . . .
I am aware of sensing . . . . .
I am aware of feeling . . . . .
I am aware of imagining . . . . .

Figure 14.2: Awareness check sheet

supervision is a rarity, and there is little counselling or support (Moscato, 1976).

I am attempting to address all this by emphasising personal awareness, individual perception, and self-analysis of moment-to-moment function. The more self-aware nurses become (I suggest), the less blind they will be to what they do professionally, and how they manage their care role.

Transactional analysis (TA), a theory of human development and relating, may help here. Eric Berne (1967), the originator of transactional analysis, suggests that as infants grow they become aware of two images of themselves. First, they are aware of their own emotions and physical needs; second, they are aware of the expectations of their parents. Their own feelings provide an impression of themselves from the driver's seat, and the social viewpoint of their parents gives them a mirror with which to assess themselves. Parents provide their children with a model of social behaviour.

Consequently the infant, in loving, respecting and imitating his parents, internalises a social perception of the world. His orientation to his parents' world causes the development of an inner **'parent ego'** of his own, while his experience of his own emotional energies, his playful fantasies and creativity form the bounds of his own **'child ego'**. Last to evolve, and very much linked with the growth of mobility, independence and questioning, is his **'adult ego'**, his view of the world as he found it and checked it out to be.

This model is illustrated in Figure 14.3. Three orientations to the world are evident. The 'parent ego' serves to relate us to the social world and 'life as taught', that is, our cultural beliefs and values. Under this is placed the 'adult ego', an exploratory and assessment mechanism that relates to everyday reality and 'life as found to be'. Below is the 'child ego' which orientates us to our vulnerable, childlike qualities – along with the creativity and energies of 'life as felt'.

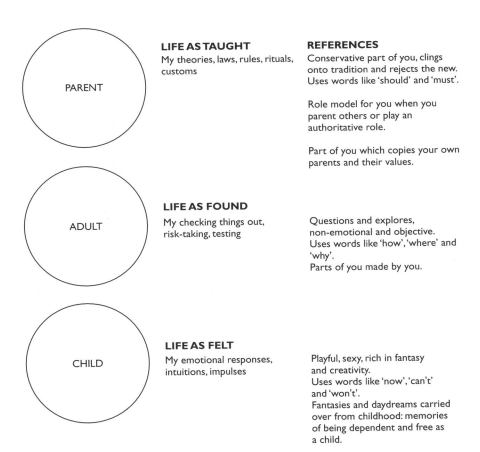

Figure 14.3: A transaction model of ego function

Taking this model into the realms of the nursing profession and the roles carers play, further insights are available. Nursing has an abundance of rules, theories and rituals; it is overtly concerned with the structuring of the care experience and the formation of care strategies. Simply, training and practice encourage the nurse to perceive him/herself primarily as a 'parent' figure. A similar process occurs in the preparation of physicians, but unlike nurses, they are taught to exercise more autonomy and to validate the reality of their experiences; their 'adult' function is more developed through 'research-mindedness'.

If we combine those experiential insights from the self-awareness exercise – Figure 14.2 – with transactional analysis and the nursing role, we observe that awareness of theories and beliefs puts us in touch with our socially construed 'parent', awareness of our observations and physical sensations relates to functional reality and our 'adult', while recognition of our feelings and fantasies places us in touch with the energies available within our 'child' (Figure 14.4).

The above egos are valuable to us and relevant to nursing, but the strengths of each ego (i.e. the social awareness and intellectual structuring of the 'parent', the reality orientation and testing of the 'adult', and creative energies of the 'child') are rarely facilitated – with conscious intent – in nurse education or in clinical practice.

It is a sad fact that most educational and clinical relationships are predominantly 'parent-to-child' ones (Moscato, 1976). That is to say, professionals tend to adopt the roles of authoritative and critical parents, the 'know bests' who seek to control and impose their will upon others. Interactively, the resulting pecking order is often that represented in Figure 14.5.

The issuing of authoritative demands, the withholding of information, and the absence of sharing, counselling and research-minded discussion leads to rigid role performance which encourages seniors to relate to juniors as childlike and naive entities, and juniors to **idealise** and **project** 'parent-like' images and personal responsibilities upon the seniors. This corresponds with Menzies' (1960) findings in her study:

'Each nurse tends to split off aspects of herself from her conscious personality and to project

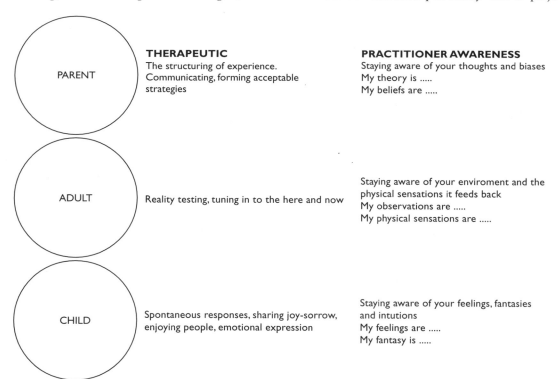

THERAPEUTIC
The structuring of experience. Communicating, forming acceptable strategies

PRACTITIONER AWARENESS
Staying aware of your thoughts and biases
My theory is .....
My beliefs are .....

Reality testing, tuning in to the here and now

Staying aware of your enviroment and the physical sensations it feeds back
My observations are .....
My physical sensations are .....

Spontaneous responses, sharing joy-sorrow, enjoying people, emotional expression

Staying aware of your feelings, fantasies and intutions
My feelings are .....
My fantasy is .....

Figure 14.4: Transactional qualities of care

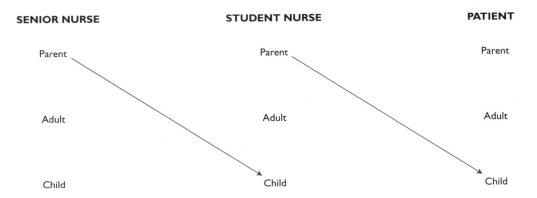

Figure 14.5: Authoritative interactions

them into other nurses. Her irresponsible impulses, which she feels she cannot control, are attributed to her juniors. Her painfully severe attitude to these impulses and burdensome sense of responsibility are attributed to her seniors. Consequently, she identifies juniors with her irresponsible self and treats them with the severity that self is felt to deserve. Similarly, she identifies seniors with her own harsh disciplinary attitude to her irresponsible self and expects harsh discipline. There is psychic truth in the assertion that juniors are irresponsible and seniors harsh disciplinarians. These are the roles assigned to them. There is also objective truth, since people act objectively on the psychic roles assigned to them'.

Interactions returning to seniors thus reinforce the original transferences and counter-transferences (Figure 14.6). In this situation, reality orientation is poor, personal awareness and self-awareness are lost and although feelings and stresses are experienced, they are denied and ignored. Burn-out and disillusionment follow naturally in such climates.

A healthier and far more therapeutic culture evolves when 'adult-to-adult' interactions are the prevailing norm (see Figure 14.7). Material stored in our 'parent' and 'child' egos is primarily archaic and serves to orientate us to our social and emotional pasts (Harris, 1973). The adult, by contrast, orientates us to everyday reality.

Too often the nursing profession has bred in its practitioners an overstrong degree of 'parenthood', along with such parental social fears as losing control, losing self-respect and the respect of others. As a consequence, nurses have tended to conform too rigidly. They have not been prepared in a way where fears may be voiced and worked through; their preparation is nearer one of 'paper-

ing over the cracks'; their superficial veneer is shallow and prone to fracture.

Nurses are taught primarily to hide their vulnerabilities from others – and themselves – but in so doing they also reduce their sensitivity.

Bump the skin and it gives, stretches and returns quickly to normal in a fluid and flexible fashion; bump a blister and – no matter how hard it appears superficially – it cracks, weeps and takes an extraordinarily long time to heal. Nurses cover the sensitive bits of themselves with blisters. Change is threatening and costly to nurses when their defences are so brittle. Change must address the individual – rather than the system in which individuals operate – and specifically, it must be felt, checked out, and evaluated experientally.

> **Reflection Point**
>
> Behaviour to facilitate your 'adult' function and ability to adapt is suggested in Figure 14.8. Try out these behaviour cues in your nursing role. Goals I have found it especially useful to work towards are 'Giving myself permission to stay with my uncertainties', and 'Allowing myself to make mistakes'. The path of your enquiry is just as sacred as mine, and your own findings are much more relevant for you.

BEING: LIVING AND CARING IN THE 'NOW'

Let us leave both 'nursing' and the 'care role' for a while and examine a little further the concept of 'existence'. The need to focus upon 'existences' rather than 'essences' was touched on earlier.

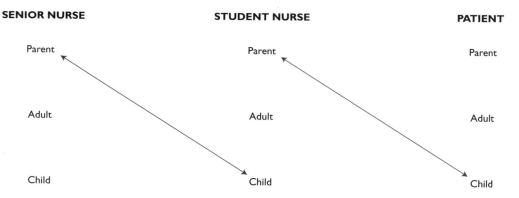

Figure 14.6: Responding to authoritative interactions

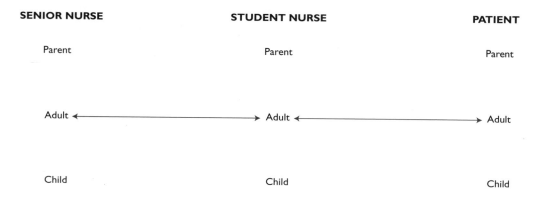

Figure 14.7: Healthy interactions (adult to adult)

When we seek out the essence of a thing we must of necessity confine, measure and define it. In doing this there is a tendency for us to fit the object under examination into a frame of reference already known to us; 'not seeing the wood for the trees' is an example of the danger in this type of thinking. Our contact with 'direct experience' is reduced by this means; for example, if I go for a walk at dusk and see in the distance an object I cannot identify, my imaginative perception runs riot. I squint to perceive the object more clearly, and tilt my head to one side to listen for any tell-tale noises to help recognition. I sense myself becoming aroused by expectancy and surprise within me. I approach the object tentatively for fear of a heaven-only-knows-what encounter. I am also truly alive.

If, as I draw nearer, I identify the object as an old tree root – suddenly my enquiring stops. 'It's only an old tree root', I repeat to myself as I walk on. Could I recognise it again or have I learnt any-

thing from it? Sadly, no. By defining what I believe it to be – the 'essence' of it – I cease to be moved.

Sometimes the same thing happens with inter-personal perception. In married life, for example, partners define and label each other with such judgements as 'they don't care', 'things will never improve', 'they'll always be the same – and they stop looking, listening, being imaginatively aware of or emotionally moved by the other. A similar process can also happen in nursing care. Definition of the 'patient' as dependent and needing, or of 'nurses' as independent and caring, can cause stereotypical perceptions that hinder the transmission of care (Stockwell, 1972). The humanity within each individual may then be lost.

Concentration upon 'definition' may increase our knowledge but at the cost of our understanding. We earlier identified four perceptive functions: thinking, sensing, feeling, and intuition. Figure 14.9 isolates what are suggested to be 'growth-inducing' and 'non-growth-inducing'

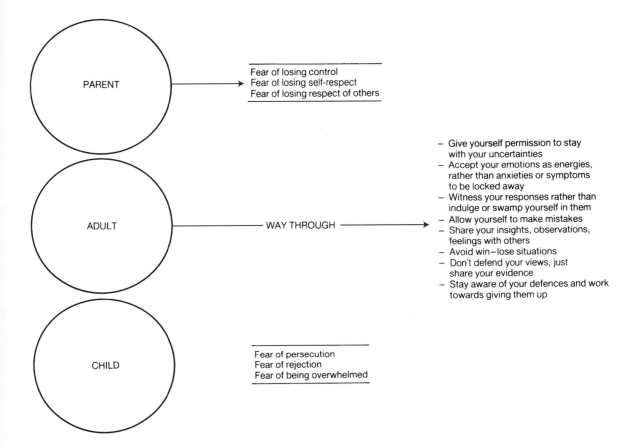

Figure 14.8: A transactional view of personal adaptation

aspects of these functions. The shaded parts of the 'thinking function' suggested to be antagonistic to healthy and aware performance are: fears of losing control (earlier related to TA); irrationality; being judgemental and critical, of shallow intent; and displaying empty niceness.

Growth-promoting orientations of 'thinking' – which are portrayed as unshaded – are order and clarity; the acceptance of responsibility and nurturing; the planning of strategies; values of right and wrong; social alertness and an awareness of relevant theory and knowledge.

Not only the quality of 'thought' but also its distinction from other functions is desirable. If the boundaries of our 'thinking', 'sensing' and 'feeling/intuition' overlap, confusion and disorientation result.

The consequences of perceptual confusion and blurring are portrayed diagrammatically in Figure 14.10. When 'thinking' overlaps with 'sensing', prejudice (i.e. unexplored and unvalidated social

bias) occurs. When 'sensing' overlaps with feelings and intuitions we become deluded, for untested feelings of the world can develop; unclear boundaries between 'thinking' and 'feeling/intuition' may flood our intellect with irrational fears. Last, profound overshadowing of all three functions is seen to relate to **psychotic** states when theories, sensory impressions and those meanings and values we attach to the world become jumbled and distorted. The more jumbled we become, the more unaware and unconscious we are of our own processes; this is denoted by increasing shade within the diagram. The more shadow you have within your personality, the less aware you are of yourself and the less able you become to make positive gains from your experiences. Growth lies in the *working through* and *resolution of your shadow*, and nursing involves the **facilitation** of this process in others.

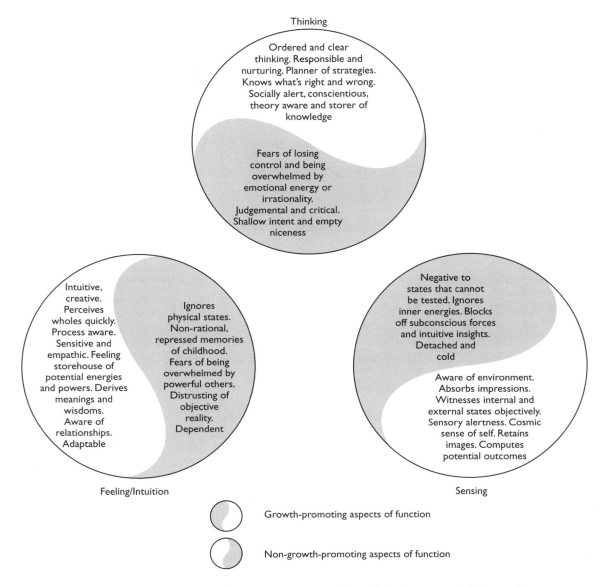

Figure 14.9: Growth-promoting and non-growth-promoting qualities of thinking, sensing, feeling and intuitive functions

Reflection Points

To broaden our perceptions and widen our appreciation we must view things in the raw, stay open and receptive and withhold those definitive judgements that get in the way of listening to and hearing others. We need to capture some of our earlier childlike enthusiasm and interest in the world and to be fully committed to our own existence and the existence of others. As an individual's self-awareness grows, so too does his sense of 'existence'.

Anything that clogs up or blocks off our perceptive machinery interferes with our ability to contact our 'existence' directly. Self-actualisers – individuals who maintain peak performance (Maslow, 1967) – demonstrate an ability to:

■ Perceive reality efficiently, and to tolerate uncertainty

■ Accept themselves and others for what they are – be spontaneous in thought and behaviour

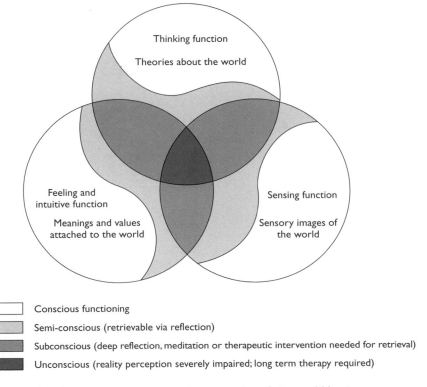

Thinking function

Theories about the world

Feeling and
intuitive function

Meanings and values
attached to the world

Sensing function

Sensory images of
the world

Conscious functioning

Semi-conscious (retrievable via reflection)

Subconscious (deep reflection, meditation or therapeutic intervention needed for retrieval)

Unconscious (reality perception severely impaired; long term therapy required)

Figure 14.10: Model of dysfunction: consequences of perceptual confusion and blurring

- Be problem-centred rather than self-centred – have a good sense of humour
- Be highly creative
- Be resistant to enculturation, although not purposely unconventional
- Demonstrate concern for the welfare of mankind – deeply appreciate the basic experiences of life
- Establish deep satisfying interpersonal relations with a few, rather than many, people
- Look at life from an objective viewpoint.

The above characteristics suggest that acceptance, spontaneity, joy and a sense of wonder are vital to growth, and provide a springboard for discovery of what to aim towards for maximum health.

- In which of the above areas do you excel?
- Where are you weak?
- How might you change your profile on the above?
- When will you know you have changed?

FACILITATING: ENABLING HEALTH TO GROW

The less shadow you carry with you the more potential you have to share. Simplistically, personal growth might be represented as a movement from darkness into light (see Figure 14.11). 'Health' is balance, growth is 'super-health'. If we relate the findings of Menzies and our earlier discussion of nursing to our model, some interesting features develop (see Figure 14.12). Here nurses are portrayed as being very 'head' motivated, intellectually stuck in issues of being right or fearing being wrong. Their orientation to reality is also seen as seriously impaired, for there is a blocking-off of intuitive insights leading to a denial of feelings and a negative response to change. There is not much fun in such nursing, nor room for enjoyment. Because feelings and intuitive functions are denied expression, the energies arising from these eventually build up to threaten objective work performance.

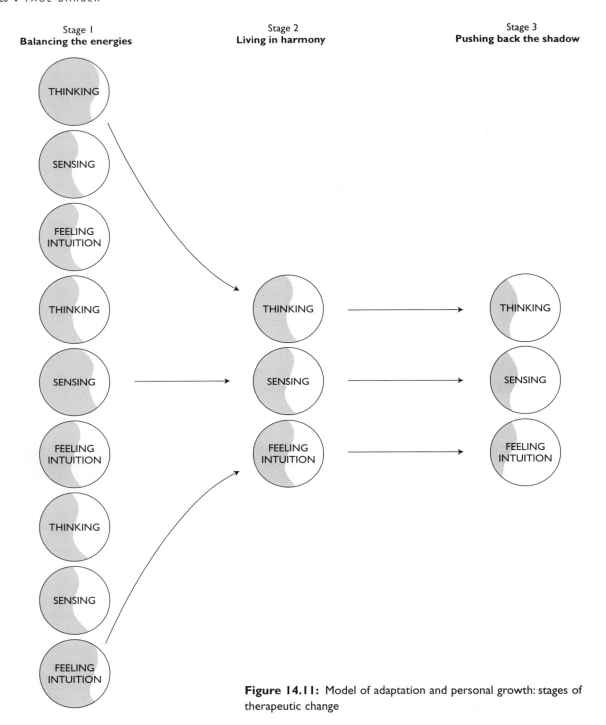

Figure 14.11: Model of adaptation and personal growth: stages of therapeutic change

Nurses judiciously exercise control of themselves and their environment, demonstrating a brusque buinesslike exterior in their performance of all those 'tasks-at-hand'. The maintenance of this facade is an expensive process, especially in terms of 'burn-out' and personal cost (Edelwich and Brodsky, 1980). To deny your emotionality leads to fear of the emotionality of others, for their anxiety in turn stimulates your own. Defensive ploys of displacing emotional energy on to work, the 'work hero' syndrome, are then commonly found.

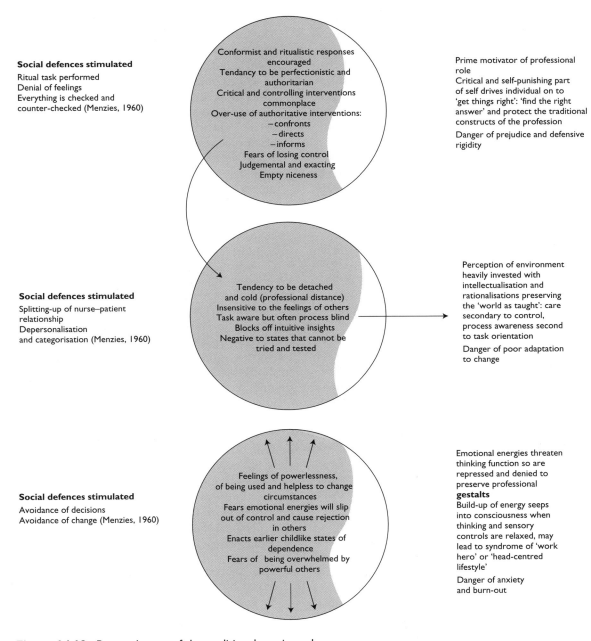

Social defences stimulated

Ritual task performed
Denial of feelings
Everything is checked and
counter-checked (Menzies, 1960)

Conformist and ritualistic responses
encouraged
Tendancy to be perfectionistic and
authoritarian
Critical and controlling interventions
commonplace
Over-use of authoritative interventions:
 – confronts
 – directs
 – informs
Fears of losing control
Judgemental and exacting
Empty niceness

Prime motivator of professional
role
Critical and self-punishing part
of self drives individual on to
'get things right': 'find the right
answer' and protect the traditional
constructs of the profession
Danger of prejudice and defensive
rigidity

Social defences stimulated

Splitting-up of nurse–patient
relationship
Depersonalisation
and categorisation (Menzies, 1960)

Tendency to be detached
and cold (professional distance)
Insensitive to the feelings of others
Task aware but often process blind
Blocks off intuitive insights
Negative to states that cannot be
tried and tested

Perception of environment
heavily invested with
intellectualisation and
rationalisations preserving
the 'world as taught': care
secondary to control,
process awareness second
to task orientation
Danger of poor adaptation
to change

Social defences stimulated

Avoidance of decisions
Avoidance of change (Menzies, 1960)

Feelings of powerlessness,
of being used and helpless to change
circumstances
Fears emotional energies will slip
out of control and cause rejection
in others
Enacts earlier childlike states of
dependence
Fears of being overwhelmed by
powerful others

Emotional energies threaten
thinking function so are
repressed and denied to
preserve professional
gestalts
Build-up of energy seeps
into consciousness when
thinking and sensory
controls are relaxed, may
lead to syndrome of 'work
hero' or 'head-centred
lifestyle'
Danger of anxiety
and burn-out

Figure 14.12: Personal costs of the traditional nursing role

When anxiety-motivated behaviours predominate over other behaviours, emotional burn-out and physical collapse easily ensue. Many nurses are able to describe first-hand experiences of burn-out; they are used to working overtime, facing stress without support, and to meeting criticism more frequently than nurture. Because of this, they end up denying their own psychological and physical needs. Such circumstances light the fuse of burn-out. Sickness rates are often high. It is no wonder that declarations of sickness are preferable to other expressions of discontent or exhaustion when the workplace is geared to the care of others, when systems of instrumental activity override person perception, and discipline takes the place of counselling – and when no one either listens to your feelings or sees the real you behind your role.

Attention was drawn earlier to the way senior nurses adopt an 'authoritative' role. Authoritative perceptions of oneself and others further the critical 'parent' role previously discussed. Authoritative interventions differ in type and kind from those **facilitative** interventions that further personal growth. A drastic reorientation is required if the nursing profession is to be kinder to its practitioners and clients. The philosophy of facilitation provides this. The philosophy of facilitation has been detailed by Carl Rogers in his many texts (see, for example, Rogers, 1967, 1983). Rogers (1983) makes the following points about the role of the facilitator:

1 *A facilitator has much to do with setting the initial mood or climate of a group's experience.* If his own basic philosophy is one of trust in the group and in the individuals who comprise the group, then this point of view will be communicated in many subtle ways.

2 *A facilitator helps to elicit and clarify the purposes of the individuals as well as the more general purposes of the group.* If he is not fearful of accepting contradictory purposes and conflicting aims, if he is able to permit the individuals a sense of freedom in stating what they would like to do, then he is helping to create a climate for learning. There is no need for him to try to manufacture one unified purpose in the group if such a unified purpose is not there. He can permit a diversity of purposes, both contradictory and complementary, to exist in relationship to each other.

3 *A facilitator regards himself as a flexible resource.* He does not downgrade himself as a resource. He makes himself available as a counsellor, lecturer and advisor, a person with experience in the field. He wishes to be used by individuals and by the group in the ways which seem most meaningful to them – in so far as he can be comfortable in operating in the ways they wish.

4 *In responding to expressions, a facilitator accepts both the intellectual content and emotional attitudes, endeavouring to give each aspect the approximate degree of emphasis which it has for the individual or the group.* In so far as he can be genuine in doing so, he accepts rationalisations and intellectualising, as well as deep and real personal feelings.

5 *He takes the initiative in sharing himself with the group – his feelings as well as his thoughts – in ways which do not demand or impose but represent simply a personal sharing which students may take or leave.* Thus, he is free to express his own feelings in giving feedback to students, in his reaction to them as individuals, and in sharing his own satisfactions or disappointments. In such expressions it is his 'owned' attitudes which are shared, not judgements or evaluations of others.

6 *In his function as a facilitator of learning, he endeavours to recognise and accept his own limitations.* He realises that he can only grant freedom to the extent that he is comfortable in giving such freedom. He can only be understanding to the extent that he actually desires to enter the inner world of another. He can only share himself to the extent that he is reasonably comfortable in taking that risk.

Facilitation puts 'people' firmly back into the care process. 'Systems' are secondary here to individual response. The above suggestions are readily applicable to those models of care collectively termed the 'nursing process'; indeed, they give the interactive foundation we need to prevent their freshness being swamped by the restraints of traditional practice.

Rogers' work on facilitation suggests a philosophy which enables the provision of a care climate in which education and care giving may be maximised. But we need to know specifically what skills are necessary to inculcate the above.

Rogers suggests that the characteristics of caring relationships are related to how well individual carers work through their own interpersonal and personal baggage, the doubts they have regarding care – for example:

- 'Can I be caring in some way which will be perceived by the other person as trustworthy, as dependable, or consistent in some deep sense?'
- 'Can I be expressive enough as a person for what I am to be communicated unambiguously?'
- 'Can I let myself experience positive attitudes toward this other person – attitudes of warmth, caring, liking, interest or respect?'
- 'Can I be strong enough as a person to be separate from the other?'
- 'Am I secure enough within myself to permit him his separateness?'
- 'Can I let myself enterfully into the world of his feelings and personal meanings and see these as he does?'

- 'Can I accept each facet of his personality that a client presents to me?'
- 'Can I act with sufficient sensitivity in the relationship, so that my behaviour will not be perceived as a threat?'
- 'Can I free him from the threat of external evaluation?'
- 'Can I meet this other individual as a person who is in the process of becoming, or will I be bound by his past and my past?'

Further analysis of what we may do in the therapeutic relationship comes from the work of John Heron (1990). Heron describes two main orientations – or, as he calls them, styles – of intervention: the 'facilitative' and the 'authoritative'. Under the heading of *Authoritative Interventions*, he places those occasions when individuals speak from the power they invest within themselves and their role; *prescriptive, informative* and *confronting* models of approach are cited here.

Conversely, under the heading of *Facilitative Interventions*, Heron stipulates those times when an individual attempts to attune to another and function in a person-centred fashion to enable that other to explore and take responsibility for himself. Under this category, Heron places *cathartic, catalytic* and *supportive* interventions. A fuller explanation of these terms is given in Table 14.1.

Six Category Intervention Analysis, as Heron calls this system, is a valuable tool for assessing professional intentions and performance. It has opened my eyes to those options I have at my disposal in education and clinical practice alike.

Most nursing models state the importance of a healthy nurse–client relationship but fail to give a reference for these skills. Now you have one. *Authoritative interventions* frame the contextual and task boundaries of nursing care; *facilitative interventions* shape the interpersonal exchange process; both dimensions are also therapeutic and help you clarify clinical intent.

'Task' orientation contains a high frequency of *prescriptive, informative* and *confronting* interventions that 'tell people what to do'. Facilitative interventions are rather at the heart of the **psychotherapies**; they are essential components of non-directive counselling.

Both authoritative and facilitative interventions are necessary in holistic care.

Hildegard Peplau, a notable nursing theorist, has made the following statement:

Table 14.1: Heron's Six Category Intervention Analysis

Authoritative		Facilitative	
1 Prescriptive	*Give advice, be judgemental/ critical/evaluative* A prescriptive intervention is one that explicitly seeks to direct the behaviour of the client, especially behaviour that is outside or beyond the practitioner–client interaction	**4 Cathartic**	*Release tensions in, encourage laughter/crying* A cathartic intervention seeks to enable the client to experience painful emotion
2 Informative	*Be didactic, instruct/inform, interpret* An informative intervention seeks to impart new knowledge and information to the client	**5 Catalytic**	*Be reflective, encourage self-directed problem-solving, elicit information from* A catalytic intervention seeks to enable the client to learn and develop by self-direction and self-discovery within the context of the practitioner–client situation, but also beyond it
3 Confronting	*Be challenging, give direct feedback* A confronting intervention directly challenges the restrictive attitude/belief/ behaviour of the client	**6 Supportive**	*Be approving, confirming, validating* A supportive intervention affirms the worth and value of the client

'Nursing is a service for people that enhances healing and health by methods that are humanistic and primarily non-invasive.'

(Peplau, 1987)

In the context of this statement, it would seem more appropriate for today's nurses to err more in the direction of facilitative interventions than of authoritative ones.

REFLECTING: THE NATURE OF NURSING CARE

The foremost duty of anyone who wishes to be an effective care giver is to work on the self; we are each our own most important therapeutic tool.

Enriched, self-aware people make good nurses; emotionally impoverished, unaware people do not.

It would appear that in the past nursing has sought to produce impoverished, unaware practitioners to benefit its traditionally rigid system (see Figure 14.9). This is now changing; there is promise of person-centred care in the implementation of nursing models, awareness training via experiential encounter in nurse education, and a political awareness in the use of advocacy as a care skill – notably in the nursing of people with learning difficulties.

With the nursing process established in general nursing, the psychosocial perspectives of psychiatric nurses have become increasingly relevant to general care. Nurses of the future could reasonably be expected to synthesise the empathic relating, political and educational awareness that nurses from the discipline of learning disability employ; the interactive skills and psychotherapeutic insights used by mental nurses; and the physiological awarenesses and cognition that general nurses incorporate in their work.

All of the above must be incorporated into our therapeutic arsenal if we desire to fulfil the ideal of 'holistic care'. Sociological insights flow from learning disabilities, psychological insights from mental illness, and physiological ones from general care.

As man is a physiological organism who correlates his world in psychological terms and defines reality in social ones, all dimensions must be combined.

Nursing is suggested in this chapter to be an interpersonal process that relates scientifically derived insights to clients in empathic humane ways, while educating these clients to ways of thinking, feeling and relating that maximise their ability to grow in a self-directed and therapeutic way. Nurses need cognitive skills to learn and understand these processes involved in health; they need empathy and an interest in the human condition; they need insight into their own unique composition, together with an ability to develop personal and interpersonal relationship skills so that they may share these insights with others. That body of theory and research findings derived from care is the *science* of nursing, while the expressive, empathic and relating aspects of nursing constitute its *art*. Therapy is both an art and a science.

Reflection Points

- List those qualities and skills you associate with nursing as a *science*.
- List those qualities and skills you associate with nursing as an *art*.

EXPRESSING: DYNAMICS OF CARE

The nursing profession needs to *develop* its therapeutic arts. It has nursing models, a bank of theory extending back some 50 years but, from examination so far, it appears that nurses have developed more instrumental skills than expressive ones.

One is reminded of the 'Nursing Procedure Books' produced by many health authorities, emphasising instrumental vision across a host of 'care' activities, respectful of which tray or trolley arrangement to use and supportive of the philosophy that care can be reduced to the memorising of appropriate rituals safeguarding 'the right way' of doing things. All tend to be devoid of expressions of care or interpersonal nurse–client exchange; procedure books are one of the profession's horror stories.

Possibly this may sound radical to some. If so, it is not inappropriate, especially if it exposes the professional sterility we incur from the use of a pseudo-scientific and reductionist vision. Nursing has produced many more sheep than goats. Sheep make poor carers and are a far from potent symbol of assertion or advocacy. Intuitively, I feel that when I am ill and low in energy I will want – and need – those who care for me to be assertive, to defend my rights and be strong enough to accept my pains, frustrations and angers, so that these may be expressed and released by me as they arise. I don't want to feel I must be on my best behaviour, scared to vent those emotions that naturally percolate from disease states; simply, I want to be able to give myself permission to be real and to express my suffering in realistic terms. Expression is therapeutic; when energies are summoned, they demand release. **Repression**, by contrast, has been linked to much somatic disturbance (Cox, 1983). Cathartic skills, that is the ability to enable a client to release his emotions, are crucial though often forgotten caring skills.

In Table 14.2, we return to the work of Heron and stipulate cathartic interventions. These take therapeutic courage to initiate, sensitivity of timing and practice to use expertly. Cathartic interventions also require a fair degree of personal maturity in the practitioner. This is a part of that future therapeutic territory nurses need to make their own. Cathartic interventions are not rarified specialist psychiatric techniques, but tools all nurses require; anxiety is common to all hospital admission (Franklin, 1984).

CREATING A WORKABLE SYNTHESIS

My dream is of a nursing profession where those we care for enter at times when life crises cause them to be patients, and as such may depend upon us and regress – if need be – and receive the nurturing they require; of a nursing profession that will encourage these individuals to share in their care as co-therapists in a regime that is primarily client-centred until, at a time preceding discharge, the recipients of our service truly become clients and care is client-directed in character.

But I'm discontent, I wish to make my dream reality. I am aware I am taking a risk in this chapter by sharing myself with an audience I have already identified as unsympathetic, namely my own profession.

Table 14.2: Examples of cathartic interventions

Giving permission:
'It's OK if you cry with me'

Removing physical blocks:
'Try taking deep breaths'/'Say that and make a movement at the same time'

Picking up physical movements:
'Exaggerate that arm movement . . . that facial expression . . . etc.'

Noting mismatches between verbal and non-verbal behaviour:
'You say you're upset and you're smiling'

Inviting earliest memory of an event or feeling:
'Whom did you first say that to?'

Repetition:
Inviting repetition of a word or phrase – 'Say that again louder'

Catching the thought:
Noting eye movements, facial expressions and inviting the verbal communication of thought. 'What are you thinking now?'

Role play:
(a) 'What would you say if she was here now?'
(b) 'Act as though you were her . . . What is she saying?'

Monodrama:
(a) Invite the client to play two or more conflicting roles
(b) Invite the client to address his feelings: 'If you could talk to your anger, what would you say to it?'

Exploring fantasy:
'What might happen if you allowed yourself to do that?'

Focusing:
Inviting the client to identify an emotion bodily. 'Where is your anxiety? . . . point to it . . . can you intensify it?'

Addressing hidden agendas:
'Who do you want to say that to?'
'What would you really like to say?'

Touch:
Gently touching a client's hand or shoulder
Massaging tense muscle groups

Taking risks arouses energy. Pulling off these risks in positive and creative ways breeds confidence. Failing, and indeed I might fail, provides one more experience to learn from and is nothing to fear. If I try my best there is nothing more in my power to be done; believing in this relieves me of much unnecessary stress.

You too can do no more than your best. It is important as a care giver to define clearly your boundaries – how much can you reasonably give? Do you know when to say no? It is imperative that you care for yourself. It is not selfish to safeguard your own resources but logical and necessary. Unless you learn to 'care' for yourself – and experience such care – how will you be able to care for others?

Finally, in this chapter I would like to share my own care orientation. My client group is composed mainly of clinical nurses, educators and managers; some come from the field of social work and a few are individuals who seek therapy. Whether I function as an educationalist or as a therapist, the same rules apply. I attune myself to my positive perceptive functions (Figure 14.9), stay cognisant of the role interactions available (Figure 14.4), am mindful of Rogers' philosophy of facilitation, note my intentions and those interactions open to me (Table 14.1) and share with my clients the insights that arise from our interaction and the rationale of my work. To evaluate my performance I employ the experiential exercise (Figure 14.2) described on page 320.

My intention is primarily an educational one and seeks to solicit growth of insight and self-directed problem-solving within clients. I view myself as a resource. As I view nursing as an interactive process, the approach outlined appears suitable for clients suffering physical, psychological or social ill health.

As a general nurse I would seek – where possible – to educate my client to self care, share the reasoning behind the specialist medical procedures and investigations performed and use the disease state as a learning experience whereby clients gain new insights into their disease process and develop physiological care skills or preventive measures to forestall their condition recurring and aggravating their lifestyle.

As a mental nurse I would seek to intervene in my client's life crisis, educate him – where possible – about his emotions and behaviours, relay insights that enable him to understand those personal and interpersonal dynamics that trigger malfunction, and help him to identify his support agencies.

As a nurse for people with learning difficulties I would concentrate on educating my client towards independent social functioning, and facilitating experiments of living where he may advance his capacity to enjoy, grow and maintain healthy modes of performance in keeping with his individual desires and abilities.

In all the above areas my attention is focused upon the here-and-now reactions that occur between us. I stand on my senses and those patterns perceived from the interactive environment, but am ever mindful of my own intellectual and intuitive resources.

Care is a feeling state besides a string of growth-promoting strategies. Figure 14.13 attempts to correlate a few of those features I have related to my work.

As a facilitator I witness myself and the environment via my senses, intellectually share my knowledge and social orientation, and allow my feeling and intuitions to suggest creative and empathic responses while using those authoritative or facilitative interventions relevant to immediate care. All is dependent on how well I can contact – and remain with – the unbreaking wave of my client's experience; if I fail to tune in and 'stay with' him, my therapeutic potential is weakened.

In this chapter I have endeavoured to share my own facilitative style. I hope it has stimulated your own creative and imaginative processes, helping you to reflect upon, and synthesise, your own unique vision.

Nursing is at a crossroads. It can go through the motions of being a profession, or it can develop its therapeutic potential. If the latter road is chosen nurses must refine their skills to the level of a therapy. Nurses are interactive agents. Whether they are concerned with physical or psychological health, their role is essentially that of a facilitator who supports, nurtures and educates others to independence. Their uniqueness lies in the therapeutic manner in which they use themselves and their interpersonal skills. All else is determined by the orientation of their discipline.

General nurses have specialist knowledge of physical disorder. Psychiatric nurses have specialist knowledge of psychological disorder. But, in the last analysis, they both need person sensitivity,

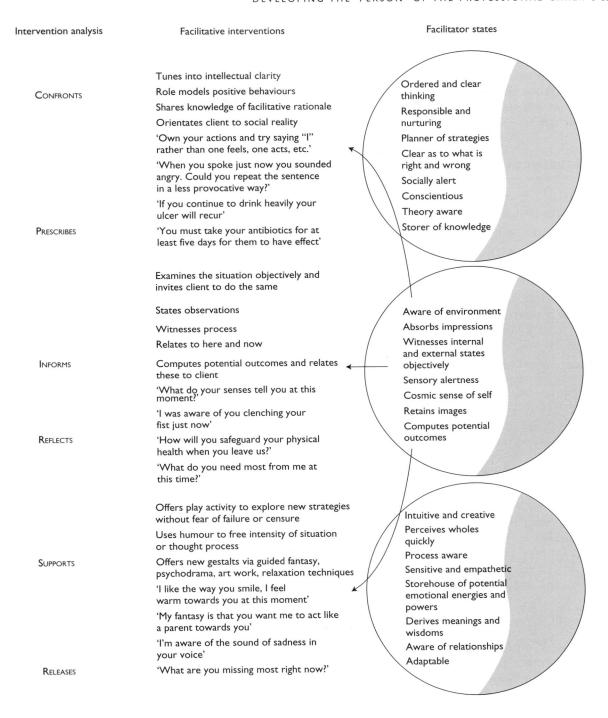

Intervention analysis | Facilitative interventions | Facilitator states

CONFRONTS

Tunes into intellectual clarity

Role models positive behaviours

Shares knowledge of facilitative rationale

Orientates client to social reality

'Own your actions and try saying "I" rather than one feels, one acts, etc.'

'When you spoke just now you sounded angry. Could you repeat the sentence in a less provocative way?'

'If you continue to drink heavily your ulcer will recur'

PRESCRIBES

'You must take your antibiotics for at least five days for them to have effect'

Ordered and clear thinking

Responsible and nurturing

Planner of strategies

Clear as to what is right and wrong

Socially alert

Conscientious

Theory aware

Storer of knowledge

Examines the situation objectively and invites client to do the same

States observations

Witnesses process

Relates to here and now

INFORMS

Computes potential outcomes and relates these to client

'What do your senses tell you at this moment?'

'I was aware of you clenching your fist just now'

REFLECTS

'How will you safeguard your physical health when you leave us?'

'What do you need most from me at this time?'

Aware of environment

Absorbs impressions

Witnesses internal and external states objectively

Sensory alertness

Cosmic sense of self

Retains images

Computes potential outcomes

Offers play activity to explore new strategies without fear of failure or censure

Uses humour to free intensity of situation or thought process

SUPPORTS

Offers new gestalts via guided fantasy, psychodrama, art work, relaxation techniques

'I like the way you smile, I feel warm towards you at this moment'

'My fantasy is that you want me to act like a parent towards you'

'I'm aware of the sound of sadness in your voice'

RELEASES

'What are you missing most right now?'

Intuitive and creative

Perceives wholes quickly

Process aware

Sensitive and empathetic

Storehouse of potential emotional energies and powers

Derives meanings and wisdoms

Aware of relationships

Adaptable

Figure 14.13: Relationship of facilitation to functions and personal awareness

an understanding of the dynamics of a caring relationship, counselling skills, and sufficient maturity and self-awareness to share of themselves, working therapeutically through, and with, the life crises of others. As agents of intervention in the crises of others, nurses must have worked through their own emotional and professional baggage.

Well, this is the theory; are you up to acting as a therapeutic agent, facing yourself and contacting the reality of a truly caring relationship? As we enter the twenty-first century, the future of the profession is dependent upon you and the quality of your self, and the sensitivity and alertness of your care.

REFERENCES

Altschul, A. (1972). *Patient–Nurse Interaction*. Churchill Livingstone, Edinburgh.

Ashworth, P. (1980). *Care to Communicate*. RCN, London.

Barber, P. (1990). *The Facilitation of Personal and Professional Growth through Experiential Groupwork and Therapeutic Community Practice*. Unpublished PhD thesis, University of Surrey.

Barber, P. (1997). Caring; a therapeutic relationship. In *Nursing: a Knowledge Base for Practice*, 2nd edn, Perry, A. and Jolley, M. (eds). Edward Arnold, Sevenoaks.

Barber, P. and Dietrich, G. (1985). The skills of the nurse, caring for people with mental handicap. In *Making Interventions. A Learning Package for Nurses*, Barber, P. and Deitrich, G. (eds). ENB, London and Sheffield.

Barber, P. and Norman, I. (1987). An eclectic model of staff development. In *Using Nursing Models: Mental Handicap – Facilitating Holistic Care*, Barber, P. (ed.). Hodder and Stoughton, Sevenoaks.

Berne, E. (1967). *Games People Play*. Penguin Books, Harmondsworth.

Cox, T. (1983). *Stress and Health*. Macmillan Press, Basingstoke.

Edelwich, J. and Brodsky, A. (1980). *Burnout: Stages of Disillusionment in the Helping Professions*. Human Sciences Press, London.

Franklin, B. (1984). *Patient Anxiety on Admission to Hospital*. RCN, London.

Harris, T. (1973). *I'm OK, You're OK*. Pan Books, London.

Heron, J. (1990). *Helping the Client: a Creative Practical Guide*. Sage Publications, London.

Holmes, P. (1986). Facing up to disfigurement. *Nursing Times*, 82(34), 16–18.

Jung, C. (1957). *The Undiscovered Self*. Mentor Books, London.

Lamond, N. (1974). *Becoming a Nurse: a Registered Nurse's View of General Student Education*. RCN, London.

Maslow, A. (1967). Cognition of being in peak experience. *Journal of Genetic Psychology*, 94, 43–66.

Menzies, I. (1960). *The Functioning of Social Systems as a Defence Against Anxiety*. Tavistock Pamphlet No. 3, London.

Moscato, B. (1976). The traditional nurse–physician relationship: a perpetuation of social stereotyping. In *Current Perspectives in Psychiatric Nursing*, Kneisl, C. and Wilson, H. (eds). Mosby, St Louis.

Olsen, V. and Whittaker, E. (1961). *The Silent Dialogue*. Jossey-Bass, San Francisco.

Peplau, H. (1987). Tomorrow's world. *Nursing Times*, 83(1), 29–32.

Rogers, C. (1967). *On Becoming a Person*. Constable, London.

Rogers, C. (1983). *Freedom to Learn for the Eighties*. Merrill, Columbus, OH.

Rogers, M. (1970). *The Theory Basis of Nursing*. F.A. Davies, Philadelphia.

Seligman, M. (1975). *Learned Helplessness*. Freeman, Oxford.

Stockwell, F. (1972). *The Unpopular Patient*. RCN, London.

Vousden, M. (1986). Talking to patients. *Nursing Times*, 82(34), 32–5.

Wilson, M. (1975). *Health is for People*. Darton, Longman and Todd, London.

FURTHER READING

Barber, P. (1997). Caring; a therapeutic relationship. In *Nursing: a Knowledge Base for Practice*, 2nd edn, Perry, A. and Jolley, M. (eds). Arnold, London.

Provides an example of care relationships and professionalism from the client perspective, while updating the relevance of Menzies' (1960) study to the 1990s.

Barber, P. (1997). *Journey Beyond the Boundaries: a Transpersonal Glossary of Terms*. Triangle Trust Publication (available from author, School of Educational Studies, Surrey University, Guildford.

Lists terms and concepts relating to transpersonal communication and personal growth. New edition in production with examples of application.

Tschudin, V. and Schober, J.E. (1998). *Developing Yourself*, 2nd edn. Macmillan, Basingstoke.

A text aimed at nurses, containing vital guidance relating to personal and career development.

UKCC (1997). *PREP and You*. UKCC, London.

The professional responsibilities of nurses relating to registration, profiling and continuing education are contained here.

CHAPTER FIFTEEN

EXPERIENCING *and* MANAGING PAIN: THE PATIENT—NURSE PARTNERSHIP

Eloise C.J. Carr

- Multidimensional nature of pain
- Incidence and prevalence of pain
- The assessment of pain
- Pain assessment tools
- The management of pain
- Multidisciplinary teams
- Conclusion

Pain control is a contemporary issue that is of immense importance due to the devastating and dehumanising effects it can have upon an individual. Nursing the patient who is experiencing pain requires contemporary knowledge, skilled interventions (pharmacological and non-pharmacological) and attitudes which convey trust, care and an honest belief in the patient.

The aim of this chapter is to describe the multidimensional nature and prevalence of pain before critically examining some of the tools available for assessing pain. Interventions which can be used in the management of pain are discussed and will include both pharmacological and non-pharmacological approaches. Finally, the role of different multidisciplinary teams is considered and the importance of teamwork for effective pain relief.

MULTIDIMENSIONAL NATURE OF PAIN

DEFINING PAIN

Pain is a subjective experience which is individual to each person and no one else can know how pain feels except the person experiencing it, rather like shoes – only the person wearing them knows how they feel. McCaffery and Beebe (1994, page 15)

define pain subjectively as originally proposed by McCaffery (1968) as:

'Pain is whatever the person says it is and exists whenever he says it does'.

A more formal definition is offered by the following statement:

'Pain is an unpleasant **sensory** and emotional experience associated with actual or potential tissue damage'.

(Merskey, 1986)

TYPES OF PAIN

Pain can be further divided into acute and chronic pain. Acute pain has a sudden onset, a foreseeable end and tends to get better. It is frequently associated with trauma, surgery, childbirth and dental work. By contrast, chronic pain may continue long after an injury has healed and may involve parts of the body not associated with the injury. Examples of chronic pain include arthritis or back pain. Chronic pain is sometimes further subdivided into malignant (cancer) and non-malignant. The rationale for diagnosing the type of pain is to form a framework for the best treatment approach. For instance, chronic low back pain which is non-malignant may involve regular visits to a pain clinic where the treatment emphasis might be on 'living with the pain' and identifying strategies to help the person cope with chronic pain. However, if the low back pain was caused by spread of a cancerous tumour, then this treatment would be inappropriate and pharmacological interventions might be more appropriate.

NEUROPHYSIOLOGY OF PAIN

Receptors which respond to harmful stimuli are **nociceptors** and are responsible for the initial transmission of pain. Sharp pain is transmitted via small diameter myelinated (fast) A-delta fibres, whereas burning dull, aching pain is transmitted via small diameter unmyelinated (slow) C-fibres (Puntillo, 1988). These impulses travel to the spinal cord and pass up along the *substantia gelatinosa*, in the dorsal horn, to the brain. Here they pass through the thalamus, reticular formation and limbic system. During this journey the impulse can be altered and its potential increased or decreased through a variety of mechanisms. The reader is strongly advised to read further on the 'neurophysiology of pain' before progressing with this chapter. An excellent chapter is to be found in Clancy and McVicar (1995).

GATE CONTROL THEORY OF PAIN

The neurophysiology of pain is frequently brought together under the **gate control theory** originally proposed by Melzack and Wall in 1965.

This theory suggested that the pain impulses travelled up the dorsal horn of the spinal cord to the brain but could be modulated by a gating mechanism. These gating mechanisms are located throughout the spinal cord and at several sites within the brain and central nervous system (CNS) and are influenced by higher centres in the brain such as the limbic system (emotion), cerebral cortex (knowledge and meaning) and brain stem (sensory input). Impulses travelling down the spinal cord may close the gate and modify the ascending impulses, resulting in reduced pain perception.

This theory enabled people to understand that pain was not unidimensional, relating just to *intensity* but multidimensional, with sensory, cognitive and emotional (affective) components. The **gate control theory** is particularly helpful in the management of pain as it offers a theoretical framework which accounts for both the individual experience of pain and provides a basis for the development of multimodal interventions, e.g. pharmacology and anxiety reducing strategies. More detailed accounts of the gate control theory can be found in Clancy and McVicar (1995) and in O'Hara (1996).

Key Points

- Types of pain are acute and chronic pain (malignant and non-malignant).
- Pain is multidimensional.

INCIDENCE AND PREVALENCE OF PAIN

Despite dramatic advances in pain control, many patients in both hospital and the community continue to suffer unrelieved pain and up to three-quarters of patients experience moderate to severe pain whilst in hospital (Commission on the Provision of Surgical Services, 1990). It has been estimated that one in 14 of the adult population (7%) in the UK has been in pain for more than 3 months. Of the people in pain, 70% are taking pain-killers (Rigge, 1990). A random sample of 5150 patients who had been recently discharged from hospital were interviewed and findings revealed that 61% cited problems experienced in relation to pain management, and 33% of those suffering experienced pain all or most of the time (Bruster *et al.*, 1994). Webb and Hope (1995) interviewed 103 patients and asked them to rank nursing activities in order of importance, and found that 'relieving pain' was ranked the second most important activity.

> **Activity**
>
> Think back to a clinical experience (hospital or community). How many people did you encounter who were experiencing pain or discomfort? Why did they have pain and had anything been done to help alleviate their suffering?

Further on in this chapter there will be a detailed exploration of the process of assessing another person's pain and will include assessment strategies for people with cognitive impairment. Certain groups of people are particularly 'at risk' of experiencing pain which may go undetected as they are unable to express it verbally, i.e. a person who has lost his or her speech due to a stroke, or may be too young to have learnt the words. Other vulnerable groups include people with learning disabilities, those with any form of cognitive impairment and those who do not have English as their first language. Two groups who have received increased attention over the past few years, in the pain literature, are elderly people and children.

PAIN AND ELDERLY PEOPLE

Pain is extremely common in those who are elderly with studies suggesting up to 50% of those living in the community having pain (Brattberg *et al.*, 1989). Pain-inducing diseases, such as arthritis, also affect as many as 80% of people over the age of 65 (Davis, 1988). Pain associated with chronic disease results in diminished sleep, loss of appetite with altered nutrition and reduced mobility. In turn, these can lead to isolation and depression, thus worsening the pain.

Elderly people often present challenges to assessment due to impaired hearing or sight which can make communication of their pain difficult. An excellent chapter, based on research with elderly people in a community setting, explores many of the factors which influence their ability to cope with pain (Walker, 1993). Another useful text is Ferrell and Ferrell (1996) who outline approaches to specific pain problems in those who are elderly and present an informative and clinically oriented text.

PAIN IN CHILDREN

Research suggests that children undergoing surgery are not given adequate pain relief, which is often due to inadequate assessment and reluctance to administer analgesia. Until recent years it was inaccurately assumed that neonates did not have the ability to feel pain, due to the immaturity of their central nervous system. They experienced painful procedures and investigations with little or no analgesia. Professionals held 'myths' about their pain experience and crying was often assumed to be due to separation from the parent, hunger or fear. Facial expression, body movement, heart rate and crying are responses which are known to indicate pain (Johnston and Strada, 1986). Current research using video material to identify neonatal behaviours, which indicated pain, enabled the development of a scoring system using eight behavioural categories (Horden *et al.*, 1996). From this a distress score was developed for use in practice which will enable interventions to be evaluated. It is essential that pain is recognised in neonates and children. Nurses need to understand the complexity of the experience if they are to manage it effectively.

> **Key Points**
>
> ■ Pain is prevalent in both the community and hospital setting.
> ■ People who cannot easily communicate their pain are vulnerable.

THE ASSESSMENT OF PAIN

WHY ASSESS PAIN?

Pain is a subjective phenomenon which is unique to each person, reflected by McCaffery and Beebe (1994) as 'whatever the experiencing person says it is and existing whenever he says it does'. A key component to the successful management of the patient's pain is an accurate assessment of the patient's situation which will form the foundation on which all intervention can be based. Without formal assessment the patient may not be given the opportunity to express his or her pain and one nurse's interpretation of someone else's experience is not only inappropriate but has been shown to be inaccurate (Seers, 1987; Zalon, 1993).

Patient Study

Peter Smith had an appendicectomy the previous day. During the first night he hardly slept at all as the pain was horrid. He felt as if someone was stabbing his side. The pain had made him feel anxious, too, as he wondered what would happen if it got worse and he was reluctant to move, so his back ached now. The staff nurse had come round late with the drug trolley but he had been dozing and she hadn't woken him to assess his pain and offer him pain-killers. He wanted them now but didn't like to ask. Surely the nurses would know if he needed pain relief and offer it to him? In the morning when the nurse on the morning shift came to give him a wash he couldn't even sit up. He felt too sore and the thought of getting out of bed terrified him ... he felt like death and wondered if he would die.

The day staff were surprised to find Peter in such a state as the night staff said he was asleep when they did the drugs at 10 pm and that he slept well. The staff nurse caring for Peter for the morning used a pain assessment chart and quickly identified the location of the pain, its intensity and how Peter felt about it. She then gave him 10 mg of morphine intramuscularly, which he had been prescribed. Peter was relieved to have someone ask him about his pain.

The patient study illustrates how poorly pain can be managed when no assessment tool is used. Casual questions about someone's pain fail to elicit detailed information and this patient had no opportunity to discuss his pain and as a consequence suffered needlessly. His pain had not been identified and certain 'factors' inhibited him from ringing his buzzer.

Activity

Thinking about this care study and other patients you may have cared for can you identify what factors these might be?

Patient Study

Ann was married with two grown children who both had young families of their own. For the past year she had suffered with low back pain which often radiated down both or one of her legs. The pain was now virtually constant and Ann found herself reluctant to go out with friends these days as she felt she spoilt the outings. Her husband, Peter, had been very understanding when she initially had the back pain but was losing patience with her and tended to brush her complaints aside. Ann felt isolated and saddened by her life. She couldn't remember the last time they made love and could see no end to this spiral of pain, anger and suffering. Each day seemed such a struggle. Finally, she went back to her GP for a third time to see if there was anything he could do. She could see he was busy and although he was very kind she didn't feel able to tell him how awful she was feeling. He suggested she try another type of pain-killer and 'take things easy'.

Regular assessment of pain contributes to the quality of communication between the patient and the nurse/doctor and the process itself may actually help reduce the patient's pain as it conveys to patients that you are concerned about their pain and believe them. Documentation of pain assessment formalises the pain assessment process and is essential to the provision of individualised care from both the legal and professional perspectives. In the patient study above it can be seen that the pain had encroached on every aspect of Ann's life – she was 'living through the pain'.

When she saw her GP there was no formal assessment and thus she had little opportunity to talk about how the pain had *affected* her and her whole life. Further on in the chapter we will discuss how chronic pain management is often focused on helping people *cope with* pain and improving the quality of their lives through the use of coping strategies. With any type of pain the first step towards effective management must always be assessment.

FACTORS AFFECTING THE ASSESSMENT OF PAIN

Pain assessment may not always be straightforward and an awareness of the factors which can affect the assessment process will help nurses to understand how an assessment may be jeopardised. Effective communication, honesty and an awareness of these influences can result in an accurate and valid assessment which then enables appropriate interventions to be used. The following section illustrates patient and nurse factors which are known to influence the assessment of pain. A more detailed discussion of these factors can be found in Allcock (1996).

Patient factors

It is important to be aware that people are individual and their pain experience will be unique to them. This is why two people who may have had the same operation can experience very different levels of pain and may express their pain differently.

Patient Study

Jane and Tracey both had surgery yesterday to remove wisdom teeth. They both hope to be going home later this morning. Both women tell you their pain is awful – 'the worst pain I've ever had' and give it a rating of 8/10. However, Jane is sitting up and engrossed in the morning TV but Tracey is lying down and appears rather withdrawn and disinterested.

Activity

Reflect on the patient study above. Who do you think has the most pain? It is tempting to think Tracey does because her 'behaviour' suggests someone in awful pain. Behaviour can be extremely misleading and is not sufficient evidence to enable us to draw conclusions about someone else's pain. Now consider the next case study.

Patient Study

William had lived alone since he was widowed 7 years ago. He had arthritis in both hips which limited his mobility considerably. Over the past few months the district nurse had been visiting once a week. Whenever she called William appeared bright and pleased to see her. When she asked him if anything was bothering him, he said 'the pain in my legs – it's excruciating'. Later that day when she called back to the surgery Margaret mentioned to William's GP that he had been complaining of pain but she didn't feel it was as 'excruciating' as he suggested.

McCaffery (1991) discovered that nurses were strongly influenced by the behaviour of patients, when making a pain assessment. It is important to be aware that pain behaviours may not always indicate the 'level' of pain a person is feeling. People experiencing pain may try to minimise their pain; they may not want to worry their family, may be embarrassed, feel it is better to bear the pain, or worry that it may stop them going home from hospital. Think back to the patient study of William. Why might he not have shown obvious 'pain behaviours'?

The experience and expression of pain are known to be influenced by many factors. Briggs (1995) presents an interesting paper which has explored the literature on patient factors which influence the expression of pain and highlights these in relation to acute pain assessment. Table 15.1 lists some of the research-based patient factors which are known to influence the experience.

Nurse factors

Table 15.2 lists some research-based nurse factors which have been found to influence pain assessment. Nurses are individuals with their own experiences, attitudes and beliefs. It is most important to be aware that these factors may influence your assessment of pain and therefore always ensure that you approach a person in pain with empathy, belief and trust.

Although the nurse may not be able to change any of these factors, it is *awareness* of them and the possible impact they may have on the pain assessment which is the key to successful outcome. The skills of assessment require nurses to have appropriate knowledge, e.g. an understanding of pain and the ability to use a pain assessment tool, effective communication skills and skills of

Table 15.1: Patient factors which influence pain experience

Patient factor	Research
Age	Closs (1994)
Cultural background	Calvillo and Flaskerud (1993)
Social conditioning	Seers (1988)
Expectations	Carr (1990)

Table 15.2: Nurse factors which may influence pain assessment

Nurse factor	Research
Professional education	Halfens *et al.* (1990)
Expectation of pain in relation to diagnosis or surgery	Halfens *et al.* (1990)
Culture	Calvillo and Flaskerud (1993)
Personal experience of pain	Ketovuori (1987)

observation. Assessment requires skilled nursing as patients may be unwilling or unable to express their pain because, for example, they fear extending their hospital stay, worry that their condition may be getting worse, do not have the vocabulary (neonates and young children) or the capacity (those who are unconscious or have cognitive difficulties).

Key Points

- Accurate pain assessment is essential for successful management.
- Patients may be inhibited to communicate their pain.
- Belief in the patient is essential.

PAIN ASSESSMENT TOOLS

Evidence suggests that nurses' assessment of pain is limited as well as often being inaccurate (Albrecht *et al.*, 1992; Jandelli, 1995). Nurses often use their own judgement and prefer to rely on physiological signs and behaviours, which can be misleading and inaccurate. Formal pain assessment tools facilitate effective communication and assessment by reducing the chance of error or bias.

It is imperative that nurses use a pain assessment tool rather than ask vague questions from the drug trolley, such as 'anything for pain Mr Jones?'. A district nurse might elicit very little information if asking closed questions, such as 'have you any pain?'. It is not a pain assessment

and may even inhibit a truthful answer as the patient may feel he or she cannot talk about their pain.

Activity

Approach a person you know who is experiencing pain or discomfort. Ask him or her about the pain and make some notes about what was said. We will revisit your notes at the end of this section.

In addition to using a pain assessment tool, further information can also be collected as part of the assessment (Table 15.3). When someone experiences chronic pain it is particularly important to gain an understanding of the meaning of this pain and how it has affected his or her life so we can increase our knowledge (Seers and Friedli, 1996).

The pain assessment tool needs to be valid, reliable, easily understood by the patient and quick to use. Pain assessment should also include the family or immediate carer. They will have valuable insights into and understanding of the patient's pain experience, especially if there is cognitive impairment, hearing or visual difficulties.

PAIN INTENSITY ASSESSMENT TOOLS (SIMPLE RATING SCALES)

The most reliable indicator of a person's pain and the distress it may be causing them is the patient's self-report. Self-report measurement scales include numerical or descriptive rating scales and the visual analogue scales (Figure 15.1). A pain intensity score is a quick way of finding out the intensity of the pain for a given individual and evaluating the effectiveness of an intervention. They are quick and simple to use and most patients are able to understand them. The disad-

Table 15.3: Elements of a pain assessment

Pain assessment questions
1 Where is the pain?
2 When did it start and for how long does it last?
3 Can you describe the pain?
4 What makes the pain better and worse?
5 What is your desired goal for pain relief?
6 What does this pain mean to you?

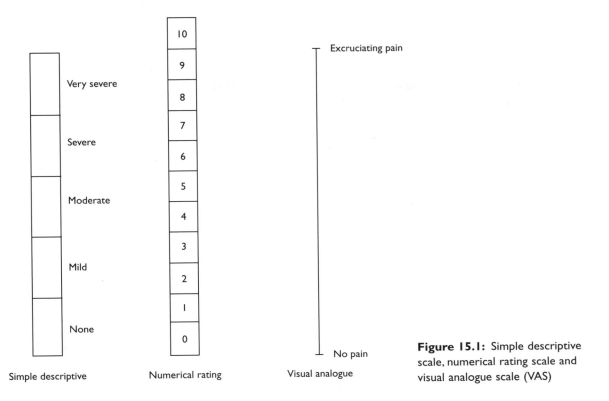

Figure 15.1: Simple descriptive scale, numerical rating scale and visual analogue scale (VAS)

vantage to these scales is that they only measure intensity and do not give a description of the pain or additional information.

A measurement tool must be both valid (measure what it intends to measure, i.e. pain) and reliable (will give the same result when repeatedly used). Baillie (1993) describes in more detail these assessment tools and the research which has evaluated their use in clinical practice.

The pain ruler (Figure 15.2) combines an intensity score (numerical rating scale) with qualitative descriptors of the pain (Bourbonnais, 1981). It enables the patient to describe his or her pain, which may help with diagnosis, and has been shown to be liked by nurses (Berker and Hughes, 1990).

PAIN ASSESSMENT TOOLS FOR CHILDREN

Measurement of pain in children has gained popularity in recent years and numerous assessment tools have been developed in an attempt to measure their pain experience. McGrath *et al.* (1995) give a detailed overview of pain assessment including self-report (what children say), behav-ioural (what children do) and biological measures (how their bodies react).

An example of a self-report scale is the poker chip tool (Hester, 1979) where several poker chips (or other objects) are put before the child and each chip is described as a 'piece of hurt'. One chip corresponds to 'a little hurt', two to 'a little more hurt', etc. The child is then asked 'how many pieces of hurt do you have?'. The answer is then confirmed. This is useful for children who understand the concept of 'more or less'.

A popular behavioural tool is the Children's Hospital of Eastern Ontario pain scale or CHEOPS (McGrath *et al.*, 1985). It rates six behaviours: crying, facial expression, verbal expression, torso position, touch and leg position. It was originally developed to measure post-operative pain in children 1–7 years old.

The literature suggests that when assessing pain in children, behavioural measurements should be used in conjunction with children's self-reports. Be aware that a child may deny any pain if the person asking the question is a stranger, or if they are fearful or frightened of having an

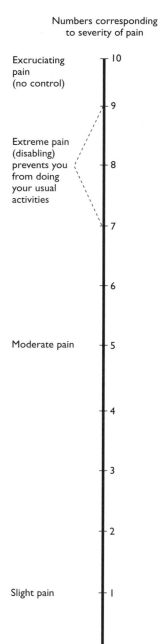

Numbers corresponding
to severity of pain

Excruciating
pain
(no control) — 10

— 9

Extreme pain
(disabling)
prevents you
from doing
your usual
activities — 8

— 7

— 6

Moderate pain — 5

— 4

— 3

— 2

Slight pain — 1

No pain — 0

Words to describe
your pain

Match the words(s)
that apply to your
pain with a number
in the ruler which
corresponds to the
severity of your pain
Draw an arrow from
the word to the
number, or tell the
nurse

tender
crushing
squeezing
stabbing
sharp
burning
feels like an electric shock
throbbing
cramping
dull
sore
aching
gnawing
feels like a weight
pressure
a discomfort

Figure 15.2: Bourbonnais pain ruler (1981)
(Reprinted with kind permission from Blackwell Science Ltd.
Source: Bourbonnais, F., 1981, Pain assessment: development of
a tool for the nurse and the patient. *Journal of Advanced
Nursing*, 6, 277–82)

injection. Wherever possible the parents should be
included in the pain assessment process.

THE LONDON HOSPITAL PAIN OBSERVATION CHART

Pain is not unidimensional but multidimensional.
Simple tools such as rating scales will not capture
all the pain and there is often a need to use a tool
which will encompass more than just the intensity
of the pain. Such tools are particularly useful for
chronic or malignant pain.

The London Hospital pain observation chart
(Raiman, 1986) was developed with the aim of
improving communication between the patient,
nurse and doctor. The chart (Figure 15.3) incorporates a body map which has been shown to be particularly useful in pinpointing the source of pain
(Latham, 1989). It also has clear instructions on
how to complete the chart and includes simple
pain interventions. It is helpful if the patient can
indicate the pain on the body map as it encourages him or her to participate actively in the pain
assessment process.

McGILL PAIN QUESTIONNAIRE (MPQ)

Melzack and Torgerson (1971) suggested that the
words people choose to express their pain could
form the basis of an pain assessment tool. It is now
one of the most utilised pain assessment tools in
both research and clinical practice and is particularly helpful across a range of painful conditions
(Melzack, 1975). It consists of 78 words which are
categorised into 20 groups that represent four
major dimensions of pain quality: sensory, affective, evaluative and miscellaneous. Each word
had a score value and the patient is asked to select
words which describe his/her pain. Having done
this, several scores can then be calculated. For
instance, the total value of the words chosen is the
pain rating index (PRI) for each of the dimensions:
sensory, affective, evaluative or miscellaneous.
These can also be added together to give the PRI
total. The total number of words chosen (NWC) is
another score and there is also the present pain
intensity (PPI) which is an intensity score derived
from from a 0–5 scale. A criticism of the MPQ is
the time required to complete it. A shortened form

DATE _____

SHEET NUMBER _____

PATIENT
IDENTIFICATION
LABEL

TIME	PAIN RATING — BY SITES								OVER ALL	ANALGESIC GIVEN (Name, dose, route, time)	MEASURES TO RELIEVE PAIN — Specify where starred							COMMENTS FROM PATIENT'S AND/OR STAFF	Initials
	A	B	C	D	E	F	G	H			Lifting	Turning	Massage	Distracting activities*	Position Change*	Additional aids*	Other*		

This chart records where a patient's pain is and how bad it is, by the nurse asking the patient at regular intervals. If analgesics are being given regularly, make an observation with each dose and another *half-way between* each dose. If analgesics are given only 'as required', observe 2-hourly. When the observations are stable and the patient is comfortable, any regular time interval between observations may be chosen.

TO USE THIS CHART ask the patient to mark all his or her pains on the body diagram below. Label each site of pain with a letter (i.e. A, B, C, etc.).

Then at each observation time ask the patient to assess:

1. The pain in each separate site since the last observation. Use the scale above the body diagram, and enter the number or letter in the appropriate column.

2. The pain overall since the last observation. Use the same scale and enter in column marked OVERALL.

Next, record what has been done to relieve pain:

3. Note any analgesic given since the last observation stating name, dose, route and time given.

4. Tick any other nursing care or action taken to ease pain.

Finally, note any comment on pain from patient or nurse (use the back of the chart as well, if necessary) and initial the record.

Excruciating	5
Very severe	4
Severe	3
Moderate	2
Just noticeable	1
No pain at all	0
Patient sleeping	S

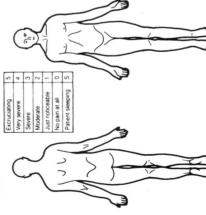

Figure 15.3: The London Hospital pain observation chart

of the MPQ (Figure 15.4) has been developed which takes less than 5 minutes to complete and is sensitive to clinical change due to pain interventions, e.g. analgesia (Melzack, 1987). These assessment tools have been used with people experiencing chronic pain and the SF-MPQ (short-form MPQ) has been successfully used with acute pain suffers.

PAIN DIARY

Another useful assessment tool is the pain diary. This can quite simply be a notebook, in which the patient keeps a record of his or her pain over a period of hours, days or weeks. It is helpful as it allows patterns of pain to be seen, causative factors identified and any coping strategies or activi-

SHORT-FORM McGILL PAIN QUESTIONNAIRE

RONALD MELZACK

PATIENT'S NAME:_____   DATE:_____

	NONE	MILD	MODERATE	SEVERE
THROBBING	0) ____	1) ____	2) ____	3) ____
SHOOTING	0) ____	1) ____	2) ____	3) ____
STABBING	0) ____	1) ____	2) ____	3) ____
SHARP	0) ____	1) ____	2) ____	3) ____
CRAMPING	0) ____	1) ____	2) ____	3) ____
GNAWING	0) ____	1) ____	2) ____	3) ____
HOT-BURNING	0) ____	1) ____	2) ____	3) ____
ACHING	0) ____	1) ____	2) ____	3) ____
HEAVY	0) ____	1) ____	2) ____	3) ____
TENDER	0) ____	1) ____	2) ____	3) ____
SPLITTING	0) ____	1) ____	2) ____	3) ____
TIRING-EXHAUSTING	0) ____	1) ____	2) ____	3) ____
SICKENING	0) ____	1) ____	2) ____	3) ____
FEARFUL	0) ____	1) ____	2) ____	3) ____
PUNISHING-CRUEL	0) ____	1) ____	2) ____	3) ____

NO PAIN |————————————————————————| WORST POSSIBLE PAIN

PPI

0   NO PAIN   ____
1   MILD   ____
2   DISCOMFORTING   ____
3   DISTRESSING   ____
4   HORRIBLE   ____
5   EXCRUCIATING   ____

© R. Melzack, 1984

The short-form McGill pain questionnaire (SF-MPQ). Descriptors 1–11 represent the sensory dimension of pain experience and 12–15 represent the affective dimension. Each descriptor is ranked on an intensity scale of 0 = none, 1 = mild, 2 = moderate, 3 = severe. The Present Pain Intensity (PPI) of the standard long-form McGill pain questionnaire (LF-MPQ) and the visual analogue (VAS) are also included to provide overall intensity scores.

Figure 15.4: Short-form McGill pain questionnaire (SF-MPQ) (Melzack, 1987) (Reprinted with the kind permission of Elsevier Science and Professor R. Melzack from Melzack, R., 1987, The Short-form McGill Pain Questionnaire, *Pain*, 30, 191–97)

Table 15.4: Example of a pain diary

Date and time	Pain description	Intensity /10	Pain-relieving activity/action	Activity associated with pain
1/10 9 am	Nagging lower back pain	7/10	Lying down on the floor with a heat pad	Hanging out the washing
Noon	Back pain radiating down legs – sharp	8/10	Two co-proxamol and resting for 30 minutes reading a book	Lifting children into and out of car

ties which were particularly helpful. In the community this is a useful approach to gathering information, as it really involves the patient, who often finds the activity of writing in the diary cathartic. An example of headings which could be helpful are shown in Table 15.4.

PAIN ASSESSMENT WITH PEOPLE EXPERIENCING COGNITIVE DIFFICULTIES

Most of the published work on pain assessment focuses on people who can respond verbally. In practice, life is different and two groups of people who often experience pain which is not managed effectively are those with learning disabilities and those with chronic brain syndrome (CBS). More than one million people in the UK are affected by CBS and 65% of these have Alzheimer's disease (Chapman and Marshall, 1993). Difficulties in assessing pain where the person may not be able to understand the question or express him/herself coherently contribute to the difficulties.

Pain is often expressed behaviourally and the nurse can elicit a great deal of information by being perceptive to the cues people give. Changes in behaviour or mood can be valuable indicators of pain. What behaviours are associated with pain? Table 15.5 reveals some of the behaviours which could be helpful in assessing pain with such individuals.

It is essential to involve family or key workers in the assessment of pain as they are often able to notice subtle changes in behaviour or mood. Documenting the assessment is imperative and a pain diary format is often very helpful to gain an understanding of the pattern of the pain.

To evaluate the effectiveness of pain interventions the diary will provide an excellent source of baseline information. Improvements in any baseline information may indicate a reduction in pain.

Simons and Malabar (1995) present an informative paper which evaluated the impact of carrying out pain interventions and observing pain behaviours in a group of elderly patients who were unable to respond verbally. They found that pain interventions changed the exhibited pain behaviours to non-pain behaviours.

Hayes (1995) wrote an informative and thought-provoking article on pain assessment in elderly people, but encountered difficulties find-

Table 15.5: Observations in pain assessment for people with cognitive impairment

Pain assessment – behavioural observations

1 Verbal response

Appropriate	Groaning
Inappropriate	Shouting

2 Facial expression

Smiling	Frowning
Impassive	Angry
Grimacing	

3 Mobility

Usual activity	Rubbing
Immobile	Rhythmic movement
Hyperactive	Lethargic

4 Mood

Smiling	Withdrawn
Crying	Agitated
Seeking comfort	Aggressive

5 Alteration in daily routine

Altered behaviours (hygiene, sleep, eating, bowel habits, self care abilities, etc.)

6 Observations from family/key worker

Change in behaviour/mood

7 Physiological changes

Blood pressure, respirations, pulse

ing literature on pain assessment in non-verbal, confused elderly people. This reflects a profound lack of interest from researchers in this area and should raise concern. This group of people are extremely vulnerable and it is essential that research helps uncover the difficulties and provides knowledge that will inform practice, as it has done with other populations.

Research suggests that people continue to suffer uncontrolled pain despite advances in pain management. The main reason for this is attributed to lack of formal assessment by health care professionals. Nurses have a central role in performing an accurate pain assessment, using formal assessment tools, skilled communication and conveying at all times a belief in the person's experience of pain.

Activity

Select one of the pain assessment tools mentioned above and approach the same person you initially spoke to at the beginning of this section. Compare the information you got this time with that collected without a structured assessment. What did you notice about the information you obtained and the nature of the interaction between yourself and the person you spoke with?

Key Points

- Pain assessment is central to the effective management of pain.
- The patient's self-report of pain must be seen as the 'true experience'.
- A formal pain assessment tool should be used wherever possible.
- Pain assessment tools give patients an active role in their pain and may promote a therapeutic relationship between the nurse and patient.
- Pain assessment must always be documented.

THE MANAGEMENT OF PAIN

In bringing together the following section there has been an intentional effort not to separate the management of acute and chronic pain (including malignant). Although some strategies are more appropriate for certain types of pain, many interventions can be used successfully for different types of pain. Where certain interventions have been shown to be particularly effective with a certain type of pain this will be indicated. The reader is encouraged to understand the principles of providing effective pain management and select interventions which are tailored to meet individual need.

Many people, living in the community, experience pain and may seek their own strategies to manage their pain but they may need to know what other interventions may be of help to them. Increasingly, for many people, there is no cure for their pain (e.g. arthritis, low back pain) and so helping them and their families cope with pain enhances the quality of their lives.

In the USA the Agency for Health Care Policy and Research (AHCPR) have produced excellent practice guidelines for the management of pain and the reader is referred to these publications for more detailed guidance on the management of acute pain (AHCPR, 1992) and cancer pain (AHCPR, 1994). For the specific management of post-operative pain the reader is referred to Jurf and Nirschl (1993) and also to McCaffery and Beebe (1994), who have produced excellent manuals which describe, in considerable depth, tools and specific techniques which the nurse and other health professionals can use in the management of pain. Some of the non-pharmacological strategies that follow, in 'the management of pain', will naturally include some complementary therapies and these have been mentioned where appropriate.

ANALGESICS FOR THE MANAGEMENT OF PAIN

This section gives an overview of the main groups of analgesics and the rationale for their use. The reader is referred to drug formularies and pharmacology textbooks for more detailed information and discussion of the routes of administration. The principles underlying the effective administration of analgesics are emphasised.

A summary of major drug groups, indication for use and example analgesics is presented in Table 15.6.

Table 15.6: Summary of major analgesic drug groups and indications for use

Drug goup	Indication	Analgesics
Strong **opioids**	Moderate to severe pain. Use post-operatively, for trauma and in cancer pain	Diamorphine Morphine Papaveretum Fentanyl
Weak opioids	Moderate pain. Used in trauma, surgery and chronic pain	Codeine Dihydrocodeine
Non-steroidal anti-inflammatory drugs (**NSAID**)	Mild to moderate pain. Used for post-operative pain and inflammatory pain (e.g. arthritis). Can be used with opioids	Diclofenac Ketorolac Aspirin
Simple analgesics	Mild to moderate pain	Paracetamol
Tricyclic antidepressants	Migraine headaches, chronic pain syndromes	Amitriptyline Imipramine
Anticonvulsants	Pain associated with chronic neuralgias and phantom limb pain	Phenytoin
Steroids and corticosteroids	Reduces spinal cord compression and raised intracranial pressure	Dexamethasone

Principles of analgesic administration

The administration of analgesia to the patient is viewed primarily as a nursing role, within the hospital setting. Evidence suggests that there are many missed opportunities for prescribed analgesia to be as potentially effective as it could be. It is imperative that the nurse takes an active role to ensure the patient achieves the maximum benefit from the analgesia. Analgesics are one of the most common types of 'over the counter' (OTC) drugs but knowledge is required for their optimal effectiveness. It is essential to teach patients about how drugs work, possible side-effects and how to minimise them. Table 15.7 identifies some of the potential opportunities to maximise analgesic effectiveness.

Patient controlled analgesia (PCA)

Patient controlled analgesia is a method of pain control which has been shown to reduce pain significantly and it provides more effective pain relief than traditional intramuscular analgesia (Ballantyne *et al.*, 1993). PCA involves patient control of a pump to self-administer analgesia, usually intra-venously or subcutaneously. The pump is pre-programmed to deliver a small bolus dose of analgesia when the patient presses the button, but a 'lock-out' period prevents the patient receiving further doses should he or she press again within, for example, 5 minutes.

PCA enables patients to receive analgesia when they need it as they do not have to ask a nurse and so it avoids the unwanted peaks and troughs associated with intramuscular administration. The plasma concentration can be kept within a minimum effective analgesic concentration (**MEAC**), as shown in Figure 15.6.

PCA may not work for all patients as some people do not feel comfortable being responsible for their own administration of analgesia. Thomas and Rose (1993) consider the wide variety of clinical settings which have used PCA and discuss some of the patient variables, such as **locus of control** and coping styles, which may affect the efficacy of PCA.

Epidural analgesia

Epidural analgesia is increasingly popular as a method of providing effective pain relief. It is often used post-operatively and during labour.

Table 15.7: Actions to maximise the opportunity for effective pain relief

Opportunities to maximise analgesic effectiveness
■ Check the prescription and ensure the dose and time interval between doses is correct. Research suggests doctors frequently underprescribe analgesia and overestimate the dose duration (Oden, 1989).
■ When the analgesia dose is prescribed as a variable amount, i.e. 10–20 mg, titrate the analgesia against the pain, rather than always giving the smallest amount possible.
■ For cancer pain use the World Health Organization (WHO, 1996) analgesic ladder. See Figure 15.5.
■ Educate patients about their analgesia and why they should be comfortable, e.g. to enable them to mobilise and prevent complications. This will make them more likely to be open about their pain and accept analgesia.
■ If an **opiate** has been prescribed then request that an anti-emetic and laxative will also be prescribed and use these pro-actively.
■ Around the clock (ATC) dosing is more effective than traditional PRN regimens. Give analgesia before the pain returns rather than after.
■ Fear of respiratory depression and addiction are often reasons why health care professionals are reluctant to prescribe and administer opioids. Research indicates these fears are unfounded as less than 1% of patients suffer these unwanted side-effects (Friedman, 1990) and every opportunity should be taken to dispel these myths.

The epidural space is located between the dura mater and the spinal canal. A fine catheter is inserted into the epidural space, between the vertebrae, enabling the delivery of analgesics. Opioid drugs can be given in small quantities as they diffuse through the dura mater, binding with **opioid receptors** in the spinal cord, thus producing analgesia. Local anaesthetic agents such as bupivacaine can also be used, but these exert their action by anaesthetising the nerves which leave the spinal cord, thus numbing pain at the area supplied by these nerves, e.g. muscle. Jaques (1994) provides an informative paper which outlines the physiology, nursing care and possible complications associated with this method.

CUTANEOUS STIMULATION

Therapeutic touch

Therapeutic touch has been reported to affect the autonomic nervous system by dampening the sympathetic response, resulting in observable relaxation (Mackey, 1995). It is postulated that in healthy individuals there is a balance of inward and outward energy but in illness the balance is altered. With therapeutic touch the healer uses his or her hands to direct energy exchange and several studies have supported the role of therapeutic touch and the analgesic properties it can produce

(Meehan, 1993). Sayre-Adams (1994) defines this therapy and summarises some of the research which has measured its effectiveness.

Massage

Massage is an important comfort measure which can be used to aid relaxation and reduce pain (Stevenson, 1994). It is thought that stimulation of the skin activates the large diameter A-beta fibres, which then close the gate and prevent pain impulses from A-delta and C fibers reaching the central nervous system. Gentle firm stroking of the foot, hand or arm are often very effective relaxation interventions for pain relief and can easily be used whilst waiting for analgesia to take effect, during a procedure or whilst washing. Family and friends often feel powerless to relieve the suffering of pain but simple massage or gentle stroking can bring pain relief and help them feel needed.

Back and body massage is also effective but cultural considerations may mean it is less acceptable for either the nurse or patient. Skilled massage requires specialist input and many health professionals are now studying additional courses to increase their skills. **Aromatherapy** is the combination of skilled massage and the use of essential oils, e.g lavender. Some patients find this combination particularly pleasant and acceptable.

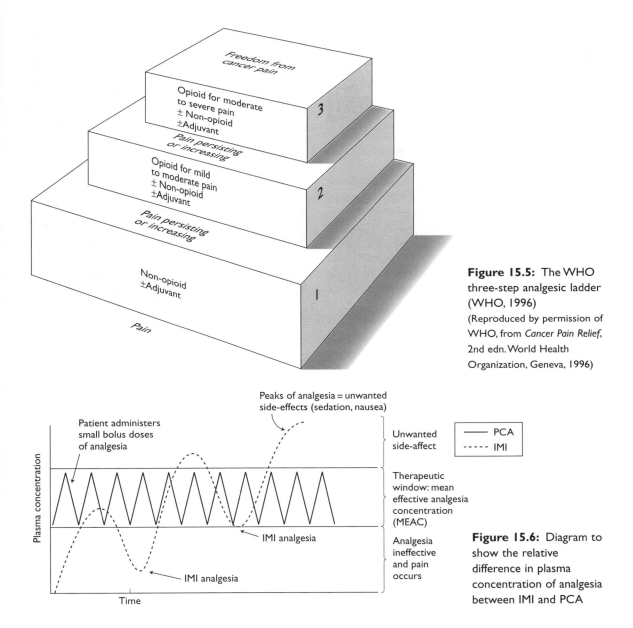

Figure 15.5: The WHO three-step analgesic ladder (WHO, 1996) (Reproduced by permission of WHO, from *Cancer Pain Relief*, 2nd edn. World Health Organization, Geneva, 1996)

Figure 15.6: Diagram to show the relative difference in plasma concentration of analgesia between IMI and PCA

Transcutaneous electrical nerve stimulation (TENS)

Transcutaneous electrical nerve stimulation (TENS) is a non-invasive method for the relief of both acute and chronic pain. It consists of a small electrical pulse generator, the size of a personal stereo, with two or four electrodes which are placed on the skin (Figure 15.7). It is battery powered and the electrical impulse discharged can be altered in intensity, duration and frequency for each individual. It is suggested that the electrical stimulation excites the large diameter A-beta fibres and closes the gate, as well as stimulating the release of **endorphins** (Hargreaves and Lander, 1989). However, a recent review of the research suggests that there is a lack of methodological rigour in the original studies (Moore and McQuay, 1997) and therefore the results of these studies studies should be treated with caution. In acute post-operative pain it should not replace conventional interventions but where patients do derive benefit from TENS its use should be encouraged.

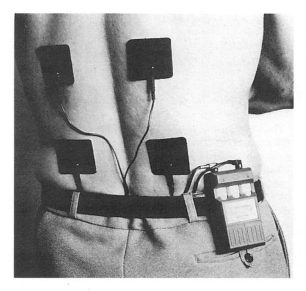

Figure 15.7: Placement of electrodes and lead wires attached to TENS

It can easily be worn beneath clothes and does not restrict mobility, which allows the patient to continue normal activities such as work or gardening (Figure 15.8).

Many companies lease the devices out to patients with simple instructions (e.g. for labour pain and muscle and joint pain associated with arthritis) and it is becoming a popular intervention. It is essential that nurses have the knowledge to use new technologies safely and confidently.

> **Activity**
>
> Find out where you might obtain a TENS machine in your hospital and/or community. Identify your own learning needs that would enable you to recommend its use to a patient or friend and teach him/her how to use it. Speak with someone who has used a machine and find out how they use it for pain relief. Physiotherapists are a good source of expertise.

Heat

Heat is a useful intervention for deep aching pain, muscle discomfort and joint stiffness. Arthritis and rheumatic disease often produce this type of pain. It is thought that the warmth increases the circulation by vasodilation and facilitates the removal of chemicals which increase pain, such as

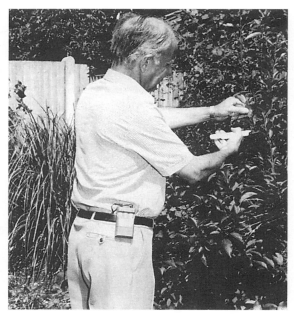

Figure 15.8: Patient is able to work in the garden whilst obtaining pain relief from TENS

prostaglandins. At home many people will naturally seek comfort from a hot water bottle or a good soak in the bath. Electric heat pads are particularly helpful as they can easily be positioned to relieve pain, e.g. in the back of a chair. An electric underblanket can be helpful in providing a warm relaxing bed and reducing stiffness. A warm bath at either end of the day may help in providing comfort to facilitate dressing or induce relaxation and comfort.

Cold

Cold therapy is reportedly more effective than heat for reducing pain but obviously lacks the appeal and comfort! It works through stimulating large fibres and 'closing the gate' as well as slowing nerve conduction. The latter reduces muscle spasm. Crushed ice wrapped in a towel (to prevent burn) can limit recent trauma damage and burn pain. Fordham and Dunn (1994) discuss in more detail physical non-pharmacological interventions for the management of pain.

Other cutaneous stimulation techniques which have been used to reduce pain are **acupressure** and **acupuncture**. A nurse might undertake specialist training to become competent in such techniques but it is also important to know how they work. It is then possible to suggest these to patients. Many people these days are keen to embrace non-pharmacological strategies and consider complementary therapies.

> **Key Points**
> - Simple massage can be incorporated into general care.
> - TENS can be used for acute and chronic pain.
> - People naturally seek pain relief through heat/cold therapy.

RELAXATION STRATEGIES

These psychological strategies are widely used for the reduction of distress and anxiety by reducing muscle tension, encouraging an inner sense of calm and diminishing the activity of the autonomic nervous system. Pain often produces muscle tension, which in turn produces anxiety and more pain. Breaking the cycle is an important way of reducing the pain or helping the person to cope with his or her pain. Helping people live with pain is tremendously important, as many types of chronic non-malignant pain are not always amenable to conventional treatment and people may feel there is no hope. Offering pain strategies which increase people's ability to cope with the pain and give them a sense of control over their pain, and thus their life, is vital. Many of these strategies are well used in chronic pain management but are also effective for acute pain (Mogan et al., 1985).

Many patients may already have their own relaxation strategies, such as listening to a certain piece of music, having a warm, fragrant bath or going to the hairdressers. These should be identified and where possible included in their care. Three simple relaxation techniques are considered which have been shown to be particularly useful in the management of pain. Where possible the environment should be warm, peaceful and have an 'air' of relaxation.

Deep breathing exercises

This involves a simple technique where the patient is positioned comfortably in a quiet and peaceful environment. The person is instructed to take a slow deep breath in through the nose, hold for 5 seconds and then gently let it out again with a focus on dissipating tension when exhaling. This can be repeated.

Progressive muscle relaxation

Usually starting at the feet and working up, muscle groups are selected and purposefully tensed for several seconds and then relaxed. Anxiety and muscle relaxation produce opposite physiological states and therefore cannot exist together.

> **Activity**
> Get in a comfortable position and bring your shoulders up towards your ears and hold the position for 10 seconds. Then slowly let your shoulders down as low as you possibly can let them go. What do you notice about your shoulders now? Were you aware of the muscle tensions before you did this exercise?

Music

Music can be used as a relaxation or distraction strategy in pain management. A detailed review of studies on the effects of relaxation and music on post-operative pain concluded they reduced the pain, especially the affective (emotional) component (Good, 1996). A personal stereo can be used to listen to music. The volume can be increased or decreased to respond to the pain and it can even be used at work or while being active. Sometimes the fear of the pain occurring at work can be particularly worrying so interventions which are discreet and easily utilised are important. This gives people a sense of control over their lives and reduces the anxiety often associated with pain.

Creating the relaxing environment

People entering hospitals or clinics immediately get a sense of the atmosphere. With increased turnover of patients and shortage of resources the pace of life can feel frenetic, which in turn can transfer itself to patients. Soothing music in the background, plants or flowers at various points and a few small bowls of pot pourri can contribute to a relaxing environment. Awareness of our own actions is important and attempts to 'look' relaxed whilst moving quickly are difficult but important, as many patients are reluctant to report pain because 'everyone is so busy'. If pain occurs at work or home try to encourage the patient to create his or her own 'small voice of calm' amid the chaos. Although this may not always be possible, there may be small changes which contribute positively, e.g. desk lamps rather than fluorescent lighting, liberal use of plants and having one part of home as a sanctuary.

> **Key Points**
> - Incorporate a patient's own relaxation strategy into his/her care.
> - Muscle relaxation and anxiety cannot exist together.
> - Create a relaxing environment.

THERAPEUTIC NURSE–PATIENT RELATIONSHIP

The nursing partnership has been viewed as a way of looking at what happens when the nurse offers expertise to a person who is experiencing a health-related experience (Christensen, 1993). This partnership can be an essential component in the management of pain. The ability to convey trust and empathy are skilled nursing actions which require a partnership in care where the patient and his or her family are central. When patients are experiencing pain they are especially vulnerable and the nurse can be instrumental in helping them cope with their pain.

This is particularly important when the person is experiencing chronic pain. Coping with pain day and night and feeling isolated, depressed and frightened is devastating. This may be compounded if no physical cause can be found for the pain and an endless round of hospital appointments have left the person feeling that no one believes him or her. Having others believe the pain has been found to be crucial for non-malignant chronic pain sufferers (Seers and Friedli, 1996). A therapeutic nurse–patient relationship has trust which conveys belief in the person's pain. This fundamental approach can help people live with their pain and cope more positively.

COMFORT MEASURES

Comfort has been identified as a central facet of nursing (Morse, 1992) and Ersser (1991) has suggested that 'comfort' is one of the five categories which describes the therapeutic approach to nursing. In a frantic world it can be easy to overlook simple strategies which can be of immense benefit. Most people have developed their own 'comfort' strategies and it is important to identify what these are and integrate them into a plan of care.

It is important to note here that these strategies may be particularly helpful with people who have learning disabilities or senile dementia. The inability to express one's pain must only contribute to the fear and dread of it getting worse. The following are three examples of simple comfort measures which reduce anxiety and pain.

Positioning

Positioning or making someone comfortable is a skilled nursing intervention and one which is essential in the management of pain. Many patients see this activity as central to nursing care but nurses may underestimate its role in pain management. Using pillows and soft blankets, patients can be positioned, so reducing muscle spasm and relief from bony prominences. Patients in pain may come to dread being moved so it is essential that positioning is carried out carefully and skilfully. If patients have favourite pillows or blankets which they find helpful at home, ask friends or family to bring them into hospital. Be creative with the environment!

Family and friends

Family and friends can be a tremendous comfort and their presence can help people cope with pain or even relieve it. Nurses may observe that a patient who had been complaining of pain is seen laughing and joking with a visitor shortly thereafter. There may be a danger of disbelieving the pain experience and nurses may feel the patient exaggerated his/her pain. What has happened is that the presence of a friend or family member provides both comfort and distraction from the pain. Nurses should optimise these strategies and work alongside the patient. In the community, leg ulcer dressings are often painful to redress. The district nurse might encourage the presence of a family member or friend during the dressing change, thus distracting and relaxing the patient.

Skilled companionship

Nurses may avoid patients who are experiencing pain if they feel there is nothing they can do or it makes them feel awkward and uncomfortable. When pain is distressing, the close company of another person can help the sufferer cope with the experience. Nurses can stay with the person and be there for him/her. When nurses have stayed with patients at this time they talk about the nurse 'knowing what I was going through' or 'I just knew that she was there and it helped me cope'. Holding the person, letting him or her talk or just sitting quietly are all important actions which should be part of the rich repertoire of nursing care. We should not fear others' pain or suffering but allow ourselves to enter their world and be there for them.

COGNITIVE INTERVENTIONS

Distraction

Distraction is a strategy which allows one's mind to focus on pleasant stimuli other than the pain or negative emotions (McCaffery and Beebe, 1994). Distraction strategies are often used routinely by patients who experience chronic pain and they can range from watching television, reading a book, listening to music or going for a walk.

Imagery

Imagery is a mental picture of reality or fantasy and usually involves all five senses. It is a technique which is relatively easy to use and can be helpful for chronic pain and short painful procedures. Like other non-pharmacological strategies it should not take the place of analgesia but complement it. Try to make sure that there will no be interruptions and that the environment is warm. Choosing a subject to explore through the senses, should be agreed between the patient and nurse – maybe a holiday or activity which was particularly enjoyed. The following activity is an example of 'guided imagery'. Imagine yourself beneath the tree ....

Activity

It is a warm summer evening and the wind gently rustles through the leaves on the trees. You are sitting beneath the oak tree and can feel the slightly damp grass beneath you and the warm rays of sun on your skin. In the distance you hear the sounds of laughter from children playing and the splash of water as they paddle and jump. The fragrant smell of warm earth and heady scents of night scented stocks mingle together ....

Patient teaching

Patient teaching is central to effective pain management. Information prior to medical procedures has long been shown to reduce pain and anxiety (Hayward, 1975; Shade, 1992). Information given prior to a medical procedure can be **sensory** (what it will feel like, smell, taste, etc.), procedural (what time events will occur and in what sequence) and instructional (deep breathing exercises and relaxation strategies). Not all patients want the same amount of information and it is necessary to assess each person and decide with them how much they want to know.

Another form of patient teaching which is important relates to the process of pain management: understanding pain, pain assessment, drugs being used to reduce pain and non-pharmacological strategies. It should also include dispelling misconceptions sometimes held by patients or their families which are barriers to effective pain relief, e.g. fear of **addiction**, not wanting to complain about their pain and the possibility that if they take pain medication now, then it might not be effective when pain is severe.

Many people will want to help themselves and nurses should be aware of literature that will help. Jan Sadler (1996) has written an informative book which aims to be a practical handbook for natural pain relief, which would serve as an excellent resource for those suffering from pain.

Key Points

■ Although acute and chronic pain are different, many interventions can be used very effectively with both types of pain.

■ Strategies which combine pharmacological and non-pharmacological interventions are more

> powerful than single strategy approaches to pain management.
> - Allowing patients to express their pain and being there with them through their pain can be an important therapeutic intervention.
> - A therapeutic nurse–patient relationship is the foundation for the effective management of pain.

MULTIDISCIPLINARY TEAMS

Various professions can make an important contribution to providing effective pain relief, both as individuals and as part of a specialist team. In the previous section a range of interventions were identified for the management of pain and in some cases, e.g. TENS, a physiotherapist may be referred to for his/her expertise and contribution. Key professions and examples of their contributions are summarised in Table 15.8.

For some client groups, e.g. surgical patients, people with chronic pain and those experiencing symptoms of cancer, there are professional teams established which offer expert advice in relation to pain management and other problems. These teams 'work together' with a unified approach and shared goals. Their effectiveness lies in their 'teamwork'. The communication between team members is often very good and each member of the team is important for the overall success.

ACUTE PAIN SERVICES

The concept of the acute pain service (APS) was originally developed by Ready *et al.* (1988) in Seattle, USA and provided a template for development in the UK. In 1990 The Royal College of Surgeons and College of Anaesthetists published their report on pain after surgery (Commission on the Provision of Surgical Services, 1990). They reviewed research on pain after surgery and concluded that the traditional methods of managing pain after surgery, e.g. PRN opioid analgesia given intramuscularly, were inadequate and recommended that acute pain services should be introduced into all major hospitals performing surgery in the UK. A national survey of UK hospitals in 1995 revealed that 42.7% had an APS (Harmer *et al.* 1995).

The acute pain service or team is usually composed of an anaesthetist(s), acute pain clinical nurse specialist and a pharmacist. Some teams may also have a clinical psychologist. The team is responsible for the day-to-day management of pain after surgery and for ensuring that adequate monitoring is available for the pain-relieving technique chosen, e.g. epidural analgesia or PCA. The teams run in-service training on analgesic techniques and on pain-related topics. In many hospital wards nurses now care for patients receiving epidural analgesia, whilst a few years ago these patients would have been nursed in an intensive care unit. The teams also undertake research related to pain and it is standard practice to be

Table 15.8: The contribution to pain management by different professions

Profession	Contribution
Nurse	Assessment, coordination of other professional input, appropriate analgesic administration, non-pharmacological interventions, skilled companionship
Doctor	Diagnosis, prescribes treatment, gives information
Occupational therapist	Assessment and facilitation of learning new skills for activities of daily living
Physiotherapist	Exercise, TENS, education, ultrasound, hydrotherapy
Psychologist	Assessment, psychotherapeutic interventions, relaxation, distraction, **biofeedback**
Pharmacist	Advice on pharmacology, instrumental in setting up protocols and guidelines regarding drug administration

auditing the service continuously to evaluate the effectiveness of these initiatives.

The role of the ward nurse is critical to the success of the endeavours of the acute pain team and it has been suggested that hospital nurses need further education to enable them to broaden their role in pain management (Mather and Ready, 1994). It is therefore essential that nurses are empowered to take responsibility for pain management and take an active role in assessing pain and evaluating the effectiveness of interventions. The following patient study illustrates the importance of the hospital nurse's role in pain management even when there is an acute pain service.

Patient Study

Mandy James returned from surgery last night following a colon resection for cancer. She had a PCA machine and was pressing the button regularly for analgesia. During the night she woke experiencing intense pain across her abdomen. Despite pressing the button several times her pain continued and Mandy began to feel anxious and frightened. Mandy waited until the staff nurse came to check the pump, She then told her that she still had pain. The staff nurse replied 'use the PCA and just keep pressing the button regularly'.

The nurse was not assessing Mandy's pain at all but rather 'checking' the pump. Both are essential if pain is to be well managed. The dose and lock-out times programmed into the pump may not provide adequate analgesia for all patients and therefore it is essential to assess the pain regularly and ascertain how many times the patient has attempted to receive analgesia against how many times the analgesia has been delivered. In the above situation it might have been necessary to increase the bolus dose or reduce the lock-out time, but the nurse needed to assess Mandy more thoroughly before being able to make a decision. Hospital policy varies across the UK regarding the role of the ward nurse with PCA/epidural, but broadening the scope of practice for ward nurses may well contribute to more effective pain relief.

CHRONIC PAIN TEAMS

The chronic pain clinic was initially set up by two enthusiastic anaesthetists in the 1960s (John Lloyd and Samual Lipton). Techniques originally used were **nerve blocks** and pharmacological interventions but clinics now utilise a range of strategies from acupuncture and exercise to **operant conditioning**, involving a range of professionals. These multidisciplinary pain clinics have become increasingly popular and have adopted a variety of formats.

Patients may be referred to a chronic pain clinic from their GP or a consultant who has been managing their care. These clinics vary greatly in their structure and management. An inpatient programme of one month is described by Crabbe (1989), but others can be accessed on a daily basis (see O'Hara, 1996, for more detail on the structure of such teams and the role of individuals).

The goal of treatment focuses upon helping the person cope with pain and facilitating coping strategies, to enable him or her to achieve this. This is termed a **cognitive-behavioural approach**. The patient is often asked not to mention the pain and avoid moaning about it (as this can do little to help). Instead, the emphasis is on positive aspects and achievements. Treatment success is measured in terms of improvement in quality of life, func-

---

Patient Study

Steven Jennings, aged 47 years, came to the pain clinic last year for the first time, having suffered chronic low back pain for 8 years. He had been through a variety of different treatments and all had failed. He gave up his job 3 years ago as he couldn't tolerate sitting down all day. His wife was the main breadwinner and he said this made him feel useless and 'worth nothing really'. He spent most of his days in bed or watching television and friends had stopped visiting. His weight had increased and he rarely slept more than 2 or 3 hours. They had discussed the possibility of divorcing last year and this prompted Steven to make a final effort to 'try and do something – anything'. The chronic pain programme focused on helping Steven cope when he experienced pain. Exercise and relaxation strategies were particularly effective in giving Steven confidence in coping with his pain. Not only could he avoid situations which triggered the pain, he could actively do something to reduce his response to the situation and pain. One year on he has a small pottery business and orders are ever increasing and life hasn't looked so good for many years!

tion and mood, rather than only reduction in pain intensity (Ralphs, 1993).

PALLIATIVE CARE TEAMS

The practice of palliative medicine was established primarily in hospices and the community, but more recently has evolved in the acute setting (Hockley, 1992). Teams are not all the same and vary with the types and numbers of professionals involved. They are usually composed of a palliative care consultant, palliative care nurse and social worker. In the community this team would draw on members of the primary health care team. If it was in the hospital setting, then members of the health care team would be involved.

The team provides specialist care related to people living with cancer and also those with life-threatening diseases, such as AIDS, multiple sclerosis and chronic respiratory diseases. This may include advice about symptom control (e.g. pain and constipation), respite care and rehabilitation. The team also incorporates a psychosocial and 'family focus' to its delivery of care.

Referral to the palliative care team is usually done by the hospital consultant or GP and the patient and his or her family/carer will be visited by a member of the team and assessed. The nurse often conducts the initial assessment and will liaise with her colleagues for further advice and discussion. In the team there is often a flattened hierarchy and communication between the members is good with each person being equally important to the effective functioning of the team.

In a busy general ward patients with cancer may experience pain and a junior doctor may be unwilling to prescribe higher does of analgesia (and nurses may be reluctant to administer these) for fear of causing the patient to become addicted or of inducing respiratory depression. Both these widely held misconceptions have been shown to be unjustified, yet they persist as a major barrier to effective pain management. See Carr (1997) for a fuller discussion pertaining to the barriers to effective pain management. A recent report on the provision of palliative care in the hospital setting reviews the provision of services and makes recommendations on good practice and future development (National Council for Hospice and Palliative Care Services, 1996).

Educating health care professionals in the palliative care approach is a vital part of the work for palliative care teams. The palliative care team is a resource for clinical staff, offering informal advice, staff support and education. Education ranges from formal lectures on specific patient problems and their management to talking through informally some of the anxieties staff may have in caring for someone with cancer. The palliative care team are often working with staff whose expertise varies widely, therefore much of their work is helping staff to develop a palliative care approach to their delivery of care.

The palliative care team will also liaise with other specialists involved with the patient's care, e.g. surgeons, radiologists, GPs and clinical nurse specialists. When a patient has complex problems the palliative care team are able to offer expert advice. Sometimes it might be necessary to admit the patient to a palliative care unit or hospice for specialist management. The patient may well then be discharged home or back to a general ward.

Activity

The next time you have the opportunity to observe a multidisciplinary team in action make some notes on the following questions:

- How did they communicate with the patient?
- Did they involve the family?
- Which members of the team asked questions?
- How did the team communicate with each other?
- What happened when the team left?
- What was documented, where and by whom?

Observe several different teams and then answer the following questions:

- Are some teams better than others?
- How did you judge a what makes a 'good team'?
- Who has overall responsibility in the team?

You might have noticed quite different styles between the teams you observed. Effective teams communicate freely with each other and you might notice that each member of the team contributes to the conversation and there is a collegiate approach. Inclusion of the patient and his or her family in the decision-making process is another hallmark of a good team.

The phrase 'terminal care' is no longer synonymous with palliative care but part of the palliative care continuum. Many people now live with cancer rather than die from it. People with cancer live at home with their families, return to work and often enjoy many months or years free from pain and symptoms. Although nursing care in the community is usually delivered by a district nurse and the GP, the palliative care team continues to be involved with the patient and family care and is an important source of expert advice to other members of the primary and community nursing team. Skilled counselling and family support augment the quality of care given by the primary heath care team or the hospital team.

When a patient is discharged from hospital the palliative care team will liaise with the primary care team. To ensure that seamless care is facilitated, good communication between the two teams is essential. Sometimes the palliative care nurse may continue to visit the patient at home. Living with cancer and coping with uncertainty, disease recurrence, active treatment regimens and unwanted side-effects requires specialist input from a range of professionals. This input may be short or long term as patients may be cured or their disease may go into remission. Palliative care teams continue to demonstrate the benefits of a multi-professional team working together to meet the needs of individuals and their families (see Chapter 27 for further descriptions of the work of palliative care teams).

Key Points

- The role of the ward nurse is critical to the success of an acute pain team.
- Chronic pain programmes help patients cope with their pain.
- People with cancer can enjoy months or years pain and symptom free.
- Good communication and patient/family involvement and the hallmarks of an effective team.

CONCLUSION

Pain is a subjective human experience which can have a devastating impact on the quality of a person's life. Due to the multidimensional nature of pain it is something which is often hidden by those suffering it, and this is compounded by a lack of knowledge and inappropriate attitudes on the part of some health care professionals.

Accurate pain assessment and documentation is central to the successful management of pain. Establishing trust and a belief in the patient and his or her pain experience is essential to establishing a therapeutic relationship. Using a formal pain assessment tool conveys genuine concern about an individual's pain and reduces the chance of bias and error. Careful questioning of patients about their pain, its meaning to them and what has made it worse or better, all complement the data collected. The assessment and positive outcomes are reliant on a genuine belief in the patient's pain experience.

For the person experiencing pain the skilled and sensitive practitioner conducts an accurate assessment before providing optimal pain-relieving strategies. As well as using a range of therapeutic interventions he/she understands the need to be with the patient (or withdraw) by providing skilled companionship or presence. A combination of interventions, which exploit the multidimensional nature of pain, is essential if pain is to be alleviated. Involving the family or close carer is also imperative as pain does not always affect just the patient but also those closest to them.

When pain does not have a foreseeable end and may have to be endured through life, the nurse can help the person and his or her family come to terms with this situation and cope with the pain. Allowing the free expression of pain, unconditionally, is important. Explaining to patients and their families about the pain and drawing on their coping skills gives them some control over their life and allows them to live through their pain and improve the quality of their life.

Summary

Pain is a multidimensional experience which potentially affects each and every person. The sensory, cognitive and emotional components of pain are individual to each person. The nurse–patient relationship forms the central pivot for effective pain management and commences with an accurate assessment. This is essential if interventions are to achieve their maximum potential. Therapeutic interventions should exploit the multidimensional nature of pain and nurses should always combine pharmacological and non-pharmacological interventions for the greatest effectiveness. Effective pain management requires collaboration with multidisciplinary teams and other health care professionals. Clear communication and team work are essential for success.

'By any reasonable code, freedom from pain should be a basic human right, limited only by our knowledge to achieve it.'

(Leibeskind and Melzack, 1987)

REFERENCES

AHCPR (1992). *Acute Pain Management*. Publication No. 92–0032. Department of Health and Human Services, Rockville, MD.

AHCPR (1994). *Management of Cancer Pain*. Publication No. 94–0592. Department of Health and Human Services, Rockville, MD.

Albrecht, M., Cook, J.E., Riley, M.J. and Andreoni, V. (1992). Factors influencing staff nurses' decisions for non-documentation of patient response to analgesia administration. *Journal of Clinical Nursing*, 1, 243–51.

Allcock, N. (1996). Factors affecting the assessment of postoperative pain: a literature review. *Journal of Advanced Nursing*, 24, 1144–51.

Baillie, L. (1993). A review of pain assessment tools. *Nursing Standard*, 7(23), 25–9.

Ballantyne, J.C., Carr, D.B., Chalmers, T.C., Dear, K.G.B. and Angellilo, I.F. (1993). Postoperative patient controlled analgesia: meta analyses of intial randomised controlled trials. *Journal of Clinical Anaesthesiology*, 5, 182–93.

Berker, M. and Hughes, B. (1990). Using a tool for pain assessment. *Nursing Times*, 86(24), 50–2.

Bourbonnais, F. (1981). Pain assessment: development of a tool for the nurse and the patient. *Journal of Advanced Nursing*, 6, 277–82.

Brattberg, G., Throslund, M. and Wikman, A. (1989). The prevalence of pain in a general population. The results of a postal survey in a county of Sweden. *Pain*, 37, 215–22.

Briggs, M. (1995). Principles of acute pain assessment. *Nursing Standard*, 9(19), 23–7.

Bruster, S., Jarman, B., Bosanquet, N., Weston, D., Erens, R. and Delbanco, T.L. (1994). National survey of hospital patients. *British Medical Journal*, 309, 1542–6.

Calvillo, E. and Flaskerud, J. (1993). Evaluation of pain response by Mexican American and Anglo-American women and their nurses. *Journal of Advanced Nursing*, 18(3), 451–9.

Carr, E.C.J. (1990). Postoperative pain: patient's expectations and experiences. *Journal of Advanced Nursing*, 15(1), 89–100.

Carr, E.C.J. (1997). Overcoming barriers to effective pain control. *Professional Nurse*, 12(6), 412–16.

Chapman, A. and Marshall, M. (1993). *Dementia: New Skills for Social Workers*. Jessica Kinsley, London.

Christensen, J. (1993). *Nursing Partnership: a Model for Nursing Practice*. Churchill Livingstone, Edinburgh.

Clancy, J. and McVicar, A.J. (1995). Pain. In *Physiology & Anatomy: a Homeostatic Approach*. Edward Arnold, London.

Closs, J. (1994). Pain in elderly patients: a neglected phenomenon. *Journal of Advanced Nursing*, 19, 1072–81.

Commission on the Provision of Surgical Services (1990). *Report of the Working Party. Pain after Surgery*. Royal College of Surgeons of England and College of Anaesthetists, London.

Crabbe, G. (1989). Crossing the pain threshold. *Nursing Times*, 85(47), 16–17.

Davis, P. (1988). Changing nursing practice for more effective control of postoperative pain through a staff initiated educational programme. *Nurse Education Today*, 8, 325–31.

Ersser, S. (1991). A search for the therapeutic dimensions of the nurse-patient interaction. In *Nursing as Therapy*, McMahon, R. and Pearson, A. (eds). Chapman & Hall, London.

Ferrell, B. and Ferrell, B. (eds). (1996). *Pain in the Elderly*. International Association for the Study of Pain Press, Seattle, WA.

Fordham, M. and Dunn, G. (1994). *Alongside the Patient in Pain: Holistic Care and Nursing Practice*. Baillière Tindall, London.

Friedman, D.P. (1990). Perspectives on the medical use of drug abuse. *Journal of Pain and Symptom Management*, 5, S2–S5.

Good, M. (1996). Effects of relaxation and music on post-operative pain: a review. *Journal of Advanced Nursing*, 24, 905–14.

Halfens, R., Evers, G. and Abu-Saad, H. (1990). Determinants of pain assessment by nurses. *International Journal of Nursing Studies*, 27(1), 43–9.

Hargreaves, A. and Lander, J. (1989). Use of transcutaneous electrical nerve stimulation for postoperative pain. *Nursing Research*, 38(3), 159–61.

Harmer, M., Davies, K.A. and Lunn, J.N. (1995). A survey of acute pain services in the United Kingdom. *British Medical Journal*, 311, 360–1.

Hayes, R. (1995). Pain assessment in the elderly. *British Journal of Nursing*, 4(20), 1199–204.

Hayward, J. (1975). *Information: a Prescription against Pain*. Royal College of Nursing, London.

Hester, N.O. (1979). The poker chip tool. *Nursing Research*, 28, 250–5.

Hockley, J (1992). Role of the hospice support team. *British Journal of Hospital Medicine*, 48, 250–3.

Horden, M., Choonara, I., Al-Waidh, M., Sambrooks, J. and Ashby, D. (1996). Measuring pain in neonates: an objective score. *Paediatric Nursing*, 8(10), 24–7.

Jandelli, K. (1995). A comparision study of patients' and nurses' perceptions of pain relief. *International Journal of Palliative Nursing*, 1(2), 74–80.

Jaques, A. (1994). Epidural analgesia. *British Journal of Nursing*, 3(14), 734–8.

Johnston, C.C. and Strada, M.E. (1986). Acute pain response in infants: a multidimensional description. *Pain*, 24, 372–82.

Jurf, J.B. and Nirschl, A.L. (1993). Acute postoperative pain management: a comprehensive review and update. *Critical Care Nursing Quarterly*, 16(1), 8–25.

Ketovuori, H. (1987). Nurses' and patients' conceptions of wound pain and the administration of analgesics. *Journal of Pain and Symptom Management*, 2(4), 213–18.

Latham, J. (1989). *Pain Control*. Austin Cornish Publications, London.

Leibeskind, J.C. and Melzack, R. (1987). The International Pain Foundation. Meeting a need for education in pain management. *Pain*, 78, 173–81.

McCaffery, M. (1968). *Nursing Practice Theories related to Cognition, Bodily Pain and Man-environment Interactions*. University of California at Los Angeles Students' Store, Los Angeles.

McCaffery, M. (1991). Pain control vignettes: how would you respond to these patients in pain? *Nursing*, June, 34, 36–7.

McCaffery, M. and Beebe, A (1994). Assessment. In *Pain: a Clinical Manual for Nursing Practice*, Latham, J. (ed.). Mosby, London.

McGrath, P.J., Johnson, G., Goodman, J.T., Schillinger, J., Dunn, J. and Chapman, J.A. (1985). CHEOPS: a behavioural pain rating scale for postoperative pain in children. In *Advances in Pain Research and Therapy*, 9, Fields, H.L., Dubner, R. and Cervero, F. (eds). New York, Raven Press.

McGrath, P.J., Unruh, A.M. and Finley, G.A. (1995). Pain measurement in children. *Pain: Clinical Updates*, 3(2),

1–4. International Association for the Study of Pain, Seattle, WA.

Mackey, R.B. (1995). Discover the healing power of therapeutic touch. *American Journal of Nursing*, 4 , 27–32.

Mather, C.M.P. and Ready, L.B. (1994). Management of acute pain. *British Journal of Hospital Medicine*, 51(3), 85–8.

Meehan, T.C. (1993). Therapeutic touch and postoperative pain: a Rogerian research study. *Nursing Science Quarterly*, 6(2), 69–78.

Melzack, R. (1975). The McGill Pain Questionnaire: major properties and scoring methods, *Pain*, 1, 277–99.

Melzack, R. (1987). The short-form McGill Pain Questionnaire. *Pain*, 30, 191–7.

Melzack, R. and Torgerson, W.S. (1971). On the language of pain. *Anaesthesiology*, 34, 50–9.

Melzack, R. and Wall, P. (1965). Pain mechanisms: a new theory. *Science*, 150, 971–9.

Merskey, H (1986). International Association for the Study of Pain – pain terms: a current list with definitions and notes on use. *Pain* (Suppl.), 3, S1–S225.

Mogan, J., Wells, N. and Robertson, E. (1985). Effects of preoperative teaching on postoperative pain: a replication and expansion. *International Journal of Nursing Studies*, 22, 267–80.

Moore, A. and McQuay, H. (eds) (1997). Does TENS Work? *Bandolier*, 4(3), 3–4.

Morse, J. (1992). Comfort: the refocusing of nursing care. *Clinical Nursing Research*, 1(1), 91–106.

National Council for Hospice and Specialist Palliative Care Services (1996). *Palliative care in the Hospital Setting*, Occasional Paper 10. National Council for Hospice and Specialist Palliative Care Services, London.

Oden, R.V. (1989). Acute postoperative pain: incidence, severity, and the etiology of inadequate treatment. *Anaesthiology Clinics of North America*, 7, 1–15.

O'Hara, P. (1996). The role of the professionals. *Pain Management for Health Professionals*. Chapman & Hall, London.

Puntillo, K. (1988). The phenomenon of pain and critical care nursing. *Heart and Lung*, 17, 262–71.

Raiman, J. (1986). Pain relief – a two way process. *Nursing Times*, 82(15), 24–7.

Ralphs, J. (1993). The cognitive-behavioural treatment of chronic pain. In *Pain Management and Nursing Care*, Carroll, D. and Bowsher, D. (eds). Butterworth-Heinemann, Oxford.

Ready, L.B., Oden, R., Chadwick, H.S. *et al.* (1988). Development of an anesthesiology-based postoperative pain management service. *Anesthesiology*, 68, 100–6.

Rigge, M. (1990). Pain research on prevalence of pain in Britain. *Which? Way to Health*, April, 66–8.

Sadler, J. (1996). *Natural Pain Relief: a Practical Handbook for Self-help*. Element Books, London.

Sayre-Adams, J. (1994). Therapeutic touch: a nursing function. *Nursing Standard*, 8(17), 25–8.

Seers, K. (1987). Perceptions of pain. *Nursing Times*, 83, 37–9.

Seers, K. (1988). Factors affecting pain assessment. *Professional Nurse*, 3(6), 201–6.

Seers, K. and Friedli, K. (1996). The patients' experiences of their chronic non-malignant pain. *Journal of Advanced Nursing*, 24, 1160–8.

Shade, P. (1992). PCA: can client education improve outcomes? *Journal of Advanced Nursing*, 17, 408–13.

Simons, W. and Malabar, R. (1995). Assessing pain in elderly patients who cannot respond verbally. *Journal of Advanced Nursing*, 22, 663–9.

Stevenson, C.J. (1994). The psycho-physiological effects of aromatherapy massage following cardiac surgery. *Complementary Therapies in Medicine*, 2, 27–35.

Thomas, V.J. and Rose, F.D. (1993). Patient-controlled analgesia: a new method for old. *Journal of Advanced Nursing*, 18, 1719–26.

Walker, J. (1993). Pain in the elderly. In *Pain Management and Nursing Care*, Carroll, D. and Bowsher, D. (eds). Butterworth-Heinemann, Oxford.

Webb, C. and Hope, K. (1995). What kind of nurses do patients want? *Journal of Clinical Nursing*, 4, 101–8.

World Health Organization (1996). *Cancer Pain Relief*, 2nd edn. WHO, Geneva, Switzerland.

Zalon, M.L. (1993). Nurses' assessment of postoperative patients' pain. *Pain*, 54, 329–34.

FURTHER READING

Ferrell, B., Wheden, M. and Rollins, B. (1995). Pain and quality assessment/improvement. *Journal of Nursing Care Quarterly*, 9(3), 69–85.

This exciting paper brings pain management into the initiatives of quality improvement in health care. It gives guidance on how to evaluate pain management in clinical practice and how and what to consider in the process.

Holritz, K.E., Racolin, A.A. and Bookbinder, M. (1995). Nursing's changing role in cancer pain management. *Pain Digest*, 5, 318–24.

This review article considers the role of nursing in cancer pain from the 1950s to the future and discusses the health care issues which shape the provision of care.

Soafer, B. (1992). *Pain: a Handbook for Nurses*, 2nd edn. Chapman & Hall, London.

An informative and very readable textbook which emphasises the nurse–patient relationship in the management of pain.

Stevenson, C. (1995). Non-pharmacological aspects of acute pain management. *Complementary Therapies in Nursing and Midwifery*, 1, 77–84.

An excellent source of information about using non-pharmacological interventions in the management of acute pain.

Thomas, V.J. (ed) (1997). *Pain – Its Nature and Management*. Baillière Tindall, London.

An interesting, informative and wide-ranging textbook from authors working in pain. Using a multidimensional approach to pain management and includes much new material.

Ward, S.E. and Gordon, D. (1994). Application of the American Pain Society quality assurance standards. *Pain*, 56, 299–306.

This illuminating study raises questions about the interpretation of patient satisfaction as an outcome in studies on the quality of pain management.

CHAPTER SIXTEEN

PROVIDING A SAFE ENVIRONMENT – *the* MANAGEMENT *and* PREVENTION *of* INFECTION

Jennie Wilson

- Introduction
- An introduction to microbiology
- Routes of microbial transmission
- Defences against infection
- Infection associated with health care
- Preventing infection associated with health care
- The management of an infectious patient
- Education and training
- Conclusion

Infection has long been recognised as a complication of health care. Micro-organisms may be introduced via tubes, catheters and cannulae or during surgical procedures and can be readily transmitted from one patient to another by staff or on equipment. Almost every contact between nurse and patient has the potential to transmit micro-organisms. However, it has been estimated that at least a third of these infections can be prevented by good infection control practice (Haley *et al.*, 1985). The prevention and control of infection forms part of the central responsibility of the nurse – to 'safeguard the interests and well-being of their patients' (United Kingdom Central Council for Nurses [UKCC], 1992). The risk and responsibilities are real; neglecting to wash hands after emptying a urine drainage catheter could result in the transmission of infection to another patient. Understanding and applying the principles of infection prevention is therefore essential to ensure that a safe environment is provided for patients receiving care. The aim of this chapter is to provide an overview of those principles of microbiology, epidemiology and immunology that provide the basis for infection control. It also explores the significance of infections acquired as a result of health care and strategies for their prevention, including routine infection prevention measures, identification of susceptible individuals and isolation procedures for patients with infectious disease.

INTRODUCTION

Epidemics of **infectious diseases** such as plague, typhus and smallpox were commonplace until the late 1800s, but since they were widely considered to be a punishment from God, little attempt was made to control them. By the mid-1700s several academics and physicians had realised the contagious nature of infection. However, their views were not widely accepted until the late nineteenth century, when Louis Pasteur and Robert Koch began the study of the micro-organisms first seen by Anton van Leeuwenhoek under his microscope in 1676.

In the hundred years that followed, our understanding of infection, the micro-organisms which cause it, and how they are transmitted has increased considerably. The implementation of simple infection control measures such as improving living conditions, food hygiene, drinking water quality and sewage disposal systems, proscribed in the Public Health Acts of the mid-1800s, were able to achieve dramatic reductions in the death rate which by 1900 had fallen from 25 to 15 per 1000 population. At the same time life expectancy increased from 40 to 50 years.

The susceptibility of hospital patients to infection has been recognised, if not always acted upon, for thousands of years. Hospitals caring for the sick were known in the civilised world 500 years before the birth of Christ, particularly in Palestine, Egypt, India, Greece and the Roman Empire. Despite a very limited understanding of the causes of infection, many of these institutions exhibited high standards of hygiene, based on religious rituals, and provided spacious and well-ventilated wards. Ancient Jewish laws, for example, included reference to the isolation of those who were infected and to the destruction of **fomites**. Other Jewish writings warned that surgeons should not touch wounds because their hands were the cause of **inflammation** (Selwyn, 1991).

The advent of Christianity saw a major increase in the number of hospitals, but unfortunately with a reduced emphasis on hygiene and ventilation. As a result, mortality due to infection was extremely high. These conditions persisted until the end of the nineteenth century when improvements in hospital design and planning began to be introduced. Florence Nightingale was an advocate of ward ventilation and small ward size and was also influential in improving the quality of nursing, establishing the first nursing training school at St Thomas' hospital in London in 1860. At the same time, marked improvements in infection prevention were brought about by, amongst others, Lister, who began to use antiseptics to remove micro-organisms from the surgical incision and Von Bergman, who introduced the concept of asepsis (preventing micro-organisms contaminating a site) by using sterilised surgical equipment. The development of antibiotics in the 1940s enabled infections to be treated easily and effectively for the first time and mortality associated with infection acquired in hospital began to decrease.

Health care in the twentieth century is associated with quite different infection problems. The simple surgical treatments of 100 years ago have now been replaced by increasingly sophisticated treatments involving more seriously ill patients who are particularly vulnerable to infection. The streptococcal infections, which in the 1800s were the major cause of **hospital-acquired infection**, especially after surgery and childbirth, have been replaced by Gram-negative **pathogens**. These micro-organisms frequently take advantage of the invasive devices inserted into highly susceptible patients receiving intensive nursing and medical care. In addition, the emergence of bacteria resistant to a wide range of antibiotics is threatening to undermine the progress made in the treatment of infection (Communicable Diseases Surveillance Centre, 1995).

It has been estimated that around 6% of patients admitted to hospital will acquire an infection as a result of their care and that up to one third of these could be prevented (Haley et al., 1985). These infections can have a major impact on those patients affected, their families and the costs associated with their treatment. All health care workers have a responsibility to minimise the risk of patients in their care acquiring an infection, whilst eliminating unnecessary or ritualistic activities practised in the name of infection control. In addition, the nurse has a key role as a health educator. Central to carrying out these responsibilities is a good understanding of the principles of infection prevention and control.

AN INTRODUCTION TO MICROBIOLOGY

This section reviews some of the basic information about micro-organisms and the techniques used to identify them in a laboratory, a knowledge of which is fundamental to understanding the principles of infection control. It is not within the scope of this chapter to examine the subject of microbiology in detail. More information can be found in other texts, including *The Microbiology and Epidemiology of Infection for Health Science Students* by Meers *et al.* (1995) and *Microbiology – an Introduction for the Health Sciences* by Ackerman and Dunk-Richards (1991), especially Chapters 4, 5 and 8.

Micro-organisms (or microbes) are living creatures that are so small that they cannot be seen with the naked eye. They are able to survive in almost any environment, can grow at temperatures as high as 95°C or as low as −10°C and can use almost any substance as a source of energy. Many are essential for our survival, forming vital links in the food chain, such as algae which convert atmospheric nitrogen into a form that plants can use, and others, called **saprophytic bacteria**, which break down dead plants and animals to release nutrients into the food chain.

The human body is populated by a wide variety of micro-organisms, each adapted to local conditions of nutrient supply, oxygen level, pH and temperature. Conditions may vary on different parts of the body so that the micro-organisms inhabiting the cool, dry environment of the skin will be different to those inhabiting the warm, moist and oxygen-free environment of the gut. The organisms which usually inhabit the body are called the **normal flora**. They are **commensals**, that is, they do not harm their hosts and may even benefit them by degrading material passing through the gut or preventing invasion by other, more harmful species.

A small proportion of micro-organisms cause disease by invading and damaging tissue in a process known as infection; these organisms are referred to as pathogens. Some micro-organisms always cause disease if they encounter a susceptible host, e.g. *Salmonella typhimurium*, although the extent of the disease they cause may vary according to the defence mechanisms of the host and the capabilities of the invading organism. Other microbes are described as **opportunistic pathogens**, because they are only able to cause disease in people whose normal defence mechanisms are impaired. For example, *Pneumocystis carinii* is a single-cell microscopic organism called a protozoon, which is normally found in the respiratory tract but only able to invade the tissues and cause disease in people with deficient immune systems. Some commensal organisms, whilst harmless in their usual habitat, may cause disease if transferred to another part of the body. For example, *Escherichia coli*, which forms part of the normal flora in the gut, may cause infection if it enters the urinary tract. Infection acquired in this way is called **endogenous infection**.

Occasionally, a pathogen may be present on or in the body without invading the tissues. In this situation, although the organism can be identified at the site, its presence will not be accompanied by symptoms of infection and it is described as colonising the body. Whilst such **colonisation** may be of no concern to the individual involved, the micro-organisms may be easily transferred to another person in whom it is able to cause infection. Infections caused by antibiotic-resistant bacteria are commonly associated with transmission from another patient who is colonised with the antibiotic-resistant strain. Infection acquired as a result of the transfer of micro-organisms from another person is called **exogenous** or cross-infection.

THE STRUCTURE OF MICRO-ORGANISMS

There are four main groups of micro-organisms which cause disease in humans: bacteria, **fungi**, **protozoa** and **viruses**. A simple description of these micro-organisms is provided in Table 16.1.

THE MICROBIOLOGY LABORATORY

The function of this laboratory is to identify the micro-organisms responsible for an infection, assist in the diagnosis and provide advice on the method of treatment. The technical staff in the laboratory use a number of methods to isolate and identify pathogens from a variety of clinical specimens. Medical microbiologists are doctors with a specialist training in microbiology, who provide

Table 16.1: The structure of micro-organisms

Type of micro-organism	Description
Bacteria	Simple, **prokaryotic cells** with few internal structures. The outer cell membrane is surrounded by a rigid cell wall. There is no nucleus; the genetic material is contained in a single **chromosome** in the cytoplasm. Some species are able to form resistant outer casings (**spores**) in adverse conditions
Fungi	These are plants which comprise either tubular filaments (moulds) or large, single cells (**yeasts**). They are more complex, **eukaryotic cells** which contain several internal structures for energy and protein production and for transporting substances around the cell. The genetic material is contained in a nucleus
Protozoa	These are microscopic, eukaryotic cells. They have a tough outer cell membrane, but no cell wall. They obtain nutrients by ingesting particles of food and have several internal structures for energy and protein production and substance transport. The genetic material is contained in a nucleus. Many species have different developmental stages in their life cycle, including the formation of thick-walled cysts.
Viruses	These are not cells, but a piece of nucleic acid surrounded by a protein coat; some also have an outer lipid envelope. They have no internal structures for making **DNA** or protein but invade the cells of animals, plants or bacteria, using the structures of the cell to replicate. Infected host cells are usually destroyed by the virus

advice on the interpretation of laboratory results and the most appropriate form of treatment.

Most hospitals have a microbiology laboratory on site, although some more complicated or unusual tests may need to be carried out at larger laboratories with specialised facilities. General practitioners may arrange to send specimens to a local NHS hospital laboratory or to one that is commercially operated. There are also 52 Public Health Laboratories throughout England and Wales which provide specialist diagnostic and advisory services for the prevention and control of communicable diseases. Their work is coordinated by the Central Public Health Laboratory in London. In Scotland, similar specialist services are provided by the Scottish Centre for Infection and Environmental Health.

Identification of bacteria

MICROSCOPY

Examination of the shape and appearance of microbes under a microscope can provide some important clues about their identity (Figure 16.1). A technique called **Gram staining** is used to colour the cells and distinguish the two main groups of bacteria: Gram-positive bacteria which stain dark blue and Gram-negative bacteria which stain pink. Microscopy can sometimes be used to provide a rapid, provisional diagnosis in life-threatening infections, particularly where the range of potential pathogens is small, for example, the examination of cerebrospinal fluid in patients suspected to have meningitis.

CULTURE

It is unusual to be able to identify bacteria solely on their appearance under a microscope. Samples of a specimen are therefore transferred on to solid media containing nutrients (**agar** plates). These are incubated at body temperature, 36°C, for about 24 hours, during which time the bacteria present will have multiplied and the clumps of cells that have formed will be visible as colonies. Some micro-organisms can be identified by the characteristic appearance of their colonies, but usually further tests on the cells in the colony are required for a definitive diagnosis.

ANTIBIOTIC SENSITIVITY

Bacteria isolated in the laboratory will be tested for their susceptibility to a range of antibiotics and this information used to advise clinical staff on the best method of treatment. Antibiotics are drugs capable of either destroying or preventing the

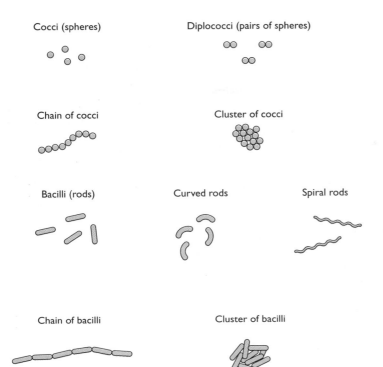

Cocci (spheres)

Diplococci (pairs of spheres)

Chain of cocci

Cluster of cocci

Bacilli (rods)

Curved rods

Spiral rods

Chain of bacilli

Cluster of bacilli

Figure 16.1: Some common shapes of bacteria cells

growth of bacteria. They have no effect against viruses and each antibiotic will have an affect on a limited range of bacterial species. Bacteria may be resistant to an antibiotic because the drug cannot penetrate their cells or the cells do not contain the protein targeted by the drug. However, bacteria previously sensitive to an antibiotic can develop resistance by acquiring extra **genes**, small pieces of DNA which enable them to resist the effect of an antibiotic or range of antibiotics. For example, the DNA may enable the cell to make a particular **enzyme** which degrades the antibiotic. These genes are often carried on small circular pieces of DNA called **plasmids** and a single plasmid can confer resistance to several antibiotics. These plasmids can be copied within the cell and then transferred to another cell along a special tube which forms between the two cells. Infections caused by bacteria resistant to many types of antibiotic are difficult, and often expensive, to treat and can cause major problems in hospitals (see Box 16.1). The emergence of resistant strains of bacteria can be discouraged by avoiding the unnecessary use of antibiotics; where their use is indicated by selecting the most appropriate antibiotic; and by using the correct dose and duration of treatment.

Box 16.1: Methicillin resistant *Staphylococcus aureus* (MRSA)

Staphylococcus aureus is a major cause of both minor and major infections. It is particularly associated with infections of the skin, for example boils and abscesses, but also causes about one-third of surgical wound infections, osteomyelitis, septicaemia, endocarditis and pneumonia (Meers et al., 1981)

Since antibiotics were first introduced in the 1940s, S. aureus has adapted to them by quickly evolving resistance mechanisms. MRSA is the term used to describe strains of S. aureus which have acquired resistance to flucloxacillin, the antibiotic most commonly used to treat staphylococcal infection (the laboratory version of the drug, used for testing resistance, is called methicillin). Usually MRSA are also resistant to several other antibiotics as well. This makes treatment of infections caused by MRSA extremely difficult, and measures to prevent patients acquiring it of paramount importance.

The widespread use of antibiotics to treat or prevent infection in hospital patients favours the survival of types of bacteria which are resistant to antibiotics over those which are readily destroyed. MRSA is therefore mostly found in hospitals and some forms of MRSA seem to be able to spread from person to person particularly easily. These epidemic strains have been known to affect large numbers of patients throughout a hospital and to spread between hospitals when affected patients are transferred (Wilson and Richardson, 1996). Both patients and staff can become colonised with the organism, providing a reservoir from which they can spread to other people (Cookson *et al.,* 1989). MRSA, like other *S. aureus*, is mostly transferred between patients on the hands of staff, although heavily contaminated uniforms, equipment or surfaces could result in transmission. Airborne spread is also possible, but in most circumstances it is an unlikely route of spread (Boyce, 1991).

Topical creams effective against MRSA are available. The key to successful control is to identify patients infected or colonised with MRSA, treat the affected sites and adhere to isolation procedures (page 385) until the organisms have been eliminated. Rigorous attention to handwashing by all members of staff who have contact with affected patients is particularly important (Hospital Infection Society, 1990).

Identification of viruses

Unlike bacteria, viruses cannot be cultured on agar plates. Some can be grown in living cells but usually their identification relies on examination of clinical specimens under very powerful electron microscopes (Figure 16.2). It can be very difficult to detect tiny virus particles in this way and a negative result should not be taken as meaning the infection is not there. Detection of specific **antibodies** made in the blood in response to infection by a particular virus is a common method used to diagnose viral illness. Different types of antibody appear in the blood during the course of an illness and the type of antibody detected in the blood can indicate whether the patient has had the infection recently or in the past (e.g. rubella, hepatitis B).

Collection of microbiological specimens

The nurse has an important role in ensuring that specimens sent to the microbiology laboratory are in the best condition for isolating the cause of infection. Bacteria can easily be recovered from almost any site on the body. Correct interpretation of the test results is more likely if accurate infor-

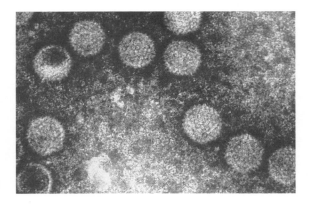

Figure 16.2: Adenovirus viewed under an electron microscope
(Source: Wilson, 1995a. Reproduced with kind permission of Baillière Tindall. Copyright 1995)

mation is provided on the laboratory request form accompanying the specimen. Information about the signs and symptoms of infection are helpful in distinguishing organisms which are harmlessly colonising from those causing an infection. Storing specimens in a cold place and arranging for prompt transport to the laboratory ensures that any bacteria present do not multiply significantly before they are examined.

Key Points

- Micro-organisms are tiny, living creatures too small to be seen with the naked eye.
- They can survive in almost any environment and many form essential links in the food chain.
- A few micro-organisms cause disease by invading and damaging tissue; these are called pathogens.
- Microbiology laboratories identify micro-organisms causing infection and advise on the best method of treatment.

ROUTES OF MICROBIAL TRANSMISSION

The key to the implementation of effective infection prevention and control measures is an understanding of how micro-organisms transfer between one host and another. This section reviews different modes of spread, how organisms enter and leave the body and common sources of infection.

Pathogens use a variety of different methods to transfer between hosts. Their preferred route depends on the point at which they enter and exit from the body and, to some extent, their ability to survive in the environment. The physical transfer of micro-organisms from an infected or colonised person to a susceptible host can occur when there is contact between the body surfaces of the two individuals. This is referred to as transmission by direct contact. Pathogens acquired by sexual intercourse, e.g. *Neisseria gonorrhoeae*, or transplacentally from mother to fetus, e.g. rubella, are examples of infection by direct transmission. Other, more common infections such as glandular fever (Epstein–Barr virus) and colds (rhinovirus) can be spread by direct contact, such as kissing.

More commonly, micro-organisms transfer to a new host indirectly by using an animate or inanimate object as a vehicle. The main vectors for the indirect transmission of pathogens are:

- Hands
- Airborne particles
- Inanimate objects (e.g. equipment)
- Food and water
- Insects.

Hands

Micro-organisms are acquired on hands by contact with contaminated substances such as secretions, excreta or infected lesions. Most of these micro-organisms can not survive on skin for long and are readily transferred to another host by touch (Mackintosh and Hoffman, 1984). Hands have been recognised as playing an important role in the transmission of infection since the mid-1800s. At this time, a doctor called Ignaz Semmelweiss demonstrated that a large proportion of the deaths from puerperal fever in the obstetric hospitals could be prevented simply by instructing medical staff to wash their hands between performing post-mortem examinations and attending women in labour. Until this policy was introduced, the streptococcus causing the puerperal fever was readily transferred from the dead bodies to labouring women on the doctors' hands. It would be easy to think that this type of problem no longer exists in modern health care. Unfortunately, the evidence suggests that hands are still commonly responsible for the transmission of infection between patients and simple infection control measures, such as those proposed by Semmelweiss, are frequently not implemented (Reybrouck, 1983, Musa *et al.*, 1990).

Airborne particles

Microbes cannot move through air on their own but are carried by airborne particles, in particular dust, water droplets and droplets expelled from the respiratory tract. Dust is largely composed of minute fabric fibres and skin squames – small, flat flakes of dead skin which are shed in large numbers from the surface of skin. Droplets of saliva are expelled from the respiratory tract during talking, coughing or sneezing. Most of these droplets are relatively large and fall to the floor rapidly but a few of the smaller droplets evaporate into minute particles of less than $10\,\mu m$ known as droplet nuclei. These can remain airborne for several hours (Rhame, 1986). Some of these airborne particles carry microbes which can subsequently cause infection by being inhaled or settling into open wounds. Pathogens on particles that have settled on to floors or furniture do not generally present a risk of infection unless they are allowed to accumulate.

For an organism to transmit on a small airborne particle it must be able to survive in the absence of moisture for a considerable time. This route of transmission is therefore more suited to pathogens which have resistant cell walls, e.g. staphylococci, *Mycobacterium tuberculosis*, or which form resistant spores, e.g. *Clostridium difficile* (Hoffman 1993). The risk of inhaling particles carrying pathogens is low and transmission of infection by this route is relatively uncommon. Many respiratory infections can also be readily transmitted though direct contact with secretions transferred onto tissues, handkerchiefs or hands during sneezing or coughing (Ansari *et al.*, 1991).

Inanimate objects and equipment

Objects or equipment used between patients can act as a vehicle for the transmission of infection, but the risk of transmission depends on the extent to which the item becomes contaminated with pathogens, how well it supports their growth and the type of contact it has with another potential host. Since body fluids are important sources of micro-organisms, objects in contact with these fluids are likely to become contaminated and, if not decontaminated between patients, are likely to transmit infection. Most organisms cannot survive in the absence of moisture, warmth or nutrients and provided equipment is kept clean and dry, very few will be able to survive on their surface. Pieces of equipment which provide a moist environment, e.g. humidifiers, are much more hazardous because they support the growth of a range of bacteria, in particular Gram-negative organisms such as *Klebsiella* and *Pseudomonas*. Equipment which only has contact with the skin, e.g. bed linen, is less likely to transmit infection than equipment used to penetrate tissues, e.g. surgical instruments.

Food and water

Some micro-organisms use food and water as a means of transmission from person to person. Some raw foods, in particular meat and poultry, are contaminated with micro-organisms which may cause disease if ingested, although most need to be consumed in large quantities before they can establish infection. Thorough cooking of food destroys most micro-organisms, rendering it safe to eat, but if food is not cooked well enough to destroy the pathogens or is contaminated after it has been cooked, it can act a vehicle for the transmission of infection. Micro-organisms can multiply rapidly in food kept at room temperature, so that if food is contaminated with only a few pathogens it can soon become unsafe. For more detailed advice and information on the safe management of food refer to a specific text such as Hobbs and Roberts (1993).

Water is an important vector of infection where purification and treatment systems are ineffective or not available. Water sources contaminated by animal or human faeces can transmit a range of pathogens including *Vibrio cholerae* (the cause of cholera), *Giardia* and *Cryptosporidium*.

An infected person may contaminate a food source if the pathogens acquired on the hands during defaecation are not removed properly by handwashing. Gastrointestinal viruses are frequently transmitted in this way. Some pathogens which mainly use food or water as a route of transmission, e.g. *Shigella sonnei*, may also transmit directly from person to person, particularly via contaminated hands.

Insects

Some micro-organisms transmit from host to host using insects as their vector. This can occur passively, as in the case of flies which can transfer pathogens such as salmonellae from faeces to food. More commonly, insects play an active part in transmission, becoming infected when sucking the blood of a host and transferring the micro-organisms to the next host to be bitten. Many insect-borne infections are caused by protozoa, e.g. malaria, trypanosomiasis, but bacteria (e.g. *Yersinia pestis*, the cause of plague), rickettsiae (e.g. typhus), viruses (e.g. arboviruses) and helminths (e.g. filariasis) can also be spread by this route.

PORTALS OF ENTRY AND EXIT

To establish infection, pathogens must be able to gain access to the tissues of the host. Different pathogens enter the body by different routes; they may be inhaled into the respiratory tract, ingested into the gastrointestinal tract or inoculated through the skin. Once the pathogen has entered the body, it may spread to cause damage elsewhere. For example, the virus which causes poliomyelitis enters the body by ingestion, but causes damage to the nervous system, rather than gastroenteritis. If the pathogen is to transmit to another host it must have a means of leaving the body. These routes of exit are usually in the excreta and secretions from the body. Body fluids are therefore an important source of pathogens and their handling forms an important part of infection prevention and control.

Susceptibility of the host

Micro-organisms may be able to gain entry to a host but not necessarily cause disease. The outcome of the invasion depends on a number of factors, in particular the number of organisms to which the person has been exposed, the general health of the person and the response of their immune system.

Virulence factors

Different strains of the same species of micro-organisms may have different capacities to cause disease. The **virulence** of an organism depends on its ability to resist the immune system and to cause damage to the tissues of the host. Methods bacteria use to protect themselves against the immune response include substances released from the cell, polysaccharide **capsules** around the cell, or structures on the cell surface. Some bacteria produce substances called **toxins** which have a harmful action on tissue cells e.g. the botulism toxin produced by *Clostridium botulinum* causes the symptoms of botulism food poisoning.

Sources and reservoirs of infection

The reservoir of a micro-organism is the place where it normally lives, providing it with nutrients, moisture and the environmental conditions that it needs to grow and multiply. The reservoir may be in the environment, another animal or another person (see Table 16.2). Reservoirs of micro-organisms are not always sources of infection. Wash basins, for example, are a reservoir for a wide range of micro-organisms, particularly Gram-negative species, but are not usually a source of infection (Levin *et al.*, 1984). Identifying sources of infection becomes important when an outbreak of infection occurs. In hospital, patients, their body fluids and skin lesions, are some of the most common sources of infection. Sometimes equipment is implicated as the cause of an outbreak, such as that reported by Davies and Blenkharn (1987), where *Klebsiella* infections were associated with the inadequate maintenance and decontamination of suction pumps.

Key Points

- Micro-organisms can transfer from host to host either through direct contact or indirectly using an animate or inanimate vehicle.
- Hands are commonly implicated in the transmission of infection in clinical settings.
- To cause infection, micro-organisms must be able to enter the body but the outcome of the invasion depends on the susceptibility of the host.
- Some micro-organisms have an enhanced capability to cause disease.
- Microbial reservoirs are places where micro-organisms usually grow and multiply.

DEFENCES AGAINST INFECTION

The body has a number of mechanisms which both protect it from invasion by micro-organisms and attack those which manage to break through the defences. This section provides an overview of these immune responses. More comprehensive information can be found in *Immunology* by Roitt *et al.* (1996) or the September 1993 issue of *Scientific American*.

The first lines of defence against invasion by micro-organisms are those general barriers to infection that protect the parts of the body where they may be able to gain entry (Figure 16.3). These barriers may be breached by medical devices such as intravascular or urinary catheters or endotracheal intubation. They may also be affected by medical treatments, e.g. disruption of the normal flora of the bowel by antibiotic therapy, drug-induced decrease in gastric acidity.

Table 16.2: Examples of microbial reservoirs

Reservoir	Site	Micro-organism	Disease
Environment	Soil	*Clostridium tetani*	Tetanus
	Water	*Legionella pneumophila*	Legionnaires' disease
Animals	Cow (gut)	*E. coli* (toxigenic strains)	Gastroenteritis
	Poultry (gut)	*Salmonella* spp.	Gastroenteritis
People	Respiratory tract	*Rhinovirus*	Common cold
	Gut	*Rotavirus*	Gastroenteritis

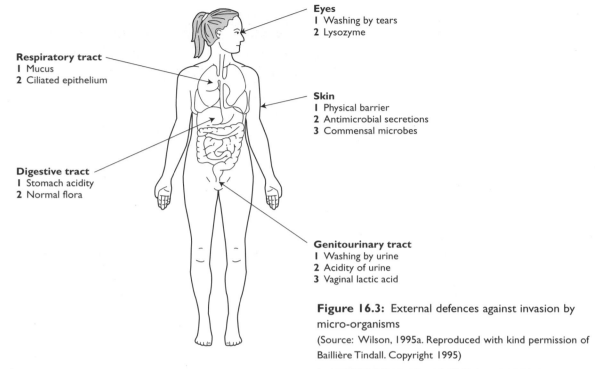

Eyes
1 Washing by tears
2 Lysozyme

Respiratory tract
1 Mucus
2 Ciliated epithelium

Skin
1 Physical barrier
2 Antimicrobial secretions
3 Commensal microbes

Digestive tract
1 Stomach acidity
2 Normal flora

Genitourinary tract
1 Washing by urine
2 Acidity of urine
3 Vaginal lactic acid

Figure 16.3: External defences against invasion by micro-organisms
(Source: Wilson, 1995a. Reproduced with kind permission of Baillière Tindall. Copyright 1995)

INFLAMMATORY RESPONSE

The inflammatory response forms the initial attack against any micro-organism which manages to invade the body. It is intended to destroy the invaders and limit their spread to other parts of the body. The effects of this response are often visible at the site of invasion (Table 16.3).

The inflammatory response attracts **phagocytes** to the area. These are special types of white blood cell which are able to engulf micro-organisms and other foreign substances. There are two types of phagocytic cells: neutrophils and mononuclear macrophages. A series of proteins, called the **complement** system, binds on to microbial cell walls and helps the phagocytic cells to recognise and engulf them. Pyrexia can also occur (see Box 16.2).

THE SPECIFIC IMMUNE RESPONSE

This is provided by a type of white blood cells called **lymphocytes**. These cells are able to recognise and bind to specific foreign proteins (**antigens**). Each time a different foreign protein is encountered, lymphocytes are generated which are able to recognise it. Once the foreign material

Box 16.2: Pyrexia

Infection is frequently associated with a rise in body temperature. This occurs through the action of pyrogenic proteins, released as a result of the inflammatory response, which stimulate the temperature control centre in the hypothalamus of the brain. It is possible that the increase in temperature may be beneficial, accelerating tissue repair by increasing metabolic rate, and it may also stimulate the immune response (Mackowiak, 1994). However, the merit of fever reduction measures is debatable. The patients' discomfort may be increased by efforts to cool them, since their symptoms of shivering and rigors may be exacerbated by further cooling (Kinmouth et al., 1992). Nursing care should therefore aim to reduce discomfort, for example, by removing some bed clothes, administering fluids to make up any excess loss due to sweating and using antipyrexial drugs such as aspirin.

has been destroyed, most of these specific lymphocytes disappear. However, a few remain, circulating in the blood. If the same foreign protein is encountered again, then these memory cells are able to respond rapidly to the invading organism, preventing it from becoming established in the

Table 16.3: The inflammatory response

Response	Mediator	Effect	Visible sign
Dilation of blood vessels	Histamine from mast cells	Increases blood flow to area	Redness Heat
Blood vessels become more permeable	Prostaglandins	Plasma cells and phagocytes migrate into tissue	Swelling
Pressure on nerve endings	Swollen tissue	Discourages movement of affected part	Pain

body. It is this mechanism which enables us to develop immunity after the first exposure to an infection in, for example, chickenpox.

There are two types of lymphocytes; **B-lymphocytes** and **T-lymphocytes**. The B-lymphocytes make Y-shaped proteins, called immunoglobulins or antibodies. Each type of antibody has a slightly different structure which enables it to recognise a specific foreign protein. At any one time there can be thousands of B-lymphocytes circulating in the blood, each carrying a different antibody. If a lymphocyte encounters a foreign protein that fits the antibody it is carrying, it binds to it and starts dividing rapidly, producing many lymphocytes all carrying the same antibody. These lymphocytes are called plasma cells and they produce large quantities of the specific antibody, which can attack and destroy the infecting organism.

There are several types of T-lymphocytes, each with different roles, but their main functions are to deal with micro-organisms which invade and multiply within the host's own cells, e.g. viruses, some bacteria and protozoa, and to coordinate the immune response. The T4-lymphocytes bind to host cells that have been invaded, start to divide and to produce substances called lymphokines. Lymphokines, such as interleukin and interferon, organise all the cells involved in the immune response, turning antibody production on and off and stimulating the activity of phagocytic cells. Cytotoxic T-lymphocytes destroy host cells which have been invaded by a micro-organism. Once the invasion has been dealt with, other suppressor lymphocytes (Ts cells) switch off the production of more T4 lymphocytes, leaving T-lymphocyte memory cells to respond rapidly should the same organism invade again (Figure 16.4).

Key Points

- Points of entry to the body are protected against infection by a range of non-specific defences such as skin, ciliated epithilium and acidic environments in the stomach, vagina and urine.
- Micro-organisms which do manage to invade the tissues trigger an inflammatory response which brings phagocytic cells to the area.
- White blood cells called lymphocytes are able to recognise and bind to specific foreign proteins.
- B-lymphocytes produce proteins called antibodies which attack and destroy the invading micro-organisms.
- T-lymphocytes recognise intracellular pathogens and play a role in coordinating the immune response.

INFECTION ASSOCIATED WITH HEALTH CARE

Infections acquired as a result of health care are a major problem, responsible for considerable increased costs. This section discusses the significance of infection control programmes in the prevention of infection.

Hospital-acquired infections are those that develop as a result of hospital treatment and which the patient did not have or was not incubating at the time he or she was admitted to hospital. Hospital patients are particularly vulnerable to infection, their external defences against micro-organisms may be breached by invasive devices or medical procedures and their illness may impair the ability of their immune system to cope with infection. In addition, at any one time around one

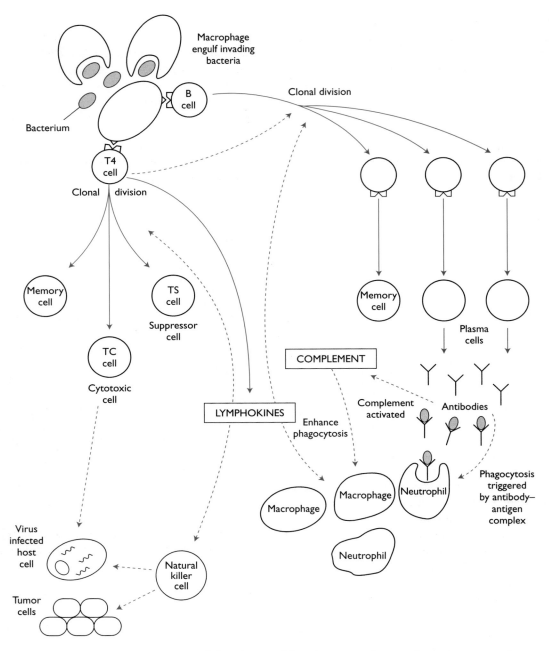

Figure 16.4: The specific immune response: B-lymphocytes, T-lymphocytes and macrophages interact to destroy invading micro-organisms
(Source: Wilson, 1995a. Reproduced with kind permission of Baillière Tindall. Copyright 1995)

in 10 patients in hospital have a hospital-acquired infection (HAI) and these patients can provide a source of pathogens which are readily transmitted to other patients (Emmerson *et al.*, 1996).

THE SIZE OF THE PROBLEM

It is difficult to calculate how many infections are acquired as a result of health care. Infections are frequently not recorded accurately in clinical records and it is time-consuming to collate and analyse information that does exist. However, studies have indicated that around 6% of patients admitted to hospital acquire an infection at some point during their stay (Haley *et al.*, 1985; Glenister *et al.*, 1992). The majority of these HAIs will be infections of wounds, the urinary and respiratory tract and occasionally the bloodstream (Haley *et al.*, 1985; Emmerson et al. 1996) (Figure 16.5).

The increasing trend for early discharge from hospital and treatment as day cases means that infections acquired in hospital are frequently not detected until after the patient has been discharged. In many provider units, as many as 50% of elective surgical procedures are now performed as day cases and even patients undergoing more major surgery are often in hospital for less than a week (Clark, 1996). Since surgical wound infections usually become apparent between 4 and 30 days after the procedure, many patients will not present with symptoms until after their discharge from hospital. Other infections acquired in hospital may also present after discharge, for example, post-operative respiratory tract infection and urinary tract infection following catheterisation. In addition, increasing numbers of patients with devices or treatments which make them vulnerable to infection, such as central vascular devices

and parenteral nutrition, are cared for in their own homes. The management of these infections and the related care of the patient become the responsibility of health care staff in the community. Patients who have developed symptoms of infection will need help and advice and concerns have been raised about the resource implications for community services of these changes in health care delivery (Stott, 1992).

Some patients will be admitted to hospital for treatment of an infectious disease. These patients need special management to ensure that the infection is not transmitted to other vulnerable patients. Occasionally, the infection control procedures break down and the infection is transmitted to other patients or staff. Fortunately, such outbreaks of infection are rare and HAIs acquired in this way probably only account for about 2–3% of the total (Haley *et al.*, 1985).

Infection has a major implication for both the patients affected and for the provision of health care. They cause considerable morbidity and mortality and many patients are anxious about the risk that they may acquire an infection in hospital. Some studies have attempted to quantify the costs associated with HAIs. These include costs of treatment, specialist care and extra days spent in hospital. In addition, they may have social costs in terms of loss of earnings, productivity and social security payments (Plowman *et al.*, 1998).

Preventing infection is therefore of considerable importance, not only to the patients themselves, but also because of resource implications for the health service as a whole. HAIs have been considered as an important indicator of the quality of care and infection control as a high priority in the planning of care provision (NHS Executive, 1996). The employment of specialists to coordinate and monitor infection control activities (see Box 16.3) is seen as fundamental to the prevention and control of infection in both hospital and community settings (DoH 1995, NHS Management Executive, 1993).

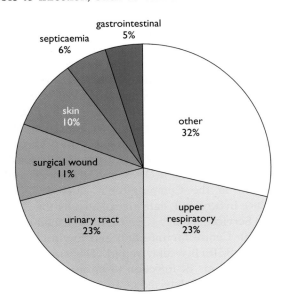

Figure 16.5: The prevalence of hospital-acquired infection: distribution of the main types of infection (Source: Emmerson *et al.*, 1996)

Box 16.3: The infection control team (ICT)

The infection control team comprises an infection control doctor (ICD) and infection control nurse (ICN). Their role includes the planning, implementation and monitoring of an infection prevention and control programme, the provision of advice and education on infection control and the development of related policies. The infection control committee (ICC) has representatives from a variety of hospital departments and provides advice and support to the ICT. Many community health care Trusts and health commissioning agencies now employ nurses to provide infection control advice to community health care workers. They will work closely with the Consultant in Communicable Disease Control who is responsible for monitoring and controlling the spread of infection in the community.

In 1985, a major American study, the Study of the Efficacy of **Nosocomial** Infection Control (SENIC), identified some of the key components of an infection control programme (Table 16.4). Infection control programmes that incorporated all of these components were reported to have substantially reduced their rates of HAI, achieving reductions of over 30% in a 5-year period, whilst in hospitals with no infection control programme the rate of HAI increased by nearly 20% over the same time period (Haley *et al.*, 1985).

The results of the SENIC study have important implications for clinical practice. They suggest that at least one-third of HAIs are potentially preventable and that, in addition to conventional control activities such as education and policy development, surveillance of HAI should be an essential part of the infection prevention and control programme.

THE ROLE OF INFECTION CONTROL IN QUALITY IMPROVEMENT

Infection prevention and control activities have a key role to play in achieving high standards of

Table 16.4: Key components of an infection control programme

Control activities	Surveillance activities
■ Detect, investigate, control outbreaks	■ Collection of data on infection
■ Policies and procedures	■ Analysis of data
■ Monitoring clinical practice	■ Interpretation of data
■ Education and training	■ Feedback of results to clinical staff

Source: Haley *et al.* (1985).

care. Improving and maintaining quality involves both audit of clinical practice and management of risk, with the former focusing on how a process occurs and its relationship to outcome and the latter on structures and staff. Risk management is the identification of actual and potential risks which could lead to mistakes and subsequent claims for damages, together with the implementation of measures to counteract such risks (Moss, 1995). In the case of infection control, risk management can include measures to avoid the risk of infectious diseases transmitting from one patient to another or systems to ensure the safe handling of equipment or body fluids and therefore minimise the risk of transmitting infection. Clinical audit involves measuring an outcome of care, for example the **incidence** of surgical wound infection, and comparing it with agreed standards (Figure 16.6). Where differences are found the reasons are investigated and attempts are made to improve practice. Monitoring for infection is described as surveillance, that is the systematic observation of the occurrence of disease in a population, with the analysis and dissemination of results. The importance of a system of surveillance for the effective control of infectious diseases was recognised in the early 1900s. As a result, the statutory requirement for doctors to notify the occurrence of certain infectious diseases was introduced. In England and Wales, these notifiable diseases are reported to the 'proper officer' of the local authority (this is usually the Consultant in Communicable Disease Control) and in Scotland, to the designated medical officer who is usually the Consultant in Public Health Medicine (Communicable Disease and Environmental Health). In England and Wales, information on these notifiable diseases is collated and analysed by the Office for National Statistics (ONS) and published weekly by the Communicable Disease Surveillance Centre (CDSC) in the Communicable Disease Report (CDR). In Scotland, data are collated by the Common Services Agency (CSA) and published in the Scottish Centre for Infection and Environmental Health (SCIEH) weekly report. This surveillance enables trends of infection to be monitored and epidemics to be detected at an early stage so that preventive measures can be planned.

In the UK, surveillance of hospital-acquired infection has, until recently, been mostly focused on infectious diseases. However, the use of sur-

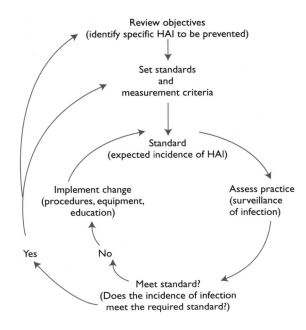

Figure 16.6: The audit cycle: role of surveillance of HAI

- are associated with considerable morbidity and mortality.
- As many as one-third of HAI may be preventable through improvements in infection control practice.
- Infection control plays an important part in quality improvement with a key role in both risk management and clinical audit.
- The infection control nurse, infection control doctor and Consultant in Communicable Disease Control have a specialist knowledge of infection control and prevention and are responsible for coordinating and monitoring infection control activity within a health care organisation.

veillance of HAI as part of a programme to improve the quality of care through clinical audit is being increasingly recognised (Figure 16.6). Surveillance data, provided to those clinical staff who are in a position to prevent infection by changing their practice, can be used to reinforce good practice and identify areas where improvements could be made (Glynn *et al.,* 1997). Purchasers of health care may demand data on rates of hospital-acquired infection as a measure of quality of care. Although such comparative data can help clinical staff to determine their performance relative to others, the data must be interpreted carefully. Differences in definition of infection, the case mix of the population and other factors affecting the risk of infection can give rise to misleading results and make the data inappropriate for comparison (Wilson, 1995a).

Key Points

- Patients are particularly vulnerable to infection whilst in hospital as a result of underlying illness which may impair their immune system and invasive devices which breach their external defences.
- Around 6% of patients acquire an infection as a result of their hospital care and these infections

PREVENTING INFECTION ASSOCIATED WITH HEALTH CARE

This section discusses some of the basic principles of infection control, practices which should be incorporated into the care of all patients both in hospital and in their own homes. These include handwashing, the use of protective clothing, disposal of waste and the decontamination of equipment and the environment. In addition, factors influencing the susceptibility of patients to infection and the use of isolation procedures for patients with infectious diseases are explored. A more comprehensive review of the principles of infection control and the research which supports them can be found in *Infection Control in Clinical Practice* by Wilson (1995b), especially Chapters 7–14 and *Infection Control. A Community Perspective* by Worsley *et al.* (1994).

All health care staff have a responsibility to minimise the risk of patients under their care acquiring an infection. Haley *et al.* demonstrated the significant effect that infection control measures can have on the incidence of hospital-acquired infection (Haley *et al.,* 1985).

There is a tendency to focus infection control efforts on patients known to have an infectious disease and a range of isolation precautions have developed as a result of this. Whilst preventing the spread of infection from such patients is undoubtedly important, it should not be forgotten that the majority of infections that result from health care occur in wounds, the urinary or respiratory tract and the bloodstream as a result of a variety of clinical treatments or interventions.

Patients cared for in the community are not exposed to the same microbiological risks as those in hospital, since they are not in contact with other patients who have infections and are less likely to be exposed to invasive procedures or devices. None the less, it is increasingly common for patients to be discharged home with long-term intravenous devices, e.g. Hickman catheters, and for a range of surgical procedures to be performed in the GP's surgery.

Infection control measures are therefore of relevance in all types of health care setting and should form part of the routine practice of all health care staff. In addition, although staff are healthy and less susceptible to infection than their patients, they also need to use practices that minimise the risk that they will acquire an infection themselves (see Box 16.4).

Box 16.4: Universal precautions

The concept of universal precautions was first developed in the late 1980s in response to the emerging AIDS epidemic and concerns that the human **immunodeficiency** virus (HIV) could be transmitted in health care settings (CDC, 1987). The risk of transmission of blood-borne viruses, such as HIV and hepatitis B, was known to be related to the inoculation of infected body fluids through the skin or on to mucous membranes. Previously, blood and body fluid precautions had been used as a category of isolation procedure for patients known to be infected with a blood-borne virus. Recognising that underlying infection with blood-borne viruses was often not evident, these precautions were recommended to be applied universally to all patients, regardless of whether they were known to be infected or not. The recommended precautions were directed towards avoiding direct contact with any body fluid by the appropriate use of protective clothing and measures to ensure the safe handling and decontamination of equipment and the environment, in particular contaminated sharp instruments which were known to be associated with the greatest risk of transmission.

As more has been discovered about HIV, it has become clear that some body fluids such as urine, faeces and vomit were not associated with the transmission of HIV (CDC, 1988). However, the widespread adoption of the principles of universal precautions as applied to all body fluids was seen to

be a useful approach to the general prevention of cross-infection of all pathogens, not only blood-borne viruses (Wilson and Breedon, 1990).

The principles of universal precautions have now been incorporated into a routine standard of practice, applicable to the care of all patients and intended to minimise the risk of transmission of both blood-borne viruses and other pathogens in health care settings (Garner et al., 1996; UK Health Departments, 1990).

Routine infection control practices are based on the principle that body fluids are a major source of pathogens and should be handled in such a way as to minimise the risk of exposure to patients and staff. In addition, non-intact skin, e.g. wounds or IV sites, and mucous membranes, are recognised as the most vulnerable points through which pathogens may be introduced.

Practices, which should be used routinely to prevent the transmission of micro-organisms between patients, from patient to staff and staff to patient, will be considered under the following headings:

- Handwashing
- Use of protective clothing
- Safe management of equipment
- Safe management of the environment
- Safe management of sharps
- Disposal of waste.

HANDWASHING

Hands are a very common vehicle for the transmission of micro-organisms (Reybrouck, 1983). Skin has its own resident microbial flora which live in hair follicles, deep crevices and sebaceous glands. These micro-organisms are not readily removed, are usually not associated with infection and are rarely involved in cross-infection. Of greater significance are the microbes which reside transiently on the surface of the skin. These are acquired by contact and readily transferred to the next object or person that is touched (Mackintosh and Hoffman, 1984). The hands simply provide a stepping stone for micro-organisms to transfer from one site to another. The hands are particularly likely to acquire pathogens when handling moist, heavily contaminated substances, such as body fluids, but microbes will still be acquired when touching apparently dry, clean surfaces, such as patients' skin, bed linen or equipment (Casewell and Phillips 1977; Ansari *et al.*, 1991; Sanderson and Weissler, 1992).

Fortunately, these transient micro-organisms are easily removed by washing with soap and water (Hoffman and Wilson, 1995). Ideally, hands should be washed between all patient contacts, but at a minimum they should always be washed *before* activities which place the patient at risk of acquiring infection, e.g. before contact with susceptible sites, and *after* activities which could have contaminated the hands, e.g. contact with body fluids. Some of the main indications for handwashing in clinical settings are illustrated below.

Indications for handwashing

- *Before* manipulation of invasive devices, e.g. urinary catheters, intravascular devices
- *Before* contact with susceptible sites, e.g. wounds, mucous membranes
- *Before* handling food
- *After* contact with contaminated items, e.g. linen, equipment, body fluids
- *After* using the toilet

Soap solutions containing antiseptics such as chlorhexidine or iodine remove the transient micro-organisms together with a proportion of the resident flora. They are designed for use in situations such as the operating theatre, where hands are in direct contact with sterile body areas and resident bacteria, if introduced, could cause infection. They are not recommended for routine use in most clinical situations because frequent application may damage the skin and as a consequence increase the number of bacteria on the surface (Ojajarvi *et al.*, 1977).

Unfortunately, a number of studies have shown that health care workers frequently do not wash their hands after contact with patients, even after dirty procedures (Gould, 1993). Hands have been implicated in the transmission of infection where outbreaks of hospital-acquired infection have occurred (Ansari *et al.*, 1991; Gormon *et al.*, 1993) and they are equally likely to be responsible for the introduction of pathogens to susceptible sites such as urinary catheters, intravenous catheters and wounds.

Alcohol handrub

- Whilst soap and water physically wash micro-organisms from the skin, alcohol can be used to destroy both transiently acquired micro-organisms and a proportion of the resident ones.
- Handrubs decontaminate hands much more rapidly than a conventional handwash since they simply involve rubbing a small amount of the solution into the skin until it evaporates.
- Handrubs are particularly useful in situations where there are poor facilities in which to wash hands or where frequent handwashing is necessary.
- They should not be used on hands which are visibly contaminated, as the alcohol will not be able to penetrate or remove **organic** material.

USE OF PROTECTIVE CLOTHING

Protective clothing should be used to reduce the risk of cross-infection following contact with substances, such as body fluids, which are likely to contain pathogens. The selection of appropriate protective clothing should be based on an assessment of the risk that the skin or clothing will become contaminated with body fluids (Figure 16.7). Most activities do not involve direct contact with body fluids and therefore protective clothing is unnecessary, for example when assisting a patient to wash or eat, recording vital signs or administering medicines.

Gloves should be worn to prevent the hands from becoming contaminated, for example when handling specimens or bedpans, and to reduce the risk that micro-organisms on the hands will be transmitted to patients during procedures involving contact with non-intact skin or mucous membranes, e.g. mouth care or vaginal examination. Micro-organisms colonising these sites can also be readily transmitted on the hands, e.g. *Candida* or herpes simplex virus (Burnie *et al.*, 1985). Hands should be washed after gloves have been removed because they may become punctured during use or the hands contaminated when the gloves are taken off (Olsen *et al.*, 1993). Protection of the clothing may be necessary when splashing of body fluid is possible, but in most circumstances a plastic apron will provide sufficient protection (Holborn, 1990).

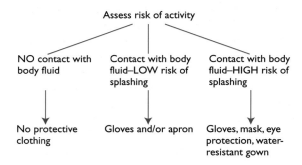

Figure 16.7: Selection of protective clothing: assessing the risk of exposure to body fluids
(Source: Wilson, 1995a. Reproduced with kind permission of Baillière Tindall. Copyright 1995)

Masks and eye protection are mainly necessary where there is a risk that body fluids may splash into the face, such as may occur during surgical procedures. Healthy people expel very few micro-organisms from their respiratory tract and masks are therefore an unnecessary precaution for most aseptic procedures (Ayliffe, 1991). Masks may be recommended for protection against inhalation of infectious droplet nuclei expelled by patients with respiratory infections, in particular tuberculosis (CDC, 1990).

If protective clothing is to contribute to the prevention of cross-infection it should be changed before contact with another patient and between dirty and clean procedures on the same patient (Patterson *et al.*, 1991).

SAFE MANAGEMENT OF EQUIPMENT

Equipment used in clinical care has the potential to transmit infection if inappropriately decontam-inated between patients. Transmission depends on the number of bacteria present on the equipment and the extent to which it has contact with susceptible sites on the patient. The risk of a particular piece of equipment acting as a source or vehicle of infection should be assessed and an appropriate level of decontamination selected accordingly (see Box 16.5). The principles used to categorise equipment as low, medium or high risk are summarised in Table 16.5.

In modern health care practice a considerable amount of equipment is intended for single-use only. Whilst there is a great temptation to decontaminate and re-use some of the equipment, this practice should be avoided: it is usually not economical, may cause the equipment to malfunction and transfers liability for the product from the manufacturer to the hospital. Although some single-use items may be easy to prepare for re-use, the process must be demonstrated to decontaminate effectively and not damage or deteriorate the material. The number of times a device can be reprocessed must be defined and proper records of re-use must be kept. If a device is reprocessed and then causes injury during re-use, both the person who reprocessed it and the user are likely to be liable to pay damages for the injury and may be held to have committed a criminal offence under the Health and Safety at Work Act, for exposing the patient to a risk of injury. What may initially be perceived as a means of reducing costs can result in the diversion of resources away from health care towards defending litigation. A risk management assessment will usually indicate that the risks and associated costs of reprocessing far outweigh any economic benefits (Pickersgill, 1988; Medical Devices Agency, 1995).

Table 16.5: Categorisation of equipment according to the risk that it will transmit infection

Category of risk	Indication	Level of decontamination	Method of decontamination
High	Item which penetrates skin/mucous membranes or enters sterile body areas	Sterilise	Autoclave and use sterile or sterile single-use disposable, e.g. surgical instruments, needles
Medium	Item which has contact with mucous membranes or is contaminated by readily transmissable micro-organisms	Disinfect or sterilise	Autoclave if possible, e.g. vaginal specula Chemically disinfect, e.g. endoscopes
Low	Item which is used on intact skin	Clean	Wash with detergent and hot water, e.g. washbowls, mattresses

There are two main approaches to destroying micro-organisms – heat and chemicals. Heat is the preferred method because it is more predictable, efficient and easier to control.

Decontamination using heat

Heat can be used in a number of ways, the level of decontamination achieved depending on the temperature and the period of exposure. The higher the temperature and the longer the exposure time, the greater the level of decontamination. Pasteurisation involves heating items to a temperature of between 80 and 65°C for between 1 and 10 minutes. This will disinfect the item, rather than sterilise, but provides a useful means of decontaminating a variety of low risk equipment. Bedpan washers use the principle of pasteurisation to disinfect bedpans, and linen is pasteurised during the wash cycle. Linen is decontaminated by both removing micro-organisms physically, using detergent, and destroying them by exposure to high temperatures. In hospitals, where linen is used repeatedly, it is particularly important to ensure effective decontamination in the laundry. All used linen should, therefore, be thermally disinfected by washing at 71°C for 3 minutes or 65°C for 10 minutes (NHS Executive, 1995). Staff in the laundry usually sort linen before it is washed. Linen that is potentially contaminated with enteric pathogens, tuberculosis or blood-borne viruses should be enclosed in a water-soluble bag and placed in a red outer bag. These bags can be segregated at the laundry and decontaminated by washing prior to sorting.

Autoclaves provide a method of sterilising items by exposing them to steam at temperatures high enough to destroy bacterial spores. Whilst water boils at 100°C at atmospheric pressure, its boiling point is raised by heating it under pressure. In an autoclave, steam at a temperature of 134°C or 121°C is generated depending on the pressure inside the chamber. At these temperature all micro-organisms, including spores, will be destroyed after exposure for between 3 and 15 minutes, depending on the temperature. In hospitals, sterilisation by autoclave is best carried out in the Central Sterile Supplies Department (CSSD) where quality control can be carefully monitored. However, a range of small autoclaves, suitable for sterilising unwrapped instruments in clinics or GP surgeries, are available (NHS Procurement Directorate, 1990).

Hot air ovens can also be used to sterilise but take considerably longer (1 hour at 171°C) because air is unable to conduct heat on to the surface of the equipment as efficiently as steam. These sterilisation methods are only suitable for equipment which can withstand high temperature without damage. Decontamination of heat sensitive equipment relies on the use of chemicals.

Decontamination using chemicals

Chemicals have a number of disadvantages as agents for decontamination. In particular, they are often corrosive, toxic or irritant, are not active against all types of micro-organism and do not penetrate organic material (Ayliffe et al., 1993). The Control of Substances Hazardous to Health (COSHH) regulation requires that the risks presented by potentially hazardous substances are assessed and guidelines on how to use them safely are drawn up (East, 1992; Health and Safety Commission, 1994). Most hospitals have a policy to describe what disinfectants are available and when and how they should be used. This policy should always be referred to before using a disinfectant.

Decontamination by cleaning

Around 80% of micro-organisms can be removed by effective cleaning (Ayliffe et al., 1967). Cleaning must involve the use of detergent, which enables grease and dirt to be more easily removed by water. Many low risk items can be safely decontaminated between uses by washing with detergent and water. However, it is also important to dry these items after cleaning to prevent multiplication of any bacteria that remain. Greaves clearly demonstrated how wash bowls could become heavily contaminated if they were incompletely dried before storage (Greaves, 1985).

Equipment destined for disinfection or sterilisation must also be cleaned since decontamination will be considerably more efficient if organic material, such as body fluid, is removed first.

SAFE MANAGEMENT OF THE ENVIRONMENT

Micro-organisms cannot survive easily on surfaces which are clean and dry. The most significant microbiological hazard is dust, which if allowed to accumulate may become a source of infection. Dust control on floors and other horizontal surfaces where dust collects is therefore the most important part of the cleaning programme in clinical areas. This is best achieved by the regular use of vacuum cleaners or dust control mops. Mopping surfaces with detergent and water is of value where soiling is likely to occur e.g. in kitchens and bathrooms. Mops themselves can become heavily contaminated with bacteria if they are not stored clean and dry and regularly laundered (Hoffman, personal communication, 1997). Chemical disinfectants are of limited value in cleaning the environment. The majority of micro-organisms will be removed by detergent; disinfectants are difficult to apply and have a very short-lived effect. Chlorine-based granules do have some advantages in that they provide a practical means of dealing with spills of body fluid, absorbing the fluid spill so that it can easily be discarded in the waste (Coates and Wilson, 1989).

HANDLING SHARP INSTRUMENTS

Sharp instruments contaminated with body fluids are particularly hazardous, since they can easily transmit infection by inoculating micro-organisms through the skin. The main risk is from blood-borne viruses, such as hepatitis B or C and HIV, although transmission of a variety of other pathogens has been reported (Collins and Kennedy, 1987). In the case of hepatitis B, inoculation of even a minute volume of infected blood is sufficient to transmit the infection. HIV is less infectious, but transmission to health care workers

as a result of an injury with a needle is known to occur (Heptonstall *et al.*, 1993).

Sharp instruments should therefore be handled as little as possible and always with extreme care. Most sharps are disposable and because of the hazard they present should be discarded in special rigid containers which are then incinerated. Research has shown that frequent causes of injury are recapping of used needles, blood glucose lancets or needles left on trolleys or bedside lockers and overfilled sharps containers (Saghafi *et al.*, 1992). Hospitals should have clear guidelines for staff on how sharp instruments should be handled. Some principles of good practice are described below.

Good sharps handling practice

- Discard sharps immediately after use into a designated container.
- Do not pass sharps into the hand of another person.
- Do not carry used sharps in the hands: bring a sharps container to the point of use.
- Do not remove the needle from a syringe.
- Do not resheath needles.
- Close sharps containers when 3/4 full.
- Seal sharps containers securely when full.

Because of the risk that they may transmit infection, injuries with contaminated sharps instruments or splashes of blood and body fluid into the eyes or mouth should always be reported to the occupational health department, where they can be properly managed.

THE SAFE DISPOSAL OF WASTE

Waste generated in health care settings that is contaminated with body fluids could expose those who handle it to a risk of infection. The responsibilities of those who generate waste, including such **clinical waste**, are described in the Environmental Protection Act (EPA) 1990 and specific advice about the management of clinical waste is published by the Health Services Advisory Committee (HSAC) of the Health and Safety Executive (HSE, 1992). A national colour coding system is used to ensure that different types of waste can be easily recognised. Clinical waste should be discarded into yellow bags and destroyed by incineration, whilst uncontaminated or household waste should be discarded into black bags for disposal on landfill sites. The EPA 1990 also encompasses the disposal of waste generated by health care workers in the homes of patients. In general this only involves small amounts of clinical waste, but employers must make arrangements for its safe disposal. Waste produced and handled by the patient or his/her family is exempt from these regulations and can therefore be discarded with the normal household waste. Needles used by people who are diabetic pose a particular safety problem; whilst their disposal is not covered by current legislation, some health authorities have made arrangements for a sharps container exchange system, operated through chemists and health centres. Local authorities only have a responsibility to collect potentially infectious waste, such as produced during home dialysis or from patients known to be infected with a blood-borne virus.

THE SUSCEPTIBLE PATIENT

Some patients are more susceptible to infection than others. By careful assessment, it is possible to identify patients who are particularly likely to acquire an infection and adapt their care either to reduce or to eliminate those risks (Table 16.6), for example, by improving their nutrition or by careful management of wounds, catheters and infusions (Bowell, 1992; Kingsley, 1992). Infection prevention takes on a particular significance in those patients identified as vulnerable, who undergo invasive procedures or have a device which compromises their external defences against the invasion of micro-organisms.

Wounds, whether they are surgical or accidental in origin or related to changes in the perfusion of blood to the skin (e.g. pressure sores, leg ulcers), are susceptible to invasion by pathogens introduced on equipment, the hands of staff or from the patients' own microbial flora. The risk of surgical wound infection is influenced by a number of factors related to the surgical technique, condition of the wound and the health of the patient (see Box 16.6).

Wounds healing by granulation, e.g. pressure sores, provide an open area of non-intact skin vulnerable to invasion by pathogens. Such wounds

Table 16.6: Factors which can increase the risk of infection

General factors	
Age:	very young or very old
Nutrition:	emaciation, obesity, dehydration
Mobility:	immobile or poor mobility
Incontinence:	urinary or faecal
General health:	debilitated
Local factors	
Oedema:	pulmonary, ascites
Ischaemia:	necrosis, thrombus
Skin lesions:	wounds, burns, ulceration, device insertion
Foreign bodies:	implants, sutures
Invasive procedures	
Intravenous cannulae:	peripheral, central
Surgery:	anaesthesia, wound
Intubation:	ventilation, suction, humidification
Cathetherisation:	intermittent, indwelling, irrigation
Drugs	
Cytotoxics	
Antibiotics	
Steroids	
Diseases	
Carcinoma	
Leukaemia	
Renal disease	
Liver disease	
Immunodeficiencies	

Adapted from Bowell (1992).

Box 16.6: Factors which increase the risk of surgical wound infection

In the wound	In the patient
Large number of bacteria present	Debility
Dead tissue present	Malnourishment
Haematoma formation	Obesity
Tissue damage during procedure	Underlying illness, e.g. malignancy
Foreign material present	Immune deficiency

are usually heavily colonised with a variety of bacteria and will heal despite their presence (Hutchinson and Lawrence, 1991). However, they will provide an important source of pathogens which can be readily transmitted to other patients. The use of aseptic technique in the management of wounds has been the traditional approach to the prevention of wound infection. This technique is often based more on ritual than science and is frequently not relevant to what we now know about promoting wound healing with the use of occlusive dressings (Walsh and Ford, 1989). The important principle is that open wounds should not come into contact with any item that is contaminated and that items that have been in contact with the wound should be safely discarded or decontaminated. The use of gloved hands is often a more practical method than forceps for cleaning away excess wound exudate and has the additional advantage of minimising the risk that hands will be contaminated with pathogens from the wound (Thomlinson, 1987).

Asepsis is also important for contact with devices which penetrate the skin or enter sterile body areas, e.g. intravascular devices or urinary catheters. Micro-organisms introduced into an intravascular device can cause septicaemia, a very serious infection of the blood with a mortality rate of between 10 and 20% (Pearson et al., 1996). Urinary catheters are responsible for most hospital-acquired urinary tract infections and approximately 10% of catheterised patients will develop a urinary tract infection (Stamm, 1991). Micro-organisms can use these devices to bypass the body defences by being carried on the device during insertion, passing along the inside of the tube or travelling along its outer surface. The problem is exacerbated by the formation of a biofilm on the catheter surface. This is a film of proteins mixed with micro-organisms which forms whenever foreign material is in contact with tissue and which protects the micro-organisms from attack by the immune system (Elliott and Faroqui, 1992).

These invasive devices should be managed in a way that minimises the risk of pathogens gaining entry as the device is inserted, from the point of insertion along the outside of the device and through the lumen of the tube. They should be inserted aseptically and hands should always be washed before and after contact with them. The insertion site of intravenous devices should be protected by a dressing and observed carefully for early signs of inflammation, the fluid administration set disconnected using a non-touch technique and access points on it kept to a minimum (Maki, 1991). Urinary catheters should be inserted as aseptically as possible, the perineum regularly cleansed to remove micro-organisms, equipment used to collect the urine should be carefully decontaminated and disconnection of the drainage system avoided to prevent the access of pathogens (Crow et al., 1986). More information on reducing the risks of infection associated with invasive devices can be found in *Infection Control in Clinical Practice* (Wilson, 1995b), Chapters 9 and 10.

Key Points

- All health care staff have a responsibility to prevent the transmission of infection to patients or colleagues.
- Body fluids are a major source of pathogens and should be routinely handled in a way that minimises the risk that other patients and staff will be exposed.
- Hands commonly act as a vehicle for the transmission of micro-organisms but these can be readily removed from the hands by washing with soap and water.
- Protective clothing should be used to reduce the risk of contamination with substances likely to contain pathogens, such as body fluids.
- Equipment must be appropriately decontaminated between patients; the level of decontamination depends on the type of equipment and the way in which it is used.
- Sharp instruments can transmit infection by inoculating micro-organisms through the skin. They must therefore be handled carefully to avoid injury both to the operator and to other staff.
- Susceptibility to infection is increased by intrinsic factors in the patient such as underlying illness, immunosuppressive therapy and extrinsic factors, such as invasive devices. Infection control practices should be particularly directed towards reducing the risk of infection in these susceptible patients.

THE MANAGEMENT OF AN INFECTIOUS PATIENT

Infections caused by micro-organisms which spread easily from person to person are called contagious or infectious diseases. Within a community they may cause epidemics of infection, spreading to any member of the population who is susceptible. Children not previously exposed to these infections are frequently the victims until, by the time they reach early adulthood, most have acquired a range of specific memory cells to help combat subsequent invasion by previously encountered pathogens. In most developed countries, epidemics of many infectious diseases are prevented by a widespread immunisation programme (DoH, 1996). The immunisation programme currently recommended in the UK is illustrated in Table 16.7.

Immunity to infection may gradually diminish with age and may also be impaired by immunodeficiency. Infectious diseases can, therefore, present particular problems in the hospital setting, where many patients may be especially vulnerable to infection. During the early part of this century, in the absence of effective antimicrobial treatment or widespread immunisation programmes, many hospitals specialising in the treatment of patients with infectious diseases, the fever hospitals, were established. Special nursing practices designed to prevent the transmission of these infections to other patients or the staff, known as 'isolation procedures', were introduced. Many of these practices are still used although there have been few studies which have evaluated their effectiveness (Garner *et al.*, 1996).

SYSTEMS OF ISOLATION PRECAUTION

Implementation of these isolation procedures has employed a variety of approaches. Many institutions group infections into categories according to their route of transmission (Control of Infection Group, 1974); the categories in common use are:

- *Strict isolation*: for highly transmissible infections, e.g. Lassa fever
- *Contact isolation*: for infections spread by direct or indirect contact, e.g. MRSA
- *Enteric isolation*: for infections spread by the faecal–oral route, e.g. salmonella
- *Respiratory isolation*: for infection spread by respiratory droplets, e.g. tuberculosis
- *Blood and body fluid isolation*: for blood-borne viruses, e.g. hepatitis B.

The disadvantage of category-specific isolation procedures is that in some situations more precautions than necessary will be used and in others the route of transmission of a particular infection can cross into more than one category. This is particularly the case with antibiotic-resistant bacteria for which the type of isolation required will depend on the site of infection or colonisation. The adoption of blood and body fluid precautions in the care of all patients, regardless of their diagnosis, has made a second tier of precautions unnecessary for some of the infectious diseases most commonly encountered in hospital patients. In addition, there is a demand for isolation precautions to be more specifically targeted, with clear rationale and decision making by staff at a local level.

Table 16.7: Immunisation schedule

Vaccine	Age	Notes
Diphtheria/tetanus/pertussis (DTP), polio, *Haemophilus influenzae* (HIB)	2 months (1st dose) 3 months (2nd dose) 4 months (3rd dose)	Primary course
Measles, mumps, rubella (MMR)	12–15 months	
DTP, polio, MMR	3–5 years	Booster dose
BCG	10–14 years or infancy	
Tetanus/diphtheria, polio	13–18 years	Booster dose

Source: DoH (1996).

THE PRINCIPLES OF ISOLATION PRECAUTIONS

Additional infection control measures are recommended for the care of patients who are known or suspected to be infected with readily transmissible pathogens, pathogens transmitted by an airborne route or pathogens considered to be of particular significance in a hospital setting. The precautions used will depend on the type of infection and should be based on interrupting its specific route of transmission. In many circumstances, adherence to the standard infection control precautions, outlined in the previous section, is sufficient to prevent the transmission of infection. For example, gastrointestinal infections, such as salmonella, are transmitted by direct contact with faeces. Correct disposal of excreta, the use of protective clothing for contact with excreta and handwashing after contact are all part of the standard approach to infection control and these precau-

tions alone, provided that they are applied correctly, would be sufficient to prevent transmission of the infection to other patients or staff. A summary of the major infections requiring isolation procedures are listed in Table 16.8.

Use of a single room

Placing infectious patients in single rooms can help to ensure that the isolation precautions are observed by staff. However, as a means of preventing transmission, physical isolation of the patient is only required for infections which have an airborne route of transmission. These are encountered relatively uncommonly in hospital, but include respiratory viruses and tuberculosis. Some hospitals have isolation rooms with negative pressure ventilation where the air pressure inside the room is reduced by extracting air to the outside. This ensures that air flows from other ward areas into the room, and that airborne micro-

Table 16.8: Infections requiring isolation precautions (some common examples)

Infections transmitted by an airborne droplet nuclei
Patient should be in single room with the door closed and preferably with negative air pressure ventilation. Their movement should be limited. Masks may be recommended.
- Measles
- Chickenpox*
- Tuberculosis

Infections transmitted by respiratory droplets
Patient should be in a single room. Special ventilation is not necessary and the door can remain open but their movement should be limited. A mask may be recommended.
- Diphtheria (pharyngeal)
- Pertussis
- Streptococcal pharyngitis, pneumonia, scarlet fever
- Adenovirus
- Meningococcal meningitis
- Influenza*
- Respiratory syncytial virus*
- Mumps

Infections spread by contact
Where possible the patient should be in a single room and their movement limited. Use protective clothing to handle material that may contain high concentration of the pathogen, avoid sharing of equipment with other patients and always wash hands on leaving the patient.
- Enteric infections, e.g. rotavirus, *Clostridium difficile*, shigella, *Escherichia coli* O157
- Skin infection, e.g. varicella zoster, major cellulitis
- Multidrug-resistant bacteria (colonisation or infection), e.g. methicillin-resistant *Staphylococcus aureus* (MRSA), vancomycin-resistant enterococcus

---

*Also transmitted by direct contact with respiratory or lesion secretions.
Adapted from Garner *et al.* (1996).

organisms in the room are expelled outside the building. This type of ventilation system can help to prevent the transmission of infections acquired by the inhalation of minute airborne droplet nuclei, e.g. tuberculosis, especially where highly susceptible, immunocompromised, patients may be exposed (CDC, 1990). However, regular monitoring of the system is essential to ensure that the correct air flows are maintained. Occasionally, physical separation of an infectious patient is indicated because there is a significant risk of environmental contamination contributing to the transmission. This may include patients with enteric infections who are vomiting or faecally incontinent, particularly where the pathogen may persist in the environment, e.g. *Clostridium difficile* (Hoffman, 1993). In paediatric units, single room isolation of any child known or suspected to have an infectious disease is recommended, because they are unlikely to be able to observe infection control precautions and other children may be particularly vulnerable to the infection.

Whilst patients with infectious diseases are under isolation precautions it is sensible to limit their movement out of the room to minimise the risk that they will transmit the infection to others. This is particularly important for infections transmitted by an airborne route but of lesser importance for those spread by contact. Some patients find isolation extremely stressful, they may feel neglected, lonely and stigmatised and can experience serious psychological effects such as anxiety, agitation or depression (Knowles, 1993). It is important to take this factor into account when planning the care of an isolated patient. Wherever possible the precautions should not interfere with any rehabilitation programme and they should not be continued any longer than necessary. Providing patients and their families with information about their condition, involving them in their treatment and making them aware of how they can prevent the infection spreading, for example by coughing into tissues or washing their hands after using the toilet, can help to ensure the isolation period is as short as possible.

Protective clothing

Many infectious diseases are spread by direct contact with body fluids and therefore the application of routine infection control precautions will min-imise the risk of spread and additional protective clothing is usually unnecessary. Plastic aprons, as opposed to cotton gowns, provide the most practical means of protecting clothing from contamination. They are impermeable, even when wet, and protect the parts of clothing most vulnerable to contamination (Babb *et al.*, 1983).

The use of masks for the care of patients with respiratory infections is controversial. There is little evidence to support their efficacy and protection of staff by appropriate **vaccination** is considered by some to be a more reliable approach (Taylor, 1980; British Thoracic Society, 1990). The use of higher efficiency masks, called particulate respirators, for prolonged contact with patients who have infectious tuberculosis has been recommended but their value is debatable (CDC, 1990).

Equipment

Equipment used on a patient with an infectious disease needs to be appropriately decontaminated before it is used on another patient. In most situations, the usual decontamination procedures recommended in local disinfection policies and summarised in Table 16.5 are sufficient, but if there is any doubt advice can be obtained from the infection control team. In some circumstances it may be more practical to allocate a particular piece of equipment for sole use by the patient and clean it thoroughly once it is no longer required, e.g. a commode required by a patient with an enteric infection. Any equipment that has not been contaminated by infectious material does not need special cleaning. This includes crockery and cutlery which are unlikely to become contaminated and can be returned to the kitchen or catering department in the usual way.

Handwashing

Hands are probably the most likely route for pathogens to be transmitted to other patients and particular attention should be given to washing hands after any contact with patients in isolation, including after gloves have been removed.

Cleaning

Most micro-organisms are not able to survive on dry surfaces for prolonged periods and the environment is not a significant factor in the transmission of most infections. The normal standard of cleaning should be maintained in isolation rooms and cleaning staff reassured about their risk of acquiring infection and what they should do to minimise the risk, e.g. use of protective clothing, handwashing. The room should be cleaned in the usual way once the patient has been taken out of isolation or discharged.

OUTBREAKS OF INFECTION

Outbreaks, or epidemics of infectious diseases, have long been recognised as a problem in any community of people, but only in relatively recent times have control measures been understood or widely implemented. In the UK, the Public Health Acts of the mid-1880s saw the beginning of a co-ordinated approach to preventing, monitoring and controlling infectious disease. In England and Wales, health authorities (HA) and in Scotland, health boards, have responsibility for controlling communicable infectious disease. Each HA appoints a Director of Public Health (DPH) to advise them. The DPH leads a public health department which will include the Consultant in Communicable Disease Control (CCDC) who has responsibility for monitoring, preventing and controlling of **outbreaks of infection** in the community and, as designated 'proper officer', for liaising with the HA and the environmental health officers at the local authority (NHS Management Executive, 1993). In Scotland, the Consultant in Public Health Medicine (Communicable Disease and Environmental Health) is the designated medical officer and has a similar role to that of the CCDC.

Effective control of an epidemic involves the identification of contacts who may require treatment or monitoring for symptoms and the investigation of the source of infection, e.g. food that may be implicated in an outbreak of food poisoning (see Box 16.7). Many CCDCs work with an infection control nurse who will provide advice on the prevention and control of infection, to health care staff working in nursing homes, general practice or other parts of the community.

In a hospital, outbreaks of infection can have particularly serious consequences because of the

---

Box 16.7: Outbreak of *Escherichia coli* O157 in Scotland, 1996

Escherichia coli is a normal and usually harmless inhabitant of the intestines. Certain strains, however, produce toxins and can cause a gastroenteritis which ranges from mild diarrhoea to bloody diarrhoea with severe abdominal pain. In outbreaks of infection caused by *E. coli* O157, up to 10% of cases can develop a form of renal failure called haemolytic uraemic syndrome (HUS), especially young children. Cattle are thought to be the main reservoir of *E. coli* O157 and infection is often associated with eating undercooked meat, milk and yoghurt (Communicable Diseases Report, 1995).

Late afternoon on Friday 22nd November 1996, a public health department in Lanarkshire was notified of 15 cases of *E. coli* O157, all from a town called Wishaw. All the affected people had eaten food supplied by a local butcher, either meat sandwiches, other cold cooked meat or steak in gravy served at a church lunch on the previous Sunday. Within 2 weeks, a total of 303 people had developed symptoms of infection with *E. coli* O157, 137 of them had the infection confirmed by laboratory tests of their stools. Samples of food from the butcher and the church lunch were also tested and the same strain affecting the patients was found in the gravy from the lunch and cooked beef from the shop. A further 87 cases of *E. coli* O157 from other parts of Scotland reported during the same period could be linked to the butcher in Wishaw either directly or through purchasing meats from other shops supplied by the Wishaw butcher and new cases continued to be reported over several weeks. In all, nearly 500 people were infected by the meat, 18 of whom died (Cowden, 1997).

E. coli O157 has been associated with particularly serious outbreaks of foodborne infection because of its ability to cause HUS in vulnerable people. Rapid identification of the source of infection is therefore essential. This requires accurate identification of cases through testing faecal specimens, recording symptoms and their time of onset, and the compilation of detailed histories of food consumption by those affected to determine the probable source of infection. In this outbreak food samples were also available which together with the food histories enabled the source of the outbreak, the butcher in Wishaw, to be clearly identified and remedial action taken to prevent further cases.

Box 16.8: An outbreak on Florence ward

Florence ward admits acutely ill, elderly patients. One Saturday, two patients in the same bay had an episode of diarrhoea. Since sporadic loose stools were not uncommon amongst these elderly patients, the cases of diarrhoea were not considered significant. However, during the night both patients reported severe abdominal pain and another patient started vomiting. By the morning, two more patients had both diarrhoea and abdominal pain and the staff strongly suspected an outbreak of gastrointestinal infection. The ward sister informed the consultant responsible for the patients and it was decided to start using isolation precautions with the affected patients and to collect stool specimens, ready to send to the laboratory first thing on Monday morning. The infection control doctor was contacted and a few hours later the infection control team came to the ward, by which time a further three patients had reported symptoms. Since the ward only had two single rooms, the infection control team advised the staff to move all the affected patients into one eight-bedded bay until their symptoms had resolved. Gloves and aprons were to be used for any contact with vomitus or excreta and hands washed by all staff leaving the bay.

Over the next few days, another ten cases of infection emerged, including four on Harold ward, the adjacent elderly care ward which was covered by the same medical and paramedical teams and occasionally borrowed nursing staff from Florence ward. Rotavirus was seen in the stool specimens from nine of the affected patients. This virus can cause acute gastroenteritis and particularly affects young children and the elderly. Large quantities of virus are expelled in the faeces and it is readily transmitted on hands and may contaminate the environment. The cases in Harold ward were probably transmitted on the hands of staff who worked in both wards.

Fortunately, all the affected patients recovered and no further cases occurred once isolation precautions had been introduced.

number of vulnerable patients who could potentially be exposed (see Box 16.8).

In addition to the range of infectious diseases which can cause epidemics in hospital as well as in the community, such as salmonella, rotavirus or influenza, outbreaks of 'hospital pathogens' may also occur. These may be opportunistic pathogens, e.g. aspergillus which would not normally cause infection in healthy people, antibiotic-resistant strains of bacteria, such as MRSA (see Box 16.1, page 367) or infections caused by contaminated equipment or faulty procedures. Control of outbreaks of infection in hospital are managed by the ICT (see Box 16.3) who will liaise closely with the local CCDC. They will investigate the source of infection, identify potential contacts, advise on control measures and monitor their implementation. Outbreaks of infection have also been reported in nursing homes. In this situation, the CCDC should be informed to advise on control measures and investigate the source of infection (see Box 16.9).

Box 16.9: Outbreak at the Mulberry

The Mulberry nursing home cares for 50 residents, many of whom were recovering from surgery or had minor clinical problems such as varicose ulcers. Mrs Ward had scalded her arm in hot water, and although only a superficial injury, after a few days it began to appear rather inflamed with an area of **erythema** spreading away from the lesion. A wound swab was taken and her GP informed who prescribed immediate treatment with antibiotics. Two days later another resident reported a painful inflamed lesion on her ankle and a nurse became concerned about an ulcer with signs of infection. The swabs taken from all these lesions grew a Group A streptococcus and on receipt of the third swab result, the manager of the nursing home decided to discuss the situation with the CCDC. Both the CCDC and community ICN visited the Mulberry the next day. They advised that affected patients should be given appropriate antibiotic therapy, but that once the signs of infection had resolved they would no longer be infectious. The patients did not need to be isolated but the affected lesions should be kept covered with a dressing and gloves and apron used for contact with wounds and discarded immediately after use. Hands should be washed after contact with any skin lesion and baths cleaned thoroughly after use by any patient, especially those with skin lesions. The CCDC also questioned the staff to establish whether any had recently had a sore throat. Two members of staff did report sore throats and swabs revealed that both were infected with Group A streptococcus. All skin lesions on other patients were carefully examined and swabs taken from those suspected to be infected. Once the infection control measures had been introduced no further cases of the infection were identified.

Early recognition and implementation of preventive measures is important for the effective control of outbreaks. The infection control personnel should be informed promptly if there is any suspicion that several patients or staff may be suffering from the same infection (see Box 16.10).

Box 16.10: Suspected outbreak of gastroenteritis

Where several patients or members of staff are affected by unexplained diarrhoea or vomiting, the following actions should be taken:

1. In a hospital:

- Inform the doctor in charge of the patients
- Inform the infection control doctor/nurse
- Ensure sufficient supplies of gloves/aprons
- Collect stool specimens from affected patients (even if no longer symptomatic) and arrange for them to be sent to the microbiology laboratory for bacterial and viral culture
- Transfer affected patients into single rooms and follow isolation precautions
- Ensure all affected members of staff attend the occupational health department.

2. In a nursing home:

- Inform the GP who has responsibility for the affected patients
- Inform the Consultant in Communicable Disease Control (see above)
- Ensure sufficient supplies of gloves/aprons
- Collect stool specimens from affected patients (even if no longer symptomatic) and arrange for them to be sent to a microbiology laboratory for bacterial and viral culture
- Wash hands after contact with affected patients and use gloves and aprons for handling their body fluids. Change gloves and wash hands between patients
- Ensure all affected members of staff consult their GP.

Key Points

- Infectious disease are caused by micro-organisms which spread easily from person to person.
- Isolation precautions are special measures designed to prevent the transmission of infectious disease to other patients or staff.

- Doctors have a statutory responsibility to notify certain infectious diseases to the proper officer or designated medical officer of local authorities.
- The management of outbreaks of infection in hospital is the responsibility of the infection control team in conjunction with the Consultant in Communicable Disease Control/Public Health Medicine.
- The management of outbreaks of infection in the community is the responsibility of the Consultant in Communicable Disease Control/Public Health Medicine.

EDUCATION AND TRAINING

Prevention of infection associated with health care depends on the principles of infection control being both understood and implemented. Studies have shown that despite knowledge of infection control, staff do not always use it in their practice (Gould, 1993). Larson (1988) identified three main obstacles to changing behaviour:

- Lack of skills and knowledge
- Lack of supplies and systems
- Lack of motivation.

However, other studies have shown that even if the level of knowledge is increased, compliance with infection control procedures is not necessarily achieved (Williams and Buckles, 1988).

Education programmes for staff who are qualified, as well as those who are in training, and written policies or standards can help to clarify local arrangements or areas of uncertainty. Systems for the provision of necessary equipment, e.g. disposable gloves, must be in place if infection control policies are to be implemented successfully.

Motivation of staff to comply with good practice is more difficult, although experience with audit suggests that the use of surveillance to feedback data on the incidence of infection can be used to improve practice and reduce infection rates (Cruse and Foord, 1980; Dubbert et al., 1990). Work by Seto (1995) demonstrates the power of information in persuading staff to improve their practice. Liaison or link nurses are being increasingly used as a means of improving the communication between ICN and clinical staff and to motivate and monitor changes in practice.

The frequent and sustained contact that nurses have with their patients places them in a unique position as a health educator. A sound knowledge of infection and infection prevention is essential if this role is to be carried out effectively and this can then be used as a means of encouraging people to become responsible for their own health.

CONCLUSION

Infection associated with health care is a significant problem, affecting at least 6% of patients admitted to hospital. Changes in the delivery of health care mean that patients are increasingly likely to be managed in their own homes with a range of invasive devices making them more vulnerable to infection. A considerable proportion of these infections could be prevented by a high standard of clinical practice and knowledge of infection prevention and control is therefore essential to achieve this, particularly as many nurses work in settings where access to infection control advice may not be readily available. Much of the practice directed at preventing the transmission of infection is based on ritual and tradition rather than scientific evidence. It is hoped that this chapter will stimulate an interest in the principles of infection control and direct the student towards a deeper understanding of practices which are fundamental to providing the patients in their care with a safe environment and meeting their obligation to safeguard their patients' well-being.

Summary

All health care staff have a responsibility to minimise the risk of patients in their care acquiring an infection; they therefore need a good understanding of the principles of infection prevention and control. Approximately 6% of patients acquire an infection whilst in hospital. These infections are associated with considerable morbidity and increased costs of care and as many as one-third of them may be prevented by good practice. Infection prevention and control is a key component in risk management and quality

assurance. The increasing trend to manage health care in the patient's home rather than in hospitals emphasises the importance of infection prevention and control in community, as well as hospital, settings.

Micro-organisms can transfer between hosts either through direct contact or indirectly by using a vehicle such as hands or equipment. Routine infection control practice should be directed towards the safe handling of material likely to contain pathogens, e.g. body fluids, and preventing the introduction of micro-organisms to vulnerable sites such as skin lesions or invasive devices. The susceptibility of an individual to infection is increased by underlying illness or therapy which diminishes the immune response, and by devices which breach the body's external defences against microbial invasion. Isolation procedures are designed to prevent the transmission of infectious diseases in hospital settings where patients may be particularly vulnerable to infection. They should be directed towards the specific route of transmission of the pathogen concerned. Outbreaks of infection, where there are several cases of infection caused by the same pathogen, can occur in both hospital and community settings. Control of such outbreaks depends on early recognition of cases and implementation of preventive measures.

REFERENCES

Ackerman, V. and Dunk-Richards, F. (1991). *Microbiology – an Introduction for the Health Sciences*. W.B. Saunders/Baillière Tindall, London.

Ansari, S.A., Springthorpe, S., Sattar, S.A. *et al..* (1991). Potential role of hands in the spread of respiratory infection: studies with human para-influenza virus 3 and rhinovirus 14. *Journal of Clinical Microbiology*, 29, 2115–9.

Ayliffe, G.A.J. (1991). Masks in surgery? *Journal of Hospital Infection* 18, 165–6.

Ayliffe, G.A.J., Collins, B.J., Lowbury, E.J.L. *et al.* (1967). Ward floors and other surfaces as reservoirs of hospital infection. *Journal of Hygiene*, 65, 515–36.

Ayliffe, G.A.J., Coates, D. and Hoffman, P.N. (1993). *Chemical Disinfection in Hospitals*. Public Health Laboratory Service, London.

Babb, J.R., Davies, J.G. and Ayliffe, G.A.J. (1983). Contamination of protective clothing and nurses uniforms in an isolation ward. *Journal of Hospital Infection*. 4, 49–57.

Bowell, E. (1992). Protecting the patient at risk. *Nursing Times* 88(3), 32–5.

Boyce, J.M. (1991). Should we vigorously try to contain and control methicillin-resistant *Staphylococcus aureus? Infection Control and Hospital Epidemiology,* 12, 46–54.

British Thoracic Society, Joint Tuberculosis Committee. (1990). An updated code of practice. *British Medical Journal,* 30, 995–1000.

Burnie, J.P., Odd, F.C., Lee, W. et al. (1985: Outbreak of systemic *Candida albicans* in an intensive care unit caused by cross-infection. *British Medical Journal,* 290, 746–8.

Casewell, M. and Phillips, I. (1977). Hands as a route of transmission for *Klebsiella* species. *British Medical Journal,* ii, 1315–17.

CDC (1987). Recommendations for the prevention of HIV transmission in health care settings. *Morbidity Mortality Weekly Report,* 36, 2S.

CDC (1988). Update: universal precautions for the prevention of the transmission of human immunodeficiency virus, hepatitis virus and other blood borne pathogens in health care settings. *Morbidity Mortality Weekly Report,* 37, 24.

CDC (1990). Guidelines for preventing the transmission of tuberculosis in health-care settings, with special focus on HIV-related issues. *Morbidity Mortality Weekly Report,* 39(RR–17), 1–29.

Clark, A. (1996). Why are we trying to reduce length of stay? Evaluation of the costs and benefits of reducing time in hospital must start from the objectives that govern the change. *Quality in Health Care,* 5, 172–9.

Coates, D. and Wilson, M. (1989). Use of dichloroisocyanurate granules for spills of body fluids. *Journal of Hospital Infection,* 13, 241–52.

Collins, C.H. and Kennedy, D.A. (1987). Microbiological hazards of occupational needlestick and 'sharps' injuries. *Journal of Applied Bacteriology,* 62, 385–402.

Communicable Disease Report (1995). Interim guidelines for the control of infections with Vero cytotoxin producing *Escherichia coli* (VTEC). Subcommittee of the PHLS working group on Vero toxin producing *Escherichia coli* (VTEC). *Communicable Disease Report,* 5(6). R77–80.

Communicable Diseases Surveillance Centre (1995). Epidemic methicillin-resistant *Staphylococcus aureus. Communicable Disease Report,* 5(35), 1–4.

Control of Infection Group, Northwick Park Hospital (1974). Isolation systems for general hospitals. *British Journal of Medicine,* 2, 41–6.

Cookson, B.D., Peters, B., Webster, M. et al. (1989). Staff carriage of epidemic methicillin-resistant *Staphylococcus aureus. Journal of Clinical Microbiology,* 27(7), 1471–6.

Cowden, J.M. (1997). Scottish outbreak of *Escherichia coli* O157 November-December 1996. *Euro Surveillance,* 2(1), 1–2.

Crow, R.A., Chapman, R.G., Roe, B.H. et al. (1986). *A Study of Patients with an Indwelling Urethral Catheter and Related Nursing Practice.* Nursing Practice Research Unit, University of Surrey, Guildford.

Cruse, P.J.E. and Foord, R. (1980). The epidemiology of wound infection – a 10 year prospective study of 62,939 wounds. *Surgical Clinics of North America,* 60(1), 27–40.

Davies, B. and Blenkharn, I. (1987). On the right track. *Nursing Times,* 83(22), 64–8.

DoH (1995). *Hospital Infection Control – Guidance on the Control of Infection in Hospitals.* Prepared by the DH/PHLS/Hospital Infection Control Group. HMSO, London.

DoH (1996). *Immunisation against Infectious Disease.* HMSO, London.

Dubbert, P.M., Dolce, J., Richter, W. et al. (1990). Increasing ICU staff handwashing: effects of education and group feedback. *Infection Control and Hospital Epidemiology,* 11, 191–3.

East, J. (1992). Implementing the COSHH regulations. *Nursing Standard,* 6(26), 33–5.

Elliott, T.S.J. and Faroqui, M.H. (1992). Infection and intravascular devices. *British Journal of Hospital Medicine,* 48(8), 496–7, 500–503.

Emmerson, A.M., Enstone, J.E., Griffin, M. et al. (1996). The second national prevalence study of infection in hospitals – overview of the results. *Journal of Hospital Infection,* 32(3), 175–90.

Garner, J.S., Hierholzer, W.J., McCormick, R.D. et al. (1996). Guideline for isolation precautions in hospitals. *Infection Control and Hospital Epidemiology.* 17(1), 53–80.

Glenister, H.M., Taylor, L.J., Cooke, E.M. and Bartlett, C.L.R. (1992). *A Study of Surveillance Methods for Detecting Hospital Infection.* Public Health Laboratory Service, London.

Glynn, A., Ward, V., Wilson, J. et al. (1997). *The Control of Hospital-acquired Infection in Nineteen Hospitals.* Surveillance, policies and practice. Public Health Laboratory Service, London.

Gormon, L.J., Sanai, L., Notman, W. et al. (1993). Cross-infection in an intensive care unit by *Klebsiella pneu-*

moniae from ventilator condensate. *Journal of Hospital Infection*, 23(1), 27–34.

Gould, D. (1993). Assessing nurses' hand decontamination performance. *Nursing Times*, 89(25), 47–50.

Greaves, A. (1985). We'll just freshen you up, dear. *Nursing Times*, Mar 6 (suppl), 3–8.

Haley, R.W., Culver, D.H., White, J.W. *et al.* (1985). The efficacy of infection surveillance and control programs in preventing nosocomial infections in US hospitals (SENIC Study). *American Journal of Epidemiologyp*, 121, 182–205.

Health and Safety Commission (1994). *Control of Substances Hazardous to Health Regulations. Approved Codes of Practice.* HSE Books, London.

Heptonstall, J., Gill, O.N., Porter, K. *et al.* (1993). Health care workers and HIV: surveillance of occupationally acquired infection in the United Kingdom. *Communicable Disease Report Review*, 3(11), R147–R153.

Hobbs, B.C. and Roberts, D. (1993). *Food Poisoning and Food Hygiene*, 6th edn. Arnold, London.

Hoffman, P.N. (1993). *Clostridium difficile* and the hospital environment. *PHLS Microbiology Digest*, 10(3), 91–2.

Hoffman, P.N. and Wilson, J.A. (1995). Hands, hygiene and hospitals. *Public Health Laboratory Service Microbiology Digest* 11(4), 211–16.

Holborn, J. (1990). Wet strike through and transfer of bacteria through operating barrier fabrics. *Hygiene Medicine*, 15, 15–20.

Hospital Infection Society (1990). Revised guidelines for the control of epidemic methicillin-resistant *Staphylococcus aureus*. Working Party Report. *Journal of Hospital Infection*, 16, 351–77.

HSE (1992). *Safe Disposal of Clinical Waste.* HMSO, London.

Hutchinson, D.U. and Lawrence, J.C. (1991). Wound infection under occlusive dressings. *Journal of Hospital Infection*, 17, 83–94.

Kingsley, A. (1992). First step towards a desired outcome. Preventing infection by risk recognition. *Professional Nurse*, 7(11), 725–9.

Kinmouth, A.L., Fulton, Y. and Campbell, M.J. (1992). Management of feverish children at home. *British Medical Journal*, 305, 1134–6.

Knowles, H.E. (1993). The experience of infectious patients in isolation. *Nursing Times*, 89(30) 53–6.

Larson, E. (1988). *Psychology of Change in Infection Control.* Proceedings of the second international conference on infection control, CMA Medical Data Ltd, Cambridge.

Levin, M.H., Olsen, B., Nathan, C. *et al.* (1984). *Pseudomonas* in the sinks of an intensive care unit: relation to patients. *Journal of Clinical Pathology*, 37, 424–7.

Mackintosh, C.A. and Hoffman, P.N. (1984). An extended model for the transfer of micro-organisms via the hands: differences between organisms and the effects of alcohol disinfection. *Journal of Hygiene*, 92, 345–55.

Mackowiak, P.A. (1994). Fever: blessing or curse? A unifying hypothesis. *Annals of Internal Medicine*, 120, 1037–40.

Maki, D.G. (1991). Infections caused by intravascular devices: pathogenesis, strategies for prevention. In *Improving Catheter Site Care.* Proceedings of a Symposium, Series 179, March 1991. Royal Society of Medicine Services, London.

Medical Devices Agency (1995). *The Re-use of Medical Devices supplied for Single Use Only.* Medical Devices Agency, Department of Health, London.

Meers, P.D., Ayliffe, G.A.J., Emmerson, A.M. *et al.* (1981). Report of the national survey of infection in hospital. *Journal of Hospital Infection*, 2(Suppl). 1–51.

Meers, P., Sedgwick, J. and Worsley, M. (1995). *The Microbiology and Epidemiology of Infection for Health Science Students.* Chapman & Hall, London.

Moss, F. (1995). Risk management and quality of care. *Quality in Health Care*, 4, 102–7.

Musa, F.K., Desai, N., Casewell, M.W. *et al.* (1990) The survival of *Acinetobacter calcoaceticus* inoculated on fingertips and formica. *Journal of Hospital Infection*, 15, 219–28.

NHS Executive (1995). *Hospital Laundry Arrangements for Used and Infected Linen.* HSG(95)18. HMSO, London.

NHS Executive (1996). *Priorities and Planning Guidance for the NHS: 1997/98.* Department of Health, London.

NHS Management Executive (1993). *Public Health: Responsibilities of the NHS and the Roles of Others.* HSG(93)56. Health Publications Unit, Heywood, Lancs.

NHS Procurement Directorate (1990). *A Further Evaluation of Transportable Steam Sterilisers for Unwrapped Instruments and Itensils.* Health Equipment Information 196. HMSO, London.

Ojajarvi, J., Makela, P. and Rautasalo, I. (1977). Failure of hand disinfection with frequent handwashing; a need for prolonged field studies. *Journal of Hygiene*, 79, 107–12.

Olsen, R.J., Lynch, P., Coyle, M.B. *et al.* (1993). Examination gloves as barriers to hand contamination in clinical practice. *Journal of the American Medical Association*, 270(3), 350–3.

Patterson, J.E., Vecchio, J. and Pantelick, E.L. (1991). Association of contaminated gloves with transmission of *Acinetobacter calcoaceticus var anitratus* in an intensive care unit. *American Journal of Medicine*, 91, 479–83.

Pearson, M.L., Hierholzer, W.J., Garner, J.S. *et al.* (1996). Guideline for prevention of intravascular device-related infections. *Infection Control and Hospital Epidemiology*, 17, 438–73.

Pickersgill, F. (1988). The case against re-use. *Nursing Times*, 84(44), 45–8.

Plowman, R., Graves, N., Roberts, J. *et al.* (1998). *The Socio-economic Burden of Hospital-acquired Infection*. Public Health Laboratory Service, London.

Reybrouck, G. (1983). Role of the hands in the spread of nosocomial infection 1. *Journal of Hospital Infection*, 4, 103–10.

Rhame, F. (1986). The inanimate environment. In *Hospital Infections*, Bennett, J.V. and Brachman, P.S. (eds), 223–50. Little, Brown, Boston.

Roitt, I.M., Brostoff, J. and Male, D. (1996). *Immunology*, 4th edn. Mosby, Times Mirror International Publications Ltd, London.

Saghafi, L., Raselli, P., Francillon, C. *et al.* (1992). Exposure to blood during various procedures: results of two surveys before and after implementation of universal precautions. *American Journal of Infection Control*, 20(2), 53–7.

Sanderson, P.J. and Weissler, S. (1992). Recovery of coliforms from the hands of nurses and patients: activities leading to contamination. *Journal of Hospital Infection*, 21, 85–93.

Selwyn, S. (1991). Hospital infection: the first 2500 years. *Journal of Hospital Infection*, Suppl A, 5–64.

Seto, W.H. (1995). Staff compliance with infection control practices. Application of behavioural sciences. *Journal of Hospital Infection*. 30(suppl), 107–15.

Stamm, W.E. (1991). Catheter-associated urinary tract infections: epidemiology, pathogenesis and prevention. *American Journal of Medicine*, 91(suppl 3B), 65S–71S.

Stott, N. (1992). Day case surgery generates no increased workload for community based staff, true or false? *British Medical Journal*, 304, 825–6.

Taylor, L. (1980). Are face masks necessary in operating theatres and wards? *Journal of Hospital Infection*, 1, 173–4.

Thomlinson, D. (1987). To clean or not to clean? *Nursing Times*, 83(9), 71–5.

UKCC (1992). *Code of Professional Conduct for the Nurse, Midwife and Health Visitor*, 3rd edn, UKCC, London.

UK Health Departments (1990). *Guidance for Clinical Health Care Workers: Protection against Infection with HIV and Hepatitis Viruses*. Recommendations of the Expert Advisory Group on AIDS. HMSO, London.

Walsh, M. and Ford, P. (1989). *Nursing Rituals, Research and Rational Actions*. Butterworth-Heinnemann, Oxford.

Williams, E. and Buckles, A. (1988). A lack of motivation. *Nursing Times*, 84, 67–70.

Wilson, J. (1995a). Infection control: surveying the risks. *Nursing Standard*, 9(15 suppl NU), 3–8.

Wilson, J. (1995b). *Infection Control in Clinical Practice*. Baillière Tindall, London.

Wilson, J. and Breedon, P. (1990). Universal precautions. *Nursing Times*, 86(37), 67–70.

Wilson, J. and Richardson, J. (1996). Keeping MRSA in perspective. *Nursing Times*, 92(19), 58–60.

Worsley, M., Ward, K., Painer, L., Privett, S. and Roberts, J. (1994). *Infection Control. A Community Perspective*. Daniels, Cambridge.

FURTHER READING

Ackerman, V. and Dunk-Richards, F. (1991). *Microbiology – an Introduction for the Health Sciences*. W.B. Saunders/Baillière Tindall, London.

This microbiology text is written for the health care professional. It provides simple explanations of all aspects of the subject and relates them to clinical situations.

Hobbs, B.C. and Roberts, D. (1993). *Food Poisoning and Food Hygiene*, 6th edn. Edward Arnold, London.

This text contains a wealth of information on the micro-organisms which cause food poisoning, how they are spread, factors which contribute to pathogenesis and measures which should be taken to ensure food is handled safely.

Hoffman, P.N. (1987). Decontamination of equipment in general practice. *The Practitioner*, 231, 1411–15.

This paper outlines the principles of disinfection and sterilisation and discusses how they should be applied in general practice, highlighting the most appropriate methods for equipment in common use in community settings.

Meers, P., Sedgwick, J. and Worsley, M. (1995). *The Microbiology and Epidemiology of Infection for Health Science Students*. Chapman & Hall, London.

Provides a description of a wide range of micro-organisms, detailing their pathogenesis, epidemiology, treatment and control. It also includes chapters on laboratory testing and antimicrobial therapy.

Roitt, I.M., Brostoff, J. and Male, D. (1996). *Immunology*. 4th edn. Mosby, Times Mirror International Publications Ltd, London.

This comprehensive text covers all aspects of the immune system in considerable detail. It is written in an accessible style with a large number of excellent illustrations to facilitate understanding of this complex subject.

Scientific American (1993). September issue.

The whole of this issue is devoted to describing current understanding of the immune system. Written in a read-able style and with many colour illustrations, the articles on 'How the immune system recognises invaders' and 'AIDS and the immune system' are particularly useful.

Wilson, J. (1995) *Infection Control in Clinical Practice*. Baillière Tindall, London.

This text provides a comprehensive guide to the principles of infection control, reviewing practices related to wounds, intravascular devices, urethral catheters, food hygiene and disinfection. It also includes an introduction to microbiology, immunology and epidemiology.

Worsley, M., Ward, K., Painer, L., Privett, S. and Roberts, J. (1994). *Infection Control. A Community Perspective*. Daniels Publishing, Freepost CB640, Cambridge CB2 1BR. Tel. 01223 467144.

This multi-author book reviews the principles and practice of infection prevention and their application in a variety of community settings, providing practical information and advice to community-based staff.

CHAPTER SEVENTEEN

WOMEN'S HEALTH

Mary Hamilton and Judy Reece

- ■ Introduction
- ■ Health care and women
- ■ Women and their specific disorders
- ■ Women as carers
- ■ Conclusion

This chapter aims to explore the roles of women in society and how these impinge upon their health, with reference to the perception of women by health care professionals. It will examine the health problems related to the various stages of womanhood and the relationship between the promotion of women's health and health-related choices. A discussion on how women influence the health care of others will be included

INTRODUCTION

The inclusion of a chapter specifically related to women's health may be viewed as inappropriate in terms of equality of the sexes and may even be questioned as irrelevant. The argument for its inclusion is important, in that women have specific health problems related not only to their specific physiology but also to how they are perceived and treated by society and health care professionals.

Nurses meet women in a variety of situations, not just those in which the women require nursing care, but also, for example, when caring for elderly people and caring for children. In these circumstances, the woman is often the person who takes responsibility for the day-to-day well-being of the primary client. In those situations, and when it is the woman herself who requires nursing care, the nurse should be aware how the various roles and responsibilities can affect the woman's behaviour, health and progress of her illness. Webb (1983) found that one of the main wor-

ries of women who are ill is the effect on their families, especially when they return home. The common myth within nursing is that, when hospitalised, many women take on totally the 'sick role', showing a reluctance to self care and placing undue demands upon the time of the nurse. If this is reality, then an understanding of why it may occur is essential for nurses to support and care for women in a meaningful way. Therefore, knowledge of the roles of women and the demands of those roles is important. As Kettel (1996) points out, women and men 'lead gender-differentiated lives'. The fact that they may live in the same environment means little. She suggests that 'from the time they rise until they go to bed, they may actually occupy and use very different life spaces, and be exposed to very different environmental illnesses as a result'.

The social role of women and how this influences health and health-related choices, along with the specific disorders associated with the different phases of their lives, are important when assessing, planning and evaluating their care. The role of women as carers, both paid and non-paid, is an important one for the nurse to consider, from a professional and personal perspective, as most carers are women.

WOMEN'S ROLE IN SOCIETY

Women are socialised into their 'roles' in a society in which women survive longer, work longer in caring roles and face a variety of conflicting messages about their place in a male-orientated system.

In the past, women were presented as the weaker sex, yet this is not always true. Around the fourteenth century, there was an abrupt halt in the development of women leaders. At this time theology determined that the healing powers of women, directed both to themselves and to and for others, were acts of demon possession and evil. This meant the removal of an important aspect of women's power. There was a gradual translation of women's leadership to a situation where their power, rather than being viewed as intrinsic to the very essence of their womanhood, was regarded with suspicion. Their psychological strengths now resided largely in their home functions, and in their abilities to be carers in relation to men.

It is only in the last 30 years that women's access to higher education has become more common, resulting in higher entries of women into many undergraduate programmes. For many years now, girls have been closing the gap in attainment and have surpassed boys in the 16–18 years age range, but the subjects studied continue to differ. According to Walby (1994), boys, in the main, still study sciences and girls the arts. Recently, Maras and Archer (1997) have suggested that women's experience of schooling from age 3 to 16 remains subject to discrimination. The manner in which girls and boys are spoken to, judged, potential achievements described and play activity encouraged, are all framed within the context of stereotypical expectations of gender. They go on to suggest that women may return to education much later in life. Increased access to higher education for older female learners is not without cost to the women, however. These costs may be social, economic or psychological in terms of personal health.

More women are entering education and, subsequently, careers that do not necessarily enhance their traditional female caring roles. Media portrayals of women still centre largely on roles to do with home management. Hence the work of Faludi (1992) is pertinent, in discussing the notion that women are now suffering a psychological backlash as a direct result of changing expectations of their roles, both outside and inside the home. Psychological distress is increased because women are working harder outside the home to further their careers, with little respite in the demands placed upon them within the home. For women who reject outside work, 'feminist inspired' pressure to be more than just a home-based mother can induce feelings of inadequacy and guilt. Whether part-time work, which women predominantly undertake, allows them to work outside and inside the home without increasing their distress, is debatable. They still have to cope with both roles and the possibility of distress and guilt if they cannot adequately cope with both. The resulting guilt of a desire to work, according to Faludi (1992), drove women to seek the therapy that was very much a feature of the 1970s and 1980s, and did not prove to be successful in relieving their guilt. She suggests that women have to learn new ways of gaining psychological strength and seek change in ways which are both appropriate and relevant to their lives and health.

The identification of women within the domestic sphere and as performers of 'natural' functions, such as child-rearing has, in the eyes of many feminists, led to women being viewed as less than full persons, or less intelligent than their male counterparts (Martin, 1989).

Some might argue that this view is no longer true, that equal opportunities for women are more apparent in modern society. While acknowledging that progress has been made in creating a more equal society for women, many feminist writers with an interest in health care highlight that within the health care system women are often viewed and treated in a subordinate manner (Doyal, 1995; Busfield, 1996). The result is that women, as consumers of the services, are often disempowered within the system and discouraged from active participation in health-related decisions.

HEALTH CARE AND WOMEN

Health care in the Western world is accused of both disregarding the needs of women

(Goudsmit, 1994) and of the over-medicalisation of their lives (Ardner, 1977; Martin, 1989). While both these views may seem contradictory, it could be argued that they are interrelated. The unique body functions of women are often ignored in the wider arena of health and health care. Abouzahr *et al.* (1996) highlight the dearth of information on the biological and social determinants and consequences of infection and disease in women. By contrast, women's reproductive systems are often the subject of intensive detail and management.

Physiology books perpetuate the view of the woman as the deviant 'other'. Details of the functioning of the body are usually related to the average man, with little acknowledgement of how female physiology may be different from that of men. For instance, there is little reference to hormone influences on factors such as water balance within the body or clearance of toxins. The acknowledgement of women is usually contained within the section related to reproduction. While their unique physiology should not be ignored, its role in total physiological response in health and illness is often disregarded. This is especially true within clinical research. Rosser (1994) details the total exclusion of women in a study of the effects of cholesterol-lowering drugs and in the use of low dose aspirin therapy in the management of myocardial infection. Oberman (1994) postulates two reasons for exclusion; the inclusion of women adds variables that make any study more costly and difficult, and the risk that drugs may cause congenital malformations should the women become pregnant. She further argues that it is not the risk of the abnormality that frightens the manufacturers, but the fear of lawsuits which could bankrupt them. Excluding women because of the variables caused by normally occurring hormonal variations may seem inexplicable. Oberman speculates that the cost of including samples large enough to take account of the variables may make the study too expensive and therefore not attractive to sponsors. Rosser (1994) warns that drugs, whose effects on women are unknown, are being marketed and subsequently used to treat women. There seems to be little acknowledgement of the effect that hormones, normal female body fat percentage, menstrual cycle changes or other less tangible female-specific factors may have on drug metabolism (Driscoll *et al.*, 1994). There is also little research on how disorders may affect women's sexuality. Tiefer (1994) argues that for every 10

studies on the effect of diabetes mellitus on men's sexuality there is one on the effect on women. This is also true of studies of the effects of antihypertensive therapy where there are 20 studies on men to every one on women.

Women are disadvantaged not only within the area of research. They are less likely to have investigations when presenting with symptoms which might suggest coronary heart disease, and are less likely to have surgery when admitted to hospital with a diagnosis of myocardial infarction (Limacher, 1996). Mastroianni *et al.* (1994) claim that there is a generally held belief among clinical researchers that responses of men and women to treatment is similar and this belief is seldom questioned by clinicians and researchers. An example of this disregard is obvious within the area of autoimmune deficiency syndrome (AIDS). Much of the information regarding the transmission and progression of the illness relates to the symptoms and signs observed in men. It is unknown whether AIDS has the same aetiology in women. Consequently, women may receive inappropriate treatment.

When it comes to disorders related to the reproductive tract or reproductive physiology, women are the subjects of intense research and treatment. The history of the medicalisation of childbirth is well documented (Oakley, 1984; Donnison, 1988) but the process is not just restricted to childbearing. Menstruation has become the focus of research and medical management. The interest in pre-menstrual syndrome has escalated, culminating in the widely held view that menstruation and its associated physiological changes is a pathological condition. The list of symptoms appears endless, from physical changes to behavioural changes (Table 17.1). The diversity of the symptoms, along with the assertions that three-quarters of all women experience some symptoms before menstruation, has led some feminist social scientists to seek a sociocultural explanation for pre-menstrual syndrome. Whilst not dismissing the symptoms that women experience, feminist literature explains that the anger, irritability and aggression women feel are based in the demands made upon them and their lives. The expression of these feelings is contrary to what is normally expected of women (cheerful, submissive and non-complaining) but they are 'given permission' to express negative feelings, provided there is an underlying explanation. Pre-menstrual syndrome

Table 17.1: Physical and psychological manifestations of pre-menstrual syndrome

Physical manifestations	Psychological manifestations
Insomnia	Irritability
Acne	Nervousness
Greasy hair	Depression
Dry hair	Inability to concentrate
Increased thirst	Paranoid thoughts
Increased appetite	Suicidal thoughts
Weight gain	Decreased motivation
Breast tenderness	Decreased efficiency
Diarrhoea	Clumsiness
Constipation	Increased libido
Headache	Decreased libido
Nausea	Exhaustion
Craving for sweets	

is not only acceptable to society, but it also sanctions a specified time when women can 'vent their anger' (Martin, 1989; Helman, 1995). Acknowledgement of pre-menstrual syndrome as a sociological phenomenon, which has a biological basis, may be difficult to accept, especially for those women who experience severe symptoms. There is also the danger that the condition is trivialised, or that women are ignored or labelled unstable. It is important to acknowledge the biological changes that occur as hormone levels alter, and that the symptoms women experience are real. Strategies to alleviate the distressing effects of premenstrual syndrome need to take into account all the contributing factors.

The menopause is also subject to the same medicalisation process. It is no longer viewed as a normal biological process but as an endocrine disorder caused by oestrogen deficiency which induces symptoms such as hot flushes, night sweats and osteoporosis (Helman, 1995). This has led to the growth of an industry, medical and pharmaceutical, to manage the menopause. The message often conveyed to women is that hormone replacement therapy will not only alleviate the symptoms associated with the menopause, but it will rejuvenate them and prevent osteoporosis. This could result in disappointment if normal signs of ageing appear. There is also the possibility that women who choose not to take HRT, and who later develop osteoporosis, may be seen as failing to take appropriate preventive measures

and therefore are, in some way, however small, responsible for their condition.

MENTAL HEALTH

The mental health of women has also been subjected to medical authority and the social definition of their roles. Showalter (1985) is helpful in elucidating the progress of women through the early years of psychiatry. The early asylums were places of control, vicious restraint and great inhumanity to both sexes. However, women's madness was often overlaid with echoes of weakness and moral instability. Even attempts by Henry Maudsley at the Bethlem hospital in London to initiate a firm research base to psychiatry may have served only to redefine the problem. English doctors took up the largely American theory of neurasthenia as a diagnosis for many symptoms of distress displayed by women and men. The term 'hysteric' was largely reserved for women alone. Hysteria, like neurasthenia, covered a wide range of symptoms from paralysis to anorexia nervosa. Women who were diagnosed as hysterics were often treated harshly within the health care system. They were seen as reacting against their role as women by over-using their minds, or objecting to the domination of men in their lives. To argue about one's position in society in the early nineteenth century was to risk incarceration in an institution. For men, according to Showalter (1985), the case was very different. Whilst they suffered from similar symptoms, these were seen as a consequence of their struggle to succeed as males in a capitalistic property-based society.

The female hysteric was the subject of much study and treatment, and Charcot (1825–1893) was one of the first people to suggest a non-physical management by his use of hypnosis. Hypnosis, he suggested, could successfully 'cure' hysterical paralysis. Looking from today's perspective, it could be interpreted that hypnosis worked because it released deep feelings in the women that were beyond their conscious control. Another pertinent point is that the women were given personal time and space, and this may have had a healing effect.

After the First World War, the demands of women for their most fundamental rights finally began to remove the notion that women were weak and subject to hysteria. This was a position forced on medicine when men, returning from war, began to display signs that resembled hysteria in women. The signs were recognised as reaction to the constant bombing to which they were subjected within the enclosed spaces of the trenches. The symptoms were labelled 'shell-shock' which is now recognised as post-traumatic stress disorder.

Demand for equality and rights for women could no longer be ignored. Showalter (1985) notes:

'Only when hysteria, under the new name it was given during the war, become a widespread malady of men did the talking cure enter English psychiatric practice. Not Feminism but shell shock initiated the era of psychiatric modernism.'

(page 164)

The search for the source of women's psychological distress has led to the exposure of the physical and sexual abuse to which women have been subjected. This is not to say that all distress is rooted in such abuse, but that the subject of abuse has, to some extent become less of a social taboo.

There are whole ranges of disorders that may be attributed to earlier abuse in childhood, which is often, although not exclusively, sexual in nature. Miller (1994) describes these as symptoms of what she terms 'trauma re-enactment syndrome' (TRS). Miller describes the women:

'They are all women who hurt their bodies because of childhood histories of interpersonal or family trauma. They re-enact the harm done to them as children and reinforce their belief that they are incapable of protecting themselves because they were not protected as children.'

(Miller, 1994, page 8)

The disorders are social, in that they are not seen as psychiatric illnesses as such. However, that is not to say that women have not acquired such a label in the past and will not continue to do so, in the future. The self-abuse can be lifelong and range from mild to severe – obesity, bulimia, anorexia nervosa, smoking, driving recklessly, exercising taken to obsessional levels of working out, are such examples with which we are all familiar.

If we are honest, we all exhibit degrees of self-harming. Some start in early life, while others start much later on. Substance abuse includes alcohol, cigarettes, and the use of recreational and prescribed drugs. These have the express purpose of making emotions less raw, or making us feel good.

ETHNIC MINORITIES

Health care professionals are often criticised for perceiving women as one homogeneous group, regardless of their ethnic status. Women who do not display stereotypical white middle-class characteristics are treated as having special needs, the meeting of which is likely to make extra demands on the services (Phoenix, 1990). Two issues here are important, the assumption that all white women share a common culture and that each ethnic group shares a common culture. Saifullah-Khan (1989) argues that using the concept of culture is a way of stressing ethnic differences, which results in avoidance or denial of the issues of class distinction within the population as a whole. When difficulties arise, the cultural differences of ethnic groups can be blamed for the problem, thus confirming the ethnic group in their subordinate position. Communication difficulties with women whose first language is not English are frequently blamed upon the women (Phoenix, 1990), most commonly for their failure to learn English, or upon their culture, which may discourage them from learning English. Health care workers do not always acknowledge that learning a foreign language can take time and resources that many women do not have. They are often totally occupied caring for their families with little opportunity to engage in a time-consuming activity. They may also lack the opportunity to practise their speaking skills if most of their friends speak their native tongue. Even when a language is learned, it can be difficult to have the confidence to speak it.

Reflection Point

In common with most children in this country, you have probably learned French at school. However, speaking French when in France can be daunting. The variations of accent and the apparent speed of the native French speaker can make comprehension difficult. There is also the consideration of your English accent that can make the pronunciation of some French words arduous. In some situations, you may persevere, but in others, it may be easier to say you cannot speak French.

It should be remembered, however, that many women from minority ethnic groups have been born in this country; therefore language is not a barrier to communication. As Torkington (1994) points out, within Britain it does not seem to matter whether the black person is first, second or third generation, being black means the automatic presumption of being from a different culture. Ahmed (1996) argues that the concept of culture is being used in an inflexible way that can impede communication and understanding. He explains:

'My argument is not that in considering the health, illness and health care of minority ethnic groups culture is not important. It is that stripped of its dynamic social, economic, gender and historical context, culture becomes a rigid and constraining concept which is seen somehow to mechanistically determine peoples' behaviours and actions rather than providing a flexible resource for living, for according meaning to what one feels, experiences and acts to change.'

(Ahmed, 1996, page 190)

Cultural stereotyping can provide health care workers with incorrect interpretations of behaviours and actions. For example, there is a belief that Asian women prefer women doctors. According to Ahmed (1996), this is not necessarily true. He found that non-fluent English-speaking Asian women, when given the choice between a female doctor who spoke only English and a male, who was fluent in Asian languages, they were more likely to choose the man.

The arguments regarding the invisibility of women within the health care system are reiterated regarding women of minority ethnic groups. Ahmed (1993) argues that black women and their health issues have largely been excluded from the work of leading British feminist writers. However, Moore (1990) argues the case of solidarity between women. She acknowledges the overlap of women's experiences, circumstances and difficulties, but in order to assert solidarity 'it is not necessary to assert that all women are, or have to be the same'.

WOMEN WITH DISABILITIES

Women with disabilities of any kind are one of the most isolated and invisible minority groups. Within society in general, they are marginalised from the normal expectations of what women should achieve – for example, having a career or being a mother. For the latter there is a reluctance to accept the reality of sexual activity in women who have, for example, quadriplegia or learning difficulties, and a pregnancy is the proof of behaviour which is not totally accepted, or acknowledged, by society. Media attention has been given to the forced sterilisation of women with learning disabilities, but the issues remain unresolved. The belief that women who are 'imperfect' may produce imperfect children, in a society where pressure to reproduce perfect babies is all too apparent, places women with disabilities in a difficult situation, to say the least. They are often treated in a way that denies them the information and choices that non-disabled women expect within the health care system (Gill et al., 1994). There is also the problem of access to health care. Many buildings lack basic amenities such as examination rooms with equipment that is accessible to those who are physically disabled. Services that may improve the encounter are also lacking, with few hospitals or clinics providing Braille signs that would benefit people who are blind, or staff with the training to assist women with a range of disabilities. Communication with women with disabilities, such as sight or hearing defects, or those with learning disabilities can be difficult if an alternative format is not available. Gill et al. (1994) remind us that women with disabilities are women with the same range of health care problems as any other woman.

SOCIO-ECONOMIC CONDITIONS

The link between poverty and ill health is well documented (Townsend and Davidson, 1987), and of the millions of people who live on the breadline, the majority are women (Reid, 1994), especially those with children. In general, poverty in women has a greater effect on their mental and physical health than poverty in men (Miller, 1992; Kettel, 1996).

For one-parent families, where women are the lone parents, earnings tend to be lower than those of an equivalent male lone parent. In 1995, 23% of families with dependent children were headed by a lone parent, most by lone mothers (Bridgewood et al., 1996); this represents a threefold increase since 1991.

Living in poverty affects physical and psychological health as it often involves living in an area with poor housing, inadequate public amenities and a deficient public transport service. This, along with lack of money, can make escape from the environment, even for a short time, difficult.

Living in poor housing increases the risk of illness, for example, upper respiratory tract infections. The cost of providing a balanced diet can also be prohibitive, as demonstrated by Charles and Walters (1994). In their study, women in South Wales identified lack of money as the most common social source of worry. Poor diet is linked to many illnesses, from gastrointestinal disorders to coronary heart disease (Gizis, 1992). Living within the confines of poverty can also result in pursuing a so-called unhealthy lifestyle (Charles and Walters, 1994), which also has negative effects on health. The stress created by constantly trying to cope with little money and few expectations of any change in circumstances can lead to increased consumption of alcohol and cigarettes. The subjects in Oakley's (1989) study explained their reasons for smoking. They saw the time taken to smoke a cigarette as their personal time, which others within the family also recognised and, in the main, respected. It also relieved the stress caused by their social conditions, for example, poor housing, living in a depressed area with few amenities and the possibility of increased exposure to crime. Promising women living in these conditions that their health will improve if only they modify their behaviour, is ineffectual. Explanation for the failure of health education strategies is rooted in the different perceptions of the health planners and the local populations (Oakley, 1989; Graham, 1994; Helman, 1995). The problem appears to lie in the differences in perception of the middle-class health planners and the people who are the targets of their advertising. The basis of health promotion strategies is that by 'investing' in yourself by healthy living you will 'profit' by not developing specific diseases in future years (Helman, 1995). This approach ignores the reality of struggling to provide the daily necessities of life that makes planning for the future irrelevant. The promise of good health, or at least reduced risk of illness, such as cancer and coronary heart disease, is meaningless, so the impetus to follow a healthy lifestyle is absent or lessened.

Women at the other end of the socio-economic scale are not immune to the effects of their social environment. Alcohol-related problems are more common in women who have a more affluent lifestyle; those in social classes 1 and 2 are more likely to consume more than 14 units per week (Bridgwood et al., 1996). Explanations include social isolation potentially experienced by women who stay at home and the social acceptability of drinking within professional, managerial and non-manual workers (Miles, 1991). A study by Filmore, in 1984 (cited by Miles, 1991), showed an increase in the likelihood of becoming a heavy drinker in women between the ages of 21 and 29 who were employed within these occupations. Women who stay within the home are most likely to be lone drinkers and hide their habit.

SUBSTANCE USE AND MISUSE

Some of the factors that influence women to smoke and drink alcohol were outlined above, but there are other substances ingested by women that may influence their health; these include prescribed drugs. In the Western world, women are twice as likely to be prescribed **psychotropic drugs** (Helman, 1995); even those suffering relatively minor mental illness are treated with drugs (Foster, 1995). Whilst not dismissing the importance of drug treatment for severe mental illness, consideration of the extent of the use of drugs to relieve symptoms of distress in women is important. The type of drugs prescribed may have changed from substances such as Valium in the 1970s to Prozac in the 1990s; the evidence remains that women are still the main recipients. Attempts to explain this phenomenon focus on the perceptions of women by their doctors and the influence of the pharmaceutical industry (Ettorre, 1994). Advertising of tranquillisers in medical literature refers directly to women in a vast majority of cases (Melville, 1984). These advertisements not only have the effect of influencing the type of drugs prescribed, but also reinforce doctors' stereotypical views of the role and coping mechanisms of women (Foster, 1995). Apart from the possible effects on the physiological functioning of psychotropic and antidepressant therapy, there is the consideration of development of dependency and the difficulties associated with their withdrawal.

There is minimal information on the use of illicit drugs by women; indeed the issue of substance abuse is minimised and research often sees all substance abuse problems as applying, in a generic way, to all women. This is regardless of class and ethnic grouping. Ettorre (1994) suggests that this is, in any case, an over-generalisation, because much research neglects the pleasure principle involved in substance abuse by women. We need, she suggests, to ask what it is that women need in order to feel pleasure, as well as pain. It may be that early on in life women already feel a lack of choice and autonomy in their lives. Youth culture has a real emphasis on women being perfect for others – parents, boyfriends, peer groups, for example. It is not surprising that young women attempt to re-establish control of themselves by acting in a way that is seen as the opposite by others around them. Ettorre (1994) suggests that women turn to substances as a way of taking something for themselves, something that gives them pleasure.

FAMILIES AND MOTHERHOOD

Just as women are pressured into particular social and gender roles, likewise they are also steered towards sexual roles. When we speak of women's health we often speak of it in terms of heterosexual health and health care needs. In fact, women who reject this pattern of existence are either ignored, or, at best, become almost invisible. Brogan (1997) points out the difficulties of acceptance within health care which can potentially lead to a late diagnosis of illness. She notes:

> 'They fear homophobia from healthcare providers; the consequences of being open about their sexuality and that if they are not, that they may not receive relevant care; may suffer physical harm; and breaches of confidentiality leading to negative consequences for family and friends, as well as for their own employment, housing and future health care. Consequently, they may delay seeking health care professions entirely, thereby adversely affecting their health.'
>
> (Brogan, 1997, page 42)

The view of women as the nurturers and carers within a traditional family, consisting of two heterosexual parents and two children, is no longer the norm within contemporary white European society. Women are increasingly delaying pregnancy and may even reject heterosexual partnerships altogether as a longstanding means of establishing a family unit. This can create severe tensions for the woman, feeling that 'the biological clock is ticking'. This is, in itself, an indication that women still feel that their personal integrity and personal validity is psychologically bound up with the notion that being a woman MUST, inevitably, mean having babies. Such prevailing attitudes present problems for the woman with an abusive background, for which the expression of sexuality may be a time of unpleasant memory recall. The guilt of having to enter such relationships can be enough to trigger a variety of self-harming behaviours. Some of these behaviours are largely distresses of adolescence, but others can and do present only when the woman enters the world of health care.

Self-harming behaviours may subtly lead the woman into relationships that are re-enactments of past abuse. The cycle of entry into abusive relationships is often hard to break. Domestic violence does not always stop when the woman leaves a violent parental family, and the woman becomes a part of a new family unit. The memories of abuse can last many years and can be very pervasive in the woman's life. Domestic violence impinges on the health of the pregnant woman, not only as a risk to the fetus, but also in the psychological responses of the woman concerned. Stewart and Cecutti (1993) suggest screening women as part of antenatal care by assessing possible risk factors. Women may need referral to counselling services, or alternative accommodation; such decisions will often require very gentle persuasion. However, accomplishment by persuasion is unlikely in an outpatient clinic, and alternative sites should be sought, for example, self-help groups or groups in local community health settings.

Women are still seen by society as being the constant figure in the family unit. There remains a taboo against women who choose to leave their children in response to many years of emotional, and/or physical abuse from their spouse. The woman who leaves her child is likely to receive more stigmatisation than the male who leaves, even if it follows many years of emotional neglect. Women who remain in abusive relationships are more likely to suffer a range of physical disorders that are a part of the double bind of emotional relationships (Waites, 1993). According to Waites, they need to acknowledge their entrapment and the hostage nature of the relationship before healing can take place. Women can begin mourning only when they have left that relationship, either physically or through therapy, and begun the exploration of the nature of power as a feature of their relationships.

For the woman, the early and excessively romantic relationship can become a cycle of love and abuse, almost without the woman realising it. In many communities, this is still held to be the norm for partnerships. In terms of relationships, the cycle may need exploration in therapy for the woman to function as an independent and psychologically healthy person. According to Waites (1993):

> 'In order for the symbiotically enmeshed woman to extricate herself from an abusive partner, she must separate from him psychologically as well as physically and mourn the loss.'
>
> (page 110)

A challenge to women's sexual and gendered roles is required if their physical and emotional health is to remain a positive experience for them.

Choosing motherhood

Motivation for parenthood is a factor about which little is known. Stotland (1994) questions whether it is a biological drive for heterosexual intercourse and conception is a byproduct, or a drive for parenthood itself. She cites the number of abortions carried out each year as evidence that conception could be viewed as an unintentional outcome of heterosexual intercourse. There are also the numbers of women who become pregnant, without conscious intention, who go on to become mothers. These are not just women who are young, immature or ignorant. It is a phenomenon across all strata of society. This does not mean that these women are irresponsible or careless, but rather that there may be 'psychological factors between the biological and social that . . . we have failed to take into account' (Stotland, 1994, page 142). Supporters of the drive for motherhood may cite the number of women who use technology in their quest, as well as the wish of some lesbian women to become mothers. For women whose quest to become pregnant has failed, choosing motherhood is not a simple decision. In recent years services to assist reproduction have grown. New reproductive technologies (NRT) cover a wide range of techniques from donor insemination to surrogacy. They have been the source of much debate and controversy. For anthropologists the use of NRT and surrogacy challenges the concepts of parenthood, family and kinship. Parenthood can be defined as biological or social, the biological parent being the one who supplies the ovum or sperm and the social parent the one who nurtures the child. These categories can be further expanded to identify the genetic mother (donor), the carrying mother (surrogate) and the nurturing mother (rearer). The complexities of family and kinship relations between these three categories and between grandparents and grandchildren who are not genetically related to each other give the anthropologists many areas to explore and compare with other societies (Helman, 1995).

Sociologists are interested in the social implications of the decisions made by the medical profession regarding who should receive these treatments. The concept of 'the fit parent' is one that causes major dissent. There is some concern that the medical profession will have the power to decide who become parents, with middle-class heterosexual couples becoming the beneficiaries (Spallone, 1994). There are also the issues surrounding **sex selection** and **eugenics**. The fear is that women who have a potentially transmissible disorder maybe coerced into accepting NRT as an alternative to choosing whether to conceive naturally and take the risk that their child will have the defect. Although many women in this position will welcome the choice of NRT, there is the argument that as a society we may totally reject individuals who are not perfect and view disability of any kind as avoidable. Consequently, the woman who produces a less than perfect child, either knowingly or by rejecting available technologies, may be viewed as undeserving of support and care of the society. Feminists have been very vocal in highlighting the effects of NRT on women as a whole (Stacey, 1991; Strathern, 1994). They challenge the notion of choice for women whether or not to have children. The pressure to undergo treatments that will result in motherhood can be overwhelming. Women can be compelled to keep on trying regardless of failure, although the success rate is relatively low (Foster, 1995). The technologies are often presented as unproblematic, but this is not necessarily true (Hanmer, 1993). Hormonal injections to stimulate the ovaries to produce ova carry side-effects. Egg collection requires the insertion of a needle into the ovary, which can be painful and carries risk of infection and bleeding. The emotional effects of failure are high. Many women find it difficult to stop the programmes; their failure is now twofold. The initial failure to conceive is compounded by their 'failure' to respond to treatment.

The use of surrogate mothers has been the source of extensive debate within the professions and the media. Anleu (1992) explores the contrasting publicity given to women who choose to carry a baby for another woman for payment and those who request no monetary reward. She suggests that surrogacy which attracts no monetary reward is more acceptable because it is based on a perceived motivation for women to have children. Such motivations 'should be based on emotion, selflessness, and caring and not self-interest, financial incentives or pragmatism' (Anleu, 1992). She warns that absence of monetary award does not, in itself, exclude the possibility of exploitation of women. In instances where the surrogate is a family member, the potential for family pressure on the surrogate mother not to change her mind can be extensive and this is more exploitative than a fee-for-service arrangement. Choosing motherhood is not just concerned with becoming pregnant; opting to continue with the pregnancy is also important. The debate between those who support women's right to choose and the **pro-life** movement shows little signs of abatement. Both groups are vocal in their contrasting views, and individual women are caught in the middle of both. Stotland (1994) points out the stressful and even traumatic nature of abortion, but warns that:

'in one sense there is little use trying to determine whether ... abortion (is) "good for" women. Women have consistently demonstrated that they will risk their lives to obtain them.'

(page 149)

Choosing motherhood is embedded in social, cultural and psychological factors influenced by the society in which women live. The complexities of choices are evident by the discussion and controversy surrounding each step in the process.

Key Points

- The effect of social conditions and pressures on women's health are important factors. Being a mother and home managers, and at the same time career women, has implications for their health. Women who do not work outside the home may be made to feel inadequate as women. Poor social conditions affect both their physical and psychological health, while the gender-specific needs of women with disabilities are often ignored or dismissed.
- Health care concentrates on their reproductive functions while ignoring the effect their specific physiology may have on the progress and management of specific illnesses. Opting for motherhood appears no longer to be a personal choice. New reproductive technologies have been accused of both controlling and redefining motherhood.
- Women's mental health is also framed within the context of the social explanation and medical interpretation of the source of their unhappiness.
- Women from minority ethnic groups are often labelled 'problems' within the health service. Ethnicity is not the same as culture, specific ethnic groups have cultures which are as varied and different as those throughout Britain.

WOMEN AND THEIR SPECIFIC DISORDERS

It is recognised that a number of diseases and illnesses are specifically related to women's physiology but, as previously stated, there are numerous disorders which are not gender-specific but their manifestation, diagnosis and progress are gender-related. This section addresses such disorders and diseases. A life-cycle approach is utilised, starting with the onset of womanhood and the early adult years, through the reproductive period to middle and old age.

ADOLESCENCE

The onset of menstruation (menarche) marks the commencement of reproductive life, and the physical onset of womanhood. In many cultures, rituals acknowledge the onset of menstruation. These celebrate the change from child to woman. Following these rites, the girl becomes a recognised adult member of her society, taking on the rights and responsibilities of the new role. In Western society, no such recognition of transition to womanhood is apparent, and menarche largely receives little attention. The transition to woman-hood constitutes two related events, puberty and adolescence. Puberty is the process of physical development; adolescence is the process of cognitive and psychosocial development (Stevens, 1993). Within Western society, the time of psychosocial development outlasts the period of physical development. The resulting long transition to adulthood influences the social behaviour of the adolescent, which in turn may affect the short- and long-term physical and psychological health status of many females.

Whilst the physical sequence of development can be identified, psychosocial maturity is less easily distinguished.

Menstruation usually commences, on average, between the ages of 11 and 16 years (Guyton and Hall, 1996). The actual mechanism that triggers the production of hormones, responsible for the onset of menstruation, is not clear. It is thought to be related to body weight or to the maturity of the hypothalamic neurones, which occurs during the adolescent years (Guyton and Hall, 1996). Once matured, the hypothalamus secretes luteinising hormone releasing factor, which stimulates the anterior pituitary gland to secrete both follicle stimulating hormone and luteinising hormone, and the menstrual cycle commences (Figure 17.1).

Nutrition

It is essential to review the nutritional needs and status of the adolescent within the context of the cultural factors that influence not only the type of foods available and acceptable, but also the acceptable female body shape. There appear to be two conflicting paradigms. Nutritionists warn of the short- and long-term damage to female bodies of restrictions in essential nutrients, while the media portray the excessively slim body as the epitome of femininity and desirability. In their review of nutrition, dieting and fitness messages in magazines aimed at adolescents, Guillen and Barr (1994) found that during the period 1970–1990 both nutrition and fitness messages emphasised weight loss. They also identified that during this time the body shape of models became progressively less curvaceous. The inducement by companies to consume and use products that enhance young women's sexual development early in adolescence becomes the means by which women actively damage their

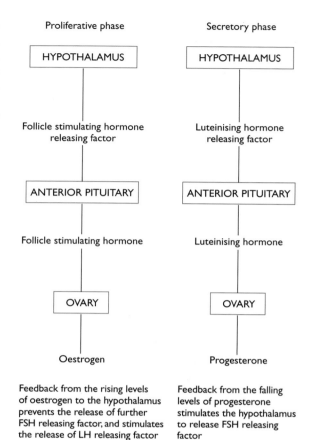

Figure 17.1: Menstrual cycle

health, often without them realising what is happening to them. The constant feeding, via advertisements, of youthfulness in the form of a slender and sexually attractive body, is an illusion that, for some, all too quickly turns into the nightmare of anorexia and substance dependence. The depression and despair that result from the feeling that a young woman is sexually unattractive leads to further abuse of the body. In her review of nutrition in women across the lifespan, Frances Gizis (1992) highlights two essential nutrients, iron and calcium, as important in the short- and long-term nutrition of the female. She identifies one of the periods when iron deficiency is likely to occur as during the rapid growth of early adolescence. In addition, once menstruation occurs, the average loss of iron during menstruation is 1.3 mg/day (Guyton and Hall, 1996). Iron deficiency anaemia is, therefore, likely to affect many adolescents if intake is not, at least, sustained during this time.

By contrast, the effects of a reduction in calcium intake occurring during the adolescent years may not become obvious until much later in life. The daily recommended dose of calcium for the average male is 800 mg, but recent research shows that this is insufficient for adolescent girls (Bonner, 1994) and a daily intake of 1200 mg is essential to ensure optimal bone mass and size.

IRON SOURCES AND METABOLISM

The normal source of iron is red meat, poultry and pulses, such as nuts, and it is found in two forms, haem and non-haem iron. The two forms of iron contained within the diet are absorbed in different ways. Haem iron, of which a greater proportion is found in red meat and poultry, is actively transported into intestinal epithelial cells and absorbed. Non-haem iron, contained within plant foods and pulses, is less easily absorbed (Guyton and Hall, 1996). Vitamin C markedly increases the rate of absorption of non-haem iron, whereas foods containing large amounts of bran or those containing polyphenol compounds, such as tannin, can inhibit the absorption of all forms of iron (Gizis, 1992).

CALCIUM SOURCES AND METABOLISM

Calcium is essential for bone and tooth formation, blood clotting and nerve impulse transmission. Absorption of calcium from the gastrointestinal tract is regulated by parathyroid hormone and requires the presence of vitamin D (Guyton and Hall, 1996). The main source of calcium is milk, milk products, such as cheese and yoghurt, and also pulses. The long-term benefits of milk consumption during adolescence are highlighted by Soroko *et al.* (1994). They found that regular consumption in adolescence is associated with better bone mineral density in older age. Wyshak and Frisch (1994) warn of the association between a high consumption of carbonated drinks and a declining consumption of milk. The rise in intake of carbonated drinks may place young women at risk of osteoporosis in later life, and this is exacerbated by the reduced intake of milk.

Substance use and misuse

The early adult years are usually the time when individuals develop their identity and begin to socialise within a wider social circle. This inevitably leads to exposure to opportunities to experiment with alcohol, tobacco and drugs. All these substances can have a detrimental effect on the teenager, both within the short and long term. The incidence of smoking in girls aged between 11 and 15 is greater than in boys of the same age (Graham, 1994). The factors that influence young women to smoke appear to be different from those that influence young men. The enticement to smoke can come from both within the teenager's social group and from the influence of the advertising industry. Charlton (1990) found that young teenage girls saw smoking in a positive way, in that it calmed the nerves, made them look more grown up and controlled their weight. He also established that advertising posters and pages within women's magazines attracted girls within the 12–13 age groups. Although advertising is banned in teenage magazines, adolescents do read magazines aimed at older women. Attempts to dissuade young women from smoking by various health promotion agencies are far from successful. One attempt by the British Medical Association focused on the premature wrinkling effect of smoking on the female skin (Foster, 1995). The use of such strategies for young adolescent women must be questioned on two fronts. First, at such a young age, the appearance of wrinkles is not particularly relevant, it is related to growing old, and most teenagers do not look far enough ahead ever to visualise themselves growing old. Second, the beauty industry bombards them with miracle cures, creams that will reduce the appearance of wrinkles. Smoking, however bad it is for health, does perform a seemingly vital function for young women, whose situation is permanently marked by various crises. The risk of addiction is clearly known to these young women, but which problem is worse?

Recent publicity regarding the use of 'alcopops' gives the impression that the incidence of alcohol consumption in children and young adults is becoming a major social and health problem. While there is some evidence that there is an increase in alcohol-related problems in women, Foster (1995) warns that sensationalising the figures gives a false impression of the prevalence of alcohol-related problems in women. What is apparent is the increase in advertising aimed at women, and this may have an impact on patterns of consumption by females (Miles, 1991). Helman (1995) highlights the relationship between sociocultural attitudes to alcohol and patterns of alcohol consumption.

Clear statistics for the use of non-prescribed drugs are difficult to obtain. Media coverage of the use of recreational drugs tends to sensationalise their use by children and young adults. Statistics available for 1995 indicate that within the 14–25 years age group 7% have admitted to taking Ecstasy and 33% cannabis (Bridgewood et al., 1996). These statistics appear surprising when compared with the media hype regarding the use of drugs, but it may be that this group is reluctant to give honest answers due to the illegal nature of drug-taking. It should be noted, however, that the high rate of those admitting to cannabis consumption may also reflect society's more liberal attitude to this drug.

It would appear, therefore, that substance use and misuse within the young adult population is a complex issue, with social factors imposing the greatest predisposition to use. Attempts to educate teenagers on risk-taking behaviour is difficult; many will avoid or disbelieve conventional strategies. The pictures of young, slim and sexually attractive women may negate the health education messages.

Sexuality

Interest in sex and sexual orientation is a normal part of development but when this interest is translated into actual sexual activity is difficult to identify. Various statistics relating to the age at first intercourse are available. In 1995, the mean age for first sexual intercourse in the female population, was 17.8 years (Bridgewood et al., 1996). An earlier study by the Health Education Authority (HEA) revealed that 31% of 16-year-olds admitted to having full sexual intercourse (HEA, 1990). The consequences of early heterosexual intercourse are well documented – the increased susceptibility to sexually transmitted diseases and cancer of the cervix are linked with early sexual activity. The reasons are many; the immature genital tract of the young woman offers decreased immunity to infection (Smeltzer and Barre, 1996). Becoming sexually active early also increases the likelihood of many sexual partners and a longer time during which exposure to infections can occur (Greenberg et al., 1992). In 1995, one-quarter of the 16–24-year-old age group reported two or more partners in the last year (Bridgewood et al., 1996).

Research into sexual behaviour is more problematic than most other research, as those willing to talk about their sexual activity may not necessarily be typical of the population. There is the added disadvantage that even when information is divulged, it may not always be totally honest because of embarrassment or not wanting to seem either promiscuous or inexperienced. For young women the conflicting messages about the role, status and value of women can be confusing. The media uses the sexuality of young women to sell many products, yet an open approach to sex education is not always welcomed. This confusion is mirrored in the attitudes of teenagers to those who are known to be sexually active (referred to as a slag) or to those who are not (referred to as a drag) (Cowie and Lees, 1987).

For those who are sexually active, there is the issue of contraception. Although there is an increase in the number of teenagers attending family planning clinics, there are many reluctant to attend for advice. This may be due to confusion regarding their rights or fears about breaches of confidentiality (Family Planning Association, 1992). According to Hepburn (1995):

'no method (of family planning) is absolutely contra-indicated for adolescents ... but protection from pregnancy and protection from sexually transmissible infections are both of vital importance and, particularly within this age group, must be clearly distinguished.'

(pages 25–6)

At a time when young women are making relationships, they often have to deal with changing bodies as well as their own sexuality. Women eventually have to make choices about the nature and orientation of their relationships. Such relationships are influenced by what has happened to them in their childhood. For the survivor of sexual abuse, guilt, love and shame may intermingle with anger and self-loathing. Anger may be directed at the mother figure for not protecting the child. Guilt may occur because the survivor feels a kind of real or misplaced love for the abuser. It is only as the individual reaches maturity that the consequences of what has happened may become apparent. Abuse manifests in self-harm, as mentioned earlier. Cutting, burning of the skin by various means and repeated overdoses is common in survivors of abuse (Van de Kolk et al., 1991).

Young women in this situation invariably carry a label of madness in some form or another. The most frequently applied label is that of **personality**

disorder. It is as if the labelling somehow places a professional gap between patient and carer. Perhaps we find it hard to realise the level of distress that can lead a woman to mutilate the same body that society invests in so much. The perceived rise in the incidence of self-harm in the last two decades has led to a rise in research, yet have we learned to listen to the distress behind the presentation? Arnold (1995) would suggest that we have not.

Scenario

Annie is a 19-year-old student, seen yet again in your accident and emergency department. This is the fifth time in the last 2 months that she has been brought to the department with cuts to her upper arm. The staff in the unit admit that they cannot understand why she does it and feel that she 'needs to be sorted out'.

Annie seems to relate to you, as you are attending to her sutures, and begins to tell you a little of how it feels for her at the time of cutting. You realise that you feel somehow disgusted by what she is describing, and at the same time, you feel overwhelmed.

Consider what help and advice you would offer and where you would seek to obtain it for her?

Where would you seek help for dealing with your feelings and reactions?

REPRODUCTIVE PERIOD

This section will deal with the health of women after adolescence and up to the menopause, and will concentrate on the major women's health issues.

Reproductive tract disorders

The most commonn disorders of the reproductive tract are vaginal infections, for which there are many causes (Table 17.2). Infections can be a source of embarrassment for women as they are often associated with sexual transmission and uncleanness. Whilst many infections can be sexually transmitted and some are exclusively so, there are other causes. Candidiasis or thrush infection can follow antibiotic therapy, occur during pregnancy and in diabetes mellitus. The causative organism, *Candida albicans*, is a normal inhabitant of the large intestine and vagina but is controlled by the acidic nature of the vagina. The normal pH of 4.5 is maintained by the action of the vaginal flora on the secretions within the vagina. Antibiotic therapy can destroy the flora and *Candida albicans* has the opportunity to proliferate. Diabetes and pregnancy increase the glycogen content of the vaginal secretions, thereby upsetting the normal balance and allowing the *Candida albicans* to grow. Organisms such as *Escherichia coli*, *Staphylococcus* and *Streptococcus* may also invade the vagina and cause discharges.

Vaginal bleeding is one of the most common signs of disorders of the genital tract and investigation of any abnormal vaginal bleeding is essential. The causes are outlined in Table 17.3. Abnormal vaginal bleeding can be a source of great anxiety for women, especially if it occurs after the menopause. Abnormal vaginal bleeding is rarely the result of uterine malignancy in young women, but in the post-menopausal period, especially if it is more than 6 months since the last menstruation, bleeding should be regarded with suspicion (Sloane, 1993). Investigations can be frightening, samples of endometrium are obtained, under local anaesthetic, by inserting a tube through the cervix into the uterus. Support by the nurse before, during and following the procedure, with adequate explanations of each step, is important.

For younger women, vaginal bleeding may be more likely to indicate cervical polyps, cervical erosion and occasionally cervical cancer. Again, the nurse has an important part to play in supporting women undergoing diagnostic procedures. The use of the colposcope, although useful in the diagnosis of abnormal cervical pathology, can be frightening to the woman, especially if she is already worried about an abnormal smear. Cervical smear and pelvic examination are the methods used to detect genital tract abnormalities. The Working Party on Cervical Cytology of the Royal College of Obstetricians and Gynaecologists (RCOG, 1987) recommended:

■ All women should be screened regularly from the age of 20
■ 3-year screening for women between the ages of 20 and 64.

These examinations are also offered to younger women if they are sexually active. Although the

Table 17.2: Vaginal infection

Infection	Organism	Signs and symptoms	Possible complications
Thrush	*Candida albicans*	Itching. White, cheese-like discharge	
Bacterial vaginosis	*Gardnerella vaginalis*	May be none. Greyish white to yellow-white discharge	Predisposes to pre-term labour
Trichomoniasis	*Trichomonas vaginalis*	Yellow-green frothy offensive discharge. Inflammation of vaginal epithelium and cervix	
Chlamydia	*Chlamydia trachomatis*	Frequently none, or occasionally mucopurulent discharge	Can cause pelvic inflammatory disease, infertility and predispose to ectopic pregnancy
Herpes genitalis	Herpes simplex	Single or multiple blister-like vesicles in external genital areas, occasionally affects the vagina	Spontaneous recurrences may occur
Warts	Human papilloma virus	Single or multiple soft, greyish-pink, cauliflower-like lesions in genital area	Human papilloma viruses 16 and 18 implicated in 90% of cervical cancers

Table 17.3: Abnormal vaginal bleeding

Site	Cause	Type of bleeding
Vagina	Infection	Intermittent, spotting
Cervix	Cervical polyps	Intermittent, streaking, post-coital
	Cervical erosion	Staining, intermittent, post-coital
	Cancer of cervix	May be none, intermittent
Uterus	Endometrial polyps	Menorrhagia. Intermenstrual bleeding, post-menopausal bleeding
	Myoma	Menorrhagia
	Endometrial cancer	Irregular bleeding, slight and recurring, may be offensive

recommendation is that 3-yearly screening occurs, in some instances it is only undertaken every 5 years. Cervical cytology gives the opportunity to diagnose abnormal changes in the cervix for further investigation. As many as 5% of all smears show some abnormality (Last, 1995). Not all changes in cervical pathology will progress to cancer, but diagnosis of tissue abnormality can allow more frequent examination to monitor the progress (Smeltzer and Barre, 1996).

The accompanying pelvic examination gives the opportunity to identify conditions such as vaginal discharges, cervical polyps, abnormal uterine size and some pelvic masses (Sloane, 1993).

Structural disorders of the genital tract often follow childbirth, although they do not usually appear until many years later when genital atrophy associated with ageing occurs. Rectocoele is caused by damage to the pelvic floor. The rectum pouches upwards, pushing the posterior vaginal wall forward. Cystocoele occurs when the anterior vaginal wall bulges downward, at the level of the bladder. Rectal pressure and constipation can accompany rectocoele. Urinary frequency and urgency along with back pain and a sense of pelvic pressure are the common signs of cystocele. Management of these conditions initially is by the use of the pelvic floor exercises, but in severe cases surgical treatment is required to repair the defect. Prolapse of the uterus may be mild to severe, and the only permanent method of correction is surgical repair.

Breast cancer

In the Western world breast cancer is the primary cause of death in women aged between 40 and 55, and the second most frequent cause of death in women over 50 (Royak-Scholer, 1994). The incidence of breast cancer has risen by over 50% in the last 40 years and despite changes in treatment and management, mortality rates have remained almost unchanged. This suggests that current treatments have produced little improvement in the prognosis of this disease (Smeltzer and Barre, 1996).

The cause of breast cancer has not been established, and many risk factors have been identified, some more controversial than others. Alcohol intake, diet and taking of synthetic hormones have all been implicated, but the attention they receive varies. Foster (1995) suggests that the evidence for implicating alcohol and diet is questionable, but that further research on the effect of hormone intake is needed. The evidence of oral contraceptive use at an early age and the risk of breast cancer is also inconclusive, but Foster (1995) warns that further research is essential. There is also controversy surrounding the use of hormone replacement therapy (HRT) and the incidence of breast cancer. Despite several clinical trials, the evidence remains inconclusive. Sloane (1993) argues that HRT taken for several years increases the risk of breast cancer, and the risk is greater if oestrogen alone is used. According to Abernethy (1997), the risk may be greatest after 10 years' use, and taking oestrogen alone does not increase risk. The familial tendency in the incidence of breast cancer has led researchers to identify a genetic link that increases the risk. Some recent evidence suggests that there may be a defect on chromosome 17, which makes the individual more vulnerable. However, it is thought to be a very small risk factor (Smeltzer and Barre, 1996).

Whatever the risk factors or causes, it remains that as many as one in eight women are diagnosed as having breast cancer and require care and treatment, and again controversy surrounds the treatment. The use of radical mastectomy as the treatment of choice has been phased out, but new treatments can have the same devastating effect on women. The combinations of surgery and chemotherapy and/or radiotherapy can have both physical and psychological consequences. Foster (1995) warns that many of the treatments, although still in experimental form, have been 'hailed as "breakthroughs" long before clinical trials have been completed and thoroughly evaluated'.

Wilkinson and Kitzinger (1994) address the psychological impact of diagnosis and subsequent management of breast cancer. Women have to come to terms with the impact on their body image. The breast, which is viewed as an essential part of femininity by society, is now defective, whether or not a mastectomy is performed. If mastectomy is undertaken, then the use of a prosthesis can actually confirm the negative feelings (Wilson and Kitzinger, 1994). Women need time and space to address these feelings.

The Health of the Nation (DoH, 1992) strategy for reducing mortality from breast cancer focuses on mammography screening. The recommendation is for a single-view mammogram every 3 years in women aged between 50 and 64. Although the use of mammography has demonstrated some success in reducing mortality, it is less sensitive in younger women and there is the risk of false negatives in all age groups (Royak-Scholer, 1994). The use of breast self-examination is still the most common method of detection of breast lumps, although many women do not perform this examination on a regular basis (Smeltzer and Barre, 1996).

The nurse is in the ideal position to educate women on the importance of breast self-examination. When caring for women in any situation the issue of breast self-examination could be raised and the opportunity used to teach women how to examine themselves correctly.

THE MIDDLE YEARS

The physical and psychological health of women during the middle years has largely been neglected or dismissed. Disturbances in both are often seen as the result of changes in hormonal activity. For many women, this is a time of re-evaluation of lifestyles and purpose. Changes in hormonal activity, commonly known as the menopause, is more accurately, the climacteric. Menopause is the actual cessation of menstruation, but is commonly used to describe the total process, and is an important social, physical and psychological process which has been the subject of much research and debate within many professional parameters as well as in the media.

The menopause

The menopause is the period in a woman's life when changes occur in the reproductive tract. As a woman ages, the ovaries' reaction to hormonal stimulation reduces and finally ceases, and the levels of oestrogen and progesterone reduce. Eventually, menstruation ceases. This occurs, most commonly, between the ages of 45 and 55 years, although the physiological changes that lead to cessation of menstruation can last about 10 years. According to Defey *et al.* (1996), the only apparent universal symptoms are hot flushes, dry skin and mucous tissue. Many other symptoms and feelings are determined by culture. The incidence of symptoms such as joint pain, palpitations and insomnia vary, even within Western society. In particular, psychological manifestations vary enormously. In Britain and the USA, mood changes, irritability, depression, **agoraphobia**, panic attacks and loss of concentration are most common. Foster (1995) suggests that before the advent of hormone replacement therapy, the medical profession accepted that peri-menopausal women who were emotionally and psychologically disturbed experienced such symptoms. The treatment of choice was often tranquillisers. The introduction of HRT changed the view of menopause as a normal life event to one that is primarily a deficiency disease and thus could be successfully treated. The original publicity of the pharmaceutical companies marketing HRT extolled the virtues of HRT not only as a treatment for the symptoms associated with the menopause, but also as a way of delaying the visible signs of ageing (Foster, 1995). Today, HRT is hailed as the preventive measure for osteoporosis and coronary heart disease (National Osteoporosis Society, 1993; King and Kerr, 1996).

There are disadvantages to taking HRT, and some of the benefits are questionable. The role of HRT in preventing osteoporosis is reviewed by Abernethy (1997). The evidence to date appears to demonstrate that long-term use, of 5 years or more, decreases the risk of hip and vertebral fracture, but there is uncertainty about the doses required by individual women. A study by Felson (1993) showed that bone mass was preserved only after 7 years of taking HRT, but that women aged 75 who had taken HRT for more than 10 years had only a 3.2% higher bone density than women who had never taken HRT. Jacobs and Loeffler (1992) suggest that it may be just as effective for women to take regular load-bearing exercise such as walking briskly for 20 minutes, three times a week.

Foster (1995) questions the link between reduction in heart disease and HRT. Whilst acknowledging the studies that correlate the protective effects of HRT, she cites a number of studies that question the accuracy of some of the epidemiological studies and the fact that the studies were on women who took oestrogen only. There is a suspicion that the use of combined HRT may negatively effect any potential benefits (Abernethy, 1997). Progesterone is included in the regimen of HRT, as oestrogen alone was found to be linked with an increased risk of breast cancer and endometrial cancer. Maddox (1992), in her review of the literature relating to the side-effects of HRT, has identified a number of physiological changes which can occur. These include alteration of the hepatic proteins in liver metabolism; this may lead to hypertension, thromboembolic disorders and gall bladder disease. Oestrogen also stimulates the synthesis of renin that can cause increased levels of angiotension and aldosterone. This may also lead to hypertension. She also cites a number of side-effects that 50% of all women on HRT experience; these include oedema, bloating, lower abdominal cramps, dysmenorrhoea and breast tenderness.

The evidence regarding many of the benefits of HRT appears, in the main, to be inconclusive. It would appear that many women are encouraged to take HRT without full knowledge of the benefits, risks and side-effects. Hailing HRT as the new cure for the ills of peri-menopausal women, at a time when they have to come to terms with the many physical and psychological changes associated with the menopause, is, in the eyes of many feminists, another sign of the medical control wielded over women.

Psychological well-being

Depression in middle age has been associated with the physical loss of children from the home. It was seen as a time when women were vulnerable mentally because of the menopause. Indeed, the diagnosis of 'involutional melancholia' which was used until relatively recently as a psychotic disorder, was associated specifically with middle age. Busfield (1996) seriously questions the extent to which depression associated with menopause has a biological basis at all.

The woman may see herself as finished in her caring role. The family for whom she made sacrifices and cared has now left home and she has to face life, maybe for the first time with no children to distract from the possible unhappiness of her life. The realisation of unfulfilled expectation can have positive and negative consequences for the woman. Negatively, she may make excessive demands on her GP and other medical and paramedical services because she cannot name the real cause of her dissatisfaction. Positively, the woman may decide that now is the time to pick up education again and begin a new life and career, in which case her demands on health services may be lessened. If the woman decides to re-enter employment then she does so at a certain disadvantage to her male colleagues who may not have experienced career breaks. This could result in loss of self-confidence and a new cycle of self-doubt and negative feelings that have to be overcome.

However, middle age is not just a picture of depression and self-doubt. Women can and do strike out into new ventures and new positive lifestyles outside the home. This may extend to the choice of new and hitherto unacceptable relationships, for example a relationship with a younger man, or lesbian or other female-centred relations (Barnes and Maple, 1992). Alongside this, for some women there is no choice. Socio-economic factors may mean that they have to maintain the role of family income manager, or remain the sole income earner in a unit. These situations may induce feelings of guilt, which may be detrimental to their psychological health. For the woman who breaks out of her previous role, the guilt may stem from the rejection of her former life. For women who are trapped, the guilt of wanting to escape has the potential to induce depression. It appears to be a case of damned if you do and damned if you don't. Alternatively, the woman may be facing an extended period of caring for an ageing relative. Kizilay (1992) noted the prevalence of depression in women in this situation:

> 'A chronic unremitting stressor for this age group is the assumption of the caregiver role for a disabled spouse or parent. Most caregivers are women between 40 and 60 years of age. To be effective in this role, previous lifestyles are often sacrificed, jobs are relinquished, and social activities changed.'
>
> (page 989)

If a woman is involved in caring for a relative after discharge from hospital, she may have to make many changes to her routine and life. The woman concerned may well have to develop routines of caring that imitate the patterns of care seen in hospitals. In fact, this may be the way in which total home care can be delivered. This is clearly a highly stressful event for all concerned. One way in which this stress can be reduced for both people, but in particular for the carer, is by the adequate provision of good quality information before discharge. The establishment of routines was seen to be a factor in stress reduction, as well as information-giving (Bull and Jervis, 1997). Psychological health in middle age can be affected by social and financial factors which are often more significant than biological factors. Middle age for women is, above all, an issue of gender. There are discernible changes in the media representation of the middle-aged woman, most commonly they are depicted as an asexual being, unhappy with their personal identity. Soap operas abound with many such characters. Psychological health can be damaged by the constant portrayal of attractiveness and sexual prowess as the central roles of women in society. The woman who is growing older can be made acutely aware of these factors in the media and feel that she must attempt to maintain her lost youth and femininity. This is not presented in the same way for men. Male pursuit of lost prowess is portrayed rather as an active process whereby they seek a new and younger partner to indicate their continuing virility. It is the lot of women either to ingest hormones or undertake physical manipulations, either internal or external, to delay the damaging consequences of ageing. If older women feel that their bodies are valueless, then their psychological well-being can be equally affected. It is not surprising, therefore, that levels of depression are higher in middle-aged women.

Recent evidence has emerged concerning the beneficial link between women's mental health and their being employed outside the home. As Doyal (1994) comments, these may not all be positive but, overall, women in full-time paid work seem to be psychologically stronger. Women are now susceptible to industrial diseases previously experienced by men. Further research is indicated to determine accurately the balance of benefit versus costs for women who work outside the home. However, for middle-aged women, where the focus is moving towards independence, the benefits of outside work could be great.

Doyal (1995) has suggested that the propensity for alcohol abuse is an issue associated with women working. This relates to work where there is an alcohol culture. Whether this applies to middle-aged women who work, as well as men, requires research. Certainly, female partners of men who use high levels of alcohol are likely to be influenced and over-use alcohol, purely out of habit, or as a result of social networks and availability.

There is, of course, the issue of black and Asian women's mental health needs, which are often absent from consideration of what constitutes happiness and role adjustment, in a largely white middle-class framework of analysis. Whilst white European writers often speak of women's mental health needs, they essentially mean white women. They clearly do not have in mind the needs of, for example, Asian women.

Reflection Point

Wheeler (1994) cites a moving account of an Asian woman who, after numerous attempts to break from her home and family, was deemed to be 'successfully treated', after she had accepted her role as wife and mother. The woman in question was still young at the time of the research.

How will her dissatisfaction influence her health in middle age?

As a nurse, what role would such factors play in assessment of health needs?

Women in middle age face not only the natural loss of children from the family home but also the loss of partners by divorce, separation or death.

Loss for the woman who comes from a childhood where loss was a feature may have all these old fears as well as the current ones to face. Loss of a partner brings with it the psychological distress of dealing with authority and learning again to live life alone. Nurses need to remember that women in same sex relationships also face losses by the break-up of relationships or death. These women are often not accorded the same status as family members, nor the same respect when their partner dies.

Positive mental health care at this time should, where possible, concentrate on the positive rather than the negative aspects. This is best summarised by Barnes and Maple (1992):

'[It] needs to go beyond helping women to adjust to loss. It also needs to be capable of empowering women to develop newly independent lives based on an awareness of their individual needs, which may have been repressed during years of caring for and supporting others.'

(page 87)

Scenario

Sharon (47) attends the health promotion clinic at her general practitioner. She is well, apart from the fact that she still feels acutely sad after the loss of her partner of 20 years. In the course of the interview, it emerges that this partnership was a same sex one, which she had succeeded in keeping to herself all her life. She now faces eviction from their home by her partner's family. Sharon states that life has now ended for her, so she is going away for a while.

As a practice nurse how would you react to this, what help could be offered and what issues might you raise in your next supervision session?

OLDER YEARS

The title of this section was chosen deliberately to reflect the fact that 'old age' now has such a wide parameter, and could be said to be relative to age. For the purpose of this chapter the official retirement age of 65 will be used as starting point of the older years. At the outset of the period that marks older years, one of the most traumatic periods an older woman may have to live through, apart from death of a partner, is the experience of retirement. This experience may be either her own, or her partner's retirement. We are entering a time when retirement covers a greater period of life. Adjustment can be positive. It may mark the time for new hobbies or taking alternative further employment that is less stressful or part-time. This will not be the case for some women who may rely on their work as a source of identity, friendship and social relationships (Brady, 1997). When planning health care needs, careful assessment has to be made of all aspects of lifestyle. Women who experience the death of their partners may well feel socially isolated. This can obviously have deleterious effects on the woman's mental health. When the partnership is a same sex one then the sense of aloneness outside the 'gay' community is all the harder, as is the invisibility. Death of the partner after retirement adversely affects the health of the surviving partner; however, the mortality figures are better for women than men, the rates in men being almost double those for women, at 48% and 22% respectively in the first 3 months after the death (Brady, 1997).

As with other age groups, total assessment of the health needs of this group is essential. This must include socio-economic factors, cultural factors, pre-existing health status, gender, sexuality, and vulnerability to suicide. The last factor is important where an unresolved bereavement is prominent in the person's life.

Finally, although women may expect to live longer into later years, they are more likely to suffer from mobility problems and longer periods of terminal illness (Scott and Wenger, 1995). Women are also more likely to have peer support in bereavement in older age. Again, attention is drawn to the ever-changing patterns of family units in the twentieth century. More women are not having children until later life, and more are living as lone parents. We have yet to see whether children will still feel obliged to care for ageing, single mothers and aunts in the same way as they have in the past. It is also necessary to remember that increasing numbers of women are opting for same sex relationships. At the time of writing, the provision of support systems and care provisions for this group is limited. Unger and Crawford (1992) draw attention to the absence of legal acknowledgement of relationships other than a married heterosexual one, and of the economic consequences for the remaining partner. She may find herself having no claim on the estate of her partner and unable to claim benefits normally received by spouses.

Against all this, however, is an increasing awareness by many institutions of the power of the older person in terms of spending power. Women are now beginning to outgrow the stereotypical older person. Older women are taking up all types of physical sport, some of which could be classed as risk sports, and in so doing are shattering myths. There are positives in becoming a single person again: women may be free to utilise their free time as they wish, without having to be constrained by the wishes of a partner.

The final step, according to Unger and Crawford (1992) is to reveal the older woman in psychological research. This is equally true of texts on caring for older people in general and women in particular. There is too great an emphasis on seeing the older woman as the sum of her old age problems, just before senility in its true sense takes over. We need to emphasise the positive aspect of the older woman's health status as against the problems of old age, which inevitably seem to focus on the loss of cognitive mental function. However, none of this can be a possibility whilst women in older age continue to live in situations of socio-economic deprivation. Such deprivation compounds the effects of old age and its inevitable chronic disorders. As life expectancy for women is now 79 years in Western society, it is inevitable that more will suffer some form of chronic disorder. Four out of five women will suffer from at least one chronic disorder such as arthritis, hypertension or heart disease.

Key Points

- While many health problems and illnesses are common to all women whatever their age, there are problems related to the stages of a woman's life. Throughout their lives some women are subjected to both physical and emotional abuse by partners.
- During adolescence, social pressures and expectations, which can influence nutritional status and encourage substance use and misuse, can be the source of many health problems for the present and future health of the individual. Sexual activity at an early age can lead to both short- and long-term health problems, and contraception is an important consideration for this age group.
- During reproductive life the specific disorders which affect the reproductive tract can be distressing to women. Breast cancer is the primary

cause of death in women between the ages of 40 and 55.

■ The middle years see physical and social changes which can affect the well-being of women. Dealing with the menopause can be both physically and emotionally demanding, as can changing family circumstances and responsibilities as children leave home. For some women, however, it is a time to re-evaluate their lives and to make positive changes.

WOMEN AS CARERS

Social and political changes have forced women into roles which can include a lifetime of caring. They care for children and then for ageing relatives. In the role of carer, women are responsible for the maintenance of health and the recovery from illness (Fisher, 1994). Health promotion literature and media advertising constantly bombard women with information on how they can improve the health of their families. This can leave women with the constant worry that the diet they provide, or the care they give, may lead to illness in their family (Foster, 1995).

Women also have to contend with social pressures that seem to blame them for many of the ills of society. Media coverage on the influence that women have on their children's educational attainment as well as their social behaviour serves only to create more stress. It can induce feelings of guilt if their children fail to achieve or they misbehave in any way.

The growing number of elderly people requiring care has grown over the last 20 years. This, combined with the changes in care provided by health and social services, means that the burden of care falls on the family, and most commonly upon women within the family (Wynne, 1994). The stress of caring for an elderly relative, with little respite, can have detrimental consequences on the carer's physical and psychological health. There is the risk of back injury if the elderly person requires assistance with mobility. The emotional effect of a confused parent or one suffering from dementia can be devastating. It is not only the distress of seeing a parent in this state; it is the time required for caring. Women may have to balance the needs of their partner and children with the needs of the elderly

relative, and there is always the worry that neither is met satisfactorily (Rutman, 1996). Regardless of these problems, women are expected to take on the role with little or no support within the community (Wuest et al., 1994).

Typical extensions of the caring role are the professions of nursing and midwifery, which, according to Fisher (1994), followed the pathway of other domestic skills into paid employment during industrialisation. Consequently, nursing and midwifery remain primarily the domain of women, mirroring the gender divisions of the Victorian family of father (doctor), mother (nurse) and child (patient) (Helman, 1995). The role of the nurse, although identified separately, is still subordinate to that of the doctor (Stacey, 1988). An interesting study by Rutman (1996) compares the feelings of powerfulness and powerlessness in unpaid care givers and nurses. Both groups identified the same causes of powerlessness and powerfulness in their role. Lack of recognition of their competence and expertise, lack of control, lack of resources and clashes between the care giver's and receiver's values and preferences equated with feelings of powerlessness. Powerfulness occurred when others valued their knowledge and opinions, when changes could be made to benefit the recipient of care, when sharing their knowledge and skills and when they had the opportunity to make time for themselves. The very things that frustrate the nurse or enhance job satisfaction are the same as those that thwart or improve the role of the non-paid carer. There are lessons for nurses from this piece of work. Just as they value being consulted by other members of the health care team, they may undervalue the importance of consultation to the non-paid carer, thereby making them feel slighted.

Key Points

■ Women are the main carers of children, partners and ageing relatives.

■ Within this caring role they take responsibility for the physical and emotional well-being of the person for whom they care, with little support from outside agencies.

■ The pressure to ensure children grow into responsible and healthy adults can be overwhelming.

■ Caring for the elderly can be stressful emotionally and cause physical injury.

CONCLUSION

The health of women throughout their lifespan is related not only to the physical and emotional changes which occur at the various stages, it is often embedded in the pressures on women to conform to the social roles expected of them. These expectations are often the source of many of their health problems. For health care professionals, not only an understanding of the physical ailments that affect women, but also an appreciation of the social and psychological factors that influence their health are essential. Whilst much has been said of these factors, it is important that the diversity of women is recognised and they are not identified as one homogenous group.

The expectations that women will stay young and beautiful by whatever means possible has a detrimental effect on their health as they take prescribed drugs and treatments in the quest to retain youth. Consequently, older women are often neglected not only by the health care industry but also by other women; for example, many nurses do not like to care for women especially those who are beyond their prime. The consequences for all women requires reflection and perhaps the words of Stern (1996) may help:

'If young girls considered themselves crones-in-training, youth would cease to be treasured above all else, sexual desirability would become a property of all women. Women would treasure their longer life as a source of power, and older women would then be consulted for the wisdom of their years. Older life would be seen as distinguished, surely the most treasured dimension of all.'

(Page 159)

REFERENCES

Abernethy, K. (1997). *The Menopause and HRT.* Baillière Tindall, London.

Abouzahr, C., Vlassoff, C. and Kumar, A. (1996). Quality health care for women: a global challenge. *Health Care for Women International*, 17(5), 449–67.

Ahmed, W.I.U. (1993). Making black people sick: 'race', ideology and health research. In *'Race' and Health in Contemporary Britain*, Ahmed, W.I.U. (ed.). Open University Press, Buckingham.

Ahmed, W.I.U. (1996). The trouble with culture. In *Researching Cultural Differences in Health*, Kelleher, D. and Hillier, S. (eds). Routledge, London.

Anleu, S.R. (1992). Surrogacy: for love but not for money? *Gender and Society*, 6(1), 30–48.

Ardner, S. (1977). *Perceiving Women.* Dent, London.

Arnold, L. (1995). *Women and Self Injury.* Bristol Crisis Service for Women, Bristol.

Barnes, M. and Maple, N. (1992). *Women and Mental Health, Challenging the Stereotypes.* Venture Press, Birmingham, UK.

Bonner, F. (1994). Calcium and osteoporosis. *American Journal of Clinical Nutrition*, 60(6), 831–6.

Brady, P.F. (1997). Mental health of the ageing. In *Psychiatric–Mental Health Nursing*, 4th edn, Johnson, B.S. (ed). Lippincott, Philadelphia.

Bridgewood, A., Malbon, G., Lader, D. and Matheson, J. (1996). *Health in England 1995.* Office for National Statistics, London.

Brogan, M. (1997). Healthcare for lesbians: attitudes and experiences. *Nursing Standard*, 11(45), 39–42.

Bull, M.M. and Jervis, L.L. (1997). Strategies used by chronically ill women and their care giving daughters in managing post hospital care. *Journal of Advanced Nursing*, 25, 541–7.

Busfield, J. (1996). *Men, Women and Madness. Understanding Gender and Mental Disorder.* Macmillan Press Ltd, Basingstoke.

Charles, N. and Walters, V. (1994). Women's health: women's voices … health concerns of women. *Health and Social Care in the Community*, 2(6), 329–38.

Charlton, A. (1990). Women and smoking. In *Promoting Women's Health*, Pfeffer, N. and Quick, A. (eds). King Edward's Hospital Fund, London.

Cowie, C. and Lees, S. (1987). *'Slags or Drags'. Sexuality: A Reader, Feminist Review.* Virago, London.

Defey, D., Storch, E., Cardozo, S., Diaz, O. and Fendandez, G. (1996). The menopause: women's psychology and health care. *Social Science and Medicine*, 40(10), 1447–56.

DoH (1992). *The Health of the Nation.* Department of Health, London.

Donnison, J. (1988). *Midwives and Medical Men: a History of Inter-professional Rivalries and Women's Rights*, 2nd edn. Heinemann, London.

Doyal, L. (1994). Waged work and well being. In *Women and Health. Feminist Perspectives*, Wilkinson, S. and Kitzinger, C. (eds). Taylor and Francis, London.

Doyal, L. (1995). *What makes Women Sick? Gender and The Political Economy of Health.* Macmillan, London.

Driscoll, M., Cohen, M., Kelly, P., Taylor, D., Williamson, M. and Nicks, G. (1994). Women and HIV. In *Reframing Women's Health*, Dan, A.J. (ed.). Chapter 16, 175–86. Sage Publications, London.

Ettorre, E. (1994). What can she depend on? Substance use and women's health. In *Women and Health. Feminist Perspectives*, Wilkinson, S. and Kitzinger, C. (eds). Taylor and Francis, London.

Faludi, A. (1992). *Backlash*. Vintage, London.

Family Planning Association (1992). *Young People: Sexual Attitudes and Behaviour*. Factsheet No. 5B. Family Planning Association, London.

Felson, D. (1993). The effect of postmenopausal oestrogen therapy on bone density in elderly women. *New England Journal of Medicine*, 329(16), 1141–6.

Fisher, S. (1994). Is care a remedy? The case of nurse practitioners. In *Reframing Women's Health*, Dan, A.J. (ed.). Sage Publications, London.

Foster, P. (1995). *Women and the Healthcare Industry. An Unhealthy Relationship*. Open University Press, Bristol.

Gill, C.J., Kirsti, L., Kirchner, J. and Reis, P. (1994). Health services for women with disabilities: barriers and portals. In *Reframing Women's Health*, Dan, A.J. (ed.). Sage Publications, London.

Gizis, F.C. (1992). Nutrition in women across the life span. *Nursing Clinics of North America*, 27(4), 971–82.

Goudsmit, E.M. (1994). All in her mind! Stereotypic views and the psychologisation of women's illness. In *Women and Health. Feminist Perspectives*. Wilkinson, S. and Kitzinger, C. (eds). Taylor and Francis, London.

Graham, H. (1994). Surviving by smoking. In *Women and Health. Feminist Perspective*, Wilkinson, S. and Kitzinger, C. (eds), Chapter 7. Taylor and Francis, London.

Greenberg, J., Magdar, M.H. and Aral, S. (1992). Age at first coitus: a marker for risky sexual behaviour in women. *Sexually Transmitted Diseases*, 19(6), 52–6.

Guillen, E.O. and Barr, S.I. (1994). Nutrition, dieting, and fitness messages in a magazine for adolescent women. *Journal of Adolescent Health*, 15(6), 464–72.

Guyton, A.C. and Hall, J.E. (1996). *Textbook of Medical Physiology*, 9th edn. W.B. Saunders Company, London.

Hanmer, J. (1993). Women and reproduction. In *Women's Studies. A Reader*, Jackson, S., Atkinson, K., Beddoe, D. *et al.* (eds). Harvester Wheatsheaf, London.

HEA (1990). *Young Adults' Health and Lifestyle: Sexual Behaviour*. MORI, London.

Helman, C.G. (1995). *Culture, Health and Illness*, 3rd edn. Butterworth-Heinemann, London.

Hepburn, M. (1995). Factors influencing contraceptive choice. In *Handbook of Family Planning and Reproductive Health Care*, Loudin, M., Glasier, A. and Gebbie, A. (eds). Churchill Livingstone, London.

Jacobs, H.S. and Loeffler, F.E. (1992). Postmenopausal HRT. *British Medical Journal*, 305, 1403–8.

Kettel, B. (1996). Women, health and the environment. *Social Science and Medicine*, 42(10), 1367–79.

King, K.M. and Kerr, J.R. (1996). The women's health agenda: evolution of hormone replacement therapy as treatment and prophylaxis for coronary heart disease. *Journal of Advanced Nursing*, 23, 984–91.

Kizilay, P.E. (1992). Predictors of depression in women. *Nursing Clinics of North America*, 27(4), 983–93.

Last, P. (1995). Screening and reproductive health. In *Handbook of Family Planning and Reproductive Health Care*, 3rd edn, Loudon, N., Glasier, A. and Gebbie, A. (eds). Churchill Livingstone, London.

Limacher, H.V. (1996). Coronary artery disease in women. Past gaps, present state and future promises. *Journal of the Florida Medical Association*, 83(7), 455–8.

Maddox, M.A. (1992). Women at mid-life. Hormone replacement therapy. *Nursing Clinics of North America*, 27(4), 959–69.

Maras, P. and Archer, L. (1997). Tracey's in the home corner Darren's playing Lego, or are they? Gender issues and identity in education. *Feminism and Psychology*, 7(2), 264–72.

Martin, E. (1989). *The Woman in the Body*. Open University Press, Milton Keynes.

Mastroianni, A.C., Faden, R. and Federman, D. (1994). *Women and Health Research. Ethical and Legal Issues of Including Women in Clinical Studies*. National Academy Press, Washington DC.

Melville, J. (1984). *The Tranquilliser Trap and How to Get Out of it*. Fontana, London.

Miles, A. (1991). *Women, Health and Medicine*. Open University Press, Milton Keynes.

Miller, D. (1994). *Women Who Hurt Themselves*. Basic Books, New York, NY.

Miller, J. (1992). *Lone Mothers and Poverty*. In *Women and Poverty in Britain. The 1990's*, Glendinning, C. and Millar, J. (eds). Harvester Wheatsheaf, Hemel Hempstead.

Moore, H. (1990). *Feminism and Anthropology.* Polity Press, Cambridge.

National Osteoporosis Society (1993). *Menopause and Osteoporosis Therapy: GP Manual.* National Osteoporosis Society, Bath.

Oakley, A. (1984). *The Captured Womb: a History of the Medical Care of Pregnant Women.* Blackwell, Oxford.

Oakley, A. (1989). Smoking in pregnancy – smokescreen or risk factor? Towards a materialist analysis. *Sociology of Health and Illness,* 11(4), 311–35.

Oberman, M. (1994). Real and perceived barriers to the inclusion of women in clinical trials. In *Reframing Women's Health,* Dan, A.J. (ed.). Sage Publications, London.

Phoenix, A. (1990). Black women in the maternity services. In *The Politics of Maternity Care,* Garcia, J., Kilpatrick, R. and Richards, R. (eds), 274–97. Clarendon Press, London.

RCOG (1987). *Report of the Working Party on Cervical Cancer Screening.* RCOG, London.

Reid, T. (1994). An unequal struggle, women living in poverty. *Nursing Times,* 90(10), 30–1.

Rosser, S.V. (1994). Gender bias in clinical research: the difference it makes. In *Reframing Women's Health,* Dan, A.J. (ed.), Chapter 22, 253–65. Sage Publications, London.

Royak-Scholer, R. (1994). Health policy and breast cancer screening: the politics of research and intervention. In *Reframing Women's Health,* Dan, A.J. (ed.). Sage Publications, London.

Rutman, D. (1996). Caregiving as women's work: women's experiences of powerfulness and powerlessness as caregivers. *Qualitative Health Research,* 6(1), 90–111.

Saifullah-Khan, V. (1988). The role of the culture of dominance in structuring the experience of ethnic minorities. In *Race in Britain,* Husband, C. (ed), 197–215. Hutchinson, London.

Scott, A. and Wenger, G.C. (1995). Gender and social support networks in later life. In *Connecting Gender and Ageing. A Sociological Approach,* Arber, S. and Ginn, J. (eds). Open University Press, Milton Keynes.

Showalter, E. (1985). *The Female Malady – Women, Madness and English Culture 1830–1980.* Virago, London.

Sloane, B. (1993). *Biology of Women,* 3rd edn. Delmar Publishers Inc., New York.

Smeltzer, S.C. and Barre, B.G. (1996). *Medical–Surgical Nursing,* 8th edn. Lippincott, Philadelphia.

Soroko, S., Holbrook, T.L., Eldestein, S. and Barrett-Connor, E. (1994). Lifetime milk consumption and bone mineral density in older women. *American Journal of Public Health,* 18(1), 32–9.

Spallone, P. (1994). Reproductive health and reproductive technology. In *Women and Health Feminist Perspectives,* Wilkinson, S. and Kitzinger, C. (eds). Taylor and Francis, London.

Stacey, M. (1988). *The Sociology of Health and Healing.* Unwin Hyman, London.

Stacey, M. (1991). *Changing Human Reproduction.* Sage Publications, London.

Stern, P.N. (1996). Conceptualising women's health: discovering the dimensions. *Quality Health Research,* 6(2), 152–62.

Stevens, S.C. (1993). Clinical application of adolescent female sexual development. *Nurse Practitioner,* 18(12), 18, 21, 25–7.

Stewart, D.E. and Cecutti, A. (1993). Physical abuse in pregnancy. *Canadian Medical Association Journal,* 149(9), 1257–630.

Stotland, N.L. (1994). Contraception and abortion: challenges now and for the next century. In *Reframing Women's Health,* Dan, A.J. (ed.). Sage Publications, London.

Strathern, M. (1994). *New Reproductive Technologies.* Macmillan, London.

Teifer, L. (1994). Women's sexuality: not a matter of health. In *Reframing Women's Health,* Dan, A.J. (ed.), Chapter 15, 151–62. Sage Publications, London.

Torkington, P. (1994). Black women and health: a political overview of British health care. In *Healthy and Wise. The Essential Health Handbook for Black Women,* Wilson, M. (ed.). Virago, London.

Townsend, P. and Davidson, N. (eds) (1987). *Inequalities in Health. The Black Report.* Penguin, London.

Unger, R. and Crawford, M. (1992). *Women and Gender. A Feminist Psychology.* McGraw-Hill, New York, NY.

Van de Kolk, B.A. *et al.* (1991). Childhood origins of self-destructive behaviour. *American Journal of Psychiatry,* 148(12), 1665–71.

Waites, E. (1993). *Trauma and Survival. Post-traumatic and Dissociative Disorders in Women.* W.W. Norton, New York, NY.

Walby, S. (1994). *Theorising Patriarchy.* Blackwell, Oxford.

Webb, C. (1983). Hysterectomy – dispelling the myths. *Nursing Times,* Occasional Papers: Paper 1, 79(47), 52–52; Paper 2, 79(47), 44–6.

Wheeler, E. (1994). Doing black mental health research observations and experiences. In *The Dynamics of Race and Gender. Some Feminist Interventions*, Afshar, H. and Maynard, M. (eds). Taylor and Francis, London.

Wilkinson, S. and Kitzinger, C. (eds) (1994). *Feminist Perspectives on Women and Health*. Taylor and Francis, London.

Wuest, J., Erickson, P.K. and Stern, P.N. (1994). Becoming strangers: the reciprocal interplay between family caregivers and victims of Alzheimer's disease. *Journal of Advanced Nursing*, 20, 437–43.

Wynne, T. (1994). The burden facing women carers today. *Health Visitor*, 67(7), 241–2.

Wyshak, G. and Frisch, R.E. (1994). Carbonated beverages, dietary calcium, the dietary calcium/phosphorus ratio, and bone fractures in girls and boys. *Journal of Adolescent Health* 15(3), 210–15.

FURTHER READING

Arnold, L. (1995). *Women and Self Injury*. Bristol Crisis Service for Women, Bristol.

An excellent study of the functions and reasons why women mutilate themselves.

Martin, E. (1989). *The Woman in the Body*. Open University Press, Milton Keynes.

A feminist perspective on how women are portrayed in health and medical literature.

Miller, D. (1994). *Women who Hurt Themselves*. Basic Books, New York.

A moving book. Essential reading for anyone interested in the subject.

Oakley, A. (1996). *Social Support and Motherhood*. Blackwell, London.

This book gives an insight into how women see their social position and the influence it has on their health behaviour. It contains some interesting quotes from the women regarding why they smoke.

Russell, D. (1995). *Women, Madness and Medicine*. Polity Press, Cambridge.

Challenges the dominance of the medical model in psychiatry in a most readable manner.

CHAPTER EIGHTEEN

MATERNITY CARE

Maureen D. Raynor

- Optimising health prior to conception
- The basis of pre-pregnancy care
- Woman as the focus of maternity care
- Care in pregnancy and childbirth
- Care during labour and delivery
- Care during the postnatal period
- Care of the newborn
- Conclusion

> The aim of this chapter is to bring the reader up to date on some of the contemporary issues affecting maternity care. The chapter begins by examining the value of pre-pregnancy care followed by a critical appraisal of recent sociopolitical reforms influencing the childbearing experience. A psychosocial theoretical framework will be used to underpin much of the debate. The reader is therefore expected to have an understanding of the physiological processes of pregnancy and childbirth.

OPTIMISING HEALTH PRIOR TO CONCEPTION

Although giant strides have been made in preventive care, the notion of pre-pregnancy care only received significant focus within the last decade (Cefalo and Moos, 1995). The terms pre-pregnancy care and pre-conception care are often used interchangeably as they signify the period before conception, when a woman and her partner make a conscious decision to take positive steps toward changing their lifestyles and generally improving their health, thus making provision for two major life events – pregnancy and parenthood.

Minimising risks and optimising health for some couples will necessitate major changes in lifestyle as they prepare themselves physically, psychologically and socially for the challenges of pregnancy and parenthood. For others who have been 'health conscious' the change will be less disruptive. In addition, this is an opportune time for prospective parents to seek guidance on pre-existing medical disorders, such as hypertensive disease and diabetes mellitus (Shorney, 1990).

The two aims of pre-pregnancy care, according to Illman (1997) are:

- To provide the developing fetus with the best possible start to life by avoiding or reducing risks associated with lifestyle, hereditary disorders and medical complications
- To promote the health of the mother.

Wynn and Wynn (1991) stressed that the quality of the spermatozoon is just as important as that of the ovum in influencing the health of the fetus. Yet, paradoxically, women bear the brunt of responsibility for the health of the fetus. The two aims of pre-conception care outlined above fail to account for the significant part that men play in planning for a healthy baby. It is necessary that men should take an active part in pre-conception care, since

Table 18.1: Factors influencing poor pregnancy outcome

- Poor socio-economic conditions, e.g. poverty and poor housing
- Maternal weight (overweight and underweight, i.e. >120% and <95% of standard height for weight ratio)
- Poor nutritional status/poor diet
- Abuse of substances harmful to health and general well-being, e.g. smoking, alcohol and other drugs
- Pre-existing medical conditions, e.g. diabetes mellitus, hypertension, renal disease, anaemia and malabsorption syndromes
- Poor obstetric history, e.g. previous intrauterine fetal death, low birth weight baby, congenital abnormality
- Frequent pregnancies at close intervals

Adapted from Doyle (1994).

potential fathers who abuse their health, and who may be exposed to toxic substances, such as radiation and smoking, are probably just as likely to be the cause of birth defects (Charles *et al.*, 1991).

Pre-pregnancy care provides an excellent opportunity to maximise health before conception, becoming the ideal precursor to antenatal care because of the crucial period of **organogenesis**. This is the period during the first trimester of pregnancy when the developing fetus is at its most susceptible to dietary deficiency and **teratogens**. Cell multiplication and differentiation are rapid during this period, as vital organs, such as the brain and nervous system, are being formed (Shorney, 1990). Pre-pregnancy care should therefore be seen as a natural extension of the midwife's role (Pownall, 1994).

There are known factors which may have deleterious effects on maternal and fetal well-being, culminating in poor pregnancy outcome. Table 18.1 highlights some of the common risk factors which may influence poor pregnancy outcome.

THE BASIS OF PRE-PREGNANCY CARE

It is outside the scope of this chapter to examine this area in depth; however, by focusing the atten-
tion of the reader on a number of selected topics it is hoped that interest will be stimulated to explore further the issues of health education and health promotion before conception. Main areas to be addressed are:

- Assessment
- Diet and nutrition
- Supplementation
- Smoking and alcohol
- Contraception
- Screening/investigations and outlets for care.

ASSESSMENT

Counselling specific to pre-pregnancy care needs to be tailored to meet the holistic needs of women and their partners within the context of sociocultural determinants influencing cultural and religious practices as well as race, ethnicity and socio-economic status.

Detailed assessment of the couple's health should, therefore, include medical and surgical history, psychosocial background, and for the woman, her obstetric history (Table 18.2).

Assessment should also include:

- Leisure pursuits and general interest
- Expectations and insights regarding lifestyle and an exploration of the couple's understanding of their risk status
- What strategies have been tried to bring about behavioural modification, how effective these have been and the couple's motivation and commitment to change.

Obstetric factors need to be carefully reviewed, especially in cases where there has been an underlying complication (e.g. pre-term delivery). Health education in such instances is highly desirable before the next pregnancy in order to identify and manage risk factors appropriately. However, these are usually the very cases which, unfortunately, may not be seen again until the next pregnancy is confirmed.

DIET AND NUTRITION

The importance of nutritional factors in reducing mortality rates influenced some of the targets set

Table 18.2: Factors that should be considered in the assessment and planning of pre-pregnancy care

Psychosocial history	Physical history	Past obstetric history
Stress factors	Medical history (e.g. hypertension, phenylketonuria, diabetes, renal and cardiac disorders)	Type of delivery
Mental health		Weight of baby
Cultural beliefs and attitudes	Menstrual history	Gestation at time of delivery (e.g. term/preterm)
Socio-economic status	Method of contraception	
Eating disorders	Known hereditary conditions	Outcome of pregnancy and delivery (e.g. complicated/uncomplicated)
Social habits (e.g. smoking and alcohol)	Relevant surgical operations	Congenital abnormalities/birth defects
Exercise taken Occupational hazards		

by the Health of the Nation report for England (Department of Health [DoH], 1992a). The report recognised that the achievement of a balanced diet and its contribution to the health and well-being of the population of England could only be achieved by adopting a new approach to sensible eating habits. The key targets that have been identified in relation to diet are:

- To reduce the average percentage of food energy derived by the population from saturated fatty acids by at least 35% by the year 2005 (from 17% in 1990 to no more than 11%)
- To reduce the average percentage of food energy derived from total fat by the population by at least 12% by the year 2005 (from about 40% in 1990 to no more than 35%)
- To reduce the proportion of men and women aged 16–64 who are obese by at least 25% and 33% respectively by 2005 (from 8% for men and 12% for women in 1986/87 to no more than 6% and 8% respectively).

A report on pre-conception care by the House of Commons (1991) claims that diet before conception holds the key to health, and may reduce the risk of perinatal morbidity and mortality. The direct link between diet and poverty has long been recognised (Wynn and Wynn, 1991), and since poor socio-economic conditions will have a profound influence on the quality of food ingested, the health status of women, especially those in poverty, needs to be raised. The DoH (1996a) published a report which made a number of recommendations aimed at targeting low income families. This is to ensure that families in

poverty have real choices of purchasing affordable and good quality food items.

As no single food will provide couples with the essential nutrients needed for health, the challenge is to find innovative ways to assess what the prospective mother and her partner's diet entails, and to educate them to eat a varied and balanced diet from a variety of food sources, if they are not already doing so. The information subsequently offered should be appropriate to cultural practices (Fieldhouse, 1995). An educational approach will be needed to bring about gradual changes in attitudes and flawed practices, resulting in benefits for the whole family. A balanced diet should include foods from the recognised four main food groups (Figure 18.1) as identified by the DoH (1994a, 1996b) and Health Education Authority (HEA, 1994).

SUPPLEMENTATION

The consumption of vitamin A and folic acid during pregnancy have been the subject of much debate over recent years because of their relationship to congenital abnormalities.

Folic acid

Folic acid is essential to the development of the nervous system, and a deficiency in dietary folate has been linked with neural tube defects (Medical Research Council, 1991; Czeizel and Dudas, 1992). Consequently, the DoH (1992b) recommends that all women who are planning a pregnancy, or who

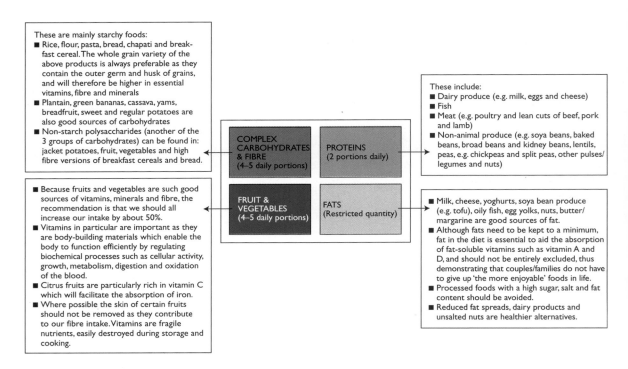

These are mainly starchy foods:
- Rice, flour, pasta, bread, chapati and breakfast cereal. The whole grain variety of the above products is always preferable as they contain the outer germ and husk of grains, and will therefore be higher in essential vitamins, fibre and minerals
- Plantain, green bananas, cassava, yams, breadfruit, sweet and regular potatoes are also good sources of carbohydrates
- Non-starch polysaccharides (another of the 3 groups of carbohydrates) can be found in: jacket potatoes, fruit, vegetables and high fibre versions of breakfast cereals and bread.

These include:
- Dairy produce (e.g. milk, eggs and cheese)
- Fish
- Meat (e.g. poultry and lean cuts of beef, pork and lamb)
- Non-animal produce (e.g. soya beans, baked beans, broad beans and kidney beans, lentils, peas, e.g. chickpeas and split peas, other pulses/legumes and nuts)

| COMPLEX CARBOHYDRATES & FIBRE (4–5 daily portions) | PROTEINS (2 portions daily) |
| FRUIT & VEGETABLES (4–5 daily portions) | FATS (Restricted quantity) |

- Because fruits and vegetables are such good sources of vitamins, minerals and fibre, the recommendation is that we should all increase our intake by about 50%.
- Vitamins in particular are important as they are body-building materials which enable the body to function efficiently by regulating biochemical processes such as cellular activity, growth, metabolism, digestion and oxidation of the blood.
- Citrus fruits are particularly rich in vitamin C which will facilitate the absorption of iron.
- Where possible the skin of certain fruits should not be removed as they contribute to our fibre intake. Vitamins are fragile nutrients, easily destroyed during storage and cooking.

- Milk, cheese, yoghurts, soya bean produce (e.g. tofu), oily fish, egg yolks, nuts, butter/margarine are good sources of fat.
- Although fats need to be kept to a minimum, fat in the diet is essential to aid the absorption of fat-soluble vitamins such as vitamin A and D, and should not be entirely excluded, thus demonstrating that couples/families do not have to give up 'the more enjoyable' foods in life.
- Processed foods with a high sugar, salt and fat content should be avoided.
- Reduced fat spreads, dairy products and unsalted nuts are healthier alternatives.

Figure 18.1: The four basic food groups of a balanced diet

are already pregnant, should take 400 µg of folic acid per day. The dose is increased for women who have had a previous pregnancy affected by neural tube defect. But the recommendation may not be applicable to all women, especially those with pre-existing medical conditions, such as epilepsy and vitamin B_{12} deficiency, as the treatment of these conditions may be adversely affected if folate supplementation is used (Enkin *et al.*, 1995).

Neural tube defects, such as **spina bifida**, occur during the period of organogenesis – conception to first 12 weeks of pregnancy when vital organs (e.g. brain and spinal cord) are being formed. This is often a period during which many women are blissfully unaware that they are pregnant. Folate supplementation 3–6 months prior to conception, and continued to the end of the first trimester of pregnancy, is therefore prudent. Theoretically speaking, the daily recommended intake of folic acid could be reached by a folate-enriched diet, achieved by eating foods which are particularly good sources of folic acid, such as yeast extract (e.g., Marmite), legumes or pulses, dark leaf vegetables (e.g. spring cabbage, spinach, callaloo – a West Indian vegetable similar to spinach but with a stronger flavour) and foods

fortified in folates (e.g. breakfast cereals, some wheat and flour products).

Even though reliable evidence now exists to suggest a direct correlation between folate supplementation and the reduction in incidence of neural tube defects (Medical Research Council, 1991), a recent study conducted by Cuskelly *et al.* (1996) highlighted the difficulties that are likely to be experienced in achieving the desired effect. The results of the research suggest that by adjusting daily dietary intake to account for folate intake may create problems because trying to calculate the amount of folic acid in food groups is very difficult; the efficacy of 0.4 mg (i.e. 400 µg) extra folate from food is questionable. Folate from food appears not to raise the plasma folate concentrations as effectively as the tablet form. Women and their families also need to be aware that folic acid may be lost from food through processing at high temperatures, leaching into cooking water, through light and through imbibing excessive alcohol.

Vitamin A

Vitamin A is essential in our diet as it regulates cell differentiation and proliferation by binding with retinoic acid, thus regulating gene expression (Rothman *et al.*, 1995). However, an excessive intake of vitamin A may result in congenital birth defects, especially cranial neural crest defects. Because of the fetotoxic effects of an excessive intake of this vitamin in the diet of pregnant women, the DoH (1990) recommends the avoidance of supplements and foods with a known elevated vitamin A content. This information should extend to couples seeking pre-conception care (Ranjan, 1991). Foods known to have a high vitamin A content are:

- Liver
- Liver pate
- Liver-based sausages.

Although caution should be exercised, an adequate intake of vitamin A in the diet is vital for good vision, healthy skin and an effectively functioning immune system.

> **Case Scenario**
>
> Michelle is 35 years old and the mother of a 10-year-old son, Matthew. She hopes to extend her family in the near future and visits the practice nurse at her local health centre to discuss a healthy eating plan. During the discussion, Michelle mentioned that she has been reading an article in her weekly woman's magazine about the dangers of excessive intake of vitamin A during pregnancy. She asks the practice nurse for more detailed information as she enjoys liver and did include it as part of her weekly diet when she was pregnant with Matthew.
>
> The practice nurse should provide relevant literature and explanation regarding the potential teratogenicity associated with an increased intake of vitamin A without being alarmist. Michelle can easily be reassured, after careful assessment of her dietary habits and likes and dislikes, that an adequate intake of vitamin A can be obtained from a food source other than liver, for example fish, dairy products and green and orange vegetables, such as spinach and carrots.

Salt in the diet should also be considered. DoH (1994a) recognised the association between dietary intake of salt and hypertension, recommending a reduction in the daily intake of salt in our diet from the level reported by the committee of approximately 9 g/day to approximately 6 g/day. This information is particularly important pre-conceptionally as the pregnant state predisposes women to hypertensive disorders. Body weight is equally important as it is considered to be a measure of health and well-being, being linked to diet and nutrition (Pickard, 1983). The body mass index (BMI) is therefore a useful guide when used as a crude indicator in assessing the average weight for height ratio (Table 18.3).

SMOKING AND ALCOHOL

Cigarette smoking before conception is an important variable affecting health and well-being, and has been increasingly cited as a cause of ill health and a major cause of premature death for both men and women (Office of Population Censuses and Surveys [OPCS], 1992); thus pre-conception education regarding the dangers of passive and active smoking should commence as early as possible, preferably during childhood education, becoming an integral part of parents', teachers' and health professionals' joint responsibility.

Maternal and paternal smoking habits are known to affect the health of the fetus, contributing to a wide range of prenatal and postnatal complications (HEA, 1993), such as:

- Ectopic pregnancy
- Miscarriage
- Antepartum haemorrhage
- Pre-term labour
- Low birth weight baby
- Stillbirth
- Sudden infant death syndrome (SIDS)
- Childhood morbidity, e.g. upper respiratory tract infections.

Additionally, a worrying trend has developed which demonstrates that while smoking prevalence has shown a sharp decline in the population as a whole, women are now the section of the population who smoke the most, especially those who are socio-economically disadvantaged (Graham, 1993). Women represent a fresh and lucrative target for the tobacco industry; therefore, the habit which had a clear male identity has firmly become a women's issue as the role of women continues to change (Chollat-Traquet, 1992). Today, women have to face increasing pressures as they struggle

Table 18.3: Body mass index

$$\frac{\text{Weight in kg}}{(\text{height in m}^2)} = \frac{58.5}{1.62 \times 1.62} = 22.3 = \text{Weight in kg divided by height in metres squared}$$

BMI	Category	Effect	Example
<20	Underweight	Increased risk of amenorrhoea and infertility. Long-term health problems	19.5 = 8 st 11 lb
20–24.9	Desirable	Best range for pregnancy and long-term health	22.3 = 9 st 3 lbs
25–29.9	Moderate obesity	Slight risk to health. May lead to severe obesity	27.5 = 11 st 5 lb
30	Severe obesity	Increased risk of menstrual problems and pregnancy complications. Long-term health hazard	30.3 = 12 st 7 lb

Examples given are for a 5' 4" (1.62 metres) woman.
Adapted from Pickard, 1983, page 424.

to juggle the demands of, for example, being career women, mothers, daughters and lovers.

Case Scenario

Julie is 27 years old and has two children from a previous relationship; the children are aged 3 and 4, respectively. Julie is pregnant for the third time by a new partner, who left her on hearing that she was expecting twins. She now lives with her children in a two-bedroomed third floor council flat, in a socially deprived area. She has no social support from her family as they do not approve of her pregnancy. Julie has always been a heavy smoker, smoking in excess of 20 cigarettes per day. She is fully conversant with the risks to her own health as well as her existing children and developing fetuses, but feels unable to change her smoking habit.

Julie's situation highlights the dilemma many women face who are socially isolated, caught in the poverty trap and who feel trapped by their financial and material circumstances. Women like Julie will need social support, understanding and carers who are non-judgemental. It will be difficult for Julie to kick the habit if she has no child care, little money and hungry mouths to feed.

For the woman who is socially disadvantaged, 'smoking provides a way of keeping going when women have little going for them' (Graham 1994; page 103), the very women who would benefit most from pre-conception care but who are the least likely to get it. The link between low income and smoking therefore throws light on the wider debate between poverty and ill health, and begs the question whether the increased morbidity and mortality associated with socially deprived families are the result of their lifestyle, rather than their material circumstances (Graham, 1993).

Details relating to pre-conception assessment of smoking habits should include:

- Past and present smoking habits
- Assessment of knowledge regarding the effects of passive and active smoking
- Knowledge of self-help groups and strategies that may help
- Assessment of socio-economic status so that families at risk can be identified and appropriate help and support mobilised
- Ability to stop and stay stopped (i.e. degree of motivation, quality of social support, previous attempts to stop, confidence and commitment towards smoking cessation).

In relation to smoking cessation, Prochaska and DiClemente (1983) identified five categories in the process of behavioural change:

- Pre-contemplation: lack of awareness of lifestyle problems with no intention of altering behaviour

- Contemplation: being aware of health risks and contemplating changes but not quite ready to take positive action
- Preparation: having an intention to alter lifestyle in the next month
- Action: successfully modifying the identified behaviour for a significant period ranging from 1 day up to 6 months
- Maintenance: remaining focused and motivated, continually engaging in new lifestyle modification for more than 6 months, and working towards preventing relapses and maximising on gains.

Different interventions will be required at each of the stages outlined, e.g. education, information, clear objectives, action plan, timescales, use of diary or other self-monitoring device, plus encouragement and support (Elford *et al.*, 1994). The framework requires flexibility and fluidity to allow for the expected relapse and cyclical progression through all five stages.

Effects of alcohol on health and well-being

Alcohol consumption is a habit that is usually established well before conception, and is often linked to smoking. The reasons for imbibing alcohol are manifold (R.G. Smart, 1991). According to Barbour (1990) couples may drink alcohol for any of the following reasons:

- Social reasons, for example to celebrate
- Psychological reasons, for example to cope with stress and internal conflict

- Intrinsic reasons, for example for the taste and to quench thirst.

However, women must be aware that alcohol consumed during pregnancy readily crosses the placenta and diffuses into the fetal circulation. In addition, alcohol may inhibit the multiplication and division of cells, resulting in fewer and smaller cells (Plant, 1990). Of concern is the fact that no one seems to know how much is too much in predisposing the fetus to fetal alcohol syndrome (FAS) and fetal alcohol effects (FAE). The former remains at the extreme end of the scale and relates to a triad of symptoms, i.e. fetal and neonatal growth deficiency and central nervous system dysfunction, including mental retardation and other major systematic **dysmorphic** features (Autti-Ramo and Granstrom, 1992). FAE, on the other hand, describes the milder form of the condition, e.g. learning difficulties, maladaptive behaviour, hyperactivity and attention deficit (Barbour, 1990). The increased use of alcohol during pregnancy may also predispose to miscarriages and low birth weight babies.

The Department of Health Interdepartmental Working Group (DoH, 1995) recommended an increased threshold in the maximum safe limits for alcohol consumption of 21 units for women and 28 units for men. However, Edward (1996) challenged the increase, suggesting that the previous rate of 14 units for women and 21 units for men would perhaps be more sensible. Hence the unit system identified by the Royal College of Physicians (RCOP, 1991) is still useful in assessing our weekly intake of alcohol (Figure 18.2). However, the safe limits must not be oversimplified by taking the limits as a cut-off point between what levels are deemed safe and what levels are deemed unsafe. Conversely, the safe limits have no way of accounting for our inherent characteristics, such as height, weight, sex, genetic background and personality, all of which

One unit of alcohol is equivalent to:

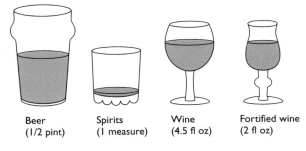

| Beer | Spirits | Wine | Fortified wine |
| (1/2 pint) | (1 measure) | (4.5 fl oz) | (2 fl oz) |

Figure 18.2: Standard units for the measurement of alcohol
(Source: RCOG, 1991)

Two Key Points

- A heavy drinker is defined as a woman who drinks 35 units of alcohol per week or a man who drinks 50 units of alcohol per week.
- A problem drinker is defined as an individual whose physical or psychosocial well-being has been harmed as a consequence of drinking.

can affect the way in which alcohol is metabolised within the body. Assessing an individual's intake of alcohol is, therefore, never easy, as questions designed to elicit information on the pattern of couples' drinking habits may be construed by the carer/counsellor as rather intrusive, and could be glossed over. Nevertheless, it is an important part of the health assessment and should be treated accordingly. Couples can be informed, in a sensitive, non-threatening and supportive way, of the benefits of using a diary to chart their drinking habits.

CONTRACEPTION

A pregnancy should always be carefully planned for the reasons previously outlined. Assessment and education around family planning and spacing during the pre-conception period should be sensitive, non-judgemental, respectful of sociocultural and religious influences, as well as the personal preferences of the woman and her partner.

Women who are using a hormonal method of contraception will need to discontinue its use 3–6 months before conception to allow the body to readjust the artificially raised ovarian hormones in conjunction with the levels of some essential minerals and vitamins, which may have been depleted. Intrauterine contraceptive devices, i.e. the coil, should be removed and barrier methods such as the sheath, Femidom or diaphragm employed, as they are more suitable alternatives from a health perspective. Table 18.4 summarises the key factors that should be considered when discussing contraception with couples.

SCREENING/INVESTIGATIONS AND OUTLETS FOR PRE-PREGNANCY CARE

Following careful assessment of the couple's health and lifestyle (which should include past and present medical, surgical and psychosocial histories, as well as the woman's past obstetric background), a number of screening tests may be performed depending on their individual case scenario, as outlined below:

- Blood group and rhesus factor
- Full blood count
- Urinalysis

Table 18.4: Pre-pregnancy care and methods of contraception – main factors to be considered

Physical
- Health and well-being
- Underlying medical condition, e.g. diabetes mellitus, hypertension
- Drugs being taken, e.g. antibiotics, anticonvulsants
- Maternal weight
- Recent rubella or hepatitis B vaccination
- Previous pelvic infection
- Parity, i.e. number of existing children
- Family/personal history of congenital anomalies
- Current method of contraception being used, if any
- Age of couple

Psychological
- Motivation
- Psychological well-being
- Choice of methods and control/ability to cope
- Aesthetically acceptable

Social
- Cultural and religious beliefs
- Accessibility of facilities
- Safe and safer sexual practices
- Desirable family size and spacing
- Cost of availability of method(s)
- Use of primary health services, e.g. well persons' clinic for men and women
- Education of the couple/ability to understand
- Lifestyle – substance abuse, e.g. alcohol, smoking, other drugs
- Supportive/unsupportive, who is responsible/irresponsible
- Research evidence regarding efficacy/risks

- Blood pressure
- Height and weight
- Cervical cytology
- Breast/testicular examination.

Specific screening/investigations

- Haemoglobinopathies for sickle cell trait and thalassaemia
- Hepatitis B surface antigen
- Human immunodeficiency virus (HIV) status
- *Chlamydia*
- **Phenylalanine** levels if woman has phenylketonuria

- The TORCH screen – this is an acronym which describes a group of infections:
  - T – toxoplasmosis
  - O – other infections, e.g. syphilis, chlamydia, group B haemolytic streptococcus
  - R – rubella
  - C – cytomegalovirus
  - H – herpes simplex group of viruses.

Possible outlets for pre-pregnancy care

Pre-conception care can be provided in a variety of different settings, and the responsibility for the provision of care not only rests with members of the primary health care team, but with society as a whole. Table 18.5 gives a summary of likely outlets for care provision in conjunction with people who may help.

Key Points

- Vitamins, minerals and trace elements such as zinc should be part of a healthy and varied diet. The diet should contain a variety of water- and fat-soluble vitamins.

- A balanced intake of vitamins, minerals and trace elements will necessitate avoidance of excesses as well as deficiencies. Vitamin A and folates are two good examples.
- Poverty, poor housing and unemployment are inextricably linked to increased morbidity and mortality.
- Smoking undermines health of mother, partner, fetus/baby and general health of other family members.
- The pre-conception period is a good time to promote health and well-being in order to bring about long-term behavioural changes.
- Couples who smoke and who are caught in the poverty trap can be helped to give up smoking by assistance with improved housing and living conditions.

WOMAN AS THE FOCUS OF MATERNITY CARE

Over a long history contemporary Western society has undergone major political and sociocultural changes in attitudes and beliefs towards child-

Table 18.5: Outlets for pre-conception care provision and possible sources of help

Outlets for pre-conception care	People who may help
- Family planning clinics - Church halls - Community centres - Youth clubs - Health centres - General practitioner surgeries - Schools - Well men's and well women's clinics - Media - Postnatal follow-up clinics	Members of the primary health care team who may consist of: - General practitioner - Midwife - Health visitor - Practice nurse - School nurse - Social worker - District nurse - Physiotherapist - Community psychiatrist nurse Significant others: - Occupational health therapist - Obstetrician - Teacher - Geneticist - Diabetic liaison nurse speicalist - Dietitian/nutritionalist - Advocacy/link workers - Television programme managers and presenters

birth (Tew, 1990). It is well recognised that the shift from home to hospital as the ubiquitous place of birth, the deskilling of many midwives and the gate-keeping presence of many obstetricians have all contributed to the stark rise in medicalisation of childbirth throughout this century (Treichler, 1990; Reissmann, 1992; Donnison, 1993).

The increase in medicalisation throughout the 1970s and 1980s contributed to an apparent confrontation between women and their professional carers. Understandably, women were becoming increasingly angry that their ability to take control, make informed choices and to experience birth as a satisfying and meaningful sociocultural event has been hijacked by the more dominant ideology of the biomedical paradigm (Davis-Floyd, 1990; Garcia et al., 1990; Jacobus et al., 1990).

The growth in consumerism coupled with women's dissatisfaction with their care heralded major reforms to the organisation of maternity care, resulting in a reformation not only in the delivery of maternity care, but a major change in the structure of the National Health Service (NHS) as a whole. The NHS and Community Care Act 1990 enshrined the principle of competition as the motivating factor in the assurance and delivery of quality health care (Harrison et al., 1992; Taylor et al., 1992). This ensures that the contemporary maternity service is constantly audited, evaluated, expert clinical advice sought and contracts given to the provider who is both cost-effective and able to ensure that a high standard of care is delivered to the users of the service (Walton and Hamilton, 1995).

Ostensibly, the last Conservative government pledged its commitment to give power to the people, resulting in a succession of publications such as *The Citizen's Charter* (DoH, 1991a), *Maternity Services Charter* (DoH, 1994c) and *The Named Midwife* (DoH 1991b). The concept of empowerment was, therefore, popularised. Gibson (1991) argues that empowerment is a complex term which attracts varying definitions, thus making it difficult to conceptualise. Nevertheless, Gillen (1995) and Hawks (1992) define empowerment as an 'interpersonal process' of providing the resources, tools and environment to develop, build and increase the ability and effectiveness of others to set and reach goals for individual social ends.

It is clear, then, that midwives cannot empower or value others unless they too feel valued. Hence, a real shift in power from service provider (mid-

wife) to service user (the pregnant woman) may be hampered if the service provider feels threatened and undermined (Chavasse, 1992; Evans, 1993). Some midwives and doctors may resist the empowerment of service users due to many factors, not least being their own socialisation and experience of medicalisation, as well as their long-standing cultural attitudes of being in 'charge' of the pregnant woman (Lovell, 1996). Clearly, then, empowerment may be limited in helping pregnant women to take control of their lives. The concept is also politically weighted, as midwives may be expected to take on an increasing workload for no extra remuneration (Wright, 1995). There can be little doubt that medicalisation has polarised two groups of women – midwives and mothers – who may be at odds with each other, thus mirroring the worst aspect of medicalisation of childbirth, user and provider divided yet strangely united in a common endeavour.

The test, then, is to try and theorise just what it is about some midwives and childbearing women that may put them at odds with each other. In part the answer lies in the process by which midwives and childbearing women are rendered powerless in the wider patriarchal society (Porter, 1990; Witz, 1992; McCrea and Crute, 1994). Because midwives are predominantly women, many are expected to give selflessly of their time to care for women, and then return home to carry on their gendered role of caring, such as attending to the demands of being a mother, daughter and lover (Kitzinger, 1989; Walton and Hamilton, 1995).

OPPOSING MODELS OF CHILDBIRTH

A further confrontation developed as a result of the medicalisation of childbirth, between two distinct models and philosophies of childbirth. In the first – the pathological model – pregnancy and birth are perceived as partially diseased processes, which are located firmly within the realms of medical or scientific discourse, with no respect for wider sociocultural influences (Oakley and Houd, 1990; Treichler, 1990; Reissmann, 1992; Donnison, 1993). The premise is that all births require expert management and control by the expert technician (the doctor), thus justifying the 'clinical gaze', i.e. surveillance by the gate-keeping presence of the obstetrician, who erroneously believes that responsibility for the care of the pregnant woman rests completely with him (Lupton, 1994). The second model is situated within a social context, being respectful of the individuality of women from diverse social settings. It acknowledges the physiological process of birth, but not at the exclusion of important psychological and cultural influences. Within this context, pregnancy and birth are seen as major life events powerfully shaped by culture, affecting every woman's psyche at a very profound level (Price, 1988; Oakley and Houd, 1990). Bryar (1988, 1995) examines and summarises the two opposing views of childbirth (Table 18.6), which is useful in helping us to understand why childbirth continues to be a site of 'contested meanings' (C. Smart, 1991).

CHANGING CHILDBIRTH

Women's dissatisfaction with the lack of information, lack of choice in the decision-making process relating to their care, and lack of power and control over the entire birth experience contributed to the publication of the House of Commons Health Committee's Report on the maternity services, commonly known as the Winterton Report (DoH, 1992c). It has been hailed as a benchmark, and heralded as the most radical review of the maternity services ever carried out within the UK (Walton and Hamilton, 1995). The three key elements of pregnancy and childbirth in relation to service users are identified as:

- Continuity of care with carer
- A woman's choice in the decision-making process regarding her care and preferred place of birth
- A woman's right to gain control over her body at all times during pregnancy and birth.

The implications of the report have far-reaching consequences, requiring providers of maternity care to shift thinking away from the comfort of conventional practices, to an emboldened service that fosters a woman-centred approach to care and committed to change. Achieving the vision of Changing Childbirth is outlined in Figure 18.3.

Table 18.6: Medical perspectives of pregnancy versus pregnancy as a normal life event

Medical perspectives	Normal perspective
■ Birth is normal only in retrospect ■ Doctor in charge ■ Choice and control denied ■ Information restricted and likely to be biased, with a tendency to scare ■ Safety is an overriding factor ■ Prevention of physical complications ■ Tendency to adopt a 'blanket approach' to care ■ Increased chance of labelling and stereotyping women, if they deviate from what is seen as the 'norm', e.g. a challenging and questioning woman is likely to be labelled as 'difficult' as she refuses to be a passive and compliant 'patient' ■ Birth likely to be more technological with increased risk of intervention ■ The usual case as interesting	■ Birth is normal in anticipation ■ Woman and family major decision makers and equal partners ■ Woman and family in control ■ Information shared and unbiased ■ Safety an important factor but not used to deny access to choice and voice ■ Development of women and their partners through the experience of pregnancy ■ Holistic care is fostered ■ Heterogeneity of women is acknowledged and respected ■ Technology and intervention only employed with maternal consent and if their use can be justified ■ No two pregnancies are the same; thus each pregnancy seen as a unique experience for each woman
Outcomes Because the issue of safety dominates then the main outcome is to have a live, healthy mother and baby	**Outcomes** Psychosocial factors are equally important to those of the physiological processes of birth. The main outcome is, therefore, concerned with realising a live mother and baby as well as the woman's satisfaction and fulfilment with the whole experience of pregnancy and birth

Adapted from Bryar, 1988.

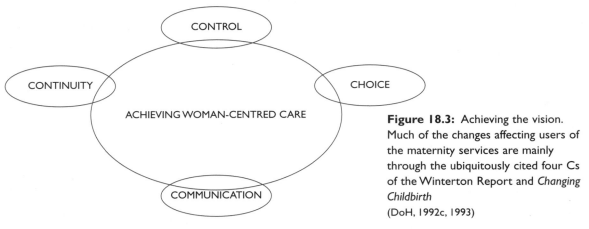

Figure 18.3: Achieving the vision. Much of the changes affecting users of the maternity services are mainly through the ubiquitously cited four Cs of the Winterton Report and *Changing Childbirth* (DoH, 1992c, 1993)

Changing Childbirth (DoH, 1993), the successor policy document to the Winterton Report, also acknowledges that in the past women have not been given the opportunity to make informed choices, to be treated as equal partners in their care, or to have a real range of facilities from which to choose. The report therefore identified 10 indicators of success which are to be achieved within 5 years of publication of the report (Table 18.7).

CHOICE

The concept of choice can be seen as the ultimate test of midwives' and doctors' commitment to a woman-centred philosophy of care. The Winterton Committee concluded:

' . . . There is a widespread demand among women for greater choice in the type of care they receive, and the present structure of the maternity services frustrates, rather than facilitates those who wish to exercise their choice.'
(DoH, 1992c, para 52)

Brook's and Black's (1994) survey also concluded that the care women wanted from the maternity service was not necessarily what they received (Table 18.8). Clearly, then, choices in childbirth are important if the individuality of women is to be respected. An understanding of the concept empowers health care professionals to be knowledgeable about the range of services that can be offered to women, and to be aware of the available evidence regarding their effectiveness (Anderson, 1996).

Since the publication of *Changing Childbirth* (DoH, 1993), a lot of work has been undertaken nationally to increase women's awareness regarding the choices available during pregnancy and childbirth. The Midwives' Information and Resource Service (MIDIRS) in conjunction with

Table 18.7: Changing childbirth: 10 indicators of success

1 All women should be entitled to carry their own notes.
2 Every woman should know one midwife who ensures continuity of her midwifery care – the named midwife.
3 At least 30% of women should have the midwife as the lead professional.
4 Every woman should know the lead professional who has key role in the planning and provision of her care.
5 At least 75% of women should know the person who cares for them during their delivery.
6 Midwives should have direct access to some beds in all maternity units.
7 At least 30% of women delivered in a maternity unit should be admitted under the management of the midwife.
8 The real number of antenatal visits for women with uncomplicated pregnancies should have been reviewed in the light of the available evidence and the RCOG guidelines.
9 All front-line ambulances should have a paramedic able to support the midwife who needs to transfer a woman to hospital in an emergency.
10 All women should have access to information about the services available in their locality.

Adapted from DoH (1993, page 70).

Table 18.8: What women want from the providers of maternity care and what they get

	Women get	Women want
Care location and environment	Hospital antenatal care and inadequate transport	Antenatal services close to home, comfortable and child-friendly
Type of care	Didactic care with little or no choice	Full involvement in care plans and decisions
Care pattern	Lack of continuity – no choice of carer	Continuity of care and choice of lead professional
Relationship with health professional	Paternalistic attitude: 'provider knows best'	Equal and respectful partnership
Appointments	Antenatal clinic visits coincide with work and family 'conveyor belt' approach	Individualised approach, humane system
Information	Poor and inconsistent	Comprehensive, clear and unbiased
Communication	Poor, impersonal care, advice and support	Care personalised, meeting individual needs with an open and trusted carer

Adapted from Brooks and Black, 1994, page 33.

the NHS Centre for Reviews and Dissemination launched their informed choice leaflets and accompanying video, at the end of 1995. This is a series of fully referenced leaflets for maternity care health professionals and parents. A range of controversial and contemporary issues of general interest to women are addressed, such as ultrasound scanning, positions for labour and delivery, alcohol consumption, support in labour, fetal heart monitoring and eating and drinking in labour. Each leaflet is produced in two forms:

- One aimed at parents, explaining key information in an attractive, accessible and unambiguous way, making the information presented easy to read. The series also caters for couples whose first language is not English.
- The second leaflet is targeted at health care professionals. The leaflets are fully referenced and provide a summary of available research evidence, promoting evidence-based practice rather than practice rooted in custom and tradition.

The project is funded by the DoH and it is hoped that a variety of topics of interest to women and their professional carers will be added to the series on a regular basis. For further information contact:

MIDIRS
9 Elmdale Road
Clifton
Bristol
BS8 1SL
Tel: 01179 251791

CONTINUITY

Continuity of care relates to the care that women receive; it should be consistent, reliable and non-conflicting, preventing duplication, confusion and fragmentation of care (DoH, 1992c). Continuity of care may take two forms:

- Continuity of care within an identified team
- Continuity of care with named carer.

The team approach to care

According to the Institute of Manpower Studies (IMPS) who undertook the research into team midwifery on behalf of the DoH:

'. . . Team midwifery, has become a broad generic term which refers to a wide range of practices. There is no agreed definition of team midwifery.'
(Wraight *et al.*, 1993, page 15)

In response to the varying definitions, coupled with working patterns of team midwifery, the IMPS Report developed a scoring system for defining an effective team approach to care – effective because the characteristics identified are the features which guarantee satisfactory results for women experiencing continuity of care. According to Wraight *et al.* (1993, page 123), these are as follows:

- Team consists of no more than six midwives
- Each team has a defined caseload
- Team provides total care for that caseload
- Team works in all areas according to client need
- 50% or more women are delivered by a midwife known to them.

Team midwifery was implemented during the 1980s in an effort to improve continuity of care for childbearing women, and describes a group of midwives and possible other health professionals, e.g. general practitioner (GP) and/or obstetrician, who provide a defined pattern of care for a group of childbearing women. The group may be large or small, users of the service may be defined or unspecified, and the care provided may embrace all aspects of maternity care or focus on certain components of that care. The concept of team midwifery, although altruistic, continues to be cloaked in problems even though many models have been tried and tested. Figures 18.4 and 18.5 attempt to compare and contrast the benefits and difficulties of team midwifery with the more traditional model of care.

CONTINUITY OF CARE WITH CARER

Continuity of care with carer has provided one of the main challenges to the reformed maternity service in recent years (Flint, 1991; Ball *et al.*, 1992; Wraight *et al.*, 1993; Page, 1995; Sandall, 1995). The DoH (1993, page 70) identified that 'at least 75% of women should know the person who cares for them during delivery'. Yet only a minority of pregnant women have real continuity of care with a professional they know and trust for the duration of their pregnancy, labour, and post-delivery period (Raynor, 1995; Sandall, 1995).

The crux of the matter is that women's expectation of care may be greater than can be achieved by named midwives, who may find that as their responsibilities and roles expand well beyond traditional boundaries they cannot meet the everyday demands of being on call 24 hours (Warwick, 1995). This means that the whole issue of service users' empowerment may pose a real contradiction for their largely female carers – midwives. Newburn (1995) poignantly reflects:

> 'Mothers and midwives have dissimilar, as well as similar interests. They are user and provider, respectively. The convenience of one, may cause discomfort for the other. There is no doubt that if women are to have care which is tailored to meet their needs, midwives will pay a price for it.'
> (Newburn, 1995, page 32)

In any case, it is questionable whether all woman want continuity of care with a named carer, as the quality of care may not always be enhanced. In a small-scale study conducted by Lee (1994), women reported that first they wanted a carer who inspired confidence, followed by a safe and competent practitioner; knowing the midwife was ranked fifth by the respondents. There is no doubt that continuity of care with a known carer will continue to be a real challenge for the midwifery service in years to come.

COMMUNICATION

All meaningful relationships are fundamentally dependent on effective communication, and since maternity care is essentially an interactive process, developing good practice through effective communication is the key to cultivating helpful and

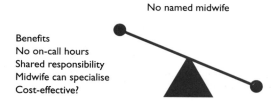

No named midwife

Benefits
No on-call hours
Shared responsibility
Midwife can specialise
Cost-effective?

Fragmented care
Several carers
Conflicting advice
Loss of control (woman)
Difficulties

Figure 18.4: The benefits and difficulties of having no named midwife
(Adapted from Wraight, 1995, page 9 and reproduced with kind permission of English National Board)

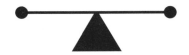

Named midwife within a team

Small team – recognised caseload – one named midwife –
other associate midwives (all known to woman) –
shared responsibility – shared on call –
team philosophy of care

Figure 18.5: The benefits having a named midwife (Adapted from Wraight, 1995, page 9 and reproduced with kind permission of English National Board)

meaningful relationships between women and their carers (Hicks, 1993). Studies have illuminated how a two-way exchange of good information is one of the major determinants of women's satisfaction with their care (Green *et al.*, 1988; Kirkham, 1992).

Part 2 of *Changing Childbirth* (DoH, 1993) is dedicated entirely to the results of a survey which gives tangible examples of good communication practice in the maternity service. Patterns of communication in the maternity service have long been flawed, because of the power imbalance between women and their carers, negating women's experience of childbirth and reinforcing the control of the health care professionals over the pregnant woman (Lupton, 1994). Essentially, then, if the woman is to choose freely from the information communicated to her about her options for care, the power in the midwife–mother and mother–doctor relationship must be

diffused. Improved communications will bring positive benefits for women, who are less likely to feel anxious and more inclined to achieve a sense of satisfaction if they receive adequate information (Kirkham, 1993). The benefits of effective communication versus the effects of ineffective communication are summarised in Table 18.9.

CONTROL

Control is the final of the four C's identified by the Department of Health (DoH, 1992c, 1993) as one of the key principles deemed a measure of good practice. Women must have control to make informed decisions about a multitude of different issues affecting their care, such as options of care, named carer(s), antenatal screening test, labour room technology and birth environment of their own choosing. There are still many hurdles to overcome in the quest to provide a more woman-centred focus for care. A number of obstacles stand in the way of progress and have far-reaching consequences for mothers and midwives. Shifting the locus of control effected through arbitrary rules, confining technological equipment, hospital protocols and rituals invoked by complete strangers, coupled with a host of other factors, continue to contribute to women's sense of disappointment and loss of control over their bodies. Finally, we must not forget that the interprofessional rivalry between midwives and doctors continues to exert tacit forms of power and control

Table 18.9: Effects of good versus bad communication practice in maternity care

Effects of good communication	Effects of bad communication
■ Less room for errors and misdiagnosis	■ More room for errors and misdiagnosis
■ Empowers woman to make informed choices and maintain control	■ Disempowers woman, denies choice and creates passivity
■ Promotes knowledge and understanding	■ Promotes poor knowledge and understanding
■ Women more inclined to ask questions	■ Woman likely to be frustrated and less inclined to ask questions
■ Woman more likely to receive care which is personalised, respectful and kind	■ Care more likely to be depersonalised, insensitive and generalised
■ Woman more likely to be treated as equal partner in her care	■ Cultivation of partnership less likely, therefore increased risk of unequal relationship
■ Woman more likely to heed health education advice	■ Increased chance of non-compliance to treatment
■ Reduced risk of litigation	■ Increased risk of litigation
■ Woman more likely to feel satisfied, fulfilled and psychologically prepared to face the challenges of motherhood	■ Greater margin for dissatisfaction and mother being psychologically ill prepared to take on the powerful role of motherhood

by means of a set of prescribed actions and limits (Annandale, 1988), even though efforts are being made nationally to combat this trend (DoH, 1996c).

Key Points

- Choice, continuity, control and effective communication are fundamental to a woman-centred approach to care.
- Health professionals should continue to increase a woman's knowledge and sense of control by providing clear, unbiased information, a balanced discussion of choices and respecting the difficult decisions that many women have to make pertaining to their care.
- All women, regardless of their cultural background, should have their special needs met in a special way.
- Doctors and midwives have a moral obligation to work together, ensuring justice and positively contributing to the health of mothers and tomorrow's generation.

CARE IN PREGNANCY AND CHILDBIRTH

This section of the chapter will focus on the psychosocial aspects of childbirth. The author has deliberately excluded relevant physiology of pregnancy and childbirth to make way for some of the important psychosocial factors during the antepartum, intrapartum and postpartum periods, which have largely been ignored in the past. For the physiological changes during pregnancy and childbirth the reader is directed to some of the more popular midwifery textbooks, and is expected to have an understanding of:

- Maternal physiological adaptation to pregnancy and the diagnosis of pregnancy
- The process of fertilisation and development of the embryo/fetus
- Minor disorders of pregnancy and relevant health education information that may be provided by carers
- The physiology of labour and the physiology of pain.

ANTENATAL CARE

Pregnancy is typically depicted as a period of heightened sensitivity as many women embark on a journey into the unknown (Oakley, 1993). This is a critical time, culminating in major upheavals in the life of the pregnant woman (Price, 1988). The aims of antenatal care should not only account for the physical needs of the woman, but should also focus on the woman's and her partner's ability to adapt to change and cope with the anxieties and worries of impending parenthood (Ball 1994). The aims of antenatal care, therefore, are manifold and are summarised in Figure 18.6.

The pattern and organisation of antenatal care

The pattern within antenatal care of seeing women once a month until 28 weeks of gestation, then every 2 weeks until 36 weeks, followed by antenatal examination at weekly intervals until the commencement of labour was started in 1929, following the recommendations of the Ministry of Health (Currell, 1990; Charles, 1992). This practice now seems rather anachronistic, in the light of a woman-centred approach to care, and has been the subject of fierce criticism, with efforts being made to adjust the pattern of antenatal visits to meet the needs of women on an individual basis. This seems sensible, as the quintessence of a woman-centred approach to care in pregnancy and childbirth is to create a service which gets rid of wastage, duplication and fragmentation of care, whilst fostering a service which enhances a woman's satisfaction with the care provided. Collaboration and cooperation are therefore needed on the part of all care providers to ensure that antenatal care is tailored to service users' needs. During the antenatal period the woman will make decisions regarding her preference in relation to the type of care she receives (Figure 18.7) and the birth environment of her choosing (Figure 18.8).

Home births

Safety is an important issue in the provision of care as the aim is to have a live and healthy mother and baby at the end of pregnancy and labour. However, safety has been the main factor used to deny many women their choice (Tew, 1990). Although safety is

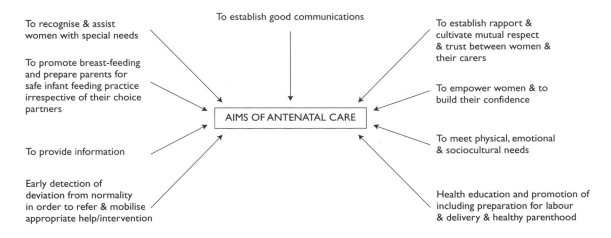

Figure 18.6: Aims of antenatal care

'part of a greater picture encompassing all aspects of health and well-being' (DoH, 1993, para 2.1.6), it should not be used as a stick with which to beat women. Approximately 98% of all births now occur within a hospital setting (Campbell and Macfarlane, 1994).

The DOMINO scheme

This scheme is sometimes offered to women who want a minimum hospital stay, i.e. a stay of 6 hours post-delivery, or those who want a home birth but who may have a poor obstetric history. **DOMINO** literally means 'domiciliary midwifery in and out'. In theory, the mother receives care with her named community-based midwife (or another midwife in the same team) during pregnancy, labour and puerperium. Once labour commences, the midwife usually assesses the woman at home before arranging for her admission to the chosen maternity unit. The midwife will accompany the woman to hospital, provide her with support and encouragement during labour, help her to give birth and then return with the woman 6 hours later back to her community, to continue the postnatal care of both mother and baby. The DOMINO scheme places a heavy burden on an already stretched midwifery service and is rarely promoted, as demand tends to outstrip supply.

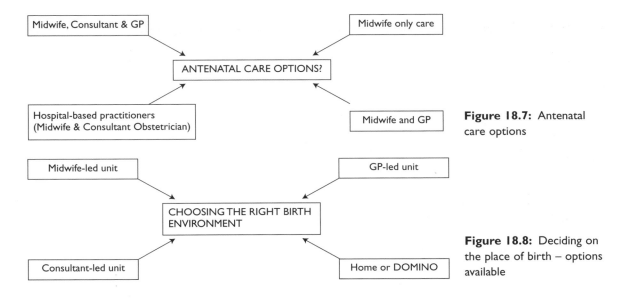

Figure 18.7: Antenatal care options

Figure 18.8: Deciding on the place of birth – options available

Consultant-led care

Care under this umbrella relates to care which comes under the jurisdiction of a named consultant obstetrician. The hospital-based midwife usually works in partnership with the identified consultant in providing antepartum, intrapartum and postpartum care. The woman will usually give birth to her baby in the hospital setting and will have a choice regarding her length of stay in the post-delivery period. This will be influenced by a variety of factors, e.g. mode of delivery, quality of social support, cultural practice, condition of baby at birth and demands for maternity beds.

Midwife-led unit

The predominant model of shared care in the UK, i.e. care divided between midwives, GPs and obstetricians, has been researched and its efficacy criticised (Murphy-Black, 1992; Hundley et al., 1994). However, a growth of midwife-led units is helping to redress the balance. In a midwife-led unit, midwives are truly autonomous, accountable practitioners; being experts in normal midwifery, they can care for women who want to experience a normal, natural birth, referring care to the obstetrician only if there is a clear indication to do so.

This may benefit the woman in many ways, as there is more chance of realising greater satisfaction for the woman, coupled with the likelihood of reduced intervention (Hundley et al., 1994). This is supported by encouraging results from a randomised controlled trial of midwife-managed care (Turnbull et al., 1996). The researchers concluded that more work needs to be done to foster more evidence-based practices, for example reducing the use of unnecessary routines and interventions, such as continuous fetal heart monitoring during uncomplicated labour.

General practitioner-managed units

These have rapidly declined since the beginning of the 1980s (Tew, 1990). Consequently, there are now only a few isolated units remaining nationally as most of them have been closed down or incorporated into larger district general hospitals, which house all the consultant-managed obstetric units. This allows easy access and transfer of care to the obstetric team should an emergency arise.

ANTENATAL SCREENING AND DIAGNOSTIC TESTS

Advances in technology have resulted in a plethora of antenatal screening and diagnostic tests. These are too numerous to examine in any depth, and so a list of some of the more common blood tests along with more invasive forms of investigation will be presented (Table 18.10), allowing examination in depth of some of the thorny issues around antenatal screening and diagnosis. Not all the investiga-

Table 18.10: Selected antenatal screening and diagnostic tests

Blood tests in pregnancy	Other probable investigations
■ ABO blood group and rhesus factor ■ Antibody titres (usually reserved for rhesus-negative woman as well as for women who have had a blood transfusion in the past) ■ Full blood count (FBC) including Hb estimation ■ Rubella titre ■ Maternal serum alphafetoprotein (MSAFP) ■ Predictive testing for Down's syndrome ■ Haemoglobinopathies – sickle cell and thalassaemia ■ Serology testing for hepatitis B surface antigen (HBsAg) and HIV (especially for at-risk groups) ■ Glycosylated haemoglobin (HBA1$_1$) for women with diabetes mellitus ■ Venereal Disease Research Laboratory test (VDRL), e.g. syphilis	■ Cervical cytology ■ Midstream specimen of urine (MSU) for asymptomatic bacteriuria ■ Titres for *Toxoplasma gondii* ■ High vaginal swab (HVS) for group B haemolytic streptococci **Non-invasive investigation** ■ Ultrasound **Invasive investigations** ■ Amniocentesis ■ Chorionic villus sampling/biopsy

tions detailed will apply to every pregnant woman. Women should be seen as individuals with clear, unbiased information forming part of the counselling process to enable them to make informed decisions. Many are still faced with a situation where they have to opt out of rather than opt in to screening programmes.

Ethical considerations

Screening for fetal abnormalities has become an integral part of antenatal care for the majority of pregnant women (Green, 1990). The author further asserts that antenatal screening tests have brought an added dimension of burden to bear on women when pregnancy, for most, is already an extremely testing time. Many pregnant women and their partners now have to make complex decisions that their mothers and grandmothers perhaps did not have to encounter. Consequently, Green *et al.* (1993) concluded that antenatal screening and diagnostic tests have opened doors that cannot be closed again.

Moral and ethical principles should, therefore, be applied to all antenatal screening tests, ranging from a simple blood test to the more invasive investigations of amniocentesis and chorionic villus sampling. With this in mind, counselling must be offered prior to screening to enable women to understand the purpose and implications of the test, and to make informed decisions based on accurate information. Green (1990, page 26) identified the main ethical issues that should underpin all prenatal screening/diagnostic tests, as follows:

- The purpose of the test, i.e. what is being investigated and/or what abnormality is being screened
- The accuracy of the test, i.e. the likelihood of predicting or diagnosing the specified abnormality
- An explanation of what the procedure involves
- Risks and benefits of the procedure
- The meaning of the results, e.g. concepts of 'high' and 'low' risk.
- Options for further investigations especially if the test is only predictive and not diagnostic, e.g. blood test for MSAFP levels and that taken for Down's syndrome
- Limitations of the test and an outline of further investigations that may be necessitated, along with their risk factors.

Main challenges

The new reproductive technologies cannot guarantee a healthy or 'perfect' baby; therefore, the concept of choice is a dubious one. Hence, prenatal screening and diagnosis will always bring difficult philosophical dilemmas in terms of choice. The danger of women becoming overwhelmed, overloaded and utterly confused as a result of the growth of antenatal screening tests is real, and cannot be ignored. At best, the very tests which are meant to put a woman's mind at rest create unnecessary anxiety, tending to frustrate rather than reassure, and may very well render the woman incapable of making an informed choice (Rothman, 1986; Reid, 1988; Richards, 1989; Green, 1994). Equally worrying is the fact that some women do not seem to realise that the ultrasound scans they favour during pregnancy, because of their visual impact, are in fact a screening tool (Green, 1990).

So although different issues will arise from the array of antenatal screening/diagnostic tests, some common findings do emerge. First, to have doubt cast upon the health of the fetus is an unwelcome stressor, especially for those women with no prior reason to consider themselves at risk. So whatever the benefits of screening, there is no escaping the fact that anxieties will be generated for a proportion of women whose fetuses, are, in fact, healthy. Second, one of the main problems of prenatal testing is that the investigations performed cannot guarantee 100% accuracy. Hubbard (1992) states:

'... All tests must be as specific as possible, that means that there must be a high degree of probability that the condition one intends to test for is the only one being tested, and that the test will not indicate that the condition is present when it is not (**false positives**), or that it is not present when it is (**false negatives**). No test satisfies these criteria perfectly, but the better the test, the closer it must come to doing so.'

(Hubbard, 1992, page 153)

Finally, there is the issue of the human gene becoming rarified. This has been one of the more recent challenges to women since the birth of the human genome project, causing the 'gene' to be making headlines (Hubbard and Wald, 1993). There are now predictions of a genetically engineered future (Birke *et al.*, 1992), creating the spectre of a sinister world where many believe that babies can be designed to order. This is not science fiction, but in reality it affects us now; we are faced with situations where the gene has become rarified (Woliver, 1991), becoming the unit of individuality (Rowland, 1992; Birke, 1994).

Reflection Points

- Rarification of the 'gene' is a very problematic and misleading stance, because the potential for human development does not lie solely within our genes.
- Could there be an eugenic argument that scientists are simply playing God and meddling in matters that do not concern them?
- The implications of this debate for those who are disabled and other vulnerable groups within our society are colossal; for example, Birke (1994) asks what is to stop the scientist who is already trying to find the gene that determines sexuality, while Hubbard and Wald (1993) ask who is to decide who is and who is not fit to make a contribution to the 'gene pool'.
- This debate blames individuals without any consideration for sociopolitical influences.

As can be seen, testing during the antenatal period presents many challenges. Of course women should be offered choice, which means respecting the decision many women have to make as to whether or not to participate in screening programmes, as well as protecting them from the potential dangers of scientific research.

IDENTIFYING WOMEN WITH SPECIAL NEEDS DURING THE ANTENATAL PERIOD

Even though it can be argued that all pregnant women have special needs, there are nevertheless minority groups of women who need to have their special needs met in special ways, in order to avoid the danger of disenfranchising women who may already be marginalised in the larger society. The following list adapted from Johnstone (1994) summarises the key issues and may be useful in focusing the attention of the reader during the maternity care experience:

- Ethnic minority groups, e.g. travellers, non-English speaking women
- The young pregnant teenager
- The pregnant lesbian woman
- Women with disability
- Women with multiple pregnancy
- The sexually abused woman
- Women in violent relationships
- Women with medical disorders (e.g., epilepsy, asthma, metabolic disorders, haemoglobino-pathies and cardiac disease)
- Diagnosis of fetal abnormality
- Diagnosis of intrauterine fetal death
- Women who have experienced previous pregnancy loss, stillbirth or sudden infant death syndrome (SIDS)
- Pregnancy complicated by obstetric conditions (e.g. antepartum haemorrhage, preeclampsia)
- Women and partners with history of infertility/subinfertility and who have sought assisted means of reproduction, e.g. *in vitro* fertilisation (IVF)
- Women with poor social support
- Women with antenatal depression/past history of postnatal depression/mental illness and indeed current mental health problems, as the latter group of women may miss out on adequate support from health care professionals and other agencies, partly because of their psychological state or poor attendance at antenatal sessions
- Previous traumatic birth complicated by intervention, women with a sense of a loss of control.

NORMAL EMOTIONAL CHANGES DURING PREGNANCY

According to Johnstone (1994) there is no standard or distinctive psychological state experienced by all women during pregnancy, as each woman's emotional reaction to her pregnancy will be different, and is the net result of influential factors such as quality of social support, socio-economic status, as well as the woman's cultural beliefs and rituals (Oakley *et al.*, 1990). Nevertheless, Johnstone (1994, page 11) identifies some common psychological responses which are experienced by many women, which can best be examined under the umbrella of all three trimesters of pregnancy as follows.

First trimester (1–12 weeks' gestation)

- Ambivalent or pleasurable feelings
- Confirmation of femininity (may have a strong cultural influence)
- Effects of tiredness, nausea and vomiting on psychological state.

Second trimester (12–28 weeks' gestation)

- Sociocultural acceptance may confirm woman's status and position with her society
- Feeling of relative well-being as nausea and vomiting usually abate
- Increased attachment to the developing fetus, which may be strengthened with use of ultrasound scan and/or fetal movements, audible auscultation of the fetal heart rate by the midwife/doctor
- A need to make preparations for the birth and withdraw from employment commitments.

Third trimester (28–42 weeks' gestation)

- Anxiety about **labour** and delivery – 'how will I cope with the pain?'
- Worries/anxieties about health of the fetus – 'will he/she be abnormal?'
- Increased vulnerability to life events, such as financial instability, separation from partner, moving house, personal loss/bereavement
- Need for social support, especially from own mother or significant others
- Psychological effects of the minor disorders of pregnancy (e.g. backache, heartburn and constipation) which may affect the woman's sleeping pattern.

An increasing understanding of these common psychological changes will enable the midwife to support women in adjusting to change, whilst recognising that pregnancy and childbirth are transitional periods culminating in major emotional upheavals for the whole family. The way in which a woman is treated during pregnancy, and her memories of this, will affect her profoundly for the rest of her life (Oates, 1989). Women and their partners need to be prepared adequately psychologically to enter labour confidently, and ready to meet the challenges of parenthood. The following case scenario examines how a midwife may assess a couple's psychological needs during the antenatal period.

Case Scenario

Yasmin is 40 years old. She and her partner John are both devout Catholics. The couple are self-employed accountants and are expecting their first child. At 12 weeks' gestation Yasmin meets her named midwife to discuss her options for care, antenatal screening tests and her feelings about infant feeding.

In meeting the psychological needs of this couple the midwife should bear in mind the following key objectives:

- The midwife should inform the couple of the options available to them and respect their wishes, and demonstrate sensitivity of the couple's sociocultural background.
- Because the couple are both self-employed the midwife should provide flexible patterns of care which inspire confidence and boost self-esteem.
- The midwife should provide appropriate support by employing counselling skills, e.g. attending, listening, conveying acceptance, genuineness, empathetic response and a general non-judgemental approach.
- The midwife should recognise that Yasmin will have 'special needs'.
- The midwife should avoid conveying disapproval of the difficult choices the couple have to make in relation to prenatal screening tests.
- The midwife should arrange parenthood education to meet John's and Yasmin's needs.
- The midwife should be honest about the demands and joys of parenthood.
- The midwife should discuss Yasmin's feelings on infant feeding, whilst remembering that her final decision should be an informed one.

CARE DURING LABOUR AND DELIVERY

Labour commonly commences at *term*, i.e. between 37 completed weeks and 42 weeks of gestation. The process usually begins with the onset of regular, rhythmic, painful uterine contractions and ends with the expulsion from the uterus of the fetus, placenta and membranes and the achievement of homeostasis in relation to bleeding from the placental site. Although labour is really one continuous process, it is divided into three stages (Table 18.11) to aid comprehension of its complex physiology.

Case Scenario

Bebe is a 17-year-old **primigravida** who is admitted to her local maternity unit following commencement of her labour at term. She is accompanied to the labour suite by her mother, who will be her birth companion. Bebe is no longer in contact with the father of her baby. The midwife discusses Bebe's birth plan in order to meet her physical, psychological and social needs.

NORMAL EMOTIONAL CHANGES DURING LABOUR

In assessing Bebe's psychosocial needs the midwife must have an understanding of the normal emotional changes Bebe and other women are likely to experience during labour. Johnstone (1994) describes a range of emotional responses during labour which are encountered by many women. These may include fear of technology, fear of the loss of self-control, helplessness and dependency on others, especially in relation to pain and the process of giving birth. It is essential that the midwife acknowledges these fears as Bebe's sensitivity will be heightened and her vulnerability increased.

Table 18.11: Definitions, descriptions and durations of the stages of labour

Stage of labour	Description	Duration
1st Stage	The onset of regular, rhythmic, painful uterine contractions to full dilatation of the os uteri	Variable: ■ **Primigravida:** 12–18 hours approx. ■ **Multipara:** 6–8 hours approx.
2nd Stage	From full dilatation of the os uteri to the birth of the baby	■ **Primigravida** May be greater than 1 hour at times, will depend on factors such as presentation, position of the fetus as well as the position of the mother, presence of maternal urge to bear down, directed versus non-directed pushing and whether mother has an effective epidural ■ **Multipara** May last for approximately 30 minutes once expulsive efforts are activated. Factors affecting delay for the primigravid woman may also cause delay for the multiparous woman
3rd Stage	From birth of the baby to complete expulsion of placenta and membranes, and control of bleeding	5–15 minutes if actively managed, may be considerably longer if physiologically managed, but not necessarily so

Psychosocial care during labour

In meeting Bebe's psychosocial needs during labour the midwife should also draw on the four Cs of 'Winterton' and *Changing Childbirth* (DoH, 1992c, 1993):

- Choice – choice of carer, pain relief, mobility and positions for labour and delivery, monitoring of fetal heart
- Control – over labour room technology/intervention. She will need a supportive, empathetic carer who listens and empowers, and supports hydration and nutrition needs. Bebe also needs control over personal hygiene to enhance comfort, e.g. care of hair, teeth, bladder and bowels, ability to shower/bathe freely
- Continuity – preferably with a midwife she knows and respects as Bebe may need advocate/spokesperson
- Communication – effective communication keeps Bebe well informed on the progress of labour, minimising anxiety, boosting confidence and probably increasing her tolerance of pain.

These issues are important to Bebe's psychological well-being, as they promote psychophysical harmony, thus facilitating the progress of labour. Green *et al.* (1988) revealed that if women were more central to the decision-making process they were more likely to feel satisfied with events around birth, as they felt in control and would more readily accept that the 'right thing' was done in relation to any ensuing intervention.

PAIN RELIEF IN LABOUR

During labour women like Bebe may choose between pharmacological and non-pharmacological methods of pain relief, although many may choose a combination of both (Figure 18.9). There are many factors that are likely to affect a woman's pain threshold which may stem from physical, psychological and social influences. The midwife should ensure that women are psychologically well prepared for the processes of labour and childbirth during the antenatal period, because they may not be in any fit state to be making informed decisions during labour. An overload of new information during an event which is already punctuated with stressors may adversely affect a woman's ability to cope with the pain of labour (Dick-Read, 1981) as depicted in Figure 18.10.

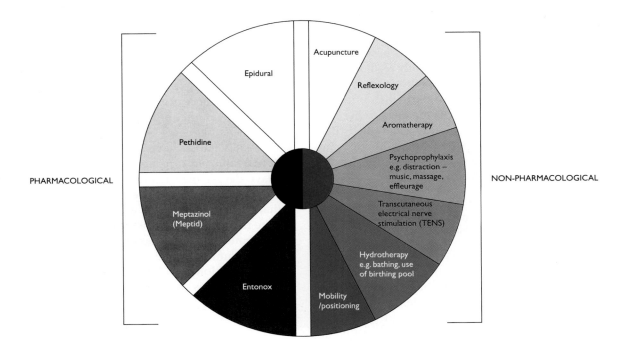

Figure 18.9: Methods of pain relief during labour

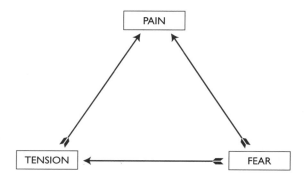

Figure 18.10: The cyclical dimension of pain in labour (Adapted from Dick-Read, 1981)

CARE DURING THE POSTNATAL PERIOD

The *postnatal* period and *puerperium* are commonly referred to as the fourth trimester (Oates, 1989; Johnstone, 1994).

The *postnatal period* is defined as:

'A period not less than ten and not more than twenty eight days after the end of labour, during which the continued attendance of a midwife on the mother and baby is requisite.'

(UKCC, 1993, page 8)

The *puerperium* is defined as a period of recuperation which extends up to 6–8 weeks post-delivery, when the mother's body physically readjusts from the physiological demands of pregnancy, major organs return as near as possible to their pre-pregnant state, the mother starts to adjust to her new role and successful lactation is established (Ball, 1994). The postnatal period brings about many changes in emotions and is a particularly stressful time, which leads Ball to assert that:

' . . . The objectives of maternity care must be as concerned with the emotional and psychological processes as they are with the physiological.'

(Ball, 1994, page 116)

It is during the postnatal period that women are at their most vulnerable, especially to the development of postnatal depression (Holden, 1991). The woman will therefore need time and patience to recover from the stresses and demands of childbirth. Post-delivery, early parent–infant interactions are important to the development of healthy relationships and successful breast-feeding. However, this must not be at the expense of women's feelings – some women will need time to reflect and space to become themselves again before reaching their arms out to comfort their baby.

In order to nurture their children women have to feel that they too are valued and nurtured (Ball, 1988; Elbourne *et al.*, 1989). In caring for the postnatal mother the midwife must also bear in mind the vital and complementary and invaluable contributions of some voluntary organisations: e.g. National Childbirth Trust (NCT), La Leche League for breast-feeding mothers, Meet-A-Mum association, Twins and Multiple Births Association (TAMBA), Stillbirths and Neonatal Death Society (SANDS), Support Around Termination For Fetal Abnormality (SATFA), CRY-SIS for crying babies, caesarean section and postnatal support groups. It is comforting for many mothers to know that others share similar experiences to their own. Voluntary organisations put women in touch with each other, thus providing excellent social support.

ROLE OF THE FATHER

Strictly speaking, a section entitled 'role of the father' may be politically incorrect, as we need to recognise that not all women have the support of a male partner, or want the support of a male during pregnancy and childbirth. This scenario can be applied to women who are separated, in single sex partnerships, or use ethnic or cultural practices where the presence of a female companion is more acceptable than that of a male. Nevertheless, the role of the father needs to be considered, because traditionally fathers have been portrayed as uninvolved with child care, and women are assumed to have deep-rooted maternal instincts, whereas no similar assumptions are made in relation to fathers (Heath, 1995).

The role of the father was never clearly defined until about 20 or so years ago, and even then remained limited at and around the time of birth (Bedford and Johnson, 1988). Indeed, for some the term 'parent' is synonymous with 'mother'. Bowlby's (1953) influential work left us with no doubt as to his views on the role of the father: one of social obligation, to provide food and financial support for his family, rather than a psychological or biological necessity.

Today the stereotype of the uninvolved father rests on contemporary interpretations of past historical events such as John Bowlby's doctrine, which suggested that the role of the mother is essential in meeting the psychological and physical needs of the infant, and that of the father inessential, apart from making a financial contribution. Yet, motherhood, like fatherhood, is a socially constructed term. The time has surely come to challenge the assumption that child-rearing is exclusively a mother's job. Such ideology only serves to confirm motherhood, as an occupation whilst fatherhood, at best, is a relationship (Lewis, 1986).

It has now been recognised that just as women become mothers, men, too, have psychophysical reactions to the experience of becoming a father (Summersgill, 1993). Men, like their female counterparts, are initiated into parenthood through cultural rites, which may be a more elaborate process in some societies than others, and the psychophysical reactions some men may experience are thought to mimic those of their pregnant spouses, as if in sympathy, which is referred to as *couvade* (Chalmers, 1990; Summersgill, 1993). Men may experience symptoms such as tiredness, headaches, backache and nausea.

More recently, the presence of men in the delivery room has caused a backlash. Fewer than 20 years ago men who attended their partners during labour and delivery were the exception rather than the rule. Could it be that the pendulum has swung too far in women's expectation that all men should be present at the birth of their offspring? Do men make an informed choice to be with their labouring partners, or is their presence the result of their partner's expectations, together with peer and media pressure? Indeed, Nolan (1996) asks whether men need to be involved with the birth of their child at all. This is an important question because we need to find out how the male presence during childbirth benefits the couple, and we should explore the disadvantages, if any, of this arrangement.

It has been suggested, by Klaus *et al.* (1993), that men are often pressured into attending the delivery of their child, suggesting that perhaps the pressure could be taken off by introducing a **doula** system. A doula is a female companion who is not a midwife, but who assumes a non-clinical role to provide social support for the woman in labour. As the debate continues to rage one thing is sure:

if midwives and other health care professionals expect male partners to take on the role of supporter and nurturer they must recognise that fatherhood is about joint responsibility, teamwork and cooperation. They will, therefore, need careful preparation for the demands of fatherhood (Donovan, 1995; Heath, 1995).

CARE OF THE NEWBORN

At birth the baby leaves the fluid, warm, nurturing and protective environment of the mother's uterus to face the challenges of the external world. Once the baby's lifeline – the umbilical cord – is severed, the baby is very much on his or her own. The body must now work independently of the placenta, which was life sustaining during intrauterine existence. The baby has to breathe, establish cardiopulmonary function, feed and eliminate without the aid of the placenta. As the major organs adjust to their new demands the baby will be thrust into a state of transition during the early weeks of life, as it takes on its separateness from its mother.

This final section of the chapter will concentrate on three key areas:

- Immediate care of the baby at birth
- Parent–infant dynamic interactions
- Promoting safe/healthy feeding practices.

IMMEDIATE CARE OF THE NEWBORN

The midwife employs the Apgar score to assess the baby's condition at birth. Apgar is used as an acronym which describes five key areas:

A – appearance
P – pulse/heart rate
G – grimace or cry
A – attitude, i.e. degree of muscle tone and general activity of the baby
R – respiration.

Each criterion is allocated a minimum point of 0 score or a maximum of 2 (Table 18.12). The scores are summated and noted at 1 minute and 5 minutes, respectively, but the midwife also notes the time taken from birth to the baby's first gasp, including the onset of regular respirations. The

Table 18.12: Apgar score

	0	1	2
Heart rate	Absent	<100	>100
Respiratory effort	Absent	Weak, or shallow cry	Good, strong cry
Muscle tone	Limp	Some flexion	Active, well flexed
Reflex/ irritability	None	Grimace	Cry
Colour	Pale/blue	Body pink, extremities blue	Pink

Apgar score gives a crude indicator of the well-being of the infant at birth but is quite limited and could be criticised for being ethnocentric. Take colour for instance: Afro-Caribbean babies cannot be described as being 'pink' at birth!

Clamping and cutting the umbilical cord

The timing of clamping and cutting the umbilical cord is usually dependent on two factors:

- Physiological management of the third stage of labour
- Active management of the third stage of labour.

With the move towards an individualised approach to care, current thinking would indicate that the midwife needs to assess each case on its own merit. It is thought that a number of cases may benefit from delayed clamping of the umbilical cord, for example the preterm baby and women who are rhesus negative (Clarke and Hussey, 1994).

Identification and examination of the baby

Since approximately 98% of births take place within an institutional setting (Campbell and Macfarlane, 1994) it is important that midwives are vigilant to secure the identity of newborn babies, to avoid adverse media attention, and more importantly, to reassure parents. To assist midwives, the Royal College of Midwives (RCM, 1992) released guidelines, intended to be used as an adjunct to the policy and procedures of maternity units.

Following birth, the midwife employs a systematic approach in performing a detailed examination of the newborn baby in the presence of the parents (Figure 18.11). The midwife then makes a detailed record of her findings in the appropriate documents. A further examination will be performed when the baby is 24 hours old, either by the hospital-based paediatrician, if the mother had a hospital birth, or the GP, if the mother had a home birth or an early transfer from hospital. As a result of *Changing Childbirth* (DoH, 1993), it is hoped that the midwife's responsibilities will be extended to include the examination of the newborn currently performed by doctors.

PARENT–INFANT DYNAMIC INTERACTIONS

The management of childbirth often reflects the controlling forces which may directly affect the parent–baby relationship. Birth, of course, is only the start of a cascade of events and an introduction to some of the thorny issues of parenting; being a rite of passage it will be subjected to covert, but stringent, social control. The first hour following birth, the healthy, full-term, undrugged baby (i.e. no narcotic analgesia was used during labour) will be at his/her most alert for the next 24 hours. Parents should be educated to maximise on this opportunity to interact with their young (Klaus, 1995). It is important that the midwife withdraws to allow both parents and their new baby as well as other siblings, to be alone together, to welcome the new addition into the family unit. Skin-to-skin contact can also be encouraged. It is thought that mutual exploration and stimulation of mother and infant can help to establish the basis of a healthy relationship and contribute to initiation of breast-feeding (DeChateau and Wiberg, 1977).

Flexibility in the above approach is required, however, as some mothers will fall in love with their baby immediately, whilst the process may be delayed for others. The mother's response may be influenced by her baby's initial reaction, appearance, expression and imagined-versus-actual features of the baby (Chalmers, 1990). The individuality of women and babies should always be considered.

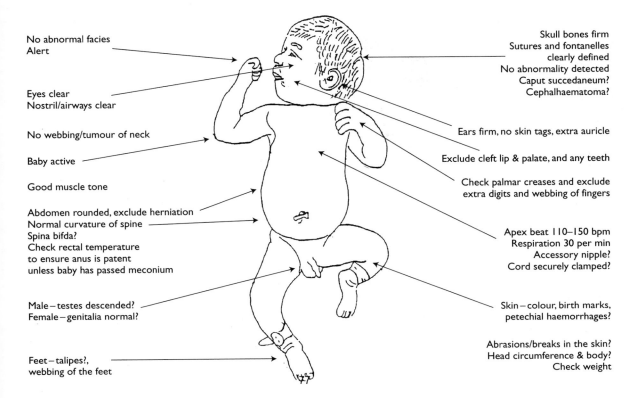

No abnormal facies
Alert

Eyes clear
Nostril/airways clear

No webbing/tumour of neck

Baby active

Good muscle tone

Abdomen rounded, exclude herniation
Normal curvature of spine
Spina bifda?
Check rectal temperature
to ensure anus is patent
unless baby has passed meconium

Male – testes descended?
Female – genitalia normal?

Feet – talipes?,
webbing of the feet

Skull bones firm
Sutures and fontanelles
clearly defined
No abnormality detected
Caput succedaneum?
Cephalhaematoma?

Ears firm, no skin tags, extra auricle

Exclude cleft lip & palate, and any teeth

Check palmar creases and exclude
extra digits and webbing of fingers

Apex beat 110–150 bpm
Respiration 30 per min
Accessory nipple?
Cord securely clamped?

Skin – colour, birth marks,
petechial haemorrhages?

Abrasions/breaks in the skin?
Head circumference & body?
Check weight

Figure 18.11: A midwife's examination of the newborn

PROMOTING SAFE INFANT FEEDING PRACTICE: BREAST VERSUS BOTTLE DEBATE

'Euch, those are for your husband!'
(Morse, 1990, page 223)

Fundamental structures and cultural values in many societies make breast-feeding particularly difficult, as poignantly depicted in the opening quote by Morse (1990), which may manifest themselves in many shapes and guises. These include specific hospital practices of offering artificial milk to breast-fed babies. A staggering 45% of babies who are breast-fed are offered breast milk substitutes in the UK, whilst still in the hospital environment, according to the results of the latest OPCS survey (White *et al.*, 1992) – a factor strongly associated with an early switch to the bottle.

Yet breast milk is undoubtedly best for babies: it is species specific (Figure 18.12), free, sterile, is delivered at the correct temperature, and contains just the right amount of proteins, vitamins and essential minerals for a developing infant. It also contains immunoglobulins and other anti-infective agents that provide the baby with natural immunity against viral infections, respiratory infections, infections of the gastrointestinal tract, as well as protecting against sudden infant death syndrome (Ebrahim, 1991). But even though the edict 'breast is best' now seems an axiomatic statement, breast versus bottle continues to represent a real dilemma for a high proportion of mothers.

Even though the decision to breast- or bottle-feed is usually made well in advance of pregnancy, labour and delivery (Thomson, 1989), all remains far from well with the current state of breast-feeding within the UK. Disturbing figures from the latest survey on infant feeding practice point out that only 63% of babies initiate breast-feeding at birth in 1990, compared to 64% in 1985 and 65% in 1980 (White *et al.*, 1992), reflecting the static rate of breast-feeding for about 15 years. Just as alarming and worrying is that less than 30% of mothers are still breast-feeding at 13 weeks, the minimum time required to provide protective immunity (WHO, 1989; DoH, 1994b).

Fat		Protein		Carbohydrate	g/100 ml	Calories
Buffaloes' milk	7.5		3.8	4.9		101
Camels' milk	4.2		3.7	4.1		68
Cows' milk	3.5		3.3	4.7		62
Dogs' milk	8.3		7.1	4.1		119
Goats' milk	4.1		3.8	4.6		69
Horses' milk	1.4	1.8		6.7		45
Human breast milk	3.3	1.5		7.0		62
Pigs' milk	8.5		5.8	4.8		118
Reindeers' milk	22.5		10.3	2.4		253
Sheep's milk	6.2		5.2	4.2		92
Yaks' milk	7.0		5.2	4.6		101

Figure 18.12: Comparison of human milk with various species
(Source: Ebrahim, 1991 *Breastfeeding: the Biological Option*. Reproduced with the permission of Macmillan Press Ltd.)

The Innocenti Declaration, signed in 1990 by 32 countries and 10 United Nations Agencies, endorsed the WHO/Unicef statement on the protection, promotion and support of breast-feeding, which states:

'As a global goal for optimal maternal and child health and nutrition, all women should be enabled to practise exclusive breast-feeding and all infants should be exclusively fed on breast milk from 4–6 months of age. Thereafter, children should continue to be breast-fed, while receiving appropriate and adequate complementary foods, for up to two years and beyond.'

(WHO, 1989)

The number of babies who are breast-fed in this way in the UK is miniscule, partly because breast-feeding is not only rooted in physiological concerns but also in behavioural and social factors (Palmer, 1991). Many mothers have to deal with the strong antagonism towards long-term breast-feeding, coupled with society's reluctance to accept breast-feeding in public spaces. Designated facilities now exist but these are not available in every shopping centre, and if they are, they may not be easily accessible, especially for the disabled mother. The National Baby Care symbol is used to identify available baby care facilities (Figure 18.13).

Breast-feeding in public may also be particularly difficult because of the way in which women's bodies are eroticised (Ramazanoglu and Holland, 1993). Within consumer culture breasts are portrayed as symbols of male desire in fashion, cinema, literature and advertisements. The role that the media and society play in manufac-turing 'perfect' breasts and generating distortions and idealised images of women's bodies is considerable. Media norms of women's breasts make impossible demands for high, firm and pointy breasts (Young, 1990). It is hardly surprising, then, that for many women breasts are an important component of body image. Women's experience of breast-feeding in public sits alongside the way in which women experience their breasts and the cultural meaning of breasts. Consequently, women are torn between the needs of their baby, needs of their partner and the needs of society at large – strange hypocrisy in a society that accepts

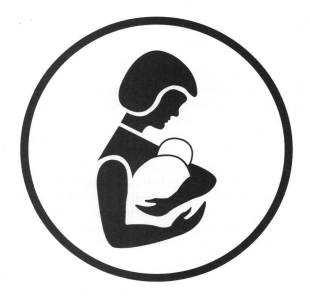

Figure 18.13: The national baby care symbol
(Source: Department of Health and Social Security [DHSS], 1988)

bare-breasted waitresses and encourages bare-breasted females in the tabloid press.

Promoting successful breast-feeding

Following the publication of successive government reports showing a steady decline in the breast-feeding rates nationally, active steps have been taken to raise awareness of health care professionals and the profile of breast-feeding generally. However, demographic factors influencing wide regional variation in breast-feeding rates means that regional targets will be more realistically achieved than national ones. A multidisciplinary approach involving midwives, health visitors, GPs, paediatricians and representatives of the voluntary organisations supportive of breast-feeding practice, e.g. National Childbirth Trust and La Leche League, have helped to form national breast-feeding working groups, which are now well established in most health districts. Their remit is to examine ways in which the preva-

lence of breast-feeding can be increased and to educate, support and nurture women who choose to breast-feed.

From an international perspective, the global campaign by the WHO and consumer groups led to the adoption of the International Code of Marketing of Breastmilk Substitutes by the World Health Assembly in 1981 (WHO, 1981). The Code was formulated to regulate the aggressive advertising and promotional techniques used to sell formula milks (Interagency Group on Breast-feeding Monitoring, 1997). Table 18.13 compares the key differences between the WHO International Code and the UK's Federation for the Manufacturer of Formula Feeds (FMF) Code. However, as can be seen, the FMF aim is to protect the interest of its manufacturers (Murray, 1996). Not surprisingly, concerned that breast-feeding was becoming an increasingly endangered practice, the United Nations Children's Fund (UNICEF) and the World Health Organization enlisted the support of governmental organisations, health professionals and

Table 18.13: Comparison of the codes of the international WHO and UK Federation for the manufacturer of Formula Feeds (FMF)

WHO code	FMF code
■ Prohibits advertising and other forms of to the general public or service	■ Permits advertising and promotion through promotion direct the health service to health workers and through the health the general public
■ Lists nine specific requirements about what should and should not be included in material for mothers	■ Lists two modified requirements to be included in material for mothers
■ Prohibits free samples to pregnant women, mothers and their families	■ Permits free samples to mothers through or members of the health service and distributed by health service staff
■ Prohibits material inducements to health service staff to promote infant formulae	■ 'Inexpensive' gifts of 'relevance' to the practice of medicine and general health care permitted
■ Donated equipment may show only the company's logo, not a product brand name	■ Donated equipment need only conform to the 'normal policies' of the health service
■ Manufacturers should disclose any fellowships, grants study tours or conference attendances that they sponsor, and so should the recipient	■ There is no requirement to disclose any such forms of financial support, for either donor or recipient
■ Prohibits company staff from directly/indirectly contacting pregnant women and mothers	■ Permits company staff to contact mothers under supervision of a health worker, and give information if a mother asks
■ Prohibits words like 'humanised' and 'maternalised' on labels and prohibits pictures of infants	■ Such words and pictures are permitted on labels
■ Requires five messages on all infant formula packages, including use by mothers in hospital	■ Requires four messages, and these only those supplied for on packages for retail sale
■ Code applies to all products used to replace breast milk, including bottle feed, weaning foods, bottles and teats	■ Code applies to manufactured infant formula only

Adapted and expanded from Hamilton and Whinnett, 1987, with permission.

charities around the globe, and launched the 'baby friendly initiative' in 1990, to challenge behaviour and attitudes actively, and to convince parents, health professionals, hospitals and health ministers that breast-feeding gives babies the best possible start in life. The now well documented 'Ten Steps to Successful Breast-feeding, (Table 18.14) are used as the criteria for meeting the standards for the award of a baby-friendly status. Many units within the UK are now working towards baby-friendly status.

Bottle-feeding

Not much space has been allocated to this method of infant feeding as the student can easily refer to other sources regarding the practicalities of preparing artificial feeds. It is important to recognise, however, that holistically bottle-feeding may not only be the best choice in some cases, but for a number of mothers a choice is not really possible at all.

So although bottle-feeding may be seen as an easy option, it may be a difficult choice. Women and their partners will need support, education and sound information to meet the baby's needs. Disapproval should never be conveyed to the mother regardless of her choice.

Key Points

■ To become equal partners in their care, women should be fully informed regarding all aspects of their care during pregnancy and childbirth.

■ Women have the right to decide whether or not to participate in antenatal screening programmes, and should be protected from the potential harm of scientific research.

■ Health professionals should ensure that women receive effective psychosocial support during pregnancy and childbirth, especially during labour, as such support is known to be conducive to the progress of labour, reducing the need for analgesia and labour interventions.

■ Psychological care during the pregnancy and childbirth is essential to enhance positive memories of a woman's childbearing experience, thus enabling her to take on the powerful role of motherhood.

■ Parent–infant dynamic attachment should be facilitated by the midwife as soon after birth as possible, but respecting the sociocultural factors which may influence such interactions.

■ Public breast-feeding practices can be fostered in many ways, starting with the media presenting women in a more positive light by creating real images of women, rather than objects of male desire.

CONCLUSION

Education and change are seen as dynamic processes. This chapter has, therefore, examined a variety of topics, ranging from the benefits of optimising health before conception, along with the

Table 18.14: The WHO/UNICEF 10 steps to successful breast-feeding

Every facility providing maternity services and care for the newborn infants should:
1 Have a written breast-feeding policy that is routinely communicated to all health care staff
2 Train all health care staff in skills necessary to implement this policy
3 Inform all pregnant women about the benefits and management of breast-feeding
4 Help mothers initiate breast-feeding within half an hour of birth
5 Show mothers how to breast-feed, and how to maintain lactation even if they should be separated from their infants
6 Give newborn infants no food or drink other than breast milk, unless *medically* indicated
7 Practice rooming-in: allow mothers and infants to remain together 24 hours a day
8 Encourage breast-feeding on demand
9 Give no artificial teats or pacifiers (dummies or soothers) to breast-fed infants
10 Foster the establishment of breast-feeding support groups and refer mothers to them on discharge from hospital or clinic

Source: WHO 1989, page iv, Reproduced with the permission of the World Health Organization.

vexed issue of antenatal screening/diagnostic tests, coupled with a critical review of current infant-feeding practices. Against the background of *Changing Childbirth*, attempts have been made to place pregnancy and childbirth in a social and political framework, where the advantages of a woman-centred approach to maternity care has been illuminated.

Finally, in considering the maternal and social conditions in which women give birth, along with their cultural beliefs, values and expectations about childbirth, some of the neglected questions and contradictions affecting the recipients of maternity care have been challenged. Hopefully, the reflective discourse presented will help the reader to recognise that pregnancy and childbirth are periods in a woman's life when her vulnerability exposes her to a significant amount of psychological pressure. Indeed, C. Smart (1991) asserts that historically, pregnancy and childbirth have been the sites of contested meanings, which of course may continue to be two of the greatest pleasures and burdens for women within our multicultural society. An understanding of these fundamental issues should enrich the maternity care experience.

ACKNOWLEDGEMENT

The author would like to thank Jenny Pallet, Desktop Publisher, University of Nottingham School of Nursing, for the illustrations included in this chapter.

USEFUL ADDRESSES

Association of Breastfeeding Mothers
26 Holmshaw Close
London
SE26 4TH
Tel: 0181 778 4769

National Childbirth Trust
(Breastfeeding promotion group)
Alexandra House
Oldham Terrace
Acton
London
W3 6NH
Tel: 0181 992 8637

CRY-SIS
(Support for mothers with crying/sleepless babies)
BM CRY-SIS
London
SW1 3XX

Support Around Termination for Abnormality (SATFA)
73–75 Charlotte Street
London
W1P 1LB
Tel: 0171 631 0285

The Association for Postnatal Depression
25 Jerdan Place
Fulham
London
SW6 1BE
Tel: 0171 386 0868

La Leche League
(Breastfeeding, help and information)
BM 3424
London
WC1V 6XX
Tel: 0171 242 1278

Foundation for Sudden Infant Death Syndrome
35 Belgrave Square
London
SW1X 8QB

UNICEF Baby Friendly Initiative
20 Guildford Street
London
WC1N 1DZ
Tel: 0171 405 8400

Twins and Multiple Births Association (TAMBA)
PO Box 30
Little Sutton
South Wirral
Cheshire
L66 1TH

Stillbirth and Neonatal Death Society (SANDS)
28 Portland Place
London
W1N 4DE
Tel: 0171 436 5881

Meet-A-Mum Association (MAMA)
14 Willis Road
Croydon
Surrey
CR0 2XX
Tel: 0181 665 0357

Caesarean Support Network
2 Hurst Park Drive
Huyton
Liverpool
L36 1TF

REFERENCES

Anderson, T. (1996). Using evidence to empower childbearing women: the informed choice initiative. *Midwives*, 109, 12–14.

Annandale, E. (1988). How midwives accomplish natural births: managing risk and balancing expectations. *Social Problems*, 35(2), 95–100.

Autti-Ramo, E. and Granstrom, M.L. (1992). Dysmorphic features in offsprings of alcoholic mothers. *Archives of Diseases in Childhood*, 67, 712–16.

Ball, J.A. (1988). Mothers need nurturing too. *Nursing Times*, 84(17), 29–30.

Ball, J.A. (1994). *Reactions to Motherhood: the Role of Postnatal Care*, 2nd edn. Books for Midwives Press, Cheshire.

Ball, J.A., Flint, C., Garvey, M., Jackson-Baker, A. and Page, L. (1992). *Who's Left Holding the Baby?* The Nuffield Institute, University of Leeds, Leeds.

Barbour, B.G. (1990). Alcohol and pregnancy. *Journal of Nurse-Midwifery*, 35(2), 78–85.

Bedford, V.A. and Johnson, N. (1988). The role of the father. *Midwifery*, 4, 190–5.

Birke, L. (1994). *Zipping up the Genes*. Perversions, London.

Birke, L., Himmelweit, S. and Vines, G. (1992). Detecting genetic diseases: prenatal screening and its problems. In *Inventing Women: Science, Technology and Gender*, Kirkup, G. and Smith-Keller, L. (eds). Polity Press, London.

Bowlby, J. (1953). *Childcare and the Growth of Love*. Penguin, Harmondsworth.

Brooks, L. and Black, M. (1994). Maternity. Local delivery. *Health Service Journal*, 104: 33.

Bryar, R.M. (1988). Midwifery and models of care. *Midwifery*, 4(3), 111–17.

Bryar, R.M. (1995). *Theories for Midwifery Practice*, Chapter 4. Macmillan, London.

Campbell, R. and Macfarlane, A. (1994). *Where to be born? The Debate and the Evidence*, revised edn. National Perinatal Epidemiology Unit, Oxford.

Cefalo, R.C. and Moos, M.K. (1995). *Preconceptional Health Care – a Practical Guide*, 2nd edn. Mosby, London.

Chalmers, B. (1990). *Pregnancy and parenthood: Heaven or Hell*, revised edn. Berev Publications, South Africa.

Charles, D., Dickson, D., Lewin, R. and Pain, S. (1991). Why men should also think of the baby. *New Scientist*, 129 (1758), 6.

Charles, J. (1992). Pregnant pause. *Nursing Times*, 88(34), 30–2.

Chavasse, J.M. (1992). New dimensions of empowerment in nursing and challenges. *Journal of Advanced Nursing*, 17, 1–2.

Chollat-Traquet, C. (1992). *Women and Tobacco*. WHO, Geneva.

Clarke, C. and Hussey, R.M. (1994). Decline in rhesus haemolytic disease of the newborn. *Journal of the Royal College of Physicians*, 28(4), 310–11.

Currell, R. (1990). The organisation of midwifery care. In *Antenatal Care: a Research-based Approach*, Alexander, J., Levy, V. and Roch, S. (eds), Chapter 2. Macmillan, Basingstoke.

Cuskelly, G.C., McNulty, H. and Scott, J.M. (1996). Effect of increasing dietary folate on red cell folate: implications for prevention of neural tube defects. *Lancet*, 347, 657–9.

Czeizel, A.E. and Dudas, I. (1992). Prevention of the first occurrence of neural tube defects by peri-conceptional vitamin supplementation. *New England Journal of Medicine*, 327, 1832–5.

Davis-Floyd, R. (1990). The role of obstetrical rituals in the resolution of cultural anomaly. *Social Science in Medicine*, 31, 175–89.

DeChateau, P. and Wiberg, B. (1977). Longterm effect on mother–infant behaviour of extra contact during the first hour postpartum. *Acta Paediatrica Scandinavica*, 66, 137–43.

DHSS (1988). *Present Day Practice in Infant Feeding*. Third report. HMSO, London.

Dick-Read, G. (1981). *Childbirth without Fear*, 5th edn. Wessel, H. and Ellis, H.F. (eds). Harper and Row, New York.

DoH (1990). *Vitamin A and Pregnancy*. PL/CMO (90) 11 PL/CNO (90). Department of Health, London.

DoH (1991a). *The Citizen's Charter: Raising the Standards*. Department of Health, London.

DoH (1991b). *The Named Midwife: Raising the Standards*. Department of Health, London.

DoH (1992a). *The Health of the Nation: a Strategy for Health in England*. HMSO, London.

DoH (1992b). *Folic Acid and Prevention of Neural Tube defects*. Report of the Expert Advisory Group on Folic Acid. Department of Health, London.

DoH (1992c). *Maternity Services*. Second Report from the Health Committee. Session 1991–1992. HMSO, London.

DoH (1993). *Changing Childbirth*, Parts 1 and 2. Second Report of the Expert Maternity Group. HMSO, London.

DoH (1994a). *Committee on Medical Aspects of Food Policy*. HMSO, London.

DoH (1994b). *Weaning and the Weaning Diet (COMA Report)*. Reports on Health and Social Subjects No. 45. HMSO, London.

DoH (1994c). *Maternity Services Charter*. Department of Health, London.

DoH (1995). *Sensible Drinking*. Report of Interdepartmental Working Group. Department of Health, London.

DoH (1996a). *Low Income, Food, Nutrition and Health: Strategies for Improvement*. A report by the low income project team for the nutrition task force. HMSO, London.

DoH (1996b). *Eat Well II*. A progress report from the nutrition task force on the action plan to achieve health of the nation targets on diet and nutrition. HMSO, London.

DoH (1996c). *Learning Together: Professional Education for Maternity Care*. Proceedings of Conference held 15 Nov. NHS Executive, London.

Donnison, J. (1993). *Midwives and Medical Men: a History of the Struggle for the Control of Childbirth*, 3rd edn. Historical Press, London.

Donovan, J. (1995). The process of analysis: a grounded theory study of men during their partner's pregnancies. *Journal of Advanced Nursing*, 21(4), 708–15.

Doyle, W. (1994). *Teach Yourself Healthy Eating*. Hodder and Stoughton, London.

Ebrahim, G.J. (1991). *Breastfeeding: the Biological Option*, 2nd edn. Macmillan, London.

Edward, G. (1996). Sensible drinking. *British Medical Journal*, 312, 1.

Elbourne, D., Oakley, A. and Chalmers, I. (1989). Social and psychological support during pregnancy. In *Effective Care in Pregnancy and Childbirth*, Chalmers, I., Enkin, M. and Keirse, M.J. (eds). Oxford University Press, Oxford.

Elford, R.W., Jennett, P.A., Sawa, R.J. and Yeo, M. (1994). Approach to lifestyle change counselling in primary care. *Parent Education and Counselling*, 24, 175–83.

Enkin, M., Keirse, M.J.N.C., Renfrew, M. and Neilson, J. (1995). *A Guide to Effective Care in Pregnancy and Childbirth*, 2nd edn. Oxford University Press, Oxford.

Evans, A. (1993). *Nurse Empowerment: Patient Empowerment*. King's Fund Centre, Nursing Development Unit, London.

Fieldhouse, P. (1995). *Food and Nutrition: Customs and Culture*, 2nd edn. Chapman & Hall, London.

Flint, C. (1991). Continuity of care provided by a team of midwives, 'the know your midwife scheme'. In *Midwives, Research and Childbirth*, Volume 2, Robinson, S. and Thomson, A.M. (eds). Chapman & Hall, London.

Garcia, J., Kilpatrick, R.and Richards, M. (eds) (1990). *The Politics of Maternity Care: Services for Childbearing Women in Twentieth Century Britain*. Clarendon Press, Oxford.

Gibson, C.H. (1991). A concept analysis of empowerment. *Journal of Advanced Nursing*, 16, 354–61.

Gillen, T. (1995). *Positive Influencing Skills*. Institute of Personnel and Development, London.

Graham, H. (1993). *When Life's a Drag: Women, Smoking and Disadvantage*. HMSO, London.

Graham, H. (1994). Surviving smoking. In *Women and Health: Feminist Perspectives*, Wilkinson, S. and Kitzinger, C. (eds), Chapter 7. Taylor and Francis, London.

Green, J., Coupland, V. and Kitzinger, J. (1988). *Great Expectations and Experiences of Childbirth*, Volume 1. University of Cambridge, Child Care Development Group, Cambridge.

Green, J.M. (1990). *Calming or Harming? A Critical Review of Psychological Effects of Fetal Diagnosis on Pregnant Women*. Galton Institute Occasional Papers, 2nd series, No. 2, 26. Galton Institute, Cambridge.

Green, J.M. (1994). Women's experiences of prenatal screening and diagnosis. In *Prenatal Screening*,

Abramsky, L. and Chapple, J. (eds). Chapman & Hall, London.

Green, J.M., Statham, H. and Snowdon, C. (1993). *Pregnancy: a Testing Time*. Report of the Cambridge pre-natal screening study. University of Cambridge, Centre for Family Research, Cambridge.

Hamilton, R. and Whinnett, D. (1987). A comparison of the WHO and the UK Codes of Practice for the marketing of breastmilk substitutes. *Journal of Consumer Policy*, 10, 167–92.

Harrison, S., Hunter, D.J., Marnoch, G. and Pollitt, C. (1992). *Just Managing: Power and Culture in the NHS*. Macmillan, London.

Hawks, J.H. (1992). Empowerment in nursing: concept analysis and application to philosophy, learning and instruction. *Journal of Advanced Nursing*, 17(5), 609–18.

HEA (1993). *Smoking and Pregnancy: Guidance for all Health Professionals Supporting Pregnant Women who want to stop Smoking*. HEA, London.

HEA (1994). *National Food Guide: the Balance of Good Health*. HEA, London.

Heath, T. (1995). New fatherhood. *New Generation*, 14(2), 11.

Hicks, C. (1993). Effects of psychological prejudices on communication and social interaction. *British Journal of Midwifery*, 1(1), 69–73.

Holden, J.M. (1991). Postnatal depression: its nature, effects and identification. *Birth*, 18(4), 211–21.

House of Commons (1991). Session 1990–1991. Health Committee 4th Report. *Maternity Services: Preconception*, Volume 1, *Report*; Volume 2, *Evidence*. HMSO, London.

Hubbard, R. (1992). *The Politics of Women's Biology*. Rutgers University Press, New Brunswick, NJ.

Hubbard, R. and Wald, J. (1993). *Exploding the Gene Myth*. Beacon Press, Boston.

Hundley, V.A., Cruickshank, F.M., Lang, G.D. *et al.* (1994). Midwife managed delivery unit: a randomised controlled comparison with consultant led care. *British Medical Journal*, 309, 1400–4.

Illman, L. (1997). Promoting healthy lifestyle. In *Women's Sexual Health*, Andrews, G. (ed.). Baillière Tindall, London.

Interagency Group on Breast-feeding Monitoring. (1997). *Cracking the Code*. UNICEF, London.

Jacobus, M., Keller, E.F. and Shuttleworth, S. (1990). *Body/Politics: Women and the Discourses of Science*. Routledge, London.

Johnstone, M. (1994). *The Emotional Effects of Childbirth*. A distance learning course for midwives, health visitors and others who care for women around the time of childbirth. Marce Society, London.

Kirkham, M.J. (1992). Labouring in the dark: limitations in the giving of information to enable patients to orientate themselves to the likely events and timescale of labour. In *Research into Practice: a Reader for Nurses and the Caring Professions*, Abbott, P. and Sapsford, R. (eds). Open University Press, Buckingham.

Kirkham, M.J. (1993). Communication in midwifery. In *Midwifery Practice: a Research-based Approach*, Alexander, J., Levy, V. and Roch, S. (eds). Macmillan, Basingstoke.

Kitzinger, S. (ed.) (1989). *The Midwife's Challenge*. Pandora, London.

Klaus, M.H. (1995). Commentary: the early hours and days of life: an opportune time. *Birth*, 22(4), 201–3.

Klaus, M.H., Kennell, J.H. and Klaus, P.H. (1993). *Mothering the Mother: how a Doula can help you have a Shorter, Easier and Healthier Birth*. Addison Wesley, California.

Lee, G. (1994). A reassuring family face. *Nursing Times*, 90(17), 66–7.

Lewis, C. (1986). *Becoming a Father*. Open University, Milton Keynes.

Lovell, A. (1996). Power and choice in birth giving – some thoughts. *British Journal of Midwifery*, 5, 268–72.

Lupton, D. (1994). *Medicine as Culture, Illness, Disease and the Body in Western Societies*. Sage, London.

McCrea, H. and Crute, V. (1994). Midwife/client relationships: midwives' perspectives. *Midwifery*, 7, 183–92.

Medical Research Council (1991). The MRC vitamin study group: prevention of neural tube defects – results of the MRC vitamin study. *Lancet*, 2, 131–7.

Morse, J.M. (1990). 'Euch those are for your husband!': examinations of cultural values and assumptions associated with breastfeeding. *Health Care for Women International*, 11, 223–32.

Murphy-Black, T. (1992). Systems of midwifery care in Scotland. *Midwifery*, 8, 113–24.

Murray, S.F. (ed.) (1996). *International Perspectives on Midwifery: Baby Friendly; Mother Friendly*. Mosby, London.

Newburn, M. (1995). Partnership with women: getting it together. In *The Challenge of Changing Childbirth*, ENB Midwifery Educational Resource Pack, No. 3, 32. English National Board, London.

Nolan, M. (1996). One labour: two different experiences. *Modern Midwife*, 6(2), 6–9.

Oakley, A. (1993). *Essays on Women, Medicine and Health*. Edinburgh University Press, Edinburgh.

Oakley, A. and Houd, S. (1990). *Helpers in Childbirth: Midwifery Today*. Hemisphere, London.

Oakley, A., Rajan, L. and Grant, A. (1990). Social support and pregnancy outcome. *British Journal of Obstetrics and Gynaecology*, 97(2), 152–62.

Oates, M.R. (1989). Normal emotional changes in pregnancy and the puerperium. *Baillière's Clinical Obstetrics and Gynaecology*, 3(4), 791–804.

OPCS (1992). *OPCS General Household Survey 1990*. HMSO, London.

Page, L. (ed.) (1995). *Effective Group Practice in Midwifery; Working with Women*. Blackwell Science, Oxford.

Palmer, G. (1991). *The Politics of Breastfeeding*, revised edn. Pandora, London.

Pickard, B. (1983). Nutritional aspects of pre-conceptional care. *Midwife, Health Visitor and Community Nurse*, 19, 424.

Plant, M. (1990). Advising on alcohol. *Nursing Times*, 86(12), 64–5.

Porter, M. (1990). Professional–client relationships and women's reproductive health care. In *Readings in Medical Sociology*, Cunningham-Burley, S. and McKeganey, N.P. (eds). Routledge, London.

Pownall, G. (1994). Pre-conception care – are midwives in danger of missing the boat? *Modern Midwife*, April, 34–5.

Price, J. (1988). *Motherhood: What it does to your Mind*. Pandora, London.

Prochaska, J.O. and DiClemente, C.C. (1983). Stages and processes of self change of smoking: towards an integration model. *Journal of Consulting and Clinical Psychology*, 51, 390–5.

Ramazanoglu, C. and Holland, J. (1993). Women's sexuality and men's appropriation of desire. In *Up Against Foucault: Explorations of Some Tensions Between Foucault and Feminism*, Ramazanoglu, C. (ed.). Routledge, London.

Ranjan, V. (1991). Vitamin A and birth defects. *Professional Care of Mother and Child*, 1(1), 3–4.

Raynor, M.D. (1995). *Changing Childbirth: Midwives' Empowerment and Women's Choice*. Unpublished MA dissertation. University of Warwick, Coventry.

RCM (1992). *Newsletter*. RCM, London.

RCP (1991). *Alcohol and the Public Health: the Prevention of Harm related to the Use of Alcohol*. Macmillan, London.

Reid, M. (1988). Consumer orientated studies in relation to prenatal screening tests. *European Journal of Obstetrics, Gynaecology and Reproductive Biology*, 28(Suppl), 79–82.

Reissman, C.K. (1992). Women and medicalisation: a new perspective. In *Inventing Women*, Kirkup, G. and Keller-Smith, L. (eds). Polity, London.

Richards, M.P.M. (1989). Social and ethical problems of fetal diagnosis and screening. *Journal of Reproduction and Infant Psychology*, 7, 171–85.

Rothman, B.K. (1986). *The Tentative Pregnancy: Prenatal Diagnosis and the Future of Motherhood*. Viking, Penguin, New York.

Rothman, K.J., Moore, L.L., Singer, M.R., Nguyen, U.D.T., Mannino, S. and Milunsky, A. (1995). Teratogenicity of high vitamin A intake. *New England Journal of Medicine*, 333, 1369–73.

Rowland, R. (1992). *Living Laboratories: Women and Reproductive Technologies*. Macmillan, London.

Sandall, J. (1995). Choice, continuity and control? Recent developments in maternity care in Britain. In *Interprofessional Relations in Health Care*, Soothill, K., Mackay, L. and Webb, C. (eds), 297–312. Arnold, London.

Shorney, J. (1990). Pre-conception care: the embryo of health. In *Antenatal Care: a Research-based Approach*, Alexander, J., Levy, V. and Roch, S. (eds). Macmillan, Basingstoke.

Smart, C. (1991). Penetrating women's bodies: the problem of law and medical technology. In *Gender, Power and Sexuality*, Abbott, P. and Wallace, C. (eds). Macmillan, Basingstoke.

Smart, R.G. (1991). World trends in alcohol consumption. *World Health Forum*, 12, 99–103.

Summersgill, P. (1993). Couvade – retaliation of marginalised fathers. In *Midwifery Practice: a Research-based Approach*, Alexander, J., Levy, V. and Roch, S. (eds). Macmillan, Basingstoke.

Taylor, M., Moyes, L., Lart, R. and Means, R. (1992). *User Empowerment in Community Care: Unravelling the Issues*. School of Advanced Urban Studies, University of Bristol, Bristol.

Tew, M. (1990). *Safer Childbirth? A Critical Review of the History of Maternity Care*. Chapman & Hall, London.

Thomson, A. (1989). Why don't women breastfeed? In *Midwives, Research and Childbirth*, Robinson, S. and Thomson, A. (eds), Volume 1, Chapter 11. Chapman & Hall, London.

Treichler, P.A. (1990). Feminism, medicine and the meaning of childbirth. In *Body/Politics: Women and the Discourse of Science*, Jacobus, M., Keller, E.F. and Shuttleworth, S. (eds). Routledge, London.

Turnbull, D., Holmes, A., Shields, N. *et al.* (1996). Randomised, controlled trial of efficacy of midwife managed care. *Lancet*, 348, 213–18.

Walton, I. and Hamilton, M. (1995). *Midwives and Changing Childbirth*. Books for Midwives Press, London.

Warwick, C. (1995). Tensions in the system. *British Journal of Midwifery*, 3(7), 358–9.

White, A., Freeth, S. and OBrien, M. (1992). *OPCS Report – Infant Feeding 1990*. HMSO, London.

Witz, A. (1992). *Professions and Patriarchy*. Routledge, London.

WHO (1981). *International Code of Marketing of Breastmilk Substitutes*. WHO, Geneva.

WHO (1989). *Protecting, Promoting and Supporting Breastfeeding: the Special Role of Maternity Services*. A joint WHO/UNICEF Statement. WHO, Geneva.

Woliver, L.R. (1991). The influence of technology on the politics of motherhood: an overview of the United States. *International Forum*, 14(5), 479–90.

Wraight, A. (1995). Organisational styles and patterns of care. In *The Challenge of Changing Childbirth*. ENB Educational Resource Pack No. 3. ENB, London.

Wraight, A., Ball, J., Secombe, I. and Stock, I. (1993). *Mapping Team Midwifery: a Report to the Department of Health*. IMS report series 242. Institute of Manpower Studies, Brighton.

Wright, J. (1995). Can patients become empowered? *Professional Nurse*, 10(9), 599.

Wynn, M. and Wynn, A. (1991). *The Case for Pre-conception Care of Men and Women*. AB Academic, Oxford.

UKCC (1993). *Midwives Rules*. UKCC, London.

Young, I.M. (1990). *Throwing like a Girl and Other Essays*. In *Feminist Philosophy and Social Theory*. Indiana Press, Bloomington and Indianapolis.

FURTHER READING

Green, J.M., Coupland, V.A. and Kitzinger, J.V. (1994). Midwives' responsibilities, medical staffing structures and women's choice in childbirth. In *Midwives, Research and Childbirth*, Robinson, S. and Thomson, A.M. (eds), Volume 3, Chapter 2. Chapman & Hall, London.

This chapter explores some of the factors which may negate a woman's choice during pregnancy and childbirth.

Moore, S. (ed.) (1997). *Understanding Pain and its Relief in Labour*, Chapters 2–6. Churchill Livingstone, London.

This text is essential reading in understanding the biophysical and psychosocial factors affecting pain perception and how these are related to the management of pain during labour.

Spedding, S., Wilson, J., Wright, S. and Jackson, A. (1995). Nutrition for pregnancy and lactation. In *Aspects of Midwifery Practice: a Research-based Approach*, Alexander, J., Levy, V. and Roch, S. (eds), Chapter 1. Macmillan, Basingstoke.

This is one of the key texts that examines the importance of nutrition during pregnancy and childbirth.

Sweet, B. (ed.) (1997). *Mayes Midwifery – a Textbook for Midwives*, 12th edn, Chapters 7–9, 12, 15–20. Baillière Tindall, London.

These chapters provide useful insights into the development of the embryo/fetus, physiology of pregnancy and the care of the pregnant woman during the antenatal period.

CHAPTER NINETEEN

FAMILY-CENTRED CARE

Norma Whittaker

- Family nursing
- The effects of illness within the family
- Family-centred care in practice
- The implications of family-centred care for practice
- Conclusion

The importance of considering the needs of families has long been acknowledged by nurses but has gained an even higher profile in recent times, following changes in the organisation and delivery of nursing and health care. The aim of this chapter is to outline the role of the family in relation to health education/promotion, health seeking behaviour and health care delivery. It also explores the effects of illness upon a family, describes how models of nursing care can be applied to the care of families and discusses the implications of family-centred care for nursing practice.

FAMILY NURSING

HISTORICAL PERSPECTIVES

Organised health care has its origins in religion, in the days when various religious orders ministered to the sick. The Parish then took over the responsibility of organised care, the task being supplemented by private philanthropists in the eighteenth century, leading to the founding of a number of charity hospitals. In spite of this, the majority of sick people were still cared for in their own homes by their families. Wealthy families paid doctors to attend them and treat their ailments, whereas poor families, by and large, were left to fend for themselves. When illness was beyond the scope of the poor **family**, the only help to be had came from neighbours, the local village 'midwife', wise woman or 'quack'. The destitute sick were likely to end up in a workhouse, where the task of caring for the sick, which family members would normally have carried out, was undertaken by other inmates.

Given the rudimentary knowledge of infection, home was probably a safer place to be nursed, but as medical knowledge increased, so did the impetus to found more hospitals. The teaching hospitals tended to be selective, choosing to treat only those patients who interested them. The voluntary hospitals only admitted patients on the recommendation of people who supported the hospital by making cash donations; thus the majority of people were still cared for at home (Baly, 1980). Despite this, the growth in the number of hospitals brought the dawning of a new era. By the end of the nineteenth century, the organisation of health care was beyond the scope of charities and was to become the concern of the state and private insurance schemes. Significantly, care was shifting away from the home and family to organised care in hospital.

THE FAMILY AS A UNIT

The family forms a basic component of society, idealistically providing individuals with love and security and protecting and nurturing those who are young. Families provide physical shelter, warmth, clothing and food, the basic material and emotional requirements which enable individuals to learn and grow in readiness for taking their place as useful members of society. Sadly, the world is not always an idealistic place and some families are unable to fulfil these roles. Poverty, for example, means that some families are unable to provide adequate shelter, warmth or food and, for some, home is a place of violence – physical, mental and sexual abuse being a frequent occurrence in some family homes.

The traditional definitions of the nuclear family, that is parents and children, and the extended family, that is parents, children, grandparents, aunts, uncles and cousins, have little relevance in the society of today; a much broader definition is necessary. In today's society, a family group or unit may, for example, constitute a re-ordered family, that is, a family where parents are no longer living together, and one or both parents may have children with new partners. There are many other kinds of families: these include lone parent families; homosexual families; single adult children living with parents and elderly parents living with an adult child and his or her partner and their children. Groups of unrelated people

may also live together and function in every way as a family, caring for each other's well being. These alternative models of the family as a unit are shown in Figure 19.1.

Although descriptions of twentieth century families may differ from descriptions of families in the eighteenth and nineteenth centuries, on closer examination, such families share a number of similar characteristics in relation to the roles that various family members undertake and the functions that the families carry out.

It is important for nurses caring for families to understand what belonging to a family can mean to different people. Just as nurses recognise that knowledge of a patient's social and cultural background is a prerequisite to the practice of individualised nursing care, so knowledge of the family is a prerequisite to the practice of **family-centred care**. Nurses must have knowledge of the usual functions of a family in order to recognise one that is dysfunctional. Such a family would have different needs to that of a well functioning family. On a micro-level, the sick individual family member from a dysfunctional family may have very different needs from someone who belongs to a well functioning family with a strong and supportive family network.

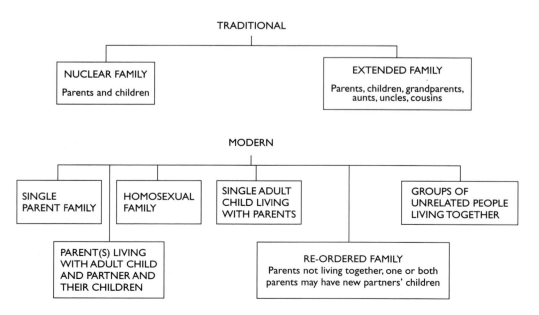

Figure 19.1: The family as unit – alternative methods

THE FAMILY'S ROLE IN HEALTH CARE

Family beliefs, values and behaviour can significantly shape the health-related behaviour of family members. Family attitudes may reflect a positive approach to health, with the family taking responsibility for health care, health promotion, health education, early diagnosis, uptake and **compliance with treatment**. Alternatively, attitudes towards health may be viewed negatively and may lead to unhealthy practices, late diagnosis and referral and poor compliance with treatment, as illustrated in Figure 19.2.

In order to appreciate the need for family-centred care, it is necessary to be aware of the role which families play in health care, in health promotion and education and in help-seeking behaviour. This knowledge should help nurses to understand the importance of the family and the need to assist relatives to fulfil their roles when care of their loved ones is transferred from them to health care professionals and, conversely, when care is returned to them following medical and nursing interventions.

LEARNED BEHAVIOUR FROM WITHIN THE FAMILY

Children are influenced by the beliefs, values and behaviour of older family members, so the family can shape the future lifestyles and behaviour of its younger members. Health promotion, for good or bad, is in part a function of the family. If certain behaviours and practices are deemed acceptable by parents, it is likely that children will also accept them. This is as true of health promoting and health seeking behaviour as it is of behaviour which poses a risk to health. Children as young as 4 years can understand and practise health behaviours (Danielson *et al.*, 1985). For example, health promoting and health seeking behaviour will be reinforced by regular mealtimes, regular sleep patterns and the adoption of strategies for coping with life's stresses by pursuing healthy leisure activities, rather than by turning to the use of alcohol and cigarettes. An early study by Mechanic (1964) found that young adults who reported fewer symptoms of illness recalled an emphasis on self care and healthy practices within their families, the influence of the mother being a significant factor. The traditional division of roles saw the woman as the main care giver and health educator. Many women today, by choice or by necessity, go out to work, so that, in some families, the father may have become the main care giver and health educator, whereas in other families the roles are shared by both parents. For nurses working with families, it is important to establish who is influential in relation to health promotion and education. The nurse may then maximise opportunities to pass on knowledge to the person most likely to influence the family.

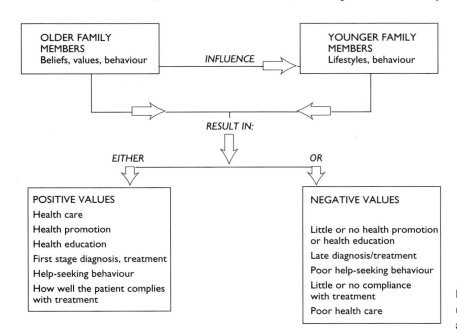

Figure 19.2: The family's role in health care – positive and negative values

LAY REFERRAL

The family acts as a **lay referral** system, which influences patterns of help-seeking behaviour. When a family member falls ill, it is often the family that responds initially by interpreting the illness, offering advice and seeking possible over-the-counter remedies. In the event of the initial advice not working, the family may then turn to outside agencies for help. The family may also decide when the sick person is fit to resume usual activities.

THE POTENTIAL FOR NURSING INTERVENTION

Nurses practising family-centred care may educate and advise family members and dispel misconceptions about healthy and unhealthy practices and their acceptability in terms of health. Different cultures, for example, have different perceptions of what is recognised as good health and bad health. Asian women may consider that, once past childbearing age, no further attention should be paid to the female reproductive organs, and may therefore ignore invitations for cervical screening (Gregory and McKie, 1990). The degenerative changes of old age may be accepted as inevitable, with no attempt to seek help in order to minimise the pain and infirmity of arthritis, deafness or failing general health. Nurses practising family-centred care can encourage a more positive approach to health by working with families, in order to ensure that the lay referral system acts swiftly in seeking professional help when appropriate.

THE FAMILY'S ROLE IN THE COMPLIANCE WITH TREATMENT

Once that help is sought, the family can be a significant influence on how well the sick individual complies with treatment. Nurses should not underestimate their influence nor the importance of gaining the trust and confidence of relatives as well as the patient. Family-centred care involves nurses in communicating with relatives; if relatives know what is happening and why treatment is being carried out, they are more likely to support and encourage the patient to comply. Implicit in such communication of information is the consent of the patient. Nurses practising family-centred care have a duty to respect patient confidentiality and that of any other member of the family who comes to be viewed as the nurse's client.

If nurses fail to establish a good rapport with the family and convince the family of the benefits of treatment, it is less likely that the patient will continue to take the prescribed medication or other treatment, once discharged from hospital. This is especially true for long-term treatment and is applicable to all branches of nursing. Parents are generally responsible for carrying out treatments for their own children, as are the parents of those with learning disabilities. If, for example, parents have no understanding or confidence in the action of nebulisers during an asthma attack or in the continued use of anti-epileptic medication, they are less likely to ensure that the treatments will be given as prescribed. Mentally ill individuals often require long-term medication, as do adults suffering from chronic illnesses and the support of family members in these circumstances is invaluable.

THE BENEFITS OF INVOLVING RELATIVES IN TREATMENT REGIMENS

Acute disorders may also benefit from family involvement and it may be more important, in some circumstances, for example, to convince the patient's partner of the need for certain treatments. If, for example, a person needs to lose weight and the partner is the person who prepares most meals, then he or she must be convinced of the value and necessity of possible changes to established eating habits. Similarly, advising a patient to stop smoking may have more chance of success if both partners smoke and both are persuaded of the necessity and positive outcomes of giving up together. The advantages of positive compliance are numerous and may include a speedier recovery, less need for further appointments with health care professionals, fewer readmissions to hospital, less distress and less cost both to the patient's family and to the National Health Service (NHS).

The financial costs to a family when a member is sick may be significant. Such costs may include prescription charges and transport costs, incurred while keeping medical appointments or when visiting relatives in hospital. The cost to the NHS is also significant in terms of wasted expenditure for the prescription of medication that is not taken and the costs of treating individuals as inpatients and outpatients. Also, a speedier recovery means less demand on services and also indirectly benefits other individuals still waiting for treatment.

FAMILY INFLUENCES ON THE HEALTH AND WELL-BEING OF INDIVIDUALS

Just as the family may have a positive influence on health and well-being, so it may also have a negative influence. Disturbed family relationships may, for example, exacerbate mental health problems. The preponderance of aetiological theories which assumed that the family played a central role in causing illness may be a reason why mental health services have taken so long to recognise the burden facing families and the extent of their specific requirements (Brooker and Towl, 1990).

Family tensions may cause psychosomatic illnesses, such as headaches, peptic ulcers, vomiting and abdominal pains. The children of re-ordered families, that is families where parents no longer live together, are more likely to experience health problems and educational and social problems than children whose families stay together (Joseph Rowntree Foundation, 1994). The increased mortality and morbidity that follows bereavement in a family is another example of how family disruption can affect the health and well-being of family members.

Key Points

Family nursing

- Most sick individuals were cared for in their own homes until the upsurge of hospitals in the eighteenth century, when care began to shift from the family into the domain of doctors and nurses.
- A family today may be described in a number of ways but the term generally refers to a group of people who are bonded in some way and who share a number of beliefs and values.
- Some families are unable to provide the material and emotional necessities expected by our society and in reality some family homes are far dif-

ferent from the place of love and safety most individuals desire.
- The family plays a significant role in health care, in health promotion and education, in interpreting health and ill health, in terms of help-seeking behaviour and in meeting the emotional and physical needs of sick family members.
- The family can also significantly influence individuals' health and well-being in a negative way.

THE EFFECTS OF ILLNESS WITHIN THE FAMILY

THE NEEDS OF RELATIVES

Most people belong to a family and most patients return to their families following treatment in hospital or, in the case of community care, continue to be cared for by family members, with or without help from outside agencies. The family's social circumstances may enhance or impede the sick person's potential for recovery and so may the way the family reacts to the illness. In some instances, illness can unite and strengthen family relationships but in other cases, the illness of one family member can be detrimental to individuals within the family or to the family as a functioning unit. In order to understand the potential effects of illness in the family, the nurse must have knowledge and understanding of the ways in which a family might function, how decisions are reached and how crises are dealt with. It is important to understand the various roles which family members take, the purpose of such roles and the nature of the interactions which can occur within a family, as these can all be factors which influence how families cope, or fail to cope, with an illness.

The potential seriousness of the illness may determine how relatives will react. Nurses should remember, however, that what might appear to be a routine hospital admission or an exacerbation of a chronic illness will not necessarily be considered in the same way by relatives.

PSYCHOLOGICAL, PHYSICAL AND SOCIAL EFFECTS OF ILLNESS WITHIN THE FAMILY

The effects of illness on the family are diverse. An overview of the effects of illness within the family and the role of the nurse are shown in Figure 19.3.

Psychological effects which an illness may have upon other family members

Relatives may experience a number of emotions when a member of the family becomes ill. Considerable anxiety may be experienced throughout the

relative's illness (Lugton, 1989) and lack of knowledge and understanding about the illness or treatment and uncertainty about the outcome will add to the anxiety (Gibbon, 1988). As previously stated, family roles include early diagnosis of an illness, referral to professional health care agencies and the provision of care for the sick person. There is, therefore, the potential for relatives to experience feelings of guilt and failure when the sick person is removed from their care. The unremitting demands of caring for a chronically sick relative at home are both emotionally draining and socially limiting. Carers' needs may become almost entirely subordinated to those of the dependant. Carers in such situations may feel

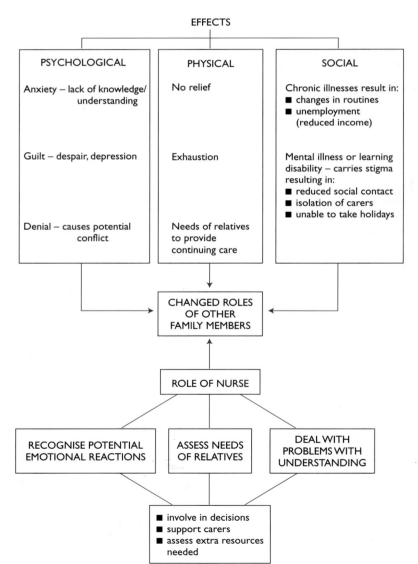

Figure 19.3: The effects of illness within the family

trapped, to the extent that they have no life outside caring, and experience guilt if they think about themselves (Nolan and Grant, 1989). In some cases, the toll of care giving can be high, giving rise to both physical and mental health problems (Baillie *et al.*, 1988). Acceptance of a poor prognosis may vary between family members (Lugton, 1989), which in turn may lead to increased stress and tension within the family. Individuals may also blame one another for a relative's illness. For example, an individual whose partner suffers a heart attack may blame the person for not following his or her advice to lose weight, give up smoking or cut down on his or her working hours, or blame their children for causing stress by their behaviour (Frost, 1970). An illness, such as a myocardial infarction, has the potential to result in the patient's partner suffering anxiety, fatigue, depression, insomnia, tearfulness, palpitations and lack of sexual interest (Thompson and Cordle, 1988).

Nurses who recognise the potential for such emotional reactions will be prepared to assess family members' needs, whether in the context of a home visit or a hospital admission.

Physical effects which an illness may have upon other family members

The physical demands of caring for a sick individual at home are great. Whereas nurses are able to go home at the end of a shift, many elderly people are left caring at home for a sick partner or a child with profound physical and/or mental disability, with no one to relieve them. The reader might find it useful to reflect that a job advertisement indicating the requirements of a typical carer may be written as follows:

- The person required must be versatile, multi-skilled and of a very patient disposition.
- Housework and nursing skills are needed, but training can be arranged.
- Hours required to be worked are 24-hour shifts, 7 days a week.
- It may be possible to negotiate one week's holiday per year.
- Payment is subject to a means test.
- Age no limit – many retired persons are carers.

These are important factors for nurses to take into consideration when practising family-centred care. Many relatives reach the point of exhaustion. The role of the nurse in these circumstances is to assess the needs of the relatives. It may well be that such relatives will be glad to hand over the responsibility of care to professional agencies when a sick relative is admitted into a hospital or nursing home. An important part of family-centred care is the nursing assessment, which will identify how the needs of relatives can be met most appropriately. Some relatives, despite their exhaustion, may need to continue to care in a physical sense for a sick relative and be involved in decision making; others will not and should not be made to feel guilty about relinquishing the caring role. If care is to be continued in the home, it may not be possible for relatives to carry out care independently. Nurses must, in this case, support the primary care givers as much as possible and make an assessment of the need for extra resources as appropriate and possible within the constraints of the current NHS.

Social effects which an illness may have upon a family

The illness of a family member can influence the social behaviour of the family group. Chronic illness, in particular, may affect the social aspects of family life in a number of ways, depending upon its nature and severity. Relatives faced with caring for a frail elderly parent, for example, may be confronted with a number of problems. These may include disturbed sleep patterns caused by the nocturnal wanderings of the dependent relative; security risks to the home when doors are left open; spoiled home furnishings due to spilled food and incontinence; extra laundry; difficulty in dealing with memory lapses; accusations of theft and aggressive behaviour which, normally, would be totally out of character. The primary carer may find it difficult to continue in paid employment and, as benefits do not usually equate to income from paid employment, the family's social activities may be constrained by the decrease in income. Also, some individuals placed in a caring role experience difficulty and embarrassment in coping with bathing and other aspects of hygiene (Bloomfield, 1986). Nurses who recognise the socially limiting nature of caring for such a relative will be better able to plan care for the family, which will allow family members time for each other, for example, by arranging for periods of respite care.

Families caring for relatives with a mental illness or learning disability have the added stress of coping with the stigma frequently associated with such problems. Some families feel a sense of shame and embarrassment and reduce social interaction because of this. Such families may appear defensive and overprotective when dealing with professional agencies. This type of reaction must be dealt with sensitively by nurses who should demonstrate understanding of the problems that these families may have experienced from other people. For other families, the constant physical and emotional demands placed upon them by the sick or disabled dependant may mean that it is difficult to arrange any social life for themselves outside the home. Even within the home, inviting friends around is not without problems. It may be necessary, for example, to use a downstairs room as a bedroom, which limits the opportunity to entertain guests. Carers may become very isolated, sometimes unable to leave their dependent relative in order to go shopping and many carers are unable to take a holiday.

The role that the sick person plays within the family is a significant factor to be taken into consideration when assessing how illness may have affected other family members. The illness of one person may mean that another member of the family may take on the sick person's role. This could mean taking responsibility for decision making or for organising family holidays or outings; some elderly relatives may even learn to drive in order to maintain a degree of independence when their partner becomes infirm. Taking control of family finances and being responsible for paying the bills may be a completely new role that has to be adopted, as may everyday tasks, such as housework, doing the shopping and preparing meals. All these role changes can add greatly to the stresses already highlighted.

Perhaps the most difficult role changes are those which take place between partners and between parents and their children. When one partner becomes chronically sick, it may mean that a previous style of relationship between a man and woman is no longer possible. The deficits may not be merely a lost physical relationship but the loss of a trusted confidant, whom the well partner previously relied upon for strength and support. It can be very difficult for some people to adapt to being the stronger partner. It may also be difficult to reverse the parent/child role. Instead of the parent looking after the child, the child may now need to care for the parent as if the parent was a child.

YOUNG CARERS

Issues concerning **young carers** are characterised by their hidden nature. This may be due to lack of targeted services and the fear of stigma perceived by parents to be a consequence of drawing attention to their needs (Meredith, 1992). Fear of being separated from their families, either by the institutionalisation of the dependent person or by the removal of the child into the care of the local authority, are further reasons for maintaining secrecy. Child carers perform all the tasks associated with adult carers, including intimate acts of personal hygiene. Sexual taboos, however, make it socially unacceptable for children to be performing such acts for a parent of the opposite sex, or for any adult. Fear of punishment may be a further inducement to a child's silence (Dearden *et al.*, 1995).

Caring can affect a child's development, physically, emotionally, educationally and socially (Meredith, 1992). Lifting can cause health problems. Children are not receiving training in lifting, perhaps because offering such training would condone and legitimise the lifting of adults by children. Friendships and socialisation are restricted; for many children, the restrictions placed upon them also interfere with their fundamental right to education (Dearden *et al.*, 1995).

Nurses are well placed to identify and support child carers. Knowledge of the family roles and dynamics will assist the nurse to identify the primary carer within the family, as it should not be assumed, where adults are part of the household, that the child is not the primary carer. Gaining the young carer's trust is crucial to the success of the nursing intervention. The nurse should be prepared to listen to the views of the young carer, recognise and respect his/her possible reluctance to give up the role, while monitoring the situation and offering extra support as appropriate. The need for accurate, intelligible information is even more crucial for young carers, who should not be expected to care without the knowledge of the implications of such caring, its possible duration and outcome. The recognition and support of young carers will improve their health and well-being and promote family-centred care (Dearden et al., 1995).

ABUSE OF ELDERLY DEPENDANTS

The stress of caring can lead to abuse of the dependant. In a 1990 study of elders admitted for respite care, 2% were found to have suffered physical abuse, 20% verbal abuse and 20% neglect. Forty five per cent of carers admitted some form of abuse (Homer and Gilliard, 1990). The only UK national abuse study to date, found a reported prevalence of 2% physical abuse, 5% verbal abuse and 2% financial abuse (Ogg and Bennett, 1992). **Elder abuse** is an escalating problem (Lynch, 1997), but dissemination of research carried out in the USA, where many studies have been undertaken on elder abuse, has been inadequate (Warren and Bennett, 1997). An awareness that elder abuse exists is a prerequisite for nurses involved in caring for families where there is an elderly dependant.

Nursing interventions focus on maintaining safety and evaluating a patient's autonomy and capacity to make decisions. The elder's acceptance or refusal of assistance is fundamental to any nursing intervention. The nurse should also support the abusers, by removing the victim from danger, thus relieving the abuser of care-giving responsibility and stress. The provision of counselling services and education are further options (Lynch, 1997).

BURN-OUT SYNDROME

Chronic illness in one partner and the resulting burden of care placed upon the other partner can lead to spouse burn-out syndrome, which encompasses both physical and emotional symptoms (Ekberg et al., 1986). In the first stage of burn-out, described by Shubin (1978), emotional and physical exhaustion occurs, with the accompanying signs and symptoms of stress. Insomnia and depression may also be evident. In the second stage, the individual develops a negative, cynical and dehumanised attitude, becomes withdrawn, experiencing feelings of futility with no opportunity to ventilate such feelings. At this stage, the individual is likely to be quick to anger and develops a paranoid-like state. In the final stage of

burn-out, all emotional feelings and concern for others have been described as being lost. Behaviour may include complete detachment, self-disgust and sourness towards oneself and humanity. Almberg et al. (1997) found that older wives and daughters were most likely to report burn-out in their lives, although some siblings and daughters-in-law also risked developing burn-out. An awareness of the adverse effects of being a primary carer and recognition of the signs and symptoms of burn-out syndrome enable the nurse to prevent it, or to recognise the first-stage signs and symptoms and plan appropriate nursing interventions.

CULTURAL DIFFERENCES

Understanding of cultural differences in family roles and communication patterns is essential for the practice of family-centred care. In Asian cultures, for example, pregnancy and childbirth may be regarded as the sole domain of women. Husbands may be excluded from the discussions and preparations for childbirth and refuse invitations to accompany their wives to antenatal classes or be present at the birth of the child. It is also common for relatives to care for children (Parmar, 1985).

Understanding such cultural characteristics avoids misunderstandings and also enables health education and the teaching of nursing skills to be directed at the most appropriate primary care giver. Poor communication patterns can lead to hostility, anger or silence and it is necessary for nurses to identify the person or persons to whom information should be given. This is particularly so in cases where language is a potential barrier to communication, and in cases where there is a recognised head of the family. It is to this person that matters requiring decisions on health care issues are best addressed. The customs surrounding life events and the values concerning life and health vary in different cultures and these should be considered and assessed when planning family-centred care.

ACCESS TO RELATIVES IN HOSPITAL

In the eighteenth century, the voluntary hospitals were quick to draw up rules and regulations to establish the roles expected of nurses, patients and relatives. Such rules gave nurses the power to enforce the behaviour of visitors. Initially, this was deemed to be good for the organisation and latterly for the good of the patient (Hawker, 1984). Restrictions on visiting continued until the middle of the twentieth century. It was common practice in the 1950s for two visiting cards to be handed to patients. Relatives were only admitted if they showed a visiting card to the porter 'guarding' the entrance to the wards. In some cases, parents were not allowed to visit their sick child unless he/she was asleep, which was traumatic both for the child and the parents. The Platt Report (Platt, 1959) drew attention to the need to encourage a more open and participative approach to the care of children in hospital and this was further reinforced by the work of Bowlby and Fry (1965), who compared the emotions experienced by children who were separated from their mothers as similar to the process of grieving which follows the death of a loved one. Yet, despite this report and the growing impact of consumerism, the strength of the hospital as an institution, with the power to resist change, is such that response to more open visiting has been slow in many cases (Biley, 1988; Griffith, 1988; Pottle, 1990).

When a sick member of the family is admitted to hospital, most relatives will wish to visit. Visiting is, for many, an expression of love for the sick person. In some settings, however, restrictions remain on visiting times, despite the benefits to be gained from open visiting. Individuals who are seriously ill derive comfort and support from the presence of those closest to them; similarly, being present at the sick person's bedside may also comfort relatives. Sick children usually respond more positively to a parent than to a nurse who is a comparative stranger. Patients with head injuries have been shown to respond better in the 'waking up period' when a relative or friend stays in the room with them (Date *et al.*, 1987). Enabling relatives to continue their caring roles can be beneficial to relative, patient and nurse.

As previously stated, the powers of the 'hospital' are slow to be eroded and patient autonomy remains secondary to the rules of the institution. The question of open visiting is often countered by the need for patients to rest, yet most relatives, when given guidance, are only too willing to respond to suggestions that the patient does need some time to rest. Open visiting can be particularly beneficial to relatives who work shifts or who have distances to travel. Elderly people, particularly, may not like using public transport when it is dark. It should be remembered that open visiting does not necessarily mean the same as all day visits. Perhaps this is the message that needs reinforcing; as one ward sister observed to the author, 'Visitors feel obliged to stay for long periods and the ward can become very noisy and patients can't rest.'

Many paediatric wards and maternity wards have noted the psychological benefits to patients as a result of extended visiting times (Pottle, 1990). It seems anomalous that the family should be excluded from visits when a baby is born, as this is a time when most families wish to celebrate and welcome the new family member and a time when a mother wants to show her new baby to the family. Extending visiting hours also helps patients who do not have many visitors. Such patients are spared the discomfiture of being conspicuous by the absence of visitors during a limited, set period of visiting.

Adequate provision for visiting by members of the extended family may be necessary. Asian cultures, for example, often express feelings of caring by their physical presence and attendance in times of illness rather than by using verbal expressions (Kozier and Glenora, 1988). In a small study I sought to determine the extent of the practice of family-centred care in six wards of a general hospital in a large East Midlands city. In relation to visiting, provision was made on all six wards for relatives to carry out customs and practices associated with death and dying and also preferred dietary requirements. Large numbers of visitors were allowed, subject to the patient's condition, and alternative areas were made available to groups of visitors on two of the wards (Whittaker, 1992).

The way that nurses view relatives may influence their views about open visiting. Beggs (1991) found that while patients and visitors preferred extended visiting, many nurses continued to doubt that it was in the best interests of the patients. Nurses felt reluctant to disturb visitors, a situation that they felt led to unsatisfactory care, but patients and visitors did not share this view. If nurses consider relatives as partners in care, such barriers would not be present; it is when nurses view their roles as distinct from the caring role of relatives that such barriers in communication are likely to arise.

On admission to hospital, the patient's relatives assume the role of visitor and in many cases are called upon to relinquish their caring role. For some this is done readily and with relief, as previously stated, but nurses cannot assume that this will apply to all relatives. Some relatives need to continue to care for the sick person and can support nurses and save nursing time by carrying out some aspects of care. They can contribute a great deal of information about the patient, as relatives often know the patient best. They have background knowledge that doctors and nurses have no access to and which may make them an invaluable resource but, unfortunately, one which is often a wasted resource. It must be emphasised, however, that meeting the needs of relatives involves an invitation to participate in care and not an assumption that care can be left to relatives. Many carers suffer from chronic physical and mental exhaustion and are themselves elderly; the nurse's role in this instance is to instil relatives with the confidence to let go and leave the care to the nursing team.

The nursing profession claims to practise holistic care, which is nursing care that embraces the whole person (this is explored more fully Chapter 11). If we accept that the majority of patients belong to a family and may be influenced by that family and that, conversely, the patient may also influence how the family adapts and copes with illness, then excluding the family from visiting and participating is a failure to practise holistic care. Holistic care, in this sense, means allowing the family to be together, to support, comfort and encourage each other. Holistic care then is synonymous with family-centred care.

RELATIVES' DISSATISFACTION

Relatives most frequently seek information about the diagnosis, treatment and prognosis of their next of kin and, if relevant and sufficient information is given, anxiety is likely to be reduced (Gibbon, 1988). There is evidence, however, that relatives are frequently dissatisfied with the information given to them (Fox, 1985; Bolger, 1986; Whalley, 1988). Such anecdotal accounts are supported by research, for example, studies by Thompson and Cordle (1988), Lugton (1989), Harrison and Smith (1990), and Newens (1995) indicated that there was a need for more effective communication with relatives. Writers such as Frost (1970) and Gibbon (1990) have focused upon the poor performance of nurses as communicators. In some cases, it may be that nurses do not have the information, or that they lack the skills and training required to exchange information effectively. Good communication skills will, according to Crossfield (1990), reduce the stress nurses can experience in relating to anxious relatives.

Gibbon (1990) points out that relatives may be reluctant to approach busy nurses, they may feel anxious about their ability to articulate the question or to understand the answer. Using jargon may enhance the nurse's power over the relative and may be used subconsciously by nurses to reduce their own stress in the relationship. This is reinforced if the onus to seek information is on the relative. Krozek (1991) further suggests that, under stress, relatives may not hear all that is said to them and information may therefore need to be repeated.

When a family member becomes ill, the whole family can be thrown into a state of crisis. The way in which family members adapt and cope with the illness can ultimately influence the outcome of the illness for the individual and the well-being of the other family members. Nurses are able to assist or hinder relatives in this process of adaptation and coping.

Nurses may underestimate the degree of anxiety that minor procedures or illnesses can generate for relatives. For example, parents who agree to their child having a tonsillectomy may be plagued with uncertainty and guilt when the time comes for the operation to take place. In recognising this potential anxiety, a planned admission could include an opportunity to express such anxieties and, at the same time, enable nurses and doctors to give full explanations of the procedure and care. This helps to reassure parents and results in satisfactory outcomes of care for all concerned.

Relatives often wish to know the diagnosis, the outcome of present treatment and the prognosis, assuming of course that the patient consents to this. This information is necessary in order for family members to adopt an appropriate coping strategy. Being told to take the patient home and contact the general practitioner in 2 weeks' time to find out if the tests show that the patient has cancer is totally unacceptable, yet such was the author's experience. A less assertive, informed relative may well have complied with the nurse's instructions and spent 2 weeks in distress, awaiting the outcome of the tests. Relatives must be spared such unnecessary stress by passing on information as soon as possible.

Complaints made to the Health Service Commissioner indicate some relatives' dissatisfaction with the information given to them. Such complainants claim that information is inadequate and contradictory, as in the complaint made by the relatives of an elderly woman who fell from her hospital bed. Complaints have also highlighted a lack of information about the cancellation of an operation; a decision not to resuscitate an elderly woman; post-mortem arrangements for a stillborn baby; failure to inform relatives of the financial consequences of transferring an 89-year-old woman (Health Service Commissioner, 1996). These complaints highlight the distress that such lack of information has caused to relatives.

Relatives may feel dissatisfied with the information given to them even though doctors and nurses have given both oral and written information, as demonstrated in a study by Thompson and Cordle (1988). They concluded that there is a need to repeat information once the acute stage of an illness is past, for if the information is given at the stage when relatives are in a state of anxiety, it is likely that they will not remember all that they have been told. This has the potential effect of leaving them feeling dissatisfied with the level of knowledge that they have about such things as the illness the relative has suffered, about the after care of the patient or his/her prognosis. The way that nurses respond to requests for information can influence relatives' satisfaction and is illustrated in Figure 19.4.

Relatives may feel reluctant to 'bother' busy staff and if requests for information are dismissed in a brusque and demeaning manner, this serves to reinforce relatives' feelings of being a nuisance. When nurses resort to the use of medical and nursing jargon, this reinforces the power of the professional and places the relative at a disadvantage. This tactic may also serve to keep relatives 'at arms' length', discouraging further approaches for information. The onus should be on staff to ensure that both relatives and patient are kept informed. It is also important that the information given should be accurate and realistic. It is distressing for relatives to be given false hope or

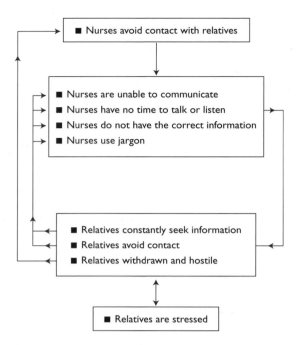

Figure 19.4: Responses to requests for information – influence on relatives' behaviour

unrealistic goals in terms of rehabilitation and similarly distressing to be given confusing and conflicting information by different members of the multidisciplinary team. It is thus imperative that good communication exists between all health care professionals involved in the care of a patient.

Dissatisfaction may also stem from relatives' lack of confidence in the health care professionals responsible for the delivery of care. For example, relatives of individuals with a learning disability will need to know that nursing staff understand the special needs of patients and, to do this, nurses must be prepared to listen to relatives. If such a partnership in care is formed, relatives will have the confidence to entrust care to the professionals who have listened and noted what they have to say, and who are prepared to adapt nursing care to meet the special demands of the patients.

INVOLVING RELATIVES IN CARE

Gibbon (1988) contends that excluding relatives from caring for the patient may act as a stressor. Relatives relinquish their caring role when a family member is admitted to hospital. While recognising the expertise of health professionals, relatives may still wish to be involved in care, as this is one way in which affection for another person can be manifested. The onus is upon nurses to assess the relatives' needs.

Involving relatives in care can be successful where the patient is very young (Parfit, 1975; Pike, 1989), and when the patient is elderly (Turner, 1989). Relatives can also be successfully involved in psychiatry (Wilkinson, 1981; Youssef, 1987) and in critical care situations (Millar, 1989).

PARTICIPATION IN CARE

Relatives' needs may be met by giving information and by allowing participation in care. Dissatisfaction with hospital care can arise when relatives are left to carry out basic nursing care. If relatives do not wish to participate and feel uncomfortable in doing so, they may be left feeling angry and resentful at nursing staff and perhaps guilty that they are not willing participants. Thrusting care upon unwilling relatives is contrary to the concept of family-centred care.

The finding of my study was that relatives were sometimes invited to participate in planning care; only one ward sister thought that this was always appropriate. She said: 'If the patient is to be discharged into the relative's care, we would probably include them.' Only two ward sisters considered that it was always appropriate to invite relatives to participate in care, although all subjects were able to confirm that relatives did sometimes participate in a number of nursing care tasks (Whittaker, 1992). Although the findings of my study cannot be generalised, given the small number of wards involved, they are significant in that they concur with Gibbon's (1988) assertion that relatives are often not involved in planning care.

Key Points

- Initially, restriction was considered to be 'for the good of the organisation', then 'for the good of the patient'.
- Restricting access is a way of exerting power.
- Sick people respond well to the presence of relatives.
- Cultural considerations must be acknowledged.
- Relatives can add to the quality of care.

- The role that relatives can play and wish to play may vary.
- Nurses may underestimate the role that relatives can play and thereby waste a valuable resource.
- Many relatives may be dissatisfied with the ways in which nurses treat them.
- Relatives are frequently dissatisfied with the information that they receive.
- Nurses may underestimate the anxiety that relatives experience.
- Information should be passed on to relatives at the earliest opportunity.
- Good communication between members of the multidisciplinary team is essential.
- Relatives must have confidence in health care practitioners' abilities to meet the needs of indivudal patients.
- Relatives should be invited and not expected to participate in hospital care.

FAMILY-CENTRED CARE IN PRACTICE

Family-centred care is a systematic approach to meeting the needs of family members, either on an individual basis or collectively as a family unit. Just as models of nursing have been developed to meet the individual needs of patients and clients, similarly models have been developed in relation to family-centred care. For example, Friedemann (1989) describes the concept of family nursing as being on three levels, as follows:

- Individual level
- Interpersonal level
- System level.

On an individual level, any family member may become the client. Individuals are seen as subsystems of the total family system. While one individual is seen as the client, the subsystems provide a supportive network. When the ill family member is the client, the nurse may provide skilled care, counselling and health promotion. Other family members become clients when they are taught how to perform caretaking tasks or when they are helped to meet their particular physical and emotional needs. This level assumes a well-functioning family system.

At an interpersonal level, the need for intervention arises when conflict occurs between individuals. The nurse's role at this level involves the use of communication techniques and addresses family processes, such as decision making, limit setting and defining family roles. The nursing goal is to achieve a harmonious environment. Nursing intervention must be based on knowledge and understanding of the family and its interpersonal processes.

Family system nursing includes all actions aimed at changes in the system process or processes. System changes are achieved through nursing interventions directed at the individuals and family interactional system and may also involve the environment within which the system interacts. Family system nursing plans personal and interpersonal changes as parts of a master system plan. When a system change is indicated, the nurse specialist negotiates with the family an approach that is tailored to the family's needs and one which is also consistent with the general coping strategies of the family (Friedemann, 1989). This is illustrated in Figure 19.5.

In the context of acute nursing situations and for those requiring day care when turnover of patients is rapid, there is less opportunity for family-centred care than in long-term care situations. However, whether in hospital or the patient's home, whenever nurses have the oppor-

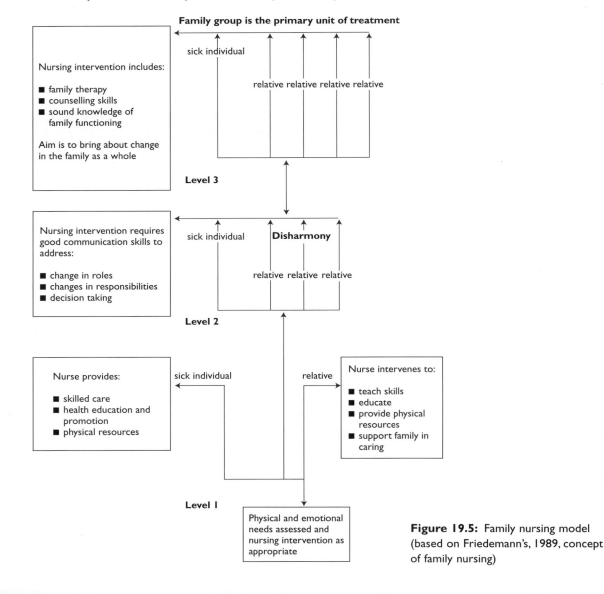

Figure 19.5: Family nursing model (based on Friedemann's, 1989, concept of family nursing)

tunity to develop rapport with relatives, there is a chance to practise family-centred care.

Identifying stressed relatives, during short-term hospital admissions, affords an opportunity to practise family-centred care at an individual level. The stressed relatives, as well as the sick individual, can become the nurse's clients. Just as a plan of care is formulated to meet the physical and emotional needs of the sick person, so nursing interventions can be systematically planned to meet relatives' needs, for example in alleviating stress. Caring for carers should have a high priority for nurses involved in community care. Many carers are themselves elderly or responsible for other dependants and can easily become depressed and physically exhausted. In such circumstances, the nurse's focus of care can be upon the patient and carers and nursing interventions aimed at meeting relatives' needs. This may include making referrals to other agencies for extra resources or increasing the level of support made available to the carer in terms of extra visits by nursing staff. Respite care for the sick person to give the carer a rest is a further option for consideration.

When illness in the family leads to changes in members' roles, such as who makes decisions, or financial hardship due to the loss of income brought in by the sick person, discord among family members can occur. It may be that the person left to pay the bills has never had control over the finances and does not deal with them very successfully, leading to family arguments and individuals blaming each other. Sometimes family members may blame each other about decisions that have been taken, or vie with one another for control of family decisions. In some cases family members become angry if they feel that they are being left to do most of the work involved in caring for the dependent person. To restore harmony, the nurse practising family-centred care at the interpersonal level can plan interventions aimed at resolving the conflict. This may be achieved by the nurse spending time with groups of family members and encouraging them to communicate with each other and to plan workable strategies to overcome the problems that they are able to identify. In order to practise at the interpersonal level, the nurse must have good communication skills and must know the family, understand how family members interact with each other and how they are likely to respond to the planned interven-

tion. Furthermore, a prerequisite to the practice of family-centred care is that the family must recognise that a problem exists and want to resolve it.

Nursing interventions at a family system level involve interventions at an individual and an interpersonal level, with the ultimate aim of causing changes in the system processes or structure (Friedemann, 1989). Family-centred care at this level, according to Friedemann, requires the nurse to have knowledge of family development, family functioning and therapy theories. Nurses need to know how family members react with each other and their environment. Although nursing at this level requires a specialist practitioner, it may be practised in any branch of nursing. Mental health nurses frequently work with dysfunctional families, with the aim of bringing about changes at a system level. Similarly, nurses with the appropriate skills from other branches working with a family in crisis may plan interventions at a system level, for example, in families where one member develops autoimmune deficiency syndrome (AIDS) or when a child becomes terminally ill. In such instances the whole family is the nurse's client.

Nursing theories developed for individualised care may also be adapted to family-centred care. Orem's self care deficit is described by Taylor (1989) as follows:

- The family may condition the patient's therapeutic self care demand and self care agency.
- The family may be the setting within which dependent care is given.
- The family is the client – in this case nurses accept responsibility for individual family members, dependent care units and the family as a unit.

Key Points

Models of family-centred care

- Family-centred care requires a systematic approach.
- Models of family-centred care enable the focus of care to fall upon the individual family member, dyads, triads or the whole family unit.
- Nursing theories based upon individualised care can be adapted to family-centred care.
- Family members need to recognise the need for nursing intervention and be prepared to accept help.

THE IMPLICATIONS OF FAMILY-CENTRED CARE FOR PRACTICE

Embracing the concepts of family-centred care does not mean that nurses are accepting something that is an entirely new idea, for nurses have always been involved with the families of those individuals who require nursing interventions. What is perhaps 'new' is the concept of adopting a systematic approach to the care of families. In essence, the patient can no longer be seen in isolation from other individuals or subsystems that make up the family system. Nurses practising family-centred care acknowledge the effects which illness has upon other members of the patient's family and how family members can influence the patient's compliance with treatment and his or her ultimate recovery.

Family-centred care needs to be integrated within the theoretical and practical components of nursing. A prerequisite to the successful practice of family-centred care is that nurses must have good communication skills. The dissatisfaction expressed by relatives about the lack of information is evident in complaints made to the Health Service Commissioner and in reports in the media. There are a number of factors to consider in relation to nursing practice and relatives' dissatisfaction with the information that they have been given. The following questions should be addressed:

- Do nurses have the relevant communication skills?
- Do nurses recognise the need to give information?
- Is the information being given at the appropriate time?
- Is the information given in a way that relatives can understand?
- Do nurses have the time to give to relatives?

IMPLICATIONS FOR NURSE EDUCATION AND TRAINING

A study by Gibbon concluded that most nurses had not acquired effective communication skills by the time that they had completed the theoretical component of the training course. When faced with a difficult question, nurses were also found to resort to the use of stock phrases (Gibbon, 1990). The onus is upon nurse education to ensure that communication skills are given a high profile in pre-registration courses and are included progressively throughout the entirety of the course. Clinical practitioners supervising students must also participate in assisting students to develop good communication skills. When practitioners have well-developed communication skills, dealing with anxious relatives will become less stressful and this will thus help both practitioners and relatives.

In order for nurses to be able to practise family-centred care, pre-registration nursing courses must reflect family issues. The curriculum should include such things as family theories, family development and function theories so that nurses can understand the ways in which families may influence matters relating to health and welfare. An integrated approach to the study of social sciences, biological sciences, psychology and nursing studies will further enhance the opportunity for nurses to practise holistic care in its fullest sense.

IMPLICATIONS FOR CLINICAL PRACTICE

A study by Newens (1995) concluded that nurses were frequently not pro-active in offering information to the relatives in the study. This is a short-sighted approach because relatives who are given adequate information can do much to reassure the patient and aid his or her recovery. Well-informed relatives are also less likely continually to seek information. Given the results of the study by Thompson and Cordle (1988), it would also seem appropriate to repeat the information that is given.

The way in which nursing moves forward depends in part on the relationships which nurses establish with relatives. Nurses may see relatives as nuisances, demanding attention, criticising and interfering with care. Robinson and Thorne (1984) suggest that interference represents the family's way of attempting positively to influence the care of the sick individual. When such interference is recognised within the context of health care relationships, family and health care professionals can negotiate in order to reach a mutually satisfying plan of care.

Family-centred care involves nurses working as partners in care, supporting relatives whether in hospital or in the community and passing on, as appropriate, nursing skills and knowledge. It requires an approach to care that recognises the need to offer relatives the opportunity to continue to be involved in care during hospital admissions, if they so wish. When care is taking place in the patient's home, the nurse's role in family-centred care will also be a partnership in care, in this case with the informal carer. It is important that nurse and carer agree the goals of care and therefore plan care together.

The effective practice of family-centred care requires a great deal of commitment from the nursing profession together with adequate resourcing.

PROFESSIONAL COMMITMENT TO THE CONCEPT OF FAMILY-CENTRED CARE

- Practising nurses must be committed to the concept of care being focused upon the family.
- Pre-registration nursing courses must adequately prepare nurses for the practice of family-centred care.
- Pre-registration and post-registration courses must reflect the principles of family-centred care.
- There must be adequate resources in terms of staff, finances and physical resources.

The latter point has significant implications in relation to practising family-centred care. Time is often at a premium and when faced with a choice, nurses' first duty must be to attend to the needs of the sick person. If staffing levels are poor, it is unlikely that nurses will have time to address the needs of the family at any level of family nursing. Busy hospital wards may be short-staffed and the number of visits to patients in the community may be limited. Providing nursing aids, such as lifting equipment, is costly and ensuring that such aids are available requires a financial commitment from central government. Nurses wishing to practise family-centred care may well find themselves frustrated by the lack of resources available for them to provide the extra help that they believe carers require. The reality of health care in the current climate of financial restraint may mean that a 'sticking plaster' approach is all that can be managed, rather than addressing the total needs of families in crisis, as nurses committed to family-centred care would wish to do.

THE IMPLICATIONS OF THE COMMUNITY CARE ACT FOR FAMILY-CENTRED CARE

A long-term aim of the Community Care reforms, which were implemented from 1993, was to allow vulnerable people to live as independently as possible in their homes. The term 'care in the community by the community' is an apt and familiar description of these reforms. It serves to highlight the reality of community care for the carers, estimated in the General Household Survey in Britain in 1990 to be in the region of 6.8 million people (the figure is likely to be much greater after the next General Household Survey, due to be carried out in the year 2000). Of these 6.8 million people, 3.7 million adults are bearing the responsibility for the care of someone. Just under one-third of these carers live with the dependent relative. A significant number of carers report a longstanding illness that limits their activities and, overall, two-thirds of carers do not receive regular visits from social services and voluntary groups (International Year of the Family [IYF] 1994). An objective of the reforms was to ensure that service providers give high priority to giving carers practical support. This was to be achieved by needs assessment of both patients and carers in a joint nursing and social services undertaking.

The burden of caring for a dependent relative can be a heavy one. Carers may find themselves virtual prisoners in their homes, unable to leave the house to go shopping, unable to socialise, take a holiday and at the same time emotionally and physically exhausted. Financial assistance is available to full-time carers through the Invalid Care Allowance. This is not available to young carers over the age of 16 years who are in full-time education (Dearden et al., 1995). The mainstay of community care, however, is adequate provision of financial resource and, by 1994, some local authorities declared that they had no funds for new cases, whilst other authorities predicted that they would face a similar situation before the end of the financial year. This had clear implications for community nurses who could be involved in decisions as to where to withdraw services. Nurses are also in the 'front line' when relatives are dissatisfied with the services provided. The Patient's Charter produced by the Department of Health (DoH, 1992) served to raise people's expectations of the standards of service that the public should receive from the NHS. Local community care charters include the following commitments:

■ To provide full and accurate information, in plain language, about available services
■ To fully involve carers in the arrangements made by the local authority, to have their views taken into account (DoH, 1994).

The above points are integral to family-centred care, so it is not a matter of choice for nurses but an expectation of those caring for a dependant. This serves to reinforce the need for a programme of education and practice that adequately prepares nurses to practise family-centred care in a manner that is based on theoretical concepts.

Key Points

Implications of family-centred care for nursing practice

■ Nurses have always been involved with families.
■ There is a need to adopt a systematic approach to family nursing.
■ Good communication skills are a prerequisite to the practice of family-centred care.
■ Nursing curricula should prepare students for family-centred care.
■ Nurses in practice should recognise and plan to meet the needs of relatives.
■ Practitioners must adopt a philosophy of forging partnerships in care with relatives.
■ The practice of family-centred care has resource implications in terms of training, staffing levels and provision of nursing aids.
■ The Community Care Act aims to assist individuals to live independently in their homes rather than in an institution.
■ Care in the community by the community.
■ 6.8 million carers in 1990.
■ Carers can become emotionally and physically exhausted.
■ Parliament recognised the need to support carers.
■ Funding needs to be sufficient to meet resource demands.
■ Carers may have raised expectations of the standards of service to be provided by the National Health Service.

■ Meeting local charter standards reflects some aspects of family-centred care.
■ The Community Care Act reinforces the need to prepare nurses for the practice of family-centred care.

CONCLUSION

The need for family-centred care has never been greater, given that people are living longer and that the number of frail and elderly people requiring assistance to live independently has consequently increased. The current government policy, to return people to the community rather than providing institutional care, means that families are, in many cases, undertaking care for elderly, chronically sick and disabled relatives. The financial implications of a competitive health service also adds a further dimension to the informal care scenario, as the trend continues to make hospital stays as short as possible. Relatives are expected to continue care after acute episodes of illness, until the sick person is able to regain independence. The nurse's role for the future will centre on family groups, assessing the needs of the patient and carers, whether in the context of community or hospital.

Funding family-centred care in the short term has financial implications but in the long term may well prove to be cost-effective, for example, in preventing carers becoming acutely ill through the stress of looking after a dependent relative, which in turn places extra demands on health services. In acute illness, nurses practising family-centred care can do so much to alleviate the stress experienced by relatives. This can be done, for example, by assessing relatives' needs; to be involved in care; by keeping relatives informed and participating in care if they so wish. Such participation may be in carrying out simple tasks or in some instances, technical and skilled tasks, such as teaching relatives to undertake renal dialysis at home for a patient. Working in partnership with relatives enables nurses to utilise a valuable resource, that is the knowledge that relatives have of the patient. It also can free nurses to carry out other tasks. If nurses fail to recognise the role of the family as a health care agency, it is unlikely that a successful partnership will be achieved.

When families are dissatisfied with care, they can exert a negative influence on the patient that can affect the patient's compliance with treatment. This in turn has financial implications on health services in terms of a more lengthy term of illness and repeated demands upon health care services.

Relatives may well have increased expectations of the health care services that should be made available to them and to the patient. They may also have expectations of nurses and other health care professionals. Whatever the family configuration, in most cases there is an underlying need to care for the sick individual, and when the family can no longer care, they want the best for the patient from the professional agencies, in whom they place their trust. When the agencies fail, trust is lost. Relatives then face conflict, they feel dissatisfied with care and fear alienation if they complain but accept the need for continued intervention from health professionals. Re-establishing trust and confidence may be difficult and forging a successful partnership in care with relatives is therefore important, in order to avoid such a situation. Indeed, failing to meet the needs of patients and their relatives may not only be in breach of the promises incumbent in the Patient's Charter but also contrary to the Code of Professional Conduct for the Nurse, Midwife and Health Visitor (UKCC, 1992). Ultimately, however, it may not be lack of commitment to families that hinders care but lack of resources.

Key Points

- The need for family-centred care has never been greater.
- Carers can become ill themselves if unsupported in their caring role.
- Nurses practising family-centred care can do much to alleviate the stress experienced by relatives.
- Funding family-centred care can be cost-effective in the long term.
- Family-centred care can be practised whenever nurses are able to develop rapport with relatives.
- Failing to meet relatives' needs may be in breach of the Patient's Charter and the Code of Professional Conduct for the Nurse, Midwife and Health Visitor (UKCC, 1992).

Summary

- Historically the majority of sick people were cared for in their own homes.
- As medical knowledge increased, the demand for more hospitals also increased and care shifted from the family to care by health professionals.
- Families have much to do with health education; the lifestyle of a family may be reflected in the future behaviour of the young.
- Families may act as a lay referral system and can influence the sick individual's compliance with treatment.
- Whatever the configuration of the family, and this is so diverse in the 1990s, the instinct to care for sick members remains true for most families.
- The illness of one family member may cause illness in other family members.
- Evidence suggests that relatives are frequently dissatisfied with care.
- Relatives are frequently excluded from care or conversely may be left to shoulder the burden of care without adequate support.
- Family-centred care is a systematic approach to meeting the needs of family members; it is much more than just giving information or allowing participation in care.
- Models of family-centred care enable the focus of care to fall upon individual family members, dyads, triads or the whole family system.
- The result of one small research study indicated that the needs of relatives were not systematically assessed or planned for.
- Nursing practice of the future may depend upon nurses' ability to form working partnerships with relatives.
- Nurse educators must ensure that nursing curricula encompass the principles and theoretical concepts of family-centred care.
- Effective communication skills should be a taught component of nursing courses that are progressively developed throughout the course and during clinical practice.
- Care in the community places the burden of care upon relatives, and without adequate support, that burden may prove too great.
- Financing family-centred care may be costly in the short term but cost-effective in the long term.
- Ignoring the needs of relatives may be seen as a violation of the promises made in the local com-

munity care charters, which have served to raise carers' expectations of the health services and resources that should be available to them.

- Failing to meet the needs of relatives may be contrary to the Professional Code of Conduct for the Nurse, Midwife and Health Visitor (UKCC, 1992).
- Nurses cannot claim to practise holistic care if they ignore the needs of relatives.

REFERENCES

Almberg, B., Grafstrom, M. and Winblad, B. (1997). Caring for a demented elderly person – burden and burnout among caregiving relatives. *Journal of Advanced Nursing*, 25(1), 109–16.

Baillie, V., Norbeck, J.S. and Barnes, L.E.A. (1988). Stress, social support, and psychological distress of family caregivers of the elderly. *Nursing Research*, 37(4), 217–22.

Baly, M.E. (1980). *Nursing and Social Change*. 2nd edn. William Heinemann Medical Books Ltd, London.

Beggs, H. (1991). Extended visiting in a surgical ward. *Nursing Standard*, 5(3), 29–31.

Biley, F. (1988). Open all hours? *Nursing Times*, 84(44), 60–1.

Bloomfield, K. (1986). Ask the family. *Nursing Times*, 82(11), 28–30.

Bolger, T. (1986). Safe in whose hands. *Nursing Times*, 84(44), 60–1.

Bowlby, J. and Fry, M. (1965). *Child Care and the Growth of Love*. Penguin, Harmondsworth.

Brooker, C. and Towl, G. (1990). All in the family. *Nursing Times*, 86(2), 26–9.

Crossfield, T. (1990). How to deal with patients' relatives. *Nursing Standard*, 4(25), 52.

Danielson, C.B., Hamel-Bissell, B. and Winstead-Fry, P. (1985). *Families, Health and Illness. Perspectives on Coping and Intervention*. Mosby, St Louis.

Date, E., Goede, G. and Werner, G. (1987). Familiar faces. *Nursing Times*, 83(37), 26–7.

Dearden, C., Becker, S. and Aldridge, J. 1995: Children who care: a case for nursing intervention? *British Journal of Nursing*, 4(12), 698–701.

DoH (1992). *Patient's Charter*. HMSO, London.

DoH (1994). *Local Community Care Charters – press release, 3 August 1994*. DoH Health Publications Unit, Heywood, Lancashire.

Ekberg, J.Y., Griffith, N. and Foxall, M.J. (1986). Spouse burnout syndrome. *Journal of Advanced Nursing*, 11, 161–5.

Fox, C. (1985). Dreaded visitation. *Nursing Mirror*, 161(14), 39–40.

Friedemann, M-L. (1989). The concept of family nursing. *Journal of Advanced Nursing*, 14, 211–16.

Frost, M. (1970). Talking and listening to relatives. *Nursing Times*, 66(supplement), 129–32.

General Household Survey. (1990). HMSO, London.

Gibbon, B. (1988). Stress in relatives. *Nursing*, 3(28), 1026–8.

Gibbon, B. (1990). Giving information to relatives. *Nursing Practice*, 3(3), 19–23.

Gregory, S. and McKie, L. (1990). Smear tactics. *Nursing Times*, 86(19), 38–40.

Griffith, D.N.W. (1988). Hospital visiting hours: time for improvement. *British Medical Journal*, 296, 1303–4.

Harrison, N. and Smith, B. (1990). Information wanted. *Nursing Times*, 86(6), 46–8.

Hawker, R. (1984). Rules to control visitors. *Nursing Times*, 80(9), 49–51.

Health Service Commissioner (1996). *Third Report for Session 1995–96. Selected Investigations Completed October 1995 to March 1996*. HMSO, London.

Homer, A.C. and Gilliard, C. (1990). Abuse of elderly people by their carers. *British Medical Journal*, 301, 1359–62.

International Year of the Family [IYF] (1994). *Families and Caring. Factsheet 4*. IYF UK Office, London.

Joseph Rowntree Foundation (1994). *Children Living in Re-ordered Families*. Social Policy Research Findings No. 45.

Kozier, B. and Glenora, E. (1988). *Concepts and Issues in Nursing Practice*. Addison-Wesley Publishing Company, California.

Krozek, C.F. (1991). Helping stressed families on an ICU. *Nursing*, 21(1), 52–5.

Lugton, J. (1989). Communicating in the hospice. *Nursing Times*, 85(16), 28–30.

Lynch, S.H. (1997). Elder abuse: what to look for, how to intervene. *American Journal of Nursing*, 97(1), 27–32.

Mechanic, D. (1964). The influence of mothers on their children's health attitudes and behaviours. *Paediatrics*, 33, 444–53.

Meredith, H. (1992). Supporting the young carer. *Community Outlook*, 2(5), 15–18.

Millar, B. (1989). Critical support in critical care. *Nursing Times*, 85(16), 31–5.

Newens, A.J. (1995). The experience of women during their partners' hospital stay after MI. *Nursing Standard*, 10(6), 223–8.

Nolan, M.R. and Grant, G. (1989). Addressing the needs of informal carers: a neglected area of nursing practice. *Journal of Advanced Nursing*, 14, 950–61.

Ogg, J. and Bennett, G. (1992). Elder abuse in Britain. *British Medical Journal*, 305, 998–9.

Parfit, J. (1975). Parents and relatives. *Nursing Times*, 71(38), 1512–13.

Parmar, M.D. (1985). Family care and ethnic minorities. *Nursing*, 2(36), 1068–71.

Pike, S. (1989). Family participation in the care of central venous lines. *Nursing*, 3(38), 22–5.

Platt, H. (1959). *The Welfare of Children in Hospital: Report of the Committee*. Department of Health and Social Security. HMSO, London.

Pottle, A. (1990). To visit – or not to visit. *Nursing Practice*, 3(2), 7–11.

Robinson, C.A. and Thorne, S. (1984). Strengthening family 'interference'. *Journal of Advanced Nursing*, 9, 597–602.

Shubin, S. (1978). Burnout: the professional hazard you face in nursing. *Nursing* 8, 23–7.

Taylor, S.G. (1989). An interpretation of family within Orem's General Theory of Nursing. *Nursing Science Quarterly*, 2(3), 151–7.

Thompson, D.R. and Cordle, C.J. (1988). Support of wives of myocardial infarction patients. *Journal of Advanced Nursing*, 13, 223–8.

Turner, K. (1989). Partners in care. *Nursing Standard*, 3(35), 30–2.

UKCC (1992). *Code of Professional Conduct for the Nurse, Midwife and Health Visitor*, 3rd edn. UKCC, London.

Warren, K. and Bennett, G. (1997). Elder abuse: an emerging role for the general practitioner. *Geriatric Medicine*, 27(3), 11–12.

Whalley, G. (1988). Death of my father. *Nursing*, 3(32), 32–4.

Whittaker, N.A. (1992). Family-centred care. Unpublished Dissertation as part of BA (Hons) Health Studies. De Montfort University, Leicester.

Wilkinson, T.R. (1981). What about the family? *Nursing*, 30, 1301–2.

Youssef, F.A. (1987). Discharge planning for psychiatric patients: the effects of a family–patient teaching programme. *Journal of Advanced Nursing*, 12, 611–16.

FURTHER READING

Ekberg, J.Y., Griffith, N. and Foxall, M.J. (1986). Spouse burnout syndrome. *Journal of Advanced Nursing*, 11, 161–5.

Ekberg *et al.* examine the stages of burn-out experienced by the subjects in their study and question whether the manifestations of the spouses were similar to indications of burn-out exhibited by health professionals. This is useful reading from two perspectives: the need for nurses to recognise behaviour that may be indicative of burn-out in carers and also burn-out syndrome in themselves.

Friedemann, M-L. (1989). The concept of family nursing. *Journal of Advanced Nursing*, 14, 211–16.

This article describes Friedemann's system-based conceptualisation of family nursing which has been referred to only briefly in this chapter but can be used as a basis for the practice of family-centred care.

Gibbon, B. (1990). Giving information to relatives. *Nursing Practice*, 3(3), 19–23.

An overview of Gibbon's study to determine how student nurses perceive their role as information givers to relatives of hospital inpatients. Its conclusions have implications for student nurses and all those involved in nurse education.

Price, B. (1987) Happy families. *Nursing Times*, 88(47), 45–7.

This is a useful article, in that it includes a comprehensive overview of the nature of the family, the effects of illness, the role of the family and the nurse in caring for a sick family member. It also includes some references in support of the text that would be useful as further reading.

CHAPTER TWENTY

NURSING'S CONTRIBUTION *to the* HEALTH CARE *of* CHILDREN *and* ADOLESCENTS: SOME PRINCIPLES *for* PRACTICE

Chris Caldwell and Katy Lee

- Introduction
- Introduction to the child: why children's health care requires a separate focus
- The child and child health nursing: philosophy, knowledge and theory
- The child as a unique individual: development and understanding
- The child and the wider environment: social constructions of childhood
- The nursing contribution to children's health care: principles and goals
- Conclusion

The aim of the chapter is to raise the reader's awareness of the diverse and unique nature of child health care needs and the ways in which any nurse who comes in to contact with children, however infrequently, can use this insight alongside their existing knowledge and skills in order to play some part in helping to meet these needs.

INTRODUCTION

Although it has recently been recognised that all nurses who have children as the main focus of their work should be qualified children's nurses (Health Committee, 1997a), this is likely to take some time to achieve and is unlikely to include all nurses who have some contact with children during their work. This chapter is therefore not solely addressed to those nurses who are registered or intend to register as children's nurses. The aim of the chapter is to raise the reader's awareness of the diverse and unique nature of child health care needs and the ways in which any nurse who comes into contact with children, however infrequently, can apply his/her existing knowledge and skills in order to play some part in helping to meet these needs. For those who are pursuing careers in child health nursing, this chapter will provide a stepping stone to more in-depth study.

Within the chapter we will make assumptions that the reader will also study much of the material in other chapters of the book, particularly those relating to the context in which nursing occurs and the chapter on family-centred care and mental health nursing. We will refer to this literature and apply it to child health nursing. We intend to draw from our own backgrounds and perspectives – health visiting and children's nursing – in order to outline what we believe are key areas of knowledge and skills, and the principles and goals of contemporary child health nursing. We realise that not everyone will agree with us, but we will strive to present a balanced perspective. Consequently, throughout the chapter we will direct the reader to other sources for more detailed information to enable you to pursue those aspects which particularly interest you.

The chapter should assist the reader to:

- View each child and adolescent as a unique developing individual who exists within a complex system with which he/she interacts in a symbiotic manner
- Consider the specific health care needs of children and adolescents within this system
- Appreciate the ways in which childhood has been constructed within our society and how this has influenced our approach to child health
- Gain insight into some health and social services with which children, both sick and well, may come into contact
- Understand some of the key principles of nursing children and adolescents
- Recognise that the goal of any nursing intervention is to assist the child to reach his/her individual potential and appreciate the knowledge which nurses caring for children need in order to achieve this goal.

Throughout the chapter, unless otherwise stated, the term 'child' or 'children' will be used to refer to all individuals residing in that diverse part of the lifespan which stretches from birth through until adulthood is reached. We will, however, explore the nature of childhood in some detail within the chapter.

INTRODUCTION TO THE CHILD: WHY CHILDREN'S HEALTH CARE REQUIRES A SEPARATE FOCUS

In the introduction to this chapter we stated that children and adolescents have diverse and unique health care needs and it is on these grounds that we argue for a separate chapter which examines the principles of providing nursing care for them. The rationale for this argument is provided through considering the following questions:

1. How do we define 'childhood'?
2. What makes children different from adults?
3. Do children have specific needs, and if so, what are they?
4. What are the implications for nurses providing health care to children?

Reflection Point 20.1

Drawing on your own experiences of childhood and children, spend a few minutes considering questions 1 and 2, and then use your ideas to brainstorm question 3. These are clearly three big questions and your response may depend to some degree on the extent of your experience with children. Try to generate a few ideas quickly and then read on.

HOW DO WE DEFINE 'CHILDHOOD'?

The term 'childhood' is in some ways an umbrella term which encompasses a number of others. Within this umbrella we talk about 'neonates', 'infants', 'babies', 'toddlers', the 'school-aged child', 'teenagers' and 'adolescents'. The terms chosen are largely dependent upon context. Definitions of childhood also vary across disciplines.

Childhood is defined biologically as the period

of physiological and anatomical development which ends with full reproductive function, i.e. biological maturity. Since this state can be reached naturally at as young as 10 or 11 years of age, this definition might exclude the period of development known as 'adolescence'. Within this definition, it is also worth thinking about how one would treat the cases of those 'children' who undergo precocious puberty and those 'adults' who have absent reproductive function. Would we consider them adults or children?

On a social level, 'childhood' can be defined in relation to the law. Reaching the age at which a range of social activities may be legally undertaken by individuals is often seen as a sign that adulthood has been reached. These activities include full-time paid work, drinking alcohol, smoking cigarettes, having sexual intercourse, getting married, voting in a local or national election and giving informed consent to health care. Clearly, however, there are a range of ages at which these activities become legal, even within the English legal system, let alone in other countries where some of them remain illegal regardless of age. Does this mean that some of these activities are more 'adult' than others?

Some define 'childhood' in relation to personal qualities which distinguish children from adults, qualities such as 'good sense' and 'responsibility' being signs of adulthood, which is somehow seen as an end state. Archard (1993, pages 36–37) analyses this perspective in more detail in relation to children's rights.

Even from this brief account, it is apparent that attempts to define 'childhood' are fraught with problems, since one's definition is likely to be influenced by one's values, beliefs, historical context, background and social situation. Childhood is also not a fixed state but incorporates a substantial period of dramatic but gradual human development. Whilst these issues are considered in more detail later in the chapter, Cherry and Carty's (1986) broad definition of childhood based on their selective review of the literature provides a useful starting point:

> 'a period of developing body size, structure, function, maturation and learning that are necessary to become a functioning adult.'
>
> (Cherry and Carty, 1986, page 421)

WHAT MAKES CHILDREN DIFFERENT FROM ADULTS?

In addressing this question it is important to accept that any differences identified are not likely to be uniform throughout childhood since they will vary according to the extent of the child's developmental progress, which is a function of many factors, including age, experience, genetic predisposition and health. Some of the many difference are identified below:

Physical differences
- Children are anatomically and physiologically immature and as a consequence of this they are usually smaller and less strong than adults and are therefore more prone to physical abuse.
- They are more prone to specific illnesses and are often more seriously affected by illness because of their immaturity.
- Their immature nervous system means that they are less able to make accurate judgements about themselves in relation to the environment and are consequently more prone to accidents.
- The consequences of inherited conditions, abnormal fetal development and perinatal trauma are usually first apparent in childhood.

Psychological differences
During childhood children gain experience in how to deal with the world which surrounds them. Lack of experience may mean that they are particularly vulnerable to stress.

Social differences
- Children are usually part of some form of family on which they depend.
- Since education is usually compulsory at some point, the school world plays a key role in children's lives.

DO CHILDREN HAVE SPECIFIC NEEDS, AND IF SO, WHAT ARE THEY?

We hope that you can now begin to see that children and adolescents do have specific needs. In attempting to describe these needs, it is helpful to refer to a paper prepared for the Department of Health and Social Security in 1975 by Mia Kellmer-Pringle, then director of the National Children's Bureau. Although now over 20 years old, we would argue that this work is still useful. Kellmer-Pringle presented a multidisciplinary perspective on child development and parenting and suggested that children have four basic needs (Box 20.1).

Box 20.1: The needs of children

According to Kellmer-Pringle (1975) children's needs can be classified as follows:

- The need for love and security
- The need for new experiences
- The need for praise and recognition
- The need for responsibility

Kellmer-Pringle rejected the view that developmental needs come into play in a hierarchical sequence. She believed that all human needs are interrelated and interdependent in a subtle, complex and continuous way. This perspective is illustrated well if one considers the behaviour of children who are experiencing sexual abuse, which is examined later in the chapter, or how a child who is experiencing stress as a result of her parents' relationship breakdown might refuse to eat, or even if she does eat, may fail to thrive. Kellmer-Pringle stressed that the four needs must all be met from the beginning of life and require fulfilment to varying extents through childhood and adulthood, with their relative importance changing through different developmental phases.

The need for love and security

A stable, continuous, dependable and loving relationship with the main carer(s) facilitates the child's realisation of a personal identity and worthwhileness, the development of the personality (including moral values) and forms the basis of all later relationships. Children must be valued unconditionally and carers should communicate this to the child through all their relations with him/her, from physical care and protection to disciplining. The need for security is met through stable, consistent and dependable 'family' relationships (including relationships between 'family' members as well as with the child); a familiar, predictable living environment; and a known individualised routine. Kellmer-Pringle argued that the development of an individual personalised routine allows the child his/her right to

individuality and self-expression and contributes to the development of a sense of worth.

The need for new experiences

New experiences and their mastery are essential for the development of the mind, motivation, learning and a sense of achievement. There is a need for the child to be able to explore the environment and try out different things. The level of stimulation must be carefully planned since too much can cause withdrawal and fear and too little can lead to apathy and boredom. Kellmer-Pringle and others have concluded that play and language are the key ingredients through which the child explores the world and learns to cope with it. This includes both the external world and the internal world of his/her thoughts and feelings.

PLAY

It is argued by some that play is possibly more important to children than work is to adults; thus there has been a tremendous amount of research and theory generated about how and why children play (see Sylva and Lunt, 1982, for an introduction to this literature). Some writers argue that the educational value of play is debatable and that play has only been elevated to a position of importance in the Western world because of the role which children occupy in our current social construction of childhood (see later in the chapter) (Hobsbaum, 1995). Hobsbaum refers to Tizard (1977), who pointed out that children (in the West) are now provided with special toys to occupy them rather than being encouraged to assist with household chores or other employment. Whatever one's viewpoint, clearly Western children do spend a considerable amount of their time taking part in play and it thus is likely to contribute to all aspects of their development (Table 20.1).

LANGUAGE

Again there is a vast literature related to language development and you are referred to child development texts for an analysis of current thinking. Briefly, language helps children to think and understand the world around them. It helps them to learn to reason, and speech facilitates the development of relationships. Verbal communication is also an important means of coping with, and coming to terms with life. Table 20.2 provides a brief summary of norms of language development.

Table 20.1: The contribution of play

The contribution of play	Aspect of play promoted
Active play encourages both gross and fine motor development	Physical development
Through active exploration of the environment and through passive play activities like watching television and reading	Cognitive development
Before a child is able to use words to decribe what he/she sees, his/her experiences with space, sound, colour and relationships help him/her to form impressions about the environment. It is these early experiences and formation of multiple images that help a child put words into use	Language development
Children can experiment in play and may then transfer learning to other situations	Stimulus for creativity
Children learn something of their abilities and how they compare with their peers	The development of self-insight
This is a lifelong learning process. Children engage in fantasy play to explore feeings, lessen fears and work through conflicts. In games of pretending, imaginary playmates are safe recipients of aggressive impulses. Experiences that have frightened or excited a child may be re-enacted in play with imaginary participants. Through such play activities a child can express those intense feelings that may not be perceived as acceptable forms of behaviour in the real world	Expression of emotions
As play becomes more bound by rules so these become enforced more rigidly and group norms of right and wrong, fair and unfair are learned	Moral standards
Sex roles are rarely taught explicitly. Play provides many opportunities for covert instruction	Learning to play 'appropriate' sex roles

Table 20.2: Norms in language development: a summary

Age range	Language ability
0–2 months	Cooing
2–6 months	Babbling
12–18 months	First words (imitation)
18 months–3 years } 3–5 years }	Rapid acquisition of vocabulary, multi-word sentences, basic language mastered by 5 years
6–11 years and onwards	Progressively complex sentences, use of propositions, pronouns and proper nouns, grammatic mastery

The need for praise and recognition

The process of growing from infanthood to adulthood requires an enormous effort and a strong incentive. The child who has a loving relationship with his/her main carers will be keen to please them. Consequently, as well as encouragement the child needs a level of expectation carefully geared to his/her capability at any particular point in time so that success is possible but not without effort (Kellmer-Pringle, 1975). Mistakes and failure should be regarded as an integral part of learning and treated separately from those behaviours which require disciplinary action (see, for example, Bettelheim, 1987, for further reading about parenting and parent–child relationships).

The need for responsibility

This need is met through allowing the child to develop personal independence and through ownership of possessions of some kind. Role modelling is crucial, as is a framework of guidance so that the child knows what is expected, what the rules are, and reasons for these. It is therefore important that carers share their values, beliefs and standards with children as well as distinguishing between disapproval of the child's behaviour and rejection of the child him/herself.

For example, in the case of a child who has smacked his/her younger sibling for no reason, it is more appropriate to tell the child that smacking was a naughty thing to do, rather than saying: 'You are a bad boy/girl!'

During adolescence the need for responsibility has a high profile. The significance of peer relationships during this period allows adolescents to practise coping with autonomy and independence in egalitarian relationships, rather than their usual relationships with adults in which they are invariably subordinate. Adults must take risks during this period to allow young people to exercise responsibility, yet many find this difficult, preferring to continue to protect them from the world. This issue is analysed later in more detail in relation to social constructions of childhood and child sexual abuse.

WHAT ARE THE IMPLICATIONS FOR NURSES PROVIDING HEALTH CARE FOR CHILDREN?

We have briefly considered the issues around defining childhood, the differences between children and adults, and the specific needs of children. It is now possible to identify some of the key areas of knowledge and skills which nurses who provide health care for children (Figure 20.1) must have themselves – or at least be aware of so that they are able to access and seek advice and support from nurses who have such abilities – when they have children in their care.

Reflection Point 20.2

Go back over the issues that you raised in Reflection Point 20.1 as well as the points raised in the text. Write down briefly what you think are the main implications for nursing.

Figure 20.2 provides an overview of what we believe are the main implications for nurses' knowledge and skills in relation to child health nursing. The rest of this chapter will focus on some of those areas highlighted. This does not mean, however, that the other issues (or indeed others that you may have thought of which we have not included) are less important. You are therefore advised to refer to the texts identified for further reading, both during and at the end of the chapter in order to extend your knowledge and thinking. Some of the issues are also covered elsewhere in this book.

THE CHILD AND CHILD HEALTH NURSING: PHILOSOPHY, KNOWLEDGE AND THEORY

When addressing the health care needs of children it would be simplistic to view that child as a static isolated entity. The child is a dynamic developing individual who exists within a complex world. Our actions as nurses and the actions of other health professionals, the families and the children we work with, are all inevitably and intricately influenced by our world and what we value, know and believe about the world.

Dominant philosophical thought over the centuries has influenced theory generation, knowledge and subsequent action by individuals and societies in diverse ways (see Gaarder, 1995, for a highly readable account of the history of Western philosophy through the eyes of an adolescent girl). Health care and nursing are no exception (see Masterson, 1995 for a more detailed examination of the impact of philosophy, knowledge and theory in nursing). Consciously or subconsciously, our theories as well as those of others guide the way we think and act as nurses (Ramprogus, 1992) and account for the diverse nature of nursing.

Many of the theories which have been proposed to explain children's behaviour, both in health and illness, and the models which have been developed to guide child care practices can be classified within four main theoretical foundations which are not necessarily mutually exclusive: systems theories, developmental theories, interaction theories and caring theories (Bellman, 1996) It is helpful for you to be aware of the theoretical as well as the philosophical origins of different approaches because it will assist you to fit the many parts of the jigsaw together, to be self-aware, to understand the actions of others, and to take a holistic perspective on the nursing care of the child.

The most commonly encountered approaches have their origins in either systems or developmental theory.

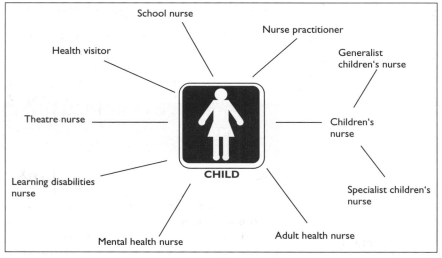

Figure 20.1: Some of the variety of nurses who provide health care to children

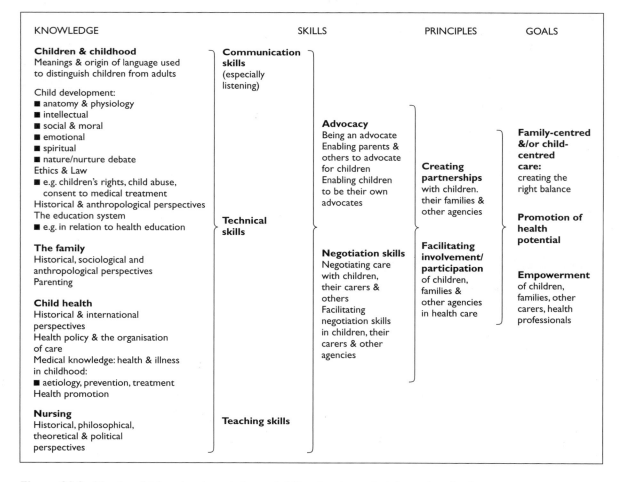

Figure 20.2: Nursing children: key knowledge and skills related to principles and goals of care

SYSTEMS THEORIES

Systems theories define both people and their environment as open systems existing in relationship to each other. A change in one system affects the others and the systems are therefore constantly evolving and adapting to change (Bertalanffy, 1968; King, 1981). Physiological theories about homeostasis (see Chapter 5) and some of the theories about how individuals cope with stress are examples of systems theories (e.g. Selye, 1976, see Chapter 8).

Within nursing, King's (1981) general systems framework and Roy's adaptation theory (Roy and Andrews, 1991) can be classified as systems theories. To help you to understand the systems approach in relation to child health nursing, you may want to refer to Mackenzie (1991) who describes the use of Roy's model in the nursing care of a hospitalised neonate. Figure 20.3 demonstrates the relationship between the three open systems (personal, interpersonal and social) within which children exist in a dynamic interacting framework. Included are some of the many systems which are influential in most children's lives.

Box 20.2: Case vignette, Alice aged 1 year

Alice is 1 year old when she is diagnosed with a malignant brain tumour. Intensive treatment is begun in a hospital 100 miles from home and has many side-effects. The pressures of caring for her three youngest siblings whilst Alice's mother is resident in hospital leads her father to lose his job and results in the end of her eldest sister's engagement. Unable to cope on state benefit, the family's home is repossessed.

Reflection Point 20.3

In this chapter some of these systems will be examined as they relate to the provision of nursing care to children. The simplified case vignette in Box 20.2 illustrates just some of the ways in which serious illness impacted on one child's personal, interpersonal and social systems. Can you identify some of the systems which were influenced in this case?

Personal systems

Alice's physiological systems which maintain equilibrium in body function have been seriously affected, not only by the malignant disease but also by the effects of the treatment, both surgery and cytotoxic drug therapy.

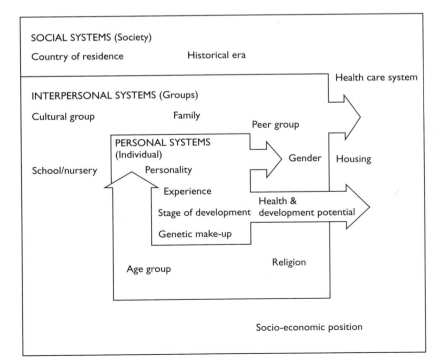

Figure 20.3: Systems theory: children and their environment as open systems (adapted from King, 1981, page 20)

Interpersonal systems

The impact of Alice's illness on her family and the many subsystems within it, such as her sister's peer relationships, are profound and likely to be longlasting.

Social systems

The family's position within society has changed as a consequence of Alice's illness, both in relation to their economic and housing status and also their role within society. Where once her father was in employment, providing for his family and contributing to society's wealth, the family is now dependent on financial support from the state and charitable sources in order to function adequately.

You may think that this case vignette was a very extreme fictitious case, made up in order to illustrate systems theory. In fact, it is based on a real scenario: even relatively minor and short-lasting illness can have a significant and enduring impact on the child's life.

DEVELOPMENTAL THEORY

Developmental theory focuses on the stage, direction and potential for human growth, motivation and change. Examples of developmental theories from child psychology include Piaget's theory of cognitive development (Piaget and Inhelder, 1969) and Erikson's (1959) theory of psychosocial development (see below). A number of nursing theorists have also been influenced by developmental theory in their construction of models for nursing. These including Orem's model of nursing (Orem, 1991), which is examined in more detail later in the chapter, and the work of Roper *et al.* (1990) in the UK. Many clinical areas caring for sick children use adapted versions of these models to guide nursing care. For example, Welch (1993) describes how she used Orem's model to assist her in the care of a child with spina bifida, whilst Wallace (1993) gives an account of how Roper *et al.*'s model was implemented to guide the care of a teenager with burns.

Casey's conceptual framework for child health nursing, based on partnership in care with the child and family (Casey, 1993), could be said broadly to use a systems approach, in that it considers the interrelationship between the child, the family and the nurse during illness. It also, however, has its philosophical origins within developmental theory and shows the interrelationship between the two theoretical approaches. It considers the child's development from conception through to adolescence and beyond and addresses the extent of dependency on others during this time (Figure 20.4). You may well be familiar with this framework, since it has become very popular in the UK as a framework to guide practice and education in child health nursing. We will return to Casey's model later in the chapter.

Reflection Point 20.4

As you read more about the concept of partnership and Casey's model and become more familiar with it in practice, try to think of other reasons why this approach has become so popular in the UK. Do you think that nurses who use it are improving the quality of care which children and their families receive? Can you think of any problems with it? The vignettes later in this chapter may help you to consider these questions (see also Fulton, 1994; Baker, 1995; Jones, 1995; Mason, 1995).

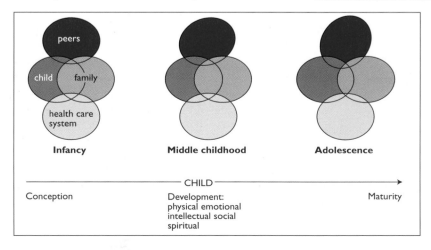

Figure 20.4: Systems and developmental theory in Casey's partnership model of paediatric nursing. (Casey, 1988)

You may also, perhaps to a lesser extent, come across approaches to child health care based upon interactional and caring theories.

INTERACTIONAL THEORY

Interactional theory emphasises relationships between people and the roles they play in society. Within this approach, there is a focus on all the individuals involved in a specific situation and their unique individual interpretations of it. For example, interactionists believe that within a health care situation, the values, beliefs, needs and roles of the nurse, the child and the family in that situation, along with their expectations of each other must all be taken into account (Jones, 1994). The interactionist approach emphasises the necessity for nurses providing health care for children to clarify their own values and beliefs as well as those of the child and family. As has already been stressed in previous chapters, our values and beliefs influence our actions even though we may not be aware of them. By being self-aware and open, and honest about what what we expect of our clients as well as what they can expect from us, we can ensure that we work alongside children and families in ways which ensure that all parties value and respect each other's contribution.

CARING THEORY

Caring theory encompasses human, moral and cultural valuing of persons and involves a personal sense of commitment and responsibility (Bellman, 1996). Some would argue that caring theories are the core of nursing (see Brykczynska, 1996). Bellman (1996) cites Leininger's model of 'culture, care, diversity and universality' (1991), as an example of a model which has caring theory as its philosophical framework.

Leininger (1991) defines care in relation to:

> 'assisting, supporting or enabling experiences or behaviours toward, or for others with evident or anticipated needs to ameliorate or improve a human condition or lifeway.'
> (cited by Rosenbaum and Carty, 1996, page 742)

The model addresses the similarities and differences amongst culturally different groups world wide in relation to how they understand the concept of 'caring'. It also provides a framework to guide nurses in their care of culturally diverse individuals and groups. The influence of the other three major theoretical frameworks already discussed is apparent, in that Leininger described care as:

> 'essential for growth and wellbeing, with social structure factors such as values, economics, religion, politics and education influencing care and health.'
> (Rosenbaum and Carty, 1996)

Leininger's model has been widely used by nurses attempting to care for clients whose cultural background is different from the dominant culture in which they reside, and more specifically, perhaps, different from the cultural background of the health care professionals charged with caring for them (see Weller, 1994). Adolescence is often described as a subculture since adolescents share a distinct lifestyle with which they identify, yet feel that neither adults nor younger children understand them (Leininger, 1978; Bibby and Posterski, 1992). Rosenbaum and Carty (1996) focused on adolescence as a specific subculture, and used Leininger's model to enable them to address Canadian adolescents' beliefs about health and care in order to make more effective decisions about health education and health care provision for this client group (Figure 20.5).

Reflection Point 20.5

Whilst there is a danger of cultural stereotyping if individual diversity is not recognised and assessed, you may want to consider further how Leininger's model and other transcultural nursing models might influence your own approach to caring for children and their families, whose cultural background is different from your own (see Dobson, 1991).

Approaches like Leininger's model encourage us to ask questions about taken-for-granted aspects of health and go some way towards ensuring that nursing care is relevant and appropriate to the individual's unique situation. We are also encouraged to challenge our own stereotypes and enter into open dialogue with clients. Such dialogue facilitates trusting relationships where clients see that their opinions are valued and can help to ensure that health service provision meets the needs of *all* users.

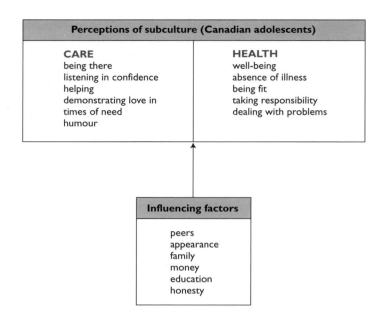

Figure 20.5: Caring theory: using Leininger's model to plan health education and care for Canadian adolescents (adapted from Rosenbaum and Carty, 1996)

Key Points

- Nurses caring for children and their families must appreciate that individuals' actions are influenced both consciously and subconsciously by their diverse and highly individualised experiences of the world, including their roles and functions within that world.

- There are many different theories and approaches which influence child care and child health nursing – these are all embedded within the beliefs and values of the individual and the society from which they emerged.

- In order to provide effective holistic health care to children, nurses must have a knowledge of, and be able to analyse, a range of theories about practice.

- Nurses must also be self-aware in order to appreciate how they themselves might influence health care encounters with children and their families.

- A critical reflective approach to nursing practice will facilitate this process (DoH, 1993; UKCC, 1995).

THE CHILD AS A UNIQUE INDIVIDUAL: DEVELOPMENT AND UNDERSTANDING

We have previously argued that the goal of nurses providing health care for children is the promo-tion of health potential through family-centred or child-centred care. The promotion of health potential requires that the promoter has insight into the individual's developmental process and how factors in their environment might be affecting him/her, positively or negatively. This knowledge can be successfully gathered through a number of sources: through effective communication with the child and his/her family, from the nurse's previous experience and from theoretical knowledge. In this way nurses working with children use their knowledge of the commonalities of human development combined with knowledge about the unique individual child as a basis for the recognition of actual and potential deviations from or alterations in growth and development. They are then able to plan and evaluate appropriate interventions (Anderson, 1989).

The development of the whole person is a highly complex and multifaceted process. Many theories have been put forward which provide different conceptual frameworks for the organisation of data about the person which allow us to some extent to describe, explain, predict and control growth and development. It is necessary to study and analyse a number of these theories because some do not cover all domains of development and several theories may explain the same phenomena differently. The choice of theory is consequently likely to influence nursing assessment and intervention. A thorough analysis of developmental theory is beyond the scope of this chapter and the reader is referred to child development texts, such as Bee (1989). Anderson (1989) provides a useful table which illustrates these differences by comparing nine theories of human growth and development.

Most texts which focus on child development assign developmental norms to individual children based on chronological divisions and associated developmental stages (see Table 20.3). This is done in an attempt to facilitate learning and, as we will discuss in more detail later, it is important that when caring for children you assess their individual behaviour and their family's perceptions in order to determine developmental ability. There is also a tendency within the literature to categorise aspects of the development of the whole person to facilitate easier understanding. Such categorising is arbitrary and can be done in many different ways. It is important to remember that the different individual developmental systems are interlinked and interact with each other and the environment (see Figures 20.3 and 20.4 and associated text).

Anderson (1989), for example, describes children's development as three facets of the self called physical, intellectual and emotional–social competencies.

PHYSICAL COMPETENCY

Physical competency refers to the child's ability to apply various aspects of biological capacities to achieve steadily more mature self care skills. This includes physical health, body size, motor skill and strength. Because physical development is observable and quantifiable, it is easily measured. There are also some age uniformities and consequently the measurement of numerous aspects of physical development is used to evaluate the child's relative health status, using standard charts which compare the child with established norms. Such measurements include growth charts which plot head circumference and body weight. Such charts are only useful if the child being assessed is representative of the sample used to collect the data on the chart.

It is only in recent years that growth charts have been introduced into the UK which are specifically developed for children from non-Caucasian British races. Prior to this, all children were measured on the same charts which resulted in inappropriate medical referrals and much unnecessary anxiety for the families of children whose racial origin meant that they were naturally smaller or larger than the Caucasian norm.

A further issue in relation to routine measurement of aspects of physical development relates to difficulties in obtaining accurate measurements over a period of time from a subject who is likely to squirm or protest and when the individual taking the measurement, as well as the equipment used, are likely to change. This is a particular issue in relation to the measurement of height in non-weight-bearing infants and children and has resulted in staff in many areas not routinely measuring infants' height. Physical measurement requires skill and the risk of error should thus be borne in mind when evaluating such measurements, to avoid unnecessary intervention yet ensure appropriate action.

INTELLECTUAL COMPETENCY

Intellectual competency involves the development of language and reasoning, perception and communication skills. This includes memory, problem-solving and academic ability. Intellectual competence is a composite of skills, behaviours and adaptive abilities that make it possible for an individual to adjust to new situations, to think abstractly and to profit from his/her experiences. Intellect is demonstrable in the way a child solves problems and the appropriateness of his/her response in any given situation. It was once believed that intelligence was genetically fixed; however, longitudinal research conducted in the 1960s established that intellect fluctuated and that both internal and external environmental factors influence intellectual development and function (Pulaski, 1971).

These findings have contributed to the rising concern for the provision of sufficient appropriate early learning opportunities for children, and has led to a specific focus on those children who might suffer some kind of sensory deprivation as a result of sociocultural or physical limitations. For sick children, whether in hospital or at home, such concern means ensuring that these children are still able to achieve learning through play and school work if at all possible. This often requires that nurses act as advocates to lobby for the provision of appropriate toys, specialist play workers

Table 20.3: Children's perceptions of illness: a summary of the stage approach based on Piaget's (1968) theory

Stage and main features	Perception of health and illness	Practical implications
Sensorimotor (0–2 years): ■ Learning mainly through senses ■ Concerned with the relationship between what they do and the consequences of their actions ■ Exploration vital ■ Develop object permanence at around 1 year old	■ Largely non-verbal; therefore little understanding of language	■ Best to communicate through parents as verbal explanations are largely inappropriate
Pre-operational (2–7 years): ■ Invest objects with life ■ Use objects and words as symbols to represent things in their world though not necessarily using the same symbols as adults ■ No conservation of objects or experiences ■ Egocentric	■ See illness as external, concrete and remote from them, it is out of their control; they may believe that it is controlled by magic (witches, monsters, etc.) ■ See illness as a punishment ■ Unable to see illness as a process; focus on one experience at a time	■ Cannot see relationship between medical procedures and cure, likely to see procedure as punishment and may believe that doctor is out to hurt them, will need reassurance ■ Due to inability to contemplate internal body, focus heavily on what they can see on body and in environment; therefore explanations need to relate to what they can see and touch
Concrete operations (7–12 years): ■ Learn to conserve ■ Can form internal pictures of actions and see relationship between things ■ See things relatively ■ Less egocentric ■ More logical but still only see things in relation to experiences they have had	■ Still see causes as external but say that child must contact illness physically or engage in harmful activity in order to develop illness ■ Still believe all illnesses have a physical cause ■ Can link concrete symptoms together ■ Illnesses seen as located inside the body; the child has some notion of internalisation of agents by inhalation or swallowing ■ Illnesses and causes described vaguely showing confusion about internal organs and their function ■ Still focus on the surface with little speculation about insides ■ Begin to see relationship between illness and treatment and that treatment is intended to help	■ Because they concentrate on the surface they do not worry about what may be going on inside
Formal operations (12 years +): ■ Think abstractly as well as concretely ■ Can reason symbolically without object or experience present	■ Illness described in terms of non-functioning of internal organs ■ Some understanding of external causes and internal responses ■ Appreciate that there are many causes of illness ■ Can imagine relationships and processes that they have not directly experienced ■ Can infer empathy and can understand that the nurse realises that procedures may be unpleasant	■ Can begin to see the effects of illness on the rest of life and may develop a pessimistic view of chronic disease, need opportunities to discuss their worries ■ Show increasing concern about the disease process, e.g. pain, may imagine sinister damage and malfunction inside

Derived from Muller et al., 1992.

and teachers for children receiving health care in a climate of dwindling public finances.

Advocating for children and their families has been identified as a key principle of child health nursing and is analysed later in relation to empowerment. It is evident from this case, however, that advocacy requires that the nurse can present a sound rationale for her case based on an understanding of theoretical knowledge and research as well as the strategic use of appropriate policy documents and case evidence. In this case there are a number of policies which could be cited, such as the NAWCH charter for children in hospital (1985) and the Audit Commission report *Children First* (1993).

Perhaps the most influential theorist in relation to intellectual or cognitive development is Jean Piaget. During the 1950s and 1960s this Swiss psychologist and his colleagues conducted a series of research studies from which they derived a stage theory about the gradual evolution of children's intellectual activity throughout childhood (Piaget and Inhelder, 1969) (see Box 20.3 and Table 20.3.) As already mentioned, understanding the child's level of intellectual thought and function, in order to establish the meanings attached to specific experiences around health care, is fundamental to their care.

Piaget's theory is perhaps so appealing as a conceptual framework for this activity because it is usually presented in a simple user-friendly way. Its appeal may also derive from the fact that other theories do not seem as easy to understand and use. Whatever the reasons, Piaget's theory continues to be widely used within child health care and

you will find it presented more fully and analysed to some extent in most children's nursing and all child development texts. There are, however, a number of potential problems which can arise from both the wholesale, uncritical adoption of one theory and the simplification of that theory, so that it is no longer a true reflection of the author's original ideas. Some of these problems will be highlighted when we examine some of the theory and research relating to children's understanding of health, illness and their bodies.

EMOTIONAL–SOCIAL COMPETENCY

Emotional–social competency concerns the development of an inner sense of security evidenced by the ability to form productive interpersonal relationships. This includes temperament, interpersonal skills, sexuality and morality. The goal of emotional–social competency, according to Anderson (1989), is a healthy adult personality: 'the capacity to love, to achieve and to become interdependent in function' (page 108). She goes on to point out, however, that it is a process competency which unfolds throughout the stages of life, with each stage having its own tasks to be mastered and resolved.

Erik Erikson, a psychoanalyst, building on the work of Freud, developed a theory of psychosocial development which illustrates the lifelong struggle for emotional–social equilibrium (Erikson, 1963) (see Box 20.4 and Table 20.4). This theory also usefully illustrates how the individual child's development occurs within the context of his/her interactive relationship with his/her social and cultural environment. When used in relation to child health care it also enables us to take into account the impact of our own and other family members' emotional–social development on each child's health and care.

Health promotion activities in well children – and nursing interventions in the care of sick children – should be planned carefully in order to support development and mastery, rather than compound further the problems of a child who is already experiencing a normal developmental crisis. A consideration of Erikson's theory or another theory of emotional–social development can assist you to gain insight into, and assess, the developmental tasks already facing the child, so that care planning is appropriate. This theory also helps to

---

Box 20.3: Piaget's theory of cognitive development: brief summary of key concepts

- There are four stages of cognitive development: sensorimotor, pre-operational, concrete operational, formal operational.
- Each stage has its own substages or phases
- Each of the major stages represents a qualitative change in the way the individual thinks or behaves
- All individuals progress through the stages in the same order and no stages are skipped.
- Each stage is built upon what occurred in the previous stage and each stage provides the basis for the next stage.

Box 20.4: Erikson's theory of psychosocial development, brief summary of key concepts

- Individual development occurs within the context of social and cultural environment.
- There are eight stages of psychosocial development (see Table 20.4).
- During each stage the individual is presented with a basic developmental task or crisis requiring him or her to resolve a conflict between two opposing forces (one positive and one negative).
- Progression to the next stage depends on resolution of the previous stage's conflict.
- Ideal resolution results in a predominance of the positive psychological attribute (ego quality) for the stage; however, there should always be at least some of the negative attribute present.
- Crisis resolution involves the acquisition of new skills and qualities, which, in turn, assist the individual to master the new task set by society and culture in the next stage.
- Healthy psychosocial development occurs if favourable mastery exists most of the time and if healthy compensations are used when mastery is not achieved.

explain why regression to a previous task level, or reversion towards the negative counterpart of the current task stage, frequently occurs in children (and adults) who are experiencing extreme stress as a result of health-related issues. Box 20.5 presents a case vignette to illustrate this issue.

Erikson's theory also enables us to understand that parents and other people involved in the child's care, including nurses and other health care workers, are also in the process of developing. Anderson suggests that nurses need to assist parents (and other carers) to:

- Build constructive relationships with each other and the child
- Feel satisfied and confident in their parenting skills
- Learn to cope with the stresses confronting the child and in knowing their responsibility in helping the child manage those stresses.

We would add that through the process of critical reflection on practice during clinical supervision, nurses caring for children can support each other

through stressful incidents, as we develop from novices into expert practitioners. Examples of this can also be seen in the case vignette.

Box 20.5: Case vignette, James, aged 10 months

James was admitted with a suspected non-accidental injury. He is, however, making a remarkable recovery. Thomas is a newly qualified staff nurse allocated responsibility for James' care under the supervision of his preceptor. When James' father, Jack, arrives to spend some time with James, he and Thomas quickly develop a friendly relationship, being of a similar age and having similar interests. James is very attached to his father, who is his main carer since James' mother works full-time. When Jack goes off to have a cigarette, James, who had previously been playing happily with Thomas and his father, screams and is inconsolable. Thomas finds this very stressful and, feeling very embarrassed that he cannot cope, eventually asks someone to find Jack who quickly returns. In the process of discussing James' behaviour, Jack explains that he finds it difficult caring for James all day because he always seems to want his mother, and confesses that it was he who is responsible for the physical injuries. Thomas is extremely shocked and upset and arranges to spend some time with his preceptor to reflect on what has happened in order to determine what action he needs to take.

FOCUS: CHILDREN'S UNDERSTANDING OF HEALTH, ILLNESS AND THEIR BODIES

As already indicated, research which expands our knowledge of children's understanding of health, illness and their bodies is extremely valuable, since it has many implications for health care practice. In health promotion, it can facilitate more effective working with children to promote positive health behaviours, both in childhood and in adulthood (Kalnins et al., 1992; Whiting, 1997) (see Table 20.5). In acute illness and hospitalisation, it can be used to enable health care professionals to alleviate illness-related stress, prepare children for medical procedures and minimise the long-term sequelae of acute illness (Muller et al., 1992). In chronic illnesses, such as asthma and diabetes mellitus, which are experienced by increasing numbers of children (Hobbs and Perrin, 1985;

Table 20.4: Erikson's eight stages of man

Age range norms	Development task	Negative counterpart of task	Significant persons	Significant supporting experiences
Infancy 0–1 year	Sense of trust	Mistrust	Primary carer	Consistent quality care
Toddler 1–3 years	Sense of autonomy	Shame & doubt	Main carers	Attaining self-control based on self-esteem
Pre-school 3–6 years	Sense of initiative	Guilt	Family	Self care based on exploration within set limits
School age 6–12 years	Sense of industry	Inferiority	Neighbourhood, peers, school, adults, idols	Success & recognition in tasks in social world
Adolescence 12–? years	Sense of identity	Role confusion	Peer group, models of leadership	Establishing purpose in society, need for independence
Late adolescence/young adult	Intimacy & solidarity	Isolation	Partner in friendship, sex, competition, cooperation	Experiencing close relationships, establishing own & others' identity
Adulthood	Sense of generativity	Self-absorption & stagnation	Spouse, children, friends, colleagues	Involvement in activities related to next generation
Late adulthood	Sense of integrity	Despair	Spouse, children, grandchildren, friends	Being acknowledged for successful life accomplishments

Derived from Erikson, 1963; Anderson, 1989.

Caldwell, 1997), the value of such research is argued for in its relationship to empowering practices, such as the promotion of self care and informed decision making (Eiser, 1990; see also the later section focusing on empowerment).

The bulk of the early research was carried out by psychologists in the late 1970s and early 1980s (e.g. Bibace and Walsh, 1981; Perrin and Gerrity, 1981; Eiser and Patterson, 1983; Bird and Podmore, 1990; Eiser, 1990), and was based heavily on the work of Piaget. This research seemed to draw consistent conclusions, demonstrating that understanding of illness parallels the development of other concepts within Piagetian theory, but appears more slowly, showing considerable consistency in relation to the type of understanding exhibited by children at different stages of development (see Table 20.3).

This early research has been the subject of crit-

icism, both in relation to its methodology (Eiser, 1989) and theoretical foundations (Eiser, 1989; Hergenrather and Rabinowitz, 1991; Burman, 1994) which is summarised below.

Theoretical criticisms

- Piaget's theory is often adopted uncritically and out of context and more recent developments of the theory are overlooked.
- Since Piaget's work is reductionist and based on data from one sociocultural group, the sociocultural background of the child and the environment in which the research takes place are often ignored.
- Stages are rigidly adhered to as a result of poor understanding or simplification of Piaget's work.

Table 20.5: Typical age-related concepts of health, cognitive level, approach to teaching and expectations for self care

Age	Health concept	Cognitive level	Age-related teaching approach	Responsibility for self-initiated care
Infancy (0–1 year)	No concept, learns to assign value to needs on the basis of how well and how consistently they are met	Egocentric	Basic needs must be fully and consistently met	None – totally dependent on caretakers
Early childhood (1–4 years)	No concept; merely imitates behaviours of role models that are satisfying and/or earn reward	Egocentric; pre-conceptual; does not question own perceptions	Continue meeting basic needs but steadily demand that child master skills of daily living; model wellness behaviours; reward his/her imitations. Play with child to learn perceptions since he/she cannot communicate them adequately	Some capacity to carry out tasks to promote own health if taught skills and allowed opportunity to take responsibility; likes to practise wellness behaviours
Middle childhood (5–8 years)	Recognises that health involves a series of health practices – (eat a balanced diet, brush teeth, stay clean, etc.)	Egocentric; concrete reality predominates	Encourage child to say what his/her health needs are, what caused any deficit, what he/she might do to resolve that need. Correct misperceptions. Use teaching techniques that provide child with tactile, visual, auditory and motor experiences	Can carry out many tasks to promote own health, seeks responsibility; practice is important. Can take independent action to identify many health needs and can identify some realistic solutions
Late childhood and pre-adolescence (9–13 years)	Concept of health as sense of physical well-being, for example 'feeling good', 'being fit'	Objective, systematic thought; questions and seeks validation and correction of own perceptions. Gradual increase in causal reasoning; still favours concrete reality	Share assessment and/or finding; this allows child to perceive changes in health status. Allow time for him/her to validate perceptions of his/her needs and what actions should be taken, respect his/her views and opinions. Give simple rationale for health practices/procedures. Make invisible processes of health real with diagrams, models. Teach the skill/procedure then give the rationale in simple terms	Can plan for and take initiative to carry out most health needs if he/she has learned trust and autonomy. Can participate actively in managing his/her own health needs. Acute interest in health education. Can consider possible risks and benefits of health behaviours if allowed to participate in problem-solving

Table 20.5: Continued

Age	Health concept	Cognitive level	Age-related teaching approach	Responsibility for self-initiated care
Adolescence and young adulthood (14–21 years)	Concept of health as physical, emotional, social stability that is long term though superimposed brief illness may cause temporary instability. Evidenced by 'feeling good', being in control of self, being able to participate in desired activities	Realises realm of possible and hypothetical as well as the real. Develops theories. Craves details primarily for egocentric purposes	Important to have people whom he/she respects as role models to overcome peer group pressure. Honesty imperative to his/her cooperation. Present all details; relate them to him/her personally. Especially likes theoretical explanations and discussions. Allow discussion of the effects of health problems and health behaviours on him/her and his/her future. Let him/her determine the possible resolutions to his/her health needs and collaborate to determine management. Begin by presenting rationale for a skill procedure, then give details of performing it	Can assume full responsibility to identify his/her health needs, determine possible resolutions and carry them out. Can use concepts of wellness constructively in decision making

Methodological criticisms

- Researchers frequently failed to check the reliability and validity of research instruments.
- There were few replication or comparison studies.
- The findings of studies which used different sample populations (sick and healthy children and those with chronic and acute illnesses) were compared inappropriately.
- The influence of being ill on ability to respond to research questions, as well as the influence of experience of illness, were often not considered.
- Health was often pre-conceptualised from an (adult) medical model perspective as the absence of disease and subsequently imposed on the children's responses.
- The research was framed in adults' perceptions of how children *should* think.

As a result of the enormous impact of this early research, there has been relatively little attention to how children perceive health and what they want to learn about health and illness (Kalnins *et al.*, 1992). In recent years, however, there has been a steep increase in nursing research related to child health care and this topic has formed the focus of numerous studies. Nurse researchers have built on the earlier research and addressed the theoretical, methodological and ethical criticisms (e.g. Longsdon, 1991; Holdsworth, 1995; Rushforth, 1996; Gaudion, 1997). Notable themes are a move away from relying solely on Piaget's theory, and instead critiquing, analysing and building on the work of Piaget, and alternative theorists, such as Vygotsky (1978) and Carey (1985). Data collection techniques other than semi-structured interviews, such as the 'draw and write technique' (Pridmore and Bendelow, 1995), are now being used in which data are collected from the analysis of children's pictures and written accounts of their knowledge of particular concepts.

Much of the more recent research is also less patriarchal. It accepts that children are competent and seeks to understand from children's own perspectives rather than imposing 'adult' ideas on them (e.g. Kalnins *et al.*, 1992). Such approaches are vital for the adoption of empowering approaches. Studies such as Kalnins' and colleagues' work, conducted in the context of everyday life, have concluded that children perceive health in relation to negotiation and interaction with events and people in their environment, and in relation to resolving conflict situations, rather than in the abstract, a presumption previously made based on ideas about 'adult' understanding. This clearly reflects normal emotional–social development as presented by Erikson. Figure 20.6 illustrates how a 6-year-old girl understands the concept of 'being alive' in relation to the human body and in the context of her current reading book, a story about trolls (mythical monsters). The dangers of overlooking children's own perceptions of illness are highlighted below.

Comparing adult and child perceptions of illness

'Chicken pox is a common and highly infectious disease but it is usually very mild in childhood.'
(Quote from medical text book)

'My last illness was chicken pox, it was dreadful. I did not just have chicken pox, I was ill as well. I think that chicken pox was the worse illness that I have ever had and I have had a lot. I still have a lot of scars. It was dreadful and I hope I never get it again.'
(Quoted by a child in Bartram, 1965)

Key Points

In this section we have provided a limited perspective on some of the key principles of child development and considered some of the nursing implications for child health care. The section will conclude with a summary of these principles. The first three principles underpin those that follow.

- The child is an open system who has adaptive potential, and who makes two-way transactions with other systems.
- Heredity and environment shape the open system into a unique human being.

- Self-actualisation (achieving one's potential) is the goal of human development.
- Development is a complex lifelong process including both growth and ageing.
- Development has direction: it is progressive, orderly and follows a sequence (see Table 20.6).
- Development is predictable: the rate of development may vary according to the individual child but the sequence is invariable.
- Children develop uniquely: each child has his or her own genetic potential that cannot be exceeded but can be deterred or modified at any point in the sequence as a consequence of transactions between the child and the environment.
- Development occurs through conflict and adaptation and involves challenge, practice and energy investment (see Table 20.7).
- Mastery of developmental tasks occurs within the context of gender, and the ethnic and cultural characteristics of the child's main carers (Levine *et al.*, 1983).
- Research which expands our knowledge of how children themselves understand health, illness and their bodies is extremely valuable since it has many implications for health care practice.

Table 20.6: The direction of human development

Human development proceeds in most (but not all) cases:

- *From simple to complex*: children are able to tolerate liquid nourishment before they can tolerate semi-solid and solid foods
- *From general to specific*: young children perceive all painful stimuli as negative and threatening, whereas with experience they are able to appreciate that some painful stimuli can have positive consequences, e.g. intravenous cannulation for the adminstration of analgesia
- *From head to toe* (cephalocaudally): for example, ossification of the bones occurs from the head downwards
- *From inner to outer* (proximodistally): the child learns to control near structures before the structures which are further away from the body centre, so that an infant who is laid under a hanging toy will reach up and strike it with his/her arm before learning to grasp it with his/her fingers.

Source: Bee, 1989; Glen and Colson, 1993.

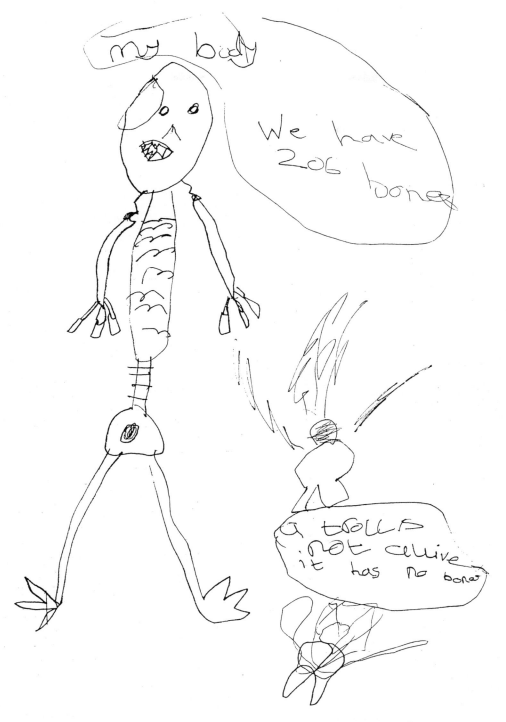

Figure 20.6: Drawing illustrating a 6-year-old child's understanding of the human body

Table 20.7: Development requires practice and energy investment

- During infancy the central focus is on sensorimotor and physical growth
- Developing a sense of self and body control are the focus of the toddler's energy investment
- The pre-school child practises language skills
- During the early school years cognitive development and social relationships take up the bulk of the child's energy
- During adolescence there is a demand for a massive investment of energy in physical growth, establishing intimate relationships and establishing social identity
- During periods of illness energy levels are likely to be diminished, any available energy may be used in coping with the illness and its consequences and development may regress, slow down or halt

Adapted from Glen and Colson, 1993.

THE CHILD AND THE WIDER ENVIRONMENT: SOCIAL CONSTRUCTIONS OF CHILDHOOD

Throughout the twentieth century children have increasingly received the attention of governments and other official organisations within Western society. Indeed, James and Prout (1990) refer to this century as the 'century of the child'. This attention has given rise to the notion that the West, in particularly, is a child-centred society where 'the child' and 'the interests of the child' are given a prominent place in the policy and practices of legal, welfare, medical and educational institutions. Consequently, much academic and popular debate has been devoted to understanding the qualities of children, and, with increasing frequency, popularised versions of these debates are presented in the mass media (Hendrick, 1990; James and Prout, 1990; Phillips, 1994).

Childhood, however, as we know it today, is a relatively new 'invention' and is constantly developing (Phillips, 1994). It is not such a fixed, natural and universal feature of human groups as many texts might lead us to believe. Historical analysis demonstrates that dominant (adult) groups within different societies throughout the world have con-tinually sought to construct and reconstruct childhood in such a way that it functions to suit the needs of that society at any given time. Indeed, the current focus in the West on children's rights, when placed into the historical context, can be seen both as a very recent perspective and one which reflects many of the dominant notions of childhood held in Britain in the past. Box 20.6 illustrates the way that childhood has been socially constructed in Britain by presenting a brief historical perspective.

Box 20.6: A historical perspective on the social construction of childhood in Britain

The way in which childhood has been constructed in Britain must be viewed in relation to the responses of different generations to the social, economic, political and religious challenges of the time.

The mediaeval child
Historical data prior to the eighteenth century would suggest that the only members of a community who were treated any different from the rest were those who were dependent on others, such as infants. If such a concept as 'childhood' existed, it referred solely to the period of infancy. Physically independent individuals were considered fully equal members of the community, with all the rights and responsibilities with which any independent member of that community was normally endowed. Young people were in no way protected from any experiences – positive or negative – and were seen as adults in the eyes of the law from a young age (under Tudor law any convicted child criminal aged 7 years or above could be hanged). Society was not divided according to chronological age but according to able-bodiedness and economical viability.

The Romantic and the evangelical child
It is argued that the idea of childhood was initiated through direct intervention as a consequence of the moral and economic dilemma created by activists lobbying on the part of orphaned or abandoned vulnerable infants, who, it was viewed, could not be considered the same as the rest of the community, since they needed to be both cared for and educated. The age range for this accepted demarcation was gradually raised, initially amongst the upper classes, and there were two main viewpoints about how these children should be treated. The evangelists (such as

Wesley) promoted the need to break the inherently evil wills of children by instilling order and obedience, whereas the Romantics (followers of Rousseau) saw children as innocent and natural and in need of gentle education and protection.

The factory child

The Industrial Revolution demanded use of the child as part of the increasing labour force and in the working-class family the working child was also a valuable source of income. There was then, therefore, little support for the Romantic notion of childhood. Lobbyists (e.g. Charles Kingsley) still spoke out about the way children were being exploited both by employers and their families, whilst members of the richer classes became increasingly anxious about the moral and social instability of the working classes. Although education for the upper-class child was now commonplace, the idea of compulsory education for all children, as a way of controlling 'delinquent' child workers, and, through them, the working classes, began to be discussed.

The schooled child

Although partial education for working class children began in the early 1800s, it required government legislation to ensure that all children received education, since this meant that these children were no longer of such economic value. Compulsory schooling, by the mid-nineteenth century was potentially able to facilitate the goal of instilling civilisation, order and obedience into the working classes from the bottom upwards and this effectively created the 'universal classless child', available always for political indoctrination. At the same time, it reconstructed the factory child as ignorant and dependent on his/her family (whose own education the child was encouraged to reject), with a reduced sense of his/her own (economic) value and therefore power, and a different (unequal) set of rights which were controlled by (more powerful) adults. Compulsory schooling also provided an ideal opportunity for the growing disciplines of psychology and medicine to use the school as a laboratory, and consequently the child welfare and development movements began in earnest during the early 1900s.

The family child and the public child

An interesting reconstruction of childhood occurred around the time of the Second World War. Child psychologists and psychiatrists had begun to stress the importance of parents, particularly mothers, in successful child-rearing. Research into the experiences of children during the war years, including evacuation from the inner cities, increased day nursery provision and raised rates of illegitimacy, was utilised after the war to reinforce the government's belief that the family (particularly the mother's presence) were the most valuable influence in the life of children (see the work of Bowlby, 1953, and Winnicott, 1958, for example). Public institutions which cared for children were heavily criticised and the (progressive) Children Act of 1948 (Ministry of Health [MoH], 1948) proclaimed the need to maintain the child's links with its natural family. Indeed, by 1960, this view of the family as the domestic ideal was so assured that the Ingleby Committee concluded that cruelty and physical neglect of children were no longer a problem.

The child of the nineties

There are a number of significant issues in contemporary British society which are influencing the way we view childhood. Most notable, perhaps, are the acknowledgement of child abuse, the Children Act (DoH, 1989), the children's rights movement (Archard, 1993), the treatment of children who commit serious crime (Morrison, 1997) and the subsequent responsibility which children are being encouraged to take for what happens in their lives. Changes in the structure of employment and education have also been influential, in that the age at which individuals are encouraged to take up full-time work has been raised, creating increasingly longer financial dependence on the family. There has also been a (perhaps) parallel increasing interest in the period of development known as adolescence. There seems to be a tension between the rhetoric of allowing children to make independent decisions about their lives and providing the kind of economic and emotional environment which supports them to do this in reality.

Adapted from Hendrick, 1990.

Although biological immaturity is the only feature of childhood which is accepted as a universal and natural feature of human groups (James and Prout, 1990), the institution of 'childhood' is no less important, since it forms a specific structural and cultural component of all societies and provides an interpretive framework for contextualising the early years of human life within those societies. Like gender, ethnicity, and social class, childhood is a variable of social analysis, and comparative and cross-cultural analysis reveals a variety of childhoods, rather than a single and universal phenomenon.

Interestingly, just as historically there have been few official social statistics regarding social class, gender and ethnicity, similarly children have largely remained absent from official social statistics (Qvortrup, 1990). That this is still the case, specifically in relation to child health, has recently been highlighted by the United Kingdom all-party House of Commons Select Committee on Children's Health (Health Committee, 1997a).

There is no doubt that during the twentieth century, a huge body of knowledge has been built up regarding the nature of childhood through the systematic study of children within a number of disciplines, including psychology, sociology, anthropology, history and medicine. This study has largely taken place in the West, using children, who represent a narrow range of society, as research subjects and adopting existing (adult-based) research approaches, which have been applied to the study of children rather than being specifically designed for this new focus (James and Prout, 1990).

Problems are now arising, however, as this stereotypical and idealised Western conceptualisation of a single and universal childhood (Figure 20.7) is promoted by dominant parties, not only as the global experience of children in the West (see Hunt and Frankenberg, 1990), but also imposed on the rest of the world (see Glauser, 1990). Such a conceptualisation remains difficult to challenge, partly because of the lack of social data about children. Thus, the fact that childhood is a social construction has been effectively concealed. Consequently, during the twentieth century an idealised conception of childhood has been promoted and exported throughout the West and to the developing world. Unfortunately, this conception labels as deviant or criminal much of working-class life and many children's activities in non-traditional Western societies.

Some researchers are now, however (as we saw, in relation to children's understanding of health and illness), beginning to challenge this traditional approach (e.g James and Prout, 1990; Burman, 1994). They argue that children must be seen as active in the construction and determination of their own social lives, the lives of those around them and of the societies in which they live, rather than just the passive subjects of social structures and processes.

Such a change in focus demands that research methodologies must be explored and used which allow children a more direct voice and participation in the production of data about themselves and their lives. Ethnography, therefore, for example, has been found to be more useful than experimental or survey methods (see, for example, the study undertaken by Rosenbaum and Carty, 1996, which was mentioned earlier in the chapter). This new approach is not without its own inherent problems, largely related to the amount of control which children have, in reality, over their own lives (Phillips, 1994). The case of child sexual abuse presented in Box 20.7 illustrates not only the numerous implications of current constructions of childhood for abused children but also the challenges facing those who seek to liberate these children.

We have examined the case of child sexual abuse, but other particularly pertinent examples might be the experiences of the ethnic minority child, the child with a chronic or life-threatening disease, the child with mental health problems or the homosexual adolescent. Some of the issues relating to these examples will be picked up within the chapter. To help you further, you might refer to the following texts: Karpf, 1988; Eiser, 1990; HEA, 1992; Egger et al., 1993; Signiorelli, 1993; Lindsay, 1994; Philo, 1994; Bedi and Gilhorpe, 1995; Kitzinger and Skidmore, 1995; Strasburger, 1995).

DEVELOPMENT
(natural universal progressive evolutionary)

CHILDHOOD

immature
dependent
irrational
natural savage
incompetent
asocial
acultural

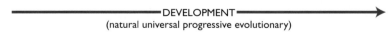

ADULTHOOD

mature
independent
rational
civilised
competent
social
cultural

Figure 20.7: The 'global childhood' stereotype (developed from James and Prout, 1990 and Phillips, 1994)

Box 20.7: The case of child sexual abuse: a crime against childhood?

Both those who seek to justify and those who condemn child sexual abuse (CSA) use images of children which are widely portrayed in the media to reinforce their positions: those who condemn frequently use images which portray the child as innocent and vulnerable, often black and white or sepia images – reinforcing 'traditional' visions of childhood; those who seek to justify sexual abuse of children use images of alluring Lolitas and cheeky minxes, including images of young girls dressed in 'adult' clothes and underwear or wearing make-up. Both types of image are commonly found throughout contemporary media, the latter becoming increasingly prevalent.

Debates about child sexual abuse draw upon discourses about sexuality, gender, class and race but they are also firmly rooted in discourses about childhood and it is the youth of the victim and images of their childish nature which predominate in media coverage.

Childhood innocence

Child sexual abuse is commonly referred to as the 'theft' or 'violation' of childhood. This implies that there is agreement about what an 'authentic' childhood should be like. The concept of childhood innocence has been used to incite public revulsion against CSA. Victims are robbed of their innocence, they are seen as blameless and helpless, and recovery from CSA often involves striving to reclaim that 'lost' innocence. This approach is problematic for three reasons:

1 The notion of childhood 'innocence' is a source of titillation for abusers.
2 Childhood innocence is a romanticised notion and this approach both stigmatises the child who responds in some way to the abuse or who does not fit in with the image, and leaves the abused child as 'damaged goods', psychologically and socially at risk of further exploitation.
3 Childhood innocence is an ideology which denies children access to knowledge and power and increases their vulnerability to abuse – they are protected from potentially 'corrupting' influences, are left ignorant about their sexuality and not in control of their own bodies.

The passive victim

Abuse victims are frequently presented as passive victims of adult demands as a consequence of the imbalance of power between adults and children and subordination of children in our society. Many children who are experiencing abuse, however, despite the imbalance of physical power, employ strategies commonly used by oppressed groups, including cunning, manipulativeness, energy, feigning illness, running away and making themselves look ugly.

Protecting the weak

Images of children as innocent and passive promote the notion that children rely on adult protection, that all children are at risk, and that the abuser could come from anywhere. Hence, there is increasing support for children to remain in the sight of their adult carer at all times, which places great strain on parents, particularly mothers, and implicitly blames parents who fail to comply with this more. It also encourages children to live in fear. Parents (and adults more generally) also have considerable control over the way in which children learn about adult life, for example, in relation to sex education (see later in this chapter). This increase in parental control may be contributing to the finding that in Western societies children remain dependent on their carers for longer than in other societies.

Child sexual abuse prevention programmes

Traditional (protectionist) approaches to CSA prevention have taken, and continue to take, the form of (largely government-led) warning campaigns (e.g. 'Say no to strangers'). More innovative (liberationist) approaches have often developed out of feminist initiatives, and try to assist children to identify abuse and seek help. Such approaches demand that images of children as innocent, passive and in need of protection are set aside. They use child-sensitive and child-centred methods including harnessing the kinds of media which are meaningful to children, in order to introduce topics in a non-threatening way, build on children's existing knowledge of topics such as bullying, unfairness and nasty secrets and encouraging children to trust their own instincts. They also listen to children's feedback to improve the programmes. There are some problems with liberationist approaches, however:

- They are often racist, classist and heterosexist.
- Approaches which seek to empower children (see later in this chapter for a more detailed discussion of this concept), to make them 'streetwise', confident and in control provoke unease in those who seek to maintain the status quo. Such traditional protectionists claim that such approaches seek to undermine parental authority; consequently such liberationist approaches may produce children

who do not 'fit in' with traditional views of children and are consequently viewed as deviant (Vallely, 1997).

- Empowering approaches locate the potential for change within the individual and do not address social structural issues within society. Thus, those who cannot resist abuse are likely to feel responsible for their failure. Indeed, it is those who are most oppressed, are most powerless and who have the lowest self-esteem who seem to benefit least from these approaches (Gough, 1989). As one child pointed out in support of this view: 'he was big, I was little, I had to do what he said' (Gilgun and Gordon, 1985, page 47).

Kitzinger (1990) argues that a more appropriate, but more radical (consciousness-raising) approach to CSA prevention would be to support children to recognise their own oppression. She suggests open discussions about power which consider how adults have used their power over children rather than focusing on 'giving' children a 'sense' of power and 'telling' them their 'rights'. Whilst not without problems, such an approach, she argues, does not, at least, gloss over inequalities or undermine the struggle against structural change.

Source: Kitzinger, 1990.

Reflection Point 20.6: Synthesising exercise

In the light of the issues addressed in this section of the chapter, consider the images of children and childhood portrayed within your society, particularly as reflected in the mass media. Identify a child for whom you have been involved in providing health care. Consider the implications for that child of living in a society which has certain beliefs about childhood and how children should behave.

IMPLICATIONS FOR CHILD HEALTH POLICY AND CHILD HEALTH SERVICES

The tension between the rhetoric and reality in relation to society's attitudes towards children can be clearly observed in the arenas of health policy and health care provision in the UK. Over the last 60 years, paralleling current social constructions of childhood, there has been a steady stream of official reports making recommendations for health policy and practice (see Darbyshire, 1993; Robertson, 1995; Watt and Mitchell, 1995; Bradley, 1996 for a fuller discussion). None of these recommendations, however, have ever been imposed by government, with the result that health services for children are extremely varied in quality across the country. This situation has recently been highlighted by the House of Commons Select Committee report on children's health (Health Committee, 1997a, b). It remains to be seen whether the hard work of this committee will result in real action rather than more hollow words.

Key Points

- There is a plethora of literature which stresses the value of children, yet there is little statutory legislation to ensure that children are accepted and valued in their own right for what they are, rather than as our stereotyped perceptions of them.
- Childhood is a socially constructed phenomenon which is neither a universal, natural, nor fixed feature of human groups.
- We know very little about the experiences of children in the UK in relation to health, since there are few official social statistics.
- More research needs to be undertaken which examines children's social relations and cultures.
- Whilst we need to encourage children to become active in decision making about their health, we must appreciate how little control, in reality, most children have over their lives to make this possible.
- Current health policy and health care provision reflect social constructions of childhood.

THE NURSING CONTRIBUTION TO CHILDREN'S HEALTH CARE: PRINCIPLES AND GOALS

Having addressed some of the areas of knowledge and skill required in the provision of nursing care to children, we will now briefly address the principles and goals of nursing care.

FACILITATING PARTICIPATION/ INVOLVEMENT

Parent's participation in the care of their hospitalised child has been a major focus of attention over the past five decades and is demonstrated in a succession of governmental reports, including the following:

- 1946 Ministry of Health (The Curtis Report)
- 1959 Ministry of Health (The Platt Report)
- 1976 Department of Health and Social Security (The Court Report)
- 1991 Department of Health (*Welfare of Children and Young People in Hospital*)
- 1993 Audit Commission (*Children First*)
- 1996 Department of Health (*Care of Children in the Community*).

It is suggested that Bowlby's work on maternal deprivation (Bowlby, 1953), and the Robertsons' films of children undergoing hospitalisation and separation (Robertson, 1962, 1970) largely stimulated the interest in this concept (Darbyshire,1993). It is now widely accepted that parent participation is a pivotal concept in the provision of contemporary child health care.

However, there seems to be confusion in the literature over what actually constitutes 'parent participation'. Coyne's (1996) analysis of the concept describes how a number of terms are 'interchangeably and indiscriminately' (page 733) used, such as 'partnership in care', 'involvement in care', 'mutual participation' and 'family-centred care'.

The concept of parent participation needs to be further examined and clarified so that it can be used more appropriately and its strengths and limitations addressed. Historically, much of the work on parent participation has focused on organisational approaches to hospital care. Mothers 'rooming in' with their children is described by Craig and McKay (1958), McCarthy *et al.* (1962) and Meadow (1969). Later, 'care by parent' units are referred to by Webb *et al.* (1985).

Sainsbury *et al.* (1986) provided an important development of the concept which involves the issue of parental responsibility in the healing process, and includes fathers and grandparents, as well as mothers, in the process. A broader philosophical view of parent participation involving consideration of community-based care is provided by Fradd (1987). She states that nurses must enable parents participating in care to retain total responsibility for the care of their child, wherever he or she is nursed, and whatever the diagnosis or treatment. Fradd clearly viewed parent participation as 'family involvement' and included siblings, fathers, step-parents, aunts, uncles and grandparents.

From a sociological perspective, Benner is critical of nurses and hospitals, referring to their role as social control agents. She sees parents as no more than 'passive ciphers' in an institutional conspiracy which seeks to control and oppress (Benner, 1984). The issues of power and control are considered in more detail when we examine empowerment. For a more detailed analysis of the many other issues around parent and family participation see Darbyshire (1993) and Coyne (1996). The case vignette in Box 20.8 illustrates the concept further.

Box 20.8: Case vignette, Sarah and Emily

Sisters Sarah, aged 7 years, and Emily, aged 5 years, both suffer with moderate to severe eczema which is controlled in the community using the 'wet wrap' technique introduced by Anne, a community paediatric nurse (Figure 20.8). The technique involves applying creams and wet tubular bandages to heal the dry, itchy and flaky skin (Bridgman, 1995). Having been taught the technique, the girls' mother, Sue, carries out the daily care each evening. She is committed to the treatment and values its benefits for the children's health, despite the large amount of work involved. Sue is due to go into hospital for a hysterectomy and will need to convalesce on her return home. Sue calls Anne to express her grave concern that there is no one else who is willing or able to manage the care while she is incapacitated and that the children's skin condition will deteriorate. How might Anne think about and manage this problem?

The key issues raised in the vignette are listed below:

- Maternal participation or family involvement?
- Who has the burden of responsibility?
- Who has control/power?
- Negotiation of care.

The use of the wet-wrap technique in the community may be seen as a perfect example of parent

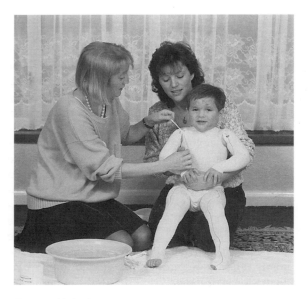

Figure 20.8: Wet wrapping

participation. The situation described in the example, however, is more akin to maternal participation than family involvement, thus landing a huge burden of responsibility on one carer, the mother. Apparent lack of family commitment to the treatment may be due to an omission in involvement. There is now a need to involve Sarah's and Emily's other carers, namely their father, childminder and grandparents, who will carry out the bathtime routine in Sue's absence.

The nurse has a high degree of control over the situation as she remains one of the few carers able to do the wet-wrapping, and Sue must go straight back to her with the first problem in the care management. The nurse may need to return to the family, admit that she applied the concept of participation too narrowly and negotiate a package of care for the children, involving the whole family, as well as perhaps herself and/or a district nurse or health visitor. In the long term this may have benefits for the family's commitment to treatment, as well as a shared sense of responsibility and greater family control.

CREATING PARTNERSHIPS

Partnerships in the care of children include both partnerships between health professionals and families, and partnerships between different professionals. Casey (1988, 1993) viewed parent par-

ticipation in terms of 'partnership' and developed the 'partnership model of paediatric nursing', which we referred to earlier and which is summarised in Figure 20.9. The nurse complements parental care and the emphasis is on the family providing care, based on an assumption that parents and families are willing and able to be effective carers, and take responsibility for the care.

The Children Act (DoH, 1989) adopted a similar model of parent participation, viewing it as a working partnership with parents and families, promoting the role of families in the care of their children. Both Stower (1992) and Dearmun (1992) have explored the boundaries of the concept 'partnership' and concluded that equality, negotiation and mutual respect were central issues.

It is not just in hospital care of sick children that a partnership model is employed. In the community, the health visitor, whose role is largely that of health educator, works in partnership with parents. 'High risk families' are identified according to local authority policy and health visitors will discuss with parents themes such as developmental expectations, child care skills and child behaviour management. Health visitors work with families experiencing stress of any kind. They are involved in family care when a child is deemed 'at risk' according to the Children Act.

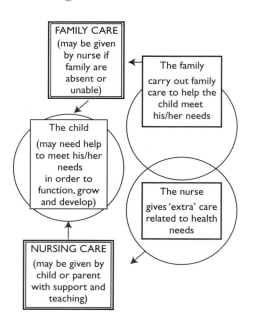

Figure 20.9: Summary of the partnership model of paediatric nursing
(adapted from Casey, 1988)

As well as partnership with families, another theme that is central to the Children Act is that of partnerships between professionals through close interdisciplinary working. The protection of children involves a close working relationship between social services departments, the police service, medical practitioners, community health workers, schools, voluntary agencies and others. In 1996 the Department of Health issued a guide to good practice in community child health (DoH, 1996), which provides further recommendations for improving partnerships in the care of children.

These include:

- Joint involvement in purchasing child health services between NHS Trusts, general practitioners, social services departments, local education authorities, voluntary bodies, and community health councils
- More emphasis on bringing primary and secondary services together through joint working parties
- Creation of more posts with duties in both hospital and community
- Widespread use of parent-held child health records which pass between all professionals involved in the child's care as well as the parents.

FAMILY-CENTRED AND CHILD-CENTRED CARE: CREATING THE RIGHT BALANCE

One of the widely documented principles of nursing children is that of family-centred nursing care (Forfar, 1989; While, 1991). Family-centred care occurs when carers and the child are involved as active partners with the health care professionals in management, decision making, treatment and care. It implies consideration of all family members in planning and providing care, whether in the home, community or in the hospital. By working with, and teaching and supporting families, the health care professional can assist acceptance of nursing care as an extension of the familiar caring role.

Vital in the study of family-centred care is a critical analysis of common and prevailing assumptions about the nature and functioning of 'the family'. (See Chapter 19 for a more detailed examination of this concept.)

Two key issues are central to child-centred nursing care: child development (which has already been touched on) and *child health rights*. The concept of children's rights, as we pointed out in relation to the social construction of childhood, is a relatively new one (Archard, 1993) and, according the Lansdown (1995), draws on both the recognition that every individual human is entitled to enjoy the full range of human rights, and the recognition that children should be treated as people in their own right and not just as the property of the adults who are responsible for them.

The Children Act (DoH, 1989) has helped to ensure that the child has a right to a say in his/her life and legal procedures. However, it is somewhat limited, in that it applies only to a relatively small number of children defined by local authorities as 'in need' under section 17 of the Act. In the autumn of 1991, soon after the Children Act came into force, the UK government ratified the United Nations Convention on the Rights of the Child. The Convention is the first real international recognition of children's rights and promotes the rights of all children and young people up to 18 years old by giving information to them and all those who care for them (United Nations General Assembly, 1991).

Article 24 of the Convention is the main article concerned with the provision of health services. It states that all children have the right to 'the enjoyment of the highest attainable standard of health' and there is also a duty to ensure this right to each child 'without discrimination of any kind' (Article 2.1). Many NHS Trusts in Britain have now signed up to the UN Convention and this is as a result, in part, of the work of the Children's Rights Development Unit (Children's Rights Development Unit, 1994; Children's Rights Development Unit & British Paediatric Association & Royal College of Nursing, 1995) and you are referred to their publications for more information about child health rights.

The case vignette in Box 20.9 illustrates the challenges for nurses of trying to strike a balance between family-centred and child-centred care. In approaching this situation, there are a number of issues which the nurse must consider. These include:

- Legal implications
- Karen's rights to privacy and confidentiality

- Parental involvement and parental rights
- Informed consent to treatment
- Health promotion implications.

> **Box 20.9: Case vignette, Karen, aged 15 years**
>
> Karen, aged 15 years, presents one evening at a family planning clinic away from her home town. She was brought to the clinic by her boyfriend who is 20 years old. She is requesting the contraceptive pill instead of the condoms she has received before from the clinic. Karen states that her parents are unaware of her visit to the clinic and that she has a poor relationship with them.
>   Karen is initially seen by a family planning nurse.

Legal implications and rights

The UN Convention on the Rights of the Child (Article 5), recognises that parental rights must be exercised in line with 'evolving capacities of the child'. In addition, although in some cases it has since been over-ruled, **Gillick competency** established that children under 16 years can give legally effective consent independent of their parents' wishes, providing they have sufficient understanding of what is proposed. The family planning nurse must use her knowledge of the child, as well as her skills in effective communication and information-giving, to assess whether she feels Karen has sufficient understanding of the contraceptive method requested. As already discussed, maturity does not necessarily depend on age.

Rights to confidentiality and parental involvement

Whilst it would be pertinent to encourage Karen to share the information about her sexual behaviour with her parents, the duty of confidentiality owed to a person under 16 years is as great as the duty owed to any other person (UN General Assembly, 1991). The nurse should also consider the right of 'protection from harm', including sexual exploitation (Article 34), in assessing whether Karen has given truly informed consent to a sexual relationship with her boyfriend.

Health promotion implications

Orem first described her model of nursing in 1959. Central to Orem's model is the concept of self care. Orem (1985) defined self care as 'the practice of activities that individuals initiate and perform on their own behalf in maintaining life, health and well-being (page 84). The concept of self care is relevant to health promotion, and applies to healthy individuals as well as those who are ill. Orr (1985) considers that the development of the self care concept will 'result in educating the individual to maintain and improve the state of well-being'(page 91). Using Orem's model the nurse would assess Karen's health behaviours relevant to her contraception, such as smoking and sexual behaviour. From this any self care deficits are determined, and can be addressed at subsequent follow-up appointments. Orem is emphatic that decisions about the need for nursing care should be made in the context of an effective relationship between the client, nurse and family, when, and if, appropriate.

EMPOWERMENT OF CHILDREN, THEIR FAMILIES/CARERS AND HEALTH CARE PROFESSIONALS

A review of the concept of empowerment indicates that, whilst there is on-going debate around a precise operational definition, it is a concept which seems to encompass many, if not all, of the key principles of child health nursing identified within this chapter, whether the nurse is aiming to provide family-centred or child-centred care. As such, therefore, empowerment can be viewed as one of the potential goals of child health nursing, and it is therefore appropriate that we end this section with a brief analysis of it.

Certainly, a crucial role of someone who is empowered or is promoting empowerment is that of advocate. Advocacy refers to the process of lobbying or speaking out on behalf of disadvantaged groups or individuals, such as dependent children, in situations where they are not able to speak up for themselves. Being an advocate also extends to the advocate seeking to enable those disadvantaged groups or individuals to speak up for themselves through the empowerment process. Thus empowerment and advocacy are inextricably linked in a cyclical process of sharing power and control.

There is no doubt that 'empowerment' is a very popular term within both nursing specifically and child health care more generally. This may be, as Keiffer (1984) points out, a consequence of it being an intuitively appealing idea because of its psychosocial, political and ethical connotations. It certainly would appear to fit well with current health care ideology. Are we, however, using the concept correctly when we refer to practices as being empowering or talk about the empowered child, carer or nurse, or is it just another poorly understood label, which conveniently and acceptably pigeonholes an action or behaviour, and thus averts the need for further analysis or evaluation of nurses' work?

The concept of empowerment has been examined at some length, from both a theoretical and an empirical perspective, within nursing and health promotion. It is worth noting that it appears that, whilst nursing has traditionally seen empowerment as an individual-focused idea, which can be equally applied to the client or the health care professional, within health promotion the concept of empowerment seems to be largely applied to groups of clients or communities (Gallagher and Burden, 1993).

Both Gibson (1995) and Fradd (1994) suggest that the main reason why empowerment is so difficult to operationalise or measure is because it is an emerging *process*, rather than simply a static outcome, and is therefore subject to constant change. There is agreement, however, that it involves the mobilisation of power and the capacity to adapt to a situation and develop and maintain a sense of control (Howkansen Hawks, 1991; Kalnins *et al.*, 1992; Fradd, 1994; Gibson, 1995). Empowerment is also associated with such concepts as coping, social support, self-esteem, locus of control, self-efficacy and motivation, which you will find referred to in other chapters of this book or more fully in the health psychology literature (see Broome and Llewellyn, 1995; Ogden, 1996 for further reading).

The process of empowerment thus has both intrapersonal and interpersonal elements and there is debate about the extent to which it is a process which individuals or groups must progress through for themselves, or which they

Table 20.8: The challenges of promoting empowerment

1 Within health care generally
- Those who are empowered must accept the burden of responsibility for their situation and its accompanying frustrations, along with the benefits of the knowledge, confidence and competence they gain and the right to be heard by those who traditionally hold the power which they achieve
- Health care professionals must feel confident in sharing their own knowledge and skills and be able to value others' expertise, in order to establish partnerships of mutual respect, open communication, active participation, collaboration and a sharing of power (this demands an organisational culture in which traditional power structures are flattened and health care professionals are themselves supported and empowered)
- All parties in the empowerment process must work as a team, with the same agenda and a commitment to a common goal
- Because empowerment is a continuous cyclical process, with individual and groups feeling more or less empowered as a consequence of the situation at any particular moment in time, those who are empowered must be protected from 'responsibility overload' (Gibson, 1995) and it must be recognised that they will need on-going support from a range of sources, particularly in 'new' situations or during crises

2 Within child health care
- We must accept that children's own views and needs are valid even if they are different from adults' views
- We must strive to understand health and illness as children see them
- We must recognise that children are competent and are able to be full partners in health care planning and decision making, both at a strategic level and individually
- We must acknowledge the ability of children of all ages to identify their problems for themselves, to exercise choice and to make decisions about action
- We must prepare children for these actions through appropriate education (e.g. life skills training) and provide support to enable them to take responsibility for their choices

Sources: Howkansen Hawks, 1991; Kalnins *et al.*, 1992; Fradd, 1994; Gibson, 1995.

can be enabled or facilitated through it by others. Certainly, within the child health nursing literature, there is a strong focus on the empowerment of others (usually mothers, though sometimes fathers and other carers, and increasingly children themselves). This process is often portrayed as a crucial element of contemporary children's nursing (e.g. Fradd, 1994). Whatever the form or extent of this facilitation, achieving true empowerment clearly provides a significant challenge to traditional beliefs, attitudes and power structures within child health care. Table 20.8 lists some of these challenges which are analysed in more depth in the papers referred to.

In conclusion, then, the concept of empowerment is clearly not straightforward. It is a complex continuous process (see Figure 20.10). Indeed, approaches which are referred to as being empowering may, in fact, exhibit few of the characteristics outlined in this section. As a nurse caring for children and their families, when analysing whether to utilise the principles of empowerment, the following questions should be considered:

- Do you and your colleagues have your own agenda in which you seek to direct or control your clients through 'empowerment' or do you truly want them to become empowered, accepting all that this process will entail?
- Does the client want to be 'empowered'? Will becoming empowered benefit him or her?
- Are you (the health professionals) and your clients ready to work together towards empowerment?
- Do you all have appropriate prerequisites for successful empowerment?

Key Points

- A number of key principles and goals have been identified in the provision of nursing care to children.
- These principles and goals, in themselves, are not necessarily exclusive to the care of children; however, their implementation may be different as a result of the specific health care needs of children.
- From a brief analysis of the literature it becomes apparent that the principles and goals are not mutually exclusive; they are related in a complex manner and this makes a separate conceptual analysis of each element problematic.
- The single most important factor in the implementation of these principles, and the achievement of the goals, is effective communication, and in particular, skilled listening (see Figure 20.2).

CONCLUSION

We stated at the beginning of this chapter that our aim was to raise the reader's awareness of the needs of children in relation to health care, so that any nurse who comes into contact with children as part of his or her nursing work might use this insight, in order to play a part in meeting children's health care needs. We also pointed out, early on, that children can come into contact with a diverse variety of nurses, depending on their health care needs.

What we hope we have achieved is to highlight that it is precisely because children have special needs that their nursing care should be provided by nurses who have all the necessary knowledge and skills to meet these needs. It is inappropriate, unprofessional and potentially negligent to dabble or make a 'stab in the dark' in relation to anybody's health. This means that nurses who do not have all the appropriate knowledge and skill, who find themselves faced with caring for children, should take heed of the need for professional accountability and consult with appropriately qualified nursing colleagues in order to ensure that such children receive appropriate care. This may involve referring the child to another nurse or working in partnership with other nurses, pooling resources to provide clinically effective, child-focused care.

There have been many changes in the UK health service since the inception of the NHS, and no less so in recent years. All these changes have been aimed at providing an improved service. Yet few nurses were surprised at the conclusions of the House of Commons' Committee on Children's Health (Health Committee, 1997b) when they stated that, within current child health services, there was poor communication and a lack of coordination, as well as a lack of specific education and training for nurses, and that services were often based on traditional custom and practice and professional self-interest, rather than the needs of children and their families (Casey et al., 1997), as highlighted in this chapter.

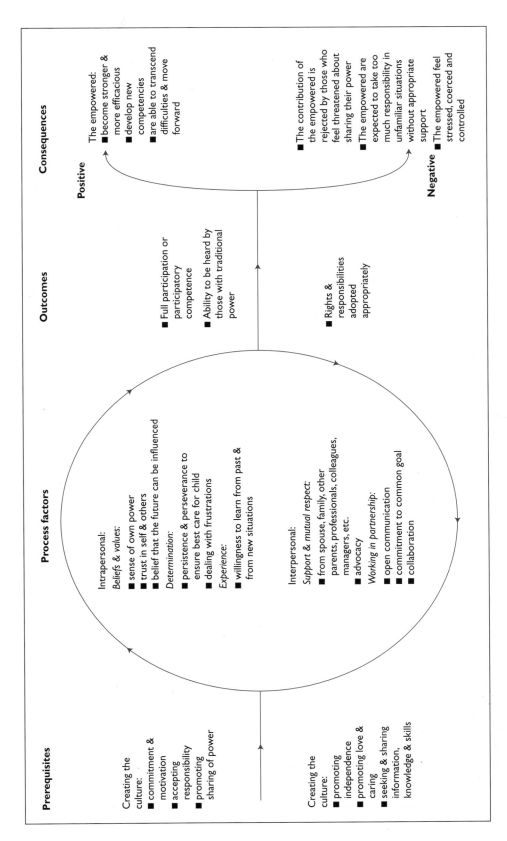

Figure 20.10: The process of empowerment (adapted from Fradd, 1994 and Gibson, 1995)

The Health Committee report stresses the importance of integrated health services for children. The Royal College of Nursing, in its response, suggested that, rather than a generic children's nurse, different nurses caring for children should bring their skills together to work as teams which function within a culture of mutual support and respect, valuing skills rather than job titles (Casey *et al.*, 1997). The Report's publication coincides with a new political era in Britain and a feeling of optimism for the next millennium. One can only hope that in this mood of optimism the recommendations of this report *will* be acted upon, because as the cynics can already be heard retorting, we have heard much of this before!

Summary

This chapter has considered how we understand children and childhood in order to identify the differences between children and adults and the special needs of children in relation to health care. In doing so we have identified and analysed the principles and goals of nursing in the provision of health care for children, as well as some of the key areas of knowledge and skills required to meet those goals.

REFERENCES

Anderson, J.J. (1989). Developing children. In *Family-centred nursing care of children*, Foster, R.L.R., Hunsberger, M.M. and Anderson, J.J. (eds), 92–130. W.B. Saunders, Philadelphia.

Archard, D. (1993). *Children: Rights and Childhood*. Routledge, London.

Audit Commission (1993). *Children First: a Study of Hospital Services*. HMSO, London.

Baker, S. (1995). Family centred care: a theory practice dilemma. *Paediatric Nursing*, 7(6), 17–19.

Bartram, A. (1965) *World of the Child*. Penguin, Harmondsworth.

Bedi, R. and Gilthorpe, M.S. (1995). The potential use of 'ethnic mass media' in health education – a case study of the Bangladeshi community. *Journal of the Institute of Health Education*, 33(2), 42–4, 52.

Bee, H. (1989). *The Developing Child*, 6th edn. Harper and Row, London.

Bellman, L. (1996). *Exploring the Art and Science of Nursing II: Study Guide*. RCN Distance Learning programme, Royal College of Nursing, London.

Benner, P (1984). *From Novice to Expert: Excellence and Power in Clinical Nursing*. Addison-Wesley, Menlo Park, California.

Bertalanffy, L. (1968). *General Systems Theory*. George Braziller, New York.

Bettelheim, B. (1987). *Good Enough Parent: a Guide to Bringing Up Your Child*. Thames and Hudson, London.

Bibace, R. and Walsh, M.E. (1981). *Children's Concepts of Health Illness and Bodily Function*. Jossey-Bass, San Francisco.

Bibby, R.W. and Posterski, J. (1992). *Teen Trends: a Nation in Motion*. Stottard, Toronto.

Bird, E. and Podmore, V.N. (1990). Children's understanding of health and illness. *Psychology and Health*, 4, 185–97.

Bowlby, J. (1953). *Child Care and the Growth of Love*. Penguin, Harmondsworth.

Bradley, S.F. (1996). Processes in the creation and diffusion of nursing knowledge: an examination of the developing concept of family centred care. *Journal of Advanced Nursing*, 23, 722–7.

Bridgman, A. (1995). The use of wet wrap dressings for eczema. *Paediatric Nursing*, 7(2), 24–7.

Broome, A. and Llewellyn, S. (1995). *Health Psychology: Processes and Applications*, 2nd edn. Chapman & Hall, London.

Brykczynska, G. (1996). *Caring: the Compassion and Wisdom of Nursing*. Arnold, London.

Burman, E. (1994). *Deconstructing Developmental Psychology*. Routledge, London.

Caldwell, C. (1997). Management of acute asthma in childhood. *Paediatric Nursing*, 9(6), 29–34.

Carey, S. (1985). *Conceptual Change in Childhood*. MIT Press, Cambridge, MA.

Casey, A. (1988). A partnership with child and family. *Senior Nurse*, 8(4), 8–9.

Casey, A. (1993). Development and use of the partnership model of care. In *Recent Advances in Child Health Care*, Glasper, A. and Tucker, A. (eds), 183–93. Scutari, London.

Casey, A., Young, L. and Rote, S. (1997). Integrated nursing services for children. *Paediatric Nursing*, 9(5), 8.

Cherry, B.S. and Carty, R.M. (1986). Changing concepts of childhood in society. *Pediatric Nursing*, 12(6), 421–4, 460.

Children's Rights Development Unit (1994). *UK Agenda for Children*. Children's Rights Development Unit, London.

Children's Rights Development Unit & British Paediatric Association & Royal College of Nursing (1995). *Child Health Rights*. BPA, London.

Coyne, I. (1996). Parent participation: a concept analysis. *Journal of Advanced Nursing*, 23, 733–40.

Craig, J. and McKay, E. (1958). Working of a mother and baby unit. *British Medical Journal*, 1, 275–8.

Darbyshire, P (1993). Parents, nurses and paediatric nursing: a critical review. *Journal of Advanced Nursing*, 18, 1670–80.

Dearmun, A.K. (1992). Perceptions of parental participation. *Paediatric Nursing*, 4(7), 6–9.

DHSS (1976). *The Report of the Committee on Child Health Services. Fit for the Future*, Volume 1 (The Court Report). HMSO, London.

Dobson, S. (1991). *Transcultural Nursing*. Scutari, London.

DoH (1989). *The Children Act*. HMSO, London.

DoH (1991). *Welfare of Children and Young People in Hospital*. HMSO, London.

DoH (1993). *A Vision for the Future*. HMSO, London.

DoH (1996). *Care of Children in the Community*. HMSO, London.

Egger, G., Donovan, R.J. and Spark, R. (1993). *Health and the Media: Principles and Practice for Health Promotion*. McGraw-Hill, Roseville, Australia.

Eiser, C. (1989). Children's concepts of illness: towards an alternative to the 'stage' approach. *Psychology and Health*, 3, 93–101.

Eiser, C. (1990). *Chronic Childhood Illness*, Cambridge University Press, Cambridge.

Eiser, C. and Patterson, D. (1983). Slugs and snails and puppy-dog's tails: children's ideas about the insides of their bodies. *Child Care: Health and Development*, 10, 233–40.

Erikson, E.H. (1959). *Identity and the Life Cycle*. Norton, New York.

Erikson, E.H. (1963). *Children and Society*, 2nd edn. Norton, New York.

Forfar, J. (ed.) (1989). *Child Health in a Changing Society*. British Paediatric Society, Harper and Row, London.

Fradd, E. (1987). A child alone. *Nursing Times*, 83(42), 16–17.

Fradd, E. (1994). Power to the people. *Paediatric Nursing*, 6(3), 11–14.

Fulton, Y. (1994). An analysis of family care. *Paediatric Nursing*, 6(10), 22–4.

Gaarder, J. (1995). *Sophie's World*. Phoenix House, London.

Gallagher, U. and Burden, J. (1993). Nursing and health promotion: a myth accepted? In *Research in Health Promotion and Nursing*, Wilson-Barnett, J. and Macleod-Clark, J. (eds). Macmillan, London.

Gaudion, C. (1997). Children's knowledge of their internal anatomy. *Paediatric Nursing*, 9(5), 14–17.

Gibson, C.H. (1995). The process of empowerment in mothers of chronically ill children. *Journal of Advanced Nursing*, 21, 1201–10.

Gilgun, J. and Gordon, S. (1985). Sex education and the prevention of child sexual abuse. *Journal of Sex Education and Therapy*, 11(1), 46–52.

Glauser, B.(1990). Street children: deconstructing a construct. In *Constructing and Reconstructing Childhood*, James, A. and Prout, A. (eds), 138–56. Falmer Press, London.

Glen, S. and Colson, J. (1993). The care of children. In *Nursing Practice and Health Care*, 2nd edn. Hinchliff, S.M., Norman, S.E. and Schober, J.E. (eds). Edward Arnold, London.

Gough, D. (1989). *Child Abuse Prevention: a Review of the Research Literature*. Research Report to the DHSS, SPORU, Glasgow University.

HEA (1992). *Teenage Smoking Mass Media Campaign: Qualitative Evaluation of TV and Print Advertising*. HEA, London.

Health Committee (1997a). *The Specific Health Needs of Children and Young People*. Health Committee second report of 1996–1997. HMSO, London.

Health Committee (1997b). *Health Services for Children and Young People in the Community: Home and School*. Health Committee third report of 1996–1997. HMSO, London.

Hendrick, H. (1990). Constructions and reconstructions of British childhood: an interpretive survey, 1800 to present day. In *Constructing and Reconstructing Childhood*, James, A. and Prout, A. (eds), 35–59. Falmer Press, London.

Hergenrather, J.R. and Rabinowiz, M. (1991). Age-related differences in the organisation of children's knowledge of illness. *Developmental Psychology*, 27(6), 952–9.

Hobbs, N. and Perrin, J.M. (1985). *Issues in the Care of Children with Chronic Illness*. Josey-Bass, San Francisco.

Hobsbaum, A. (1995). Children's development. In *Child Health Care Nursing. Concepts, Theory and Practice*, Carter, A. and Deamun, A. (eds). Blackwell Science, Oxford.

Holdsworth, K. (1995). Age-related differences in the organisation of children's knowledge of illness: a British perspective. *British Psychological Society Proceedings*, 4, 2.

Howkansen Hawks, J. (1991). Power: a concept analysis. *Journal of Advanced Nursing*, 16(3), 754–62.

Hunt, P. and Frankenberger, R. (1990). It's a small world: Disneyland, the family, and the multiple representations of American childhood. In *Constructing and Reconstructing Childhood*, James, A. and Prout, A. (eds), 184–95, Falmer Press, London.

James, A. and Prout, A. (eds) (1990). *Constructing and Reconstructing Childhood*. Falmer Press, London.

Jones, L.J. (1994). *The Social Context of Health*. Macmillan, London.

Jones, S. (1995). Managing pain using the partnership model of care. *Paediatric Nursing*, 7(1), 21–4.

Kalnins, I., McQueen, D.V., Backett, K.C., Curtice, L. and Currie, C.E. (1992). Children, empowerment and health promotion: some new directions in research and practice. *Health Promotion International*, 7(1), 53–8.

Karpf, A. (1988). *Doctoring the Media: the Reporting of Health and Medicine*. Routledge, London.

Keiffer, C. (1984). Citizen empowerment: a developmental perspective. *Prevention in Human Sciences*, 3(2/3), 9–36.

Kellmer-Pringle, M. (1975). *The Needs of Children*. Hutchinson, London.

King, I.M. (1981). A theory of goal attainment. In King, I.M. (ed.) *A Theory for Nursing: Systems, Concepts, Processes*. Wiley, New York.

Kitzinger, J. (1990). Who are you kidding? Children, power and the struggle against sexual abuse. In *Constructing and Reconstructing Childhood*, James, A. and Prout, A. (eds), 157–83. Falmer Press, London.

Kitzinger, J. and Skidmore, P. (1995). Playing safe: media coverage of child sexual abuse prevention strategies. *Child Abuse Review*, 4(1), 47–56.

Lansdown, G. (1995). The United Nations convention on the rights of the child. In *Child Health Care Nursing*, Carter, B. and Dearmun, A.K. (eds), 537–9. Blackwell, Oxford.

Leininger, M. (1978). *Transcultural Nursing: Concepts, Theories and Practices*. Wiley, New York.

Leininger, M. (1991). *Culture Care Diversity and Universality*. National League for Nursing Press, New York.

Levine, M. *et al.* (1983). *Developmental Behavioral Pediatrics*. W.B. Saunders, Philadelphia.

Lindsay, B. (1994). Influencing development: the media. In *The Child and Family: Contemporary Nursing Issues in Child Health Care*, Lindsay, B. (ed.). Baillière Tindall, London.

Longsdon, D. (1991). Conceptions of health and health behaviours of pre-school children. *Journal of Pediatric Nursing*, 6(6), 396–406.

McCarthy, D., Lindsay, M. and Morris, I. (1962). Children in hospital with mothers. *Lancet* 1, 603–8.

Mackenzie, H. (1991). Caring for a neonate in hospital using Roy's adaptation model. In *Caring for Children. Towards a Partnership with Families*, While, A. (ed.). Edward Arnold, London.

Mason, G. (1995). Conceptual frameworks for planning care. In *Child Health Care Nursing: Concepts, Theory and Practice*, Carter, B. and Dearmun, A.K. (eds). Blackwell Science, Oxford.

Masterson, A. (1995). *Exploring the Art and Science of Nursing I*. RCN Distance Learning programme, Royal College of Nursing, London.

Meadow, S.R. (1969). The captive mother. *Archives of Diseases of Childhood*, 44, 362–9.

Ministry of Health (1946). *Report of the Care of Children Committee* (The Curtis Report). HMSO, London.

Ministry of Health (1948). *The Children Act*. HMSO, London.

Ministry of Health (1959). *The Welfare of Children in Hospital* (The Platt Report). HMSO, London.

Morrison, B. (1997). *As If*. Granta, London.

Muller, D., Harris, P.J. and Taylor, J.D. (1992). *Nursing Children: Psychology Research and Practice*, 2nd edn. Chapman & Hall, London.

NAWCH (1985). *A Charter for Children in Hospital*. NAWCH/Action for Sick Children, London.

Ogden, J. (1996). *Health Psychology: a Text Book*. Open University Press, Milton Keynes.

Orem, D. (1985). *Nursing: Concepts of Practice*, 3rd edn. McGraw-Hill, New York

Orem, D. (1991). *Nursing: Concepts of Practice*, 4th edn. Mosby, St. Louis.

Orr, J. (1985). Assessing individual and family health needs. In *Health Visiting*. Luker, K. and Orr, J. (eds). Blackwell Scientific Publications, Oxford.

Perrin, E.C. and Gerrity, P.S. (1981). There's a demon in your belly: children's understanding of illness. *Pediatrics*, 67, 841–9.

Phillips, L. (1994). Children and power. In *The Child and Family: Contemporary Nursing Issues in Child Health Care*. Lindsay, B. (ed.). Baillière Tindall, London.

Philo, G. (1994). The impact of the mass media on public images of mental illness. *Health Education Journal*, 53(3), 271–81.

Piaget, J. (1968). A theory of development. *International Encyclopaedia of the Social Sciences*. Crowell Collier Macmillan, New York.

Piaget, J. and Inhelder, B. (1969). *The Psychology of the Child*. Routledge and Kegan Paul, London.

Pridmore, P. and Bendelow, G. (1995). Images of health: exploring beliefs of children using the 'draw-and-write' technique. *Health Education Journal*, 54, 473–488.

Pulaski, M.S. (1971). *Understanding Piaget: an Introduction to Children's Cognitive Development*. Harper and Row, New York.

Qvortrop, J. (1990). A voice for children in statistical and social accounting: a plea for children's rights to be heard. In *Constructing and Reconstructing Childhood*, James, A. and Prout, A. (eds), 78–98. Falmer Press, London.

Ramprogas, V. (1992). Developing nursing theory. *Senior Nurse*, 12(1), 46–51.

Robertson, J. (1962). *Hospitals and Children: a Review of Letters From Parents to 'The Observer' and the BBC*. Victor Gollancz, London.

Robertson, J. (1970). *Young Children in Hospital*, 2nd edn. Tavistock, London.

Robertson, L. (1995). Professional perspectives. In *Child Health Care Nursing: Concepts, Theory and Practice*, Carter, B. and Dearmun, A.K. (eds). Blackwell Science, Oxford.

Roper, N., Logan, W.W. and Tierney, A. (1990). *The Elements of Nursing*, 3rd edn. Churchill Livingstone, Edinburgh.

Rosenbaum, J.N. and Carty, L. (1996). The subculture of adolescence: beliefs about care, health and individuation within Leininger's theory. *Journal of Advanced Nursing*, 23, 741–6.

Roy, C. and Andrews, H.A. (eds) (1991). *The Roy Adaptation Model: the Definitive Statement*. Appleton & Lange, Norwalk, CT.

Rushforth, H. (1996). Nurses' knowledge of how children view health and illness. *Paediatric Nursing*, 8(9), 23–7.

Sainsbury, C.P.Q., Gray, O.P., Cleary, J., Davies, M. and Rolandson, P.H. (1986). Care by parents of their children in hospital. *Archives of Disease in Childhood*, 61, 612–15.

Selye, H. (1976). *The stress of Life*, 2nd edn. McGraw-Hill, London.

Signorielli, N. (1993). *Mass Media Images and Impact on Health*. Greenwood, Westport, CO.

Stower, S. (1992). Partnership caring. *Journal of Clinical Nursing*, 1(2), 67–72.

Strasburger, V.C. (1995). *Adolescents and the Media: Medical and Psychological Impact*. Sage, Thousand Oaks, CA.

Sylva, K. and Lunt, I. (1982). *Child Development: a First Course*. Blackwell Scientific, Oxford.

Tizard, B. (1977). Play: the child's way of learning? In *Biology of Play*, Tizard, B. and Harvey, D. (eds). Heinnemann, London.

UKCC (1995). *Registrar's letter 4/95: Clinical Supervision for Nursing and Health Visiting*. UKCC, London.

United Nations General Assembly (1991). *UN Convention on the Rights of the Child*. UNICEF, Geneva.

Vallely, P. (1997). How street-wise can a nine year old be? *The Independent*, 6 January, 6.

Vygotsky, L. (1978). *Mind in Society: the Development of Higher Psychological Processes*. Harvard University Press, Cambridge, MA.

Wallace, E. (1993). Nursing a teenager with burns (using Roper's model of nursing). *British Journal of Nursing*, 2(5), 278–81.

Watt, S. and Mitchell, R. (1995). Historical perspectives. In *Child Health Care Nursing: Concepts, Theory and Practice*, Carter, B. and Dearmun, A.K. (eds). Blackwell Science, Oxford.

Webb, N., Hull, D. and Madelay, R. (1985). Care by parents in hospital. *British Medical Journal*, 291, 176–7.

Welch, L. (1993). Applying Orem's model. *Paediatric Nursing*, 5(6), 14–16.

Weller, B. (1994). Cultural aspects of children's health. In *The Child and the Family*, Lindsay, B. (ed.). Baillière Tindall, London.

While, A. (ed.) (1991). *Caring for Children. Towards a Partnership with Families*. Edward Arnold, London.

Whiting, L. (1997). Health promotion: the role of the children's nurse. *Paediatric Nursing*, 9(5), 6–7.

Winnicott, D.W. (1958). *Collected Papers: Through Paediatrics to Psychoanalysis*. Tavistock, London.

FURTHER READING

A number of suggestions for further reading have been made throughout the chapter and details of these texts can be found in the main reference list. In addition, there are now a number of British textbooks of children's nursing which cover in much more detail many of the issues that we have touched upon or not covered at all. Two of these are:

Carter, B. and Dearmun, A.K. (eds) (1995). *Child Health Care Nursing: Concepts, Theory and Practice*. Blackwell Science, Oxford.

Campbell, S. and Glasper, E.A. (eds) (1995). *Whaley & Wong's Children's Nursing*. Mosby, Philadelphia.

Since most textbooks are already out of date by the time they are published, you are advised to read an appropriate journal to remain up to date with the evidence-base of child health nursing practice. If you are only able to read one journal regularly, *Paediatric Nursing*, published by the Royal College of Nursing Publishing Company, is probably the most appropriate.

CHAPTER TWENTY-ONE

MENTAL HEALTH NURSING

Stephen Firn, David L. Parker and Gregory Philip Rooney

- Psychiatric or mental health nursing?
- A brief history of mental health care and mental health nursing in the United Kingdom
- Contemporary mental health nursing values
- The health–illness continuum
- Skills of the mental health nurse
- Severe and enduring mental illnes (SMI)
- Clinical scenario – care of person with serious mental illness (SMI)
- Psychosocial interventions
- Organisation and delivery of mental health care
- Legal issues relating to mental health nursing
- Incidence and description of most prevalent mental health problems
- Caring for specific client groups with mental health problems
- Conclusion

In order to understand fully the contemporary role of the nurse in mental health, it is important to be aware of the historical roots of mental health nursing and learn lessons from the rich and sometimes chequered history of the treatment and care of people with mental health problems in the UK. This chapter focuses initially on the development of mental health nursing up to the present day and highlights challenges for the new millennium.

An ethical framework and contemporary values of mental health nursing are proposed and the core skills discussed. The main body of the chapter discusses the application of evidence-based interventions and the development of the therapeutic nurse–client relationship with clients experiencing a range of mental health problems. In keeping with the recent emphasis on meeting the needs of people with severe and enduring mental illness, the role of the mental health nurse in providing care to people with schizophrenia is explored in most detail. In particular, the utilisation of skills such as psychosocial interventions is discussed along with the mental health nurse's role in case management and the implementation of the Care Programme Approach and the Mental Health (Patients in the Community) Act 1995.

The chapter concludes with an overview of specialist areas of mental health nursing practice including substance misuse, forensic mental health nursing and the care of people with eating disorders.

The emphasis throughout this chapter is on the practice of mental health nursing based on the involvement of users, collaboration with other professionals and agencies, and evidence.

The chapter will be valuable to those undertaking pre-registration mental health nurse education and an attempt has been made to avoid the use of jargon and to explain any technical terms. It is also intended that practising mental health nurses and educators will find the focus on the latest developments in the skills and role of the mental health nurse both thought-provoking and informative.

PSYCHIATRIC OR MENTAL HEALTH NURSING?

The terms psychiatric nurse and mental health nurse are often used interchangeably but a number of authors have suggested a distinction. Hally and Hardy (1997) associate the term *psychiatric nurse* with the more traditional nursing role of working in a hospital setting within a medical model of care. This model is predominantly based around a diagnosis of the mental illness, made by a psychiatrist, and the treatment and care prescribed in response to this diagnosis. Whilst this model of care still predominates and the term psychiatric nurse is still widely used, in this chapter the more contemporary title *mental health nurse* is used as this reflects the current emphasis on promoting mental health and formulating positive interventions in collaboration with the client, as well as providing care in a diverse range of settings. The title *community psychiatric nurse (CPN)* is used to refer to nurses working in the community, however, as this term is in widespread use and represents one part of the multifacted role of modern mental health nursing.

A BRIEF HISTORY OF MENTAL HEALTH CARE AND MENTAL HEALTH NURSING IN THE UNITED KINGDOM

Mental disorder has been recognised for many thousands of years. Ancient writings in the Old Testament include references to disorders of the mind including depression and self-harm and the Ancient Greeks, such as Plato, gave advice about the care of people designated as insane. In mediaeval Europe, mental disorder was often linked to witchcraft or evil. Beliefs about the various causes included individuals having lost their souls, being possessed with evil spirits or having committed great sins (Hedlund and Jeffrey, 1993).

Care for those who were mentally ill in public institutions in the UK was first recorded in the fourteenth century at the Priory of St Mary of Bethlehem (Russell, 1997). At this time, the majority of 'lunatics' were still cared for within their own homes or communities but those without the social support of friends or relatives were often banished and became outcasts. Russell (1997) records how those who were mentally ill were often compared to animals. He cites medical staff describing the 'mad' as violent wild beasts, lacking in reason and oblivious to heat or cold. Viewed as animals, it was common practice for those in mental institutions to be chained and the public fascination with these 'creatures' is evident in the establishment of viewing galleries where members of the public paid to observe the lunatics in 'Bedlam' (a corruption of Bethlehem and a word which is still used today to describe chaos or uproar).

The late eighteenth century saw more enlightened approaches being adopted, pioneered by William Tuke's Retreat at York, where chains were removed and a regime introduced that was based on the concept that madness would respond to kindness, strict moral discipline and an escape from the stimuli of the outside world. This was quite literally a place of asylum. These reforms also propagated the belief that people with mental illness could be helped to reassert self-control over their symptoms, which is a crucial principle in mental health nursing today.

The nineteenth century witnessed a vast expansion in institutional care for people who were mentally ill, resulting from Victorian legislative and moral reforms. The Poor Law Act of 1834 legislated for the collection of taxes for the treatment for those in need within each Parish, including those who were mentally disordered. The Lunacy Act of 1890 gave local authorities the responsibility to provide care for patients certified as insane, resulting in a rapid expansion of the number of asylums and 'inmates'. These self-contained and self-supporting institutions were typically built outside conurbations, effectively separating patients from their family and friends. Many remained in asylums for the remainder of their lives (Hally and Hardy 1997).

DEVELOPMENT OF MENTAL HEALTH NURSING

Those providing day-to-day care of people who were mentally ill were called by various titles including 'keeper' and 'attendant'. Russell (1997) notes that from the mid-nineteenth century female staff began to use the title 'nurse' although male staff (who tended just to care for male patients) continued to be referred to as attendants into the twentieth century. Throughout most of the nineteenth century the attendant's role entailed maintaining order in wards, which were frequently home for more than 60 patients, and assisting in the work of the self-contained communities in the kitchens, laundries and farms. Physical strength and practical skills were therefore the prime attributes for these Victorian equivalents of today's mental health nurses. During the early twentieth century physical treatments began to be developed and attendants' roles became more akin to those of nurses in general hospitals of the time, such as acting as doctors' aides and monitoring and reporting on the effects of treatments.

A national certificate for asylum attendants was first introduced as early as 1890 but by 1934 only 30% of staff in mental hospitals had this qualification. In 1919 the Nurses' Registration Act created a supplementary register for mental nurses under the auspices of the General Nursing Council (GNC) and two qualifications were available until 1951 when the education and training of mental nurses became the sole responsibility of the GNC. Nevertheless, the status of mental nursing remained below that of general nurses with Hally and Hardy (1997) noting that a 1965 advertisement for nursing barely mentioned mental nursing except to point out that it was the preserve of male nurses, suggesting that the profession had not shaken off the image of the Victorian asylum attendant.

Academically and conceptually, however, mental health nursing was beginning to mature. The seminal work of Peplau (1952) on the theory of interpersonal relationships in nursing made a major contribution to theory-based practice. This was one of the first 'grand theories' of nursing and is still widely practised in mental health nursing today. Peplau (1952) conceptualised individuals as unique beings with internal needs which generated tensions. She believed individuals capable of new learning and that the nurse and client can form therapeutic relationships in which they both experience growth and the client can learn and adapt to tensions created by his or her needs (Beard and Johnson, 1993).

Since the 1960s there has been a considerable increase in the understanding and management of mental illness. This has resulted in a substantial growth in the treatment and care options available to people with mental health problems. Contributory factors include drug therapies which have relieved or reduced some of the major symptoms of psychosis (e.g. hallucinations and delusions) in a significant number of people (albeit not without side-effects) and the increasing range of therapeutic interventions including psychosocial care, group and individual therapies and family interventions. Alongside these developments were the identification of potential debilitating effects on patients of long-term care in institutions resulting in loss of self-identity and the adoption of rigid behaviour patterns in response to the need to conform to the rules of life within institutions (Goffman, 1961).

Leff (1994) asserts that changing attitudes amongst those professionals caring for people who are mentally ill provided the main impetus towards the reduction in beds in psychiatric hospitals. This was, however, facilitated by the introduction of neuroleptic medications which helped contain the most debilitating symptoms. These were first introduced in 1954, the year in which the number of beds in psychiatric hospitals reached a peak of 148 000 and thereafter declined.

Many of the large Victorian mental hospitals in England and Wales have now closed and it is current governmental policy to close as many as possible by the end of the century (Department of Health, 1993a). Leff observes that this revolution in the way mental health care is provided is not based on research evidence that care in the community improves the mental health or the quality of life of people with mental health problems. His 1-year follow-up of clients discharged from long-term care in two psychiatric hospitals, however, suggested that most people preferred living in the community and experienced improvements in their quality of life, such as increased freedom and social network of friends.

The *Spectrum of Care* (Department of Health, 1996) outlines a comprehensive range of care in home settings, day care and residential settings (including hospitals). Mental health nurses have increasingly moved, some with trepidation and

	best possible care for people with mental illness'
90%	'Increased spending on mental health services is not a waste of money'
81%	'Best therapy for many people with mental illness is to be part of the community'
67%	'People with mental illness are far less of a danger than most people suppose'

Source: Department of Health (1996).

ambivalence, from hospital-based posts to roles in community mental health teams, day hospital, day care settings and 24-hour nursed care residential settings.

Public attitudes

There is some evidence that public attitudes towards mental illness are changing as the findings from a study carried out in 1994 on behalf of the Department of Health demonstrate (Table 21.1). Despite these encouraging indicators, which are far removed from the traditional beliefs about madness, the authors' experience of discussing plans to provide residential care for people with mental health problems indicates that many people are still initially suspicious and hostile if the plans involve their neighbourhood.

Table 21.2: Pressures on London's mental health services

- Increasing bed occupancy rates reaching 125%
- Unacceptably high levels of assaults and cases of sexual harassment on inpatient wards
- Lack of beds leading to high admission thresholds for people with serious disorders
- Poor liaison services
- Delays in providing services including median wait of 7 days for allocation to a community psychiatric nurse (CPN) or social worker
- Limited provision of day care, long-term care and employment schemes
- Lack of residential care places and high intensity 24-hour community services

munity is a positive development, a number of recent reports have suggested that mental health services are extremely stretched and, in particular, are struggling to meet the needs of those with severe mental health problems. For instance, the King's Fund (Johnson *et al.*, 1997) warn of an impending crisis in the provision of mental health services in London with the main concerns identified as shown in Table 21.2.

Key Points

- Clearly much has been achieved and much needs to be done both in the provision of care and the development of the potential of mental health nursing.
- The foregoing brief overview of mental health care in the UK details how knowledge and attitudes towards mental illness and the treatment and care of those with mental health problems has changed dramatically.
- There is little doubt that modern facilities and approaches to care are more humane and more able to respond to individual mental health needs.
- It would be easy to classify the past as cruel whilst failing to recognise that there is still much work to be done in identifying the most effective ways of providing nursing care and ensuring patients are always treated with dignity and respect.

CONTEMPORARY MENTAL HEALTH NURSING VALUES

Mental health nurses care for some of the most vulnerable people in society and, as professional practitioners, occupy a position of power by dint of their assumed knowledge and status when providing care for clients. A number of inquiries have highlighted how, in the absence of factors such as clinical supervision and strong professional leadership, abuse of patients can occur (Department of Health, 1992). In addition, the United Kingdom Central Council for Nursing Midwifery and Health Visiting (UKCC) has recently highlighted concerns about the number of mental health nurses reported for allegations of sexual misconduct (UKCC, 1996).

Whilst we cannot always ensure that every client's mental health needs will be met, we need to ensure that the potential for clients experiencing further distress and indignities whilst receiving mental health care is minimised. This reflects the fundamental principles of striving to do good (beneficence), whilst doing our utmost to prevent harm (non-maleficence).

Within this ethical framework the following principles are fundamental to the delivery of optimal mental health nursing care:

- Involving users in their care
- Working collaboratively with other professionals and agencies
- Basing practice on best available evidence
- Promoting privacy and dignity of clients.

INVOLVING USERS IN THEIR CARE

Working in Partnership was a comprehensive review of mental health nursing commissioned by the Department of Health (1994). This concluded that the work of mental health nurses fundamentally rests on the relationship they have with people who use services and their carers. The main recommendation was:

> 'Mental Health Nursing should re-examine every aspect of its policy and practice in the light of the needs of the people who use services. Nursing services should be designed and developed to meet the needs of people who use services; people should not be expected to conform to the convenience of the service.'

This presupposes a relationship between the mental health nurse and the client which is characterised by respect and concern for human dignity, as well as an orientation towards growth of all parties concerned, including families and significant others. This relationship will be influenced by the skills and attitudes of the nurse, as well as by the insight and motivation levels of the client.

In order to meet the challenge, mental health nurses must be committed to ensuring patients and their carers are fully involved in the assessment, delivery and evaluation of their care. This will mean that, on occasions, nurses will act as advocates for patients to empower them to make informed choices about their care and where they receive it. Examples of how these principles are applied in practice are described in the clinical scenario later in this chapter.

COLLABORATIVE CARE WITH OTHER PROFESSIONALS AND AGENCIES

Mental health nursing care must not only incorporate users' views, as far as possible, but must also include a commitment to close collaboration with other professionals and agencies. There are a multiplicity of factors which contribute to mental illness and how people experience these illnesses, including physical, psychological, social, spiritual and intellectual factors (Landrum *et al.*, 1993). Thus, factors such as stress, employment, housing, physical well-being and levels of social support may all contribute to how mental health problems are experienced and to rates of relapse. Responding to all these concerns necessitates a multi-professional and multi-agency approach to provide the necessary psychosocial support and respond rapidly in times of crisis. Rivalry between professionals and agencies and poor communication can be disastrous for a client's quality of care and the outcomes of his or her illness (Blom-Cooper *et al.*, 1996).

EVIDENCE-BASED PRACTICE

Simply stated, evidence-based practice entails ensuring clinical care is based on practices which have been shown to be most effective in providing health gains and are also cost-effective. There are few who would disagree with this principle and it may seem unnecessary to have to make it explicit at all. There is, however, a history of nursing practice being based on assumption or because 'we've always done it that way'. A frequently cited example is the 5–10-year delay between identification that talcum powder was not effective – and may even be harmful when used for pressure area care – and its discontinuation in common practice. Mental health nurses need to question constantly why they do things the way they do, and involve users and colleagues in evaluating their practice, in order to ensure practice is evidence-based. Evidence does not need to be drawn exclusively from published research, although clearly this is the gold standard, but can be obtained from other sources, including patient satisfaction surveys, observations and audit.

PROMOTING PRIVACY AND DIGNITY

The mental health *Patient's Charter* (NHS Executive, 1997) places particular emphasis on ensuring the privacy of inpatients is respected and that they are treated with dignity. It emphasises the importance of choice for patients along with the need for increased awareness of individual needs regardless of gender, race, sexual orientation, religious or cultural background. Thus, the Charter suggests patients should be given choices around diet and culturally appropriate meals; name or title by which they are addressed; access to quiet areas and women-only spaces. Mental health nurses are in an ideal position to ensure that patients' privacy and dignity are maintained and promoted.

THE HEALTH–ILLNESS CONTINUUM

Mental health can be conceptualised as a continuum stretching from extreme mental debilitation to a state of complete mental well-being. Maslow (1968) calls this latter state 'self-actualisation'. He believes that to attain this ultimate state individuals need to have fulfilled their highest ambitions and potential and be completely free from any concerns relating to their physical, emotional, intellectual and spiritual needs. Most people would question whether this state can ever be reached, much less sustained. The concept of the health–illness continuum suggests that, in reality, most people move along an axis between health and ill health during their lifetimes and this is influenced by a range of factors including inherited biological characteristics, upbringing and environment, physical and spiritual well-being, and major life events and stressors.

In the experience of one of the authors, the notion of each of us experiencing some degree of mental illness is not one to which the majority of people readily subscribe. This is evidenced at introductory sessions to the area of mental health for nursing students when the lecturer enquires as to the students' experience of physical illness. A large majority of students indicate that they have experienced physical illnesses and are happy to describe these. When the same question is posed regarding mental illness, the position is reversed, with a very small proportion describing experi-

ence of mental illness. When their responses are explored in more depth, it appears that they do not link experiences of anxiety and low mood to mental illness, and thus mental illness somehow lies outside their experience. This may be a reflection of the stigma attached to mental health problems and thus an unwillingness to recognise them in oneself. People with mental health problems are therefore conceptualised as 'different' from ourselves and we feel less vulnerable. This is an important point since in order to establish a therapeutic nurse–client relationship it is essential to listen to clients and to try to understand their experiences. This includes acknowledging when these connect with our own experiences.

SKILLS OF THE MENTAL HEALTH NURSE

Recent debates about mental health nursing indicate that it is difficult to define the conceptual framework and skills that are specific to mental health nursing alone (Carson *et al.*, 1995; Gijbels and Burnard, 1995). As a conceptual model for mental health nursing, Peplau's (1952) interpersonal framework is most frequently cited, although the application of 10 nursing models to the care of people with mental health problems is described in detail in Collister (1987). The value of conceptual nursing frameworks for mental health nursing, however, has not been demonstrated (Gijbels and Burnard, 1995) and there have been recent criticisms that their 'untested' application can conflict with evidence-based interventions. Indeed, one professor of psychiatric nursing has called for the abandonment of these 'millstones' because, in his view, they mitigate against the utilisation of evidence-based practice, such as the psychosocial interventions described elsewhere in this chapter (Gournay, 1995).

Some authors have argued for the introduction of a generic mental health worker, who would combine the skills of the mental health nurse and the mental health social worker with the potential to meet both the health and social needs of patients. The Mental Health Nursing Review Team (Department of Health, 1994) rejected the notion of the 'generic' nurse and came down strongly in favour of retaining mental health nursing as a specialist qualification at pre-registration

Table 21.3: Skills of the mental health nurse

- Establish a therapeutic relationship which rests in a respect for others and skilled therapeutic use of self
- Sustain such relationships over time and respond flexibly to the changing needs of those with mental health problems
- Construct, implement and evaluate a care programme
- Provide skilled assessment, on-going monitoring
- Make risk assessments and judgements
- Monitor the dosage, effects and contraindications of medication
- Detect early signs of deteriorating mental health including potential self-harm and suicide risk, worsening physical conditions and potential threats to others
- Prioritise work in order to respond to those most in need
- Collaborate with all members of the multidisciplinary team
- Network effectively, setting appropriate boundaries to the professional input

Source: Department of Health, 1994.

level. They identified a list of skills (Table 21.3) which, when combined with the values and practices common to all branches of nursing, form the unique expertise and role of mental health nurses.

There is insufficient space in this chapter to explore all these aspects of the mental health nurse's role in detail. The practical application of many of the skills listed in Table 21.3 are explored in the clinical scenario. It is helpful at this stage, however, to discuss the core skills of observation and data collection, interviewing and risk assessment and management.

OBSERVATION AND DATA COLLECTION

Observing is a key skill in information collection which is crucial to developing understanding of the client's needs and evaluating outcomes of care. A great deal of knowledge can be obtained from carefully observing a patient's appearance and behaviour. The nurse should observe the patient's body language, including voice, speech and physical state. For instance, someone who is low in mood is likely to look unhappy in terms of facial expression. Movement is likely to be restricted and slow, with stooping of the shoulders. Speech is likely to be curtailed. Any words spoken are likely to be lacking in expression and of a low pitch. Physical state may well appear neglected with unkempt, unwashed hair and lack of care in dressing and general physical appearance. The patient's behaviour in relation to others is likely to show avoidance of interaction, the individual lacking the energy and drive to make interpersonal contact.

How others react to the individual is also part of the nurse's observations, particularly relatives or friends, since depression not only leads to hopelessness and social isolation, but also to altered family processes and inability to fulfil usual social and family roles. The skilled mental health nurse will always seek to compare observations with the clients pre-morbid ('usual') mood and behaviour by speaking to relatives and significant others. It is also important to be aware of the factors which may lead to misunderstandings and false perceptions, such as different cultural health beliefs, practices and use of language.

In addition to measurements indicated by skilled observation, data collection is central to the assessment process. There are multiple sources of data, including the individual patient, if he or she is able to verbalise difficulties. Previous health records and notes may contain crucial information about factors precipitating a relapse or acts of aggression or self-harm.

Mental health nursing is carried out within a multidisciplinary context and teamwork ensures that reliance is not only on one professional's interpretations of phenomena and events. Professionals draw upon each other's knowledge, skills and observations prior to a diagnosis being made and a care plan devised.

INTERVIEWING

Interviewing is an extremely important skill in mental health nursing which incorporates both the collection of information as well as the foundation for the nurse–client therapeutic relationship. Newell (1994) points out that without effective interviewing skills, which generate accurate information and mutual trust, subsequent nursing interventions cannot be fully successful. The interview is set up to take account of the patient's individuality and the context in which the interview is to take place. Key interviewing skills are: establishing rapport; listening and attending; interpreting verbal and non-verbal communications; questioning; drawing out and checking for accuracy; enabling self-expression; responding and, above all, being receptive and accepting (Department of Health, 1994). There are many different approaches and models. One widely used model is that of Heron's (1990) Six Category Intervention Analysis. He subdivides interventions into the authoritative and the facilitative. Each of these modes of intervention is useful when used appropriately, but the nurse must be skilled in their use and know which approach to choose at any one time.

Box 21.1: Heron's (1990) Six Category Intervention Analysis

Authoritative
- Prescriptive: offering advice and giving instructions
- Informative: providing information and teaching
- Confronting: challenging the patient's perceptions or behaviour

Facilitative
- Catalytic: enabling further progress or exploration
- Cathartic: enabling the patient to express feelings or relieve tension
- Supportive: helping the patient to recognise own self-worth

---

Nurses have been shown to be most comfortable using the prescriptive and informative skills whilst finding the cathartic and confronting skills most difficult to utilise (Burnard and Morrison, 1991). This may be a reflection of social norms in that the open expression of emotions and the challenging of others are not encouraged in everyday interactions. It is crucial, however, that mental health nurses do have the skills to challenge clients' beliefs and behaviours in a positive manner, which does not affect the therapeutic relationship, whilst also feeling comfortable and competent to facilitate the expression of deep emotions. Newell (1994) offers an excellent 'how

to' guide to interviewing skills for nurses with particular emphasis on the cognitive–behavioural approach.

RISK ASSESSMENT AND RISK MANAGEMENT

Risk assessment and risk management are key areas of practice for the mental health nurse in order to predict and prevent danger towards others and self. Risk factors for assessment are shown in Box 21.2.

Box 21.2: Risk assessment and risk management

- Potential for suicide/self-harm
- Potential for assault/violence
- Potential for substance misuse/withdrawal
- Potential for allergic reaction/adverse drug reaction
- Potential for convulsion/seizure
- Potential for falls/accidents
- Potential for absconding
- Potential for physiological instability

The potential for suicide and self-harm is particularly important, since 90% of people who commit suicide have previously sought help for a mental health problem, 66% have seen their GP in the previous month and 25% are attending psychiatric outpatients (Department of Health, 1993a).

Grounds (1995) emphasises that individual risk assessments must be grounded in history. Whilst he acknowledges that the vast majority of people with active symptoms of mental illness are not violent, research studies have demonstrated that people with a history of violent behaviour whilst expressing psychotic illness (e.g. delusions and hallucination) pose an increased risk of violence. He advocates a thorough assessment which includes an examination of all clinical records, plus interviews with clients and other relevant informants. This should include specific questions such as context of violent behaviour; who was the target; which methods were used; and precipitating factors. This approach is also relevant to assessment of other risks.

According to Thompson and Mathias (1994) it is difficult to draw the line between reasonable risk and potential danger. They advocate the establishment of a check system within the service, which could include quality review teams or client-focused meetings to ensure that self-determination is not subverted on the premise that clients cannot reason and make real informed choices.

Over-reaction and excessive supervision can have adverse effects on the nurse–client relationship. This relationship is crucial to long-term monitoring of clients' mental health. Those at greatest risk may benefit from commitment to long-term collaborative care offered in the intensive case-management approach described elsewhere in this chapter. An excellent collection of papers on assessing and managing risk among clients with mental health problems is contained within Crichton (1995).

Key Points

- Mental health nursing must take place within an ethical framework which strives to do good and prevent harm to clients.
- The core values of contemporary mental health nursing must include the full involvement of users in their care; close collaborative working alongside other professionals and agencies; practice based on best available evidence; and practices which seek to promote the and maintain the privacy and dignity of clients.
- There is no one conceptual framework which adequately encapsulates mental health nursing or distinct set of individual skills which are the sole preserve of mental health nursing.
- A range of skills are discussed, which, when considered alongside practices common to other branches of nursing, formulate the unique role of the mental health nurse.

SEVERE AND ENDURING MENTAL ILLNESS (SMI)

In recent years there has been an increasing emphasis on ensuring services focus upon the needs of people with severe and enduring mental illness (Department of Health, 1993a, 1996). This term is not well defined, but is typically used to describe people with schizophrenia or major affective (mood) disorders such as severe depression or mania, which affects their well-being and social functioning over many years.

SCHIZOPHRENIA

Gournay (1996) welcomes the increased emphasis on the care of people with severe mental illness and notes that 1.6% of the total NHS budget is devoted to care of people diagnosed with schizophrenia.

> 'although there is, of course, no clear definition of serious or enduring mental illness, schizophrenia represents the biggest single challenge in mental health care . . . there is no doubt that schizophrenia accounts for more pain and suffering than any other group of mental health problems, both in those afflicted and in their families and carers.'
>
> (pages 7–8)

Critics suggest this focus is an inappropriate reaction to media-fuelled fears about people with schizophrenia committing acts of violence, but there is also evidence that this client group has not received the level or quality of services from mental health professionals that the severity of their needs indicates. A number of studies have shown that community psychiatric nurses (CPN), particularly those attached to general practice, have focused more on the needs of people with anxiety and less severe forms of depression. One study showed 24.5% of CPNs had caseloads which contained no clients with schizophrenia (White, 1990). Table 21.4 lists the key issues relating to schizophrenia.

Gournay (1996) suggests that whilst there continues to be a debate about the label 'schizophrenia', there is increasingly clear evidence of a group of syndromes caused by brain abnormalities of *neurodevelopmental origin*, i.e. occurring before birth. He predicts that in the not too distant future the aetiology of the disorder will be fully understood and we can develop evidence-based prevention interventions and treatments. Gournay asserts that this research has major implications for mental health nursing education and practice.

Table 21.4: Key issues related to schizophrenia

- Affects approximately 1% of population (higher in urban areas)
- Peak age of onset is 16–24 years
- 15% commit suicide
- 50% lose contact with specialist mental health services
- Only 20% have a CPN

Adapted from Strathdee *et al.*, 1996.

For instance, he says that nurses need an understanding of neuroanatomy, genetics and brain imaging in order to educate families effectively about the condition and to be involved in genetic counselling of families with schizophrenia and other mental disorders. He further predicts that an increased emphasis on cognitive deficits in schizophrenia will assist the future development of cognitive rehabilitation for people with the condition, which entails training people to overcome their deficits in a similar way to a person who has experienced a stroke. He goes on to suggest that there is sufficient scientific evidence for nurse educationalists to include in their curricula neuroanatomy, molecular genetics and the various methods of brain imaging.

Others have argued that viewing mental illness as discrete occurrences which need to be addressed by one specific 'scientific' intervention places a barrier between the nurse and the client which could adversely affect the therapeutic relationship (Barker, 1995). Barker has advocated that the starting point for mental health nurses should be the recognition that the client is experiencing a human response to complex situations and nurses need to empathise and understand this experience before prescribing *a priori* a set of interventions.

Dawson (1997) suggests that Professor Gournay and others are promulgating a myth that biological psychiatry will be able to provide an unambiguous model of the nature of mental disorder. He asserts that a closer examination of the evidence reveals a confused and unconvincing set of results to date and claims no significant progress has been made in the last 30 years towards understanding the biological basis of mental functioning. Thus, Dawson (1997) argues that supporters of Gournay are reductionist in the sense that their assumption that serious mental illness is due to brain disorders means that all other factors contributing to the illness are disregarded.

However, such criticisms of Gournay do not acknowledge that whilst he maintains the aetiology of schizophrenia occurs before birth, he also acknowledges other factors:

> 'this is not to say that social and psychological factors are unimportant. Indeed, there is also a large amount of evidence that shows that social and psychological factors are major determinants of long-term outcomes.'
>
> (Gournay, 1997)

Table 21.5: Symptoms of schizophrenia

Positive symptoms	Negative symptoms
Hallucinations	Withdrawal
Delusions	Decreased social skills
Thought disorder	Blunted mood and emotions
Paranoia	Decreased drive and energy

It is these social and psychological factors which are the focus of the psychosocial interventions discussed later in this chapter.

Symptoms are typically divided into positive and negative; the principal ones are listed in Table 21.5.

People with schizophrenia are more likely to be single, living in depressed areas and homeless. It is not clear if this is due to the fact that people with schizophrenia migrate to socially deprived areas because the effects of the condition lead to poverty and poor social functioning, or whether the condition can be triggered by low social status and poor living conditions. Some studies suggest people of Afro-Caribbean origin are between four and eight times more likely to be diagnosed with schizophrenia. Reasons for this have not been clearly established but suggestions include bias in using diagnosis due to racism or cultural ignorance; increased number of people of Afro-Caribbean origin with low socio-economic status; and the different ways mental health problems are perceived and expressed in different cultures (Gray and Smedley, 1997).

Schoen Johnson (1997) suggests that the major goals for nursing the person with schizophrenia include promoting trust, establishing a non-threatening environment, encouraging social interaction, increasing self-esteem, validating perceptions, clarifying and reinforcing reality, ensuring physical safety, promoting independence, meeting physical needs, administering antipsychotic medication and coordinating treatment and education with the client's family or significant others.

Key Points

- Whilst there are still significant gaps in our understanding of schizophrenia and, therefore, problems with the validity of the concept, most authors agree that recognising that there is an overall syndrome of signs and symptoms that can be referred to as schizophrenia is important. This allows communication between professionals, users and carers from widely varying backgrounds about the framework of symptoms we call schizophrenia, as well as allowing the implementation and evaluation of interventions which address multiple needs and not just individual, discrete symptoms (Birchwood and Shepherd, 1992).
- Mental health nurses must recognise, however, that each individual diagnosed with the condition will experience and interpret the symptoms in a unique manner. Responses must therefore be based on an empathic and trusting relationship as well as the utilisation of those interventions shown to be most effective.

CLINICAL SCENARIO – CARE OF PERSON WITH SERIOUS MENTAL ILLNESS (SMI)

The clinical scenario detailed below (Box 21.3) is suggested in order to illustrate a collaborative approach towards providing care and the development of the therapeutic nurse–client relationship. It is not a care plan as such, but a description of the various approaches and skills used by the mental health nurse in the care of a person with serious mental illness.

Box 21.3

A 33-year-old single man is discharged from hospital after a 3-month stay. He was first admitted to hosptial aged 21 when he was given a diagnosis of schizophrenia and has been in hospital at least once each year since then, often for long periods. He has not worked since his first admission, but is able to remain at home and, with the support of his parents who live nearby, lives independently. He has never had an intimate relationship and has no close friends. His only social contacts are with his professional workers, his parents and members of the local church which he attends regularly. Prior to his last discharge he was referred to a new community mental health nurse.

Table 21.6: Initial nursing goals

- To establish a trusting relationship with the client and engage him/her in his/her care
- To make an assessment of the client's needs and goals, taking into account the client's views, his/her parents and those who have cared for him/her in the past
- To monitor the client's mental health and participate in on-going risk assessment
- To provide the client's oral medication and administer his/her depot neuroleptic injection, as well as monitoring effects and side-effects
- To provide education about illness to client and family/significant others

INITIAL NURSING GOALS

When planning care for a person with a serious mental illness, such as described in the clinical scenario, the initial nursing goals are as shown in Table 21.6.

COLLABORATIVE ASSESSMENT

In order to begin to work with the client to identify needs and develop a therapeutic relationship, a collaborative assessment is undertaken. This explores problems, needs, goals and, indeed, strengths from the user's and the family's perspective as well as from the nurse's perspective. The priority is to establish a supportive and trusting rapport so that the client is able to discuss his/her illness and other problems, and to share his/her views on how best to tackle his/her problems. In addition, the mental health nurse has a crucial role in harnessing the views, experiences and suggestions from others, including the client's family, and his/her other professional workers including social worker and psychiatrist. It follows, therefore, that the mental health nurse requires an expert level of interpersonal skills.

The objective of collaborative assessment and care planning is *not* to reach a consensus on the cause of the problems – though that may well happen. The main benefits are that there is a shared understanding of the problems and goals of intervention, and an agreed strategy on meeting those goals and overcoming the problems. The 'pooling' method can be used by encouraging the client and

Table 21.7: Collaborative assessment – stage 1

Examples of what the main problem areas may be viewed as:				
Client	**Parents**	**Social worker**	**Psychiatrist**	**CPN**
■ Lonely ■ Voices ■ Beliefs about food ■ Beliefs about television	■ Depressed ■ No friend ■ Voices ■ Rituals, especially about food ■ Our burden	■ Parents' burden ■ Requirements of Mental Health Act ■ Benefits and budgets	■ Delusions ■ Hallucinations ■ Forensic risk ■ Needs medication	■ Voices ■ Strongly held beliefs and consequent rituals ■ Strained relations with parents ■ Prone to relapse

others to share their thoughts about the main problems. These are written as a brainstorm during sessions and are not prioritised at this stage. The whole process may take several sessions with the client as well as discussions with his/her parents and his/her other professional carers (Table 21.7).

By harnessing the views from the key people involved, the mental health nurse is able to broaden his/her understanding of the client's problems and needs. The next step is to discuss with the client each of the views put forward. This enables the client to conceptualise his/her problems as others see them. This approach places the mental health nurse in a prime position as the client's care coordinator, since he/she has actively involved other carers in the construction of the care plan. The aim is to reach a consensus on the most pressing problems and sharing ideas about how these problems may be managed (Table 21.8).

The mental health nurse must ensure that any jargon words are understandable to the client, since any language which is not understandable will render the process both less accessible and less useful. Furthermore, a care plan which is written in language that the client uses is more likely to be accepted as personal to him/her and reinforces the concept that he/she is an active participant in assessing, planning and evaluating his/her care.

Table 21.8: Collaborative assessment – stage 2

Agreed problem areas	Some of the things that can be done
Voices	Psychosocial interventions
Lonely, no friends	Confidence building, arrange activity, introduce new interests
Depressed	As above, psychosocial interventions
Rituals, especially about food	Psychosocial interventions
Parents' burden	Offer practical and emotional support, carers' groups
Requirement of Mental Health Act	Sharing of information of our rights and responsibilities
Benefits and budgets	Benefits advice, budget skills work
Forensic risk	Sharing of information of our rights and responsibilities
Needs medication	Share each others' knowledge on benefits and consequences
Strongly held beliefs	Psychosocial interventions
Strained relations with parents	Family work
Prone to relapse	Look for triggers for relapse, contingency planning

SHARING THE EXPERTISE OF ALL CARE PROVIDERS

The plan of action has to be elaborated to include specific interventions and strategies, and include ways in which progress may be evaluated. The mental health nurse's contribution is crucial in that, although the client is undoubtedly the expert in his/her own condition and experience, the mental health nurse is knowledgeable with regard to the provision of psychosocial nursing care. In short, *both* contribute to the care process, *both* have areas of expertise but *neither* has all the answers. Many of the mental health nurse's interventions will be new to the client and will need careful planning and implementation. For instance, the client may have limited experience in considering stimuli that may affect the nature, frequency or impact of his/her voices.

PROBLEM-SOLVING, GOAL-ORIENTED APPROACH

Just as it is important to assist the client to participate in defining the main problems it is crucial to seek the client's involvement in identifying the appropriate methods to alleviate those problems and the desired goals or outcomes. Goals that are defined by the client are likely to be unique and personal to him/her and will increase his/her commitment and motivation in working towards those goals. Often these goals are very different from those of the professional workers. He/she may wish to make friends with his/her voices or be able to tell them to be quiet, where the nurse may feel that elimination of hallucinations is an appropriate goal. On the other hand, he/she may have unrealistic goals such as to be completely free of all problems and get married by the end of the month. The mental health nurse has an important role in negotiating goals that both can see as realistic and agree upon them.

COLLABORATION, NEGOTIATING AND SERIOUS MENTAL ILLNESS

Using this approach with people affected by serious mental illness can be complex and challenging, especially when the individual feels that he or she does not have any problems at all. Often, individuals may define the problem as 'my neighbours belong to the Mafia, spy on me, talk about me and want to harm me'. Many nurses and doctors have defined this problem as 'the patient suffers from delusions' and the potential for the beneficial effects of establishing a therapeutic relationship are nullified with regard to this symptom. One approach the mental health nurse can use focuses on the *impact* of those beliefs so that both can agree on a common understanding. Consequently, an agreed problem may be defined as 'feeling very frightened and anxious whenever I think that the neighbours are around'. The mental health nurse can then explore ways to help the client feel less frightened and ways to manage anxiety.

Evaluation

It is also important to agree ways of knowing that progress is being made towards the agreed goals. This may be the feedback gained from using outcome measures, in the same way that a temperature chart gives the nurse feedback on how much progress has been made in reducing the temperature of a pyrexic patient. Verbal feedback from each other as well as from parents and other carers will also provide invaluable feedback. Discussed within the context of a trusting therapeutic relationship, the client and the mental health nurse can both feel in control of the care that is being provided.

PSYCHOSOCIAL INTERVENTIONS

Psychosocial interventions is the collective term for a range of techniques designed to tackle the symptoms of mental illness, usually psychoses, as well as the resultant problems. The theoretical basis is the cognitive behavioural theories and, in particular, the stress vulnerability model (Zubin and Spring, 1977), which assumes that stress is a determining factor in the development of symptoms and that all individuals have a certain vulnerability to the illness. Highly vulnerable individuals require less stress to push them into illness or relapse. People with a very low level of vulnerability can withstand high amounts of stress and remain well.

The potential effectiveness of these interventions was first recognised in the 1970s but they are still not used routinely in practice by mental health nurses. This may reflect a lack of awareness among mental health nurses, limited inclusion in mental health nurses' education, or the realities of service provision which frequently means that many CPNs carry high caseloads containing a mixture of people with severe mental illness plus clients referred from primary care settings with very different needs.

Psychosocial interventions are often grouped together under the following headings shown in Box 21.4 and these will be briefly described.

Box 21.4: Psychosocial interventions

- Coping enhancement strategies
- Stress reduction activity
- Prodromal monitoring
- Family interventions
- Psychosocial support

COPING ENHANCEMENT STRATEGIES (CES)

These interventions are also known as symptom management. The emphasis is on assessing and building on the individual's own (perhaps idiosyncratic) methods of managing his or her symptoms and encouraging the development of new ones. Assessment includes thorough investigation of patterns, modifiers and enhancers. Voice hearing may be more troublesome during particular times of the day or in particular contexts, e.g. when in the bath, or following an argument. Knowledge of these patterns can lead to methods of reorganising daily activities to reduce the impact.

Stimulus control is a CES which refers to identifying the stimulus that leads to the exacerbation of particular symptoms as well as strategies to control that stimulus. For example, wearing personal hi-fi headphones may reduce voice hearing or avoiding certain stimuli may reduce the impact of disturbing beliefs (delusions).

Self-awareness is an essential prerequisite in the client who may need assistance to enable this to develop. Lack of acceptance of mental health problems is often the case with clients who may have had long experiences of being infantalised by being labelled as mentally ill and incapable.

The CES approach acknowledges that it is often not possible to eliminate symptoms and the aim is therefore to recognise that many symptoms and resultant problems have been resistant to other interventions (usually medication) and that an alternative strategy is to assist the client to attempt to bring him or her under some personal control. Clearly, it is essential that the nurse and client have a trusting relationship for such interventions to be possible.

STRESS REDUCTION ACTIVITY

This involves a thorough assessment with the client of actual and potential challenging life events as well as vulnerability factors. The approach utilises a whole range of stress and anxiety management activities including relaxation tapes, activity scheduling, assertiveness and problem-solving training. Once again, the mental health nurse must recognise and accept that some methods of relaxation may be idiosyncratic and some may be of limited long-term utility.

PRODROMAL MONITORING

This aims to identify cues and triggers that occur before a person experiences a relapse, but they are often extremely difficult to define. Parents and experienced nurses who know the clients very well will often say 'I don't know why, but I *feel* that he's becoming unwell.' A sudden increase in stress or other activity is often implicated, as is poor compliance with prescribed medication. Birchwood and Shepherd (1992) review studies that show that early interventions at the first signs of relapse, which may include stress reduction strategies and a review of medication, are effective in preventing relapse.

Hirsch and Jolley (1989) found that clients complaining of 'a fear of going crazy' was the prodrome in 70% of clients who relapsed, which they postulate is an indication that the client knows that he/she is becoming unwell but can't articulate or define this. Also significant may be the onset of pre-symptomatic levels of worry, tension, fear and anxiety. The role of the nurse includes doing detective work such as trawling through past notes, speaking with others from the person's past, as well as talking with the client and his or her longstanding carers. It is important to disregard nothing. For instance, one of the authors cared for a client who had a fixed belief about the power of September and, as a result, the majority of his relapses occurred within an 8-week period around this time of year.

FAMILY INTERVENTIONS

Family interventions involve the formation of positive alliances with families, sharing of information about the illness to help them recognise and respond to problems, discussing the treatments available and, crucially, enabling the family to tell of their experiences. They may have some of the answers that have eluded the professionals. In reality, many people with serious mental illness are not in close contact with their families, particularly in inner city areas. These interventions may therefore relate to work with significant others in the client's life, if they have a caring role.

Families often need practical advice and therapeutic support to develop realistic expectations of the client's functioning and to help promote positive change. Consequently, some of the stress management and coping enhancement work has been shown to be useful with families. The Cochrane Centre has published a systematic review of the literature on family interventions in schizophrenia and concluded that:

- The risk of relapse (including those lost to follow-up) was significantly reduced at 12, 18 and 24 months
- Compliance with medication was improved
- Hospital admissions were reduced at both 12 and 18 months
- There was some evidence that people stay in employment longer (Mari and Streiner, 1996).

PSYCHOSOCIAL SUPPORT

Improvements in the social functioning of people with serious mental illness is one of the targets in the *Health of the Nation Key Area Handbook Mental Illness* (Department of Health, 1993a). It is considered that, apart from poor compliance with medication, poor social integration is the most important factor in relapse. Psychosocial support is a term for a broad range of interventions which may improve social functioning, such as helping clients build social networks and gain employment.

The role of the nurse in respect of psychosocial support includes looking holistically at all the patient's needs. It often means using social skills learning, role play and rehearsal, as well as activities that would not usually be described as 'nursing' such as accompanying a person to the shops to give feedback on how he or she interacted and used practical skills such as budgeting. This can help build confidence, reduce feelings of stigmatisation and improve social functioning.

ORGANISATION AND DELIVERY OF MENTAL HEALTH CARE

Clients with severe and enduring mental health problems may lack insight into the nature of their problems and have little motivation to engage in treatment or activities. Many of the psychosocial interventions described in the previous section, such as prodomal monitoring, must be linked to a rapid response to the client and support for carers who may experience considerable stress themselves if the client is relapsing. This is dependent on mental health services remaining in contact with clients and being accessible.

CASE MANAGEMENT

Case management (see Box 21.5) developed in the USA in the 1970s as a means of focusing on the needs of the severely mentally ill by allocating

---

Box 21.5: The six main elements of case management (Intagliata, 1982)

1 Comprehensive assessment of individual needs
2 Development of an individualised package of care
3 Ensuring service is accessible, continuous, comprehensive and flexible
4 Monitoring quality of service
5 Evaluating levels of need and providing flexible levels of support
6 Long-term commitment

a single professional who is responsible for monitoring care with a commitment to a long-term supportive relationship with the client (Burns, 1997).

Although different models have evolved, the clinical case management has shown most encouraging outcomes, including reduced admissions to hospital, compliance with treatment, improved social networks and increased patient or carer satisfaction compared with 'local standard care' (Burns, 1997). Clinical case management is characterised by small client caseloads (often around 10–12) with the key worker working with the client to address a broad range of concerns, including benefits and finance; medication; daily living skills; coping mechanisms; physical well-being; and occupation and leisure (Firn, 1997). Although this role crosses the traditional boundaries of a number of professions, including social work and occupational therapy, Firn (1997) argues that the mental health nurse is particularly suited to the role because of his/her experience of maintaining long-term therapeutic relationships despite potentially challenging behaviour, involving clients and carers in all aspects of care, responding rapidly to crises, and a practical and flexible approach to day-to-day problems.

LEGAL ISSUES RELATING TO MENTAL HEALTH NURSING

The 1983 Mental Health Act and the role of the mental health nurse has been extensively discussed elsewhere (Gostin, 1993) and will not be repeated in detail in this chapter. Instead, the focus will be on recent legislation regarding the care programme approach along with the implications for mental health nurse, and the Mental Health (Patients in the Community) Act 1995.

CARE PROGRAMME APPROACH

The care programme approach (CPA) was introduced by the Department of Health (1990) with the intention of ensuring that everyone with severe mental illness cared for by specialist mental health services has a full assessment followed by a systematic package of care. It builds on the principles in Section 117 of the Act to ensure that these apply to both formal and informal clients.

The main components of CPA are:

- A care plan which, ideally, has been put together with the input of all relevant professionals and agencies, as well as the user
- A nominated 'key worker' for each client to ensure that the care package is implemented
- Regular review dates as well as a contingency plan should the client suffer a relapse, not comply with the agreed plan of care, or lose contact with services.

The aim is to prevent people with severe mental illness from 'slipping through the net' but also to ensure that the client and all involved in his/her care fully understand the plan of care and their individual responsibilities. If sensitively implemented, therefore, the care programme approach should increase client involvement in their care.

Although the key worker may belong to any discipline, in reality the community psychiatric nurse most frequently undertakes this role and this has increased the mental health nurse role to include:

- Coordinating implementation of clients' care plans and liaising with other agencies and professionals
- Working alongside the client and his or her significant others to monitor care and observe and evaluate outcomes.

SUPERVISION REGISTERS

The establishment of supervision registers was aimed at identifying clients with severe mental illness who require a high level of supervision following discharge from hospital. This is to try and ensure that contact is maintained with mental health services and that any indicators of relapse are identified early and contingency plans put into place to try and prevent harm to the client or others.

As well as the comprehensive care package required as part of the CPA, the care plan for clients on the supervision register must also include:

- Client's full name, aliases and all addresses which client is known to use
- A risk assessment including nature of any risks and prodromal indicators
- Details of key worker and others involved in care.

MENTAL HEALTH (PATIENTS IN THE COMMUNITY) ACT 1995

The 1995 Act inserted new clauses into Section 25 of the Mental Health Act (1983) to allow for 'supervised discharge' of those clients most vulnerable to relapse in their mental illness after discharge. The intention is to provide 'aftercare under supervision' for clients who have a history of being admitted to hospital and being successfully treated for the acute phase of their illness, only to experience a psychiatric breakdown after discharge because they lost contact with services or ceased taking medication. These clients experience repeated admissions and are often called 'revolving door patients' and should have been assessed as presenting a serious risk of harm to themselves or others if they do not receive continuing care (Coffey, 1996).

The Act allows for clients to be discharged with a named community responsible medical officer (RMO) and supervisor on condition that they comply with certain aspects of treatment which may include:

- Attendance for treatment, education or training (can be 'conveyed' by their supervisor)
- Allowing the supervisor into their home for assessment and treatment.

If a person refuses any part of the treatment plan their care is reviewed and they can be returned to hospital. In practice, it is anticipated that the community psychiatric nurse will usually act as supervisor although others can be nominated, such as police officers, to act on the nurse's behalf if he/she is concerned about issues such as the safety of conveying a person back to hospital.

The Royal College of Nursing (RCN, 1996) has expressed concerns about the possible damaging effects this more coercive role may have on the nurse–client relationship as well as the vulnerability of the mental health nurse whilst carrying out some of the roles of the supervisor. The RCN emphasises the importance of a rigorous approach to risk assessment and management; accurate and comprehensive record keeping; and maximising patient engagement.

Despite concerns about putting the Act into operation, others such as the National Schizophrenia Fellowship have welcomed continued supervision and treatment in helping to relieve the enormous burden on relatives and in offering a compromise between institutional care and no care in the community (Coffey, 1996). Change may nevertheless be in the offing as the outcomes of the government's review of mental health services emerge.

Key Points

- Mental health nurses need to develop and maintain an up-to-date understanding of the legal and ethical issues relating to their practice, including the provisions of the Mental Health Act (1983).
- This section has briefly discussed the most recent legislation, which has had the effect of expanding the role and responsibilities of the mental health nurse and created new challenges and tensions with regard to the nurse's role in enforcing legislation alongside the need to maintain trusting and open therapeutic relationships with clients.

INCIDENCE AND DESCRIPTION OF MOST PREVALENT MENTAL HEALTH PROBLEMS

It is very difficult to identify accurately the levels of mental illness in the UK due to factors such as the lack of recognition of mental health problems in both primary care and general medicine, as well as under-reporting due to stigma (Freeman *et al.*, 1997). Nevertheless, the Department of Health estimates that mental illness accounts for 14% of NHS inpatient costs and 14% of certified sickness. Suicide has risen 75% amongst young men under 21 between 1982 and 1991 and accounts for 8% of lost working days (Department of Health, 1993a).

The Health of the Nation Mental Illness Key Area Handbook (Department of Health (1993a) estimated the prevalence of mental illnesses within a health authority covering a population of 500 000, which includes around 70 000 individuals over 65, would be as detailed in Table 21.9.

There is not the space in this chapter to go into detail about the nature of each of these mental health problems and the range of treatments and interventions which may be practised by the mental health nurse. Schizophrenia has already been discussed in detail and therefore the following

Table 21.9: Estimated prevalence of mental illness in population of 500 000 (70 000 over 65s)

Anxiety	8000–30 000
Depressive disorders	10 000–25 000
Dementia	3500
Schizophrenia	1000–2500

discussion focuses on the other most common mental health problems in Table 21.9 along with suggestions for further reading.

ANXIETY

This term refers to a whole range of conditions (Table 21.10) which affect cognition (thinking), physical well-being, emotions and behaviour. Theories about the causes of anxiety include the psychodynamic perspective that anxiety is an expression of nervous energy resulting from repressed fears and conflicts in the unconscious – whilst those who adopt a behavioural perspective view anxiety as an inappropriate learned response and favour interventions that focus upon learning new responses (Freeman *et al.*, 1997).

More women than men are diagnosed with anxiety and identified risk factors include divorce, bereavement, job loss, relationship problems and children leaving the family home (Beck and Emery, 1985). The mental health nurse's role includes interventions such as helping the client identify and understand the causes of his or her anxiety; utilising interventions such as cognitive behavioural therapy (CBT) which focuses on help-ing clients give up negative thoughts (cognitions) and develop positive thoughts; assisting clients to expose themselves gradually to the source of their anxiety and learn to control and overcome their fears (see Ash's [1997] clearly written accounts of behavioural interventions which can be practised by mental health nurses in the care of a person with anxiety).

DEPRESSIVE DISORDERS

Many of the symptoms of depression are common to everyday life and therefore diagnosis depends largely on the severity of the symptoms, the length of time they are experienced and the nature of any precipitating events. Symptoms include:

- Changes in mood such as feelings of sadness and tension
- Changes in thinking such as loss of self-worth and guilt
- Changes in drive such as apathy and fatigue
- Changes in physical well-being such as loss of appetite and sexual drive, and disturbed sleep pattern.

Freeman *et al.* (1997) identify the following four main categories of depression:

1 *Adjustment disorders* – these are reactions to major life events such as bereavement, divorce, being made redundant, or being diagnosed with a life-threatening condition such as HIV.
2 *Dysthymic disorders* – depression lasting more than 2 years in which symptoms such as negative outlook on life, lack of energy and social withdrawal become chronic and fixed

Table 21.10: Anxiety disorders

Mental health problems	Description
Generalised anxiety	Inability to relax, tense, frightened, shortness of breath, palpitations, sweating and trembling
Phobias	Fear of an object or situation disproportionate to the probability and degree of harm
Panic attacks	Characterised by episodes of intense fear
Obsessive compulsive disorders	Strong compulsion to act in manner which client recognises is irrational, but cannot resist
Post-traumatic stress disorder (PTSD)	Intense reaction to a distressing experience Often involves reliving the experience

3 *Major depression* – overwhelming depressed mood with significant 'clinical' symptoms such as weight loss

4 *Major depression with melancholia* – most severe form of depression in which a person may experience total loss of interest in his or her surroundings and become stuporose.

Freeman *et al*. (1997) estimate a lifetime risk of depression in Western developed countries to be 12% for men and 25% for women. Client groups at risk include women who have given birth, where up to 22% experience postnatal depression, and older people, among whom 16% have symptoms of depression. Burleigh (1997) emphasises that symptoms of depression may present differently in those who are elderly, such as conversation which is focused entirely in the past, complaints of multiple physical pains, and irritable responses to questions. Mental health nurses working with this client group need to be alert to these symptoms and not presume they are simply part of the ageing process.

A previous or family history of depression is a major predictor of risk. Victims of sexual abuse in childhood are also at increased risk of developing depression along with those who have experienced poor parenting, particularly following the loss of a parent. Thus mental health nurses have a role to play in working with other professionals, including health visitors, to identify individuals who may be at risk of mental health problems in the future and working with them and their carers to help prevent this development.

Freeman *et al*. (1997) cite cognitive behavioural therapy (CBT) as the favoured treatment for all kinds of depression, with medication being considered as an adjunct for major depression. Counselling is frequently offered to people with adjustment reactions and dysthymic depression although its efficacy is unproven. Electroconvulsive therapy (ECT) is used more commonly with elderly people although Burleigh (1997) warns that its effects need to be carefully monitored to prevent the person becoming elated (characterised by elevated mood and disinhibited behaviour).

DEMENTIA

This term covers a wide range of conditions, but is characterised by progressive cognitive deficiencies affecting intellectual functioning and memory loss caused by diseases of the brain such as Alzheimer's or vascular disease due to the ageing process. Dementia affects 6% of over 65s and up to 45% of over 85s (Detweiler, 1997).

The proportion of people over 65 years of age in the UK has been growing throughout the twentieth century and approximately one in four adults over 65 will be admitted to a psychiatric unit (Burleigh, 1997). The importance of a holistic approach to care for this client group cannot be overemphasised, and should include interventions aimed at meeting psychological needs such as low mood, disorientation, hallucinating and delusional experiences plus physical needs such as hydration, nutritional and elimination needs.

Dementia care mapping is an observational method, which provides a detailed evaluation of care given by members of staff to dementia sufferers. This process maps the behaviour and responses of the person over a period of time and highlights deficits in practice, which may then be rectified. It promotes care planning based on individual needs rather than an assumption that everyone with dementia has the same needs. The Dementia Care Group believe the way that individuals experience dementia is a result of the interaction between a person's personality, biography, physical health, neurological impairment and social psychology (Burleigh, 1997).

One specific intervention practised by mental health nurses caring for older people with dementia is validation therapy. This assumes all behaviour has meaning and, however confused and disoriented an elderly person may seem, the act of validating the feelings behind their behaviour is beneficial. For example, if an elderly person is pleading with a nurse to take her home, rather than stating that the client no longer has a home or avoiding the question, the nurse seeks to validate feelings behind this request by enquiring 'What do you miss about your home?' This approach has been criticised for colluding with false beliefs but validation therapy does not entail agreeing with the older person's beliefs, but acknowledging the reality of what the person is feeling and how this is affecting him/her.

CARING FOR SPECIFIC CLIENT GROUPS WITH MENTAL HEALTH PROBLEMS

There are many areas of client care that have undergone major changes in the past few years, either because of major expansion of services or through new and innovative approaches in nursing intervention. These include:

- Substance misuse and dual diagnosis
- Forensic mental health nursing
- Nursing children and adolescents with mental health problems
- Nursing people with eating disorders.

SUBSTANCE MISUSE

The area of substance misuse is particularly challenging for mental health nurses by virtue of the fact that a high proportion of patients admitted to acute inpatient services have coexistent mental illness and substance misuse problems. Menenzes *et al.* (1996), in a survey of people with psychosis, found that 47.4% had coexisting substance misuse or dependence. The term dual diagnosis refers to the overlap between mental illness and drug or alcohol misuse in the same client. A recent publication outlining guidelines for good practice in this field (ENB, 1996) suggests that non-specialist mental health nurses come into contact with people with substance misuse more often than do specialist nurses. It is clearly not possible, or indeed necessarily desirable, to refer all these people to specialist substance misuse teams.

Illegal drugs are increasingly available in society and more people with mental health problems are being cared for in the community. Besides these obvious reasons, it may also be that people with mental health problems in the community are using drugs as a coping mechanism or to provide themselves with a sense of group identity (Gournay *et al.*, 1996). According to Sinclair (1997), many areas of intervention can be delivered by nurses in all settings, provided that they receive appropriate training and clinical supervision. The most important intervention with people who have coexisting mental illness and substance misuse problems is skilled assessment to ensure the problem is recognised and addressed. This is a multidisciplinary process but the nurse may take a key coordinating role and be pro-active in identifying the problems affecting someone experiencing substance misuse.

Sinclair (1997) suggests that, once an understanding of a patient's drug use and related factors has been established, nurses are able to match a range of interventions to identified need. These interventions include: prevention and screening – a high profile national target; brief interventions, such as patients keeping a drink diary and using information booklets as a basis for assessment and education sessions; support during pregnancy; and teaching harm minimisation techniques such as safer injecting. Specialist substance misuse nurses, many of whom have a background in mental health, may utilise skills such as teaching the five stage model of change which includes precontemplation, contemplation, planning, creating change and new behaviour; motivational interviewing – a specific co-counselling process designed to develop motivation to bring about change; relapse prevention; cognitive behavioural interventions; and solution-focused therapy which concentrates on the search for ways of solving problems.

One model proposed for increasing the quality of the care provided to people with dual diagnosis is to facilitate closer liaison between generic mental health nurses and specialist substance misuse nurses who can advise on assessment, care planning, interventions and services available to clients after discharge when mental health problems have been stabilised.

FORENSIC MENTAL HEALTH NURSING

Forensic mental health nursing became a distinct area of practice with the building of the special hospitals in the UK in the nineteenth century. At its simplest, forensic psychiatry can be defined as that part of psychiatry which deals with patients and problems at the interface of the legal and psychiatric systems (Gunn and Taylor, 1993).

Although the core mental health nursing skills are fundamental to the role of the forensic mental health nurse, the need for risk assessment skills are crucial. Tarbuck (1994) has identified six key competencies of the forensic psychiatric nurse (Box 21.6).

The behaviour and presentation that the client manifests is the challenge that nurses of this client group address, since often the behaviour is harmful to others and is contrary to the law. The nurse, as part of the wider multi-professional team, is responsible for both the well-being of the client and for assessing the risk and potential risk that the client poses to society, either generally or specifically. This need to 'balance' often causes a conflict for the team and can only be resolved by discussion and consensus decision making, that is primarily based on effective risk assessment strategies.

Today forensic mental health nursing takes place in areas of high, medium and low security as well as community settings. These include:

- Prisons
- Special hospitals
- Medium secure units (MSUs)
- Long stay MSUs
- Low secure forensic units
- Community hostels
- Court diversion schemes.

CHILD AND ADOLESCENT MENTAL HEALTH

Specialist nursing practice in the area of child and adolescent mental health is a relatively recent development with the first inpatient unit in a psychiatric hospital opening in 1947 (Bakrania and Sampson, 1997). There are two broad groups of children with mental health concerns: those with conduct disorders (behavioural problems) and those with specific mental health problems, such as autism and developmental disorder. However, children can experience a number of mental illnesses associated with adults, including depression, obsessive–compulsive disorders, eating disorders and deliberate self-harm or suicide.

The Health Advisory Service (HAS) stated 'there is nothing more important than maintaining the mental health of children and young people. Happy, stable young people are more likely to become happy, stable parents' (HAS, 1995).

There is increasing evidence that children who experience distress, such as sexual abuse or poor parenting, are at greatly increased risk of developing mental health problems in adulthood. Thus, child and adolescent mental health nurses have a key role in helping parents to acquire the necessary skills to be 'good enough' parents, which are crucial in the development of well-adjusted young adults. In addition, mental health nurses have a key child protection role in both identifying and working with those children who are the victims of abuse.

The prevalence of mental illness among children may be as high as 25% (Bakrania and Sampson, 1997) and child and adolescent mental health nursing has a specialist post-registration preparation (ENB 603) which helps the mental health nurse to meet the challenges of caring for children and adolescents.

EATING DISORDERS

The term eating disorders covers a wide spectrum of conditions characterised by psychological and behavioural disturbances associated with weight, food and eating (Myers et al., 1993). Eating disorders usually refers to two conditions: anorexia nervosa and bulimia nervosa. Anorexia nervosa usually takes hold during adolescence. It can persist throughout life and may cause death and is therefore considered a serious health problem. It is characterised by a marked loss of weight or failure to gain weight and a fear of being a normal weight for age and height (Cremin and Halek, 1997). Weight loss causes physical, behavioural and mental state changes, many of which are as a result of starvation. In addition to food restriction, people with anorexia may abuse laxatives, induce vomiting, over-exercise or use drugs such as diuretics or amphetamines in attempting to control their weight. Approximately 10% of people with anorexia nervosa will die as a result of their condition (Cremin and Halek, 1997).

Bulimia nervosa is characterised by a loss of control over appetite and eating with a preoccupation about food, weight, bingeing and then how to get rid of the food which has been ingested.

Most treatments for people with eating disorders are carried out in community settings although specialist inpatient treatment or medical admission may be necessary when the client's mental or physical state places him or her at great risk. People with bulimia nervosa respond well to cognitive behavioural therapy, medication or counselling and psychotherapy (Fairburn and Wilson, 1995). Treatment for anorexia nervosa usually involves dietary and weight management, individual and family therapy and motivational work.

The role of the nurse in eating disorders has generally been acknowledged to be of primary importance to this client group. Establishing a therapeutic relationship is considered by Halek (1997) to be the single most important factor in the nursing care of people with eating disorders. Key elements within this relationship are reliability and consistency, clarity and structure, honesty, managing anxiety and managing boundaries. The mental health nurse caring for people with eating disorders requires a wide range of skills and confidence in managing the high levels of anxiety with which these clients may present. Therefore clinical supervision and support systems are essential to facilitate the management of anxiety related to working with this client group and to ensure that clinical interventions remain therapeutic.

ETHNIC MINORITIES AND MENTAL HEALTH

Over the last 20 years there has been an accumulation of evidence which suggests that the experience of people from ethnic minorities in using the mental health system is fraught with inequalities in a way that is not the case with their white counterparts. Research studies show that black people are several times more likely to receive different treatment, which includes drug therapy and ECT rather than counselling and psychotherapy (Cochrane, 1979; Francis, 1989; Littlewood and Lipsedge, 1989; Crowley and Simmons, 1992). The rate of suicide in Asian females aged 15–24 is more than double the national levels and at ages 23–34 it is 60% higher. The higher levels of diagnosis of schizophrenia among Afro-Caribbean males is discussed elsewhere in this chapter.

The Mental Health Nursing Review Team (Department of Health, 1994) observed that people from ethnic minorities are consistently treated differently within mental health services because of their belief systems. Mental health services have therefore been charged with being insensitive to the cultural as well as the social needs of ethnic minorities (Jennings, 1995).

The above evidence has led to a growing demand for alternative treatment which is effective as well as culturally appropriate. This should include more accessible services, providing useful, clear information in appropriate languages, active involvement in service planning groups, greater attention to individual needs, independent advocacy and greater collaboration and joint working with local ethnic minority voluntary groups.

The mental health nurse should also contribute to the development of ideal services for this client group which Moodley (1993) describes below:

'An ideal service for ethnic minorities is one which the majority will use voluntarily because it is a place they can trust to provide them with care when they need it. It will have a racial and cultural mix of staff which will enable them to feel understood (not black staff in inferior positions). If the languages they speak are not spoken by the staff interpreters will be easily available.'

The role of the mental health nurse is significant when working with people from an ethnic minority group. He/she must first recognise, understand and respect the cultural and religious beliefs and practices of clients belonging to minority ethnic groups. Core care plans on meeting religious and cultural needs should be developed which use checklists to improve the quality of services offered to minority ethnic groups (Gunaratnam, 1993; Chandra, 1996). The mental health nurse should also confront racist attitudes which may contribute to inadequate care for people from minority ethnic groups and adhere to the UKCC's Code of Professional Conduct which places a responsibility on nurses to recognise and respond to the need of care irrespective of ethnic origin or religious belief (UKCC, 1992).

CONCLUSION

During the twentieth century mental health nursing has emerged and matured as a profession and moved from the role of keeper and practical handyman to one which incorporates evidence-based interventions and is founded on a therapeutic relationship which seeks to involve users and carers in all aspects of treatment. In addition, mental health nurses have developed specialist knowledge and skills in the care of a range of client groups in a variety of residential and community settings, frequently acting as care co-ordinators for clients with severe mental health problems.

Despite these advances, it is nevertheless true that mental health nursing cannot lay claim to an exclusive knowledge base or set of skills and the needs of people with mental health problems can only be met if we are prepared to work openly and creatively to share knowledge and expertise with colleagues, including psychiatrists, psychologists, social workers and occupational therapists.

This chapter has sought to demonstrate that it is axiomatic that users and their carers must be fully incorporated into all aspects of care, a view espoused by the review of mental health nursing (Department of Health, 1994). A practical example of this approach is contained in the clinical scenario, but the challenges of fully involving users should never be underestimated.

The need to generate evidence about the effectiveness of mental health nursing interventions is crucial – be this from research, audit or patient satisfaction surveys – if we are to further define our roles, demonstrate our value and ensure we are meeting patients' needs. There is, however, a debate in the contemporary literature which appears to be nothing less than a struggle for the soul of mental health nursing (see Gournay, 1996; Dawson, 1997). In essence, this is between those who wish to see a focus on people who are seriously mentally ill and interventions based on research evidence, and others who fear 'cookbook' nursing whereby nurses simpy select their interventions *a priori* from a prescribed list depending on presenting symptoms, to the alleged detriment of the therapeutic relationship between nurse and client.

It has to be possible that mental health nurses can both maintain their therapeutic relationship with clients – based on principles such as empathy, honesty, openness and respect for the individual – with a commitment to utilising and critically evaluating only those interventions which have been shown to be effective. These two aims do not have to be mutually exclusive. Understandably, the success of this approach depends on a range of factors, including the skills and knowledge of the mental health nurse and the insight and motivation levels of the client. Nevertheless, mental health nurses have been sufficiently dedicated, innovative and flexible when faced with such challenges in the past and must once more demonstrate these attributes if the goal of user-focused and clinically effective mental health care is to be achieved.

REFERENCES

Ash, J. (1997). Behavioural psychotherapy. In *Stuart and Sundeen's Mental Health Nursing: Principles and Practice*, Thomas, B., Hardy, S. and Cutting, P. (eds). Mosby, London.

Bakrania, J. and Sampson, K. (1997). Child, adolescent and family mental health nursing. In *Stuart and Sundeen's Mental Health Nursing: Principles and Practice*, Thomas, B., Hardy, S. and Cutting, P. (eds), 337–56. Mosby, London.

Barker, P. (1995). Mental health. Psychiatry's human face. *Nursing Times*, 91(18), 58–9.

Beard, M. and Johnson, M. (1993). Nursing theorists approaches. In *Mental Health – Psychiatric Nursing: a Holistic Life-cycle Approach*, Rawlings, R.P., Williams, S.R. and Beck, C.K. (eds). Mosby, St Louis.

Beck, C.K. and Emery, G. (1985). *Anxiety Disorder and Phobias: a Cognitive Perspective*. Basic Books, New York.

Birchwood, M. and Shepherd, G. (1992). Controversies and growing points in cognitive-behavioural interventions for people with schizophrenia. *Behavioural Psychotherapy*, 20, 305–42.

Blom-Cooper, L., Grounds, A., Guinary, P. *et al.* (1996). *The Case of Jason Mitchell: Report of the Independent Panel of Inquiry*. Duckworth and Co., London.

Burleigh, S. (1997). Care of the elderly. In *Stuart and Sundeen's Mental Health Nursing*, Thomas, B., Hardy, S., and Cutting, P. (eds). Mosby, London.

Burnard, P. and Morrison, P. (1991). Nurses' interpersonal skills: a study of nurses' perceptions. *Nurse Education Today*, 11, 24–9.

Burns, T. (1997). Case management, care management and care programming (editorial). *Lancet*, 349, 393–95.

Carson, J., Fagin, L. and Ritter, S. (1995). *Stress and Coping in Mental Health Nursing*. Chapman & Hall, London.

Chandra, J. (1996). *Facing up to Difference: a Toolkit for Creating Culturally Competent Health Services for Black and Ethnic Communities*. King's Fund, London.

Cochrane, R. (1979). Psychological and behaviour disturbance in West Indians, Indians and Pakistanis: a comparison of rates among children and adults. *British Journal of Psychiatry*, 134, 201–10.

Coffey, M. (1996). Supervised discharge. *Nursing Times*, 92(26), 50–3.

Collister, B. (ed.) (1987). *Psychiatric Nursing: Person to Person*. Edward Arnold, London.

Cremin, D. and Hallek, C. (1997). Eating disorders: knowledge for practice. *Nursing Times Learning Curve*, 1(5) 5–8.

Crichton, J. (ed.) (1995). *Psychiatric Patient Violence: Risk and Response*. Duckworth, London.

Crowley, J. and Simmons, S. (1992). Mental health, race and ethnicity: a retrospective study of the care of ethnic minorities and whites in a psychiatric unit. *Journal of Advanced Nursing*, 17, 1078–87.

Dawson, P.J. (1997). A reply to Kevin Gournay's 'Schizophrenia: a review of the contemporary literature and implications for mental health nursing theory, practice and education'. *Journal of Psychiatric and Mental Health Nursing*, 4, 1–7.

Department of Health (1990). *The Care Programme Approach for People with a Mental Illness Referred to the Specialist Psychiatric Services*. Department of Health, London.

Department of Health (1992). *Report of the Committee of Inquiry into complaints about Ashworth Hospital*. HMSO, London.

Department of Health (1993a). *The Health of the Nation Key Area Handbook Mental Illness*. Department of Health, London.

Department of Health (1993b). *Ethnicity and Health: a Guide for the NHS*. Department of Health, London.

Department of Health (1994). *Working in Partnership: A Collaborative Approach to Care*. HMSO, London.

Department of Health (1996). *The Spectrum of Care. Local Services for People with Mental Health Problems*. Department of Health, London.

Detweiler, C. (1997). Cognitive disorders. In *Psychiatric-Mental Health Nursing: Adaptation and Growth*, Johnson, B.S. (ed.), 487–508. Lippincott, Philadelphia.

ENB (1996). *Substance Use and Misuse: Guidelines for Good Practice in Education and Training of Nurses, Midwives and Health Visitors*. ENB, London.

Fairburn, C.G. and Wilson, G.T. (1995). *Binge Eating: Nature, Assessment and Treatment*. Guildford Press, New York.

Firn, M. (1997). Developing nursing skills in an intensive care management service. *Journal of Psychiatric and Mental Health Nursing*, 4, 59–60.

Francis, E. (1989). Black people and psychiatry in the UK. *Psychiatric Bulletin*, 2(13), 482–5.

Freeman, R., Gillam, S., Shearin, C. and Plamping, D. (1997). *COPC Depression and Anxiety Intervention Guide*. King's Fund, London.

Gijbels, H. and Burnard, P. (1995). *Exploring the Skills of Mental Health Nurses*. Avebury, Aldershot.

Goffman, E. (1961). *Asylums, Essays on the Social Situation of Mental Patients and Other Inmates*. Anchor Books, New York.

Gostin, L. (1993). *Mental Health Services: Law and Practice*. Shaw & Sons, London.

Gournay, K. (1995). Mental health nurses working purposefully with people with serious and enduring mental illness: an international perspective. *International Journal of Nursing Studies*, 34(4), 341–51.

Gournay, K. (1996). Schizophrenia: a review of the contemporary literature and implications for mental health nursing theory, practice and education. *Journal of Psychiatric and Mental Health Nursing*, 3, 7–12.

Gournay, K. (1997). The biological content of mental health nursing. In *Mental Health Nursing: Principles and Practice*, Thomas, B., Hardy, S. and Cutting, P. (eds). Mosby, London.

Gournay, K., Sandford, T. and Ishnion, S. (1996). Double bind. *Nursing Times*, 92(28), 28–9.

Gray, R. and Smedley, N. (1997). Nursing interventions with acutely ill clients. In *Stuart and Sundeen's Mental Health Nursing*, Thomas, B., Hardy, S. and Cutting, P. (eds), 253–70. Mosby, London.

Grounds, A. (1995). Risk assessment and management in a clinical content. In *Psychiatric Patient Violence: Risk and Response*, Crichton, J. (ed). Duckworth, London.

Gunaratnam, Y. (1993). *Health and Race Checklist: a Starting Point for Managers on Improving Services for Black Populations*. King's Fund, London.

Gunn, J. and Taylor, P. (1993). *Forensic Psychiatry: Clinical, Legal and Ethical Issues*. Butterworth-Heinemann, Oxford.

Halek, C. (1997). Eating disorders: the role of the nurse. *Nursing Times*, 93(28), 63–6.

Hally, H. and Hardy, S. (1997). Competent caring: role of the mental health nurse. In *Stuart and Sundeen's Mental Health Nursing: Principles and Practice*, Thomas, B., Hardy, S. and Cutting, P. (eds). Mosby, London.

HAS (1995). *Child and Adolescent Mental Health Services: Together We Stand. The Commissioning, Role and Management of Child and Adolescent Mental Health Services*. HMSO, London.

Hedlund, N. and Jeffrey, F. (1993). Overview of psychiatric nursing. In *Mental Health – Psychiatric Nursing: a Holistic Life-cycle Approach*, Rawlins, R., Williams, S. and Beck, C. (eds). Mosby, St Louis.

Heron, J. (1990). *Helping the Client: a Creative Practical Guide*. Sage Publications, London.

Hirsch, S. and Jolley, A. (1989). The dysphoric syndrome in schizophrenia and its implications for relapse. *British Journal of Psychiatry*, (suppl 5), 46–50.

Intagliata, J. (1982). Improving the quality of community care for the chronically mentally disabled: the role of case management. *Schizophrenia Bulletin*, 8, 655–74.

Jennings, S. (1995). *Complementary Therapies in Mental Health Treatment*. King's Fund, London.

Johnson, B.S. (1997). *Psychiatric Mental Health Nursing: Adaptation and Growth*. Philadelphia, Lippincott, Philadelphia.

Johnson, S., Ramsay, R., Thornicroft, G. *et al.* (1997). *London's Mental Health: The Report for the King's Fund London Commission*. King's Fund, London.

Landrum, P.A., Beck, C.K., Rawlins, R.P. and Williams, S.R. (1993). The person as a client. In Williams, S. & Beck, C. (eds) *Mental Health – Psychiatric Nursing. A Holistic Life-cycle Approach*, 3rd edn, Rawlins, R., Williams, S. and Beck, C. (eds). Mosby, St Louis.

Leff, J. (1994). Care in the community. *Clinician*, 12(5), 2–7.

Littlewood, R. and Lipsedge, M. (1989). *Alien and Alienists: Ethnic Minorities Psychiatry*. Unwin Hayman, London.

Mari, J.S. and Streiner, D. (1996). *Family Interventions for Those with Schizophrenia*. The Cochrane Library. Issue 3.

Maslow, A. (1968). *Towards a Psychology of Being*. Van Nostrand Reinhold, New York.

Menenzes, P., Johnson, S., Thornicroft, G. *et al.* (1996). Drug and alcohol problems among individuals with severe mental illnesses in South London. *British Journal of Psychiatry*, 168, 612–19.

Moodley, P. (1993). Setting up services for ethnic minorities. In *Principles of Social Psychiatry*, Bhugra, D. and Leff, J. (eds). Blackwell, Oxford.

Myers, S., Davis, M.P. and Treasure, J. (1993). *A General Practitioner's Guide to Eating Disorders*. Institute of Psychiatry, London.

Newell, R. (1994). *Interviewing Skills for Nurses and Other Health Care Professionals: a Structured Approach*. Routledge, London.

NHS Executive (1997). *The Patient's Charter: Privacy and Dignity and the Provision of Single Sex Accommodation*. EL (97) 43. HMSO, London.

Peplau, H. (1952). *Interpersonal Relations in Nursing*. GP Putnams Sons, New York.

RCN (1996). *Mental Health Nursing Newsletter*. Spring Edition.

Russell, D. (1997). *Scenes from Bedlam: a History of Caring for the Mentally Disordered at Bethlem Royal Hospital and the Maudsley*. Baillière Tindall, London.

Sinclair, M. (1997). Drug and alcohol nursing. In *Stuart and Sundeen's Mental Health Nursing: Principles and Practice*, Thomas, B., Hardy, S. and Cutting, P. (eds). Mosby, London.

Strathdee, G., Kendrick, T., Cohen, A. and Thompson, K. (1996). *A General Practitioner's Guide to Managing Long-term Mental Health Disorders*, The Sainsbury Centre for Mental Health, London.

Tarbuck, P. (1994). *Buying Forensic Mental Health Nursing: a Guide for Purchasers*. RCN, London.

Thompson, T. and Mathias, P. (1994). The provision of care for people with enduring mental health problems. In *Lyttle's Mental Health and Disorder*. Thompson, T. and Mathias, P. (eds). Baillière Tindall, London.

UKCC (1992). *The Code of Professional Conduct*. UKCC, London.

UKCC (1996). *Issues Arising from Professional Conduct Complaints*. UKCC, London.

White, E. (1990). *The Third Quinquennial National Community Psychiatric Nursing Survey*. Department of Nursing, University of Manchester, Manchester.

Zubin, J. and Spring, B. (1977). Vulnerability: a new view of schizophrenia. *Journal of Abnormal Psychology*, 86, 260–6.

CHAPTER TWENTY-TWO

CARE *of the* PERSON *with a* LEARNING DISABILITY

David Sines

- Introduction
- The nature of learning disability
- The care context
- Health and social care
- Biological causes of learning disability
- Other causes of learning disability
- Prevention and intervention
- The social context of care provision
- Philosophy of care
- Maintaining valued and integrated lifestyles
- Views of service users
- Nursing people with a learning disability
- Intervention strategies
- Behavioural approaches to caring
- The multi-agency context of care
- Access to generic health care services
- Conclusion

The chapter aims to provide an overview of the key issues that shape and influence the lives of people with learning disabilities. In so doing it aims to review the social policy and political influences that impact on the context of care provision. The chapter also outlines the main approaches to learning disability and reviews a number of intervention strategies that may be employed to enhance the quality of life for this client group and their families. In particular, an overview of causation and presentation of learning disability is provided, the principles of learning theory are introduced and readers are challenged to consider the role of consumer advocacy, independence, the promotion of client rights and risk taking. Nursing skills for clinical practice and relevant research are also discussed within the context of normalisation theory, individual programme planning and care management strategies.

INTRODUCTION

Changes in the care of people with a learning disability have been influenced by political, social and economic factors and by new demands for responsive care and treatment by informed users of public services and their carers in the community (Sines, 1995). This chapter will provide a framework that presents a series of introductory competences for nursing people with a learning disability. It will emphasise the importance of working in partnership with service users and their carers and will describe a range of intervention strategies within the context of holistic and multi-agency care approaches.

People with a learning disability are similar to many other members of the society within which they live; they have similar **needs**, wants and ambitions; the majority are not ill and all have a basic right to participate in the everyday life of their neighbourhood (Towell and Beardshaw, 1991).

Over the years learning disability has been associated with a number of misconceptions which range from stereotypes which assume that people with learning disabilities are 'all the same', that 'they can do nothing for themselves' and that 'they are unable to learn new skills or make progress towards independence'. The titles that have been attributed to this client group (for example mentally handicapped people, subnormality and mental deficiency) reflect, in part, the different perceptions that the general population and professional carers have had towards people with learning disabilities. A challenge, therefore, exists for students of nursing to consider the actual needs of people as individuals rather than in accordance with subjective stereotypes which may have been produced as the result of negative associations or 'labelling'.

This chapter introduces a rather different approach and emphasises the more positive role that nurses may assume as they work in partnership with people with learning disabilities and their families, to promote valued lifestyles for service users in the community. The contribution made by various agencies involved in the provision of care and support for this client group will also be critically analysed.

THE NATURE OF LEARNING DISABILITY

Learning disability may present in a number of ways but is always associated with difficulties in learning new skills and competences in society. Some users of services have received responses from their families and carers that foster unnecessary dependence and which make assumptions about the limitations that may be made as new learning opportunities are presented. Some people with a learning disability, for example, have also been exposed to a sense of failure in their lives which may be the result of inappropriate learning situations and high expectations by society.

So what is learning disability? The term itself has only recently been acknowleged as an official designation in the UK. One other term, 'learning difficulty', has also been adopted for generic use by the client group themselves. However, the latter term is imprecise since we all have a learning difficulty of one sort or another, but when minor difficulties are compounded by a variety of other needs, society prefers to attribute a label that serves to offer some explanation for the way in which its members behave. The need to categorise does not always receive the support of the people it serves to include in the group and consequently when people with learning disabilities are asked the question 'how would you prefer to be addressed?' one receives the expected response of 'as Peter or Mary'.

There is no simple way of explaining or defining learning disability since it is not restricted to any one clinical entity or another. It is a euphemism for a collection of conditions, needs, symptoms and problems that are often grouped together and described as 'clinical types' or 'syndromes', e.g. Down's syndrome. Causes may be linked to genetic defects, birth injury or to the presentation of a variety of causes after birth. In many cases it is not possible to offer a firm diagnosis.

The definition of learning disability is also culturally determined. In some societies to refer to those of 'normal' intelligence may include a number of people who would be thought in 'other societies' to lack the functional and social skills required to be identified as core members of a valued social order. In other cases, the background of the professional making the diagnosis may influence the initial label that may be apportioned to the individual. Since people who may be described as having a learning disability are not the responsibility of any one professional group, there may be different interpretations depending on the perceived cause of the disability. Doctors, nurses, social workers, psychologists, occupational therapists, physiotherapists and speech and language therapists may be involved in the diagnosis and definition of each presenting problem, and the interdependence on a multidisciplinary approach to **assessment** and planning to meet the needs of people with learning disabilities is emphasised.

This approach is most important when diagnoses are first made. Take, for example, a young child who exhibits speech or language delay and who has demonstrated difficulty in walking. A diagnosis of learning disability might be premature unless a full range of developmental assessments have been carried out to determine the extent, severity and range of disabilities that are actually present. In many cases an isolated area of development such as 'language delay' may be attributed to developmental delay rather than a long-term disorder (Shanley and Starrs, 1993).

All people with learning disability have the capacity to learn and the majority appear (with regard to physical appearance) as other members of society, but the majority lack some degree of social competence. Perhaps the most important thing to acknowledge (Collins, 1994) is that people with learning disabilities have normal feelings. Our task, therefore, is to ensure that opportunities are presented that allow these feelings to be explored and developed appropriately and to enable people to acquire a range of skills to assist them to function to their maximum ability.

THE CARE CONTEXT

The concept of learning disability is now accepted as being mainly a social condition associated with social competence and social skill development. The majority of people who fall into this care group will, in fact, live in their own homes with their families and will not require residential support services. Eighty per cent of people (DoH, 1994) who have attended some form of 'special' educational provision fall into this category and of these very few will need skilled nursing support for anything other than ordinary ailments or illnesses (as for other members of the population).

During the course of their training students of learning disability nursing will have the opportunity to develop a number of specific competences which have been identified in response to the needs of people with learning disabilities. Learning disability nurse practitioners receive in excess of 80% of their training in community and domi-

ciliary family-based settings outside of hospital (Thompson and Mathias, 1997). During this time they are encouraged to foster close links with the primary health care team, with the local authority social services department and with the voluntary and independent sectors. Opportunities to share learning experiences with informal carers, social workers and with other professionals provide excellent opportunities to collaborate with others during the learning process. It is this opportunity for collaboration that provides the learning disability nurse with the basic tools to develop a clear framework within which he/she can work in partnership with the local authorities and to develop his or her own process of coordination at local level between his or her skills and those of social workers. Nurses may offer nursing skills in a variety of ways, but access is usually determined by the actual needs of the person concerned.

No single definition of learning disability covers all the people who may require access to specialist services at some time in their lives. There is, however, likely to be some degree of accord amongst lay and professional people about what constitutes either more severe or milder forms of learning disability. The number of people in the latter category usually presents problems for social scientists and statisticians, since the criteria for inclusion are less well defined. Many of their needs may be of a social nature and relate to competence in that area. Examples include persons who may have attended schools for people with mild learning disabilities, of whom the majority wll be semi-literate and able to seek employment in the ordinary labour market. Most will adjust normally to adult life and may enjoy ordinary social relationships. A minority may require ongoing support to assist in the acquisition of appropriate social skills.

Conversely, for the former group there may be an associated physical cause with attributes which provide easier diagnosis for both service assessment and for the specification of service responses. The person with severe learning disability will also require more intensive (and often lifelong) support, which should be offered by a variety of professional (and lay) supporters at different intervals in their lives. The majority will not acquire total independence or competence in a range of basic self-help skills and will require supervision in most areas of daily life. Examples include those persons with multiple disabilities and profound learning disabilities.

The actual needs of people with learning disabilities will often determine the kind of service response that they receive.

HEALTH AND SOCIAL CARE

Following the publication and introduction of the National Health Service and Community Care Act (HMSO, 1990) local authorities have assumed responsibility for the assessment and coordination of services for people with learning disabilities. For the majority, care will be provided in the community and clients will receive their services from generic health and social care practitioners in health centres and social service departments. For many, their needs will be similar to any other member of the population and the approaches required to provide individualised nursing care to meet their specific needs will require minimal (yet sensitive) adaptation.

However, for a small, yet significant, group of people (between four and six per thousand population in the UK) (DoH, 1996), additional health care needs may be present in addition to the social needs mentioned above. Such needs may be physical, behavioural, emotional or psychological, in both cause and nature, and in most cases specialist nursing care will be required as part of a multidisciplinary support service. The health context of care usually has a physical or organic origin that demands an intensive and often specialist response from professional staff (Fraser et al., 1997).

In some cases the requirement for specialist services may be transitory and there may not be a long-term requirement for support (e.g. for people with challenging behaviours who require some intensive support to determine more appropriate coping or learning behaviours, compared to a person who has a severe behavioural problem that persists over time). Most people who fall into this category have accumulated a history or biography that has been influenced by physical or psychological behaviours or needs, and in turn these have been influenced by life experiences received in the context of their family, care agency or from the society within which they live. The need for health care may be determined by a variety of factors relating to their social world and by the responses that are demanded by society which are in turn translated in the form of government policies that determine the way in whcih services are provided (DoH, 1994).

Emerson et al. (1994) have also reported that people whose behaviour challenges the skills of staff and carers often require considerable specialist intervention and support. The intensity of their behavioural presentation will determine the extent to which services are provided and will differ from person to person. Typical examples may be used to illustrate the problems presented by people who challenge the coping abilities of carers and these excessive behaviours may be summarised as:

- Kicking, biting or spitting
- Self-injurious behaviour
- Aggressive outbursts and violent displays
- Shouting and swearing.

To date the extent to which relevant services have been received has been largely determined by fitting people into services rather than by designing specific services to meet the needs of individuals. The NHS and Community Care Act (HMSO, 1990) advocates a rather different approach – the care management approach.

CARE MANAGEMENT

Care management places an emphasis on providing individualised services for people and requires that we design systems that are sensitive enough to take account of each person's needs (Piling, 1992). The government requires that each local authority should provide an effective, flexible and responsive framework within which individual care needs can be assessed, services delivered and evaluated by service users.

Care management requires that each person with significant social or health care needs has access to a named person who will be designated as their care manager. Care managers will usually be social workers, nurses or other community workers and they will be responsible for getting to know each individual consumer and their family. They will 'map' the person's day-to-day needs and requirements and formulate a clear action or care plan to take account of his or her needs, wants and ambitions.

The care managment system requires that service users and their families are actively engaged in the identification of their needs; it does not necessarily restrict individual choice to the current range of services on offer at the time the assessment is made. Care managment is essentially a way of ensuring that individuals are connected to all the services that they require, irrespective of the source. It is a model based on the principle of providing the widest range of choice possible to clients, without reliance on any one service agency.

Once the care manager has agreed a package of care to meet the needs of each individual, contracts will be assigned to one or more service providers who may be selected from statutory, voluntary or independent sector agencies. Contracts identify the exact nature and cost of services to be offered and delivered and contain clear statements of responsibility and accountability (see Table 22.1).

Each care package is also costed and paid for from a complex system of allowances which will be coordinated by the local authority social service department. Care packages are evaluated against a set of common standards and their effectiveness is judged in accordance with the extent to which they meet the actual needs of users (Sines, 1995).

In order for care management to operate successfully, it will be necessary for health and social care agencies to work closely together at both a planning level (where major service decisions and strategic plans are made) and at the point of service delivery. In support of this approach it will also be necessary to demonstrate that multi-agency systems are in place to assess client needs and to measure their effectiveness. Shared training opportunities for nurses and social workers and for joint participation in the design of both care packages and service systems will become an important feature of provision for people with learning disability in the future (Thompson and Mathias, 1997).

The principles of care management rely on the promotion of individually designed packages for people and, as such, this replaces traditional models of fitting people into existing services (such as hostels, day services and long-stay learning disability hospitals). It requires that a range of opportunities are provided to service users based on the principle of integration within normal communities and requires that people have the right to adopt and to maintain an ordinary life and have personal relationships and friendships.

Table 22.1: The multi-agency context of care provision

Social services
Hostel provision
Home help service
Day services
Home adaptations
Respite care
Social work support

Health services
Community learning disability teams
Specialist therapy services
Respite care
Specialist residential care
Assessment and intervention services
Acute care
Primary and secondary health care provision

The voluntary sector
Employment schemes
Residential provision
Parent and client support schemes
Respite care
Neighbourhood support
Community relations (e.g. Citizens Advice Bureau)
Social support (clubs and befriending schemes)

The independent sector
Residential provision
Private health care

THE NATURE OF NURSING

The nature of nursing for this client group has undergone major revision during the past 10 years, in recognition of changes in social and public attitudes about the definition of health and social care referred to previously. Learning disability nurses follow their own branch programme which aims to provide students with a competence-based model of training which includes an appraisal of specialist responses that will be required by users of services in both hospital and the community (ENB, 1989; Shanley and Starrs, 1993).

Nurses work with individual clients and in groups and adapt their interventions to suit the needs of the people concerned (the versatile nature of the nursing model adopted provides for assimilation into the care management model, outlined in the last section of the chapter). The activity of nursing needs to involve different kinds of knowledge, ranging from biological sciences to interpersonal behaviours, which acknowledge the importance of affective and psychomotor responses to need. Other aspects of the nurse's role require more personal knowledge of both the nurse and the client. Such skills involve an appreciation of feelings, and the development of self-esteem and personal growth. These attributes, from mechanistic to humanistic, may be demonstrated as intersecting continua, and are represented in Figure 22.1. The model of learning disability nursing is made up of scientific aspects of nursing; interpersonal aspects of nursing; social aspects of nursing; and political awareness. Although they may not have equal importance, the contributions of the various quadrants of the model occur in all nursing situations.

An understanding of personal and group psychology and the application of learning theory should enhance the quality of care given to people with learning disabilities. Similarly, an awareness of the importance of physical and sociological concepts can promote an holistic appraisal and intervention strategy to meet the various needs of clients wherever they live.

Nurses are becoming politically aware as they recognise that essential to their perception of nursing care is a knowledge of the social structures and policies that shape our environment. An understanding of the economic cost and social policy context that determine the way in which health care is delivered is important.

As one might imagine, there are various ways in which nursing care may be delivered to people with learning disabilities. These may be described as being instrumental, interpersonal, educational or organisational.

Instrumental nursing interventions

Instrumental nursing interventions include, for example, the use of instruments, appliances, techniques and schedules that have the potential to be administered impersonally. In this field these may include the provision and appropriate use of special seating or mobility aids, the use of non-verbal communication systems such as **Makaton** and the use of toys and equipment used to shape and encourage the learning of new skills (Cornforth *et al.*, 1976). Other instruments may be used to screen or test intellectual function, and these range from traditional measures of intelligence to

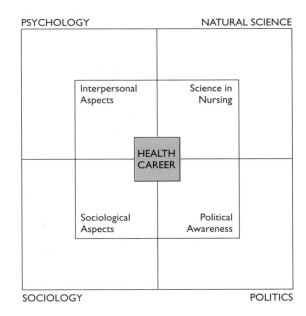

Figure 22.1: The health career matrix (simple form)

more sophisticated and applied tests of cognitive and social functioning.

Interpersonal nursing interventions

Interpersonal nursing interventions form the most important element of care provision for people with learning disabilities. These include the use of a range of therapeutic interventions which range from applied **family** or **personal psychotherapy** to the development of social skills training programmes.

Educational nursing interventions

Educational nursing interventions involve the use of educational opportunities to promote and maintain positive health, to enable people to develop appropriate behavioural responses and to facilitate new learning. Examples include one-to-one teaching in the acquisition of self-help skills or social skills training in the community (teaching somebody to use public transport).

Organisational nursing interventions

Organisational nursing interventions include referral processes which enable advice and specialist skills to be transferred to parents and to other carers. In such situations nurses may not be directly involved with clients but they may teach individuals or groups to respond appropriately to the needs of people with learning disabilities, e.g. through the provision of parent teaching sessions or group teaching for day centre staff on the management of people with epilepsy.

Nursing is quintessentially future orientated and concerned with the person in a social context. Intervention, including counselling, education or information giving, needs to take account of the physical needs and other attributes that impinge on health. Equally, psychological attributes (in terms of attitudes, beliefs, motivation, personality, cognition, perception, group processes and relationships, the dynamics of the family or network of friends) should also be taken into account.

In respect of social needs, the nurse should be aware of the norms, values and social pressures that relate to such concepts as social class and culture and their influence on the concept of health and well-being. These factors remind practitioners that the delivery of nursing care operates within a framework of politically inspired policies that need to be understood (if not challenged). These social policies construct the systems within which care is provided and determine how clients will access the particular skills of nurses; nurses should, therefore, acquire skills associated with political awareness. Accessibility of clinics, provision and allocation of resources and the ethics of any intervention, all fall within the political arena of policies that shape the human environment.

BIOLOGICAL CAUSES OF LEARNING DISABILITY

Some refer to this approach as the 'clinical syndrome' approach and most particularly it refers to a biological cause for slow learning. Developmental screening is undertaken from birth and involves health visitors, doctors and educational psychologists to identify developmental delay as an indication of potential learning disability, and to institute further investigations or interventions. This assessment approach is described by Fraser *et al.* (1997).

The presentation of a range of signs and symptoms may be grouped together to form syndromes; there are a large number of syndromes

but they actually account for very few definite diagnoses of learning disability. Whilst it is helpful to understand the cause of certain conditions, this knowledge rarely assists in the determination of relevant responses to meeting the needs of people with learning disabilities.

Down's syndrome is the most common syndrome and arises as the result of an extra chromosome (number 21 on the *karyotype*) which may be in the form of ordinary trisomy 21, *mosaicism* or translocation of a number 21 chromosome. In mosaicism the problems have arisen during the mitotic stage of embryo development and as a result some cells have an extra chromosome and some have the normal complement, the degree of disability being related to the number of abnormal cells. Down's syndrome accounts for one in 900 live births; this is a significant reduction in the incidence (from one in 600 in the 1970s). This is the result of genetic counselling, screening high risk pregnancies by amniocentesis, biopsy, testing for alphafetoprotein and selective abortion. There is an increased incidence of trisomy with maternal age: below 20 years, the chances are 1 in 2300, but at 45 years the incidence is one in 40 (Fraser *et al.*, 1997).

The physical characteristics of Down's syndrome have been well recorded and the social, physical and psychological attributes of the condition do not appear to influence the care provided to any great extent. The typical features are present at birth. The person is usually shorter in stature, has poor muscle tone that gives hyperflexibility of joints and enables contortions with the tongue. The strong facial resemblance that one person with Down's syndrome has to another enables instant recognition of the condition. The corollary is that the similarities may lead to encouraging others to disregard the uniqueness of each person as an individual in acknowledgement of their different needs and wants (Table 22.2).

Although there is not a particular heart defect with Down's syndrome, common cardiac anomalies occur with increased frequency. The discolouration (cyanosis) of the face associated with this condition is a common feature and poor peripheral circulation also occurs in many instances.

People with Down's syndrome are predominantly mouth-breathers and they appear to have a reduced capacity to combat infection as a result of poor immunological response. This sometimes results in frequent and episodic respiratory infec-

Table 22.2: Features and characteristics of Down's syndrome

- Short stature
- Poor muscle tone and hyperflexibility of joints
- Tendency to be overweight
- **Epicanthic skin folds** of the eyelids
- Rounded head and facial structure
- Low set ears
- Eye socket typically slopes forward
- Small nose with a poorly developed bridge
- High arched mouth palate
- Long and mobile (occasionally protruding) tongue
- Poor or delayed dentition
- Square-shaped hand with short digits that show deviance in shape and length
- The dermal ridges of the hands and feet have a **pathognomonic** pattern
- **Syndactyly** may occur
- Chromosomal abnormality (trisomy 21)
- Possibility of cardiovascular abnormalities and poor immunological response (leading to recurrent infections)

tions. Perhaps one particular clinical indication is worthy of note. A significant number of children with Down's syndrome have associated congenital heart disease (Walker and Kelleher, 1985). Not all of these are severely affected. The most common type of congenital heart disease is found in the atrioventricular canal, where there may be a low atrial septal defect or a common (i.e. single) atrioventricular valve. Babies born with this condition may be cyanosed when crying during the first few days of life because there is a mixing of blood between the two sides of the heart. Heart failure may result in severe cases, but many young children recover spontaneously, so that later in life the problem may be much reduced. However, there is always a risk that the child may develop secondary pulmonary vascular disease as he or she grows older. This may be evident as persistent cyanosis which may become most disabling.

The symptoms of cardiac failure in young people with Down's syndrome include poor feeding and breathlessness. The signs are tachycardia, enlarged liver, pallor, sweating and cyanosis. Treatment includes avoidance of exertion, rest and (occasionally) the administration of minor sedatives. Diuretics may also be used to reduce oedema, and medicines such as digoxin are usually successful in regulating the heart rate and, as

a result, myocardial function may improve. In some cases surgical correction may be offered.

Much research has been carried out in relation to the causes and presentational patterns of Down's syndrome but all conclusively point to the need to provide responsive and individual approaches to care provision, based on an acknowledgement of the enhanced health risk that may occur from time to time (i.e. chest infections, dyspnoea, congestive heart disease) (Shanley and Starrs, 1993). In response to these needs, nursing care should be delivered in much the same way as care would be provided for other client groups. When health risks are identified additional support will be necessary, but this rarely interferes with the pattern of daily living that is to be encouraged for all people with learning disabilities.

The provision of nursing care demands that appropriate (and sensitive) communication is developed with service users in response to their perceived level of intelligence (the level of intelligence may follow a normal distribution although all have degrees of learning disability). Nurses should also have regard to each person's potential for independence in areas where the individual can perform activities of daily living unaided (such as dressing, feeding, washing and shaving). Through the introduction of sensitive (and discrete) behavioural strategies, e.g. behaviour modification, new skills may be encouraged and others enhanced towards independence. The concept of behaviour modification will be discussed later in this chapter.

Of equal importance will be the need for socialisation and the development of relationships with others. The approach adopted by many nurses is more commonly known as 'normalisation' which aims to offer a range of ordinary life experiences and choices which prompt new and appropriate responses from clients. The maintenance of age-appropriate friendships and behaviours underpins the basic philosophy of nursing care practice (Sines, 1995).

CEREBRAL PALSY

Cerebral palsy is a term used to cover a family of conditions that have a multiplicity of causes and a variety of manifestations. The cause may be genetic, the result of birth injury, infection or other injury. Cerebral palsy is characterised by disorders of posture and movement that are highly visible and by perceptual anomalies that may be unnoticed.

A particular challenge exists for nurses in respect of the degree of learning disability that actually exists; in some cases the level of intelligence may even be above average.

The clinical signs of disorders of the motor system are *spasticity*, *ataxia*, uncoordinated movements, tremor and rigidity, dependent on the site of the brain lesion. Spasticity may affect one limb, both limbs on one side (hemiplegia) or all four limbs (paraplegia), or cause diplegia if the legs are affected to a greater extent than the arms. Other manifestations are athetosis characterised by uncoordinated rhythmic movement of the body, in particular the limbs, and ataxia in which the person has a wide-based gait, diminished muscle-joint sense and disturbances of speech and eye movements.

The classification of cerebral palsy provides some insight into the multiple ways in which this condition may be manifested. Either associated with or without learning disability (43% have an intelligence level of above 70 (Clarke and Clarke, 1985)) it will be necessary to provide responsive (and individual) services to people and their families in accordance with the motor and sensory needs that may result. One of the most commonly associated needs is to enable people to live as independently as possible and for 29% to learn to live with the secondary handicap of epilepsy (Spastics Society, 1991). Epilepsy affects one person in three but there is no consistent pattern to determine when the condition emerges. Some people develop seizures when they are infants and others not until they reach adult life.

Through the use of anticonvulsant medicines it is now possible to provide excellent control for people with epilepsy without necessarily requiring them to alter or to inhibit their lifestyle. The promotion of healthy patterns of living requires that assistance is provided to enable the person concerned to assess the degree of risk that they encounter in their environment and, like others with epilepsy, common sense is required to avoid those situations that might be hazardous during the course of a seizure.

Nursing care will also require that individuals and their carers are skilled in first aid (in particular in managing the actual process of the seizure and its after-effects) and the importance of recording seizure pattern and of taking medicines regularly must be emphasised.

The person with cerebral will require the services and support of a team of specialists. Physiotherapy facilitates coordinated movement, enhancing the capacity to explore and thus learn through the manipulation of objects, and to become independent in terms of mobility through exercises and adaptations to the environment or appliances. Speech therapy will be essential in most situations to improve communication skills and to facilitate interpersonal relationships. The combined talents of both professionals may also be witnessed in the formulation of feeding programmes that promote growth. Passive movements under the supervision of a physiotherapist and the active encouragement of movement are essential for the promotion of positive health gain.

Recently, much interest has been shown by the profession in the use of a range of alternative therapies such as **reflexology**, **aromatherapy** and **deep massage**. For those people who do not appear to respond well to external stimuli through normal channels of communication, such as verbal reinforcement, touch, smell and physical contact may be alternative routes for stimulation. Nurses are now engaged in the use of a variety of therapies for people with multiple handicaps (such as cerebral palsy) and also with people who require additional assistance to relax (for example people with hyperactive behaviours).

OTHER CAUSES OF LEARNING DISABILITY

Many theories have been generated to account for the causes of learning disability. So far this chapter has considered two specific conditions, Down's syndrome and cerebral palsy. Whilst they may be very different in respect of their cause, the care that people will require may be very similar and they serve as exemplars of care practice and provision that will be typical of many people with learning disabilities.

There are, however, other conditions that may be caused by environmental factors. These are summarised in Table 22.3.

Learning disability may be caused by a variety of factors before birth, at birth or during infancy.

Table 22.3: Environmental factors causing or contributing to learning disability

Prenatal	Natal	Postnatal

Infections
■ Rubella
■ Cytomegalovirus
■ Toxoplasmosis
 	
Trauma
■ Irradiation
■ Rhesus incompatibility
	Trauma
	■ Hypoxia
	■ Anoxia
	■ Mechanical damage
	■ Cerebral haemorrhage
	■ Hyperbilirubinaemia
	  (arising from rhesus
	  incompatibility)
	■ Hypoglycaemia
		Infections
		■ Meningitis
		■ Encephalitis
		■ Septicaemia
		■ Pneumonia
		■ Influenza
		■ Pertussis
		
		Trauma
		■ Anoxia
		  (near suffocation, near drowning,
		  post-status epilepticus)
		■ Head injury
		  (road traffic accident,
		  cerebrovascular incident)

Such factors include infections, trauma, malnutrition and understimulation.

Although not directly causal, an increased risk occurs in babies who are small-for-dates, arising from unfavourable conditions *in utero*, prematurity, multiple births and low birth weight. Some of these may be attributed to maternal malnutrition, smoking, drug abuse or excessive abuse of alcohol while pregnant. Obstetric hazard is not a major factor.

There also appears to be a relationship between learning disability and poverty (Malin, 1995). The incidence of learning disability, particularly mild disability, amongst populations with a low socio-economic status is higher than would be expected from a random distribution. Genetic causes such as Down's syndrome are non-selective in this respect; on the other hand, cerebral palsy and non-specific or undifferentiated disabilities are more prevalent. The situation may thus be the result of biological, psychological, social or political determinants (Table 22.4).

The remedy may be educational in terms of diet (for young persons with metabolic disorders such as **phenylketonuria**, a genetic condition resulting in abnormalities in the metabolism of phenylanaline), child development strategies, changes in lifestyle to promote greater use of services or the general raising of living standards. Nurses have a social and professional responsibility to develop awareness amongst members of the community to adopt positive health promotion strategies and need to be aware of factors affecting

Table 22.4: Social factors contributing to the presentation of learning disability

■ Poor nutrition
■ Understimulation (absence of play and parental interaction)
■ Social class differences in the pattern of child–parent interaction
■ Differential use of health and social resources
■ Inequalities in health provision and health promotional activities
■ Class bias of school selection
■ A combination of these factors

the health of the population as well as the specific nursing needs of individuals.

PREVENTION AND INTERVENTION

Primary conditions relate to those factors that are an intrinsic component of the condition and are potentially disabling. The restricted movement found in cerebral palsy is an example of this. In most cases the primary conditions are unlikely to respond completely to remedial intervention.

Secondary conditions relate to those factors that arise from the interaction of the primary disability with the environment. In many instances these may be of a social nature and may be experienced in the form of social stigma, such as the inability of some people with learning disability to form personal relationships with members of the general public because of their facial characteristics or behavioural responses.

Further examples of secondary handicaps would be the manner in which restricted mobility reduces the opportunity to learn from the environment, or reduced manipulative ability. Secondary conditions are, by contrast, potentially avoidable. One of the difficulties is that most of the adjustments have to be made by the person him- or herself, who may have a limited range of coping strategies from which to choose.

A consideration of handicapping conditions, such as those factors that are inhibiting or preventing normal functioning, is more important than the cause of the dysfunction itself. Children with cerebral palsy may have both restricted and/or reduced mobility. The problem, however, is the lack of mobility, not the clinical cause. The nursing intervention should concentrate on the possible: on overcoming the functional deficit of lack of mobility.

As in all forms of nursing care, prevention is an essential part of any intervention strategy. Prevention may be described as primary, secondary or tertiary (see also Chapter 4). In the learning disability field prevention refers to the use of a range of measures or processes that aim to minimise the effects that the disability may have on the person's lifestyle and level of independence.

There are, however, a number of instances when prevention may assume more traditional forms, such as in the case of primary prevention. One example relates to the provision of extensive immunisation programmes aimed at protecting mothers and their unborn children (e.g. rubella immunisation programmes) and through the development of awareness amongst pregnant mothers with regard to alcohol use and smoking. Pre-conceptual counselling, genetic counselling, good antenatal care, health education, special diets and improved social conditions are other examples.

Nurses who work with people with learning disabilities and their families will also have a major role to play in the prevention of secondary handicaps. Secondary prevention refers to the identification of conditions in susceptible people before they themselves are aware of the problem and involves making interventions aimed at preventing (or reducing) the effects of the condition on the person's health or lifestyle. Examples include the early diagnosis of phenylketonuria (through the use of universal screening programmes), special diets for people with phenylketonuria and the use of thyroid supplements for hypothyroidism, a condition that has virtually disappeared, although it was previously a cause of potential learning disability.

Learning disability nurses most often engage in tasks that aim to limit the effects of existing disabilities. Examples are the use of early intervention programmes to facilitate the development of individuals and to assist the family and other carers to provide a stimulating, growth potentiating environment. Other examples are social education programmes, skills development strategies, educational provision, interpersonal skill-awareness training, survival skills and rehabilitation. Without doubt, tertiary prevention is the major arena where nurses have a positive contribution to make to the health of individuals and their families.

THE SOCIAL CONTEXT OF CARE PROVISION

Following the publication of the National Health Service and Community Care Act in 1990, responsibility for the provision of services has been divided between the NHS (for health care needs) and social service departments (for social care needs). In the past, access to services was conditional upon the extent to which the needs of service users were met by existing resources. The key to whether services were provided by health or social agencies was usually linked to client ability (or lack of ability as the case may be). The reliance on assessment schedules to determine the level of dependence (some of which were biased and subjective in their formulation and administration) often restricted choice for people with learning disabilities (Malin, 1995).

Hogg and Raynes (1987) refer to the 'plethora of assessment instruments' (page 2) available to people working in the field and they conclude that disability is increasingly viewed as an outcome of an interaction between a person and the environment in which he or she lives. Consequently, a person who has lived a stable life in the family home may find that major changes have to take place when his/her family dies or when a new home is chosen. Perhaps the most important criterion for change will be the degree of support that the person will require in his or her new life and whilst parents and informal carers have often learnt to provide a 'tailored' service, professional agencies have tended to differentiate between high and low levels of support.

The latter has usually been seen to be the responsibility of the social services department, thus leaving the more dependent person to the health services (and consequently to care practices provided predominantly by nurses). The problem relating to placement has also been linked to unreliability in the assessment phase (Hogg and Raynes, 1987). This may be attributed to bias on the part of the professional involved in the administration of the tests or to major fluctuations that can occur in respect of the person's behaviour on the day of the assessment.

All these difficulties point to the need for a radical revision of the way in which nurses, doctors, social workers and psychologists assess people and plan to meet their needs. The care management process mentioned earlier in this chapter has been one attempt to improve the way in which we match services to people's needs. This approach requires that sensitive information is collected about individual choices and wishes and demands that an individual care package is designed in response. This is a very different approach from one which recommends a residential placement on the basis of service user's assessed intelligence level or on the extent to which they 'fit' prescribed criteria for access to health or social service facilities.

The needs of people with learning disabilities have never been a great priority within the health and social service departments in the UK (Malin, 1995). Services have often been provided in response to crisis situations or may be limited in the extent to which they meet the total needs of clients. The government has attempted to correct this imbalance and during the 1980s and 1990s priority was given to providing more money to establish a broader range of comprehensive services for this client group. The extent to which this objective has been achieved has been dependent upon the philosophy that local service providers have used in valuing and acknowledging the actual needs of people with learning disabilities and their families. For example, in 1994 a voluntary group, Values into Action, undertook a survey of health service provision and found that a significant number of people with learning disabilities were still waiting for transfer to community-based services outwith the long-stay learning disability hospitals in Great Britain (Collins, 1994).

It is the wide variation in service provision that led the government to encourage health and social service departments to move their services away from an institutional base to the community.

CARE IN THE COMMUNITY

In an excellent review of social policy development in the community, Walker (1989) argues that the Conservative governments of the 1980s commenced the introduction of a new (and deliberate) process of decentralisation for service provision for groups such as people with learning disabilities. Walker notes that care initiatives in the community have been sponsored by the government in an attempt to transfer responsibility for care from the NHS to families and to the voluntary and private sector, and in so doing, reduce the actual burden of costs for the treasury. Political influence cannot, it seems, be distanced from the quality and range of services that people with learning disabilities receive and the organisation of services will depend upon public influence and social policy.

As a result of government policy there is an increasing pattern of change in the way in which residential care is provided for people with learning disabilities. Many of the large, outdated hospitals are closing and over 80% are actively engaged in contracting their numbers as people are transferred to live in community residential facilities (Collins, 1994). These facilities may be provided by a variety of social and health care agencies and together they form what is now regarded as the 'mixed economy of care' (National Health Service and Community Care Act, 1990). The mixed economy of care refers to the broader context of care by the voluntary and private sectors who are now responsible for making a major contribution to the provision of residential care for people with a learning disability (Malin, 1995).

Service provision and its corresponding pattern of nursing care must be viewed in the context of the policies and uses of power that shape the world in which we all live. This includes the legislative framework (the NHS and Community

Care Act 1990 is an example), social policy and administration, decision making on behalf of people with learning disabilities (and the extent to which individuals are involved in discussions that determine their own futures) and power relationships in caring teams that influence care.

Policies may be simple (the way in which staff members respond to a person's physical needs) or complex (relating to the philosophy of care to be provided in a new community home). The way in which these policies are enacted may well be in the hands of the nurse in terms of how much the policy aims are respected or adhered to. Take, for example, a policy that states 'people with learning disabilities will have the same rights as other members of society'. A statement such as this requires that services are designed in such a way as to enable users to participate in ordinary life experiences and to receive opportunities to make decisions about their lives. However, participation in decisions may be limited (Sines, 1995) and there are a number of local service strategies continuing to fail to promote ordinary living experiences to the full (Malin, 1995).

Nurses should acknowledge the influence and control that they may impose when providing their clients with access to information about their rights and choices when selecting their support services. Nurses should always be alert to the potential misuse of power afforded to them by the nature of their relationship with their clients (Sines, 1994). As such it should always be remembered that people with learning disabilities are potentially vulnerable to abuse and thus health authorities and social services departments are encouraged to provide guidelines for their protection and to educate and train their staff in appropriate relationship building and client empowerment.

The UKCC have also cited concerns regarding the number of allegations (and proven cases) of abuse aginst people with learning disabilities and have agreed to issue guidelines to assist learning disability nurses to regulate their practice. All nurses are, of course, obliged to uphold the rights of their clients at all times, and to ensure that their dignity is respected (UKCC, 1992).

Learning disability does not, by itself, attract any particular social legislation but the presence and severity of the condition will determine access to support services and to social security benefits, e.g. attendance allowance, mobility allowance and community living grants. The Disabled Persons (Services, Consultation and Representation) Act (HMSO, 1986) does, however, offer some degree of support to uphold the rights of people who have special needs. Like its counterpart for school aged children, The Education Act (HMSO, 1994), local authorities are empowered to provide service users and their carers with access to information about their rights and services and also to receive regular reviews that determine their future care needs. However, whilst legislation is certainly moving in the right direction the government has failed to offer an independent advocacy service for clients who require representation when they are unable to speak for themselves.

PHILOSOPHY OF CARE

The philosophy of nursing care is based on the principle of normalisation (Wolfensberger, 1972). The characteristics of ordinary living underpin this approach, which aims to offer to people with learning disabilities a range of choices and opportunities from which they may be enabled to participate in real life experiences.

Community care is based on this principle and refers to the extent of the number of shops, public houses, leisure facilities and opportunities provided to the clients in the context of local neighbourhoods. The proximity of access to main public transport routes and the presence of community centres and local community groups also influence local perception of the community and its inhabitants.

The Oxford and Chambers dictionaries provide the following definitions of the term 'community':

'Joint ownership or liability; state of being held in common fellowship; organisational social body; body of people living in the same locality; body of people with the same needs and interests in common.'

(Oxford Concise, 1996)

'Common agreement; people having common rights; a body of people living in the same locality.'

(Chambers Concise, 1996)

In order to translate the principle of normalisation into everyday practice, local services should publish a set of general principles which underpin the philosophy and values of their community provision. A common philosophy of care is necessary; the key working principles are summarised in Table 22.5.

In order to achieve these aims nursing staff and client relationships should be developed to maximise the concept of 'life sharing' to:

- Diminish rather than accentuate distinctions between staff and residents (as fellow human beings)
- Ensure that staff and residents share space, activities, toilets, meals, recreation, holidays and interests
- Encourage nursing staff to demonstrate appropriate behaviours and attitudes that promote social acceptance and community integration.

MAINTAINING VALUED AND INTEGRATED LIFESTYLES

All nursing services should aim to develop services which are as fully integrated into local neighbourhoods as possible. Staff care practices should emphasise the importance of involving service users in the planning of their lives and should aim to promote the concept of advocacy to encourage their participation in all decision-making processes.

Essentially, most people's lives revolve around their homes, friends, work and families. The ways in which they choose to spend their time depend on their personal choices and the demands made on their 'free time' by others.

Many nursing staff are also aware of the need to ensure that clients engage in leisure pursuits that are integrated with other members of the community. This contrasts with outdated policies that encouraged people to spend a significant part of their lives in segregated activities with people with similar needs.

Wherever possible nursing staff are now discouraging such activities in favour of integrating and sharing leisure time with friends and neighbours. Use may be made of the local swimming pool and riding clubs, and visits to the local pub and restaurant to celebrate birthdays or to entertain friends are common features of the range of opportunities offered to clients. As a result, nursing staff now find that they are receiving positive feedback from neighbours and members of the community regarding the integration of people with learning disabilities in local neighbourhoods. Through the use of shops, cafés and public houses a high profile in the local community may be maintained.

Staff are also expected to ensure that people are provided with maximum control over their finances, and although many people still appear to have less money than the average unemployed person, integrated social and leisure activities are

Table 22.5: Key principles involved in the formualtion of a value statement

- People with a learning disability are entitled both to the same range and quality of services as those available to other citizens, and to services designed to meet their special needs
- Services for younger people should recognise their distinctive needs
- In order to be effective, the services must be readily available and acceptable to individuals and the families who need to use them
- Services should be able to adapt to meet the needs of each individual
- The philosophy must be to provide maximum opportunities for the residents to experience an ordinary lifestyle
- Emphasis must be on encouraging the development of new skills and staff are expected to allow or assist residents to experience life for themselves, rather than to do things for them
- Residents are encouraged to integrate within their local communities and neighbourhoods; every opportunity is taken to encourage the use of local facilities for recreation, leisure, education, shopping and employment; people will therefore be supported to contribute to the local community
- Individuals are encouraged to define their own lifestyle and individuality
- People will be encouraged to develop friendships and to form personal relationships of their choice in order to enhance the quality of their lives

Adapted from Sines, 1990; Towell and Beardshaw, 1991.

now much in evidence. One particularly important contribution made by nurses to encourage integration was that more staff were employed in small houses in the community (compared to the resident staff ratio in hospitals), which enabled many residents to experience a range of leisure or work pursuits. This in turn required a commitment from their carers to give time, energy and imagination in the design and realisation of local opportunities (Sines, 1995).

WORK PRACTICES AND OPPORTUNITIES

Nursing time and resource allocation is, in most cases, planned flexibly to facilitate the use of leisure activities which did not always fit neatly into ordinary staff shift patterns in hospital. One other important feature of the new services is the recognition that people with learning disabilities have the right to form relationships with others and to have the opportunity to feel valued and needed. Nurses are now noting the need to provide opportunities to form friendships and relationships with people of their choice from within older friendship networks and from within the wider community within which people now live.

The rapid extension of adult education programmes to people with learning disabilities has assisted in the acquisition of new social skills and leisure opportunities. Clients may attend a range of classes in photography, cookery, literacy and design. In some cases the projects have enabled people to form new and varied friendships with members of the local community and the advantages of such activities are obvious to staff. New skills are acquired, new friends made, ordinary members of the local community are demonstrating their willingness to share learning with people with disabilities. Support is provided without undue attention being drawn to the 'special learning needs of the individual'.

Taking risks has formed a central part of the debate and it should be acknowledged that an environment which allows an appropriate degree of personal choice and privacy can never be risk-free. From the author's experience it would appear that staff consider that this was one of the most difficult challenges for them to accept. Life in hospital offered protection from 'risks' and opportunities were restricted to avoid accusations being made against staff. In many services 'risk-taking' policies have been written to assist staff in calculating the risks that naturally appear to accompany life in the community. Examples of some of the principal risks are:

- Fear of pregnancy
- 'Bullying' by the 'caring' community
- 'Getting lost'
- Accidents when encouraging people to acquire new skills, e.g. crossing the road.

Work practices will also be determined by the extent to which staff offer opportunities to service users to have certain rights.

The right to choose

People must be offered the opportunity to receive individually tailored services to meet their needs based on the principle of providing real choices, e.g. where to live, work or where to go on holiday. The right to choose also implies the right to refuse to accept the offer of some or all of the facilities on offer.

The right to dignity and respect

Nurses should also aim to present a positive image for their clients by ensuring that they present themselves in an appropriate manner to the general public. Staff must make efforts to signal the respect and dignity that they give their clients to members of the general public, in order to encourage the transfer of a valued image to the community.

The right to a home of their own

Services must aspire towards the offer of a tenancy agreement to their clients. Homes should be selected in partnership between staff and residents and should be in ordinary dwellings, in ordinary streets, as close to the resident's family homes as possible. People should also have the right to have a room of their own and to have their right to privacy respected.

The right to a meaningful occupation

Evidence of a range of opportunities for daily occupation and leisure is also to be found in many services. Some people are engaged in paid employment (Malin, 1995) whilst some participate in voluntary activities – thus serving the local community – and others still attend more traditional day centres. It appears that wherever possible people are now being offered choice, from a range of available opportunities.

The right to experience personal and sexual relationships

Each service should publish a policy statement advising clients of their rights to form personal and interpersonal relationships. Some degree of privacy must be afforded to develop personal friendships and practical assistance and counselling should be available to support people to form and to maintain relationships of their choice. Safeguards will also be necessary to avoid unwanted pregnancy and health-related risks.

The right to independence

The right to self-assertion and direction is a requirement in all services. Nursing staff should encourage people to participate in all decisions affecting their lives and many provide assistance for residents to become more autonomous in their everyday lives.

The right to advocacy and representation

Services are also encouraging and providing opportunities for people to have a right to speak and to have their point of view taken seriously. It was stated that this was evident at all levels of the service from planning decisions to specific domestic decisions about daily life, work or leisure.

Many services now recognise the possibility that conflicts might occur between the expressed wishes of service users, their families and their carers. On such occasions it may be necessary to acquire the services of an independent advocate or representative to provide an objective opinion of the needs of each person.

The right to make mistakes

Rather than adopt a punitive approach when service users make mistakes or exhibit antisocial behaviour, service staff should provide support and encouragement in order to demonstrate appropriate behaviours for clients to learn new ways of dealing with situations. Staff should respond to such situations as learning opportunities for service users and should offer support to each person and encourage them to 'try again'. This approach is markedly different from the punishment models used in some hospitals where residents were rarely given the opportunity to apologise for their mistakes or encouraged to try again. Rather they were labelled as difficult and either ignored or rejected.

VIEWS OF SERVICE USERS

The following three extracts of consumer views in respect of their new service are presented to illustrate some of the points raised in the last section (these are abstracted from a research thesis; Sines, 1990). They provide a client-focused perspective of the way in which services are provided in the community and reinforce a range of issues raised throughout the chapter.

ILLUSTRATION ONE

'I now live in a house with three friends in ******. When I first moved in I enjoyed going out with my staff friends to get the carpets and the TV. My dad provided the furniture for my bedroom and we got some furniture from an old house in the next town. I was really excited when I first moved in. I enjoyed going out shopping and to the launderette and I go to Scrabble classes once a week. On Saturdays I go into town and I have a bus rover ticket for £1.75. On Tuesday nights we go to the local club where I can draw, play darts or enjoy a disco. On Fridays we have a raffle and I won this basket of fruit for the house. I went on holiday to Germany on a coach with my friends and staff, it was great fun. On Sunday I go to church in the town and on Saturdays I have lunch at the British Home Stores. I visit my friend's house sometimes and I also spend some weekends with my parents. It is much better than the hospital. Here people make me feel wanted and I can share things with them.'

ILLUSTRATION TWO

'Let me introduce the "family". There is John, Mary, Peter, Paul, Sharon and me (and the dog). We are proud because we have something to be proud of. We have had our problems, like other people do when they move into a new house. They were not terrible problems, but we got over them and now we are all going along the same path. What have we achieved?

Well! We are all a bit older and wiser, we have all got a bank account at Lloyds bank and we are learning to understand and to appreciate what it costs to buy things and that sometimes we have to wait for things. We all choose our own clothes with our staff; we have learnt to mix with ordinary people and to be part of crowds of people without fearing them. The luxury of having a bath when we want one and to linger in it if we wish.

We know that we have the right to go to our own rooms if we so wish and to be on our own when we want. We know our possessions are kept safe and respected, as are our views. We are all going to Greece for our holidays next year. We have passports and this summer we voted!

We go out a lot and we are all members of hobby clubs and we go to adult education classes in town. We had a 'Tupperware' party in the house last week. I go to sewing and embroidery and two of the men go to pottery and photography. We also have a residents' association that we go to. Life has been good to us and for us; some people, not many, seem frightened of us, but they have to learn as we had to learn. There is nothing to be frightened of! There is some rain but there is an awful lot of sunshine!'

ILLUSTRATION THREE

'It is not just the physical surroundings that are different, for example, having your own bedroom instead of a dormitory is great, but it is even better to be able to do what you want to. I have my own guinea pig in the garden, I call him "Toby". I used to be locked in a ward because I got angry sometimes. Now I only get cross if they upset me. The staff are OK here, they only make me do things I don't want to sometimes, but not often. I peel the potatoes and weed the garden, I don't like the washing up. The front room's nice, we can all use it, you know. We had one at home before I came into hospital, we were only allowed in it on Sundays. People no longer rush in or out of the house for meetings and the telephone is quieter. There are no real routines here, just some orders for the house. The neighbours are friendly, the man next door cuts the grass. I used to wet the bed, I don't now.

I like Janet, she is my girlfriend. She and I want to get married, John (a member of staff) said maybe one day!'

People with learning disabilities now receive increased opportunities to receive their care in response to the principle of 'normalisation' and efforts have been made to provide access to enable service users to enjoy ordinary lives. This aim requires some degree of commitment from staff to enter into contracts with service users to provide specific services in respect of their individual needs. A partnership in care is beginning to emerge in the services, based on a genuine concern for the welfare of individuals.

NURSING PEOPLE WITH A LEARNING DISABILITY

Nursing care for people with learning disabilities may be categorised in much the same way as general nursing: instrumental, educational, interpersonal and organisational.

Instrumental activities involve doing things for people. With people with more severe disabilities nurses may undertake the daily living activities that the person would do for him/herself if he/she were able: basic hygiene, dressing, prevention of pressure necrosis by changing position, feeding or the monitoring of medicines for people with epilepsy, for example. For some people, the presence of secondary handicaps may necessitate continued nursing care to prevent recurrent infections from causing irreparable damage, or in the case of people with multiple disability to ensure that nutritional needs are balanced and met – these needs have often been neglected as witnessed in research studies undertaken by Mamel (1989) and Patrick et al. (1986).

One of the primary goals of nursing is to assist the person to care for him- or herself or to teach the primary carer to carry out these simple nursing activities and procedures. The educational role of the nurse is essential and is of major importance in the encouragement of independence in all activities of daily living and in developing functional skills. These range from personal safety, maintenance of continence and personal hygiene to facilitating the learning of socially acceptable behaviour and reducing inappropriate behaviours, as well as learning social survival skills such as cooking, cleaning, budgeting, shopping and promoting personal growth.

Interpersonal relationships may pose particular problems for people with learning disabilities, as interpersonal skills are usually learned through modelling. The difficulties surround the inherent learning disability and the shortfall in role models arising from the segregation of schooling and recreational activities. The nurse has an important role in the development of interpersonal skills, the promotion of advocacy, self-awareness, self-assertion and the promotion of positive health.

The nurse may also have a useful role to play in the organisation and mobilisation of a range of support services for the individual and the family. The support of various community groups may also be enlisted and opportunities extended for collaboration with other nurses and members of the multidisciplinary team.

The role of the learning disability nurse is more concerned with education and social functioning than with clinical aspects of care, but the learning disability branch programme for pre-registration nurse training ensures that the learning disability nurse is proficient and competent to provide holistic care in response to a multiplicity of needs, (Shanley and Starrs, 1993).

PLANNING TO MEET INDIVIDUAL NEEDS

The problem-solving approach associated with nursing is incorporated within a framework known as **individual programme planning**. Wilcock (1987) emphasises the importance of planning for people within the context of service management structures and supports:

'The increasing emphasis on providing individualised services for people with a learning disability demands the development of service systems that will help identify the person's needs and plan to meet them . . . approaches are designed to ensure that staff make decisions that are relevant to a person's life and which emphasises the need to relate the process of individual life planning to service management.'

(Wilcock, 1987, page 57)

The individual programme planning (IPP) system has become as much a part of care for nurses working with people with a learning disability as the nursing process has for their colleagues working in other specialties. There are many parallels between the two systems. Both require:

- A systematic framework and approach
- A detailed method to assess and to identify needs
- The involvement of clients and their carers in the planning and implementation of care programmes
- A method of recording and evaluating outcomes.

Perhaps the most appropriate place to start is to consider the work of Houts and Scott (1978) who described the process of goal planning with this client group. They presented their work in a format which lent itself to adaptation by parents and carers, from which it was possible to construct teaching plans which used the principles of behaviour modification (Fraser *et al.*, 1997).

The following principles underpin the IPP system:

- People with learning disabilities should be involved in planning their own futures
- Desirable futures should be planned for people with learning disabilities
- All relevant people should be involved in the planning process
- Services should be coordinated to meet people's real needs
- Service deficiencies should be identified and used in the planning of future services.

Whilst personal planning systems were admirable in their time, and enabled people to think coherently about people's needs, they failed to provide an holistic framework in respect of the importance of considering relationships between clients, their friends and carers. Brechin and Swain (1987) provide an opportunity to address this imbalance and introduce the concept of

shared action planning which emphasises the importance of relationships 'being the heart of the matter' (Brechin and Swain, 1987, page 3).

They start their analysis of shared action planning with the following quote:

'Let us start from where you are: you are already a skilled person. The skills discussed and explored in this book are not just for "experts", though many professionals would see them as crucial to their work. These skills are part and parcel of day to day living. They are used in friendships, family living, relationships at work and in mutual helping and caring. Such skills grow and develop through and within personal relationships. Relationships are, in this sense, the heart of the matter.'

(Brechin and Swain, 1987, page 3)

They introduce a new dimension into the personal planning process which is based on the principle of the importance of the interactions that take place between the client and the carer (and his/her friends). They talk of compassionate and supportive caring relationships with reference to their place in determining the context of successful care planning and life experiences. They describe the shared action planning approach as having a focus on communication and building relationships, which are central to the process of growth and human development. It involves the sharing of key relationships and involves joint decisions and the pooling of ideas with the service user, in order to challenge the suitability of the environment by constructing an agenda of positive action. This agenda involves the formulation of shared plans of action about identified needs and includes safeguards to ensure that action plans are carried out:

'Shared Action Planning happens when there is co-ordination, organisation and people know who is responsible for doing what.'

(Brechin and Swain, 1987, page 131)

Consequently, individualised approaches to care should provide a framework for people to express their wishes and desires through a shared process with named workers, which in turn should lead to valued outcomes for the individual. Individual programme planning uses the same four stages as the nursing process (assessment, planning, action and evaluation); however it is not a purely nursing method, but incorporates inputs from every relevant discipline and carer, on the basis of equality. It pays particular attention to clarifying the client's unique needs as he/she sees them.

Shared action planning, like all other intervention techniques, will only be successful if the principles underpinning the approach are understood and practised to a standard of proficiency by the workforce. Perhaps one criticism is that it reads as a 'DIY' manual and there is an inherent danger that people will be enthused by its readable style and cartoon illustrations. As a teacher, one must ensure that such systems are introduced within the context of a structured teaching programme which must commence with a foundation course on the principles of individualised approaches to care and goal planning.

RISK-TAKING

An element of risk will always be associated with the needs assessment and care management processes (Royal Society, 1992). As individuals are encouraged to exercise their right of autonomy and quest for independence, they may naturally be exposed to a range of risks out of their immediate control. Take, for example, a person with a learning disability with epilepsy, who wishes to use public transport unaccompanied. The decision to empower the person to use public transport (a goal aimed at increasing the individual's dignity, rights and independence, rather than providing social services transport) may be associated with a risk of injury should the person fall during a seizure. Whilst it would be impossible to list every possible risk which service users might take, since risks depend upon the interaction of a number of factors (e.g. the service user's ability, past experience, support networks, previous position to specific health related conditions, age), all reasonable steps must be taken to assess risks in order to identify potential consequences of action or inaction.

The categories at risk which might be considered include:

- Embarrassment, distress, annoyance or demonstration of anger to service users or others
- Physical harm to the service user
- Physical harm being caused to other significant persons

- Damage to property
- Actions leading to law infringement.

Whenever nurses identify potential risks they should convene an interprofessional team meeting and complete a risk assessment form. The interprofessional team meeting will provide the forum whereby service users and professionals meet to consider the degree of risk that any potential intervention might present. Once the form of risk (or potential risk) has been identified, the next step is to consider how likely it is to occur and its level of impact on the individual and others. It is often difficult to judge and staff must be guided by past experience with particular clients in similar settings. The next step would be for the care plan to be implemented under carefully controlled and monitored conditions. This will, of course, be informed by the extent to which the multidisciplinary team considers the consequences of implementing this strategy outweigh the potential benefits for the user.

In such cases the following steps should be taken:

1 Staff should (within the context of a multidisciplinary team) identify the specific risks involved, taking care to complete the task analysis and highlighting and recording areas where the team believes potential risks might exist.
2 Assessment of the risk should be made, i.e. how the benefits to the service user outweigh the potential risks. It is impossible to safeguard against all possible accidents or risks, but active decisions which involve higher than normal levels of risk should be related to the importance of the objective to the person concerned.
3 The interprofessional team should decide if the risk can be eliminated or minimised by implementation of appropriate means.
4 Written records of all decisions should be maintained. These should be included in the client's personal record. Any dissensions or minority views presented by members of the multidisciplinary team should also be recorded.
5 The resources required to minimise the risk should be identified and implemented, and the implementation phase should be supported by a written action plan.
6 The action plan should be systematically monitored and reviewed and target dates set for the evaluation of the proposed programme.

APPLICATION OF NURSING MODELS

Any of the nursing models, suitably applied and adapted to meet the needs of clients, may be applied to the provision of nursing care for people with learning disabilities. Roy's adaptation model (Roy, 1976), for example, would appear appropriate, as people in this category may have problems in adapting to their physical and social world. Orem's self care model (Orem, 1980) may also be useful in some situations, as the person will have therapeutic self care deficits and may need to learn to become proficient in self care activities. Roper *et al.* (1983) also provide a useful model, as the problems experienced by people with learning disabilities may manifest themselves with problems of daily living (nursing models are also examined in Chapter 11).

Whatever model is used, the importance of application within a shared action planning framework will be of primary importance and the use of holistic models of nursing will be of great assistance to nurses involved in the assessment of need and in the design of responsive packages of care.

INTERVENTION STRATEGIES

The intervention strategy adopted will depend on the assessment of the person in their social context. Nurses must ask two questions:

- What intervention will enhance the health potential of the individual?
- What knowledge would support this intervention?

This requires an examination of those factors that impinge upon a person's needs and lifestyle from the natural sciences, social, interpersonal and political domains. This involves a retrospective examination of the person's biography and speculation about future health needs, which should aim to provide for maximum independence.

BEHAVIOURAL APPROACHES TO CARING

Behavioural approaches to caring are based upon the principle of learning theory, in particular classical and operant conditioning. In **classical conditioning** (Clarke and Clarke, 1985) behaviour is influenced by cues from the environment (as in people preparing to go home 5 minutes before the factory whistle blows). Using cues and physical prompts are an important teaching mechanism, whereby people with learning disabilities may learn new skills. Physical and verbal prompts are reduced as people become progressively competent in the required behaviour being taught at the time.

Operant conditioning (Shanley and Starrs, 1993) relies on the rewarding of appropriate behaviour when it occurs, whatever prompted the behaviour to occur, thereby reinforcing that positive behaviour and increasing the likelihood of its recurrence. In behavioural terms, if behaviour exists then something somewhere must be reinforcing it. Rewards may be physical (for example food or drink), social (in the form of praise), or intrinsic (as in the simple mastery of a task). The intention in teaching is to progress from physical to social self-fulfilment, although such a progression may be hard for any human!

BEHAVIOURAL SHAPING

Behavioural **shaping** involves progressively rewarding behaviour that approximates to the required behaviour. If the intention is that a person should learn to eat with a spoon, then a system could be devised by which a reward is given whenever the spoon is grasped, with no reward being given whenever the spoon is rejected. This may progress to rewards being given for touching the spoon for a split second, to 1 second, to 5 seconds and so on until the spoon is grasped. The rewards continue in the form of verbal praise until the spoon is eventually moved to the mouth, loaded with food, and the food is swallowed. The establishment of the behaviour depends on the reinforcer – what the student finds rewarding – and the skill of the teacher in breaking the task down into discrete and small steps that can be

taught incrementally at the level required for teaching.

The whole process of behavioural change and modification requires skill, patience and perseverance. A series of skills-based teaching packages have been introduced to assist potential teachers in this process and the **Bereweeke** skills teaching system (Mansell *et al.*, 1983) is one such example. This system provides opportunity to break tasks down into short-term goals and offers a systematic approach to writing weekly teaching targets, through the use of activity charts or plans (Figure 22.2).

The common approach to the teaching of new behaviours is to model the behaviour to be learned. This also applies to reducing those behaviours that we find to be either challenging or undesirable.

The term challenging is sometimes attributed to behaviours that we regard as being antisocial or 'disturbing' in respect of the pattern of our everyday lives. Screaming, hitting or self-mutilation are examples. Rather than aiming to encourage total conformity in our world, nurses must respond positively to people who exhibit these forms of expression, since they may be an indication that other means of communication have failed.

INTERPERSONAL ASPECTS OF NURSING	SCIENTIFIC ASPECTS OF NURSING
Challenging behaviours Solitary Limited speech Speak if prompted Attention span Frequency Boredom Absence of interpersonal skills Manipulative Will work when in a group Disrupted family life Inconsistency of management	12 years Male Epileptic – major seizures – increasing – treatment: carbamazepine 2 × 400 mg
Secondary gain Stigmatism Treated age inappropriately Patient career Life chances Council house	Epilepsy – complacency of the doctor about treatment Respite care Play area: fencing Benefits – attendance allowance Funding from Rowntree Trust Individual programme plan School
SOCIOLOGICAL ASPECTS OF NURSING	POLITICAL ASPECTS OF NURSING

Figure 22.2: David Snow: case history set out in the form of the health career matrix

The principles of operant conditioning suggest that any behaviour that is reinforced is likely to occur again given the same opportunity and circumstances. Consequently, people who learn that to behave in an unsociable manner gains them a reward are likely to repeat that behaviour again. The application of behaviour modification as a response to such problematic situations may be effective in reducing the association that occurs between the action and the subsequent attention the person experiences. Take, for example, a person who screams for attention. If a positive response is received every time then it is likely that screaming will become associated with attention. However, if attention is not given on every occasion, it is likely that the association will be weakened and the behaviour may reduce in frequency or intensity.

Since most behaviours signify some form of communication with the world, it is important that new, appropriate behaviours are taught at the same time as we aim to reduce undesirable ones. This technique is known as differential reinforcement and offers an excellent opportunity for nurses to promote appropriate learning for people with learning disabilities.

A consistent approach to care (which is so important for people with learning disabilities) is facilitated by the meticulous keeping and use of objective records.

THE MULTI-AGENCY CONTEXT OF CARE

Following the publication of the NHS and Community Care Act in 1990, health and social care agencies have been charged with the responsibility to work together to assess, plan, provide and evaluate services for people with learning disabilities.

Learning disability nurses have been preparing themselves for the emergence of a new partnership in care and many nurses work as integral members of community teams. The concept of the **community learning disability team** developed in the 1970s with the explicit aim of providing a coordinated range of support to people and their families in the community. These teams have gradually permeated every health district and board throughout the UK and may consist of community learning disability nurses (trained to a specialist level, following completion of university diploma or degree level education programmes in community learning disability nursing [UKCC, 1991] within the higher education sector), social workers, psychologists, psychiatrists and other health care staff working together to provide comprehensive packages of care for people with learning disabilities and their families.

Following the success of domiciliary support for users of services, nurses and social workers have also confirmed their intention to promote opportunities for interprofessional training and shared learning (Thompson and Mathias, 1997).

Throughout the UK, health and social service departments are actively engaged in the formulation of joint strategies to provide a 'seamless' service for people with learning disabilities and their families. The service of the future will cease to be dependent on outdated service structures, such as the adult training centre, the learning disability hospital and the social service hostel. In their place will be a comprehensive, local network of services, designed to promote ordinary living in local neighbourhoods.

Integration will demand that people with learning disabilities access further education colleges, leisure centres and live in ordinary houses. One might well wonder whether all of this will be possible, and if so, how might it happen and what role will nurses play in this new 'world'?

In 1991 the four chief nursing officers of the UK published a report (The Cullen Report) that offered a new future for learning disability nursing practice (DoH, 1991). In this report, Cullen recommended that learning disability nurses would be most useful in the context of the emerging community model of care identified in this chapter. He saw their skills as being independent of buildings or facilities and recommended that learning disability nurses should deploy their skills flexibly in the community.

The 'facility-independent' model that followed suggests that learning disability nurses will provide specialist care to people with special needs (people who have multiple handicaps, people whose behaviour requires specific attention and intervention, people with superimposed mental health needs, people with medical and sensory impairments and others who require intensive nursing care). Nurses will offer their skills on a contractual basis to their clients, either through domiciliary support teams or by working with them in their new homes in the community. New opportunities for people with learning disabilities, therefore, offer nurses a range of fresh challenges to provide appropriate nursing care in integrated settings in the community (Sines, 1995).

A new partnership with social workers will also emerge. Social workers will be particularly involved in the provision of social care for people, leaving nurses to meet the health requirements of their clients. The context within which care will be provided may be different in the future; for example, many nurses and social workers will work with people who live in accommodation managed and owned by the independent and voluntary sector and in some cases people may receive intensive care in their own homes. Care management processes (mentioned earlier in this chapter) will determine the skills that learning disability nurses will be expected to provide for their clients. Care managers (learning disability nurses may be ideal applicants for these positions) will coordinate the assessment of needs and will assist nurses and socil workers to differentiate between their unique contributions to meeting the needs of individual clients and their carers.

ACCESS TO GENERIC HEALTH CARE SERVICES

The government has recommended that, for the major part, people with learning disabilities should have access to generic health care services through primary health care teams and in general hospitals. People with learning disabilities are not immune from the trials and tribulations of day-to-day life, and as such are as likely as the next person to require access to general health services. In certain circumstances two areas might require specific attention whenever people with learning disabilities are admitted to hospital:

- The person as a patient may have anxieties
- The family at home may be concerned that the nurses will not be able to provide appropriate care.

People with learning disabilities often like consistency and order and may become anxious when confronted with changes in their routine (even those of a minor nature). The problems raised will be much more to do with the shortfall in the coping mechanisms of the nurse than in the nature of the disturbed behaviour. A noisy or distressed person may be an unfamiliar sight or experience for some nurses. At times of crisis an increase in attention is sought by all of us, and avoidance of people in distress is seldom helpful. Like any person in a situation of acute stress, the individual may exhibit behaviour usually associated with an earlier age, and this needs to be recognised with warmth and understanding. The situation should be responded to tactfully, firmly and with compassion. The client's behaviour may be unintelligible to the uninitiated but it is likely to follow a particular pattern. Violence very rarely occurs but aggressive outbursts are occasionally witnessed.

Avoidance of many of these problems can be achieved if sufficient time is allowed to take a full history from family members or carers. Normal patterns of behaviour can be predicted and if nurses are prepared in advance, precautions can be taken to ensure that the patient is settled in a manner that minimises anxiety and uncertainty. In particular, nurses should understand any form of communication system that the person uses. Communication will often be the most important aspect of care and people with learning disabilities may have developed elaborate systems of communication, in the absence of verbal reasoning or speech. In such situations, reassurance and positive body language may be most helpful and may reduce anxiety. Conversely, vacillation and ambiguity on the part of the nurse are unhelpful and the situation needs to be managed with confidence, decisiveness and sensitivity.

CONCLUSION

Care for this client group is essentially a multi-agency and interdisciplinary responsibility. The future of learning disability nursing will depend on the extent to which it responds to meet the actual needs of service users in partnership with other professionals. This chapter has outlined the role that nurses play in enabling people with learning disabilities to engage as full members of their local communities as equal citizens. Key skills such as client advocacy, user empowerment, therapeutic interventions and care management have been identified as some of the main tools employed by professional carers. In particular, nurses aim, through care management and the process of shared action planning, to respond to the needs of people with learning disabilities (and their carers) in a variety of settings. In so doing nurses are required to adapt their skills and competences to meet new demands and responses presented by their client group. Finally, the ordinary life model presented in this chapter is recommended as a framework for the provision of support to this client group and their families.

REFERENCES

Brechin, J. and Swain, A. (1987). *Changing Relationships – Shared Action Planning for People with a Mental Handicap*. Harper and Row, London.

Chambers (1996). *Concise English Dictionary*. Chambers, London.

Clarke, A.M. and Clarke, A.D. (1985). *Mental Deficiency – the Changing Outlook*. Methuen, London.

Collins, J. (1994). *Still to be Settled – Strategies for the Resettlement of People from Mental Handicap Hospitals*. Values into Action, London.

Cornforth, A.R.T., Johnston, K. and Walker, M. (1976). *The Revised Makaton Vocabulary*. Makaton Vocabulary Project, Farnborough.

DoH (1991). *Mental Handicap Nursing in the Context of the White Paper 'Caring for People in the Next Decade and Beyond'* (The Cullen Report). HMSO, London.

DoH (1994). *The Future of Learning Disability/Mental Handicap Nursing*. CNO PL (1994) 7. HMSO, London.

DoH (1996). *Statistical Bulletin*. Bulletin 2/96. HMSO, London.

Emerson, E., McGill, P. and Mansell, J. (1994). *Severe Learning Disabilities and Challenging Behaviours – Designing High Quality Services*. Chapman & Hall, London.

ENB (1989). *Project 2000: Mental Handicap Nursing Branch Programme*. ENB, London.

Fraser, W., Kerr, M. and Sines, D.T. (1997). *Hallas' Caring for People with Learning Disabilities*. Butterworth-Heinemann, Oxford.

HMSO (1986). *Disabled Persons (Services, Consultation and Representation) Act*. C.33. HMSO, London.

HMSO (1990). *National Health Service and Community Care Act*. HMSO, London.

HMSO (1994). *The Education Act*. HMSO, London.

Hogg, J. and Raynes, N. (1987). *Assessment in Mental Handicap – a Guide to Assessment Practices, Tests and Checklists*. Croom Helm, London.

Houts, P.S. and Scott, R.A. (1978). *Planning for Client Growth: a Guide to Selecting Meaningful Goals for Developmentally Disabled Persons*. University of Pennsylvania, Philadelphia.

McCarthy, M. (ed.) (1989). *The New Politics of Welfare – an Agenda for the 1990s?* Macmillan, London.

Malin, N. (ed.) (1995). *Services for People with Learning Disabilities*. Routledge, London.

Mamel, J.J. (1989). Percutaneous endoscopic gastrostomy. *American Journal of Gastroenterology*, 84(7), 369–77.

Mansell, J., Felce, D., Flight, C. and Jenkins, J. (1983). *The Bereweeke Skill Teaching System, Programme Writers Handbook*. NFER–Nelson Publishing Company, Windsor.

Oxford Concise English Dictionary (1996). Oxford University Press, Oxford.

Orem, D. (1980). *Nursing: Concepts of Practice*. McGraw Hill, New York.

Patrick, J., Boland, M., Stoski, D. and Murray, G. (1986). Rapid correction of wasting in children with cerebral palsy. *Developmental Medicine and Child Neurology*, 28, 734–9.

Piling, D. (1992). *Approaches to Case Management for People with Disabilities*. Jessica Kingsley, London.

Roper, N., Logan, W. and Tierney, A. (1983). *Using a Model of Nursing*. Churchill Livingstone, Edinburgh.

Roy, S.C. (1976). *Introduction to Nursing – an Adaptation Model*. Prentice Hall, Englewood Cliffs, New Jersey.

Royal Society (1992). *Risk: Analysis, Perception and Management*. The Royal Society, London.

Shanley, E. and Starrs, T.A. (1993). *Learning Disabilities – a Handbook of Care*, 3rd edn. Churchill-Livingstone, London.

Sines, D.T. (1987). *Towards Integration – Comprehensive Services for People with a Mental Handicap*. Harper and Row, London.

Sines, D.T. (1990). *Valuing the Carers: an Investigation of Support Systems Required by Mental Handicap Nurses in Residential Services in the Community*. PhD Thesis, University of Southampton, Southampton.

Sines, D.T. (1994). The arrogance of power: a reflection on contemporary mental health nursing practice. *Journal of Advanced Nursing*, 20, 894–903.

Sines, D.T. (1995). *Community Health Care Nursing*. Blackwell, Oxford.

Sines, D.T. and Bicknell, J. (1985). *Caring for Mentally Handicapped People in the Community*. Harper and Row, London.

Spastics Society (1991). *What is Cerebral Palsy?* The Spastics Society, London.

Thompson, A.T. and Mathias, P. (1997). *Standards in Mental Handicap Nursing – Keys to Competence*, 2nd edn. Baillière Tindall, London.

Towell, D. and Beardshaw, V. (1991). *Enabling Community Integration – the Role of Public Authorities in Promoting an Ordinary Life for People with Learning Disabilities in the 1990s*. King's Fund, London.

UKCC (1991). *Report on Proposals for the Future of Community Education and Practice*. UKCC, London.

UKCC (1992). *The Code of Professional Conduct*, 3rd edn. UKCC, London.

Walker, A. (1989). Community care. In *The New Politics of Welfare – An Agenda for the 1990s*, McCarthy, M. (ed.). Macmillan, London.

Walker, P. and Kelleher, R. (1985). Support for families with pre-school-age children. In *Caring for Mentally Handicapped People in the Community*, Sines, D.T. and Bicknell, J. (eds). Harper and Row, London.

Wilcock, P. (1987). Individual programme planning. In *Towards Integration – Comprehensive Services for People with a Mental Handicap*, Sines, D.T. (ed.). Harper and Row, London.

Wolfensberger, W. (1972). *The Principles of Normalisation in Human Services*. National Institute on Mental Retardation, Toronto.

FURTHER READING

Kinsella, P. (1993). *Supported Living for People with Learning Disabilities*. National Development Team, London.

A key text describing the importance of developing responsive residential services for people with learning disabilities.

O'Brien, J. and Lyle, C. (1987). *Framework for Accomplishment*. Responsive Systems Associates, Decatur, Georgia.

An essential reader that provides an internationally accredited framework for monitoring and evaluation of services for people with learning disabilities.

Ovreveit, J. (1993). *Coordinating Community Care – Multidisciplinary Teams and Care Management*. Open University Press, Buckingham.

A key text describing the importance of inter-professional teamwork in the community.

Papadopolous, A. (1992). *Case Management in Practice*. Winslow, Oxford.

A useful text that outlines the main issues to be addressed in the implementation of care management in the community.

Welsh Office – NHS Directorate (1992). *Protocol for Investment in Health Gain – Mental Handicap (Learning Disability)*. Welsh Office Planning Forum, Cardiff. HMSO, London.

A key publication that provides insight into the key determinants for the investment in health and social gain for people with learning disabilities.

CHAPTER TWENTY-THREE

FIRST LINE CARE

Marion Richardson

- Emergency care in the UK
- Pre-hospital care
- The organisation of the A&E department
- Aspects of 'first line' nursing
- Legal and ethical aspects of first line care
- The special needs of children in A&E
- Elderly patients in A&E
- Caring for relatives and friends
- Patients who may present problems
- Aggression and violence
- Stress
- Emergency situations
- Conclusion

The aim of this chapter is to introduce the reader to the first line care of patients when they initially present in hospital following an accident or trauma or with acute medical or psychiatric symptoms.

This chapter covers the following topics:

- Introduction to emergency care in the UK
- The organisation of the A&E department
- Working as a team
- Aspects of first line care
- The scope of practice of the A&E nurse
- The special needs of children and elderly people
- Dealing with relatives and friends
- Patients who may present problems
- Violence and aggression
- Legal and ethical aspects of first line care
- Stress
- Emergency situations
- Preparing for a major accident

The traditionally held view of first line care nursing – and certainly the one potentiated by current television series – is of constant drama – doors flung wide, trolley being rushed in by ambulance personnel, patient dashed into the resuscitation bay, on to the hospital trolley and immediately surrounded by a team of doctors and nurses busy initiating life-saving treatment – drips, drains and monitors everywhere.

Such incidents happen in Accident and

Emergency (A&E) departments throughout the world every day of the year and it is this urgent, life-saving nursing response which makes first line nursing different from nursing in other areas of the hospital and community. It is certainly the sort of situation which every nurse new to this speciality fears and yet hopes to become competent in dealing with. It is, however, by no means definitive of the work of the nursing provision in an A&E department or minor injury unit. The work is very varied – large numbers of patients and their relatives pass through the department and all types of problems are dealt with. The variety of the work is endless. It is possible to be comforting a frightened child who has a dried pea stuck up his nose one minute and caring for a patient who has suffered severe burns in an accident the next. It is impossible to know at the start of a shift what will be achieved by the end of it. Sometimes the work is exciting and provides a sense of achievement, while at other times it can be mundane or involve situations which leave the staff feeling sickened or wishing that they could have done more. Some nurses thrive in this type of atmosphere and work at their best when faced with the sort of challenge that A&E provides; others find the lack of continuity and the inability to plan their day extremely frustrating. It is natural to feel some trepidation when beginning A&E nursing but the area will have a good complement of qualified and experienced staff who will always be close by. The biggest challenge may be finding something useful to do when a very sick patient arrives as the room suddenly fills with a competent, busy team of nurses, doctors and other health professionals.

A written philosophy of care in the department will clarify for staff, patients and visitors alike the rationale of care within the area. The philosophy will reflect the beliefs of the nursing staff as to the needs and rights of their patients and of their own approach to caring for patients and their relatives or friends. It may also reflect the importance placed on the role of the nurse as a health educator and of the department as a learning environment. Such a philosophy will underpin the approach to patients and their care which is demonstrated in the department or unit.

EMERGENCY CARE IN THE UK

The nature of A&E provision in the UK has changed in recent years in response to a number of issues – financial, political, managerial and consumer demand amongst them. The term 'Casualty' has largely been abandoned in favour of the title Accident and Emergency department, which indicates the types of conditions that these departments are intended to deal with.

'TRADITIONAL' A&E DEPARTMENTS

Many district general hospitals still have a traditional A&E department offering first line care 24 hours every day to anyone who is brought in, is referred by another health care professional or who decides that A&E is the best place for their problem and walks in. They care for those who are seriously injured and the casual attender alike and are staffed by a team of doctors and nurses of all grades. These departments require the on-site support of other units and services such as paediatric services, an intensive care unit, an orthopaedic team, theatres, laboratory services and 24-hour X-ray facilities, to name but a few, if patient care is to be of the optimum standard.

MINOR INJURY UNITS

A large percentage of the patients seen in A&E departments have minor injuries and ailments and do not need the full range of A&E services and this has led (along with many other constraints) to the development in some areas of minor injury units (MIU), often staffed by nurses without medical staff or with general practitioners' services instead of the traditional hospital medical team. Some of these units have replaced A&E departments which have been closed, others have run unofficially in community hospitals for years and are now being more formally established, whilst more units are being established as satellite sites to traditional A&Es to offer the public a more comprehensive, local service. In each of these units staff have access to immediate medical advice, should they require it in an emergency, either by telephone or, more recently, through telemedical and video links with nearby

A&E departments. Most MIUs do not offer a night-time service and do not have the support services available on site which a traditional A&E department would require. The service which they offer is aimed at patients with minor injuries and ailments and allows them to be seen and treated without the long delays that they might experience in an A&E department where priority is given to those who are seriously ill and injured.

TRAUMA CENTRES

In 1988 a survey by the Royal College of Surgeons showed that 20% of deaths in trauma patients admitted to hospital were preventable. They stated that critically injured trauma victims need to be seen by the most experienced medical staff and not by the junior doctors who staff most A&E departments.

As a result, a number of centres specialising in trauma care were developed, including a centre in Stoke on Trent where the Department of Health ran a pilot trauma evaluation project.

- Trauma centres need to be easily accessible from a wide catchment area and often have the support of a helicopter to bring injured victims to the centre as rapidly as possible.
- To function optimally, trauma centres must have a senior A&E doctor in attendance 24 hours a day and be supported by neurosurgical, cardiothoracic, orthopaedic and general surgeons available immediately at all times – this is in addition to the wide range of support services required by any A&E department.

Trauma care is well established in the USA where there is much more violence as a result of the possession of firearms and the more developed gang warfare culture. In the UK there are fewer patients who require the services of a trauma centre but the value of a planned, reasoned approach to trauma care has been recognised and many A&E doctors and nurses have undertaken training in trauma life support in order to provide the best possible care at a local level where no designated trauma centre is available. The principles of advanced trauma life support (ATLS) are discussed on page 585.

THE FUTURE

A NHS Executive consultation document published in 1996 looks to the future with a more primary care led NHS. It suggests that clinical roles will be further expanded with first line care being more freely available in the community. The way people arrive at first line care may well change and people may be expected to consult a community-based telephone triage service for advice rather than simply present at their local A&E or MIU.

First line care will always be needed and the majority of this chapter aims to discuss some of the many issues surrounding the planning and delivery of such care.

PRE-HOSPITAL CARE

The ambulance service provides a remarkable link between the community and the A&E department. Ambulance crews are highly skilled and many have now undertaken intensive paramedical training and can stabilise a patient by giving drugs, interpreting cardiac rhythms, defibrillating, intubating and setting up intravenous infusions. They are expert at administering first aid in the most awkward and dangerous situations and the care which they provide for the patient before he or she arrives at the hospital may well save life and prevent further injury or deterioration.

The development of the 999 service to enable criteria-based despatching of personnel has been possible with operators trained to ask relevant questions and to give first aid advice over the telephone until an ambulance arrives. Further developments have been made in the setting up of audio and video links with hospital A&E or coronary care units, which mean that therapeutic measures can be determined by hospital consultants as a result of information relayed by the paramedic who will then administer the treatment before arrival at hospital. This additional information may also mean that the crew can be advised to bypass the nearest hospital and go instead to a specialist centre.

A system of pre-hospital trauma life support has been devised which closely follows ATLS (see above) and aims to conduct a primary survey at the scene and the treatment of life-threatening problems connected with airway and breathing before rapid transfer to the most appropriate hospital. Kilner (1996) points out that the pre-hospital environment is not the place for attempting definitive treatment for trauma victims.

THE MOBILE TEAM

If a serious or major incident occurs, a team of doctors and nurses may be called out to assist. This is common practice where a trauma unit has the services of a helicopter as this can fly a team to the scene of the incident and return with the trauma victims in the minimum time. Experienced A&E doctors and nurses can offer more than paramedics in these incidents but are generally unused to working in the pre-hospital environment with a large team from many services and are often unfamiliar with the equipment provided. As a result, many find the experience both exhilarating and traumatic at the same time. Post-traumatic stress in carers is now well recognised and will be discussed later in the chapter.

The overall aim of the pre-hospital period is to provide seamless care between the site of the incident and the hospital by stabilising patients' conditions at the scene and transferring them as quickly as possible to hospital for definitive care.

THE ORGANISATION OF THE A&E DEPARTMENT

LAYOUT

Every A&E department is different in terms of layout, but all have some features in common, whether they are modern, purpose-built departments or old units which have been altered and adapted over the years.

An emergency treatment area or 'resus' (resuscitation) room will be identified. This area is used for caring for those who are acutely ill and injured requiring, or likely to require, resuscitation and will contain equipment necessary to monitor the condition of seriously ill patients and to save and sustain life if necessary. The area may be a room or rooms with several trolleys or simply a designated bay within the unit. In areas where more than one room is available, it is customary to specify the patient groups that will be cared for in each room; for example, those with acute medical problems in one, trauma victims in another, or adults in one area, children in the other. The A&E nurse must familiarise him/herself with the location and working methods of the equipment within these areas to ensure that he/she is ready to care for the patients who are nursed there.

Most A&E patients are seen and treated, not in the emergency room, but in the cubicles or bays within the department which enable them to sit or lie down. The bays may be divided by curtains or may be rooms with doors to afford greater privacy.

Bays may be designated for the care of specific patient groups such as children or elderly people, those with eye problems or gynaecological complaints. This means that specific equipment can be appropriately stored and readily available.

One or more theatres may be available and may be used for the administration of treatment under local, regional or general anaesthesia. Wherever possible, one theatre will be kept for 'clean' procedures such as suturing and another for 'dirty' ones, for example draining abscesses or applying plaster casts.

Many departments have an observation or short-stay ward attached to them where patients who require observation for up to 48 hours may be made comfortable and cared for without being admitted to other ward areas unless this becomes necessary. Examples of patients who might be admitted to a short-stay ward are those who have suffered head injuries causing a period of unconsciousness and who require observation for 24 hours to ensure there is no concussion. Patients who have taken a drug overdose may be admitted to the short-stay ward following treatment so that they can be monitored and any adverse drug effects noted and promptly treated. Others might include those who have been given a general anaesthetic, perhaps to reduce a fracture, and who are unfit to go home. This type of unit is advantageous in that it allows patients to be cared for by the same group of nurses throughout their stay and it does not 'block' the longer-stay beds on the other hospital wards.

The waiting room is the area of A&E where many patients and their relatives spend most of their stay within the department. It is an excellent place for passing on information to the patients about the management of care within the department, about the likely waiting times and on health education and promotion. Some waiting areas house a television or video in addition to a selection of reading material. It is important that the patients waiting to be seen can, in turn, be observed by the nursing staff and constantly reassessed so that any deterioration in their condition is noted and acted upon – a role often fulfilled by the triage nurse.

WORKING AS A TEAM

Teamwork is vital if the care of acutely ill patients is to be carried out expertly and efficiently. The A&E team consists not only of doctors and nurses but also of many other personnel from both within and outside the hospital (Figure 23.1). Liaison and effective communication within this team is essential to ensure optimum patient care. The traditional medical and nursing roles are often blurred in the first line care setting as the most appropriate professional (doctor or nurse) assumes responsibility for a particular aspect of patient care.

Hospital staff

A&E nurses are trained to cope with emergency situations and will be able to assess priorities of need, plan and give care to meet those needs almost without thinking – there is no time for writing detailed care plans in an emergency! Each team member must trust and recognise the skills of all the other members of the team but each must be clearly aware of his or her own role in an emergency situation. Many advanced care courses are now run jointly for doctors and nurses so that the importance of a focused team approach is apparent.

A doctor will usually direct the team caring for a particular patient. This may be the A&E consultant or one of his/her team or another senior doctor if he/she has been asked to attend. An anaesthetist may also be present if needed. Normally the most senior doctor will make decisions about treatment in consultation with his or her medical and nursing colleagues. There may be times, however, when a nurse assumes the role of team leader because of his/her specific practice experience, for example ATLS training – see page 585.

Other hospital personnel who are likely to be involved in a patient's care are listed in Table 23.1.

Ambulance personnel

In most areas the local crews are well known to the departmental staff and may be involved in the emergency care of the patient within the

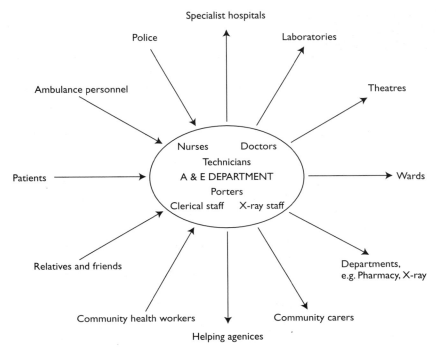

Figure 23.1: The first line care team

Table 23.1: The caring team

- Reception clerks who ensure that the patient's details are documented and any previous hospital notes and X-rays located
- X-ray staff. Many large A&E departments have X-ray facilities with radiographers available at all times; others will have trained staff available 'on call'
- Theatre staff – who must be prepared to receive emergency cases within minutes
- Staff in the intensive care unit (ICU) who must be prepared to do likewise
- Technicians and laboratory staff who may be required to perform electrocardiograms (ECGs), analyse specimens of body fluids and crossmatch blood
- Security officers and porters
- Chaplains and priests who may be asked to perform the last rites for a dying patients or talk to distressed relatives

department. Their information and history sheets provide important information about the patient's condition since the time of the incident and they often provide vital details about how an incident occurred. They provide an essential link in the patient care chain and every effort should be made to maintain their friendly cooperation.

The police force

The police also liaise closely with emergency department staff and will usually attend the hospital following any road traffic accident. They will provide assistance in identifying individuals, will check details such as whether a given address is correct and will convey information to the next of kin if requested to do so. They will provide an escort if a rapid ambulance transfer of a patient to another specialist hospital is needed and will remove patients from the department at the request of staff or give assistance in difficult or violent situations. Again, maintenance of collaborative relations with members of the police force will enhance the effective, all-round care of the patient.

The primary health care team

General practitioners, district nurses, practice nurses, health visitors, social workers and other community workers have important links with the A&E department. Many patients are referred by them and will return to their care once they leave the hospital. Communication with them is essential if continuity of patient care is to be achieved.

ASPECTS OF 'FIRST LINE' NURSING

THE SCOPE OF NURSING CARE

Nurses working in A&E departments and MIUs must be prepared to see patients of any age, at any point on the health-illness continuum and with ailments and injuries ranging from trivial to severe. In most instances there will be no prior knowledge of the patient and a rapport must be quickly established so that a trusting relationship can be fostered.

Learning to nurse patients in some specific emergency situations is important but will not form the bulk of the A&E nurse's work. He or she must learn how to do things quickly but without taking dangerous short-cuts. It is important to be able to deal sensitively and competently with a wide range of people, some of whom will speak no English and many of whom may come from a totally different ethnic and cultural background. Not all the patients will be polite, clean and friendly and the importance of interpersonal skills and means of communication other than the spoken word will soon become apparent.

There are new skills to learn, new techniques to master and the pressure of the work may reveal facets of the nurse's character and coping mechanisms of which he or she was previously unaware.

Accident and Emergency departments exist primarily to provide care for people who are acutely ill or injured. This category includes those with acute medical conditions such as **myocardial infarction**, cardiac arrest, **cerebrovascular accident**, hypoglycaemia, asthma and **pneumothorax**. It also includes those who have suffered traumatic injury, for example burns, fractured bones, head injuries, stab wounds or severe lacerations. There may also be patients who are acutely mentally ill and who may be deluded or hallucinating. Whilst the nurse may have had experience of nursing patients with these conditions, he or she may never before have seen a patient in the acute stage of the illness – actually experiencing the pain of a myocardial infarction or in the acute phase of an asthmatic attack. Many nurses assist at their first cardiac arrest during their allocation to A&E and most find it rewarding to help establish a diagnosis and initiate effective care when a patient is brought in unconscious.

Hospitals in inner cities have seen an increase in the number of patients with stabbing and shotgun injuries in recent years but tend to receive fewer patients with major traumatic injury because of the relatively slow traffic speeds in such locations, but any department situated near a major road will frequently receive the victims of road traffic accidents. All these patients can sustain severe and multiple injuries which sicken even the most experienced staff members.

The mentally ill patient may pose particular problems, especially if none of the staff members on duty is qualified in this branch of nursing. One such patient can quickly disrupt the entire department if not managed appropriately. (The nursing care of patients with acute psychiatric disorders will not be covered in this chapter – the reader is referred to Chapter 21 for further information.)

With all acutely ill patients, assessing priorities of care is vitally important. The nurse will need to work quickly and accurately and must monitor the patient's condition constantly so that any deterioration is noted early, reported and dealt with at once.

Patients who are acutely ill are not, however, the largest group of patients seen in most A&E departments. Most patients will have sustained minor injuries such as sprains, small burns or lacerations which will not necessitate their admission to hospital. Some may require treatment under local anaesthetic, for example to suture a wound or drain an abscess, others will be X-rayed or have their injuries cleaned and dressed or be given an anti-tetanus injection. Some A&E departments will have follow-up clinics where patients are seen again to check healing, re-dress wounds, remove sutures or re-apply bandages or plaster casts. Caring for these patients forms the bulk of the A&E nurse's work in most departments. For some nurses, these relatively simple treatments are a disappointment and can appear less than rewarding. It is important to remember that what appears to the professional carer to be just another cut finger needing a suture is a painful, perhaps frightening, injury to the patient and one which

may affect his or her life substantially for the next few days or weeks.

Many people, particularly in large towns and cities which attract visitors and people seeking work, are not registered with a general practitioner and use the A&E department as a substitute. These are one section of a much larger group of patients who might be termed 'inappropriate attenders'. These include patients who use the A&E department because it is convenient to their home or work or because they think they will be seen by a doctor without the need to make an appointment or at whatever time of day or night they choose to present themselves. Many of these patients would be more appropriately dealt with elsewhere. Seeing and treating them in such a specialist department may mean that waiting times for treatment may be delayed for others with more acute problems. Many A&E departments now have a policy to which they adhere strictly with regard to which patient groups will be seen and treated. Those whom they consider to be attending inappropriately are urged to visit a general practitioner or are directed to other applicable agencies such as the Samaritans or a pregnancy advisory service (a list of such agencies is provided at the end of the chapter).

RECEPTION OF PATIENTS

The Accident and Emergency department has been described as the 'shop window of the hospital'. For some patients it will be the only time they have been in a hospital and for others first impressions of the hospital are gained in the department. This means that the maintenance of high standards of care is particularly important since the rest of the hospital's nursing staff may be judged by the standards of those in this small area.

- The nurse working in the A&E department must learn to hide any feelings of fear, horror or uncertainty from patients. If these are allowed to surface it may be impossible to win the patient's confidence and trust. It behoves him or her to remember always that the patient's feelings are usually far stronger than his/her own.
- The reception of patients must be carefully managed. An impression of quiet, friendly efficiency must be conveyed in the first few

seconds of the encounter with each new, strange patient. The patient who feels at once in safe, caring hands is far more likely to co-operate with and respond to any treatment.

- The priorities of care in A&E are to save life, relieve pain and detect deterioration in the patient's condition as soon as possible so that remedial action may be taken.
- Patients should be kept fully informed of what is happening as this helps to relieve their anxiety. Terms that can be readily understood should be employed and information may need to be repeated more than once if the patient is anxious or in pain.

NURSE TRIAGE AND INITIAL ASSESSMENT

Nuttall (1986) demonstrated that waiting times in A&E are universally lengthy and this may prove dangerous for those who are severely ill. It also means that a poor service is provided for those with more minor injuries (Blythin, 1988) whom Cliff and Wood (1986) found represented 76% of patients attending A&E.

The system of triage was developed by the armed forces as a means of categorising those who were wounded in battle into priority order for treatment. It was not until 1960 that the system was adopted in a wider context in the USA and it was not formally introduced into the UK until the 1980s. The introduction of *The Patient's Charter* (DoH, 1992b) made nurse triage mandatory practice by stating that patients would be seen by a nurse immediately upon arrival (later defined as within 5 minutes).

- The aim of nurse triage is the immediate or early assessment of all patients to determine the urgency of the situation so that appropriate care can be instigated.
- Triage also helps avoid unnecessary and harmful delays and reduce waiting times for high priority patients. Crouch (1994) points out that triage is an integral part of providing a quality service and of establishing communication between patient and nurse.
- Pain assessment should form an integral part of nurse triage. The subject of pain is dealt with in Chapter 15 to which the reader is now referred. Early assessment and treatment of pain are a vital part of optimum first line nursing care and

the A&E nurse should utilise all appropriate relief methods, both pharmacological and non-pharmacological, to alleviate patients' pain.

All patients presenting in the department will be seen as soon as possible by the triage nurse who will have received guidance and training in this aspect of A&E management. The nurse's role is to elicit the relevant history, give any first aid treatment required and give the patient a priority rating before asking him/her to wait to be seen. Differing numbers of categories are used in different departments (usually between three and five) though recently a national triage scale (see Table 23.2) has been developed by the Manchester Triage Group (1997). Patients given a 'blue' priority rating may be advised to seek help elsewhere if the wait is long.

Mallett and Woolwich (1990) demonstrated that whilst overall waiting times within the department were not reduced, those patients who were given high priority ratings were seen and treated more quickly. In addition, the triage nurse is able to communicate with patients and their relatives within the department and constantly reassess the needs of patients within the waiting area, changing their priority rating if necessary. All information gleaned and advice given by the triage nurse is documented in the patient's notes.

TELEPHONE ADVICE

Many telephone calls are received each day from members of the public seeking medical advice, information or reassurance.

In some areas this service has been formalised into a telephone triage system with an advertised direct telephone line. In the USA, telephone triage has been practised for many years and Glasper (1993) and Janowski (1995) describe the use of well-researched guidelines when giving clinical advice over the telephone. A British study (Dale *et al.*, 1995) recommended the use of written, researched protocols and the allocation of an identified nurse to this service.

THE EMERGENCY NURSE PRACTITIONER

Some patients with minor ailments and injuries may be given the option of being seen and treated

Table 23.2: National triage scale

Priority number, colour and target time	Priority name	Example presentations
1 RED 0 minutes	IMMEDIATE	Cardiac/respiratory arrest Major multiple trauma Stab or gunshot wound to trunk with shock Acute airway obstruction Major burns
2 ORANGE Within 10 minutes	VERY URGENT	Cardiac chest pain Continuing fits Hypoglycaemia GCS <9 Unconscious poisoning Any very severe pain
3 YELLOW Within 60 minutes	URGENT	Eye trauma Limb ischaemia Acute phychiatric disturbance Poisoning, suspected toxicity Acute abdomen – less severe pain
4 GREEN Within 120 minutes	STANDARD	Recent injury – no threat to life or limb Minor acute condition
5 BLUE Within 240 minutes or redirect	NON-URGENT	Long-term symptoms (with no exacerbation) Non-acute rashes Prescription Certification (sick notes)

GCS, Glasgow coma scale (see Chapter 25).

by a nurse rather than a doctor. The role of the emergency nurse practitioner (ENP) has attracted much recent debate and was endorsed by the 1992 and 1996 Audit Commission reports as an alternative approach to delivering health care (National Audit Office, 1992, 1996).

An ENP is defined by Walsh (1995, page 5) as 'a nurse who is practising in an autonomous but accountable way, providing care to patients independent of direct medical supervision'. The role grew partly in response to a reduction in junior doctors' working hours which generally resulted in increased waiting times in A&E departments and partly as a result of the UKCC (1992a) *Scope of Professional Practice* document which set out the principles on which role expansion should be based. ENPs assess, treat, diagnose and prescribe care for a variety of minor ailments and injuries (see Table 23.3) within agreed protocols, though there are no nationally agreed parameters.

They can request, and usually interpret, X-rays and other diagnostic tests and can prescribe a limited range of drugs, again within agreed protocols. At present there is some debate as to the legality of this activity but the impending review of the 1968 Medicines Act will ultimately clarify the position.

ENPs may practise alongside doctors in traditional A&E departments or in MIUs (see page 566).

To be competent to undertake this role ENPs need not only considerable relevant clinical experience but also additional training in those aspects of the role which are not generally considered part of first line nursing care. There has been some debate about the confusion of accountability in these roles (Dowling *et al.*, 1996) and it would appear that in a legal case such nurses would be required to exercise a medical standard of care (Tingle, 1993).

Table 23.3: ENP framework for practice guidelines

- Assessment and treatment of minor musculoskeletal injuries
- Assessment and treatment of minor wounds and burns
- Removal of foreign bodies
- Assessment and treatment of minor ophthalmic conditions
- The use of diagnostic aids such as X-rays or blood tests
- The redirection of certain patients to more appropriate forms of care
- Health education and accident prevention

Source: RCN, 1992.

LEGAL AND ETHICAL ASPECTS OF FIRST LINE CARE

A number of legal issues affect the first line care nurse in the course of his or her work and these are discussed below.

INFORMED CONSENT

A person is regarded in law as able to give consent if he or she is able to understand what is being said and to make a decision based on that information. There is no predetermined age limit but, in practice, 16 years is generally regarded as the minimum age for consent to hospital treatment, though a House of Lords ruling in 1985 established the principle of **'Gillick competence'**, intimating that a child could give consent to treatment if he or she fully understood the nature and purpose of the proposed treatment and the likely consequences.

Failure to gain the consent of a mentally competent adult before touching him/her or even intending or threatening to touch may lead to legal action on charges of trespass, assault or battery (Dimond, 1995a). Consent may be implied, verbal or written, though the first two may be difficult to prove at a later date.

Most employers require written consent from the patient to any invasive procedures. The procedure(s) involved should be explained to the patient by a doctor, whose responsibility it is to ensure that written, informed consent is obtained.

In the case of those under the age of 16, consent is generally obtained from an adult with 'parental responsibility' for the child (see Chapter 20) who should be contacted and asked to come to the department as soon as possible. In an emergency a doctor may decide to treat a minor having received verbal consent over the telephone from a responsible adult, or may accept the child's own consent. The medical team may legally assume consent out of necessity for any treatment necessary to save life or limb or to alleviate great pain. They may also act despite refusal of consent from a patient's relative in these circumstances (Young, 1991). They have a duty of care to act out of necessity in the best interest of the patient if he or she is mentally incompetent either permanently or temporarily, for example because of pain, shock or the influence of drugs.

REFUSAL OF TREATMENT

Any mentally competent adult and any Gillick competent child has the right to refuse treatment even if their refusal will cause their death. The UKCC (1992b) Code of Professional Conduct reminds nurses that it is their duty to respect patients' autonomy at all times but refusal of treatment can lead to some difficult choices for the A&E nurse. Dimond (1994) suggests that the following principles might help:

'1. Every effort should be made to persuade a patient of the necessity to receive life-saving treatment.
2. If, despite these efforts, the patient refuses, it is the duty of the doctors and nurses to assess the competence of the patient to refuse life-saving treatment.
3. The more significant the decision being made, the greater the capacity required to refuse treatment which is life-saving.
4. If time permits, an application can be made to the court to decide if treatment can be given.
5. If the situation is an emergency, treatment could be given under the principles of ... the common law powers of the professional to act out of necessity in the best interests of the patient.

If there is doubt and no time to obtain a court ruling, err on the side of saving life.'

(Dimond, 1994, page 52)

Suicide is no longer a crime in the UK but it is a crime to assist with the suicide or attempted suicide of another and the nurse must be sure not to become involved (Dimond, 1994).

If the patient wishes to leave the department and is mentally competent, there are no powers to detain him or her but it is always wise for staff to obtain from him/her a signature that responsibility is taken by the patient for discharge against medical advice.

CONFIDENTIALITY

It is the nurse's duty to maintain his/her patient's confidentiality in respect of any information obtained in the course of his/her professional practice (UKCC, 1992b, 1996) and this must always be borne in mind. This duty is not, however, absolute and the nurse may, or may be required to, disclose information in the following circumstances:

- With the patient's consent
- In the best interests of the patient (for example, where child or elder abuse is suspected)
- In the public interest (if the patient poses a threat of serious harm or death to others)
- Where there is a statutory duty to disclose,
  e.g. Road Traffic Act
  Prevention of Terrorism Act
  Misuse of Drugs Act
  Public Health Acts
- Where there is a Court Order requiring disclosure.

The House of Lords ruling in the Gillick case (see above) made it clear that the duty of confidentiality owed to a 'competent' person under the age of 16 is just as great as that owed to any other person. If a competent young person does not wish parents informed of the visit to A&E, that confidence should be respected.

A nurse who breaches a patient's confidentiality with no good reason could face disciplinary proceedings and possibly legal action (Korgaonkar and Tribe, 1994).

NURSING NOTES

The medical and nursing notes of a patient may be used as legal evidence if necessary, as may any other documentation which can shed light on what happened, should a case come to court. This should be borne in mind when making any entries in these documents – information should be accurate and precise and each entry dated, timed and signed in accordance with UKCC guidelines on record-keeping (UKCC, 1993). Abbreviations should be avoided. Any extra sheets of documentation, such as fluid balance sheets, head injury charts and drug charts, must be clearly marked with the patient's name and kept together with his or her notes. It is all too easy to lose loose pieces of paper when a patient is being transferred around the hospital.

PATIENTS' PROPERTY

In the rush and excitement of emergency care, it is vital not to neglect or mislay any patient's property. Often the patient does not realise something is missing until ready for discharge some weeks later and difficulties can arise unless accurate records are kept. It is always wise to keep together all the property of a patient and to list it in detail as soon as possible. This is particularly important if there are valuables such as money or jewellery. Note, too, if a patient is *not* wearing a watch or carrying any money so that there is a written record should any confusion arise. If the patient is unfit to make a decision, any valuables should be stored in a safe place in accordance with hospital procedure. Otherwise the patient should be advised that the hospital authorities disclaim responsibility for personal property and that it should be deposited in the hospital safe. The patient should always be given a receipt for anything that is taken from him/her. Property should not be handed to relatives other than at the patient's specific request and written documentation of this should be kept. When a patient leaves the department, all personal property should go with him or her, preferably in one large bag clearly labelled with name and destination. Receipts for any items taken into safe custody should be firmly attached to the notes or given to the patient if he or she is in a fit state.

INFORMING THE POLICE

Often police officers will arrive with the casualties of a road traffic accident and will be aware of the circumstances and of the injuries sustained. There is a statutory duty to report to the police the names of persons involved in a road traffic accident in which injuries were sustained. The police do not normally have the right to medical information contained in a patient's notes without permission. They have no right to interview a patient unless they wish to arrest him/her and may only do so when the patient is medically fit to be seen. Most patients will, however, agree to be interviewed by a police officer and relevant information will normally be made available to them.

Nurses should not try to detain patients for police interview once they are ready to be discharged from the department, though anyone can make a citizen's arrest and hold a person until the police arrive, so long as he/she believes an arrestable offence is being committed or about to be committed.

In general, friendly relationships with the police force are easily maintained and police officers will often assist with the removal of troublesome individuals from the department.

THE CORONER

A coroner is a doctor or lawyer with a special role in investigating suspicious deaths. Deaths which must be reported to the coroner include those where the death was violent or unnatural and those where death was sudden or the cause unknown (see Dimond, 1995b). Individual coroners may have additional requirements such as wishing to be informed of any death which occurs within 24 or 48 hours of emergency admission.

If a death is reported to the coroner, all possible clues should be left in place – clothes should not be removed, drips and drains should be left *in situ*. The body is under the coroner's jurisdiction until a decision to release it is made and the coroner's consent is needed before relatives may view it. Furthermore, the relatives have no right to refuse a coroner's post-mortem examination, even on religious grounds. This can be very distressing for relatives at a difficult time and a special role is played by the coroner's officer who may be a police officer or a layperson who supports and informs the relatives – he or she will often visit the A&E department to talk to the relatives immediately after the death.

The coroner may issue a death certificate, hold a post-mortem examination and then issue a certificate, may hold an inquest or, in the case of a suspicious death, may hold an inquest with a jury. Any nurse involved in the care of the deceased may be called on to give evidence to the coroner's court.

LIVING WILLS

A living will or 'advance directive' is a document in which a person outlines the sort of health care and/or life-saving interventions they would wish to receive should they be unable to take responsibility for directing that care. In the USA most states have now recognised the legally binding nature of these documents, but the situation is less clear in the UK. It is accepted that patients have the right to refuse treatment so long as they are competent, even if this refusal will cause their death. It follows that patients who have expressed their wishes in a living will should be afforded the same degree of autonomy, so long as the caring professionals are reasonably sure that the patient was competent at the time of writing the directive, was not coerced and has not changed his/her mind. If there is any doubt, Dimond (1995b) suggests erring on the side of acting through necessity and saving life. A living will cannot be a direct request for assistance to commit suicide.

DONOR CARDS

It is not uncommon to find a donor card among the possessions of a seriously ill patient in the A&E department. Such a card expresses the wish of the patient to donate organs for transplant if possible in the event of death. At present British law states that these organs may be harvested only with the permission of the next of kin, despite the clear wishes of the patient. In some European countries, including France, Austria and Belgium, the patient is assumed to have agreed to donation unless expressly opting out of the system and there is current debate in the UK surrounding the legally binding nature of wishes expressed in donor cards.

Many patients brought into A&E departments close to death are not suitable donors but if the nurse is aware of the patient's wish to donate organs then this possibility should be explored. It is difficult to approach relatives with a request for organs at what is already an immensely difficult and painful time, but it could be argued that the nurse should act as the patient's advocate and take all reasonable steps to ensure that his or her wishes are respected. The hospital's appointed transplant coordinator may be contacted and will often attend the department to discuss the situation with the relatives.

THE SPECIAL NEEDS OF CHILDREN IN A&E

Approximately 3 million children attend first line care departments every year in the UK (Action for Sick Children, 1991). Most of them have little or no experience of hospitals and particularly of the emergency care areas. Caring for children in A&E can present problems for all concerned unless forethought is given to their special needs.

There is usually very little time to prepare ill or injured children for the fact that they are going to A&E and inappropriate handling of such a child can heighten his fear. Laing (1988) argues that all children should be given a higher priority rating at the point of triage so that their waiting time is minimised. Others have found this to be unacceptable or unnecessary within their departments.

Many departments have part of the waiting area specially adapted to provide facilities for children in an attempt to reduce the child's stress and provide a means of distraction. This may involve decorating the walls with colourful posters or providing suitable toys for the children to play with or a selection of videos which they may watch. Such an area should be within clear view of the staff since the condition of small children is prone to rapid change. It is now common practice to have a treatment area which is suitable for children within the department. Again this could be appropriately decorated so as not to look too clinical and unfamiliar. Harris and Cummings (1992) suggest that wearing tabards over uniforms and removing white coats may further help to alleviate a child's fear.

A family-centred care model (see Chapter 19) is advocated when dealing with children and the A&E department should be no exception. The benefits of allowing a parent or guardian to remain with a child whenever possible are well recognised. This can provide a familiar face and comfort in an otherwise unfamiliar setting. If appropriate, the accompanying adult should be encouraged to help as much as possible in caring for the child. Explanations of any necessary treatments should be given in terms that both can understand and such treatments carried out efficiently and quickly. The child may be given a 'bravery award' of some sort when treatment is concluded – perhaps a sticker or badge or a certificate to keep.

Unless emergency care is required, the child should be given time to settle into the new surroundings before treatment is carried out. This should be done quickly and efficiently by a skilled nurse. Examinations should be made as much fun as time permits, allowing the child to hold or use equipment if applicable. Any equipment needed should be prepared out of the child's sight and explanations about what will happen should be brief and given immediately prior to the event so that the child does not have time to worry. If possible, the child should sit on a parent's or a nurse's knee though sometimes restraint will be necessary. Wrapping babies or small children securely in a blanket whilst treatment is carried out can save time and tears in the long run.

There has been extensive debate about who should care for children in the A&E department. Should it be a nurse whose name appears on Part 8 of the UKCC Register and who is recognised as a sick children's nurse, or is an experienced A&E nurse best? It would clearly be ideal if the child could be cared for by a nurse appropriately qualified and expert in both fields of clinical practice but such nurses are not always available. Many departments now have a children's nurse among their complement of staff and make use of his/her expertise in a variety of ways. Webb and Cleaver (1991) argue that the presence of a children's nurse in A&E should be considered a necessity rather than a luxury, a fact supported by the charity Action for Sick Children (1997). The primary responsibilities of such a nurse would be to assess the needs of children and their families following their arrival in the department and to ensure that good practice continues in his/her absence through an agreed philosophy and written standards of care.

Whether there is a designated nurse within the department or not, there are certainly some nurses who are naturally adept at dealing with children and others who are not. The choice of the correct nurse to deal with a child may help to make them less fearful during their stay and in the future.

The condition of a sick child can deteriorate very quickly and many who are brought in are acutely ill on arrival. Speed, calm and efficiency are essential when dealing with such children. They will have no wish to play games or look at posters until they feel better. Again, the carer's help should be enlisted wherever practical, though the nurse must be constantly aware of the concern the carer will feel for the child's welfare and of the fact that there may be other pressing factors which need to be dealt with (other siblings at home, for example). Both child and carer should be encompassed in the nurse's care perspective.

THE CHILDREN ACT

The Children Act (DoH, 1989) makes it plain that the welfare of the child is paramount. It implies that nurses should listen to children, give them appropriate, adequate information and take into account their feelings and wishes. The A&E nurse should also be aware of the court orders that may be served under the Children Act and of the concept of 'parental responsibility' enshrined within the Act since this will affect the right to consent to treatment for the child (see Oates, 1993 for a resumé).

CHILD ABUSE

Nurses involved in first line care may be the first to come into contact with a child 'in need' or whom they suspect of being abused – either mentally, physically, sexually or emotionally – or who is suffering neglect. A further discussion of child abuse is found in Chapter 20 but the A&E nurse should be prepared to voice her concerns about the child to senior staff and be aware of how to contact the local authority. Many departments have written policies which should be followed in order to ensure the best possible care for the child.

ELDERLY PATIENTS IN A&E

The Office of Population Census and Surveys (OPCS) indicated that in 1990, 15.5% of the population of Great Britain was over the age of 65 (OPCS, 1991). This percentage has been rising gradually over the years and no decline is envisaged. Attendance rates at A&E departments have been shown to increase as people get older (Wood, 1992). The most common reasons for attending are falls, faints, confused states, hypothermia, wandering or simply inability to cope. Fractures are common in elderly people following trauma. Wood further notes that many elderly patients, particularly those who live alone, use A&E departments as a primary care provider because of the perceived difficulties of accessing more appropriate channels.

Much has now been written about the physiological changes of ageing and the special needs of those who are elderly but, whilst there are often special facilities for children in A&E departments, most make little or no specific provision for the elderly patient – the beds are generally hard and high, there are no comfortable chairs in which to sit and wait and because everyone is so busy, there is often no-one to talk to. Many elderly patients have hearing problems which can lead to communication difficulties if not adequately addressed. The department can appear unfriendly and frightening with everything happening at once and can increase the elderly patient's confusion, disorientation and agitation. Ryan (1996) suggests that a room for nursing elderly patients should include:

- A clock telling the correct time
- A poster with the name of the department, hospital and the name of the named nurse
- A calendar showing the correct date
- A call bell
- A bed with a pressure relieving mattress
- Magnifying glass, pen and paper
- A loop system for hearing aids
- A walking frame.

Elderly people tend not to make a fuss about their discomfort or the length of time they have waited in A&E and if their needs are not specifically addressed it is easy for them to spend longer in the department than other patients. In addition, it is sometimes difficult to discharge these patients even though there is no medical reason for detaining them. This is particularly true at night and when the elderly patient lives alone.

Because of their relatively frail nature, the effects of food and water deprivation and enforced immobility (for example on a hard trolley waiting to be seen by medical staff) and lack of privacy quickly begin to have a detrimental effect on elderly patients and it is vital that the A&E nurse addresses these basic needs at an early stage in the care of this patient group.

ELDER ABUSE

Vernon (1995) comments that the plight of the elderly abused patient is often unnoticed in A&E, despite the key position of the staff for intervention. Elder abuse can take a number of forms (DoH,1992a) :

- Physical, e.g. hitting, punching, shaking, pushing
- Psychological, e.g. verbal abuse, aggression, threatening behaviour
- Financial, e.g. extracting money, taking bank or pension book
- Sexual
- Neglect – failure to meet basic needs for shelter, warmth and food.

Those particularly at risk have been identified (DoH, 1992a) as 'white English', females, 80 years and over, those with poor mobility or physical or mental impairment or who need help with everyday tasks such as eating. Elderly people are most commonly abused by adult close family members, often the principal carers and often with financial or social problems of their own. More recently, the abuse of elderly people in residential nursing homes has been highlighted.

The complex pathological changes of ageing in addition to a tendency to confusion in an A&E surrounding may make the signs of abuse difficult to spot and confront. Confrontation will commonly lead to denial by both parties (DoH 1992a) and sometimes the only apparent course of action is to return the elderly patient to the abusive situation. The relevant social services department will take steps to investigate if they are informed, and elderly patients may be given the telephone number of the Elder Abuse Response Line (see 'Useful Groups and Organisations' at end of chapter).

CARING FOR RELATIVES AND FRIENDS

Many patients will be accompanied to the A&E department by a relative or close friend. The relative may be able to provide useful information about what has happened to the patient, particularly if the latter is drowsy, confused or unconscious. It is all too easy to forget waiting relatives in the hustle and bustle of caring for or treating casualties but the nurse must make every effort to keep them informed of what is happening to the patient. Whenever possible, relatives should be allowed to sit with patients or, if this is inadvisable, they could be informed of the likely wait and advised to go for a cup of tea or a meal in the interim. Relatives can provide the patient with a vital link with the real world at a time of great distress.

Imparting information to visitors is particularly important if the patient is seriously ill or gravely injured. It is unfair to be other than truthful about the patient's condition. Whenever possible, such relatives should be allowed to remain in the department, in a separate room if one is available, where they can talk together and make tea or coffee. If the patient is likely to die, every effort should be made to warn the relatives in advance. Parkes (1985) and Pisarick (1981) concluded that even the shortest period of warning of the impending death of a loved one is better than none at all. It is not always possible to allow relatives to be with a dying patient and some may not wish to be present. Relatives should always be warned about how the patient will look when they are taken to see them, whether alive or dead, and special mention should be made of any intravenous infusions, monitors or other equipment attached to or beside them.

WITNESSED RESUSCITATION

There has been recent debate as to whether relatives should be allowed into the resuscitation room whilst resuscitation attempts are taking place. A small, early study at the Foote hospital in Michigan (Doyle et al., 1987) showed a positive response from families who were allowed to be present. Staff stated that it increased their stress levels but most endorsed the practice. Witnessed resuscitation has become more common in recent years in the UK and is regarded as good practice by the Working Group of the Royal College of Nursing and British Association for Accident and Emergency Medicine (1995).

Arguments in favour of allowing relatives to be present are that it enables them to see that everything possible was tried, that nothing more could be done, it prevents the pain of being apart and the belief that a loved one died alone and ultimately assists the grieving process. It can, however, be a traumatic experience and may itself haunt the relatives.

A&E nurses need to be able to respond appropriately when relatives ask to be allowed into the 'resus' area – this will include ensuring that an appropriately trained staff member stays with them to support and explain proceedings to the relatives. Some may feel it appropriate to offer relatives the option of watching, but there should not be any attempt to persuade them to be present if they have no wish to be.

IN THE EVENT OF A PATIENT'S DEATH

If a patient dies, either in the department or before arrival there, the family and friends should be taken to a quiet room away from the main working area. Most departments have a designated room which is sensitively decorated with comfortable seating and access to a telephone and facilities for making drinks. Studies by Wright (1989, 1991) have identified the provision of a private waiting area as one of the most helpful activities following the death of a loved one.

The news will be broken by a doctor or a qualified nurse and ambiguous terms such as 'passed away' or 'left us' should be avoided, since they are open to misinterpretation. The words 'died' or 'dead' should be used so that there can be no misunderstanding.

Some departments have a trained bereavement counsellor available but in many areas it is part of the nurse's role to stay with and support the relatives at this time. Wright's 1989 study showed that the nurse who stays with the relatives is always remembered, especially if she deals with the situation skilfully and sensitively. Sitting down with relatives and showing empathy with them are seen as highly significant and contribute to the quality of support.

Relatives who have had no time to prepare for the sudden death of a loved one will need to talk and ask questions about exactly what happened and about the last minutes of their loved one's life. This is recognised as a normal part of adjustment to the news of sudden death and every attempt should be made to answer honestly and truthfully, stressing any positive aspects, such as the fact that death was instant and probably without pain or that all the correct things were done. In some departments, relatives will be invited back to the department or contacted by one of the staff a few weeks after the death so that any questions can be answered or to give them an opportunity to 'talk it through'.

Reactions to sudden bad news vary widely and the nurse should be prepared for any reaction from verbal abuse through uncontrolled weeping to hysterical laughter. Occasionally, relatives will refuse to believe the truth and may even deny it once they have seen the body. A nurse should remain with the family to offer comfort and to answer their questions and allow them to assimilate the facts. A cup of tea or coffee may be appreciated. The nurse should aim to accept reactions to shock and to allow the grieving process to begin.

If the dead patient is a child, the experience may be a particularly traumatic one for all concerned and the nurse may find herself weeping openly with the parents. This is a natural reaction to a tragedy and should not be thought of as unprofessional.

Viewing the body as soon after death as possible was shown by Wright (1989) to be of positive benefit to grieving relatives. This was valuable not only so that they could say goodbye but so that they could see the reality of the situation. There are clearly instances when this is not possible or advisable, but it should be allowed whenever possible. The relatives must always have the final right of choice as to whether or not to view the body but sensitive guidance from the A&E staff may help them in their decision.

The nurse who has spent time with grieving relatives who were previously total strangers to her will need time to recover her own thoughts and emotions once they have left and should try to talk over the event with a trained staff member as soon as possible (see also Chapter 27). A counselling service may be available within the hospital or locality, of which the A&E nurse can avail herself.

PATIENTS WHO MAY PRESENT PROBLEMS

Not all patients who attend the emergency department are pleasant or polite and the nurse may be exposed to a number of groups of people with whom she has had no previous contact.

ALCOHOL ABUSERS

Many road traffic accidents, assaults and other violent incidents are alcohol-related and the A&E nurse will regularly find herself dealing with patients who have had too much to drink.

Alcohol affects people differently and some patients may be very happy and eager to laugh at anything, including the injuries they have sustained. They usually feel little or no pain because of the analgesic effect of the alcohol and are only too keen to oblige with any necessary treatments. The best policy is usually to laugh along with them whilst trying to keep them on the couch or in the cubicle. The problem is more likely to be one of convincing them that something is wrong, particularly if surgery or hospital admission is indicated.

Other patients who have abused alcohol will be aggressive or perhaps even violent. If allowed to remain in the general waiting area they may quickly disrupt the entire department, hurling abuse and sometimes furniture at anyone within reach. Many feel 'trapped' in hospital and are anxious to escape, particularly if they think the police are likely to arrive to interview them. These patients are usually male and if possible should be dealt with by males who should be firm and persuasive. In general, whilst queue-jumping is not to be advocated, such patients are best dealt with promptly and ushered off the premises as soon as possible. Dealing with those who become violent will be discussed later in the chapter.

Some persistent alcohol abusers will be well known to the staff as regular visitors. These people will drink anything alcoholic and it is vital to ensure that any suitable substances, particu-larly methylated spirit, are locked away securely. It is not uncommon for these visitors to arrive in pairs so that one can keep the staff occupied whilst the other seeks out any unlocked cupboards in out-of-the-way areas. Such patients can be very devious and may become verbally or physically abusive if challenged.

DRUG ABUSERS

Drug abusers are also frequent visitors, particularly in large towns and cities, and many will be known to the staff by name. They are commonly found unconscious by a member of the public, often in a public convenience, following their latest 'fix' and are brought in by ambulance. Most departments have their own policy guidelines for dealing with this group of patients which usually entails placing them in the recovery position on a mattress on the floor, to ensure a clear airway and minimise the danger of falling, and observing them discretely whilst allowing them to 'sleep it off'. Naloxone (Narcan) is not generally used to reverse the effect of the opiates unless there is cause for concern about the patient's condition or any doubt as to the cause of his/her unconsciousness. When they waken, drug abusers are usually eager to leave and go out to find their next 'fix'. A careful record should always be kept of any property removed from their clothing and its disposal. It is also essential to ensure that all hospital drugs are kept locked in appropriate cupboards.

The nurse dealing with drug abusers should bear in mind that the risk that they are carriers of hepatitis or the human immunodeficiency virus (HIV) is greater than with the general population and should take all necessary precautions when caring for them (see Chapter 16).

These individuals often spend night after night in various A&E departments and, sadly, little can be done for them in the long term unless they decide to seek help for themselves.

SOLVENT ABUSERS

The sniffing of solvents used in glues and cleaning agents, lighter gas and gas from aerosol cans tends to occur in the younger age groups (12–16). McGrath and Bowker (1987) describe two phases of mood which follow glue solvent inhalation: first, intoxication with euphoria and exhilaration and sometimes hallucination, and then a period where cerebral depressant effects are noticeable as slurred speech, ataxia and drowsiness. These effects are achieved quickly and fade quickly but bizarre behaviour may occur and lead to accidents or render the inhaler unconscious. Care consists of ensuring that a clear airway is maintained and of treating any other symptoms which arise. The patient should be detained in the department until the intoxicating effects of the substance have worn off (unless admission to a ward is indicated). An interview with a social worker may be offered if this seems appropriate but, regrettably, these young people commonly resent all forms of authority including that of their parents and it is often impossible to help them.

MUNCHAUSEN'S SYNDROME

Patients with this condition present in A&E with fictitious disorders (Holmberg, 1993) in an attempt to gain either drugs or hospital admission or both. McGrath and Bowker (1987) list the most common presenting complaints as abdominal pain, usually colic, haemorrhage, neurological symptoms, myocardial infarction or pulmonary embolus. The patient will generally give an extremely convincing performance. Others will swallow objects such as coins or open safety pins in order to obtain surgical treatment.

These patients are often difficult to identify and assess since they tend to travel all over the country visiting different A&E departments and may only visit a particular area once a year or so. Something in their behaviour or medical history may arouse the suspicions of the more experienced staff and analgesic drugs should be withheld until further enquiries are made. Such patients may become aggressive if questioned in detail and most will leave the department quickly if they realise they are suspected. Many departments have a list of such patients with description, names used (they usually have a number of aliases) and presenting symptoms. Other hospitals in the area should be contacted and given relevant details so that as little time as possible is wasted in dealing with these people. Psychiatric help is generally refused when offered and these clients continue to suffer.

A less common presentation of Munchausen's syndrome is that 'by proxy' where the sufferer repeatedly inflicts harm on another individual or individuals, often children (Holmberg, 1993). Again, expert staff may have an instinctive feeling that the circumstances of attendance are unusual but Munchausen's syndrome by proxy is often not recognised until serious harm has occurred.

VAGRANTS

Vagrants and other persons of no fixed abode will also be regular visitors to inner city A&Es, particularly in winter when nights are cold and sleeping rough is difficult. It is not uncommon to find them sleeping on chairs in a quiet corner of the department in the middle of the night. Heartless as it may seem, they should be removed, by the security staff or police if necessary (it rarely is), or word will soon spread that a blind eye is being turned and the department will be full.

Those who are ill must be seen and treated. Many vagrants do not wash themselves or their clothes regularly and may be infested with lice. It is wise to wear protective clothing when caring for these patients and to be alert for head lice, body lice and pubic lice ('crabs'). The use of protective clothing should be explained sensitively to the patient and he or she should be accorded the same dignity and respect as every other patient.

Many are extremely apologetic and embarrassed about their state; others will be rude and abusive. It is important, if these patients are undressed, that their clothing and property are searched carefully before being tied securely in a plastic bag or bin sack as they sometimes carry large amounts of money. If patients are to be admitted to the ward, it is usual to bathe them and wash their hair with appropriate disinfectant solutions in the A&E department, some of which have special bath or shower rooms for this purpose. If possible, the clothes should be sent for incineration once the patient's written consent has been obtained. New clothes will be supplied by the social work department prior to the patient's discharge.

The cubicle in which they have been examined will require fumigation once the patient has left the department and, for this reason, a room with a door should be used in preference to a curtained cubicle.

AGGRESSION AND VIOLENCE

A number of factors lead to aggressive behaviour in the acute care environment and aggression, if mishandled, can soon turn to violence. It is not always the patient who becomes aggressive but often the relatives or friends who accompany him. Long waiting times, a sudden crisis situation, unrealistic expectations, lack of information about what is happening, fear, alcohol or drugs and a wish to look 'big' in front of others are some of the reasons identified as precipitating aggressive behaviour. Staff may unwittingly display judgemental attitudes which compounds the situation. What begins as verbal abuse may quickly turn into disruptive or physically violent behaviour if not rapidly defused.

Aggressive outbursts in A&E are rarely without warning (Neades, 1994) and with experience it is usually possible to identify those persons who are likely to become aggressive before the situation actually arises. Jones and Littler (1992) suggest that people may display signs of impending aggression such as:

- Appears tense and agitated
- Volume and pitch of voice increase
- Abrupt replies to questions; may be accompanied by abusive gestures
- Pupils may dilate
- Muscular tension in face and limbs – body posture changes
- Make fists with hands
- Bang fists on palm of opposite hands or other objects within reach
- Obscene and sarcastic when talking about staff.

Communication is vital, whether it be a general announcement in the waiting room about the cause of any delay or individual explanations to patients and their relatives about what is happening and how much longer they are likely to have to wait. The triage nurse is usually in an ideal position to disseminate information of this sort as he or she is aware of who is waiting to be seen and of the overall workload of the department.

The guidelines for dealing with aggression in the A&E department produced by the Accident and Emergency Nursing Association of the Royal College of Nursing (RCN, 1987) stress the importance of preventing violence from occurring by all means possible.

If an individual begins to get aggressive or argumentative, good communication skills using a calm, confident and non-threatening approach will be needed and help should be sought before the individual is confronted. Every effort should be made to find the cause of his/her discontent so that the problem can be addressed. If he/she is sitting, the nurse should sit beside him/her and not remain standing as he/she may perceive this as a threatening posture. It is inadvisable to touch an angry patient since it may provoke physical violence in return – an arm's length away is the generally recommended distance. Direct eye contact should be avoided – focus on the larynx area – and ensure that no objects which might be used as weapons (e.g. stethoscope or scissors) are within reach. In addition, always make sure you can reach an exit if needed.

Help should be sought at once if the patient refuses to calm down once explanations have been given. He/she should be removed from the department if this is appropriate or 'guarded' by a security officer or police officer if he/she requires medical attention.

Groups of youths may accompany an injured friend and become rowdy and disruptive. They should be approached at once with a friendly but firm warning that their behaviour is unacceptable. If this tactic fails, the ringleader should be identified and isolated as the other group members will often calm down when leaderless. The situation must not be allowed to get out of hand before the hospital security officers or the police force are called to remove them – it is not unknown for violent fights to occur inside an A&E department.

Should violence erupt within the department, help must be summoned immediately – Neades (1994) suggests a minimum of four staff as a show of strength. In many inner city hospitals nurses carry alarms and have emergency call bells to summon security or police officers. In places renowned for their violent patients, security officers will be on duty within the department. Nurses should aim not to become involved in the fighting and not to become the victim of an attack. It is advisable to remain in the main well-lit area of the department at night and certainly not to leave this area without a colleague.

If the aggressive patient is in a room or cubicle for observation the nurse should ensure that he/she does not become trapped inside with the patient. The nurse should always make sure he/she has an escape route and that the patient cannot place him/herself between the nurse and the door. Someone who is angry can display extreme strength and if physical restraint is necessary it is advisable to wait until sufficient help (preferably male) arrives. When restraint is attempted, the patient's fists, feet and head should be avoided.

SELF-DEFENCE

Attacks do sometimes happen in spite of all preventive measures being employed and in these circumstances the nurse has no choice but to defend him/herself. More injuries than necessary may be inflicted if the nurse is unable to put aside his/her caring role immediately and consider his/her own safety first. The following simple guidelines are recommended for those who find themselves in the position of being attacked:

1 Shout loudly for help.
2 Attempt to release the attacker's grip by causing him/her acute pain in one or more sensitive areas (see below).
3 Run away as soon as the patient's grip is released.

If attacked from the front, any of the following may help to secure the victim's release:

- Kneeing the assailant in the groin with maximum force
- Pushing fingers up the assailant's nostrils
- Pinching the inside of the assailant's thigh as hard as possible
- Kicking the assailant's shins. Aim should be made for any vulnerable areas within reach – this will, in part, be dictated by the position in which the victim is held.

If attacked from behind it is best to aim for the assailant's shins. He/she should be kicked hard with the heel of the victim's shoe which can then be scraped down the lower part of the assailant's leg.

There is no place in such a situation for gentle action. The first attack should be intended to secure release from the assailant and strength, speed and surprise will all help to achieve this. As soon as the grip is released, the victim must run. No attempt should be made to try and reason with the patient.

Following the occurrence of any violent incident a detailed account should be written and signed by victim and witnesses and any appropriate hospital documentation completed. The victim should be seen by a doctor as soon as possible and the incident reported to senior staff. The police force, if called to the incident, will advise on any further steps to be taken.

STRESS

The stress experienced by those working in an A&E department can be intense. Waters (1996) reports that causes include too few staff, an increasing workload and dealing with violent patients. Anyone can present through the doors, including those who are severely injured, dead and dying, and the nurse has only seconds to prepare to deal with the situation. Sudden, tragic death is commonly encountered and comforting bereaved relatives can be one of the most difficult duties of a nurse. The department can become extremely crowded and busy, resulting in long waits to see the doctor so that the nurse feels he/she has no time to do anything properly and little time to spend getting to know the patients. There is little continuity of care in the long term and unless one makes an effort to find out how a particular patient is progressing there is not the reward of seeing his or her condition improve. Violence and aggression are frequent occurrences in many departments and the nurse may feel very threatened, particularly during the night. Hodgkinson and Stewart (1991) note that physical and emotional fatigue and dealing with sudden death or breaking bad news are additional causes of stress for the staff in A&E.

Stress only becomes a problem if it is not addressed. Since 1980 post-traumatic stress disorder has been recognised as a legitimate diagnosis (Bamber, 1994) and efforts have been made to support staff following stressful situations in order to avoid long-term psychological trauma. Whitfield (1994) discusses the importance and the practicalities of effective 'debriefing' following such incidents and recommends that such sessions are used as a framework to confront stress.

First line care is not always exciting and whilst some may enjoy the challenges it poses and the tension of not being able to predict events, others will find the lack of planning and the constant uncertainty daunting and unsettling. The maxims which direct and instruct the work of A&E nurses have been identified by Sbaih (1997a, b) in her recent work. These maxims help to explain how A&E nursing differs from other types of nursing. Sbaih maintains that the 'A&E nurse' is regarded, amongst other things, as able to:

- Act upon impressions
- Work out the work – that is, to get on with the job without being given instructions
- Take risks when necessary
- Enjoy doing more than one job at any one time.

These are not the maxims which direct nurses and their work in other hospital areas and some nurses may not wish to embrace them. First line care *is* different and not everyone enjoys it.

EMERGENCY SITUATIONS

RESUSCITATION

Resuscitation is a term used to describe the restoration of adequate blood and oxygen supplies to the vital organs of the body. It includes the use of cardiopulmonary resuscitation, drugs and defibrillation.

Coronary artery disease is the most common cause of cardiac arrest though there are many others which need to be considered including other heart diseases, trauma, asphyxia, drowning, poisoning, hypothermia and electrocution. Once the circulation stops the tissues become hypoxic and cells cease to function efficiently and eventually die. There is damage to all body organs especially the heart, brain and kidneys – the 'vital organs'. Rising levels of carbon dioxide in the body quickly cause **acidosis**.

An electrocardiograph (ECG) recording will most commonly show the patient's heart is in **ventricular fibrillation** (VF) – producing rapid, uncoordinated and ineffective movements of the heart muscle. If uncorrected, ventricular fibrillation usually becomes asystole within 8 minutes and the patient has little chance of survival (Quinn and Ord, 1996).

In recent years the European Resuscitation Council (ERC) (1996) and the Resuscitation Council (UK) (1997) have issued guidelines to ensure standardised, prompt and appropriate interventions for patients in need of resuscitation. These are generally divided into basic life support skills, advanced life support and defibrillation. Any nurse involved in first line care of patients must be fully conversant with these guidelines and aware of the location and use of any equipment and drugs which may be needed during resuscitation attempts. The reader is referred to these guidelines for details of resuscitation measures.

ADVANCED TRAUMA LIFE SUPPORT

In 1988 the Royal College of Surgeons working party report on patients with major injuries indicated that 30% of patients with major injuries died unnecessarily. A systematic approach to the care of such patients had been developed by the American College of Surgeons and has subsequently been developed in the UK into what is known as advanced trauma life support (ATLS). Training is available for doctors and for nurses (the Advanced Trauma Nursing Course and the Trauma Nursing Core Course – details of these and other A&E nursing courses are available through the A&E Nursing Association at the Royal College of Nursing).

ATLS is a systematic approach to care aimed at reducing deaths in the so-called 'golden hour' following injury. It involves a rapid initial assessment followed by the immediate restoration of the body's vital functions. Following this, a thorough evaluation is performed to ensure that no injuries are missed (Toulson, 1993).

Mechanism of injury

A full history of the incident which produced the patient's injuries will help the trauma carers to anticipate and diagnose traumatic injuries. Many hospitals now have a designated trauma team who may be summoned at any time – the team will initially include four doctors, five nurses and a radiographer (Driscoll and Skinner, 1996) each of whom must be familiar with his/her own role within the team and with the roles of his/her colleagues. These roles are generally clearly defined and prompt cards are available in the designated trauma area of the department. Typical roles for the five nurses on the team would be:

- Nurse team leader
- Protect airway and cervical spine
- Monitor circulation and insert intravenous lines if necessary
- Ensure documentation accurate and up to date
- Support, comfort and explain situation to relatives.

Further specialists, for example cardiothoracic and neurosurgical specialists, may also be part of the team in hospitals where they are available. As a general rule, no more than six people at a time should be touching the patient (Driscoll and Skinner, 1996).

Criteria for summoning the trauma team will be based on the mechanism and type of injury (for example, impact at 20 mph or more without a seatbelt, death of an occupant of the same car) and a revised trauma score based on the patient's respiratory rate, systolic blood pressure and **Glasgow coma score**. The objectives of the trauma team are:

- Identify and correct life-threatening injuries
- Resuscitate the patient and stabilise the vital signs
- Determine the nature and extent of other injuries
- Categorise the injuries in order of priority
- Prepare and transport the patient to a place of definitive care (Driscoll and Skinner, 1996).

Primary survey

This aims to identify life-threatening conditions so that effective resuscitation can be given. A rapid examination of the patient is undertaken using the ABCDE system in strict order:

- A Airway maintenance with cervical spine control
- B Breathing and ventilation
- C Circulation with haemorrhage control
- D Dysfunction of the central nervous system
- E Exposure (the patient is fully undressed).

All trauma patients are assumed to have a cervical spine injury until it is medically excluded and neck immobilisation is maintained with a stiff neck collar and sandbags on either side of the head with tape across the forehead. During this phase, vital signs are recorded every 5 minutes.

Resuscitation phase

During this phase any life-threatening conditions identified in the primary survey are constantly reassessed. In addition, the management of shock is initiated, haemorrhage control and patient oxygenation are re-evaluated. As a general rule, any patient who is cool and **tachycardic** should be assumed to be in **shock** until proven otherwise (Toulson, 1993).

Secondary survey

The objectives of the secondary survey are:

- Examine the patient from head to toe and front to back
- Ascertain a complete medical history
- Gather all clinical, laboratory and radiological data
- Determine a management plan for the patient (Driscoll and Skinner, 1996).

A thorough and systematic head to toe examination is now undertaken and all vital signs recorded. Each area of the body is examined in turn to ensure that nothing is missed. X-rays of cervical spine, chest and pelvis are taken and the patient will be **log-rolled**, ensuring his spine is totally immobile, so that his back can be examined.

Definitive care phase

All injuries are managed at this phase – fractures stabilised, necessary operative interventions undertaken and transfer to a ward or specialist unit organised. As in previous phases, any life-threatening conditions are constantly monitored.

PREPARING FOR A MAJOR INCIDENT

An incident is categorised as 'major' when the location of the incident or the number, severity or type of live casualties require extraordinary NHS arrangements (Advanced Life Support Group, 1995). Such incidents are rare but every hospital which has the potential to receive casualties from such an incident needs to have a plan, sufficient equipment and personnel trained to deal with the emergency.

The equipment is generally kept in a dedicated cupboard or room and should be checked frequently. Equipment should include protective clothing for the mobile team (see above) and additional equipment (e.g. fluids, splints, airways, cannulae) stationary for use in the department when casualties arrive.

'Action cards' should be available for each key member of the hospital team and these should list the individual's responsibilities, immediate action to be taken and priorities during the incident. Senior staff will generally act as coordinators and will ensure that sufficient staff are recruited to staff all areas of the department.

There is generally very little warning of a major incident and the initial priorities are to:

- Clear the department as much as possible ready to receive the casualties
- Clear beds on the wards and departments so that casualties can be transferred as soon as possible
- Allocate staff and resources to all necessary areas.

Training should be undertaken regularly for departmental staff and may take the form of a paper exercise or a simulation practice in the hospital or an incident simulation undertaken with other emergency services.

Following any such training exercise, plans should be reviewed and updated.

CONCLUSION

This chapter has addressed, very briefly, some of the issues involved in first line care of patients. It has highlighted the unpredictability of this aspect of nursing and the need for a calm, efficient and structured approach to the care of patients, whatever their presenting symptoms or complaint. The need to be prepared for any eventuality has been stressed as has the need constantly to monitor situations to anticipate deterioration and allow early intervention.

Helping patients and their relatives to come to terms with acute illness or injury without feeling they have lost control is an important skill for any nurse involved in first line care and it is hoped that this chapter has helped to prepare the reader for the wide variety of patients with whom he or she is likely to come into contact.

USEFUL GROUPS AND ORGANISATIONS

Resuscitation Council (UK)
9 Fitzroy Square
London W1P 5AH
Tel: 0171 388 4678

British Heart Foundation
14 Fitzhardinge Street
London W1H 4DH
Tel: 0171 935 0185

Chest, Heart and Stroke Association
Tavistock House North
Tavistock Square
London WC1N 9JE

ATNC contact: Gabbie Lomas
Tel: 0161 787 4841

TNCC contact: Barts City Life Saver Officer
0171 601 8888

Elder Abuse Response Line: 0181 679 7074

Other groups which may provide help for those who do not require hospital admission are:

- Alcoholics Anonymous
- British Pregnancy Advisory Service
- Relate (formerly the Marriage Guidance Council)
- Salvation Army
- Samaritans

There may also be local hostels for battered women, day centres for those who are lonely or homeless and support groups for victims of rape or those suffering from a wide variety of illnesses. The numbers should be readily available in all first line care areas so that patients can be advised how to contact them or appropriate referral made.

REFERENCES

Action for Sick Children (1991). *Children in Accident and Emergency Departments* Key point 17. Action for Sick Children, London.

Action for Sick Children (1997). *Emergency Health Services for Children and Young People*. Action for Sick Children, London.

Advanced Life Support Group (1995). *Major Incident Medical Management and Support: the Practical Approach*. BMJ Publishing Group, London.

Bamber, M. (1994). Providing support for emergency service staff. *Nursing Times*, 90(22), 32–3.

Blythin, P. (1988). Triage in the UK. *Nursing*, 3(31), 16–20.

Cliff, K.S. and Wood, T.C.A. (1986). Accident and emergency services – the ambulant patient. *Hospital and Health Services Review*, 82(2), 74–7.

Crouch, R. (1994). Triage: past, present and future. *Emergency Nurse*, 1 (2), 4–6.

Dale, J., Williams, S. and Crouch, R. (1995). Telephone triage: extending practice. *Nursing Standard*, 9(21), 34–36.

Dimond, B. (1994). Attempted suicide in the accident and emergency department. *Accident and Emergency Nursing*, 2, 50–3.

Dimond, B. (1995a). *Legal aspects of Nursing*. Prentice Hall, London.

Dimond, B. (1995b). Death in accident and emergency *Accident and Emergency Nursing*, 3, 338–41.

DoH (1989). *The Children Act 1989*. London, HMSO.

DoH (1992a). *Confronting Elder Abuse*. London, HMSO.

DoH (1992b). *The Patient's Charter*. London, HMSO.

Dowling, S., Martin, R., Skidmore, P., Doyal, L., Cameron, A. and Lloyd, S. (1996). Nurses taking on junior doctors' work: a confusion of accountability. *British Medical Journal*, 312, 1211–14.

Doyle, C.J., Post, H., Burney, R.E., Maino, J., Keefe, M. and Rhee, K.J. (1987). Family participation during resuscitation: an option. *Annals of Emergency Medicine*, 16(6), 7–9.

Driscoll, P. and Skinner, D. (1996). Initial assessment and management – I: primary survey and II: secondary survey. In *ABC of Major Trauma*, 2nd edn, Skinner, D., Driscoll, P. and Earlham, R. (eds), 1–10. BMJ Publishing Group, London.

European Resuscitation Council (1996). *Guidelines for Resuscitation*. ERC, Antwerp.

Glasper, A. (1993). Telephone triage: extending practice. *Nursing Standard*, 7(1), 15–16.

Harris, A., Cummings, J. (1992). An environment fit for child care: setting standards for children in A&E. *Professional Nurse*, 7(7), 461–4.

Hodgkinson, P.E., and Stewart, M. (1991). *Coping with Catastrophe: a Handbook of Disaster Management*. Routledge, London.

Holmberg, S.K. (1993). Pain. In *Mental Health – Psychiatric Nursing: a Holistic Life-cycle Approach*. Rawlins, R.P., William, S.R. and Beck, C.K. (eds). Mosby, St Louis.

Janowski, M.J. (1995). Is telephone triage calling you? *American Journal of Nursing*, 95(9), 59–62.

Jones, D. and Littler, A. (1992). *Management of Violent or Potentially Violent Persons*, 2nd edn. South Glamorgan Health Authority, Cardiff.

Kilner, T. (1996). Pre hospital care delivery. *Emergency Nurse*, 4(1), 16–18.

Korgaonkar, G. and Tribe, D. (1994). Confidentiality, patients and the law. *British Journal of Nursing*, 3(2), 91–3.

Laing, G.S. (ed.) (1988). Children in the A & E department. *The A and E letter*, 3, 1–7.

McGrath, G. and Bowker, M. (1987). *Common Psychiatric Emergencies*. Wright, Bristol.

Mallett, J. and Woolwich, C. (1990). Triage in accident and emergency departments. *Journal of Advanced Nursing*, 15, 1443–51.

Manchester Triage Group (1997). *Emergency Triage*. BMJ Publishing Group, London.

National Audit Office (1992). *NHS Accident and Emergency Departments in England*. HMSO, London.

National Audit Office (1996). *By Accident or Design? Improving A&E Services in England and Wales*. Audit Commission, London.

Neades, B.L. (1994) How to handle aggression. *Emergency Nurse*, 2(2), 21–4.

NHS Executive (1996). *Developing Emergency Services in the Community – for Consultation*. DOH, London.

Nuttall, M. (1986). The chaos controller. *Nursing Times*, 82(20), 66–8.

Oates, M. (1993). Children Act 1989: the essential issues. *Emergency Nurse*, 1(1), 21–2.

OPCS (1991). *Britain's Elderly Population*. OPCS, London.

Parkes, C.M. (1985). Sudden death prolongs mourning period. *Nursing Mirror*, 161(14), 10.

Pisarick, G. (1981). Psychiatric emergencies and crisis intervention. *Nursing Clinics of North America*, 16, 85–94.

Quinn, T. and Ord, L. (1996). Cardiopulmonary resuscitation. *Nursing Times*, 92(45,46 & 47), Supplements.

RCN (1987). *Guidelines for Dealing with Aggression in the Accident and Emergency Department*. Royal College of Nursing Association of Nursing Practice, Accident and Emergency Nursing Forum, London.

RCN (1992). *Emergency Nurse Practitioners: Guidance from the Royal College of Nursing*. RCN Accident and Emergency Nursing Association, London.

Resuscitation Council (UK) (1997). *The 1997 Resuscitation Guidelines for Use in the United Kingdom*. Resuscitation Council, London.

Royal College of Nursing and British Association for Accident and Emergency Medicine (1995). *Bereavement Care in A&E Departments*. RCN, London.

Royal College of Surgeons (1988). *The Management of Patients with Major Injuries*. Royal College of Surgeons, London.

Ryan, N. (1996). The right track. *Nursing Times*, 92(50), 41.

Sbaih, L. (1997a). The work of accident and emergency nurses: Part 1. An introduction to the rules. *Accident and Emergency Nursing*, 5(1), 28–33.

Sbaih, L. (1997b). The work of accident and emergency nurses: Part 2. A&E maxims: making A&E work unique and special. *Accident and Emergency Nursing*, 5(2), 81–7.

Tingle, J.H. (1993). The extended role of the nurse: legal implications. *Care of the Critically Ill*, 9(1), 30–4.

Toulson, S. (1993). A guide to advanced trauma life support. *Professional Nurse*, 9(2), 95–7.

UKCC (1992a). *The Scope of Professional Practice*. UKCC, London.

UKCC (1992b). *Code of Professional Conduct*, 3rd edn. UKCC, London.

UKCC (1993). *Standards for Record Keeping*, UKCC, London.

UKCC (1996). *Guidelines for Professional Practice*, UKCC, London.

Vernon, M. (1995). A&E – why so complacent? *Nursing Times*, 91(42), 28–30.

Walsh, M. (1995). NPs: why are they so successful? *Emergency Nurse*, 3(2), 4–5.

Waters, J. (1996). News review. *Nursing Times*, 92(16), 3.

Webb, J. and Cleaver, K. (1991). The child in casualty. *Nursing Times*, 87(15), 27–9.

Whitfield, A. (1994). Critical incident debriefing in A&E. *Emergency Nurse*, 2(3), 6–9.

Wood, J. (1992). Elderly people in A&E. *Nursing Times*, 8(3), 62–5.

Wright, B. (1989). Sudden death. Nurses' reactions and relatives' opinions. *Bereavement Care*, 8(1), 2–4.

Wright, B. (1991). *Sudden Death: Intervention Skills for the Caring Professions*. Churchill Livingstone, Edinburgh.

Young, A.P. (1991). *Law and Professional Conduct in Nursing*. Scutari Press, London.

FURTHER READING

Cooper, M. and Robb, A. (1996). Nurse practitioners in A&E: a literature review. *Emergency Nurse*, 4(2), 19–22.

Dimond, B. (1993). Disclosure of information to the police and the accident and emergency department. *Accident and Emergency Nursing*, 1, 108–10.

Dolan, B., Dale, J. and Morley, V. (1997). Nurse practitioners: the role in A&E and primary care. *Nursing Standard*, 17(11), 33–8.

Raphael, B. (1986). *When Disaster Strikes: a Handbook for the Caring Professions*. Hutchinson, London.

Wright, B. (1988). *Management and Practice in Emergency Nursing*. Chapman & Hall, London.

CHAPTER TWENTY-FOUR

PRINCIPLES *of* ADULT NURSING

Nick Salter and Ruth Beretta

- Introduction
- Perceptions of adult patients
- The use of perception whilst caring
- Relationships
- Reassurance
- Advocacy
- Assertiveness
- Patient control and empowerment
- Holism
- Conclusion

This chapter aims to provide an insight into the role of the nurse caring for patients who are adults. Some concepts, which have been introduced elsewhere in this book, are discussed in terms of what the nurse actually does. How the nurse performs her/his psychomotor tasks and what drives her/his attentions towards patients are explored. More importantly, as it is the attitude of the nurse that dictates her/his intentions, interpersonal interaction is an underlying theme. The chapter also highlights the nature of the partnership between nurses, patients and their families. The special, individual nature of nurses' caring actions and patients' responses is also a theme.

INTRODUCTION

Patients/clients (hereafter referred to as patients) who are adults respond to illness, disease, disability, and indeed health in many and varied ways. What patients want, is not to be ill. Patients' desires were succinctly summarised by Kidel (1986, page 15) as: '...The hope of "cure" and the fastest possible restoration of "business as usual".' The variety of responses is only governed by the variety of individuals who make up the 'adult' population; 'Variety is the spice of life.' So a variety of adults are nursed by a variety of adult indi-viduals called nurses. This produces endless possibilities for different relationships between individuals. Some patients will be in need of caring, comfort and understanding. Unfortunately, these people might stereotypically be perceived as passive, demanding and dependent, in other words, patients. Patients' care should be determined by their nursing, medical and social needs, carers should not deliver care based on imagined labels. This is why accurate assessment of needs is central to the organisation of patient care. We will first investigate some of the attributes of adults that could be misperceived.

PERCEPTIONS OF ADULT PATIENTS

Many aspects of adulthood are common amongst most adults. Adults are not, however, a homogeneous set of people. Nurses might have to relinquish their preconceptions about adults in an attempt to understand that variety is normal between adults. Nurses need to be able to interpret information in relation to an individual's responses to their health care needs. We will look at some variations that exist and some links with nurses and nursing care in an attempt to highlight the importance of directing care towards individuals.

AGE

To state the obvious, nurses and adult patients have a lot in common. Young adult patients at the lower end of the accepted range of adulthood, i.e. 16 years of age, are only slightly younger than the youngest possible student nurse who could be between 17 and 18 years old. Nurses are also aged up to 65 years. All adult nurses, will therefore, care for patients who will be of a similar age to them. Not all old people act the same and not all young people act the same either. Some carers are in fact children. Disabled parents may rely on their children to do household tasks like the shop-

Box 24.1: Scenario, David Milne

David is 20 years old. He is contemplating surgery to repair a collapsed lung due to a spontaneous **pneumothorax**, which has occurred twice previously. David is very anxious about having surgery but hopes that the operation will prevent it from happening again. However, the cause of David's anxiety may not be simply the surgery. The strange surroundings of the hospital ward, being away from home, away from his wife might cause worry. When his admitting nurse has spent several short sessions talking and listening to David he reveals that he has only recently become a father. He has become acutely aware that his new role as a parent may be interrupted. He has discovered that he will have to relax for several weeks after the operation. He may not fully enjoy his new child because he will not feel fit enough. This is now causing him the most frustration and worry.

ping, cleaning and doing the laundry, in addition to the personal cleansing of their parents.

Not all adolescents are troubled by peer pressure, stress, drugs and sex. Studying and work of a positive nature might be high on their personal agenda, including nursing students. Young adults might also be parents or preparing for parenthood. Situations and relationships that do not conform to stereotypes often confront nurses. The example in Box 24.1 illustrates that little should be taken for granted.

In this situation, the nurse took time to build up a relationship and David felt able to discuss the reasons for his anxiety. The nurse might not have assumed, from his age, that he might be a parent and have associated worries.

MATURITY

With age usually comes maturity. However, this might not be the case as people 'grow up' at different speeds. Maturity might mean behaviour that is exhibited by wiser, more experienced adults. Some people, it is claimed, act like children when they are influenced by alcohol, letting their inhibitions 'go'. It is also the case that sick adults might prefer to act like dependent adults as opposed to independent adults. This is a way of adopting the sick role as described by Parsons (1951) and nurses must not perceive such an adult as weak or helpless. It might be that the patient's way of coping with such a change to his/her life is to decide to let others make decisions for him. This coping strategy needs to be recognised and through the operation of a therapeutic relationship (see Chapter 8), the nurse should be able to re-empower the patient, thus helping him/her redefine his/her locus of control and sense of dignity and independence.

SOCIAL CLASS

Even though there are many different ways of considering class in this and other societies (income, parental occupation, own occupation, Registrar General, social status, home ownership, etc.), there is a danger that nurses might apply their own measure to patients' likely class (see also Chapter 3). The danger is that a nurse might believe that the attention a patient requires is related to the patient's class. The job of a nurse is to remember that patients/clients who might not be able to attract attention might be in greater need for that attention. Stockwell (1972) pointed out it is possible to ignore patients for many reasons and give more attention to some patients to the detriment of others (see also Chapter 11). The important point is that patients have an equal right to attention from nurses despite any imagined unequal claim to attention.

INTELLECT

Patients occasionally complain that they are talked down to by an apparently patronising nurse. This may be a symptom of the nurse misunderstanding the patient's level of understanding. This could be a result of the chance that when a patient experiences a lot of uncertainty they may display helplessness and recede to a form of behaviour which belies their true demeanour. Ill health does not necessarily change the ability to reason. It is important that nurses acknowledge the patient's changing self-concept and self-esteem as a result of their illness and not assume that their intellect has altered. The patient would benefit from a nurse who develops an understanding of the patient's perception of his/her experiences in an attempt to understand his/her level of understanding. This will help the nurse to adjust her/his quality of conversation, to that which will be of greatest use to the patient.

LANGUAGE

It could be said that the English language, generally, is becoming corrupted with phrases that do not express true meanings. This contributes to confusion. An important part of the nurse–patient relationship involves deciphering what each is trying to say either verbally or in writing. Nursing students could inadvertently cause confusion in patients by using too many recently learned words which patients do not understand.

Learning new professional clinical, technical language could be exciting. Fellow students will use it in everyday conversation and doctors use it. Many situations serve to produce challenges to student nurses. Pleasure and enjoyment are often

in short supply for students. However, let the warning bells sound! Patients may not understand the jargon. Students and nurses should not use abbreviations and technical terminology to impress (French, 1994). Plain speaking is what they need. They need answers to questions. They need time, time to adjust, time to be alone, time to talk. Nurses need to listen and to talk but on the same 'wavelength' as the patient.

English might not be the patient's first language. If the patient can speak English though, time will have to be given to allow the patient try to make him/herself understood. Translators are often used to help conversation along with the patient's family. However, this can cause problems. The exact meaning and emphasis of a message might be lost during translation. The words used in this situation will have to be chosen with care so that an interpreter can understand sufficiently to enable an accurate translation.

LIFESTYLE

As we all have a 'lifestyle', a way of living that is similar to some but different from others, why should a nurse make judgements about the lifestyle of a patient or family? If there is a difference between a family's way of life who live in a detached house which has four bedrooms and another family who live in a two-roomed council bed-sit, this is not the nurse's concern. Should the nurse attempt to influence the life of either family differently? The answer should be only as it is relates to a health-related need and only if it is within the realms of possibility. A nurse should not believe that admitting a person to a hospital would solve all his/her problems; there is not the time and professionals can do only so much. Patients and their families can only be enlightened as to the possibilities that face them and how these changes might affect their lifestyle.

DISABILITY

There are two areas of importance with respect to disability. First, stereotypes of mentally and physically disabled adults perpetuate in society and there is a danger that nurses might act in response to these. Physical ability exists on a continuum from being paralysed and unconscious at one end and physically fit at the other. The operationalisation of this description is complicated. Where would a fit athlete who is blind, or who has *one arm or leg* be placed? Note the phraseology. It does not say 'only one arm or leg'. There is a danger of accentuating the negative. Of course it is possible to be physically fit and an amputee. It is also possible to be physically fit and have difficulty with vision, hearing or speaking. However, it is so easy to fall into the trap of stereotyping people as for example, 'blind' as if incapable of coping with life; or 'deaf', a 'stroke patient' as a lesser being, an amputee as being on the proverbial scrap heap! These are social injustices in which nurses should play no part. One only has to see the athletes competing each year in the Special Olympics held in Leicester to see their enthusiasm for sport, a triumph over learning difficulties. Moreover, the athletes who compete in the Para-olympics have overcome physical deformity and disability to show their capability and capacity for achievement. These achievements over adversity show how individuals with disability can be very fit and active even to an extent that exceeds the abilities of people who are not disabled in any way.

Second, people who have disabilities, for example difficulty seeing or hearing, pose special challenges to nurses. The patients might have already adapted to their difficulties. The nurse may still have to adapt her/his helping skills according to patient needs. Special ways of directing and informing such patients need to be found. Again, if these special needs are missed at assessment or are not given just priority during the process of caring, not only will the nurse–patient relationship be adversely affected but ultimately the patients' recovery could be affected.

PERSONALITY

When prospective students of nursing are interviewed for pre-registration nursing courses their personalities tend not to be tested or objectively analysed. Yet experience has shown that if patients are asked what they remember about the nurses after they have been discharged they do not comment on the tasks that were performed. The comments are about the way the tasks were performed. Statements like: 'They were very kind'; 'They made time to listen'; 'The team of nurses looking after me always seemed to be there'; 'My named nurse sat with me a lot, she seemed to care' (Morrison, 1994).

Expressions of this nature are related to the manner in which nurses carry out the tasks of nursing. However, if patients appear to appreciate a nurse's attitude and behaviour so much, this raises the question: does personality play a part in the delivery of patient care? It almost certainly does. We all work with people whom we 'get on with'. There are also people with whom we do not 'get on'. This is simply human nature. In a professional arena, 'getting on with' others is behaviour that can be learned, that is also an essential prerequisite to helping and caring for others. The nurse may have to try very hard at 'getting on' with some patients.

An important issue worth considering here is that patients usually don't have a choice about which nurse is to be theirs. They will probably have to disclose private information to a stranger. The nature of the information might also extend to that which is related to their family. So as there is little time given to patients to build up a trusting relationship with nurses, nurses must use their professional and interpersonal skills in an effort to establish a rapport quickly to help patients feel confident with their carer. Personality plays an essential role in this development of trust (Sundeen *et al.*, 1994).

One of the foundations of nursing, not just the nursing of adults, is that nursing is performed by individuals to individuals:

- Individuals need to feel that they are cared for as a person with individual needs; this means

---

Box 24.2: Reflection Points

- What do you do when you are caring for a patient and your involvement makes you feel uncomfortable?
- What do you do when you are caring for a patient and your involvement appears to make the patient uncomfortable?
- Can the physical tasks of nursing be separated from the personal approach used to perform those tasks?
- Should these two tenets be considered to be separate or integrated?
- Put another way: is clinical care given without projecting a personal manner?

that their needs are special and distinct from another's.

- Patients and their families need to know to whom they can talk about their needs.
- Nurses must aim to help patients and their families feel satisfied with the care they receive.
- A high quality personal service will ensure the patient feels important, self-confident and that he/she will be happy with the level of control he/she is able to exert over his/her care (see also Chapter 11).

MAKING ASSUMPTIONS

Simply labelling people as 'patients' can mean that others see them as dependent, stripped of status and role. This should not be the case. A patient can often be unconsciously seen in a submissive role with little or no control. This is not effective nursing care of adults.

Nurses are also in need of attention and understanding. It should never be forgotten that patients could comfort nurses and nurses can learn from patients, as they are adults with interpersonal abilities similar to those of nurses. Adult nurses probably have life experiences similar to those of their patients. It might be easy to fall into the trap and make assumptions about his/her patient's reactions to illness to believe that he/she understands the reactions. Moreover, his/her thoughts about experiences that the patient might have had could be assumed to be similar to those the nurse has experienced. Nurses must be above making assumptions. It cannot be assumed that the patient understands the health care situation he/she is in at that moment. It cannot be assumed that the patient wants to be there or that he/she even wants to undergo the treatment regimen that has been prescribed by medical and nursing staff. It should also be remembered that patients are mostly voluntary 'guests' and can opt out at any time. They bring with them their own abilities and intentions that should be utilised when planning interventions that contribute to their care and the resultant outcomes of their care.

Knowledge about interactions will help the nurse to adjust her/his approach to giving information to and getting information from the patient.

Key Points

- Adult nurses have a lot in common with their adult patients but there is a danger that similarities and differences could be assumed or taken for granted.
- The patient population exhibits a normal variation of physical, psychological and behavioural abilities. Nurses must accept disability as normal variant because many patients will adapt and live contentedly. Others will need help to adopt a different body image and self-confidence.
- Nurses should attempt to discover how a patient communicates so they can understand each other. This task may not be easy. The problem may be a simple one of language or one that will require time and patience from the nurse or patient.

THE USE OF PERCEPTION WHILST CARING

Perception is the product of our mind's interpretation of the messages it receives from our senses. Neuronal impulses from our five senses – sight, smell, hearing, taste and touch – are combined within our brains to inform us of our place within our world. The mind interprets the messages from our senses and selects those which are most important to us at any one time.

The mind has the vital facility to be selective; it allows us to concentrate our attention. How attentive we are to a situation will influence our perception of a situation. Professional caring involves being aware of this faculty because this leads to the understanding that selective attention to a situation or an issue which is thought to be important to a nurse but which might not be so to the patient or vice versa. Try this next reflective exercise.

Box 24.3: Reflective Exercise

Pause for a minute. Read these instructions, then close your eyes. Be aware of the messages you are receiving from your senses.

- What sounds do you hear?
- What can you smell?
- What can you taste?

- Think about the position of your limbs and your body generally.
- Are you comfortable?
- Can you feel the texture of the clothes you are wearing?
- Is anything tight or loose?
- **Open your eyes at this time.**
- Look at the colours surrounding you.
- Look at the shapes, furniture.
- Do you feel hungry or thirsty?

You may have noticed that it is difficult to focus on all your senses at the same time.

To put this knowledge into a clinical scenario: when feeling a patient's pulse it is possible to sense much more than a rhythmic pulsation of the radial artery. It is possible to:

- Feel the temperature of the skin
- Feel the dryness/wetness of the skin's surface
- Feel the hairs on the skin
- Feel the elasticity of the skin
- Feel the relative thinness/thickness of the wrist
- Smell possible body odour
- Hear if the patient is talking or making noises
- See the non-verbal signals given by the patient's facial expressions
- See the colour of the skin.

These senses may help the nurse to make assumptions and inferences, which affect perceptions that might affect problem-solving and decision making with or for the patient. For example:

1 If a patient's skin is hot, is he/she pyrexial?
2 If he/she is cold, is the peripheral circulation 'shut down' as in heart failure?
3 If it is dry, is he/she dehydrated?
4 If it is wet, is he/she perspiring; is he/she worried?
5 If he/she is hirsute, the nurse might need to remind the doctor to shave the skin before inserting a venous cannula, or recording an **electrocardiogram**?
6 If there is a loss of skin turgor, is this through the ageing process or is the patient dehydrated?
7 Does the thinness of the wrist signify a loss of weight; does a relative thickness represent muscle mass or fat and obesity?
8 Does body odour represent stress or a lack of personal cleansing?
9 What inferences can be made from the verbal and non-verbal communication received during this procedure of taking a pulse?
10 What may be the causes of **cyanosis**, pallor or jaundice?

The relatively simple procedure of taking a patient's pulse involves responding to a range of interpersonal cues, which can influence the judgements that the nurse makes. If the nurse can sense body odour, he/she could believe the patient is generally unkempt and this could lead to stereotyping the patient as one who might not comply with the therapeutic regimen. This of course would be wrong but it might happen if the nurse is not conscious of the fact that the *way he/she* thinks can affect his/her judgements.

Your attention is dependent on your interest, this is important also when you are interviewing a patient. Interviewing patients is a complex task. Patients perceive events differently from nurses and it can be a difficult endeavour to perceive events from a patient's perspective. The case of Fred Law illustrates this issue.

Box 24.4: Scenario, Fred Law

Fred has been breathless for some time and on admission, he appears acutely anxious. He is fidgeting around the bed and his eyes are looking in all directions as if he has lost something. Nurse Holmes initially attributed his anxiety to the fear which she thinks is usually induced by the unfamiliar hospital environment and his medical condition so she dismisses it as expected, understandable and not an issue that requires further questioning.

This could have been a mistake. Nurse Holmes should have clarified her perception with Fred. Fred might have accepted his breathlessness but is actually worried about the dog that he had to leave at his home as he did not have time to arrange anyone to look after its needs. If Nurse Holmes does not discover Fred's worries he might become increasingly anxious and his breathlessness might become worse.

Box 24.5: Reflection Points

- Is it easy to see events from the patient's perspective?
- How could patients' perceptions affect the way they behave?
- What affects nurses' perceptions of patients?

Box 24.6: Reflective Exercise

Try to think about these questions during your clinical practice. It is not easy because tasks of nursing tend to take priority at work. To overcome this, make a few notes in a diary, you could start with the questions above. On a couple of days each week make an effort to address your noted issues and make reflective notes in answer to your own questions.

Patients' awareness of their surroundings is often heightened in hospital because their consciousness is focused, for example, on strange events, sights and smells. If they hear their name mentioned even in the distance, their attention will focus on it. This can increase the stress the patient feels. If the nurse is aware of this effect, he/she can interpret for the patient, explain sights and smells and help the patient to understand what he/she might expect to see, feel, smell and hear. A patient's fear and anxiety will be reduced if he/she knows what is about to happen: he/she will be able to prepare him/herself for something new or feared.

Getting used to a new environment can be tiring at the best of times. Moreover, patients are usually in an environment they do not wish to be in. If they are in pain or at least a situation of expectancy, this will almost certainly be exhausting. Patients also find themselves surrounded by strangers and when all the routines are new, it is a wonder how patients cope. Of course, some do not cope very well. Again, the mind does filter out events, sights and sounds that do not hold any interest for the patient. This often leaves him/her wondering and worrying about a few issues that his/her mind will have made priorities. These will often form the basis for his/her questions. The nurse must be prepared for the fact that once the important questions (important to the patient) have been answered there will certainly be more to come.

When nurses become used to an environment, it becomes more difficult to appreciate it from a new patient's perspective. A ward might seem busy to a nurse but to a patient, who has not received much attention, the same ward may not seem busy. The patient might feel frustrated that his/her questions are met with an 'I'll be back later we can talk then' response. Not surprisingly, the patient loses interest, often becomes increasingly agitated, becoming less trusting, and can appear to be awkward. The following example illustrates the importance of recognising needs from the patient's perspective.

Box 24.7: Scenario, David Freeman

In his forties, David Freeman was a regular patient on the medical ward. He suffered with **emphysema** and frequently needed intravenous antibiotics, nebulisers, oxygen therapy and **postural drainage**. David was very popular with all the ward staff, always laughing and joking and would help out other patients whenever he could.

However, it was obvious with each admission that David was taking longer to respond to treatment and his wife and family were increasingly anxious about him.

During one of David's admissions, he was given oxygen overnight and his capillary blood was monitored for its oxygen concentration (**capillary blood oxygenation**). Despite the oxygen mask and monitoring equipment, he slept well and awoke bright, breezy and cracking his usual jokes. David's consultant recommended that he try using oxygen each night at home, as it might improve the respite between admissions. David's wife was also enthusiastic, but David refused and became very quiet. He was discharged home the following day.

However, David was not home for long. He was readmitted 2 days later, extremely short of breath and cyanosed. He was obviously upset and close to tears. 'It's no good,' said David, 'I'm just not going to make it.' The staff nurse explained again to him that using oxygen overnight at home might make all the difference to him and he would sleep more easily, wake refreshed which would reduce the strain on his heart.

'I know all this,' said David, 'and you're right but what about my wife? She won't want to sleep with me wearing that great big mask in bed.' He burst into tears.

In this situation, all the ward staff learned how important it was to see their patients as individuals. No-one had even thought of how an oxygen mask would interfere with David's sexuality, let alone considering David's right to a sex life. His problem was overcome by wearing nasal cannulae at night, which his wife also found much more acceptable.

You should understand the patient's needs, from the patient's perspective. Clarify your own interpretation so you understand as well as possible.

Prepare the patient, and apply nursing care specifically, individually, with thought and a positive attitude. Work with the patient to achieve the best possible results. They might not be what were first intended and you might not solve all the problems. The patient should be happy and contented about the care he/she has received. Evaluation of the care with the patient will show where success has been achieved and hopefully both parties will have benefited from their experiences.

These issues highlight the fact that nurse–patient interactions should occur in a relevant fashion. The nurse needs to ascertain what the patient is likely to need and this is not simply in a physical sense. Clarification of the nurse's perceptions should be sought from the patient to reassure the nurse that he/she perceives the needs as the patient does.

There also needs to be recognition that the patient may not know what is best for him/her at any given time. This lends power to the argument that nurses need knowledge, not just knowledge about health and illness, though the acquisition of these is never ending, but knowledge about interactions themselves.

To do all this, there needs to be a relationship between the nurse and patient. In some respects, this could be seen as the most important adjunct to successful nursing.

Key Points

- Caring can involve the five senses.
- We see what we want to see.
- Selective attention allows focussing.
- Nurses' perceptions can be wrong.
- Interpretations and clarification help the nurse to gain an understanding of the patient's concerns.
- Patients are all different.
- Patients need to be perceived without the bias of labels.
- An understanding of perception is essential to facilitate an:
    - appreciation of the uniqueness of people,
    - accurate assessment of needs on which to base care,
    - improvement in patients'/clients' compliance,
  because:
    - patients perceptions determines their reactions,
    - patients have equal rights to the highest standard of care possible.

RELATIONSHIPS

Communication is the vehicle of relationships. See also Chapter 8. However, for communication to help both the patient and the nurse the patient has to be willing to form a relationship (Sundeen et al., 1994). The nurse might have to work hard at helping the patient feel that he/she can talk to the nurse. Communication is not however *the* relationship. Communicated thoughts and feelings are the relationship. There is often a physical side to a relationship, which might be important, but this is not essential for a relationship to exist – after all relationships do exist between people who have never physically met, for example, pen pals. This is borne out when someone dies. A relationship existed whilst the person was alive because it could be communicated in some way, even if this was in a tactile fashion. However, after the death of the person the relationship ceases to be. The relation to the dead person remains, but the interpersonal relationship dies as the thoughts and feelings cannot be communicated to or from the deceased.

The very presence of a nurse and a patient produces a relationship. On the one hand, there may be simply a social relationship if the nurse has no professional interest in the patient. A therapeutic relationship is that which nurses develop as part of his/her caring role to provide an environment conducive to the maintenance and improvement in the patient's health state. Rapport must exist between the two or more partners in care. Purtilo (1984) underlined the need for nurses to understand the dynamics of the different types of relationships. The therapeutic relationship will succeed only if nurses interpret their perceptions and the perceptions the patient holds.

A social relationship is that which is linked to helping another. Providing general information, directions, assisting their movement around the hospital and assisting the patient and family to access the facilities provided by the services. These might be the bank, shop and toilets, etc.

Table 24.1 represents the factors that develop during relationships. Nurses must prepare themselves not only to recognise the dynamics of relationship-building but also that relationships end. The end of nurse–patient relationships should be the recognition that the goals set for patient care have been met. Patients should be helped to adapt

Table 24.1: Correlation of concepts during helping relationships

	Beginning phase	**Working phase**	**Termination phase**
Purpose	Unclear – sharing of perceptions	Developing, identifying goals	Clarity – review of goals
Trust	Limited – based on past experiences	Growing, testing out	Falters, they can grow stronger
Empathy	Difficult due to lack of awareness	Occurs more frequently due to more successful communication	Helps the termination – allows more accurate expression of feelings
Caring	Initially non-specific and superficial	Grows steadily	Shared by both if successful
Autonomy	Both act autonomously – unsure of what each can give	Sharing means some autonomy is given up by each	Enhanced autonomous behaviour through mutual learning
Mutuality	Limited – tentative sharing because they are unaware of each other	High – sharing of feelings and information	Given up – each regains independence

Adapted from Sundeen *et al.*, 1994, page 221.

to the changes they have experienced and nurses hopefully will have learned and developed as a result of meeting and caring for them.

Key Points

- The basis for relationships is communication.
- The nurse needs to become expert in forming and concluding relationships.
- Relationships are fragile and essential to the outcome of care.

REASSURANCE

Trusting relationships can develop through the use of reassuring actions performed by nurses. Reassurance is one of the most abused and misunderstood words in nursing vocabulary. Student nurses internalise its importance very early in their education. They learn to use the word in conversation and in essays, yet they find it very hard to explain what it is, let alone how to do it and how it involves patients.

Nursing students' essays sometimes contain the words: 'I will reassure the patient.' What is the student trying to say? These words explain nothing of the nurse's approach, attitude or appearance to the patient, nor do they indicate exactly how the nurse hopes to reassure the patient or how the nurse would know whether the patient had been reassured.

Registered nurses are expected by society to know the rationale for care, how to practise to produce the best possible outcome for the patient. Simply to write 'Reassure the patient' in a care plan possibly shows a lack of awareness of what the patient requires, when the patient requires it, and why the patient requires it.

Analyses of the concept of reassurance have been performed in the past. In 1955, Gregg (cited by French, 1979) saw the need to examine the concept and 24 years later French (1979) investigated the practice of reassurance. A decade later, Teasdale (1989) identified three ways of using the word reassurance:

1 As a noun, a renewed or repeated assurance (a reassurance)
2 As a verb, a purposeful attempt to restore confidence (giving reassurance)
3 As a noun, a state of mind (producing reassurance).

To gain an understanding of what reassuring does to patients the following words used in a similar context can be useful:

- To cheer, to gladden, warm the heart, comfort, console, encourage, give confidence
- Being kind or gentle or benevolent, friendly affectionate
- Being calm, self-confident
- Being efficient, competent
- Being caring, show concern or interest (expressed or implied), having regard for, showing concern
- Being supportive, keep from failing, give strength to, encourage, supply with necessaries, and provide for
- Being honest, sincere in speech and action
- Being comforting, consoling, saving trouble, soothing (Dutch, 1966).

When nurses attempt to reassure they should:

- Have a positive attitude towards the patients
- Perceive patients as valuable people
- Exhibit positive interpersonal skills towards or on behalf of patients
- Possess knowledge related to the cause of anxiety.

The case in Box 24.8, involving Mr Sharp, is an example of reassuring a patient.

Box 24.8: Scenario, Henry Sharp

Mr Sharp is an elderly man who is being supported by his named nurse Pauline Yates whilst walking to the toilet. Henry complains that he thinks he will not be able to walk all the way. Nurse Yates believes that he can walk that far and offers Henry some encouragement, saying that she will not let go of him. Nurse Yates offers Henry a chance to sit down midway to rest but he declines, saying that he feels that he will make it now as he knows she will help him.

Nurse Yates clearly offered reassurance to Henry; she offered him physical and psychological support in her encouragement. Henry felt confident as a result, confident enough to refuse the rest.

A similar example is described in Box 24.9.

The point here is that Nurse Shah might not be aiming to achieve a state of reassurance in Joan but this has been achieved somewhat because of the impression gained. Joan gained a sense of trust in the nurse not by design but by abstraction. A trusting relationship between patient and nurse

Box 24.9: Scenario, Mrs Joan Bloom

Joan feels very apprehensive about being admitted to a hospital ward. She wonders if the nurses will treat her as an individual or just a number as that is what happened to her mother a few years ago. Nurse Shah is attending to a patient in the next bed. She is sitting beside that patient, talking quietly, calmly and smiling as she attempts to get to know the patient. Joan sees that the Nurse Shah is smartly dressed, knowledgeable, polite and is interested in her patient. This helps Joan to relax, she now believes that nurses will not only care for her but also care about her and she feels more confident and trusting.

may be the key to the beliefs held by the patient and the success of reassuring actions by the nurse (Price, 1965). Furthermore, nursing care is goal-orientated but the state of reassurance, although being a goal, might not necessarily be achieved; it depends entirely on the disposition of the patient.

The state of reassurance the patient experiences (the noun reassurance) occurs when increased self-confidence is believed or internalised. A state of reassurance is something different from reassuring actions, in that a state of mind cannot be given to someone; it has to be experienced by the patient. Patients may feel reassured if they:

- Feel happy with their predicament
- Feel more secure
- Feel at ease with situations and surroundings
- Feel less anxious, less uneasy, less worried about the present and the future.

An example of *this* reassurance is illustrated in Box 24.10.

In this example, care and assistance achieved the goal, the state of reassurance. Initial assurance had been given, reassurances were given and

Box 24.10: Scenario, Tony Brooks

When the plaster cast on Tony's fractured ankle had been removed his primary nurse, Julie showed him how to move the injured ankle and the physiotherapist helped by instructing him in the use of a walking stick. Tony used to be worried that he might not walk again but Julie had previously assured him that he would. He now feels more confident; he feels that Julie was right because he can walk again.

eventually the state of reassurance was achieved. This was manifested by Tony's increased trust in the staff because he realised that their earlier assurances were correct and he proved to himself that he could walk; together they had produced the state of reassurance.

As this example illustrates, it is important for teams of nurses to be aware of the messages each individual gives to individual patients. Patients will make judgements about the consistency of the messages they receive, in this case in relation to whether they feel reassured by those messages.

Key Points

- An assurance is an optimistic statement not necessarily aimed at producing a state of reassurance.
- An assurance may be given even if a patient's confidence or anxiety is not seen as a matter of concern to either patient or nurse.
- An assurance can be repeated in which case it (academically) becomes a reassurance.
- A nurse might reassure a patient intentionally or not, by his/her actions or merely by his/her professional presence.
- Nurses should at least consider whether the patient has attained a state of being reassured to know that they have been successful, because actions may need to be changed during the reassuring process.
- A nurse can give reassurances to a patient but it is the patient's belief in those reassurances or reassuring behaviours that will determine their success, it is only the patient who can confirm a state of reassurance.

ADVOCACY

When nurses and patients are involved in discussions aimed at promoting reassurance they might not be discussing facts or beliefs, but giving and receiving incidental conversation unrelated to the patient's health. They might be attempting to help the patient feel at ease. When patients trust nurses, nurses will be in a better place to act on their behalf of the patient. This is patient advocacy.

The nurse acting as an advocate for his/her patients has become a popular theme and almost a catch phrase for nursing in the 1990s. The Web-

ster Universal Dictionary (1975) defines advocacy as 'the act of pleading the cause for another.' The RCN (1995) suggests advocacy is the process of acting for, or on behalf of, someone. The word advocacy is not specifically used in the UKCC Code of Conduct (1992). It is implied in the first clause where nurses, midwives and health visitors exercising professional accountability must:

> '... act always in such a manner as to promote and safeguard the interests and well-being of patients; (advocacy) ... Advocacy also involves providing support if the patient refuses treatment/care or withdraws their consent.'
> (UKCC, 1996, page 13)

Although a fairly new concept in nursing, the literature demonstrates there are established advocacy movements outside nursing:

1 *Legal advocacy*: related to legal practice and may involve tribunals and court cases.
2 *Self-advocacy*: Gates (1994) identifies that in self-advocacy the advocate or facilitator shifts the focus of control to people he is working with to enable them to speak for themselves. This model has been used successfully in working with people with learning disabilities.
3 *Collective or class advocacy*: This is a large, well-organised group who speak out on behalf of a category of people. Their work may involve fund raising, information giving and lobbying parliament and include such groups as SCOPE and MENCAP.
4 *Citizen advocacy*: These are trained, selected advocates who act on behalf of those unable to defend their own rights. Some authors suggest nurses are citizen advocates to patients, although the RCN (1995) sees nurses as professional advocates, in the same way as social workers or case workers.

Advocacy is an important principle in nursing adult patients because it makes it clear that generally, adults are rational. Adults are capable of making choices and making decisions; however, some illnesses and situations they are in, may mean they lose a certain amount of autonomy and need a person to speak for them. That person might be a nurse. The example in Box 24.11 demonstrates this point.

Patients are sometimes treated in ways which undermine them as adults, and doctors and nurses

Box 24.11: Scenario, Miss Hanson

Miss Hanson was a retired headmistress of a primary school admitted to the medical ward following a stroke that had left her unable to speak, although she understood everything said to her. Sandra, one of the student nurses on the ward, recognised Miss Hanson and remembered her from school as a particularly organised lady, who took a lot of pride in her appearance. She was a teacher who had always commanded the attention of her pupils.

Sandra thought it was very sad to hear the nurses call Miss Hanson 'a good girl' when she obediently took her medication, even though Miss Hanson obviously disapproved. Sandra wished she had the courage to tell the other staff what Miss Hanson was really like and how she thought she would really like to be treated.

Box 24.12: Scenario, Mr Smithers

Mr Smithers had been admitted to the medical ward with **congestive cardiac failure**. He was very ill when he arrived; he needed oxygen and intravenous diuretics to help rid him of pulmonary and systemic **oedema**. He was attached to a cardiac monitor which caused him to be very frightened. Part of his management was a strict oral fluid restriction of 750 ml per day.

On his third day on the ward, one of the auxiliary nurses overheard some of his conversation with his wife, who was visiting. She was trying to reassure him that the nurses really did care about him and he was imagining that they were ignoring him.

'Oh how can you say that?' asked Mr. Smithers indignantly. 'The drinks trolley has been round four times today and I have only had one drink – they didn't even ask me if I wanted one at the other times. And I haven't even got a glass of water left here!'

None of the nurses or medical staff had explained to Mr and Mrs Smithers the fluid restriction or the reasoning behind it, because no one had thought they would understand. The auxiliary nurse rushed over to tell Mr Smithers' nurse so they could remedy the situation.

assume they would not understand about their condition, its care and management even if they were told, so do not bother to tell them. The case of Mr Smithers (Box 24.12) is such an example.

It is easy to see how the nurse acting as an advocate was acting to promote and safeguard the interests and well-being of Miss Hanson and Mr Smithers. However, other authors suggest the advocate has another role, and that is 'to inform the client and support him in whatever decision he makes' (Gadow, 1980). So, in this instance, the nurse should give the patient information and where possible, the patient decides if and how to act upon it. The case of Mrs Jones (Box 24.13, page 602) will show this.

In the case of Mrs Jones, it would have been easy for Sister Brown to try to persuade her to accept treatment, saying it was her only option. In acting as her advocate, Sister Brown was making sure Mrs Jones and her family knew all the relevant facts before leaving them to decide what to do next, without feeling pressurised into accepting treatment.

In health care terms, patients wish to receive information to help them to make decisions about the choices that they are going to encounter. A patient requires an estimate of how much time will be required for the procedure or test(s). The nurse may be asked to describe the experiences that are about to occur, for example, is there going to be any pain or discomfort? Is the patient going to be asked to do something different from what

has become normal for him/her? Treatment might necessitate a bandage or dressing that needs to be kept dry. A shower might need to be taken rather than a bath for the following week. A period off work might be prescribed, but for how long and are there going to be any restrictions on the patient's normal way of life?

Disease and illness do change people and their outlook on life (Cribb *et al.*, 1994). Moreover, families as a whole need to adapt to change often for undetermined times and there may need to be permanent changes and the likely benefits to the patient and the family may be unknown.

Now consider the points raised in Box 24.14 (page 602).

Acting as a patient's advocate involves difficulties that may be of a legal, ethical or professional nature. Acting for or on behalf of someone has the tendency to be paternalistic. It may be that the best the nurse can achieve is to make sure his/her patient has sufficient information and then lets him/her decide on a course of action.

It may also be difficult to advocate for the patient who is advised to quit smoking, or to follow a low fat diet, or to take more exercise for a healthier

Box 24.13: Scenario, Mrs Jones

Mrs Jones was a 64-year-old grandmother of three girls, and had been admitted to the medical ward for investigations of a persistent cough. Her chest X-ray demonstrated a sizeable shadow and further investigations revealed an inoperable tumour. The medical staff told Mrs Jones that she had a lung cancer, which could be treated by chemotherapy and radiotherapy.

Mrs Jones was obviously shocked by the news. She had been widowed 12 years earlier when her husband was killed in an industrial accident, and since then, she had busied herself with her daughters and granddaughters. She was unsure what to do now. She asked Sister Brown if she would explain the treatment again to her, whilst her daughters were present. Sister Brown readily agreed and set up the meeting.

Sister Brown told Mrs Jones and her daughters how often the chemotherapy would be given, what it would make her feel like and the possible side-effects. She explained that blood tests would need to be taken regularly to check the effect of the chemotherapy and that this would continue over a considerable period. One of Mrs Jones' daughters asked Sister Brown if this was a definite cure for her mother. Sister Brown had to reply that although many previous cases had had successful outcomes, it could not be guaranteed as a cure. She left the family to discuss the situation.

On the following doctors' ward round, Mrs Jones asked to be discharged home. She said she now knew the significance of her condition, and what the treatment for the cancer involved. She now wanted time to be at home with her family to decide whether to proceed.

Box 24.14: Reflection Points

- How does advocacy differ from good patient education or good patient care?
- Is the nurse in the best position to act as advocate to her/his patients?
- Can nurses truly be advocates for their patients if they choose a course of action that is clearly not in their best interests?

ASSERTIVENESS

Speaking up for patients involves communication with many other nurses, doctors, physiotherapists, occupational therapists, medical social workers and many other health care professionals. This is not always as simple as it may seem. Nurses might experience differences of opinion, differences of knowledge or experience that can affect advice or assistance that is given and the nurses' feelings of satisfaction. The ability to be assertive will help to maintain mutual respect and help to lead the discussions towards a conclusion, which leaves each party satisfied with the decisions.

Assertiveness training can be found in many nurse training programmes, and qualified nurses are attending post-registration courses aimed at 'asking for what you want'. Nurses have traditionally been seen as doctors' 'handmaidens'. This is a view perpetuated by the fact that, particularly in the care of adults with physical illnesses, the majority of nurses have been female. They were seen as subservient to medical staff who in the past have been mostly male (Salvage, 1990).

However, many people wrongly assume that being assertive equates with being aggressive and that undergoing training in using an assertive approach will somehow change their personalities. Some nurses have even been accused of 'jumping on the feminist bandwagon' when asking assertively for something they want or standing up for themselves. The point is, though, that being assertive means that we should be able to respect our own rights and, at the same time, respect those of other people (Bond, 1986).

Bond (1988) outlined twelve rights and responsibilities of an assertive stance. It is important to realise that everyone as equals have these rights.

lifestyle, if he/she decides not to take this advice. The nurse then might consider it necessary to tell the patient which is the best course of action.

Key Points

- Illness and disease might reduce the autonomy or self-control of the patient.
- There are times when patients' best interests are served by the nurse acting on their behalf.
- Giving patients information will help them to make their own decisions.
- Being an advocate might not be easy and can involve difficult decisions and dilemmas.

1   I have the right to express myself provided I do not set out to hurt or put others down in the process ... So does everyone else.

2   I have the right to be treated with respect as an intelligent, capable human being ... So does everyone else.

3   I have the right to state my own needs and priorities as a person whatever other people expect of me because of my roles in life ... So does everyone else.

4   I have the right to deal with people without having to make them like or approve of me ... So does everyone else.

5   I have the right to express my opinions and values ... So does everyone else.

6   I have the right to express my emotions when I decide the time and place is right for me to do ... So does everyone else.

7   I have the right to ask for what I want ... So does everyone else.

8   I have the right to say 'yes' or 'no' for myself ... So does everyone else.

9   I have the right to be fallible (wrong) ... So does everyone else.

10 I have the right to change my mind ... So does everyone else.

11 I have the right to say, 'I don't understand' ... So does everyone else.

12 I have the right to decide for myself whether I am responsible for finding a solution to another person's problem ... So does everyone else.

Nurses often feel that they should stand up for the rights of their patients, but are unsure about standing up for themselves or confessing to uncertainty. The UKCC Code of Professional Conduct (UKCC, 1992) makes it quite clear that nurses have the right to state when they are unsure of an aspect of practice and should not be belittled when they do so. Nurses should:

'Acknowledge any limitations in your knowledge and competence and decline any duties or responsibilities unless able to perform them in a safe and skilled manner.'

(UKCC, 1992, Clause 4)

Likewise, not only must nurses always demonstrate accountability for their own practice, but credit individual patients with their own rights. Again, nurses should:

'Recognise and respect the uniqueness and dignity of each patient and client, and respond to their need for care, irrespective of their ethnic origin, religious beliefs, personal attributes, the nature of their health problems or any other factor.'

(UKCC, 1992, Clause 7)

An obvious example of this occurred in the case of Mr Ahmed (Box 24.15).

For nurses to need to respect the rights of their patients reinforces the implication that people could lose these rights simply by virtue of them becoming patients. On admission to a hospital ward, patients are often instructed to change out of their clothes and wear clothing which would

---

Box 24.15: Scenario, Razack Ahmed

Razack had lived in Britain since 1966, but as his family all spoke English and carried out the weekly shopping, he and his wife had never needed to learn the language.

Razack was admitted to the medical ward for stabilisation of his high blood pressure. He had been prescribed medication by his GP, but because he felt well, he never thought it necessary to continue with the tablets. He was now starting to experience double vision and it was considered to be in his interests to admit him for rest, observation and to make sure he complied with his prescribed treatment.

Razack was in a bay of five other patients, but no one spoke his language. One of the night staff nurses and a radiographer could communicate with him, but otherwise he would spend many long, lonely hours waiting for his visitors. He was not resting and his blood pressure remained high. Not only that, hospital meals were scarcely able to meet Razack's strict dietary requirements.

When chatting with Razack in the early hours of the morning, the night staff nurse Brenda, identified how unhappy he was. She arranged through consultation with day staff and Razack's family, for a member of his family to come to visit him each mealtime. They would bring food from home with them and take time out away from the ward to stroll around the hospital.

Razack was very pleased at the outcome. He felt staff had taken time and trouble to consider him and his particular needs. His wife was pleased because she could continue to provide his meals. Razack rested in between visits and made good progress.

normally only be worn in bed at night and seen only by their nearest and dearest. Routines are imposed, such as times for meals, time to go to bed, and times to wake up and bath or shower. Visitors may be given access at restricted times and patients may be subjected to medical and nursing ward rounds, may be required to answer intimate questions and may be exposed to what is often frightening, medical jargon.

The Patient's Charter (DoH, 1991) has made the protection of patients' rights much more explicit. Like any other service, the Charter informed the public of what they could and should expect of the National Health Service and the action to take if this is unsatisfactory.

Box 24.16: Reflection Points

- How easy is it for nurses to use an assertive approach in their day-to-day work?
- To what extent do you think people expect to keep their rights as individuals when admitted to hospital as patients?

Key Points

- Being assertive means that we should be able to value our own rights and, at the same time, respect those of other people.
- Patients' rights can be eroded on admission to hospital; nurses should strive to minimise this.
- Patients should be encouraged to become assertive, to ask for what they believe they need.

PATIENT CONTROL AND EMPOWERMENT

A recent definition of empowerment suggests it to be:

'The notion of people having power to take action to control their own lives, and the processes of enabling them to do so.'
(Grace, 1991, cited in Porter, 1994)

In one of the best known and often-quoted definitions of nursing, Virginia Henderson (1977) alluded to patient control and empowerment:

'The unique function of the nurse is to assist the individual, sick or well, in the performance of those activities contributing to health or its recovery (or to a peaceful death) that he would perform unaided if he had the necessary strength, will or knowledge. And to do this in such a way as to help him gain independence as rapidly as possible.'
(Henderson, 1977, page 4)

Henderson (1977) identifies nursing, not as something nurses do to patients, but that which is done with patients, so that they can take an active part in their recovery and strive to maintain their own health. Therefore, patients must have a certain amount of knowledge and control over their care. The UKCC (1992) states in Clause 5 of the Code of Professional Conduct that nurses, midwives and health visitors should:

'Work in an open and co-operative manner with patients/clients and their families, foster their independence and recognise and respect their involvement in the planning and delivery of care.'

There are many reasons for promoting patient empowerment:

- *The Health of the Nation* initiative (HMSO, 1992), now referred to as 'Our Healthier Nation' (England, 1997, page 152), aims to improve the health of the population by developing the Alma-Ata Declaration of 'Health for All by the Year 2000' (WHO, 1978). Its aim is that life expectancy be increased and premature death reduced by targeting five key areas: cancer; heart disease and stroke; mental illness; HIV/AIDS and sexual health; and accidents. Issues such as smoking, diet, exercise, drug misuse, stress, high blood pressure and high risk sexual activity have been drawn to the public's attention to encourage them to act to reduce deaths by these means. Leaflets were sent to every household with information on healthy eating, the dangers of smoking and excessive use of alcohol, the benefits of regular exercise, etc. The public is being encouraged to take an active part in health maintenance (DoH, 1986).
- The Patient's Charter (DoH, 1991) sets out patients' rights and expectations within the National Health Service. The public are being encouraged to see themselves as consumers of health care – and to treat the service as they would the telephone or gas company and complain if dissatisfied.

- Internal changes within the NHS have meant that patients are being discharged home much more quickly, often after day surgery, rather than endure a protracted stay in hospital after surgery. This means there are greater pressures within the NHS in terms of not only efficiency and effectiveness in hospitals, but also the reliance on community health services because of earlier discharges.

Many of these reasons can be seen to be political and rooted in economics. Aiming to make the patient/client take more responsibility for his/her own health may also help to reduce the ever-increasing burden on the NHS:

'Moving from a sickness service to a health service, professionals have to move from being paternalistic providers to becoming health facilitators.'
(Greenwell, cited in Soothill *et al.*, 1995)

This has had a huge impact on the way the nurse caring for adults carries out his/her role. There is a heavy emphasis on making sure patients have enough information about their condition. This often involves a chronic condition, which means that if a patient wants to take control of his/her life and illness, there might have to be a lot of family-centred care within the community, as can be seen in the case of Susan Kershaw (Box 24.17).

Box 24.17: Scenario, Susan Kershaw

Susan was almost 20 when diagnosed as an insulin-dependent diabetic. She was due to be married in the next month and she and her fiancé had been busily decorating the small terraced house they had bought. Susan thought her tiredness was due to all the hard work of decorating and the running around organising the church, flowers, bridesmaids' dresses and myriad of other things for the wedding.

A routine urine test at her health screening appointment arranged through work found glucose in her urine, and Susan was quickly diagnosed. She was admitted to the medical ward to begin insulin injections and to be taught how to manage her diabetes at home. This included how to manage her diet and insulin injections, how to test her blood and urine and how to recognise hypoglycaemia. It was important for Susan and her nurse to get on well so that Susan could learn as quickly as possible how to be independent and get on with her life.

Patients like Susan are often only admitted to hospital for initial education or if they develop complications. Most of their management is carried out at home with regular visits to the clinic and the diabetic nurse specialist. These patients usually get to know more about their condition than most nurses and medical staff, and can decide when to make adjustments in their diet and insulin dosages to manage their lives effectively, and without complication. They are very much in control.

This concept of partnership between the nurse and patient is part of what Salvage (1990) has identified as the 'New Nursing'. Nurses are no longer seen as 'experts' and in authority over patients, who have traditionally been passive and obedient. Nursing development units (NDUs), such as the one at Burford (Johns, 1994), identified nursing philosophies that developed around partnerships and power-sharing with patients. NDUs invite cooperation of patients during the process of policy making and the process of care giving. Patients' involvement can be challenging to professionals. If professionals do not feel that they have to be perfect, they are less challenged by patient involvement, complaints and ideas can be better managed and the outcomes better tailored to meeting individual patient needs (Wright, 1995).

IS EMPOWERMENT ALWAYS BEST?

It should be remembered that not all patients wish to be or can be empowered. Some, such as those in intensive care units, may simply not be well enough to take control of their own care. Others are not capable of understanding what is required. Moreover, some patients may not want to take control, believing that 'nurse knows best'.

Malin and Teasdale (1991) argue that empowering patients may be contradictory to caring for them. They suggest that some patients may find it frightening to know everything about their condition and care. The nurse may face a dilemma in deciding how much information and power to hand over to such patients, and how much information to withhold to 'protect' them.

Box 24.18: Reflection Points

■ To what extent do patients want to be partners in their care?

■ Are nurses always able to empower their patients?

Key Points

■ Nursing entails working with patients and families for the good of the patient and his/her family.

■ Patients require knowledge to help themselves.

■ The public through the Health of the Nation (HMSO, 1992) is encouraged to take an active part in health maintenance.

■ The reliance on services in the community will be reduced if patients can become more self caring.

■ Some patients are not in a position to become empowered or are unwilling to become empowered.

■ The nurse has to decide how much information to give to the patient and how much to withhold for the 'patient's good'.

■ Nurses may not have sufficient resources, or even have power themselves to hand over to patients.

HOLISM

We decided to address the topic of holism here to facilitate the amalgamation of many of the concepts and practices that have been discussed earlier in this chapter. It is not our belief that holism should be the byword for all nurses of adult patients; indeed, there are times when holistic nursing practices are not possible or are irrelevant. There are also many constraints to practising holistic nursing. The link between holism and this chapter is that the nursing of adults requires of the nurse skills, knowledge and attitudes: skills to communicate, relate, appreciate and perform actions with and for patients; knowledge of what to do, how to do it and why to do it, when to do it and where it can be done; an attitude that patients have equal rights to attention and, more importantly, are the centre of attention. Nurses do not care alone: they are but one spoke in the proverbial wheel of caring personnel. Patients and their families also play a major part in recovery. If nurses were to internalise the issues highlighted in this chapter, patients would be

valued more, will be better cared for and nurses will gain more satisfaction from the outcomes of their care.

To investigate holism we will first look at the root meaning of the word to 'nurse' which is to 'nourish'. Nightingale defined a nurse as 'Anyone who cares for the sick' which was usually a member of the family.

She would have liked another word for the concept of nursing;

'I use the word Nurse for want of a better, it has been limited to signify little more than the administration of medicines and the application of poultices. It ought to signify the proper use of fresh air, light, warmth, cleanliness, quiet and the proper choosing and giving of diet, all at the least expense of vital power to the patient.'
(Nightingale, 1859)

Florence Nightingale's concern was for the 'whole' patient: mind, body and spirit. She placed most emphasis on the patient's environment and the nurse's observation of the patient: 'We must put the patient in the best condition for nature to act upon him' (Nightingale, 1859). In this way, Nightingale was probably one of the first people to have a *holistic view* of patients. Holism is the theory that living matter, or reality, is made up of organic or unified wholes that are greater than the sum of their parts (Barry, 1996). It is a term originating from Smuts (1926, cited in Ham-Ying, 1993) who was a South African philosopher.

We are therefore more than our anatomy and physiology. We are affected by and react to our environment. Interactions with others can also affect the way we feel and behave; therefore, these relationships can be seen to be part of our being. This has become known as the holistic view of patients (Ham-Ying, 1993).

The nurse should be able to appreciate now that when caring for adults he/she needs to consider more than the physical effects of the patient's illness. How the patient feels about his/her illness; social and economic implications of the illness; and the impact on family and friends of the person's illness become equally important. Sister Doctor Callista Roy (1991), in her model for nursing, emphasised this by identifying the person as a 'bio-psycho-social being'.

Nancy Roper (1994) uses examples of nursing care to illustrate influences on the patient's well-being. She describes how nurses caring for adult patients in the 1950s were responsible for laying a tray for each patient's meal, complete with cutlery and a glass of water. Patients were positioned comfortably for eating prior to the serving of individually sized portions by the ward sister. Nurses collected in the plates at the completion of the meal, noting how much of a meal each patient had taken, alerting them to patients with possible inadequate nutritional intake. Most patients now receive meals of standard portion size, taken by a health care assistant to the bedside from a heated trolley, without a nurse even giving assistance to remove a plate cover. The quality or type of food and amount of diet a patient consumes is, therefore, often unknown. If a patient is not sufficiently motivated, or is physically unable, he/she may actually eat nothing. Yet taking adequate nutrition is essential for healing processes to take place, as well as mealtimes forming social events (Association of Community Health Council for England and Wales, 1997). Furthermore, some patients may have very special and different dietary needs that might only be met by the family providing the food. For example, a patient who does not feel like eating might be enticed by the provision of his/her favourite meal cooked at home, which is then brought into hospital. A similar situation might arise when, for example, a Jewish patient is rightly hesitant at eating hospital food and the family would be asked to bring food from home. These examples show an element of *holistic nursing* through the consideration of alternatives to routine arrangements and the involvement of a patient's family.

The consequence of this holistic view of people is that when considering the meaning of the illness, hospitalisation, treatment and recovery, the nurse must also consider the constellation of people with whom the patient interacts. As mentioned earlier, many factors make people different from each other and, therefore, individuals. There are even more reasons why patients' families should be considered as different and therefore as having different needs.

Nurses' ability to provide holistic care within adult nursing in reality is probably questionable. Nursing models, many of which use assessment tools such as the Activities of Living model of Roper *et al.* (1990), consider aspects of patients' needs. Planning care by individual components, such as maintaining breathing, eating, drinking, and eliminating, splits the focus of assessment

Box 24.19: Reflective Exercise

Can you think of what factors make you different from a friend of yours?

You could think of the obvious like race, colour of skin, gender, age, etc. The real task is to discover what differences these factors make to how people live and how they affect the way people relate to each other within a family group.

into separate functions (see also Chapter 11). This has advantages for systematic planning, record-keeping, goal evaluation and care audits, etc. Rose and Marks-Maran (1997) suggest that even in considering all aspects of a person, such as biological needs, psychological needs and social needs, all parts are considered, but not in a holistic way. They consider that any system which separates a person into parts, or systems, is reductionist rather than holistic. In some literature holism is labelled as being a positive perspective, whilst particularism is often viewed as negative. Conceptualising holism as good and particularism as negative is a simplistic and impractical way of addressing many nursing phenomena. Indeed, a point to make here is that nurses do need to concentrate on particular aspects of a patient's illness at times. For example, a patient who is breathless should be observed for signs of infection, dehydration, respiratory failure and cardiac failure; these physical signs emanate from interrelated physiological systems. Importantly, however, there is a danger that, whilst a nurse assesses according to systems or activities, etc., if the information remains isolated and disconnected, care will remain fragmented, task-orientated and less than holistic.

However, assessments of function, interaction, etc. could be linked and related to the patient's feelings, thoughts, spirit, relationships and physical functioning. The result would be that nursing has a chance to serve the 'whole' patient. Priority interventions are so important that in practice it is difficult and often irrelevant to focus on how treatment might be carried out by the family or, for example, how the patient's illness might affect his/her employment status. The point is that these factors might be a worry for the patient or his/her family in the future so at some stage during the patient's care these points should be considered.

Holistic nursing taken to the absolute degree is that which entails everything possible and misses nothing out of the care scenario. However, the nurse should strive for something manageable, feasible and realistic. For example, when a nurse is assessing a patient's needs, the nurse might not utilise all his/her questioning techniques and abilities (Griffin, 1983) (cited in Malin and Teasdale, 1991). Some questions within an assessment document might be irrelevant at the time, for example, or information might be gained from medical records or from his/her observations. The nurse could make some assumptions that can be clarified later with the patient. When choosing interventions the nurse might engage in some lateral thinking and choose therapy agents and treatments other than orthodox nursing procedures. The use of complementary therapies such as aromatherapy, massage, relaxation techniques, etc. is increasing (Which, 1992). Many patients are finding relief from symptoms using these adjuncts and a greater knowledge of their use and effects would be helpful.

Many adults also require intervention from members of different professions within the health care team. For example, following a stroke, it is not unusual for patients to receive care from doctors, specialist nurses, physiotherapists, occupational therapists, dietitians, chiropodists, speech therapists and medical social workers within a short space of time. The nurse will need to coordinate caring activities on behalf of the patient and for the good of the patient thus engaging in the role of the patient's advocate.

One of the principles of care is to be prepared, so the nurse should try to predict events for all concerned, foresee situations, prepare patients' friends and families for change to help the adaptation process leading to a resolution of illness and the resumption of their new normality.

Key Points

- People are more than the interaction of mind and body; the whole person also consists of interactions with the physical environment and other people; the person is a 'bio-psycho-social being'.
- Nurses need to focus on interrelated systems when physical symptoms become a priority for attention.
- Nurses should rule nothing out of the care scenario. The nurse needs to find out what could be relevant to his/her patient's care and who could help.
- The nurse's own awareness, skills and attitude play

a critical part in the success of patient care, not the model or documents or management, but the nurse's personal motivations and commitment to caring.

Conclusion

This chapter has described some of the pitfalls and the positive approaches that can be used to enhance the care process for adults. You have gained an insight into patients' needs and responses, which you can use to leave the patient and yourself satisfied with the process of nursing care. The words and phrases such as individualised, holistic, patient and family-centred care, advocacy and assertiveness are part of accepted jargon in nursing today. Actual adult nursing is about the professional use of interpersonal and practical skills, directed by personally held attitudes that are underpinned by the knowledge of caring, adults and illness. These are the real principles of adult nursing.

References

Association of Community Health Councils for England and Wales (1997). *Hungry in Hospital?* Association of Community Councils for England and Wales, London.

Barry, P. D. (1996). *Psychosocial Nursing: Care of Physically Ill Patients and their Families*, 3rd edn. Lippincott, Philadelphia.

Bond, M. (1986). *Stress and Self-awareness: A guide for Nurses.* Heinemann, London.

Bond, M. (1988). Assertiveness training: understanding assertiveness No.1. *Nursing Times*, 84, 9.

Cribb, A., Bignold, S. and Ball, S.J. (1994). Linking the parts: an exemplar of philosophical and practical issues in holistic nursing. *Journal of Advanced Nursing*, 5, 233–8.

DoH (1986). *The Health of the Nation: a Strategy for Health in England.* Summary booklet of Government's white paper. HMSO, London.

DoH (1991). *The Patient's Charter.* HMSO, London.

Dutch, R.A. (ed.) (1966). *Roget's Thesaurus.* Penguin, Aylesbury, Bucks.

French, H.P. (1979). Reassurance: a nursing skill? *Journal of Advanced Nursing*, 4, 627–34.

French, P. (1994). *Social Skills for Nursing Practice*, 2nd edn. Chapman & Hall, London.

Gadow, S. (1980). Existential advocacy. In *Nursing Practice: the Ethical Issues*, Jameton, A. (ed.). Prentice Hall, Englewood Cliffs, New Jersey.

Gates, B. (1994). *Advocacy: a Nurses' Guide*. Scutari Press, London.

Ham-Ying, S. (1993). Analysis of the concept of holism within the context of nursing. *British Journal of Nursing*, 2(15), 771–5.

Henderson, V. (1977). *Basic Principles of Nursing Care*. International Council of Nurses, Geneva.

HMSO (1992). *The Health of the Nation*. HMSO, London.

Johns, C. (1994). *The Burford NDU Model: Caring in Practice*. Blackwell Scientific Publications, London.

Kidel, M. (1986). The meaning of illness. *Holistic Medicine*, 1(1), 15–25.

Malin, N. and Teasdale, K. (1991). Caring versus empowerment: considerations for nursing practice. *Journal of Advanced Nursing*, 16, 657–62.

Morrison, P. (1994). *Understanding Patients*. Baillière Tindall, London.

Nightingale, F. (1859). *Notes on Nursing*, revised in 1980. Churchill Livingstone, London.

Parsons, T. (1951). *The Social System*. Routledge and Kegan Paul, London.

Porter, S. (1994). New nursing: the road to freedom? *Journal of Advanced Nursing*, 20, 269–74.

Price, A.L. (1965). *The Art, Science and Spirit of Nursing*, 3rd edn. W.B. Saunders, Philadelphia.

Purtilo, R. (1984). *Health Professional and Patient Interaction*. W.B. Saunders, Philadelphia.

RCN (1995). *Advocacy and the Nurse: Issues in Nursing and Health*. No.22. RCN, London.

Roper, N. (1994). Definition of nursing: 1. *British Journal of Nursing*, 3(7), 335–57.

Roper, N., Logan, W. and Tierney, A. (1990). *The Elements of Nursing*, 3rd edn. Churchill Livingstone, London.

Rose, P. and Marks-Maran, D. (1997). A new view of nursing: turning the cube. In *Reconstructing Nursing: Beyond Art and Science*, Marks-Maran, D. and Rose, P. (eds). Baillière Tindall, London.

Roy, C. (1991). Lovette R. Johnson Lutjens (author) *An Adaptation Model: Notes on Nursing Theories*, Volume 3. Sage Publications, Newbury Park.

Salvage, J. (1990). The theory and practice of the 'New Nursing'. *Nursing Times, Occasional Paper*, 86(4), 42–5.

Soothill, K., Mackay, L. and Webb, C. (1995). *Interprofessional Relations in Health Care*. Arnold, London.

Stockwell, F. (1972). *The Unpopular Patient*. Royal College of Nursing Research Series. RCN, London.

Sundeen, S.J., Stuart, G.W., Rankin, E.A.D. and Cohen, S.A. (1994). *Nurse–Client Interaction: Implementing the Nursing Process*, 5th edn. Mosby, St Louis.

Teasdale, K. (1989). The concept of reassurance in nursing. *Journal of Advanced Nursing*, 14(6), 444–50.

UKCC (1992). *Code of Professional Conduct for the Nurse, Midwife and Health Visitor*, 3rd edn. UKCC, London.

UKCC (1996). *Guidelines for Professional Practice*. UKCC, London.

Webster Universal Dictionary (1975). Harver Educational Services, New York.

Which (1992). *Alternative Medicine* Nov, 45–9. Which Consumers Association, London.

WHO (1978). *Report of the International Conference on Primary Care, Alma-Ata, USSR*. WHO, Geneva.

Wright, S. (1995). *We Thought we Knew… Involving Patients in Nursing Practice: an Executive Summary*. King's Fund Nursing Developments Programme, London.

FURTHER READING

Ham-Ying, S. (1993). Analysis of the concept of holism within the context of nursing. *British Journal of Nursing*, 2(15), 771–5.

Explores the concept of holism and relates it to the practice of nursing.

Porter, S. (1994). New nursing: the road to freedom? *Journal of Advanced Nursing*, 20, 269–74.

Discusses the relationships between nurses and their patients: the balance of power and constraints faced by nurses in developing partnerships.

Rodwell, C.M. (1996). An analysis of the concept of empowerment. *Journal of Advanced Nursing*, 23, 305–13.

A discussion of how nurses use empowerment processes.

Teasdale, K. (1989). The concept of reassurance in nursing. *Journal of Advanced Nursing*, 14(6), 444–50.

Critically analyses the concept of reassurance using concept analysis framework.

UKCC (1996). *Guidelines for Professional Practice*. UKCC, London.

Examples from practice embracing use of Code of Conduct and issues such as autonomy, advocacy and professionalism.

Wade, E. (1995). Partnership in care: a critical review. *Nursing Standard*, 9(48), 29–32.

A literature review relating theory to current practice in terms of patients as partners in care.

CHAPTER TWENTY-FIVE

CARE *of* ADULTS *in* HOSPITAL

Sharon L. Edwards and Kim Manley

- Introduction
- The Burford model
- Assessment of interventions in the adult hospitalised patient
- Documentation using the Burford model
- Conclusion

INTRODUCTION

An assumption is made that the adult person cared for in hospital in the future is likely to be acutely ill or experiencing an acute exacerbation of chronic illness, such as asthma, angina or chronic obstructive pulmonary disease. This trend and assumption can be supported by a number of visionary documents which highlight some benchmarks in relation to hospital care (Bull *et al.*, 1993).

Generally, there has been a move away from advocating only the biologically related aspects of care which usually predominate in the hospital setting. However, this chapter is directed towards observations, measurements and interviewing the patient and identifies the close interrelated concepts of physical, psychological and social well-being, as disruption in any one of these aspects will have implications for the others (Monat and Lazarus, 1985). It is for this reason that this chapter addresses psychological and social influences on nursing care. The aspects of monitoring parameters have been considered in some detail as accuracy in measurement and interpretation is an essential prerequisite for effective nursing care of an adult patient.

Self-assessment questions are included to assist with learning, and are identified by shaded boxes. Finally, in the last part of the chapter some assessment tools which aid comprehensive assessment in the acute setting are incorporated to enhance the care of the adult patient.

Before proceeding to these principles, the values and beliefs concerning the nature of the Burford Nursing Development Unit (NDU) model (Johns, 1991, 1994) which underlies the chapter are first stated. This model has been chosen as it encompasses reflection and caring, it is holistic in nature and advocates nursing as a human science. It is utilised to emphasise care of the adult in hospital and can be used as a framework to incorporate a number or elements of other nursing models, and as such serves to introduce nurses to how they can further articulate and understand the full potential of their practice.

THE BURFORD MODEL

The Burford NDU model was developed from clinical practice by clinical practitioners who were identifying their need for a more focused model to incorporate into the care of their patients (Johns, 1994). The main concepts central to the model are: reflection; caring, which encompasses holism, the nurse–patient relationship and situational meaning; environment of practice; and social viability. Also contained within the model are ways of knowing and learning domains, which strive to achieve defined and effective work, and will be discussed in more detail within the chapter, as they are used to elaborate particular areas that are central to first and second level assessment.

REFLECTION

Reflective practice involves the practitioner paying attention to 'significant' aspects of experience in order to make sense of them within the context of their work (Johns, 1994). By reflecting on and taking action to resolve the contradictions that occur in practice, practitioners come to know themselves and, as a consequence, learn to become increasingly effective in achieving desired work. Reflection within the Burford model focuses on reflective questions that emphasise caring for the adult patient (Johns, 1994).

It is recommended that while reading this chapter you incorporate your reflective practice skills and attempt to link certain experiences from your practice to the theory. This will serve to assist your understanding of certain aspects contained within the chapter, and build on your current knowledge in relation to your present practice setting.

CARING

Caring is increasingly becoming the foundation and essense of nursing (Dunlop, 1986; P. Morrison, 1989; Watson, 1989; Boykin and Schoenhofer, 1990; Forsyth *et al.*, 1990). A number of discrete caring concepts are central to the Burford philosophy. These caring concepts are shown in Table 25.1. This table illustrates the conceptual framework of the Burford model and how the various concepts within the model relate to each other within the total experience of caring in nursing. Further discussion of concepts central to nursing are discussed in Chapter 11.

Holism

The core assumption of holism is the recognition that patients are whole people and cannot be viewed in reductionist terms, that is, as parts, systems or mind–body–spirit. Hence the whole cannot be understood merely by isolating and examining its parts (Kramer, 1990). Holistic nursing moves beyond disease management and requires that the nurse and patient collaborate towards health (see also Chapter 24). Collaboration mandates a focus on the whole person, including the environment within which individuals live.

People do not live in vacuums; they are active members of cultural and social communities. Within these communities people have networks of relationships and roles with others, most notably, within the family. Therefore, it is important that nurses do not see patients in a reductionist way, but try to understand their experiences as members of their communities and with a network of family (see also Chapter 19), community roles and relationships.

Each health experience is unique for both the person receiving care and for the caregiver. Within the context of Burford's practice these are the patient and the nurse. Whilst they may both have similar experiences, each experience can never be the same (Kramer, 1990). Holism is a word that encompasses many of the concepts that are found within the Burford philosophy for practice, for example that care is centred around the needs of the patient and the nurse works with the patient from a basis of concern and mutual understanding. The concept of holism, therefore, moves nurses away from the perspective of seeing the patient from the previously dominant reductionist medical model.

Situational meaning

The notion that a person is more than a patient in terms of his or her social and cultural world means that the patient's perspective on the meaning of the health event that brings him or her into contact with nursing will, to some extent, be determined by the patient's accumulated experiences. In understanding 'who the person is' the nurse will immediately place the person into the context of what the situation means to the person. Only by coming to 'know' this 'situated meaning' can the nurse understand the perspectives and needs of the patient and hence effectively help.

People do not put their lives on standstill whilst in hospital. Their lives continue. Understanding the situated meanings of patients may not be easy for the nurse. Nurses have to determine their own concerns and meanings from the patient in order to come to a common understanding of the patient's situation. The difficulty with this is the tendency to impose the nurse's own meaning on other people's experiences (Johns, 1994). This can lead to labelling and stereotyping behaviour by the nurse that is antithetical to therapeutic work.

Table 25.1: Caring concepts identified by Johns (1994)

Concept	Definition
On being a patient	
Holism	The core assumption of holism is the recognition that patients are whole people and cannot be viewed in reductionist terms, that is, as parts, systems or mind–body split. Hence the whole cannot be understood merely by isolating and examining its parts. Holistic nursing moves beyond disease management and requires that the nurse and patient collaborate towards health. Holism is a word that wraps up many of the key concepts that are found within the Burford model, for example, 'that care is centred around the needs of the patient', 'the nurse works with the patient from a basis of concern and mutual understanding' and 'as a consequence the nurse comes to understand the situational meaning and the patient's significant social network'.
Situational meaning	A person is always more than a patient in terms of his/her social and cultural world; the patient's perspective on the meaning of health event that brings him or her into contact with nursing can be seen in terms of their accumulated experiences. Only by coming to 'know' this 'situated meaning' can the nurse understand the perspectives and needs of the patient and hence effectively help. Understanding the situated meaning of patients may not be easy for the nurse. Nurses have to explicate their own concerns and meaning from those of the patient in order to see the patient clearly.
On the nurse–patient relationship	
The nurse–patient relationship must be based on 'what it means to be human' understanding of each other. This relationship is a two-way process.	
'Working with'	For the nurse, 'working with' a patient is based on the holistic recognition of the patient and other members of their social world. In this collaborative relationship, care is always negotiated as appropriate to the situation.
Concern	The significance of concern is that what the patient is experiencing is important to the nurse as a person. This assumes that caring matters to the nurse. Concern also subsumes empathy but is much more than empathy. Therefore, concern is a way of being that determines how the person will act in the world.
Being available	This identifies that the nurse is available to work with the patient. Being available to patients therefore involves communicating this fact. The nurse can do this by giving the patient cues. It is saying to the patient, 'I am here for you when you need me.' This is not necessarily easy as the nurses struggle to manage the workload and meet the needs of all their patients. In this sense availability has to be negotiated with the patient. This is achieved through a sense of involvement.
Being involved	Working with patients within the nurse–patient relationship requires the nurse to become involved with the patient and family.
Mutual understanding	This is a sense of knowing what arises out of knowing the other person, who they are, what expectations each has, and of sharing concerns. This can only be achieved when each person is able to be open and authentic with each other. This is described as showing and being your real self, and opens the way for the patient and the family to care for the nurse. Clearly to be able to care requires a supportive and legitimate environment to work in.

Adapted from Johns, 1994, by courtesy of Blackwell Science Ltd.

The nurse–patient relationship

The nurse–patient relationship is the vehicle for caring, where one person, the nurse, is designated to help another, the patient. This relationship needs to be based on 'what it means to be human' and an understanding of each other. In other words, this relationship, like all relationships, whether labelled professional or personal, is a two-way process. Within the context of the nurse–patient relationship there are five areas which are integral (see Table 25.1):

- Working with
- Concern
- Being available
- Being involved with patients
- Mutual understanding and trust.

ENVIRONMENT OF CARE

Caring takes place within the context of a practice setting. There are many factors in the environment that act to limit nurses' commitment and motivation to caring for people, the patients and their families, and colleagues. If nurses are to make their adopted beliefs and values a reality then they need to understand these environmental factors and be able to take action to create an environment conducive to defined therapeutic work (Johns, 1994). The influences and constraints that impinge on the practice situation are described as the external and internal environment (Table 25.2).

SOCIAL VIABILITY

Society generally values nurses as kind, competent and caring people, the overall impression being that nursing is not itself a significant therapy but rather a support to medicine (Kramer, 1990). This impression is supported by many medical sociologists. Part of the difficulty for nursing in being viewed by society in this way is a perceived lack of professional identity shared by nurses themselves.

The Burford model aims both to challenge and raise society's expectations of nursing's role within hospitals, whilst helping nurses to develop a strong image of themselves as nurses, in order to act with greater confidence.

LEARNING DOMAINS

Johns (1994), through analysing practitioners' experiences, revealed patterns of similarity in learning to achieve defined and effective work. These patterns or 'domains' are outlined as:

- Becoming patient-centred – 'knowing' oneself
- Being therapeutic with patients and families – 'knowing' therapeutic work:
  - ethical decision making
  - involvement with patients
  - responding with appropriate and skilled action
- 'Knowing' responsibility and 'knowing' others
  - giving and receiving feedback
  - coping with work in ways that sustain therapeutic work.

These learning domains are integrated into the first and second level assessments, which frame the central part of the chapter.

RECORDING AND COMMUNICATING NURSING ACTIONS

Throughout the Burford NDU model the importance of accurate record-keeping is highlighted. This is in accordance with the UKCC (1993) who state that 'record and record keeping is an essential and integral part of care and not a distraction from providing that care'. There is substantial evidence to indicate that nurses are often guilty of keeping inadequate, inappropriate and even poor records concerning the care of patients and clients (UKCC, 1993). The UKCC state that records should be utilised as a means of:

- Communicating with others and describing what has been observed or done
- Identifying the discrete role of the nurse
- Disseminating information among members of the team
- Demonstrating the chronology of events, the factors observed and the response to care and treatment
- Demonstrating the properly considered clinical decisions relating to patient care.

In addition, any document which records any aspect of patient care can be required as evidence

Table 25.2: The external and internal environment of practice (Johns, 1994)

The external environment of practice

The external environment of practice relates to the context and function of the particular nursing setting. These are generally framed as a range of factors that establish boundaries to possibilities. As such they need to be understood by nurses in order to manage the tension between espoused values and what is achievable.

The internal environment of practice

The internal environment of practice is a complex world. It is concerned with interpersonal dynamics; with roles and relationships between nurses and between nurses and other health care workers, with attitudes, with skills and knowledge, with how nursing is organised, with how nurses are supported in their own work, and with the management of change and conflict.

Concept	Definition
Organisation of nursing	A crucial factor within the internal environment of practice is how the delivery of care to the patient is organised. Clearly this should be organised in a way that is compatible with the philosophy for practice. Primary nursing is recommended, as the model will have a greater impact where the delivery of care is organised in such a way to facilitate the caring concepts.
Tradition	The tradition of nursing or culture of nursing practice can present a formidable barrier to implementing a preferred philosophy into practice.
Nurse–doctor relationships	One particularly difficult barrier is the traditional relationship between nurses and doctors. Traditionally nurses are perceived by themselves, by doctors and by society as subordinate to doctors, yet reorientation of practice around the needs of the patient will inevitably lead to a need to reorientate the relationship between the nurses and the doctor. This will lead to a move towards professional equality where nurses work with doctors in a collaborative relationship towards achieving therapeutic outcomes.
The physical environment	The internal environment is also concerned with the physical environment in which care is practiced. Comfort is a holistic concept and has physical as well as psychological aspects.

From Johns, 1994, courtesy of Blackwell Science Ltd.

before a court of law or before the Professional Conduct Committee of the Council or other similar regulatory bodies for the health care professions including the General Medical Council. To maintain patient safety it is essential for nurses to keep accurate records throughout the patient's stay in hospital.

ASSESSMENT OF INTERVENTIONS IN THE ADULT HOSPITALISED PATIENT

Assessment facilitates appropriate intervention, but can also be an intervention in its own right. The focus for all interventions is related to the person's health in a holistic sense, rather than a narrower focus on medical diagnosis and symptoms (Johns, 1994). The assessment strategy is simply to obtain valid and relevant information to be able to nurse the person. It consists of one core question and a series of cue questions that tune the nurse into the philosophical concepts of the model (Table 25.3). In the context of the adult patient in hospital, the Burford model consists of two assessment levels: the first level assessment and the second level assessment (Garbett, 1994). The first level assessment focuses on physiological and some psychological aspects of measurement and observations by nurses, whereas the second level assessment consists of interviewing the patient and determining in more depth the psychological and social status and includes the use of additional assessment tools. However, if a patient is

Table 25.3: The core and cue questions (Johns, 1991, 1994)

Core question
■ 'What information do I need to be able to nurse this person?'
Cue questions
■ Who is this person?
■ What health event brings the person into hospital?
■ How must this person be feeling?
■ How has this event affected their usual life patterns and roles?
■ How does this person make me feel?
■ How can I help this person?
■ What is important for this person to make their stay in hospital comfortable?
■ What support does this person have in life?
■ How can they view the future for themselves and others?

From Johns, 1994, courtesy of Blackwell Science Ltd.

admitted to hospital as a booked admission and does not require immediate nursing interventions, the second level assessment can be undertaken first.

FIRST LEVEL ASSESSMENT

Before the core question 'What information do I need to be able to nurse this person?' can be answered, the nurse needs to have achieved understanding of the two learning domains: 'knowing' self, and 'knowing' therapeutic work (Johns, 1994). Encompassed within 'knowing' therapeutic work is: ethical decision making, which is about prioritising workloads, managing situations as they arise and includes the nurse's own needs as well as the needs of colleagues; and being able to respond with appropriate and skilled action, which encompasses the ability to respond appropriately to situations (Johns, 1994). These are, therefore, the prerequisites necessary to achieving well-defined and effective nursing intervention. The core question identified above and in Table 25.3 can be answered by including nurse observations and measurement, but measurement is more extensively considered.

Observation

Accurate observation is an important means of collecting information about a person's physical and mental status. This intervention requires the nurse to observe for particular warning signs, which may indicate improvement or deterioration, e.g. a patient's skin colour or mucous membranes may be observed to be: pale, but pink after a blood transfusion; blue, but following oxygen therapy, pink.

The nurse might observe that the patient is being admitted on a trolley or in a wheelchair or, if walking, is using a stick or has a limp or an unsteady gait. On admission, details may be observed such as: facial colour – pallor, flushed or cyanosed; any respiratory difficulty – rapid or shallow breathing; cool moist or dehydrated skin; ischaemia of the eyelids, lips, gums and tongue; facial expressions; oedema; increased or decreased body weight; pulsating neck veins; posture and dry mucous membranes. The person's psychological and emotional state too can be observed (Binnie *et al.*, 1988), signs of anxiety or distress, evidence of confusion, disorientation, apprehension, restlessness, agitation or calm. In addition, accurate observation depends on other senses such as hearing, touch and smell. Such observations will direct the nurse's subsequent, more systematic approach to data collection and measurement including further observation of specific factors.

Measurements

Measurements may involve psychological factors, such as anxiety or stress, but within acute hospital settings these may be predominantly physical in nature, for example: the Glasgow coma scale, central venous pressure, temperature, peripheral pulses, pulse rate which can be done by palpating the wrist, electrocardiograph, blood pressure, weight, urine output, urinalysis, blood analysis, and arterial oxygen saturation via a finger probe, pain. These measurements may be undertaken to substantiate further information obtained from observing the person.

Such measurements may also incorporate assessment tools to enhance the reliability and validity of the measurement. A tool can be defined as an implement or instrument used to do a job. Assessment tools are instruments used to guide

Table 25.4: Points to consider when using any assessment tool

- Does the person using the tool understand it?
- In what context was the tool designed and for what purpose?
- When should the tool be used?
- It is realistic to use?
- Is the tool being properly used?
- Does the person need training to use the tool?

patient assessment. Certain points need to be considered when using any tool and these are listed in Table 25.4. The use of assessment tools encourages the nurse to be organised and systematic in his/her approach to assessment. Such tools also have benefits for patients and students in that they can be used as teaching aids. In addition, if they are reliable and valid, they can increase objectivity and facilitate precise measurement, accurate record-keeping and evaluation. The measurement tools incorporated and/or mentioned in the first level assessment are: the Glasgow coma scale; anxiety measurement scales and pain assessment scales.

AUTONOMIC NERVOUS SYSTEM (ANS)

To determine the mental state (both physiological and psychological) of an acutely ill patient, it is necessary to have knowledge of the autonomic nervous system as it underpins many acute measurements. The ANS has two subdivisions: the sympathetic nervous system is active in response to stressors, and is responsible for stimulating smooth muscle fibres to contract (i.e. excitation) and the adrenal medulla to release the hormones adrenaline and noradrenaline, and is active in response to stressors; and the parasympathetic nervous system which causes relaxation (i.e. inhibition) and is most active during sleep and rest, having a 'conserving' effect on body resources (see Chapter 14 of Marieb, 1995) (see Table 25.5).

These responses, under the control of the central nervous system, regulate other areas of the body to maintain **homeostasis**. Recognition of an increase or decrease in either sympathetic or parasympathetic activity in the hospitalised person can often be reflected in other observations such as the blood pressure or heart rate. By working through learning check 1 (Box 25.1, page 619) the essential signs of increased sympathetic activity can be deduced. A general assessment of the

patient's ANS may be necessary to determine these activities, as they can alert the nurse to impending neurological overstimulation or deterioration. The assessments available to assess the ANS are the Glasgow coma scale and, more recently, anxiety measurement tools such as the linear (LAS) or visual analogue scale (VAS), the graphic anxiety scale and the hospital anxiety and depression scale.

The Glasgow coma scale The Glasgow coma scale is an example of a specific tool designed to produce a uniform method of determining and recording conscious level and therefore the activity of the ANS or mental state. The advantages of using this tool are that it increases the objectivity and reliability of neurological assessment, reducing the use of ambiguous descriptions of consciousness level. It is also quick and easy to use (Rowley and Fielding, 1991).

The Glasgow coma scale focuses on the evaluation of three parameters: eye opening, motor response and verbal response (Watson *et al.*, 1992). The person's best achievement is recorded for each parameter from a predetermined choice of options:

- Eye opening is divided into four different options: spontaneous opening; opening to speech; opening to pain; and no eye opening.
- Verbal response is described from a choice of five options: orientated in time, place and person; confused conversation; inappropriate words; incomprehensible sounds (for example, groans); no verbal response.
- Motor response is described using one of six options: obeys commands; responds to pain; localises to pain; flexion response; extension response; no response to pain.

These motor responses are further illustrated in Figure 25.1. Each of the parameters can be recorded as a graph, which will demonstrate changes visually. Alternatively, each parameter can be scored separately and then a total given as an overall numerical value which can be used as a baseline against which later changes can be compared (Sullivan, 1990). The total can range from a maximum score of 15 – where a person is fully alert and orientated – to a minimum score of 3 – where a person is completely unresponsive. In addition to providing a neurological assessment,

Table 25.5: Effects of sympathetic and parasymapthetic stimulation on various organs and tissues

(a) Organs and tissues with both sympathetic and parasympathetic nerve supplies

Organ	Effect of sympathetic stimulation (or parasympathetic inhibition)	Effect of parasympathetic stimulation (or sympathetic inhibition)
Eye	Pupil dilates	Pupil constricts
Salivary glands	Viscous saliva	Thin watery saliva
Bronchial tree	Dilates	Constricts and increases mucus production
Heart		
■ Rate	Increases	Decreases
■ Atrial excitability/conductivity	Increases	Decreases
Gut		
■ Tone	Decreases	Increases
■ Motility	Decreases peristalsis	Increases peristalsis
■ Sphincters	Constriction	Relaxation
Bladder		
■ Tone	Relaxation	Contraction
■ Internal sphincters	Increased tone	Decreased tone

(b) Organs with predominantly sympathetic innervation

Organ	Minimum or no sympathetic activity	Maximum sympathetic activity
Heart		
■ Ventricular excitability	Decreases	Increases
■ Ventricular contractility	Decreases	Increases
■ Coronary arteries	Constriction	Dilation
Blood vessels		
■ Systemic	Dilation	Constriction
■ Skin	Dilation	Constriction
■ Skeletal muscles	Constriction	Dilation
Sweat glands	No sweating	Increased sweating
Liver	—	Glucose release
Kidney	Normal urine formation	Decreased urine output
Blood glucose	Normal	Increased
Basal metabolic rate	Normal	Increased by up to 50%
Adrenal medullary secretion	—	Increased
Mental activity	—	Increased

(c) Organs with predominantly parasympathetic innervation

Organ	Increased parasympathetic activity
Exocrine glands	
■ Stomach	Increased secretions
■ Pancreas	Increased secretions

NB: Sympathetic effects may occur indirectly due to reduced blood supply to secreting glands during excessive sympathetic stimulation.

Box 25.1: Learning Check One

Self-assessment question one

What are the signs of increased sympathetic drive?

You may find that considering your own body when you are frightened may help you to list them

Answer

- Increased pulse rate/heart rate
- Increased blood pressure
- Peripheral shutdown so the limbs feel cool to the touch
- Sweating
- Dilated pupils
- Reduced urinary output
- Dry mouth
- Contracted muscles (increased muscle tone)

Self-assessment question two

When considering a patient who is stressed physiologically, e.g. following haemorrhage, following major surgery or myocardial infarction, which signs of increased sympathetic drive may be reversed and why?

Answer and rationale

Blood pressure and heart rate. The *blood pressure* may be low following large blood loss resulting in reduced circulating volume which cannot be compensated for by the body. The blood pressure may also be low if a patient has had a large left ventricular myocardial infarction, the ventricle having insufficient functioning muscle to eject the volume of blood necessary to maintain the cardiac output and blood pressure. The *heart rate* may be reduced because of interruptions or blockages in the heart's conduction system following inferior myocardial infarction which can subsequently also produce a drop in blood pressure. Three other important exceptions to the typical stressor response of increasing blood pressure also exist and these relate to the following situations:

- Patients receiving beta-blocking drugs which inhibit the actions of the sympathetic nervous system
- Drugs which affect the muscle tone of blood vessels, producing vasodilation which causes a subsequent drop in blood pressure
- Septicaemia, which also affects the tone of peripheral blood vessels, causing vasodilation and hence reduced blood pressure, even when other signs of increased sympathetic drive are evident

Self-assessment question three

If increased sympathetic arousal is sustained and large amounts of noradrenaline and adrenaline are continually circulating in the body, what changes may occur other than those identified in self-assessment question one?

(Studying Table 25.5 may help you)

Answer

- Decreased peristalsis potentially leading to paralytic ileus
- Hyperglycaemia
- Perceptual inaccuracies
  - memory alterations
  - communication difficulties

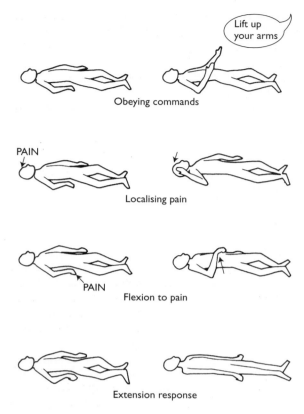

Figure 25.1: Motor responses
(reproduced by kind permission of the *Nursing Times*, in which this figure first appeared in an article by Teasdale on 12th June 1975)

this tool might also have the benefit of indicating the level of patient dependency and, possibly, the subsequent need for nursing interventions.

Anxiety A person's response to anxiety is due to activation of the sympathetic nervous system, potentiated by adrenaline and noradrenaline from the adrenal medulla, stimulated by the hypothalamus (McCance and Huether, 1994). There are many factors in everyday life that provoke anxiety, and hospitalisation can be counted as one of them. Anxiety is difficult to define (Walding, 1991), mainly because it is often explained as a vague, uneasy feeling, the source of which is often non-specific or unknown to the individual (Kim *et al.*, 1991). However, Swindale (1989) defines anxiety as:

'a fear of the unknown, as disproportionate to the threat involved and directly related to the future events in the life of the individual.'

Anxiety has been identified as both positive and negative, positive in relation to learning ability, as in this situation a high anxiety level may have a motivating function, and negative in relation to particular experiences, e.g. hospitalisation. When anxiety is longstanding it is known as a steady state, whereas transitory anxiety comes and goes and is known as an anxiety state (Walding, 1991). The response to hospitalisation and related events is usually to produce an anxiety state (Swindale, 1989).

Coping with the anxiety of hospitalisation can sometimes lead to aggressive behaviour as a result of anger and frustration (Walding, 1991). Alternatively, the coping may take the form of escape from the anxiety-provoking situation, resulting in withdrawal due to the person's feelings of helplessness and the inability to gain control over events.

Anxiety is a recognised nursing diagnosis and is present in at least some hospitalised patients. This means there is a need for nurses to be able to make an accurate assessment. Wilson-Barnett and Batehup (1988) recommended rigorous and continuous efforts to assess negative moods or the effects of anxiety.

The assessment of anxiety relies on listening and talking to patients, questioning, and discussion through interview, observation or the use of tools. There are a number of psychological tools to measure anxiety (Shuldham *et al.*, 1995). These include the linear (LAS) or visual analogue scale (VAS; Wewers and Lowe, 1990), the graphic anxiety scale (Lo Biondo-Wood and Haver, 1986) and the hospital anxiety and depression scale (HAD; Zigmond and Snaith, 1983). Nurses may already be familiar with their use.

Stress Stress (see also Chapter 8) is seen in terms of an individual's interactions with events, rather than as a univariate, unidirectional concept (Monat and Lazarus, 1985; Harvey, 1989). Thus, the whole concept of 'stress' is seen as a dynamic interactional process, between the individual and his or her environment, rather than a single event or set of responses. Stressors, therefore, make physical and psychological demands, which require individuals to assess and understand the situation and then to respond to it. In situations when a person can understand and react to the circumstances in a satisfactory manner it is unlikely to be perceived as stressful by that individual. However, if the stressors demand new responses or ones which are undeveloped, then it is likely that the experience will lead to stress. Hence 'stress' is taken to be an absence of, or a deficiency in, the individual's ability to cope with current environmental demands (Harvey, 1989). The resulting illness caused by stress is linked to increased sympathetic nervous system arousal (Marieb, 1995).

The body's response to a stressor is reflected by a reaction which involves the whole body and generally consists of three distinct response phases. The first phase is termed the **alarm reaction** and consists of a widespread physiological response which includes a large outflow into the bloodstream of adrenal hormones in an attempt to defend the body from the stressor. If the individual survives then the second phase is entered, the stage of **resistance or adaptation** where an attempt is made by the body to re-establish equilibrium and to regain control to maintain homeostasis. If the body is unable to re-establish homeostasis because of persistent exposure to the stressor then the third phase of **exhaustion** will result, ending in death. The causative agents producing this response are termed 'stressors'.

Although it is well recognised that some stress is necessary for normal healthy living and optimal functioning, the acutely ill individual in hospital is exposed to many stressors simultaneously. These act synergistically rather than cumulatively. There are a number of events that make significant emotional demands upon the person while in hospital. For example, hearing the initial diagnosis may be a difficult and stressful process. The fear and anxiety generated by the news may be disruptive and debilitating to its recipient, making it more difficult to absorb further information or to make informed choices (Harvey, 1989).

Some people react to a given situation differently from others depending on how they have perceived a stressor. Perception itself is an intricate concept which may in turn be affected by past experiences, genetic predisposition, values and beliefs, self-concept and the level of anxiety at the time the stressor is perceived.

Over and above this, some treatments use powerful drugs, accompanied by side-effects which may include nausea and vomiting. However, once treatment decisions and choices have been made, stress may still be important. The general process of hospitalisation and surgery is known to be stressful, and for the acutely ill patient, continued exposure to stressors can result in the development of stress ulcers, reduced wound healing, cardiac function, and a reduced immune response to infection, amongst other physiological and psychological sequelae.

In addition, stress can be caused by the individual being unable to cope with specific life events. These may be significant changes which may occur through choice (marriage or divorce) or they may be totally unforeseen (bereavement, redundancy, accidental injury or long-term illness). Sociologists and health psychologists consider that most people will undergo at least one such significant event and probably more within a lifetime (Harvey, 1989).

Therefore, the implications of stress for the nurse in caring for a patient in hospital is that they understand the relationship between the individual and his or her environment, life events and acute illness, and as such take the following into consideration:

- Assessment of recent and current major life events and/or crisis, as these may have accumulated to predispose to the acute illness
- Assessment of the individual's normal coping mechanisms and support networks, so that these can be enhanced, reinforced and/or improved
- Recognition that the present acute illness may cause stress in itself, particularly with regard to:

  – potential impact on employment
  – dependent family members
  – financial insecurity,

  thus making the patient more vulnerable to infection, depression and slower recovery
- The need to assist the patient's family members with positive coping mechanisms in a situation that may be perceived as stressful for them.

The ANS controls many other body functions and as such can influence the measurements frequently undertaken by the nurse during his or her daily work. Therefore, when performing measurements such as temperature, pulses, electrocardiogram, blood pressure, central venous pressure, respiration, urine output, blood analysis, oxygen saturation and pain, the nurse needs to be aware that ultimate control lies with the brain, and as such they can be affected by a reduced level of consciousness, anxiety and/or stress, which can lead to inaccurate measurements. These measurements will now be discussed.

TEMPERATURE

Temperature measurement may seem a simple procedure, but it is in fact fraught with problems which may lead to inaccurate recordings. Nursing and medical interventions are commonly based on temperature recordings which, if erroneously made, can lead in extreme instances to an elevated temperature being unrecognised. A sound understanding of temperature measurement and influencing factors is essential for nurses who care for patients in hospital.

Temperature usually fluctuates within a **circadian rhythm**, being highest in the evening and lowest at about 6 a.m. There are normal circadian fluctuations of the core temperature which can vary between 0.5° and 0.7°C, this diurnal variation in body temperature in humans will affect readings.

When taking the temperature, it is the temperature set by the hypothalamus which is attempted to be determined. The pulmonary artery temperature measurement is suggested to be the most accurate way of measuring hypothalamic set point temperature (Henker and Coyne, 1995). This form of temperature measurement is only available in critical care settings, and as such it is not feasible to use in the ward situation.

Therefore, those temperature sites which are in close proximity to the brain (axilla, oral, eardrum) and tympanic membranes best reflect the brain's thermal environment. The rectal temperature is proposed to be the most accurate tympanic membrane measure of hypothalamic temperature. Fulbrook (1993) suggested that rectal temperatures are inaccurate as they are affected by heat generated by the faecal bacteria, but Hinchliff et al. (1996) disagree, saying that rectal temperatures give a much closer approximation of the body's core temperature because of the heat produced in the rectum from the waste substances of **metabolism**.

The measured rectal temperature is consistently higher than oral or axilla temperatures (Henker and Coyne, 1995). The difference is usually in the region of 0.3–1°C, oral temperature being about 0.5°C, and axillary temperatures are up to 1°C below the core temperature (Guiffre et al., 1990). Rectal temperatures are useful as long as the probes are placed correctly, but are often uncomfortable and embarrassing for patients (Holtzclaw, 1992), and as such are only performed in acutely ill situations whereby the person is unconscious or the use of a glass thermometer in the mouth is contraindicated (Closs, 1988).

The axilla temperature is more convenient, but is generally not commonly used. This is because the axilla temperature is thought to be considered a skin temperature and not adequate as an indicator of core temperature (Holtzclaw, 1993). However, peripheral skin temperatures can be useful in determining vasoconstriction or vasodilatation to help assess adult patient's circulation status. This method is generally used in critical care areas where they have the instrumentation and technology. However, nurses can incorporate peripheral skin temperatures as a method of assessing adult patient's thermal status by just touching a toe or a foot (Braddy, 1989).

However, the most common and accessible of the routes is the sublingual route (Henker and Coyne, 1995). Oral temperature readings may seem simple, but variations with regional placement do exist (Holtzclaw, 1992). A study by Erickson (1980) indicated that for the greatest accuracy, the bulb of the thermometer should be placed to the right or left of the mouth, and not the area in the middle of the tongue, since recorded temperatures are significantly higher in these positions than in the area at the front of the mouth. Durham et al. (1986) reviewed the literature on temperature measurement and summarised a variety of factors which will affect the accuracy of oral and rectal temperature measurement. These are summarised in Table 25.6.

The most common thermometer in use to measure axilla and oral temperatures is the glass thermometer containing mercury. These are cheap but require disinfection after use, their accuracy declines with increased use or long-term storage (Abbey et al., 1978), errors can occur with cleaning and resetting, and they are likely to break, potentially exposing people to mercury vapour. There is a significant risk of cross-infection from other patients when inadequately disinfected thermometers are used (Fullbrook, 1993).

Glass thermometers should be in the mouth for 8 minutes for men and 9 minutes for women at room temperatures of 18–24°C (Nichols and Kucha, 1972). Nichols and her colleagues (cited by

Table 25.6: Factors affecting the accuracy of oral and rectal temperature measurement (Durham et al., 1986)

Oral temperature	Rectal temperature
Mouth breathing	Presence of stool
Smoking	Placement of thermometer at different sites in the rectum
Recent ingestion of hot or cold liquids	
Local inflammatory processes	
Placement of thermometer at different sites in mouth	
Time thermometer left in position	
Oxygen administration	
Tachypnoea	

Table 25.7: A summary of insertion times when measuring oral temperature

Minutes	Group	Environmental temperature
8	Men	18–24°C
9	Women	18–24°C
7	Adults	24.5–30°C
6	Febrile adults	Not noted

Baker et al., 1984) investigated this and their results are summarised in Table 25.7.

The electronic thermometer is becoming increasingly popular in clinical practice to replace the traditional mercury-filled device. Electronic thermometers are more expensive, use disposable cover slips over the probe and give a digital reading. In addition, single-use chemical thermometers are available, which work by using a chemical that changes colour with increasing temperature (Buswell, 1997). Moorat (1976) studied the use of the three types of thermometers (mercury, electronic, chemical) to find out which was most cost-effective and concluded that electronic thermometers were preferable. The debate continues as to which type of thermometer is most appropriate for ward use (Closs, 1988).

A tympanic membrane closer to the brain is the ear, a temperature site that is becoming increasingly popular in the hospital setting. It uses tympanic membrane thermometry and is known as the infrared light reflectance thermometer. It detects the temperature within the eardrum. This site of measurement has clear advantages: the close proximity of the measurement site to the hypothalamus, convenience, comfort, rapidity and acceptance by the patient (Koziol-McLain et al., 1996). It registers in a matter of seconds with little inconvenience and no discomfort to the patient (Erickson and Yount, 1991). Inaccurate

readings usually occur due to inconsistent measurement techniques by clinicians (Holtzclaw, 1992).

A temperature is recorded to determine if it is normal, high or low. It is often assumed that when it is high, the person has an infection, but this is not always the case (Cunha et al., 1984). There are three general states of increased body temperature:

1 Hyperpyrexia (fever) – involves a condition whereby the thermoregulatory mechanisms remain intact, but the body temperature is maintained at a high level. It generally has an infective aetiology, but there are other non-infectious causes of a hyperpyrexia. These include acute myocardial infarctions, haemolysis (seen in reactions to blood transfusions) and thyrotoxicosis.
2 Hyperthermia – occurs when there is hypothalamic injury, due to neoplasms, surgery or central nervous system problems, and overheating overwhelms the heat loss mechanisms.
3 Malignant hyperthermia – is caused by certain drugs commonly used in patients, e.g. diuretics, antiseizure therapy, analgesics, some common anaesthetics, antiarrhythmics and antibiotics.

All three cause an increase in body temperature, but hyperthermia and malignant hyperthermia do not respond to antipyretic therapy (Gurevich, 1985).

Hyperpyrexia is defined as a core temperature between 41° and 43°C. A temperature is most likely to be elevated at the peak of the circadian cycle which is between 5 p.m. and 7 p.m. The results of a study by Angerami (1980) indicated that the time at which body temperature should be taken is between 7 p.m. and 8 p.m.; this is the time at which pyrexia, if present, is most likely to register.

There are conflicting opinions in the literature as to the best way to treat a hyperpyrexia and it becomes difficult to decide what to do in the best interests of the person. On the one hand a high temperature is a normal body response and so should not be treated (Hart and Dennis, 1988). On the other, this natural response can be detrimental to the person (Cunha *et al.*, 1984), suggesting the temperature should be treated because prolonged temperatures of 41°C and over can lead to unconsciousness, brain damage, acute multisystem failure and haemorrhage. Yet, treating a fever by cooling and tepid sponging can only serve to increase temperature further, causing the patient discomfort and possible harm (Bruce and Grove, 1992).

Therefore, it is suggested that the best nursing intervention for a hyperpyrexia (fever) and the non-infective state caused by a myocardial infarction is by the use of antipyrexial drug therapy. For non-infective hyperpyrexias caused by haemolysis or thyrotoxicosis, treatment of the underlying condition is recommended (Krikler and Dodge, 1987). Yet, for a hyperthermia or malignant hyperthermia, cooling methods are proposed to be the most effective, to reduce the risk of cell and organ damage and potential death.

A drastic decrease in body temperature is known as hypothermia, and is characterised by a marked cooling of core temperature, and is defined as a core temperature below 35°C. Progressive temperature reduction below this level will result in reduced metabolism and risk of cardiac arrest. At 28–30°C, loss of consciousness will ensue. Low temperatures cause compensatory shivering and vasoconstriction, to shunt the blood to vital organs, and prevent excess heat loss from skin surfaces, causing metabolic and cardiorespiratory stress to ill patients (Holtzclaw, 1992). Hypothermia can be accidental or therapeutic:

- Accidental hypothermia is a temperature below 35°C and is a result of sudden immersion in cold water or prolonged exposure to cold environments. It can be associated with alcohol and some sedatives and narcotics which diminish concious perception of cold. Healthy subjects who experience hypothermia often survive profound hypothermia with medical support.

- Therapeutic hypothermia is used to slow metabolism and preserve ischaemic tissue during surgery. It can occur through exposure of body cavities to the relatively cool operating room environment, irrigation of body cavities with room temperature solutions, infusion of room temperature intravenous solutions, and inhalation of unwarmed anaesthetic agents.

The nurse needs to be aware of any patient at risk of hypothermia and take notice of how long the patient has been exposed in theatre. Rewarming methods are divided into three groups:

1 Passive external rewarming (removal of wet clothes, blankets, warm room)
2 Active external rewarming (radiant lights, convection air blankets)
3 Active internal rewarming (warmed gases to respiratory tract, warmed intravenous fluids).

The process of rewarming should proceed at no faster than a few degrees per hour (Murakami, 1995). If a patient is rapidly rewarmed, oxygen consumption, myocardial demand and vasodilatation increase faster than the heart's ability to compensate and death can occur. By working through learning check 2 (Box 25.2) the causes of a high temperature and a hypothermia can be deduced.

PULSE

The rhythmic contraction of the left ventricle of the heart results in transmission of a pressure impulse through the arteries. This pulse is customarily palpated at the radial artery in the wrist. The important factors to consider in relation to the radial pulse are:

- Rate
- Rhythm
- Pressure (volume)
- Deficits with apex rate.

The pulse rate is an important component of cardiac output. Fluctuations of pulse rate in the well individual normally occur together with fluctuations in **stroke volume** to maintain optimum cardiac output for the activity being performed, for example, rest or exercise. In the resting adult, the pulse rate would normally be about 70 beats per minute. A rate greater than 100 beats per minute is termed a tachycardia, and a rate less than 60 beats

Box 25.2: Learning Check 2

Self-assessment question four	Answer	Rationale
List some possible causes of an increased core temperature in an acutely ill person	1 Infection: ■ wound ■ urinary tract ■ intravenous cannula site ■ chest infection ■ septicaemia	The temperature regulating centre in the hypothalamus is 'reset' at a higher level due to the effects of pyrogens
	2 Reduced cardiac output due to ■ myocardial failure ■ hypovolaemia	Increased sympathetic activity produces severe peripheral vasoconstriction which then prevents the dissipation of heat produced from metabolism. Heat is, therefore, retained within the core circulation. Adrenaline release also increases the metabolic rate which results in greater heat production
	3 Tissue damage/destruction or inflammation (for example, deep vein thrombosis, myocardial infarction)	Local inflammatory responses produce heat
	4 Atropine poisoning	Atropine blocks the sympathetic nerves to the sweat glands, therefore preventing heat loss via sweating
Self-assessment question five		
What examples can you think of that are likely to cause hypothermia in patients admitted to acute care areas?	1 Accidental exposure to cold	For example: – elderly people due to poor socio-economic conditions – accidental immersion in cold water
	2 Prolonged anaesthesia	– due to reduced metabolic rate
	3 Elective cooling	– for example, for the purposes of reducing metabolic demands in patients undergoing cardiac surgery and neurosurgery
	4 Endocrine disorders ■ myxoedema ■ hypopituitarism	People with these medical problems are unable to increase their metabolic rate in response to exposure to cold
	5 Barbiturate overdose/acute alcohol poisoning	These drugs cause gross vasodilation and, therefore, excessive heat loss
	6 Spinal cord injury	Loss of vascular tone can result n gross vasodilation of peripheral vessels with corresponding heat loss

per minute is termed a bradycardia. By working through learning check 3 (Box 25.3) some reasons as to why the heart rate may deviate from its norm can be deduced.

If an altered pulse does not produce signs of haemodynamic changes it is not necessary to treat it, but if the patient does show such signs, e.g. volume depletion, immediate treatment is indicated. This may include drug or intravenous infusion therapy or non-pharmacological measures can be used, such as the Valsalva manoeuvre or the physician may perform **carotid sinus massage** (Dennison, 1994).

The rhythm of the pulse may vary normally with respiration, especially in young adults, so that the pulse is irregular, speeding up at the peak of inspiration and slowing down with expiration; this is termed sinus **arrhythmia**. An irregular pulse is commonly categorised into the following rhythms:

- Regularly irregular
- Irregularly irregular.

A regularly irregular pulse is most likely to be caused by ectopic beats (beats originating from a site other than the sino-atrial node) which occur prematurely. Occasionally, odd ectopic beats may occur in healthy individuals. If, however, they are found to persist in an acutely ill person, the medical staff will require notification as they can be indicative of increased cardiac irritability due to ischaemia or drugs (such as digoxin), increased sympathetic activity as a result of stressors (for example, hypoxia), or they may be related to potassium imbalance, all of which require further investigation.

An irregularly irregular pulse usually indicates **atrial fibrillation** where atrial behaviour is chaotic and disorganised and the transmission of impulses to the ventricles is irregular.

The pressure or volume is determined by the pulse pressure. The pulse pressure is a wave of pressure caused by a sequence of distension and elastic recoil in the wall of the aorta which forces blood rapidly down the systemic arterial system. It determines the strength of force of the pulse and it can be defined as the difference between the systolic and diastolic blood pressures.

When the pulse pressure is low, the strength of the pulse may be feeble and thready. This may occur when hypovolaemia exists, because the

---

Box 25.3: Learning Check 3

Self-assessment question six

Can you think of reasons why the heart rate may deviate from its norm in an acutely ill person?

Answer

Causes of tachycardia (i.e. pulse rates higher than 100 beats/min) include:

1 Increased sympathetic activity due to stressors, whether biological (for example, hypoxia) or psychological (for example, pain, anxiety)

2 Infection

3 Cardiac failure (The stroke volume is limited and so the heart rate increases to maintain cardiac output)

4 Cardiac arrhythmias (i.e. abnormal rhythms) resulting from electrolyte imbalance or myocardial ischaemia following infarction

5 Thyrotoxicosis

6 Drugs
 - particularly those that mimic the sympathetic nervous system, such as inhaled, nebulised salbutamol

7 Anaemia

Causes of bradycardia (i.e. pulse rates below 60 beats/min) include:

1 Increased parasympathetic activity due to anaesthesia or excessive vagal stimulation (for example, following myocardial infarction, spinal shock, surgery)
 - also vaso-vagal attacks/fainting

2 Hypothermia
 - accidental or elective

3 Dysfunction or disease of the cardiac conduction system

4 Intermittent or continuous interruption of the conduction system of the heart (i.e. atrioventricular block), or damage to the sino-atrial node (following myocardial infarction, for example)

5 Raised intracranial pressure when associated with an increase in blood pressure

6 Drugs
 - for example, digoxin or beta-blockers (which inhibit receptors in the sympathetic nerve pathway) e.g. propranolol, labetalol, atenolol

stroke volume ejected by the left ventricle into the circulation is greatly reduced. When the pulse pressure is high, the pulse strength may be bounding and the person experiencing this may feel palpitations or hear his/her heart pounding.

The pulse deficit is the difference between the heart rate counted at the apex of the heart using a stethoscope and the pulse rate counted simultaneously at the wrist. For the majority of patients the heart rate and pulse rate will be the same, but for those who are in atrial fibrillation, or who are having multiple ectopic beats, there will be a deficit which it is important to monitor by recording both apex and radial rates.

It is interesting to note that the importance of using the pulse as an early reliable indicator of physiological change is often overlooked and a greater significance put on the blood pressure (BP). Yet, the pulse rate is less invasive and less time-consuming and the pulse is measured more accurately than the BP (Burnip, 1991). In some surgical wards, it is common practice to measure BP only once on return from theatre and, if it is satisfactory and the patient is not in a high risk group, only record the pulse at regular intervals during the post-operative period.

Peripheral pulses As previously discussed, the pulse pressure is a wave of pressure which can be palpated near the body surface where large arteries are superficially located or where they pass over underlying bone. There are many pulses in the body where an artery surfaces over a bony protrusion. The main pulses are apical, radial, carotid, femoral, brachial, aortic, popliteal and dorsalis pedis (Braddy, 1989). The femoral and carotid pulses are important when establishing the adequacy of cardiac output, for example in someone who has suddenly lost consciousness due to possible cardiac arrest; the brachial pulse is used to measure blood pressure; and the pulses of the lower limbs, the popliteal pulse located behind the knee and the dorsalis pedis and posterior tibial pulses in the feet are important in determining adequacy of perfusion to the lower limbs (Figure 25.2).

Suggested methods of palpating these foot pulses are illustrated in Figure 25.3 as they can often be difficult to locate – especially when perfusion to limbs is severely reduced (for example, in peripheral vascular disease or where there is extreme vasoconstriction due to the increased activity of the sympathetic nervous system).

By feeling these pulses a nurse can determine if a pulse is present, absent, strong and equal, or faint and equal (Braddy, 1989). The force can be recorded using the scale shown in Figure 25.4 (page 629). Any weakness or a bounding feeling as if there is a great pressure within the artery, whether it is fast or slow or irregular, will all give the nurse indications as to whether perfusion is inadequate or oversupplied, each giving the nurse clues to the overall circulation of each individual area of the body.

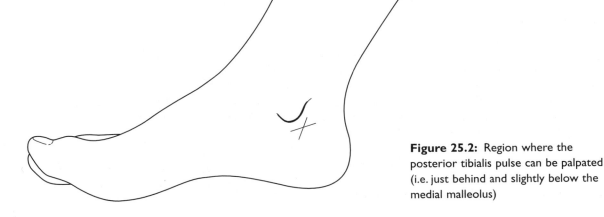

Figure 25.2: Region where the posterior tibialis pulse can be palpated (i.e. just behind and slightly below the medial malleolus)

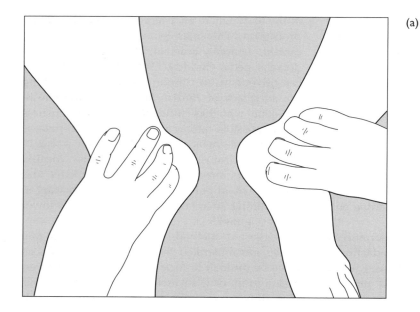

(a)

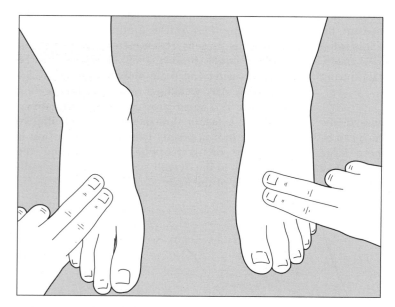

(b)

Figure 25.3: (a) Palpation of the posterior tibialis pulse. (b) Palpation of the dorsalis pedis pulse

THE ELECTROCARDIOGRAM (ECG)

The ECG is a record of the changes in electrical activity occurring within cardiac muscle. The cardiac cells involved in the contraction are specialised and are unlike any other cells in the body, as each individual cell can initiate its own electrical impulse. Although cardiac muscle has this special property, hormones and chemical transmitters are important in producing the finer control of the heart and maintenance of homeostasis.

The electrical charges within the cardiac cell are detected by bipolar and unipolar electrodes, pro-

viding an ECG rhythm known as the PQRST wave (Figure 25.5). The ECG can provide information about the heart rate and rhythm, the effects of electrolytes or drugs on the heart and the electrical orientation of the cardiac muscle. The normal ECG trace should record between 60 and 100 complexes (PQRST) per minute.

During a period of acute illness the sequence of the ECG can be affected. The rate may increase due to heart failure, hypertension, blood loss, pain, stress or anxiety or reduce its rate due to overprescription of certain drugs (digoxin) or a

```
0= impalpable
+1= feeble, thready, barely palpable
+2= decreased
+3= full
+4= bounding
```

Figure 25.4: Scale for recording pulse pressure

lack of oxygen supply. Abnormal rhythms can occur from heart failure, coronary artery disease, myocardial infarction, fluid overload and fluid and electrolyte imbalance.

BLOOD PRESSURE (BP)

By definition, blood pressure is the force exerted by the blood on the walls of the vessels in which it is contained (Jolly, 1991). It is determined by a number of factors, most significantly cardiac output, peripheral resistance, elasticity of vessels and hormonal and chemical control mechanisms (O'Brien and Davidson, 1994). Maintenance of an

adequate blood pressure is essential to permit perfusion of the brain, and the coronary arteries, and the production of urine by the kidneys.

However, in the person admitted to hospital, the homeostatic mechanisms responsible for maintaining optimum blood pressure may be stretched to their limit, fail to function, or be interfered with by drugs. The consequences of not being able to maintain an adequate blood pressure may lead ultimately to **cerebral hypoxia**, cardiac failure, acute renal failure and multi-system failure. These states occur as a result of prolonged hypotension (a low BP) or hypertension (a high BP).

Hypotension may occur in hypovolaemia where there is a diminished circulatory fluid volume (Meyers and Hickey, 1988). **Hypovolaemic shock** is the state that results from hypovolaemia and is a further decrease in the circulating fluid volume so large that the body's metabolic needs cannot be met. The principal aetiologies of hypovolaemic shock can be classified as haemorrhage,

---

Box 25.4: Learning Check 4

Self-assessment question seven

| | A low blood pressure in the acute situation is usually the result of a low cardiac output resulting from hypovolaemia. What other signs would indicate that cardiac output was low in this instance? |

Answer

Rationale

(a) Reduced peripheral perfusion

Peripheral vasoconstriction will occur secondarily to the increased sympathetic arousal found in hypovolaemia, so that the circulating volume is available for the vital organs. As circulating volume increases from transfusion of blood or blood products, cardiac output and blood pressure will improve. Perfusion to the limbs will subsequently increase; this can be felt by the nurse as the warming up of previously cold limbs.

(b) Reduced urinary output

The urinary output will fall to below 1/2 ml/kg body weight/hour for more than two consecutive hours. If the blood pressure is persistently too low to perfuse the kidneys (for urine formation) then acute tubular necrosis can result.

(c) Angina pectoris or ECG changes

If cardiac output is persistently low then the blood pressure will be inadequate to perfuse the coronary arteries with oxygenated blood and so ischaemia can result, presenting as angina and/or changes in the S–T segment on the ECG (Figure 25.5).

(d) Other signs of increased sympathetic arousal

Refer to Box 25.1.

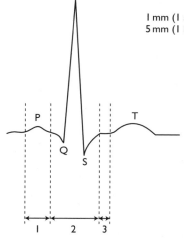

PAPER SPEED

When recording ECGs the paper speed
should be set at 25 mm/s then:

1 mm (1 small square) = 0.04 s
5 mm (1 large square) = 0.20 s

IMPORTANT LANDMARKS

Baseline
between
T wave and
P wave   : isoelectric line indicating
             no electrical activity

       P wave : atrial depolarisation

QRS complex : ventricular depolarisation

       T wave : ventricular repolarisation

ECG TERMS

Sinus rhythm   Normal ECG where the
impulse originates in
the sino-atrial node

All waves are present. All
intervals are normal
Rate 60–100 per minute
Complexes are regular (i.e.
distances between consecutive
R waves are constant)

Sinus tachycardia   Complexes are normal
but occurring 100/min to 160/min

Sinus bradycardia   Complexes are normal but occurring more slowly than 60/min

IMPORTANT INTERVALS/SEGMENTS

(1) P–R Interval 0.12–0.20 s

Represents time taken for impulse
to reach the ventricular
myocardium from the sino-atrial node

(2) QRS Interval 0.08–0.12 s

Represents time taken to
depolarise the ventricles

(3) S–T segment

Deviation of this segment above
or below the isoelectric line
may indicate myocardial ischaemia
or injury

Figure 25.5: The electrocardiogram

plasma loss and dehydration. By working
through learning check 4 (Box 25.4) signs of
hypovolaemia can be deduced.

Hypertension is consistent elevation of systemic arterial blood pressure. This can be equally

harmful to the patient in the acute setting, especially if it results in the breakdown of a recent surgical anastomosis or increases the work of a
damaged myocardium. The generally agreed values for the upper limits of a normal BP is 140 sys-

tolic and 90 diastolic. Hypertension can affect the circulation by damaging the wall of the systemic blood vessels, stimulating the vessels to thicken and strengthen to withstand the stress; this gradually narrows the lumen of the blood vessels, and can lead to heart disease (Fox, 1996) or intracerebral haemorrhage (stroke) (Shephard and Fox, 1996).

Increasing hypertension can also be indicative of raised intracranial pressure (when combined with a simultaneous decrease in pulse rate). The increasing blood pressure in this instance is a protective measure to maintain cerebral perfusion if the intracranial pressure increases (Figure 25.6) following head injury, anoxia or space-occupying lesions.

Monitoring blood pressure is an important facet of the nurse's role as systolic pressure reflects the adequacy of cardiac output, and diastolic pressure reflects the peripheral resistance exerted by the arterioles, measured in millimetres of mercury. Measuring the BP remains one of the most important and widely used assessment tools in hospital, as from this one test much information can be gleaned about the patient's state of health (Henneman and Henneman, 1989; Bardwell, 1995). Many nursing and medical staff regard this task as simple and straightforward, when in fact it is complex (Burroughs and Hoffbrand, 1990).

The technique of monitoring BP is subject to many sources of error (Venus et al., 1985; Bardwell, 1995). This is mainly because measuring and monitoring blood pressure is frequently performed, but often incorrectly. The major sources of errors are caused by the many variables involved which may mean wrong decisions being made in blood pressure management, thus compromising care (Bardwell, 1995). These errors relate to three distinct areas (Table 25.8):

- The patient
- The observer (doctor or nurse)
- Equipment.

Some of the errors identified in Table 25.8 cannot be minimised, but other variables affecting measurement can be eliminated. Strategies to achieve this include being taught the same method of taking a blood pressure (O'Brien et al., 1995) during undergraduate courses and continuing updates at postgraduate level, so that all nurses take blood pressure recordings in a standard way (Kemp, 1994). In an attempt to standardise blood pressure measurement, recommendations on how to take an accurate blood pressure are explained in Table 25.9.

CENTRAL VENOUS PRESSURE (CVP) MONITORING

The measurement of the central venous pressure (CVP) provides important haemodynamic information to guide the therapy of patients (Potger and Elliott, 1994). Central venous pressure normally reflects the volume of blood returning to the heart which exerts a pressure on the walls of the right atrium or venae cavae and measuring it can provide information about:

- The adequacy of the body's blood volume in relation to circulatory capacity
- The effectiveness of the right side of the heart as a pump
- Vascular tone
- Pulmonary vascular resistance.

A fall in CVP can indicate moderate hypovolaemic shock in patients who are bleeding, or can be due to profound vasodilatation, whereby the capacity of the circulation is increased but the circulating volume remains constant, as in patients with a pyrexia or from the excessive use of vasodilator drugs (Manley, 1991).

Often in the acute care setting the CVP is used as a guide to determine severity of loss and the fluid required to replace it (Potger and Elliott, 1994). However, CVP levels are not completely

Cerebral perfusion pressure is the difference between the mean arterial blood pressure and the intracranial pressure and represents the pressure necessary to perfuse the brain. Normally the cerebral perfusion pressure lies between 75 and 90 mmHg; if it should fall below 50 mmHg then the cerebral blood flow is severely affected.

A rise in intracranial pressure will reduce the cerebral perfusion pressure unless there is a subsequent increase in blood pressure.

CEREBRAL PERFUSION PRESSURE = MEAN ARTERIAL BLOOD PRESSURE − INTRACRANIAL PRESSURE

Normal intracranial pressure = 12–15 cm of cerebral spinal fluid (measured at lumbar puncture)

OR= 3–15 mmHg measured using an intracranial pressure monitor

Figure 25.6: Cerebral perfusion pressure

Table 25.8: The source of error when taking a blood pressure (BP)

The observer

- Observer bias – prior recording viewed by the nurse or a preference for a specific figure
- Cognitive deficits – education, inadequate training, no up-dating on the technique or principles
- Lack of understanding of the correct procedure, e.g. incorrect positioning of the patient sitting/standing, support of the arm, positioning of the cuff bladder over the centre of the brachial artery, the equipment not level with the heart
- Lack of concentration
- Hearing problems/deficit
- Sight problems

The equipment

- Cuff bladder size
- Maintenance – BP machines should be recalibrated and assessed every 6–12 months
- The level of mercury not at zero level
- Defective control valves caused by leakage, making control of the pressure release difficult
- Leaks from cracked or perished tubing
- The stethoscope should be in good condition and have clean and well-fitted ear pieces

The patient

- The patient may be suffering from exessive heat, cold, be wearing constrictive clothing, have a full bladder, recently exercised, been smoking, just had a meal or there may be a distraction, all of which will serve to either increase or decrease the BP
- Older patients have calcified/rigid arteries or anaemia which can all influence the BP reading
- A patient suffering from a high temperature may have a low BP due to vasodilatation, causing BP to fall
- In all patients the general consensus now is that disappearence of sounds (phase V) is the most accurate measurement of diastolic pressure with the stipulation that, if sounds persists to zero (e.g. in pregnant women, children or patients suffering from anaemia), the muffling of sounds (phase IV) should be used and documented on the patient's chart.
- In conditions where BP is low there may be distal vasoconstriction and it is common to underestimate the BP
- In some patients the white coat syndrome (caused when doctors appear at the bedside) affects BP, giving an inaccurately high BP reading
- Patient BP does vary during the day – higher systolic in the evening and a low recording in the morning
- Fear, anxiety, apprehension, pain can all raise the BP and these can be apparent on admission. It is recommended in this instance to wait at least 1 hour following admission to take the BP

Courtesy of Macmillan magazines.

reliable in estimating fluid needs, as the normal CVP range is from 5 to 10 cmH$_2$O when measured at the 4th intercostal space mid-axilla, yet many patients with CVP levels of 16 cmH$_2$O respond well to further fluid and blood administration. This is because CVP monitors the volume that the right myocardium can manage without failing, and this differs from patient to patient. In addition, it may take nearly 24 hours for events occurring in the left side of the heart to be transmitted through the lungs into the right ventricle, atria, and superior vena cava, and be mirrored as an increased CVP reading. Therefore, when using CVP to measure fluid replacement, the adequacy of treatment should not only be determined by the CVP but also be interpreted in conjunction with other clinical data.

A CVP can also be used to determine if fluid replacement is causing concern about overload and cardiac failure, represented by an increase in CVP. This is where the pressure on the walls of the right atrium causes increased tension to bring about an augmented CVP. This can lead to circulatory collapse, with the consequence of the heart becoming unable to pump the blood out, giving rise to a low cardiac output and an increase in

Table 25.9: How to take an accurate blood pressure

- If possible the patient should not have eaten, exercised or smoked for at least 30 minutes prior to undertaking a BP.
- The patient should be sitting or lying down in a quiet environment with his/her arm resting at heart level on a table or pillow (the antecubital fossa should be level with the fourth intercostal space). An arm that is below this level results in a falsely high reading and vice versa.
- A rest period of at least 3–5 minutes should be allowed before the reading is taken.
- Measure the circumference of the arm and use the appropriate-sized cuff. However, it is possible with modern BP cuffs to take an accurate BP even if the cuff is not an accurate size by placing the bladder centre over the brachial artery (an arrow on the actual cuff generally marks the spot) (Nolan and Nolan, 1993).
- A gap of 2–3 cm should be left between the antecubital fossa and the bottom of the cuff.
- The sphygmomanometer should be placed near to the observer (no more than 3 feet away) on a flat surface with the mercury level at zero. If the mercury is not at zero it can produce false high or low readings.
- Locate the brachial artery by palpation.
- Assess the maximal inflation level of inflating the cuff, to prevent causing pain to the patient. This is achieved by inflating the cuff and palpating the radial pulse at the same time; when the pulse disappears, the maximal inflation level will be 20–30 mmHg higher than at the level the pulse disappeared.
- The patient should not cross his/her legs as this will give a falsely high reading.
- Place the stethoscope over the brachial artery, being careful not to use too much pressure, as this lowers the diastolic pressure reading. Release the valve slowly and gently.
- The cuff should be rapidly inflated at 2 mmHg/s and deflated slowly. A slow inflation and a rapid deflation both result in inaccuracies.
- Note the systolic pressure at the onset of the first clear repetitive tapping sound of 2 beats or more (phase I Korotkoff sounds).
- The diastolic blood pressure should be recorded at the cessation of sound (phase V) for all patients, unless the recording is zero, in which case the muffling of sound (phase IV) should be used. If phase IV is used, it should be documented on the chart.
- The blood should be measured to the nearest 2 mmHg.
- The procedure should take no less than 5 minutes (Nolan and Nolan, 1993).
- If the procedure is rushed, this will result in an underestimation of the systolic pressure and an overestimation of the diastolic pressure.
- The measurement should be recorded on the patient's chart. If it is not possible to achieve optimum conditions, this should also be noted with the blood pressure reading, for example, 'BP 145/95, L arm, phase V (patient very anxious)'.
- If the reading needs to be repeated, at least 1–2 minutes should elapse before reinflating the cuff.

Courtesy of Macmillan magazines.

right and left ventricular pressures. In addition, a high CVP can depict exposure to profound cold. This causes severe vasoconstriction, returning more blood to the heart and, as the veins are already filled, causing the heart to dysfunction. In addition to measurement, the CVP catheter can also be used for rapid infusion of fluids and blood, or withdrawal of blood for laboratory samples. Table 25.10 gives examples of raised and lowered CVP.

Measurements are usually made using a water manometer which is connected to a venous cannula, usually placed within the subclavian vein or internal jugular vein (Figure 25.7). The water manometer's zero point is then aligned (using a spirit level) with a point on the patient's chest which corresponds to the right atrium. Two points are widely used as reference points:

- The sternal angle which is directly above the right atrium when the patient is lying flat.
- The 4th intercostal space mid-axilla which is anatomically in line with the right atrium.

It is imperative to use the same reference point for consecutive recordings, as normal ranges vary according to the reference point selected (Table 25.11). However, the most reliable reference point to take the CVP is the 4th intercostal space or mid-axilla, as it has been anatomically shown to be a

Table 25.10: Causes of raised and lowered central venous pressure (CVP)

	Rationale
Raised CVP	
Overtransfusion	The blood volume has increased in relation to the size of the circulation, so more blood is returning to the right atrium
Cardiac failure	The heart is impaired in its function as a pump and cannot cope effectively with the blood returning to the heart
Pulmonary embolus	The right side of the heart has to pump against a greater resistance due to thrombus occluding part of the pulmonary circulation
Tamponade	Due to fluid/blood in the pericardial sac the ventricles cannot fill properly. The back pressure is transmitted to the atria
Lowered CVP	
Hypovolaemia ■ Burns ■ Pancreatitis ■ Diabetes mellitus Haemorrhage	The circulating volume is reduced so once the venous reservoir is filled there is little blood left to return to the heart
Gross vasodilation ■ Septicaemia ■ Vasodilatory drugs	Vasodilation increases the capacity of the circulation (or the size of the reservoir) so that the circulating volume is no longer adequate both to fill the veins and provide enough volume to return to the heart.

true external point for identifying the right atrium (Callow and Pieper, 1989; Kee *et al.*, 1993). For either reference piont, the patient needs to be in the supine position. If breathlessness occurs when lying flat, the CVP readings may need to be taken with the patient lying at a greater angle, no more than 30 degrees, in which case the angle used should always be indicated alongside the recorded CVP measurement.

It is not the single CVP reading that is important but the trend demonstrated by a series of readings over time. Therefore, each time a CVP measurement is made, it is essential that it is made under identical conditions so that all possible variables (such as patient position) remain constant. How to perform a CVP measurement is illustrated in Figure 25.7, and some important precautions are identified.

All lines used to measure CVP are central venous lines and thus present the inherent danger of air embolism. All intravenous administration equipment should, therefore, possess **Luer lock** connections to minimise accidental disconnection. Another hazard pertinent to subclavian and internal jugular intravenous lines is damage to anatomical structures such as the arteries or the apices of the lungs, leading to **pneumothorax** or damage to the ventricular muscles of the heart causing ventricular arrhythmias (Darovic, 1987). Additionally, there is the risk of infection and subsequent septicaemia, so the cannula site should be treated as a minor surgical wound requiring the meticulous maintenance of asepsis.

RESPIRATION

Respiration is an essential body function necessary for the diffusion of gases between the alveoli and blood, as well as the maintenance of blood pH (Marieb, 1995). Ventilation is the mechanical movement of gas or air in and out of the lungs. The respiratory rate is the ventilatory rate, or the number of times gas is inspired and expired per minute (see Chapter 23, Marieb, 1995).

Effective respiration is dependent on many factors, both nervous and chemical in nature, but which generally include the chemoreceptors and lung receptors (McCance and Huether, 1994). The structures involved in respiration are illustrated in Figure 25.8 (page 636) together with possible causes of malfunction.

When asserting respiration there are other important observations to make (in addition to

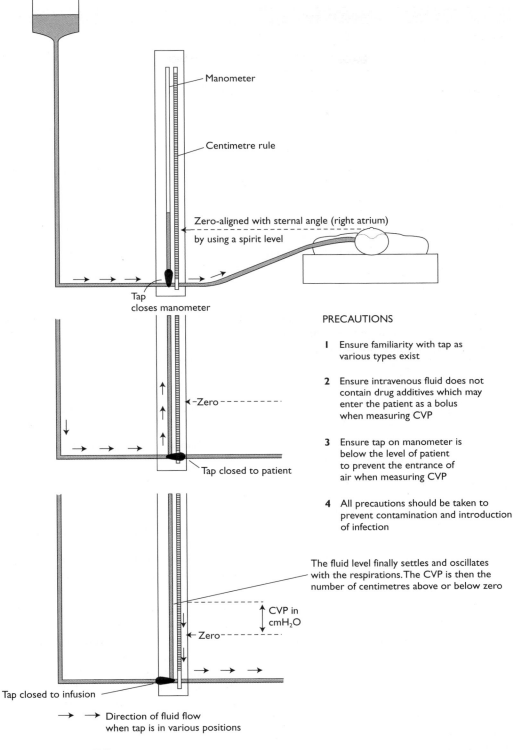

Manometer

Centimetre rule

Zero-aligned with sternal angle (right atrium)
by using a spirit level

Tap
closes manometer

Tap closed to patient

-Zero

PRECAUTIONS

1 Ensure familiarity with tap as
   various types exist

2 Ensure intravenous fluid does not
   contain drug additives which may
   enter the patient as a bolus
   when measuring CVP

3 Ensure tap on manometer is
   below the level of patient
   to prevent the entrance of
   air when measuring CVP

4 All precautions should be taken to
   prevent contamination and introduction
   of infection

The fluid level finally settles and oscillates
with the respirations. The CVP is then the
number of centimetres above or below zero

CVP in
cmH$_2$O

Zero

Tap closed to infusion

→ → Direction of fluid flow
         when tap is in various positions

Figure 25.7: Measuring CVP using a water manometer

Table 25.11: Normal CVP ranges

	Normal CVP ranges
Sternal angle	0–5 cmH₂0
Mid-axilla	5–10 cmH₂0
4th intercostal space	

rate) which will help identify the effectiveness of breathing. Observation of respiration itself can be considered in terms of quality, rate, pattern and depth.

The respiratory rate in adults is normally between 8 and 18 breaths per minute. Counting should be over a minute and take place when the patient is resting and unaware of the observation, since conscious awareness of breathing can lead to alteration in rate and pattern. This is because breathing is under the control of both the involuntary and voluntary nervous systems. Closely related to rate is respiratory pattern. Many terms are used to describe various patterns and rates; those used most commonly are set out in Table 25.12 together with the possible causes.

The depth of respiration relates to the tidal volume, i.e. the volume of air moving in and out of the respiratory tract with each breath. The depth of respiration can be specifically measured using a spirometer, or observed by inspecting chest expansion for depth or shallowness at the same time as observing for equality and uniformity of movement.

The quality of normal, relaxed breathing in any position is effortless, automatic, regular and quiet except for the occasional sighing, yawning and coughing which should be noted by the nurse. Noisy, gurgling and wheezing respirations are abnormal and imply an obstruction in the upper respiratory tract. The louder the noise heard at the mouth during inspiration, the greater the degree of airway obstruction present.

Noisy breathing must, however, be separated from other sounds superimposed on a normal breathing pattern which are usually heard through a stethoscope. The noises are termed **crackles** (or râles) and wheezes. Crackles are heard as 'crackling' or 'popping' sounds and result from the explosive opening of collapsed alveoli in deflated parts of the lungs. **Wheezes** are musical sounds often associated with asthma which result

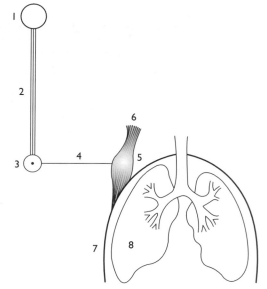

KEY NOS	STRUCTURE	CAUSES OF MALFUNCTION
I	Respiratory centre	Direct trauma Raised intracranial pressure Drugs; Hypoxia; *Hypercapnia*
2	Spinal cord	Trauma
3	Anterior horn cell	*Poliomyelitis*
4	Peripheral nerve	*Polyneuritis*
5	Neuromuscular junction	*Botulism* Muscle relaxant drugs
6	Respiratory muscles	*Tetanus*
7	Chest wall	Trauma Pneumothorax
8	Lungs & airways	Pneumonia

Figure 25.8: Structures involved in respiration
(Adapted from Sykes *et al.*, 1976 and reproduced by permission of the publishers, Blackwell Scientific Publishers)

from opposing bronchial walls oscillating or rapidly opening and closing (Harper, 1981).

In addition, observations should include: the ability to talk, as shortness of breath will inhibit conversation; and the use of accessory muscles, such as **pectoralis** or **sternomastoid** muscles used to increase thoracic size in attempts to improve ventilation where breathlessness is present. How to recognise ineffective breathing in an acutely ill person can be deduced by working through learning check 5 (Box 25.5, page 638).

Table 25.12: Variations in respirations with possible causes found in acute hospital settings

Name	Definition	Possible cause
Tachypnoea	Normal respiratory pattern with a rate greater than 20/min	Fever Hypoxia associated with cardiac/respiratory failure
Bradypnoea	Normal respiratory pattern with a rate below 8/min	Metabolic disorders (for example, drug overdoses, alcohol intoxication, abnormal brain function)
Dyspnoea	A feeling of shortness of breath (a subjective sensation)	Cardiac, neurological or respiratory dysfunction Anxiety
Hyperventilation	An increase in respiration rate and depth over and above the body's actual metabolic requirements	Pharmacological Nervous Metabolic } origins Pulmonary Psychological
Hypoventilation	When respirations are unable to match the body's metabolic demands	Any damage or malfunction in the structures involved in breathing. See Figure 25.8
Cheyne–Stokes	Period of apnoea alternating with shallow, progressively deeper, and then shallow respirations	Congestive heart failure, uraemia, brain disease
Kussmaul's respiration	Deep rapid respirations associated with diabetic ketoacidosis ('air-hunger')	Diabetic ketoacidosis
Apneustic respirations	Uncontrolled gasping respirations with pauses at full inspiration and full expiration	Damage to the pons

URINE OUTPUT

The kidneys receive about 25% of the cardiac output and the glomerular filtration rate (GFR) depends on adequate renal perfusion determined by the blood pressure; when adequate the production of urine will exceed 0.5 ml/kg per hour. Therefore, the average urinary output should be between 30 and 70 ml or more per hour (Marieb, 1995).

In an acutely ill person kidney function can be monitored by a catheter or by measuring urine output. If urine output falls below 0.5 ml/kg per hour for more than 2 hours, the medical team should be informed as it may be necessary to increase fluid administration (Dries and Waxman, 1991) or to prescribe diuretics. The measurement of urine output at hourly or regular intervals should be accurately recorded (Kee and Kayes, 1990). Interpretation of urine output should also consider overall fluid balance, and the quality of urine. Thus, it is often necessary to measure urine osmolarity and monitor electrolyte content.

URINE TESTING

The kidney has a prime role in maintaining normal healthy life and many early changes that occur in the body may be reflected in the urine well before they become clinically obvious. Therefore, by taking note of some of the areas measured in a routine urine test a person's fluid balance may be evaluated. It can aid diagnosis, assist in monitoring circulatory status, and help provide valuable clues to the effectiveness of treatment (Bowker et al., 1986). It is unfortunate that urine testing is described as 'routine' and devalued (Cook, 1995).

The significance of the urine test strip results can be found in the specific gravity, pH or whether blood, protein, bilirubin and urobilinogen, nitrates, glucose and ketones are present (Table 25.13). Some clues suggesting a preliminary urine test may be required can be viewed in Table 25.14 (page 640).

The results of ward or clinic testing of urine should be recorded accurately in the patient's or

Box 25.5: Learning Check 5

Self-assessment question eight

How would you recognise that breathing was ineffective in an acutely ill person?

Answer

1 Central cyanosis of the lips and tongue
 – in persons with normal haemoglobin levels (NB. Peripheral cyanosis only indicates local perfusion problems – for example, cold or local ischaemia)
2 Pallor of the skin
 – particularly in patients who are anaemic
*3 Increased respiratory rate (or decreased rate)
*4 Use of accessory muscles of respiration, laboured breathing and flaring of the nostrils
5 Anxiety, restlessness and confusion and loss of consciousness in extreme cases
6 Evidence of increased sympathetic activity i.e. tachycardia and irregularities in pulse
 – increased blood pressure (if patient is not hypovolaemic or in left ventricular failure)
 – sweating
 – peripheral shutdown
7 Changes in posture and facial expression (for example, hunching over a bedtable, furrowed brow, tired and drawn expression)

* Points 3 and 4 would only apply if breathing had not been affected by damage to nerves or by drugs which suppress respiration

client's records, as soon as possible after testing. A negative test result may not only point to an alternative diagnosis, but it is also a valuable baseline indicator to be referred to later in evaluating the progress of a patient during the course of his or her illness. A negative result should always be recorded even if at the time it appears unimportant or irrelevant.

BLOOD ANALYSIS

Taking a blood sample is often the role of the doctor or phlebotomist, but the results of blood tests have a prime place in assisting the nurse to gain a full detailed assessment of his or her patient. Those which the nurse may be interested in are haemoglobin, plasma osmolarity and haematocrit levels, and can be viewed in Table 25.15 (page 641).

OXYGEN SATURATION TO DETERMINE HYPOXIA

The nurse is frequently the first to observe the presence of hypoxia and the one who can intervene to correct the problem (Masasi and Keyes, 1994). Most cells require oxygen to survive, function correctly, and maintain organ function. Hypoxia can occur from a blockage and reduced blood flow, as in arteriosclerosis; or from the loss of red blood cells which carry oxygen to the cells, often observed in haemorrhage; or from the inability to get oxygen into the circulation, seen in patients with impaired respiratory function.

A nurse can observe for hypoxia in a number of ways. There may be changes in a person's behaviour and/or level of consciousness. Very early signs of cerebral underperfusion are the inability to think abstractly or perform complex mental tasks, restlessness, apprehension, uncooperativeness and irritability. Short-term memory may also be impaired. This is because the brain continuously needs a steady supply of oxygenated blood flow.

There may also be changes in BP, pulse and the colour of mucous membranes (Masasi and Keyes, 1994). This may lead the nurse to extend his/her assessment of hypoxia, by obtaining an oxygen saturation measurement. This requires placing a probe on the patient's finger and attaching it to an oxygen saturation monitor; the normal is between 98 and 100%. However, a patient may experience a large drop in oxygen supply, but with minimal effect on oxygen saturation. Therefore, caution should be taken when using this method alone to determine hypoxia, and the nurse should use his/her observational skills to complement such measurements.

PAIN

The presence of pain can interfere with obtaining accurate and reliable measurements, which can lead to false inaccurate readings. Therefore, pain needs to be assessed early (Hollinworth, 1994) and is, thus, incorporated into the first level assessment. Regular assessment of pain contributes to the quality of communication between nurse and patient, and regular pain assessment can be a contributory factor in reducing pain (Pearce, 1993). Baillie (1993) suggested that because of the subjective nature of pain, only patients can measure their own pain accurately and so nurses should provide tools to help them assess and communi-

Table 25.13: The clinical significance of urine test results

Specific gravity (SG)

Is measured to determine hydration and the amount of waste products excreted. As urine is mostly water with a variable quantity of substances dissolved in it, the concentration of these substances, diluted in water, will depend on the body's state of hydration and the amount of waste products to be excreted. Therefore, testing the urine for specific gravity can be one way to determine whether hydration is adequate.

The SG of urine will give a good indication of the net fluid balance and is of particular value in patients where there is an unquantifiable loss, such as in burns cases, breathing difficulties, diarrhoea or fever. In healthy adults, SG varies between 1.005 and 1.035 (pure water is the standard, with SG of 1.000). Urine with a persistently low SG is suggestive of diabetes insipidus or renal damage; due to the normal concentration power of the kidneys being lost, the urine passed will tend to be rather dilute. An increase in specific gravity will indicate dehydration, perhaps due to bleeding, vomiting, diarrhoea, reduction in fluid intake or fever.

The pH

The pH of urine should reflect the acid–base balance of the body, as excess hydrogen or bicarbonate ions are excreted by the renal tubules to maintain the normal status. Under normal circumstances, the urine has a pH of around 6 but it can range from about 5 to 8.5. Metabolic acidosis from starvation, high protein diets or diabetic ketoacidosis will lead to an acid urine, but diets including a lot of vegetable, mild or even bicarbonate-based antacids can cause an alkaline urine, when the pH will rise. Knowing the urinary pH can be of use when attempting to diagnose a patient's symptoms. If a urinary tract infection is suspected, proteinuria combined with an alkaline pH is highly suggestive of bacterial infection but less likely if the urine is acid.

Blood

The presence of blood is a potentially serious sign and needs a rapid investigation. Asymptomatic haematuria is usually the earliest sign of cancer of the bladder which can be treated if detected early enough. It can also be due to trauma, infection or stones. False positive results may occur, from containers contaminated with bleach, skin preparation with povidone iodine, or from the use of stale urine.

Protein

In early renal disease, the glomerulus and tubules may leak small amounts of protein into the urine. As renal disease progresses, detectable levels of protein will be found in the urine. There are a number of systemic diseases associated with proteinuria including renal disease, urinary tract infection, hypertension, pre-eclampsia and congestive heart failure. Transient positive tests are not always significant, however, and normal urine contains small amounts of albumin and globulin, although generally not enough to give a positive result on a reagent strip. Thus, when testing for urinary protein, a morning specimen of urine is recommended to ensure sufficient concentration. Proteinuria can be an early sign as well as a means of monitoring the progress of disease or its response to therapy.

Bilirubin and urobilinogen

In normal health, bilirubin is found in the urine but the majority is excreted via the bile duct into the gut. When the liver is diseased or there is obstruction to the flow of bile into the gut, bilirubin or its metabolites are likely to be found in significant quantities in the urine. Urobilinogen is normally present in urine, but elevated levels may indicate liver abnormalities or excessive destruction of red blood cells, such as in haemolytic anaemia.

Nitrates

Urine normally contains nitrates from dietary metabolites, and some of the common bacteria responsible for urinary infections will convert these nitrates to nitrites. Nitrites are not normally present in urine, but are produced in increasing numbers when Gram-negative bacteria such as *Escherichia coli* convert dietary nitrates (found in the preservatives in meat products and cheese and smoked food) to nitrites. As *E. coli* is responsible for 80% of urine infection, the presence of nitrites is strongly suggestive of urinary tract infection (UTI). A reagent strip will detect nitrite in urine and can confirm a bacterial presence.

The specimen for testing should have been present in the bladder for 4 hours before voiding, to allow sufficient time for the nitrate/nitrite conversion. Visible signs may be, for example, is the specimen clear or

Table 25.13: continued

> cloudy? If the specimen is clear and blood, protein, leucocytes and nitrites are not present, there is no UTI. If the specimen is turbid and one or more of the four tests are positive, there is a chance of a UTI.
>
> **Glucose**
>
> Glucose is not normally found in urine. The presence of glucose may be due to raised blood glucose levels (hyperglycaemia). It can be associated with many medical conditions such as diabetes mellitus, stress, Cushing's syndrome and acute pancreatitis. There is a case for screening middle-aged and older people when admitted to hospital as they may, at an early stage, be relatively asymptomatic before more serious symptoms present. Once a diagnosis is made, urinalysis for glucose can be a valuable method of monitoring the disease, particularly as diabetic retinopathy, kidney disease, peripheral vascular and cardiac disease are secondary to prolonged hyperglycaemia.
>
> There are two categories of urine tests for glucose, the Clinitest, and the impregnated test strips. The Clinitest is quite cumbersome, but provides an accurate measurement. Test strips, however, do not measure so accurately the quantity of glucose in the urine and therefore are probably only adequate for screening purposes.
>
> **Ketones**
>
> When the body metabolises fat waste, the breakdown products are the ketone bodies, which are excreted in the urine. In good health they are not detectable in urine. Usually ketones may be found in people who are fasting, but they can also be present in excessive amounts in people with uncontrolled diabetes. There are two tests available for ketones: acetest which is a tablet test, and a strip test which is available either as a single test, Ketostix, or incorporated into one of the combined multiple-strip sticks. Ketones are acidic substances and when present in excess can lead to metabolic acidosis, which, if untreated, can cause death. Early detection is therefore of value.
>
> **Appearance**
>
> The appearance of the urine should be noted for colour and clarity. Colour changes may be due to endogenous pigments such as haemoglobin (red or red/brown colour), bilirubin (yellow) or intact red cells (smoky red). Exogenous pigments may also cause colour changes: a red-coloured urine may be due to eating beetroot or to contamination with menstrual blood. A negative result should always be recorded even if at the time it appears unimportant or irrelevant.

Table 25.14: Clues to suggesting a preliminary urine test

Symptom or sign	Possible diagnosis	Tests to consider
Weight loss, perhaps with an increase in thirst	? Diabetes	Look for glucose and ketones
Frequency of micturition	? Infection	Test for bacteria (i.e. nitrites) or protein
	? Renal disease	Test for specific gravity and protein
Yellow tinge to skin	? Jaundice	Test for urobilinogen and urine bilirubin

cate their pain. Thompson (1989) considered that assessment tools can be invaluable in aiding accurate pain assessment.

There are many simple pain assessment tools. The visual analogue scale is one of the most popular (Latham, 1989). The scale consists of a straight line, usually 10 centimetres in length, with one extreme marked 'no pain at all' and the other end marked 'worst possible pain' (Schofield, 1995).

The scale may be used vertically or horizontally and descriptive words may be added to a vertical scale. Numerical rating scales are marked between 0 and 10, with 0 signifying 'no pain' and 10 meaning 'unbearable pain' (Baillie, 1993). Verbal rating scales or verbal descriptors consist of a list of adjectives that describe levels of pain intensity by extremes ('no pain', 'mild', 'moderate', 'severe', 'very severe').

Table 25.15: Some useful blood tests and their significance

Haemoglobin levels

The haemoglobin (Hb) level is the amount of red blood cells in the blood. It is contained in the erythrocytes' cytoplasm and is primary responsible for carrying oxygen and carbon dioxide to the body's tissues. The normal concentration of haemoglobin in the blood is between 12 and 15 g/100 ml of blood. When considering the Hb it is important to include the patient's age, general state and the rate of fall of the haemoglobin concentration. A low Hb will indicate that red blood cells are being lost, not being produced by the body, or the patient is haemodiluted. A haemoglobin concentration may fall suddenly, due to acute blood loss and/or overinfusion of fluids/colloids, or gradually over weeks or months, e.g. in iron deficiency anaemia, megaloblastic anaemia, renal failure and anaemias associated with chronic disorders.

In addition to determining Hb levels, other signs may be present to confirm findings, e.g. in white skin when haemoglobin is poorly oxygenated, both the blood and the skin appear blue (cyanosis); in black people, cyanosis of the skin does not appear, but can be observed in the mucous membranes and nail beds.

Plasma osmolality

Osmolality is a measure of the number of milliosmoles per litre of solution, or the concentration of molecules per volume of solution. When solute is added to water, the volume is expanded and includes the original amount of water plus the volume occupied by the solute particles (e.g. sodium, potassium, calcium, etc.). So, by taking notice of the plasma osmolality the volume of water in relation to added solutes can be determined. Therefore, when there is an increase in osmolality there is a reduction of water in relation to the solutes contained within it, as the solute concentration has not changed.

The osmolality of intracellular and extracellular fluid tends to equalise and so provides a measure of body fluid concentration and thus the body's hydration status. The normal osmolality of body fluids is 280–294 mOsm/l. Thus, a serum osmolality less than 280 mOsm/l will generally indicate an excess of fluids in the vessels indicating overhydration or hypervolaemia. An increased serum osmolality, greater than 295 mOsm/l, indicates a loss of fluid and dehdration or hypovolaemia may be present. With an increase in osmolality, thirst and a dry mouth are often experienced and may hint to the nurse to consider finding or suggesting a result for this blood measurement be investigated.

Haematocrit levels

A factor which influences blood flow is the consistency of the blood. Flow varies inversely with the viscosity of the fluid. Thick fluids move more slowly and cause a greater resistance to flow than thin fluids. The greater the percentage of red blood cells in the blood, the more viscous the blood. The relationship is expressed as the haematocrit, the ratio of volume of red blood cells to the volume of whole blood. The haematocrit is a useful guide for determining whether whole blood or some other intravenous fluid should be used for volume replacement in the haemorrhagic shock patient.

A high haematocrit reduces flow through the blood vessels, particulary the microcirculation (arterioles, capillaries and venules). Conditions in which the haematocrit is elevated, for example, dehydration, haemorrhage, anaemias, leukaemias, cyanotic congenital heart disease or polycythaemia, can lead to increased cardiac work as a result of increased vascular resistance. The viscosity of blood also increases if blood flow becomes very slow or stagnates. This condition is called anomalous viscosity.

The Bourbonnais pain assessment tool (Bourbonnais, 1981) consists of two pain assessment tools designed to complement each other, one for the patient and one for the nurse. Both tools are suitable for use with acutely ill people. The nurses' pain assessment tool was developed as a concise and systematic guide. The tool (Table 25.16) includes five sections. The first two focus on visual observations which may be exhibited by a person experiencing pain. These include non-verbal signs and evidence of any autonomic response, either sympathetic or parasympathetic. The remaining three sections focus on questions which the nurse can ask the patient and questions he/she should consider him/herself.

The patient assessment tool was tried by Bourbonnais (1981) with a limited number of patients in a variety of acute settings ranging from a coro-

Table 25.16: A pain assessment tool for nurses

1 Observe for skeletal muscle response
(a) Body movements
   ■ immobility
   ■ purposeless or inaccurate body movements
   ■ protective movements including withdrawal reflex
   ■ rhythmic or rubbing movements
(b) Facial expression
   ■ clenched teeth
   ■ wrinkled forehead
   ■ biting of lower lip
   ■ widely opened or tightly shut eyes
 	
2 Autonomic nervous system response
(a) Sympathetic nervous system activation
   ■ increased pulse
   ■ increased respirations
   ■ increased diastolic and systolic blood pressure
   ■ cold perspiration
   ■ pallor
   ■ dilated pupils
   ■ nausea
   ■ muscle tension
(b) Parasympathetic activation in some visceral pain
   ■ low blood pressure
   ■ slow pulse
For example: in pain involving the bladder, colon or rectum
Remember: patients with chronic pain usually do not display the intensive skeletal muscle and autonomic nervous system responses
 	
3 Verbal report of the patient
Questions to ask the patient
   ■ location of pain
   ■ intensity of pain
   ■ onset and duration
   ■ precipitating and aggravating factors
   ■ nature of pain (e.g. sharp, dull)
 	
4 Questions the nurse should ask herself
(a) How long has it been since the immediately post-operative patient was medicated for pain?
(b) How fatigued is the patient?
(c) Is the patient in an environment of sensory restriction?
(d) Are you reaching the true cause of the patient's pain?
(e) Are you aware of your biases?
(f) Is the patient anxious?
(g) What is the patient's past experience with pain?
(h) Does the patient have an altered level of consciousness?
 	
5 Nursing history questions (Mayers, 1972)
(a) Have you had pain or discomfort recently?
(b) If yes, what did you do to relieve the pain or discomfort?
(c) If you have pain or discomfort while in the hospital, what would you like the nurse to do to relieve it?

Reproduced from Bourbonnais, 1981, by kind permission of Blackwell Scientific Publications.

nary care unit to an orthopaedic ward. She found that patients were able to use the tool easily and that it helped them to tell the nurse about the pain they were feeling. An additional benefit was that patients found it less tiring to point to a scale than

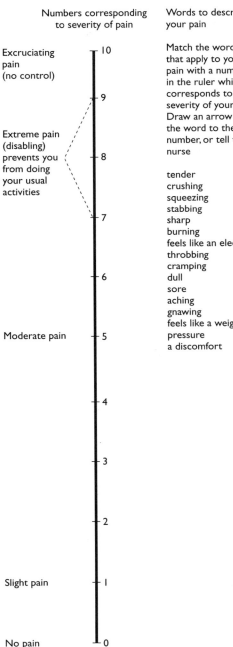

Numbers corresponding to severity of pain	Words to describe your pain

Excruciating pain (no control) — 10

Match the words(s) that apply to your pain with a number in the ruler which corresponds to the severity of your pain Draw an arrow from the word to the number, or tell the nurse

— 9

Extreme pain (disabling) prevents you from doing your usual activities — 8

tender
crushing
squeezing
stabbing
sharp
burning
feels like an electric shock
throbbing
cramping
dull
sore
aching
gnawing
feels like a weight
pressure
a discomfort

— 7

— 6

Moderate pain — 5

— 4

— 3

— 2

Slight pain — 1

No pain — 0

Figure 25.9: Patient pain assessment ruler
(reproduced from Bourbonnais, 1981, by kind permission of Blackwell Scientific Publications)

to try to describe the pain they felt. The tool (Figure 25.9), a 'pain ruler', consists of two parts: a scale ranging from 0 (reflecting no pain) to 10 (reflecting excruciating pain), and a list of adjectives which describe different perceptions of pain. The person experiencing pain is then asked to match the word or words that describe his or her pain to the number which corresponds to the intensity of the pain. This tool, therefore, enables patients to communicate their pain, which allows for easier evaluation of the effectiveness of relief, and has the further benefit of allowing continuity of pain assessment from one set of staff to another when shifts change.

A more recent pain assessment tool was devised by Raiman (1986) and is known as the London pain chart. The chart comes with specific instructions for use and includes a body chart to record the site of pain(s), a verbal descriptor scale for intensity and measures to relieve pain (Baillie, 1993). For further information on pain assessment tools, factors affecting pain assessment and nurses' attitudes towards pain the reader is referred to Chapter 15.

The first level assessment has determined that within the Burford NDU model the nurse requires both observation and measurement skills. The discussion has included psychological factors, but has focused more on the physiological measurements due to the importance of these during the acute phase of illness. Having explored in depth aspects of the first level assessment for acute adults admitted to hospital, the second level assessment can now be explored.

SECOND LEVEL ASSESSMENT

The second level assessment focuses on the cue questions outlined in Table 25.3. Before asking the cue questions, it is necessary to identify further aspects of the learning domain 'knowing' therapeutic work (Johns, 1991, 1994). The dimension of therapeutic work relating to this level is involvement with patients, and is about learning to establish and maintain the therapeutic relationship necessary to achieve a well-defined and effective interview with patients. It involves asking the cue questions identified by Johns, and includes a more detailed history relating to factors that may influence care.

Interview

A good nursing assessment relies heavily upon the nurse's skills at interviewing patients and so a good interviewing technique is important. Observational skills play a part in interviewing, because information is forthcoming from patients' non-verbal communication, in addition to what they actually say (Binnie *et al.*, 1988). Whether or not non-verbal cues support or contradict verbal communication may be important. The admission of a patient includes an interview and it is from this structured discussion that much crucial information can be obtained.

To assess the individual needs of the patient, a health history is necessary. This includes asking some of the relevant cue questions (identified in Table 25.3). The cue questions do not require specific written answers. They are designed to help the nurse most effectively expand on the core question. In addition, they serve to identify certain areas with regard to the patient and the nurse–patient relationship and incorporate the concepts identified by the model described at the outset of this chapter.

Assessment of the patient's needs may be made on the basis of a nursing history. For this, not only must the nurse be able to communicate well, but he/she must also be skilled in interviewing techniques. Through learning how to ask the right questions, and using him/herself to convey care, knowing how to encourage the patient to give information and, perhaps most importantly, to recognise non-verbal cues given by the patient, the nurse can get to know his/her patient, and vice versa. Getting to know the patient will imvolve exploring his or her health status, identifying the role of the family or important others, determining his or her level of stress and sleeping patterns, amongst other aspects of their individuality.

COMMUNICATION

Communication can be defined as all the processes, verbal and non-verbal, conscious and unconscious, by which one mind may affect another (Blattner, 1981). It is an essential activity of living, which can be as important as physical support. Many investigators (Cartwright, 1974; Spelman, 1967; Ley, 1988) have identified patients' dissatisfaction with communication during their hospital stay. This dissatisfaction relates to the quality and amount of information received (Ley, 1988), and to insufficient, confusing and contradictory information being given by different health care professionals. These areas are identified by the Health Service Commissioner, and various consumer organisations, as the main areas of complaint (DoH, 1993).

Boore (1978), Wicker (1987), Wong (1990), Radcliffe (1993) and Nelson (1996) have demonstrated how nurses, by giving active information, can speed up recovery, reduce the number of complications and the need for pain relief, particularly in post-operative patients. Yet, in the acute care setting, the development of verbal skills, the giving of information and the additional use of listening skills, although they improve the quality of care given, are insufficient on their own. What is needed is for the nurse, in addition, to increase his/her proficiency at monitoring and interpreting non-verbal cues from physically dependent patients who are unable to communicate verbally, due to speech loss or factors affecting speech, such as breathlessness or pain.

Non-verbal communication is the term used to describe all forms of human communication not controlled by speech (Kacperek, 1997) and it can be used therapeutically by nurses. Argyle (1988) suggests that the non-verbal component of communication is five times more influential than the verbal aspect. The components of non-verbal communication are illustrated in Figure 25.10. Stress in acutely ill patients can be actively reduced, using relaxation and soothing techniques, and caring can be conveyed through touch (Green, 1996). Verity (1996) made some interesting observations with regard to the use of touch in general hospital settings. In her article she suggested that touch is a means of giving and gathering information but consideration should be given to the fact that people are individuals, so interpretation of tactile communication will differ from person to person.

However, some health care members find it difficult to provide emotional support through touch, because they are often busy with the technical aspects of stabilising the patient's condition, leaving insufficient time to provide the emotional support necessary. However, Biley (1996) noted that in situations where patients were under intense personal stress, feeling isolated and vulnerable, no other method of communication compared to the comforting and quieting effects of therapeutic touch.

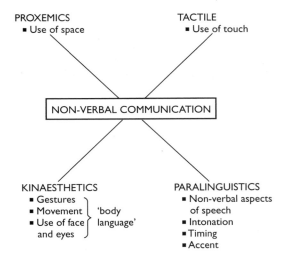

Figure 25.10: Components of non-verbal communication

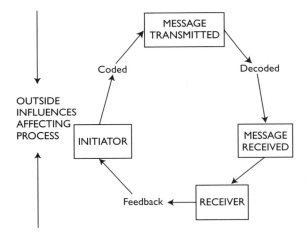

Figure 25.11: The communication process

The communication process (Figure 25.11) itself comprises five elements:

1 The sender or encoder of the message
2 The message itself
3 The receiver or decoder of the message
4 Feedback that the receiver conveys to the sender
5 The environment in which the message is transmitted.

When planning to meet patients' communication needs, Ashworth's (1979) classic six essential areas in relation to the patient in intensive care are old but remain relevant to the acutely ill patient in hospital today:

1 Orientation to the time, day, date, place, people, environment and procedures
2 Specific patient teaching on any aspect of care
3 Adopting methods to overcome patients' sensory deficits
4 Comforting patients who are confused or hallucinating
5 Communications which maintain the patient's personal identity
6 Helping the communications of voiceless patients.

Resources, nursing actions and aids which can be used in connection with these six areas are suggested in Table 25.17.

Having communicated information to patients, it is important to remember that the information may not be remembered, especially by acutely ill patients whose drugs may interfere with information processing and storage. These memory disorders are generally due to inadequate acquisition or inadequate recall. Inadequate acquisition relates to the circumstances at the time the information was acquired – the patient is unable to assign meaning to or organise the information at the time of exposure to it. This can lead to confusion and lack of memory with regard to the event.

With inadequate recall of information, the triggers for information retrieval become distorted. A patient who is depressed is more likely to have inadequate recall and generally recall unpleasant matters, and as such it may be difficult for him or her to focus on happier and more pleasant feelings and memories. Amnesia refers to the inability to recall events which have occurred, and this may be the consequences of drugs used to sedate patients during unpleasant procedures and investigations.

Barriers to, and interference with, communication can occur at any point in the process. A summary of potential problems relating to the patient's reception of messages from the nurse in acute hospital settings is provided in Table 25.18 (page 647).

HEALTH STATUS

The tool used to determine health status was developed by Campbell *et al.* (1985) out of the need to assist nurses in the identification of human responses and to provide the basic data necessary to plan holisitic care, as well as to enable the nurse to model the client's world, i.e. to interpret rela-

Table 25.17: Resources, aids and nursing actions when planning to meet the communication needs of acutely ill patients

Essential areas of planning	Resource/aid/nursing action

Orientation in time, place, person, people, environment and procedures	■ Information regarding
	  − treatment
	  − care
	  − progress
	  − how patient can help himself
	■ Visible clock and calendar
	■ Daily newspaper
	■ Day and night lighting
	■ Positioning near windows
	■ Use of glasses, hearing aids (if needed)

Communication which maintains patient identity	■ Talking about normal life, home, family interests, preferences, concerns ■ Offering as many choices affecting the environment as possible ■ Enable the patient to maintain control of his own body − choices, decisions
Special patient teaching	■ Rehabilitation programmes following myocardial infarction ■ Patient information booklets ■ Breathing/limb exercises
Overcoming sensory deficit	■ Has aids he usually needs ■ Aids are functioning and effective ■ Verbal descriptions of environment if the patient can't see ■ Tactile manipulation of equipment
Comforting patients who are confused or hallucinating	■ Acknowledge and accept the patient's delusions or hallucinations while stating that you do not see or believe the same thing
Helping communication of voiceless patients	■ Communication bells to attract attention ■ Communication cards ■ Pen and pad ■ Alphabet cards ■ Work out a system with patient and ensure continuity ■ Speaking appliances for tracheostomy tubes

tionships and develop a mirror image from his/her perspective. It covers the following areas:

■ The description of the situation
■ Expectations
■ Support resources
■ Health status
■ Strength
■ Geographical data.

The tool (Table 25.19, page 648) is composed of questions to ask the patient which serve to determine health status. These question can be used in conjunction with the cue questions to guide the nurse to help determine family history; episodes of fatigue, restlessness, **syncope** or confusion; cur-

rent medications, risk factors, such as diabetes, a high fat/cholesterol diet, smoking/exercise regimen; coping strategies; religious beliefs or preferences; sleeping and eating patterns; social status, to determine stress levels, diet, income, family concerns and job status.

THE ROLE OF THE FAMILY

A family can be defined, in the broadest sense, as a group of persons either related by birth or who are significant to one another and who share intimate and routine day-to-day living. Almost every patient has been, or is, a member of a family and a change in one family member has the potential to affect other family members. If the patient is to be

Table 25.18: Factors affecting the patient when receiving information/messages in acute settings

Environment

Distortion of message
- noise
- poor/bright light
- vibration
- temperature

Distractions
- other activity
- competing messages

The patient

Psychological
- perception altered by drugs and/or pathology
- motivation/interest in message
- attitudes/values/beliefs
- anxiety/fear
- emotions/mood
- intelligence
- self-image

Physical
- conscious level
- sensory deficits, e.g. hearing impediments/tinnitus; sight (short/long sighted diplopia, hemianopia, blindness); movement (paralysis/paresis); sensation (loss); speech (dysarthria/dysphasia/aphasia)
- constraints to movement position/infusions/equipment)
- pain

Social
- language
- culture/lifestyle
- isolation

viewed from an holistic perspective, it is important to understand the immediate social context in which he/she is situated. For most individuals that social context is the family.

Every family will vary in its behaviour and reactions to acute illness in one of its members, and it is important to remember that a crisis for one family would not necessarily be a crisis for another family. Regardless of the family response, there will be a significant effect on the situation as it relates to the nurse; this needs to be recognised.

Wright and Leahey (1984) suggest that, in order to foster health care at family level, it is useful for nurses to consider two functions:

1 The impact of illness on the family
2 The influence of family interactions on the 'cause' or 'cure' of problems.

Several other studies have considered how relatives of patients in hospital perceive their needs. These studies suggest that some factors are perceived to be more important than others (Manley, 1988; Blakemore, 1996). The factors considered most and least important to relatives are illustrated in Table 25.20 (page 649). Information that is useful to the acute care nurse about the family can therefore be listed under the following headings:

- Structure and function of the family
- Roles fulfilled by the patient within the family unit
- Expectations of family members
- Coping abilities of family members.

The cue questions, combined with Campbell *et al.*'s (1985) health status tool allow the nurse to obtain a greater insight into family strengths and problems relevant to the care of a hospitalised individual. In addition, by developing and maintaining the therapeutic relationship, family meetings with staff from the start can set a precedent for the future, contributing to holistic family care instead of fostering splintered family involvement.

Other benefits from increased family involvement include a greater insight into the patient's personality, character, culture, religion, spirituality and sexuality, enabling staff to have an opportunity to know the patient better and encourage the use of the family as the natural support system for the patient. However, Meerabeau (1991) suggested that nurses are rarely approached by patients on a spiritual level, as they are often either embarrassed or afraid. In addition, Webb (1987) highlighted the need for greater consideration of the sexuality of the individual within the context of viewing the person as an holistic being. When using the Burford model these areas need to be considered to encompass the full meaning of holism.

To understand the family's boundaries and composition, several simple tools exist which can convey a great deal of information visually. Examples of these include the **genogram** and the **ecomap**. A genogram is particularly helpful in outlining a family's internal and external struc-

Table 25.19: Health status of clients

Primary source (patient)	Secondary source (nurse and family)
Description of situation In your own words, can you tell me how you see your situation? What do you think caused the situation to occur? What do you think will improve the situation?	**Nursing observation analysis** Describe the patient and the situation **Family:** How does the family view the situation? Do they feel drained or have the energy to handle the situation? **Family:** What does the family think will improve the situation?
Expectations What do you think will happen over the next few days? What do you expect to accomplish in this hospitalisation? What is important to you at this time in your life? Is this hospitalisation affecting your long-term goals?	**Nurse:** What is patient's feeling state? Are there incongruences between what the patient says and non-verbal data? **Family:** What do they expect to occur over the next few days? During this hospitalisation?
Support resources Who do you usually talk things over with? Are they available to you while you are in the hospital? How often? How is the hospitalisation affecting the people who are important to you?	**Nurse:** Does the family appear supportive? Does the patient need help interacting with health team members? **Family:** How is the patient's hospitalisation affecting the family?
Health status How do you describe your general health? Previous health problems? Current health problems? How do you usually handle stress?	**Nurse:** Describe patient's general appearance. Describe any pertinent alteration in physical systems **Family:** How does the family describe the patient's health?
Strengths What do you see as the healthy or positive aspects of yourself? Is there anything that you will need help with in caring for yourself? Is there anything else you would like us to know about you?	**Nurse:** Additional strengths identification by the nurse **Family:** What does the family see as the patient's strengths? Anything they will need help with? Anything they would like us to know?
Demographical data Age Religion Allergies/sensitivities Contact in case of emergency Patient's report of use of medications Name Dose Frequency Last dose Patient's reason for taking medication Date Time Unit Signature	

Reproduced from Campbell *et al.*, 1985, by kind permission of Blackwell Scientific Publications.

ture. The symbols used are illustrated in Figure 25.12. Family members are placed on horizontal lines according to generation. An example of a blank genogram is included in Figure 25.13. An ecomap is a diagram portraying important connections between the family and others outside the family.

Table 25.20: The least and most important needs of relatives of acutely ill patients as perceived by the relatives themselves (Manley, 1988)

Most important needs	Least important needs
Needs for hope (Molter, 1979; Norris and Grove, 1986)	To talk about negative feelings (Norris and Grove, 1986)
To feel that hospital personnel cared for patient (Molter, 1979; Norris and Grove, 1986)	To talk about own feelings (Norris and Grove, 1986)
To be assured that the best possible care is being given to the patient (Irwin, 1973; Norris and Grove, 1986)	To change visiting hours for special conditions (Norris and Grove, 1986)
To have questions answered honestly (Irwin, 1973; Norris and Grove, 1986)	To talk about the possiblity of the patient's death (Norris and Grove, 1986)
To receive as much information as possible about the patient (Hampe, 1979)	Personal concerns (Hampe, 1979)
To receive information which would alleviate anxieties (Hampe, 1979) The need to be with the patient (Hampe, 1979)	

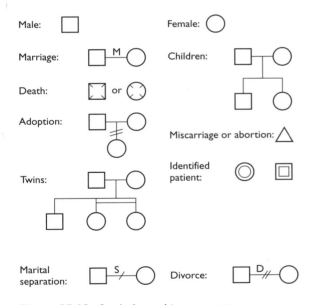

Figure 25.12: Symbols used in genograms (from Wright and Leaney, 1984)

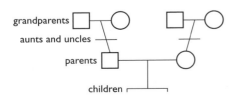

Figure 25.13: Blank genogram

SLEEPING PATTERNS

Sleep can be defined as an altered state of consciousness from which a person can be aroused by stimuli of sufficient magnitude (Hill and Smith, 1985). The function of sleep is far from clear. Historically, it has been considered as restorative and energy conserving (Canavan, 1984). McGonigal (1986) supports this theory and suggests that protein synthesis and cell division for the renewal of tissues takes place predominantly during the time devoted to rest and sleep. In addition, sleep is needed to avoid the psychological problems resulting from inadequate sleep, which might hinder recovery.

During an average night's sleep individuals pass through four or five sleep cycles, each cycle lasting about 90–100 minutes (McGonigal, 1986). Within the sleep cycle, five successive stages have been defined by their distinctive characteristics (Table 25.21). The first four stages of sleep are called collectively non-rapid eye movement sleep (NREM) and demonstrate a progressive increase in the depth of sleep. Stage five is called rapid eye movement sleep (REM), or paradoxical sleep, and is associated with dreaming, learning and memory.

If the function of sleep is correctly assumed, then sleep deprivation in the acutely ill person could be considered as an additional stressor, over and above those physical and emotional traumas already suffered.

Table 25.21: Sleep stages within one sleep cycle

	Stage	Duration	Characteristic	EEG pattern	
NON-REM SLEEP	0 Awake Eyes closed				Alpha waves (8–12 cycles/s)
	1 Light sleep	Few minutes	A feeling of 'drifting' aimless thoughts. *Myoclonic* jerks, easy awakening		Alpha waves replaced by slower low voltage waves (4–6 cycles/s)
	2 Medium sleep	10–15 min	More difficult to wake		Slower, higher voltage waves with short bursts of waves called sleep 'spindles'
	3 Deep sleep 4 Deepest sleep	Approx 70–100 min	Decreased muscle tone ↓Blood pressure ↓Heart rate ↓Respiratory rate		Slow waves (1–2 cycles/s); slow high voltage waves (1–2 cycles/s)
	5 REM sleep (dreaming)	25% of total sleep time	Muscle twitching of face and extremities, complete relaxation of lower jaw (often producing snoring) and skeletal muscle tone. Rapid eye movements which can be observed. Associated with dreaming		Similar to stage 1 but accompanied by rapid eye movements

Prolonged REM sleep deprivation is considered by some authors as exerting no adverse psychological effects (Ganong, 1983; Canavan, 1984). On the other hand, perpetual awakening and sleep interruption has been associated with increased anxiety, irritability and disorientation (Closs, 1988). Anxiety has already been indicated as a cause of increased sympathetic action which may then have a negative influence on recovery.

In addition, total sleep deprivation of 48 hours can result in changes such as behavioural irritability, suspiciousness, speech slurring and minor visual misperceptions. These may be accompanied by a reduction in motivation and willingness to perform tasks which could include mobilisation and other aspects of self care. Other detrimental psychological effects of sleep deprivation in hospital patients include lethargy, irritability and disorientation and confusion, and later, delusions and paranoia (Closs, 1988).

Fabijan and Gosselin (1982) have made several recommendations for minimising sleep interruption in patients in intensive care units. Such recommendations (listed in Table 25.22) are equally applicable to any acute care area.

SENSORY DEPRIVATION

The normal conscious state requires a minimum level of sensory stimulation and/or variation in type of stimuli received. The normal type of sen-

Table 25.22: Recommendations for reducing sleep interruption in acutely ill patients

- Turn off maximum number of lights especially at night
- Keep noise to a minimum (for example – switch off suction equipment following use; reduce talking and whispering)
- Offer cotton wool balls for patients' ears
- Continually reassess the need to interrupt patients' sleep to perform observations
- Perform as many nursing interventions as possible together
- Chart amount of uninterrupted sleep per shift and evidence of sleep stages
- Communicate the patients' need to sleep to other professionals
- Use knowledge of
  (a) patients' normal sleeping patterns and
  (b) supportive family relationships
  to optimise environment for sleep
- Administer analgesics and sedatives according to patients' felt needs and monitor events. (Care is necessary with some drugs that may interfere with sleep patterns)

Adapted from Fabijan and Gosselin, 1982.

sations received by the reticular activating system would include auditory, visual, olfactory, tactile and kinaesthetic stimuli (i.e. stimuli that relate to the position of joints in space and the degree of contraction of muscles). Sensory deprivation itself is not a syndrome associated merely with a reduction in these stimuli but is a more complex concept (McGonigal, 1986).

Studies into sensory deprivation show that when normal healthy individuals are deprived of all sensory input (i.e. auditory, visual and touch), there is a detrimental effect on the functioning of the individual (Glide, 1994). Such individuals become bored, restless, irritable and emotionally upset. Visual hallucinations, poor concentration and problem-solving difficulties also result.

Moore (1991) identified five main types of alterations to sensory input which may cause deprivation. These include:

1 A reduction in the amount and variety of stimuli
2 No reduction, but there is little variation and it is meaningless (sometimes known as perceptual deprivation)
3 Isolation – physical or social
4 Confinement – immobilisation or restriction of movement
5 Increased sensory input (sensory overload).

By working through learning check 6 (Box 25.6) contributory factors to sensory deprivation using the above five causes can be derived. Glide (1994) suggested seven points which it is useful to consider for reducing sensory deprivation in acutely ill people. These are identified in Table 25.23. Some suggestions are common for the prevention

Box 25.6: Learning Check 6

Self-assessment question nine

Can you identify possible contributory factors to sensory deprivation in acutely ill patients using Moore's causes of deprivation?

Answer

(1) Reduced variety and intensity of stimuli
   - impaired sight, hearing, sensation, taste or smell due to trauma, pathology, drugs
   - inability to communicate verbally, e.g. if unable to speak English; dysphasia

(2) Perceptual deprivation
   - sedatives, analgesics
   - reduced conscious level
   - not having hearing aids/glasses
   - pathology

(3) Social isolation
   - barrier nursing
   - the 'unpopular patient' (Stockwell, 1972)
   - cubicles
   - language barrier

(4) Confinement/immobility
   - bedrest
   - traction/plaster casts
   - pain
   - paralysis

(5) Increased sensory input/overload
   - alarms/monitors
   - frequent neurological/other observations
   - persistent disturbance
   - telephone ringing
   - smells

Table 25.23: Suggestions for reducing sensory deprivation

Create an environment with a minimum of sensory deprivation or overload ■ Maintain diurnal rhythm, by orientating the patient who is confused to day and night ■ Limb exercises to maintain proprioceptive feedback (i.e. information from the joints to the brain relating to position in space) ■ Reduce unnecessary noise, disturbance ■ Disperse unpleasant odours as soon as possible ■ Reduce 'crowding' of patient **Familiarise the environment for the patient** ■ Photographs of family members of favourite scenes ■ Position the patient to look out of a window ■ Radio and television ■ Encourage family visiting ■ Tapes of favourite music and programmes **Assist the patient to interpret incoming stimuli** ■ Wearing of glasses and hearing aids ■ Explain all nursing procedures and interventions beforehand ■ Explain unfamiliar alarms and sounds ■ Explain effects of drugs which alter sensory perception ■ Prepare patient for situation/treatments which may result in sensory deprivation	**Orientate the patient to the reality of the moment** ■ Orientate in time, place and person ■ Orientate to physical condition ■ Give patient access to a watch, clock or calendar ■ Dim lights at night ■ Use touch to assure the patient that the nurse cares **Provide the patient with an active role in his care** ■ Encourage patient to make decisions about his/her environment ■ Ask patient's permission prior to invading his/her privacy ■ Ensure maximum privacy ■ Spend time communicating with patient **Encourage the patient to use the highest form of cognitive functioning possible** ■ Encourage questioning and discussion ■ Ascertain patient's perception of situation ■ Involve him/her in care planning and decision making **Provide the patient with uninterrupted rest periods** ■ Make a contract with patient for specific rest periods ■ See recommendations for encouraging sleep

After Worrell, 1977.

of sleep deprivation with which there is a close relationship.

Additional assessment tools

The preceding sections have considered areas that are relevant to the person in hospital. In this section the need for additional assessment tools is highlighted as the basis for a more comprehensive patient assessment. The specific tools discussed here focus on a single area (such as pressure areas, wound care or nutrition) and are therefore reductionist in approach – i.e. they consider parts of a person only, and must always be used with this in mind. A range of tools have already been discussed in relation to the person in hospital; other tools that nurses can use to obtain a more comprehensive patient assessment are considered below.

PRESSURE AREA RISK ASSESSMENT

Pressure sore prevention and management is a major concern for nurses caring for the acutely ill patient, as he or she may have numerous medical and surgical problems, be malnourished, have some degree of immobility or may be elderly.

The pathogenesis of pressure sores is complex, since it is affected by so many predisposing factors. However, there are three major factors identified as significant (Johnson, 1986):

1 Pressure greater than 25 mmHg will occlude capillaries. The tissues are thus deprived of their blood supply, and if the pressure is maintained for a sufficient length of time, the ischaemic tissues die.

2 Friction is a combination of pressure and friction caused by dragging patients up the bed, which seriously damages the microcirculation.

3 Shearing forces are caused by pressure and strain to structures so great that they tear the

muscle and skin fibres from their bony attachments.

A patient suffering from a combination of predisposing factors is more susceptible to developing pressure sores. Predisposing factors can be subdivided into two main groups (Figure 25.14):

1 Intrinsic factors – aspects of the patient's condition, mental, physical and medical states, e.g., malnutrition, age, altered consciousness, immobility
2 Extrinsic factors – external effects of drugs, treatment regimens, patient-handling techniques, personal hygiene, weight distribution.

Those patients at greatest risk from developing pressure sores may be identified using a pressure sore prediction scale (Johnson, 1986). The Waterlow scale (Waterlow, 1985) is the most widely used pressure sore risk assessment calculator in the UK. The Braden scale is often preferred because it is generally more reliable and valid (Bergstrom *et al.*, 1987), as the Waterlow scale tends to overpredict risk (Dealey, 1991; Wardman, 1991). The other risk assessment calculators currently in use (Douglas score, Norton score) to determine pressure sore development have been widely criticised because of lack of research (Flanagan, 1995; MacDonald, 1995), as few have been tested for reliability and validity (Watkinson, 1997).

A recent study has been undertaken to determine the validity and reliability of a new pressure sore risk assessment scale (Watkinson, 1997). The new Watkinson pressure sore risk assessment scale was developed to encourage an accurate calculation which is both reliable and valid. The assessment of special risk factors is placed first on the scale and urinary continence separated from faecal continence to eradicate previously complicated descriptions. The Watkinson scale has not yet been thoroughly tested for reliability and validity as has the Braden scale, as it is relatively new. Only one study so far has indicated that it might be as reliable as the Braden scale at predicting at-risk patients.

However, both scales are overcautious and potentially overpredict pressure sore risk, a criticism made of both the Norton and Waterlow. Yet, it is argued that the predictive value of the Braden and Watkinson scales is high. To reduce this risk, on the Watkinson scale, the parameters could be changed and a higher cut-off point introduced,

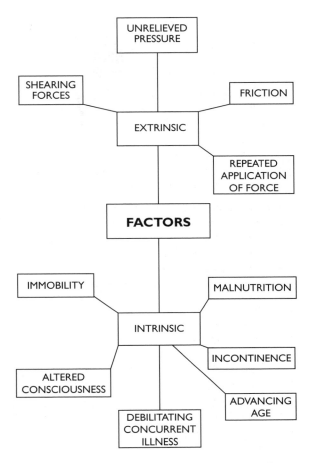

Figure 25.14: Intrinsic and extrinsic factors significant in the development and delayed healing of pressure sores

which may reduce the tendency to overpredict risk, but this could be at the expense of sensitivity and a false-negative rate (Watkinson, 1997). It is better to overpredict than underpredict risk, as the cost of treating pressure sores is high, whilst the cost of preventing them is considerably less (Hunt, 1993).

It is suggested that all patients admitted to hospital should be assessed for risk of pressure sore development within 2 hours of arrival. However, it is important to realise that a risk assessment score is not a definitive answer to the question of whether an individual will develop a pressure sore. The calculator is an aid to professional and clinical judgement in determining what resources are needed by whom. If used effectively, the calculator can be used to justify a request for resources (Watkinson, 1997), e.g. specialised beds and/or efficient moving and handling equipment.

WOUND ASSESSMENT

Wound assessment is a complex task that requires concise information before deciding on a strategy for treatment. In the literature there is a wide range of information relating to wound assessment and wound care generally, mostly in nursing journals and, more recently, in specialist wound-care journals. However, nurses have varying levels of knowledge about wound assessment, and information relating to a wound's condition can be ignored because of poor assessment skills (Guilding, 1993). Yet, using a measurment tool to assess wounds would encourage consistent intervention irrespective of who assesses the wound at any time (Lockyer-Stevens, 1995).

Where tissue damage has occurred, a body diagram is used to record the patient's wound sites and in the case of multiple wounds these should be numbered individually (Lockyer-Stevens, 1995). The site of each wound should be determined by a separate assessment sheet and/or the number identified from the initial body diagram. The next step is to ask 11 major questions relating to the condition of any wound (Morrison, 1989a). In addition, the maximum dimensions should be traced and recorded, giving the length, width and depth of the wound in centimetres, in order to have a standard method of measurement. Charting wound healing facilitates accurate recording of observations and wound treatment. Table 25.24 includes all the areas that should be included in a wound assessment.

Which wound assessment documentation tool used is largely a matter of personal preference, so long as the user is aware of the tool's limitations (Morrison, 1989b), but it is of paramount importance that the patient's wound(s) are assessed as soon as possible after admission, and that the risk is reassessed whenever there is a significant change in his/her condition.

Accurate and on-going wound assessment is a prerequisite to planning appropriate care and to evaluating its effectiveness (Young, 1996). This process identifies the expanding nature of nursing practice, not only in the realm of wound assessment but in nurse prescribing of wound-care dressings. The full implementation of the prescribing powers for nurses in 1998, announced in the White Paper (DoH, 1996), is to review nurse prescribing practices to include all health professionals. These legislative changes are necessary for nurse prescribing to find full expression appropriate to the demands of today's health services (Jones, 1997).

NUTRITIONAL ASSESSMENT

Following major injury, whether in the form of accidental trauma, burns, severe illness or major surgical intervention, the body responds with specific endocrine and metabolic changes designed to protect it. The duration of the response relates to the severity and extent of the injury

The major energy source in the body is glucose. Glucose is obtained from nutrients to carry out vital functions to sustain life, to form new body components or to assist in the functioning of various body processes, such as breathing and physical activity. To produce a constant supply of energy, the body must be constantly replenished with food to sustain physical life (see Chapter 25 of Marieb, 1995). The patient in hospital not only has an increased demand for energy, but often, due to periods of reduction or cessation of nutritional intake, has a reduced supply of energy-containing nutrients. As a result, undernutrition, or in severe cases malnutrition, may occur.

Table 25.24: Areas to consider in wound assessment/documentation

Record of wound sites	Condition of wound	Dimensions/drawing	Documentation
Body diagram from different angles	Wound dimensions	Length	All these points need to be taken into consideration when documenting nursing observations and wound treatments in relation to wound care
■ back	Nature of wound bed	Width	
■ front	Exudate	Depth	
■ legs	Odour	Outside tracking	
■ front	Pain (site, frequency, severity)	Healthy granulating tissue	
■ back	Wound margin	Sloughy areas	
■ medial	Erythema of surrounding skin		
■ lateral	Condition of surrounding skin infection		

Undernutrition – and to a greater extent malnutrition – reduces the body's ability to:

- Heal wounds and increases the risk of pressure sores
- Produce haemoglobin, which reduces the oxygen carrying capacity of the blood
- Produce white blood cells, causing suppression of the immune response and exposing the patient to the risk of infection
- Maintain adequate respiratory drive due to reduction in pulmonary diaphragmatic muscle mass and strength, predisposing the patient to respiratory failure.

Despite the importance of nutrition, Hickey (1986) reported a high priority being placed on management of the physiological measurements, e.g. blood pressure and pulse, but other areas of care such as nutritional adequacy having a lower priority. In addition, it appears that there is also a shortfall in the assessment and determination of nutritional status (Raper and Maynard, 1992; Garrow, 1994; McWhirter and Pennington, 1994; Dickerson, 1995). By working through learning check 7 (Box 25.7), how an acutely ill patient's nutritional needs would alter following a physiological insult can be deduced.

Nutritional assessment can be as simple or as complicated as desired, but should encompass both subjective and objective elements (Bishop *et al.*, 1981). Information should be based on nurses' observations of the patient and on the collection of an essential core of material, e.g. patient history, psychological and social status, physical examination, diet history and appraisal of current nutritional intake, **anthropometric measurements**, biochemical and laboratory data (Goodinson, 1986) (Table 25.25).

The second level assessment has included aspects that relate to interviewing the patient, which requires effective communication to determine the health status of the patient, the role of the family, sleeping patterns and to evaluate sensory deprivation. It incorporates the use of additional assessment tools as a basis for a more comprehensive patient assessment. It is recommended that if the first level assessment is undertaken initially, then the second level assessment should take place no later than 24 hours following admission.

Table 25.25: Areas to consider in a nutritional assessment

Patient history, psychological and social status	**Diet history**
Recent bereavement	Questions about the likes and dislikes
Bad experience	Changes in weight
Ill at home for a long time	Type, quantity and texture of food eaten since the
Age	onset of illness (disease often alters appetite)
Income support	Have there been any changes in taste
Type of accommodation	The ability to obtain and prepare food
Does the patient look thin	All factors should be noted and recorded
Appearance of skin (colour, condition)	
Loose clothing	**Biochemical measurements**
Do their dentures fit?	Serum albumin (level less than 35 g/litre being
Any recent loss of weight	indicative of protein-energy malnutrition)
	Serum transferrin levels (highlights the presence of
Physical examination	anaemia)
Oral cavity	Haemoglobin levels
Sore mouth	
Dysphagia	**Anthropometric measurements**
Difficulty in chewing and swallowing	Weight
Any physical difficulties with feeding	Changes in body weight
Any nausea, vomiting, diarrhoea or constipation	Height
Simple respiratory function tests to determine	Height and weight (BMI)
respiratory muscle strength	Body fat content estimated from skinfold thickness
	measurements:
	■ triceps skinfold thickness (TSF)
	■ mid-upper-arm circumference (MUAC)

Box 25.7: Learning Check 7

Self-assessment question ten

Can you identify how an acutely ill patient's nutritional needs would alter following a physiological insult?

Answer and rationale

- More calories would be required to meet the metabolic rate if excessive depletion of body stores was to be avoided

- More amino acids — to prevent tissue proteins such as skeletal muscle and plasma proteins from being broken down (catabolism)
  - to permit protein synthesis for repair of body tissues (anabolism)

- More K^+ to compensate for loss through the kidney which may otherwise lead to hypokalaemia and cardiac irritability

- Avoid Na^+ supplements, because large amounts of Na^+ are reabsorbed in the kidney

DOCUMENTATION USING THE BURFORD MODEL

A key nursing action within the Burford NDU model is the way in which nursing is communicated. The final learning domains focus on 'knowing' responsibility and 'knowing' others. This involves giving and receiving feedback and recognises that practitioners do not work as individuals, but need to work together to ensure patients receive consistent and congruent care. Second, it involves coping with work in ways that sustain therapeutic work; this enables practitioners to understand the dimensions of coping with stressful situations.

NURSING PROCESS

The nursing process refers to a framework for organising and providing care through a prescribed sequence of unalterable steps. Most commonly, these steps involve patient assessment, planning care, implementation of interventions, and evaluation of the process of a patient status (Barnum, 1987).

The nursing process is applied in the Burford model to document information to the relevant member of staff, to initiate support and continue observations and measurements to ensure the effectiveness of interventions. Using the nursing process format works well in communicating and evaluating physical needs or where interventions are of a technical nature.

CONCLUSION

In this chapter, the Burford NDU model has been used to structure a wide range of assessment interventions that are necessary to the effectiveness of nursing care. The interventions relevant to the care of the adult patient admitted to hospital have been described. These included observations; measurements; interview and additional assessment tools required to deliver optimum care. The often neglected psychological and social factors have been included in addition to the biological ones that usually predominate in the acute setting. However, the biologically related aspects of monitoring parameters have been considered in some detail, as accuracy in measurement and interpretation is an essential prerequisite for any nurse caring for an adult patient.

Hopefully, after reading this chapter, the needs of the hospitalised patient will be more easily and accurately identified, both in breadth and depth, and in doing so the nurse will evaluate the effectiveness of his/her decisions and actions. This is achieved through seeking valid feedback and reflection.

By incorporating the Burford NDU model, multidisciplinary, integrated caring-healing practice values and activities that seek to both integrate and transform the nurse's personal and professional values, are recognised. The model reminds us of our social mandate to improve our practice and come of age as a health and human caring profession firmly grounded in the existent world of practice.

By incorporating the Burford NDU model, conditions have been created to facilitate desired practice, thus enabling practitioners to recognise, understand and respond to the multiple influences and events that impinge upon practice and to move towards achieving effective, defined care.

REFERENCES

Abbey, J., Anderson, A. and Close, E. (1978). How long is that thermometer accurate? *American Journal of Nursing*, 78(8), 1375–6.

Angerami, E. (1980). Epidemiological study of body temperature in patients in a teaching hospital. *International Journal of Nursing Studies*, 17(2), 91–9.

Argyle, M. (1988). *Bodily communication*, 2nd edn. Methuen, London.

Ashworth, P. (1979). Sensory deprivation 2: the acutely ill. *Nursing Times*, 75(7), 290–4.

Baillie, L. (1993). A review of pain assessment tools. *Nursing Standard*, 7(23), 25–9.

Baker, N.C., Cerone, S.B. and Gaze, N. (1984). The effects of type of thermometer and length of time inserted on oral temperature measurements of afebrile subjects. *Nursing Research*, 33(2), 109–11.

Bardwell, J. (1995). For good measure. *Nursing Times*, 91(27), 40–1.

Barnum, B.J. (1987). Holistic nursing and the nursing process. *Holistic Nursing Practice*, 1(3), 27–35.

Bergstrom, N., Demuth, P.J. and Braden, B. (1987). A clinical trial of the Braden scale for predicting pressure sore risk. *Nursing Clinics of North America*, 22(2), 417–28.

Biley, F.C. (1996). Rogerian science, phantoms, and therapeutic touch: exploring potentials. *Nursing Science Quarterly*, 9(4), 165–9.

Binnie, A., Bond, S., Law, G. *et al.* (1988) *A Systematic Approach to Nursing Care: an Introduction*. The Open University, Milton Keynes.

Bishop, C.W., Bowen, P.E. and Ritchley, S.I. (1981). Norms for nutritional assessment of American adults by upper arm anthropometry. *American Journal of Clinical Nutrition*, 34, 2530–9.

Blackmore, E. (1996). The needs of relatives during the patient's stay in intensive care following routine cardiac surgery. *Nursing in Critical Care* 1(5), 230–6.

Blattner, B. (1981). *Holistic Nursing*. Prentice-Hall, New Jersey.

Boore, J.R.P. (1978). *Prescription for Recovery*. RCN, London.

Bourbonnais, F. (1981). Pain assessment: development of a tool for the nurse and the patient. *Journal of Advanced Nursing*, 6, 277–82.

Bowker, C., Jelphs, K., Nattrass, N., Boylan, A. and Brown, P. (1986). Focus on urinalysis. Part 1. *Nursing Times*, 82(17), suppl. 1–6.

Boykin, A. and Schoenhofer, S. (1990). Caring in nursing: analysis of extant theory. *Nursing Science Quarterly*, 3(4), 149–55.

Braddy, P.K. (1989). Cardiac assessment tool. *Critical Care Nurse*, 9(9), 71–72, 74, 76–81.

Bruce, J. and Grove, S. (1992). Fever: pathology and treatment. *Critical Care Nurse*, 12(1), 359–62.

Bull, M.P., Jarvis, A., Moores, Y. and Haughey, M.A. (1993). *The Challenges for Nursing and Midwifery in the 21st Century: the Heathrow Debate*. Welsh Planning Forum, Cardiff.

Burnip, S.J. (1991). Why do nurses take blood pressures postoperatively. *Surgical Nurse*, 4(2), 15–19.

Burroughs, J. and Hoffbrand, B.I. (1990). A critical look at nursing observations. *Postgraduate Medical Journal*, 66, 370–2.

Buswell, C. (1997). Comparing mercury and disposable thermometers. *Professional Nurse*, 12(5), 359–62.

Callow, L. and Pieper, B. (1989). Effects of backrest on central venous pressure in paediatric cardiac surgery. *Nursing Research*, 38, 336–8.

Campbell, J., Finch, D., Allport, C. and Erickson, H. (1985). A theoretical approach to nursing assessment. *Journal of Advanced Nursing*, 10, 111–15.

Canavan, T. (1984). The psychobiology of sleep. *Nursing*, 2(23), 682–3.

Cartwright, A. (1964). *Human Relations and Hospital Care.* Routledge and Kegan Paul, London.

Closs, J. (1988). Patients' sleep–wake rhythms in hospital. *Nursing Times,* 84(1), 48–50.

Cook, R. (1995). Urinalysis. *Nursing Standard,* 9(28), 32–7.

Cunha, B., Digamon-Beltran, M. and Gobbo, P. (1984). Implications of fever in the critical care setting. *Heart and Lung,* 13, 460–5.

Darovic, G.O. (1987). *Hemodynamic Monitoring: Invasive and Noninvasive Clinical Application.* W.B. Saunders Company, Philadephia.

Dealey, C. (1991). The size of the pressure sore problem in a teaching hospital. *Journal of Advanced Nursing,* 16, 663–70.

Dennison, R.D. (1994). Making sense of haemodynamic monitoring. *American Journal of Nursing,* 94(8), 24–32.

Dickerson, J. (1995). The problem of hospital induced malnutrition. *Nursing Times,* 91(4), 44–5.

DoH (1993). *A Vision for the Future: the Nursing, Midwifery and Health Visiting Contribution to Health Care.* NHS Management Executive, London.

DoH (1996). *Primary Care: Delivering the Future.* HMSO, London.

Dries, D.J. and Waxman, K. (1991). Adequate resuscitation of burn patients may not be measured by urine output and vital signs. *Critical Care Medicine,* 19(3), 327–9.

Dunlop, M.J. (1986). Is a science of caring possible? *Journal of Advanced Nursing,* 11(6), 661–70.

Durham, M.L., Swanson, B. and Paulford, N. (1986). Effect of tachypnoea on oral temperature estimation: a relication. *Nursing Research,* 35(4), 211–14.

Erickson, R. (1980). Oral temperature differences in relation to thermometer and technique. *Nursing Research,* 29(3), 157–64.

Erickson, R. and Yount, S.T. (1991). Comparison of tympanic and oral temperatures in surgical patients. *Nursing Research,* 40(2), 90–3.

Fabijan, L. and Gosselin, M. (1982). How to recognise sleep deprivation in your ICU patient and what to do about it. *Canadian Nurse,* 78(4), 20–3.

Flanagan, M. (1995). Who is at risk of a pressure sore? A practical review of risk assessment systems. *Professional Nurse,* 10(5), 305–8.

Forsyth, D., Delaney, C., Maloney, N., Kubesh, D. and Story, D. (1990). Can caring behaviour be taught? *Nursing Outlook,* 37(4), 164–6.

Fox, K. (1996). Hypertension and heart disease. *Nursing Standard,* 10(23), 52.

Fulbrook, P. (1993). Core temperature measurement in adults: a literature review. *Journal of Advanced Nursing,* 18, 365–9.

Ganong, W.F. (1983). *Medical Physiology,* 11th edn. Lange Medical Publications, Stamford, Connecticut.

Garbett, R. (1994). Applying the BNDU Model in an acute medical unit. In *The Burford NDU Model: Caring in Practice,* Johns, C. (ed.). Blackwell Science, Oxford.

Garrow, J. (1994). Starvation in hospital. *British Medical Journal,* 308, 934.

Glide, S. (1994). Maintaining sensory balance. *Nursing Times,* 90(17), 33–4.

Goodinson, S.M. (1986). Assessment of nutritional status. *Nursing,* 7, 252–8.

Green, C.A. (1996). Case study. A reflection of a therapeutic touch experience: case study 1. *Complementary Therapies in Nursing and Midwifery,* 2(5), 122–5.

Guiffre, M., Heidenreich, T., Carney-Gersten, P., Dorch, J.A. and Heidenreich, E. (1990). The relationship between axillary and core body temperature measurements. *Applied Nursing Research,* 3(2), 52–5.

Guilding, L. (1993). Dimensions of nursing knowledge in wound care. *British Journal of Nursing,* 2(14), 712–16.

Gurevich, I. (1985). Fever: when to worry about it. *RN* 48(12), 14–19.

Hampe, S.O. (1979). Needs of grieving spouse in a hospital setting. *Nursing Research,* 24, 113.

Harper, R. (1981). *A Guide to Respiratory Care.* J.B. Lippincott, Philadelphia.

Hart, L. and Dennis, S. (1988). Two hyperthermias prevalent in the intensive care unit. *Focus on Critical Care,* 15, 49–55.

Harvey, P. (1989). Stress and health. In *Health Psychology: Processes and Applications,* Broome, A.K. (ed.). Chapman & Hall, London.

Henker, R. and Coyne, C. (1995). Comparison of peripheral temperature measurements with core temperature. *AACN Clinical Issues,* 6(1), 21–30.

Henneman, E.A. and Henneman, P.L. (1989). Intricacies of blood pressure measurement: reexamining the rituals. *Heart and Lung,* 18(3), 263–73.

Hickey, J. (1986). *The Clinical Practice of Neurological and Neurosurgical Nursing.* J.B. Lippincott, London.

Hill, L. and Smith, N. (1985). *Self-care Nursing: Promotion of Health.* Prentice-Hall, Englewood Cliffs, New Jersey.

Hinchliff, S., Montague, S. and Watson, R. (eds) (1996). *Physiology for Nursing Practice*, 2nd edn. Baillière Tindall, London.

Hollinworth, H. (1994). No gain! *Nursing Times*, 90(1), 24–7.

Holtzclaw, B.J. (1992). The febrile response in critical care: state of the science. *Heart and Lung*, 21, 482–501.

Hunt, J. (1993). Application of a pressure area risk calculator in an intensive care unit. *Intensive and Critical Care Nursing*, 1, 1–6.

Irwin, B.L. (1973). Supportive measures for relatives of the fatally ill. *Community Nursing Research*, 6, 126.

Johns, C. (1991). The Burford Nursing Development Unit holistic model of nursing practice. *Journal of Advanced Nursing*, 16, 1090–98.

Johns, C. (ed.) (1994). *The Burford NDU Model: Caring in Practice*. Blackwell Science, Oxford.

Johnson, A. (1986). *Blueprint for the Prevention and Management of Pressure Sores*. Squibb Surgicare Limited, London.

Jolly, A. (1991). Taking a blood pressure. *Nursing Times*, 87(15), 40–3.

Jones, M. (1997). Nurse prescribing – why has it taken so long? *Nursing Standard*, 11(20), 39–42.

Kacperek, L. (1997). Non-verbal communication: the importance of listening. *British Journal of Nursing*, 6(5), 275–9.

Kee, J.L. and Hayes, E.R. (1990). Assessment of patient laboratory data in the acutely ill. *Nursing Clinics of North America*, 25(4), 751–9.

Kee, L.L., Siminson, J.S., Stotts, N.A., Skov, P. and Schiller, N.B. (1993). Echocardiographic determination of valid zero reference levels in supine and lateral positions. *American Journal of Critical Care*, 2, 72–80.

Kemp, F. (1994). How effective is training for blood pressure measurement? *Professional Nurse*, 9(8), 521–4.

Kim, M.J., McFarland, G.K. and McLane, A. (1991). *Pocket Guide to Nursing Diagnosis*, 4th edn. Mosby Year Book, St Louis.

Koziol-McLain, J., Oman, K. and Edwards, G. (1996). Ear temperatures: making research-based clinical decisions. *Journal of Emergency Nursing*, 22(1), 77–9.

Kramer, M.K. (1990). Holistic nursing: implications for knowledge development and utilisation. In *The Nursing Professions: Turning Points*, Chaska, N.L. (ed.). C.V. Mosby, St Louis.

Krickler, J.A. and Dodge, G.H. (1987). What to do about temperatures. *Nursing Standard*, 14(25), 37–8.

Latham, J. (1989). *Pain Control*. Austin Cornish Publishers Ltd, London.

Ley, P. (1988). *Communicating with Patients*. Croom Helm, London.

Lo Biondo-Wood, G. and Haver, J. (1986). *Nursing Research: Critical Appraisal and Utilization*. C.V. Mosby, St Louis.

Lockyer-Stevens, N. (1995). Nurse prescribing of wound-care dressings. *Professional Nurse*, 10(11), 697–9.

McCance, K.L. and Huether, S.E. (1994). *Pathophysiology: the Biologic Basis for Disease in Adults and Children*, 2nd edn. Mosby, St Louis.

MacDonald, K. (1995). The reliability of pressure sore risk assessment tools. *Professional Nurse*, 11(3), 169–72.

McGonigal, K.S. (1986). The importance of sleep and the sensory environment in critically ill patient. *Intensive Care Nursing*, 2(2), 73–83.

McWhirter, J.P. and Pennington, C.R. (1994). Incidence and recognition of malnutrition in hospital. *British Medical Journal*, 308, 945–8.

Manley, K. (1988). The needs and support of relatives. *Nursing*, 3(32), 19–22.

Manley, K. (1991). Central venous pressure: what, why, how? *Surgical Nurse*, 4, 10–13.

Marieb, E.N. (1995). *Human Anatomy and Physiology*, 3rd edn. The Benjamin/Cummings Publishing Company, Redwood City.

Masasi, R.S. and Keyes, J.L. (1994). The pathophysiology of hypoxia. *Critical Care Nurse*, 14(4), 55–64.

Mayers, M.G. (1972). *A Systematic Approach to the Nursing Care Plan*. Appleton-Century-Crofts, New York.

Meerabeau, L. (1991). The presentation of competence in health care. *Journal of Advanced Nursing*, 16(1), 63–7.

Meyers, K.A. and Hickey, M.K. (1988). Nursing management of hypovolaemic shock. *Critical Care Nursing Quarterly*, 11(1), 57–67.

Molter, N. (1979). Needs of relatives of critically ill patients: a descriptive study. *Heart and Lung*, 8, 332.

Monat, A. and Lazarus, R.S. (1985). *Stress and Coping: an Anthology*, 2nd edn. Columbia University Press, New York.

Moorat, D.S. (1976). The cost of taking temperatures. *Nursing Times*, 72(2), 767–70.

Moore, T. (1991). Making sense of sensory deprivation. *Nursing Times*, 87(6), 36–8.

Morrison, M.J. (1989a). Early assessment of the pressure sore risk. *Professional Nurse*, 4(9), 428–31.

Morrison, M.J. (1989b). Pressure sores: assessing the wound. *Professional Nurse*, 4(11), 532–5.

Morrison, P. (1989). Nursing and caring: a personal construct theory study of some nurses' self-perceptions. *Journal of Advanced Nursing*, 14(5), 421–6.

Murakami, W.M. (1995). External rewarming and age in mildly hypothermic patients after cardiac surgery. *Heart and Lung*, 24(5), 347–58.

Nelson, S. (1996). Pre-admission education for patients undergoing cardiac surgery. *British Journal of Nursing*, 5(6), 335–40.

Nichols, G.A. and Kucha, D.H. (1972). Oral measurements. *American Journal of Nursing*, 72(6), 1091–2.

Nolan, J. and Nolan, M. (1993). Can nurses take an accurate blood pressure? *British Journal of Nursing*, 2(14), 724–9.

Norris, L. and Grove, S. (1986). Investigation of selected psychosocial needs of family members of critically ill adults. *Heart and Lung*, 15(2), 194–9.

O'Brien, D. and Davison, M. (1994). Blood pressure measurement: rational and ritual actions. *British Journal of Nursing*, 3(8), 393–6.

O'Brien, E.T., Beevers, D.G. and Marshall, H.J. (1995). *ABC of Hypertension*, 3rd edn. British Medical Journal Publishing Group, London.

Pearce, C. (1993). Formal measurement of pain by nurses. *Nursing Standard*, 7(21), 38–9.

Potger, K.C. and Elliott, D. (1994). Haemodynamic monitoring. *Heart and Lung*, 23(4), 285–99.

Radcliffe, S. (1993). Preoperative information: the role of the ward nurse. *British Journal of Nursing*, 2(6), 305–6, 308–9.

Raiman, J. (1986). Toward understanding pain, and planning relief. *Nursing*, 3(11), 411–13, 418–23.

Raper, S. and Maynard, N. (1992). Feeding the critically ill patient. *British Journal of Nursing*, 1(6), 273–8.

Rowley, G. and Fielding, K. (1991). Reliability and accuracy of the Glasgow coma scale with experienced and inexperienced users. *Lancet*, 337, 535–8.

Schofield, P. (1995). Using assessment tools to help patients in pain. *Professional Nurse*, 10(11), 703–6.

Shephard, T.J. and Fox, S.W. (1996). Assessment and management of hypertension in the acute ischaemic stroke patient. *Journal of Neuroscience Nursing*, 28(1), 5–12.

Shuldham, C.M., Cummingham, G., Hiscock, M. and Luscombe, P. (1995). Assessment of anxiety in hospital patients. *Journal of Advanced Nursing*, 22, 87–93.

Spelman, M.S. (1967). How do we improve doctor–patient communication in our hospitals? In *Communicating with the Patient*, Ley, P. and Spelman, M.S. (eds). Staples Press, London.

Sullivan, J. (1990). Neurologic assessment. *Nursing Clinics of North America*, 25(4), 795–809.

Swindale, J.E. (1989). The nurses' role in giving preoperative information to reduce anxiety in patients admitted to hospital for elective minor surgery. *Journal of Advanced Nursing*, 14(11), 899–905.

Sykes, M.K., McNicol, M.W. and Campbell, E.J.M. (1976). *Respiratory Failure*, 2nd edn. Blackwell Scientific Publications, Oxford.

Thompson, C. (1989). The nursing assessment of the patient with cardiac pain on the coronary care unit. *Intensive Care Nursing*, 5(4), 147–54.

UKCC (1993). *Standards for Records and Record Keeping*. UKCC, London.

Venus, B., Mathru, M., Smith, R. and Pham, C. (1985). Direct versus indirect blood pressure measurements in critically ill patients. *Heart and Lung*, 14, 228–31.

Verity, S. (1996). Communicating with sedated ventilated patients in intensive care focusing on the use of touch. *Intensive and Critical Care Nursing*, 12(6), 354–8.

Walding, M.F. (1991). Pain, anxiety and powerlessness. *Journal of Advanced Nursing*, 16, 388–97.

Wardman, C. (1991). Norton vs Waterlow. *Nursing Times*, 87(13), 74–8.

Waterlow, J. (1985). A risk assessment card. *Nursing Times*, 81(48), 49–55.

Watkinson, C. (1997). Developing a pressure sore risk assessment scale. *Professional Nurse*, 12(5), 341–8.

Watson, J. (1989). *Nursing: Human Science and Human Care*. Appleton-Century-Croft, Norwalk, CT.

Watson, M., Horn, S. and Curl, J. (1992). Searching for signs of revival: uses and abuses of the Glasgow coma scale. *Professional Nurse*, 7(10), 670–4.

Webb, C. (1987). Sexual healing. *Nursing Times*, 86(4), 29–30.

Wewers, M.E. and Lowe, N.K. (1990). A critical review of visual analogue scales in the measurement of clinical phenomena. *Research in Nursing and Health*, 13(4), 227–36.

Wicker, P. (1987). Putting ideas into practice. *Senior Nurse*, 7(4), 22–4.

Wilson-Barnett, J. and Batehup, L. (1988). *Patient Problems: a Research Base for Nursing Care*. Scutari Press, London.

Wong, C.A. (1990). Pre-operative patient preparation. *Journal of Post Anaesthetic Nursing*, 5(3), 149–56.

Wright, L. and Leahey, M. (1984). *Nurses and Families: a Guide to Family Assessment and Intervention*. F.A. Davies, Philadelphia.

Young, T. (1996). Prevention and management of pressure sores: role of education. *British Journal of Nursing*, 5(15), 941–6.

Zigmond, A.S. and Snaith, R.P. (1983). The hospital anxiety and depression scale. *Acta Psychiatrica Scandinavica*, 67(6), 361–70.

Garvey, A., Hibbert, A. and Manley, K. (1994). *Nutrition and Nursing*. RCN, London.

Johns, C. (1990). Double dilemma. *Nursing Times*, 86(50), 47–9.

Perry, A. and Jolley, M. (1990). *Nursing: a Knowledge Base for Practice*. Edward Arnold, London.

Schamroth, L. (1990). *An Introduction to Electrocardiography*, 7th edn. Blackwell Scientific Publications, Oxford.

Sutherland, L. (1991). The Burford model. *Nursing*, 4(25), 19–21.

Watson, J. (1988). *Nursing: Human Science and Human Care – a Theory of Nursing*. National League for Nursing, New York.

Williams, S.R. (1994). *Essentials of Nutrition and Diet Therapy*, 6th edn. Mosby, St Louis, California.

FURTHER READING

Burnard, P. (1985). *Learning Human Skills*. Heinemann, London.

CHAPTER TWENTY-SIX

CARE *of the* OLDER PERSON

Hazel Heath

- Views on ageing and older people
- Ageing – a biographical approach
- Theoretical approaches to the study of ageing
- Theories of ageing
- Older people today
- Perceptions of older people
- Health in older age
- Illness and disability in older age
- Health and social policy and older people
- The history and development of nursing older people
- Working with older people – fundamental values and principles
- Building relationships with older people
- Assessing older people
- Promoting health in older age
- Dying and bereavement
- Conclusion

This chapter aims to enhance understanding of older people, older age and the processes of ageing. Through a **biographical approach** it explores the influences of life experiences on how individuals, particularly those from different generations, interact. It acknowledges broad demographic characteristics of older people in the UK today, and highlights current debates about their health and social care needs. The chapter traces the development of gerontological nursing as an emerging specialty. It discusses fundamental values and principles which can guide nurses in working with older people. It describes the distinct and additional considerations for assessing older people and highlights key elements of the nursing role, particularly in health promotion.

VIEWS ON AGEING AND OLDER PEOPLE

In modern Western societies, and indeed in health and social care, older people are generally viewed as a group with common characteristics and common needs. Older age is usually viewed as a state, a stage or an event (Johnson, 1985). These views derive from the bulk of research into older age which has traditionally sought to understand it through objective and observable means. In fact older age, like any age, is a subjective experience lived by individual people.

In reality, older people are not a homogenous group, but highly diverse individuals. The only factor common to all older people is an accumulation of more numerous life experiences over a greater period of time than those of younger people and, as life experiences interact with individual personalities, it could be argued that people become more unique, more idiosyncratic (Johnson, 1985), and that older age is the 'zenith' of individuality (Garrett, 1983).

Older age, like any other age, is the summation of events and experiences which occur during one's lifetime. These subjective experiences have shaped life and led to the individual's present position. Each individual person has a unique life history. Johnson (1985) highlights that the process of ageing is not a single dimension progression, but 'a complex of strands, or paths of concern, continuing for differing lengths of time throughout a life biography and moulding its individuality'. These strands may include relationships or occupations. Johnson suggests that ageing and older age are thus 'the continuing of an intricate pattern of life careers'. Each individual experiences his or her own unique biography, with hopes, fears, achievements, failures, fond memories, satisfactions, frustrations and pride in the past. All these self-estimates are part of each person's cumulative self-image and all are 'non-objective' (Johnson, 1985, pages 109–111).

Using this approach can help nurses to work with older people because they will be better able to understand the older person's self-perceived state, self-image, needs and aspirations at that point in their lives (Johnson, 1986).

AGEING – A BIOGRAPHICAL APPROACH

'To understand a man, you must first understand his memories.'

(Ancient Proverb)

Throughout each person's life history, events interact with us as individuals to form our self-perceived state. Adams' (1991a) biographical model suggests three dimensions in which these events may be experienced (Figure 26.1).

Public events, such as the millennium celebrations or Queen Elizabeth II's Golden Jubilee, are shared with many people. They may not have any direct effect on individuals but reflect in some way on each personal history.

Significant events and *personal milestones* also occur in each person's life. These may be events such as going to school, starting work, getting married, having children, moving home or losing a partner.

Personal memories are the individual's interpretation of, and attribution of meaning to, events and experiences. People may not be aware of the meaning of the memories, and they may be difficult to share with others. The interpretation and meaning of personal memories can be revisited, and can change over time.

Our beliefs and values are shaped by our backgrounds, culture, individual and shared life experiences, and Adams (1991a) suggests that these act as a 'filter' through which we view other people.

Consider the effects of the experiences shown in Table 26.1 on the three different birth cohorts. From Table 26.1 it can be seen that, even when public events are shared, they are shared at different times in individual lives, and impact differently on personal experiences. Between older people and younger people, the differences can be vast. Rabbitt (1984) describes people now in very old age as 'time travellers, exiled to a foreign country which they now share with current twenty year olds'. He describes how these groups have been fed, housed, and educated very differently, have received, or failed to receive, different medical treatment for different conditions, have been taught to prize different skills and attitudes, and have been shaped by dramatically different experiences.

It can be difficult for some older people to understand changed values and ways of living. Seabrook (1980) highlights that:

'many of the old grew up in a world where they had to be disciplined, frugal, stoical, self-denying, poor; and what this taught them, often in bitterness and pain, appears to be of no use to their children and grandchildren, who have been shaped for different purposes by changed circumstances.'

It can also be difficult for young people to empathise with the experiences and views of older people. In many years of working as a teacher trying to nurture the enthusiasm of young students for working with older people, the author was constantly reminded of the challenges which can arise in working towards intergenerational understanding. As one student nurse wrote in her essay:

'We are taught about the concept of empathy, and I try to empathise with my patients but this is very difficult to do. How can I as a young person

Table 26.1: How different generations might view world events

	World events	Personal memories Born 1915	Personal memories Born 1940	Personal perceptions Born 1975
1920s	Depression/ unemployment King George's Jubilee Flappers/charleston Wall Street crash			
1930s	Abdication of Edward VIII Start of the Second World War Depression/ unemployment	My family needed food and we had no money. I walked miles with only a cup of tea in my belly to get a job only to be told it had gone. We queued for hours and had to call the counter clerk 'Sir' before we got our dole money. I hope I never again suffer the indignity of having to ask for money!		
1940s	War years Welfare state Rationing Marriage of Princess Elizabeth	I worked as a plater's helper in the docks for most of the war and the East End got its fair share of bombings. We had some laughs in the air raid shelters and D day was a great celebration. My daughter had diphtheria but, thanks to the welfare state, she was alright.	My few memories of the war are very vivid. When the air raid sirens went, my mother would grab me and my baby brother, bundle us under the stairs and crouch over us. The noise was frightening but my mum always felt so warm and she smelled of soap.	I don't know much about the war – only what I've seen on TV, like on the VE celebrations. Grandad says that they never knew who would die next – it might be him or Grandma. I haven't a clue how that was, or why they didn't just go to live somewhere else.
1950s	Coronation End of rationing Suez Korean War			
1960s	Kennedy assassination Beatlemania/flower power Man on the moon	They sang that 'The times they were a-changing' – they certainly were. Young people seemed to want so much freedom that we hadn't had, but then, with men on the moon, life's horizons seem endless. Sad about Kennedy – such a young man and with so much promise.	I must have looked ridiculous in all that hippie gear saying 'love and peace, man' to everyone I met, and giving them flowers, but it felt like the dawning of a new age ... I was at a psychedelic party when I heard about Kennedy – it was like one of my friends dying – he carried the hopes of our generation.	I've seen pictures of the Beatles but can't really understand what all the fuss was about. Their music's still good though – I'm collecting their CDs. And some of the clothes are really fashionable now – I'm going to a 60s night next week!

Table 26.1: continued

	World events	Personal memories Born 1915	Personal memories Born 1940	Personal perceptions Born 1975
1970s	Three-day week/miners' strike Vietnam War Watergate Britain joins the EEC			
1980s	Margaret Thatcher Falklands Chernobyl Reagan/Gorbachev			
1990s	IT explosion City crash/recession Genetic engineering HIV and AIDS Channel tunnel	These computers are marvellous but I must admit I don't know what they're talking about. All this hardware, software, networking, downloading – it's like a foreign language. They use them at the GP surgery now.	I was devastated when I was made redundant. We're really struggling financially and it seems I'm too old to be wanted by another company. They say computer skills will help so the kids are teaching me. I might try to start my own business but it seems so risky.	I loved IT at school. My mate's on the Internet and we spend hours on the chat-up lines! Because I haven't got a job I've been placed on a youth employment scheme. It's not much money but better than nothing!

Adapted, with permission, from Adams, 1991a.

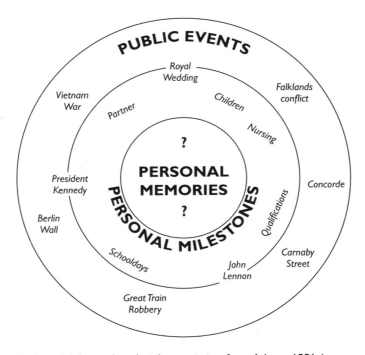

Figure 26.1: A biographical model (reproduced with permission from Adams, 1991a)

have empathy with a person who has lived for so many more years, and lived through world wars, and had so many experiences that I have not had. It's hard.'

(Heath, 1993)

Reflection Point

When you formulate your opinions, how different do you consider they would be were you to have the life experiences of someone now in their 80s?

THEORETICAL APPROACHES TO THE STUDY OF AGEING

Compared to many other disciplines, gerontology, the study of ageing, is relatively young, and some would say immature. Much of the early research was concerned with mapping the 'problems' of older age, along with their medical, psychological and social correlates (Johnson 1985). These have tended to reinforce the perspective of older age as decline.

In addition, the predominant use of cross-sectional methodologies has resulted in a general picture of ageing as declining physical and mental functioning. In cross-sectional studies different age groups, or cohorts, are studied at the same time. For example, the blood pressure of cohorts of people aged 50, 60 and 70 might be measured. If this was highest in the 70-year-olds and lowest in the 50-year-olds, it might be concluded that blood pressure increases with age. In fact, this may be due to factors specific to that group of people, such as smoking, eating habits and amount of exercise taken.

Longitudinal studies take one group or cohort of people over a period of time. Using this methodology, the blood pressure of one group of subjects would be taken when they were aged 50, 60 and 70. It thus gives a better indication of the progress of the same individuals over time and, to a greater extent, removes the influences of the other variables.

Recent work using longitudinal methods demonstrates that some of the earlier results suggesting that ageing brought decline were, in fact, characteristics of different lifestyles and illness experiences of the cohort samples used, rather than the true effects of ageing (Grimley Evans *et al.*, 1992).

Longitudinal studies are more complex to conduct. It can be difficult to maintain continuity with the research subjects, researchers and research finance. Further challenges to studying older age are presented by the inherent complexities of health in later life. Physiologically, no two individuals age in the same way and the range of 'normal' is greater in older age than younger age. In addition, many factors impact on health, such as genetic, environmental, psychological, social and general lifestyle. For example, some people over 80 remain physically generally well, active and contributing to life, whilst others are more sedentary.

What is clear from the research is that chronological age is a poor predictor of either health or functional level in individuals (Brouwer, 1990), and age is therefore not a useful label, for example, when health and social service provision is being rationed on the basis of age alone.

THEORIES OF AGEING

One of the earliest approaches in gerontology resulted in the *disengagement theory* (Cumming and Henry, 1961). This maintains that society and individuals mutually withdraw or disengage, in order to allow the ageing individual to focus on him- or herself in preparation for death. Critics of the disengagement theory suggest that, in fact, the opposite was true. *Activity theory* states that older persons need and want to become involved with a variety of activities. The new involvements substitute for changes that come with growing older and the roles that are lost with retirement (Berger, 1994). With *continuity theory*, each person copes with the later years of life in much the same way as they coped with the earlier period. In this sense, ageing is seen as a continuation of the earlier life rather than as a separate period (Berger, 1994).

Developmental theories focus on life tasks to be accomplished at particular stages. Older age is encompassed within one or two stages. Erikson's stages of development (1950) are widely cited as a way of viewing development across the lifespan with the eighth stage, integrity versus despair, used to describe older adulthood. Erikson admitted to being surprised at the creativity and generativity of older adults and, particularly in view of increasing life expectancy, Erikson suggested that the entire life cycle should be re-examined rather than adding another stage toward the end (Erikson *et al.*, 1986).

Havinghurst (1952) also described older adulthood as one stage beginning around age 55, which was termed later maturity. Later maturity was seen as a time during which the older adult was faced with adjusting to retirement and reduced income, adjusting to decreased physical strength, adjusting to the death of a spouse, establishing alliances with others of the same age, and adapting to changing social roles.

Butler (1963) proposed the process of life review, which involves integrating past life experiences in an attempt to believe that life has had meaning. Life review is characterised as a universal process that occurs at any point in life when a person is forced to confront his or her mortality. Perceiving that life has had meaning enables the individual to prepare for death without fear.

BIOLOGICAL THEORIES

In biological as well as psychosocial terms, there is no specific group which can be accurately described as 'older' or 'the elderly'. The biological ageing process is continuous throughout life and there are no particular points at which older age begins. Biological ageing occurs through an interaction of various intrinsic and extrinsic processes. Intrinsic processes are largely governed by an individual's genetic inheritance. Extrinsic factors derive from an individual's lifestyle and environment (Grimley Evans, 1994).

Biological theories have generally summarised ageing as a loss of adaptability over time. The homeostatic mechanisms which normally enable humans to adapt to challenges within the environment become impaired with increasing age. This loss of adaptability increases until the challenges can no longer be overcome.

One of the oldest biological theories is the *wear-and-tear* theory. This theory maintains that just as parts of machines wear out, parts of the human body also deteriorate with each year of use. According to this theory, we wear out our bodies just by living (Berger, 1994).

The *cellular interaction* theory suggests that an organism's individual cells are influenced by other cells. Unless the cells are functioning in har-

mony, the feedback mechanisms will fail and the cells will degenerate (Berger, 1994).

The *somatic mutation theory* states that as cells divide, they develop spontaneous mutations. These mutations eventually lead to death (Kane *et al.*, 1994).

The *error catastrophe theory* proposes that errors occur in deoxyribonucleic acid (DNA), ribonucleic acid (RNA), and protein synthesis (see page 128). Each error augments the other and culminates in an error catastrophe (Kane *et al.*, 1994).

The *disposable soma theory* suggests that ageing and death occur for evolutionary reasons. Throughout life, the body's cells are damaged by factors such as radiation, chemicals or free oxygen radicals generated by the body's own metabolism. Unrepaired cell and tissue defects gradually accumulate, and there comes a point where the amount of biological resources required to repair this damage and maintain the cells is not worth the expenditure of resources, given that death by accident will occur sooner or later and that, in the wild, survival would be unlikely (Kirkwood, 1994).

Individual theories of ageing can be helpful in providing a framework within which to understand a particular aspect of ageing, or within which to work with an individual older person. However, ageing is a holistic experience, which integrates biological, psychological, social and many other factors. The subjective experience of growing older is ultimately unique to each individual.

In addition, both biologically and in terms of life experience, there are aspects which distinguish older people. Older people are the survivors, in that they have survived when their contemporaries have not. Precursors to survival may lie in characteristics of personality (see later discussion), or in biological factors. For example, older people have been found to have a higher prevalence of the genes that protect against cardiovascular disease (Grimley Evans, 1994).

In addition, there are cohort effects, and each cohort of individuals, as it becomes older, will bring the influences of particular lifestyles and other influences on health. For example, people who are currently old may have worked in areas of high environmental pollution, with exposure to chemicals, dust or asbestos. In addition, smoking, eating and exercise habits will exert their influences on health.

OLDER PEOPLE TODAY

The only characteristic common to all older people today is a relatively greater accumulation of life experience. In all other respects they are possibly the most diverse group of individuals to be described under a collective label.

People described as 'older', 'old' or 'elderly' may be aged 55 or 105 – a span of five decades! Older people derive from all social groups, backgrounds, social classes and income levels. Their living circumstances and lifestyles are similarly widely diverse, as is their health status.

For distinction, older people are sometimes categorised into two subgroups:

- People in the third age are those who have retired from mainstream paid employment and people who have completed family raising, and some others who do not fall into either of these categories. The third age can begin at around 50, and generally includes people who are physically and mentally healthy.
- The fourth age usually encompasses people in their 80s and 90s who experience temporary or permanent illness or disability (Grimley Evans et al., 1992).

In Great Britain today, 12.8 million people are aged 55 and over, and 11.6 million are aged 60 and over. This represents approximately 21% of the population, and has increased by 8% since 1981. The increase is almost entirely in the older age groups, where the number of people aged 85 and over has increased by 50% between 1981 and 1991. Two million people are currently aged 80 and over, and more than 7000 are more than 100 years old (OPCS, 1993). In both absolute and relative terms, the increase in the older population is projected to continue. Between 1989 and 2026, the number of people aged 65 and over is expected to increase by 30%, and the number of people aged 85 and over by 66% (DoH, 1992). By the year 2025, the proportion of pensioners in the population is projected to be around 22% (OPCS, 1993), and the number of people aged 75 and over around 2.9 million (CSO, 1991).

The increase in the older population is occurring for two reasons. First, the reduced death rate overall means that more people are reaching older age. Second, the reduced birth rate results in fewer younger people. However, the Medical Research Council (1994) urges caution in interpreting population projections because of the dearth of research into projection methodologies and detailed analysis of later life trends.

There are more females than males in the older age groups. Women comprise 58% of people aged 60 and over, 67% of those aged 85 and over (OPCS, 1993) and 79% of those aged 90 and over (DoH, 1992). It has been suggested that, because this female predominance in the older age groups is not appreciated, their needs are often neglected in policy and planning, and they are among the most disadvantaged people in our society (Bernard and Meade, 1993).

THE LIVING CIRCUMSTANCES OF OLDER PEOPLE

Older people live throughout the UK, but the proportions differ. In some parts of the country less than 10% of the population is over pensionable age, whilst other areas are almost retirement centres, with up to 35% of the population over pensionable age (Warnes and Law, 1985). The subjective experience of older people will be influenced by the age mix of their local community, but also how well the community recognises and caters for the needs of the older population.

Currently, over 95% of people over 60 years of age in Britain today live in private households (OPCS, 1993), and approximately half of people aged 65 and over own their own homes (Institute of Actuaries, 1993). A small percentage live in privately rented accommodation, particularly those aged 70 and over, elderly women, and those who live alone (Smythe and Browne, 1992). Older people more commonly live in older housing than younger householders, and particularly if the accommodation is rented (DoE, 1988).

The homes of older people, and particularly those aged 75 and over, are more commonly in poor condition, or even unfit for habitation, lacking in amenities, and with substandard heating (OPCS, 1990). In successive general household surveys, only about half of elderly households had central heating (OPCS, 1980, 1990), and Hunt's (1978) survey found that approximately 8% of older people were not warm in bed or in their living room, and 12% were not warm in their kitchens. This raises concerns about the effects of poor housing on the health of older people, and inadequate housing has been cited as a contributory factor in the admission of older people into residential care (Phillips, 1992).

There has been an increase in the number of very old people living alone. It is estimated that 41% of older people, some 3.4 million, live alone (Help the Aged, 1995). One survey of over 1000 adults aged 65 and over found that, although older people chose to live independent lifestyles, thousands had little or no social contact, and many did not receive the help and support they needed to lead fulfilling lives (Help the Aged, 1995). There are positive aspects in living alone, and people who live alone do not always perceive themselves to be lonely. Indeed, some individuals who are married and living with a spouse have described themselves as feeling lonely (Barron et al., 1994). However, studies have identified that loneliness can not only be unpleasant, but is also linked to various health problems (Berg et al., 1981; Schultz and Moore, 1984; Holmen et al., 1992). Living alone is also the largest demographic risk factor, after age itself, for admission to hospital or entry into long-term care (Laing and Hall, 1991).

ECONOMIC CIRCUMSTANCES

The economic circumstances of older people vary considerably. Some media emphasis has been given to images of 'woopies' (well-off older people), 'jollies' (jet setting oldies with loads of loot), and 'opals' (older people with affluent lifestyles) (Victor, 1991). However, the predominant image, and that which more accurately reflects the circumstances of the majority of older people, is one of poverty. Well over half of pensioners live in or on the margins of poverty, and the numbers of pensioners with an income below half of the national average has nearly trebled since 1979. Older people are more likely to live in poverty over a long period of time than any other age group (Walker, 1990). Ageing itself can be associated with a loss of the social and economic resources available to younger people. This has direct implications for the extent to which older people are able to cope with illness or disability, and it is generally the oldest and most disabled who are the poorest (McGlone, 1992).

Poverty in older age arises partly from the economic redundancy enforced on older people by retirement (Fennell et al., 1988), and partly from the progressive reduction of the relative value of the state pension on which a high proportion of older people are dependent (Walker, 1981). It has been suggested that poverty in older age has gone unchallenged and has thus become accepted as an inevitable part of growing older (Walker, 1981). This has reinforced society's view of older people as economically and socially redundant, and has legitimised their marginalisation (Fennell et al., 1988).

OLDER PEOPLE FROM DIFFERENT LANDS

The population of older people from minority ethnic groups is small at present: only 1–6% of people within each of the minority ethnic groups overall are currently post-retirement age, about 93 000 people (Jones, 1993). It is estimated that about 5% of West Indians, 4% of Indian, Chinese and Arab peoples, 2% of Africans and Pakistanis, and 19% of the white population is currently over pensionable age (Hasky, 1995). However, within the next 10–20 years, these proportions will increase (DoH, 1992). It has been suggested that little attention has been paid to the needs of these groups of people, and there is a dearth of information about them. What information there is suggests that older people from minority groups are more disadvantaged than the white population in terms of social class, income, health and housing (Norman, 1985; Hasky, 1989).

Here again, biographies are significant. Adams (1991b) describes how some people came to the UK during the Second World War to escape Nazi persecution and others came during the 1950s from the New Commonwealth. Adams uses Perks' (1984) research to illustrate the acclimatisation of subsequent generations of people who immigrated from the Ukraine.

First generation Ukrainian, aged 74:
'I born for Ukraine country, I like my country, I want to go back to my country. If my country free.

Second generation Ukrainian, aged 34:
Q You have an English passport and you have got English nationality; do you still see yourself as Ukrainian? A I do, it sounds odd, but I really do: I would never say anything against the British and I mean they have given me everything, and they have given me an education and so on and so forth, but in my heart I just feel Ukrainian.

Third generation Ukrainian, aged 10:
Q Do you think you will ever go back to the Ukraine? A Yes, when I'm older . . . I have never seen it, and I'm kind of part of it, so I'd like to go and see it, and see my relations there.

Adams (1991b) highlights how the third generation migrant may be influenced predominantly by the British culture in which he spent his formative years, the second generation migrant is influenced by both Ukrainian and British culture, but that older man still sees himself as being Ukrainian. His lifestyle, and his beliefs about health and health care will likely derive from his own cultural traditions.

The older generations from immigrant populations may face particular difficulties if they have spent more formative years in their own culture and had limited opportunity to socialise and to learn the English language (Cameron *et al.*, 1989).

PERCEPTIONS OF OLDER PEOPLE

Western cultural images and perceptions of older people have resulted in a number of ideologies which significantly influence not only health and social policy, but also the subjective experiences of older people who need health or social care.

Common assumptions are:

- That there is a 'rising tide' of older people which could potentially overwhelm other age groups
- That older people are not economically productive and therefore do not contribute to society
- That there are now fewer younger people to support the non-productive or 'dependent' older population
- That the majority of older people are ill, disabled and dependent, and therefore consume large amounts of resources.

These perceptions are specific to Western cultures, as distinct from many other societies around the world where older people are venerated as the repositories of cultural heritage and wisdom. Negative Western perceptions arise for many reasons such as linking older age with physical decline, biological inferiority and a fear of death. In a society which exalts youth and beauty, people who are less youthful or less 'beautiful' may be seen as less valuable. The structure and organisation of modern societies can also contribute to these negative views. For example, rapid developments in industrial and technological processes can render the skills and knowledge of older generations less relevant. In addition, the Western consumer culture renders those with most resources as most powerful. The devaluing and marginalisation can thus become 'structured' into societal functioning.

One way in which this works is through mandatory retirement, which removes from older people the opportunity to work and to continue to update their work skills, and reduces their income and thus their consumer power. Society thus forces them into this 'non-productive' category, in which they can be viewed as socially dependent. So pervasive and powerful can be this process, that a cycle of dependency is created, which becomes a self-fulfilling prophecy.

Kuypers and Bengston (1984) applied Zusmann's (1966) concept of a social breakdown syndrome to older people (Figure 26.2).

Examples of this structurally induced dependence abound in many aspects of health social policy, alongside the assumption that it is accept-

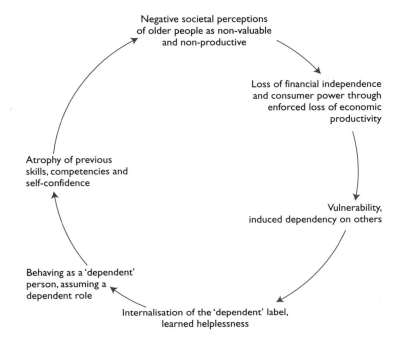

Figure 26.2: The cycle of structurally induced dependence (adapted from Kuypers and Bengston, 1984)

able for older people to be offered lower standards of service than younger people. For example, because older people are expected to be ill and disabled, they are denied benefits such as mobility allowance and other disability benefits unless they claim for these before reaching pensionable age. If they become disabled after retirement age, they are not eligible to claim. Thus younger people are deemed worthy of some financial help to cope with disability whilst older people have to cope without (Evandrou and Falkingham, 1989).

Partially due to the negative assumptions and prejudices which underpin much of Western society's treatment of older people, the undervaluing and marginalisation of older people has historically continued largely unchallenged. However, there are exceptions. In 1991 Bury and Holme's study of people aged 90 and over clearly demonstrated that older age did not inevitably bring greater dependence and suggested that it was not older age as such, but death, that was the resource-consuming event in later life. In addition, in 1986 Falkingham re-examined the impact of an increasing number of older people on society and concluded that 'it is not necessarily the case that a change in the age profile of the population will lead to a greater burden of dependency'. Falkingham suggested that, in fact, a

breathing space exists with respect to increasing age dependency until around the year 2020, and that current and short-future problems regarding dependency levels are likely to relate to the state of the economy rather than to age pyramids. She added:

> 'that is not to say that we should be complacent over future dependency levels, but rather that the degree of scaremongering over the ageing of the population that has been prevalent in the last few years has been unfounded.'
>
> (Falkingham, 1986, page 230)

HEALTH IN OLDER AGE

In recent years there has been an increasing emphasis on positive health, yet health is usually measured in negative indicators such as mortality or morbidity.

Functional ability is increasingly being used as an indicator of general health. Activities of daily living (ADL) scales usually focus on basic activities such as eating and washing. Instrumental ADLs include activities such as shopping and cooking.

Sources of statistics on the health of older people include the general household survey (GHS), which reports longstanding illness in the general population, excluding people living in care homes or institutions, and the Office of Population Censuses and Surveys (OPCS) surveys on disability in Great Britain, which include more specific details of disability. These surveys generally suggest that the incidences of both chronic illness and disability increase with age. However, the Medical Research Council (MRC) suggests that, because older people may be excluded from major studies, or the questionnaires structured in such a manner which does not highlight key indicators of their health status or needs, data sources such as the GHS are not adequate for comprehensively monitoring the health of older people.

As a result, according to the MRC, the current health status of older people as a group, and changes in their health status over time, remain largely unknown. The MRC therefore raises doubts about whether the increase in average lifespan achieved during this century has, in fact, resulted in an increase in illness and disability in older people, or the total 'burden' of dependence. The MRC urges that the eligibility criteria of studies should ensure that older people are not excluded, and thus services may be more appropriately planned to meet their real health status and needs.

Reflection Point

When you formulate a view about an older person, or older people in general, would your view be considered prejudicial if applied to another group of people, such as one gender, a racial or religious group, people of a particular sexual orientation or those with a physical or learning disability?

ILLNESS AND DISABILITY IN OLDER AGE

There are many myths and stereotypes about illness, incapacity and dependency in older age. In addition, definitions of dependency vary, which makes direct comparison difficult.

Of people aged 60 and over, about 38% report having a limiting long-term illness (i.e. any health problem or handicap which limits their daily activities). One in eight of these people with limiting long-term illness live in a communal establishment, such as a communal home (OPCS, 1993). Major causes of limiting long standing illness are arthritis and rheumatism, which affect around 18% of males and up to 30% of females aged 75 and over, other bone and joint problems, hypertension, heart problems and cataracts (DoH, 1992).

There are estimated to be 6.2 million disabled adults in Great Britain of whom more than two-thirds are aged over 60. The proportions and severity of disability increase steadily with age, becoming particularly marked over 80. Over 90% of disabled adults live in private households (McGlone, 1992).

General household surveys illustrate that the percentage of people unable to perform self care and household tasks independently increase with age, particularly at ages over 80 years. For most tasks at all ages, the proportion of women unable to do them independently is greater than the proportion of men. This may arise because there are more women than men in the older age groups, but may also be due to differences in muscle strength (Medical Research Council, 1994).

The later a disease develops, the greater the likelihood of it being fatal. This means that the longer a disease can be avoided, the shorter should be the period of disability (Medical Research Council, 1994). The MRC also highlights that, although there is an assumption that an increased lifespan will automatically be accompanied by an increase in disease and dependency, there are, at present, no theoretical or empirical grounds to support this idea. In fact, the data suggest that, in terms of dependency, the longer an individual can live in an independent state, the shorter the period of dependency subsequently (Medical Research Council, 1994). This highlights the importance of preventive strategies and their implementation at an early age.

HEALTH AND SOCIAL POLICY AND OLDER PEOPLE

Policies affecting older people are consistent across Europe, with moves towards the care of older people in the community and the more cost-effective use of scarce health resources. There is generally increased emphasis on family care, despite changes in traditional family structures, divorce, remarriage and employment patterns (Nolan, 1996).

Health policy, and the planning and provision of health and social care services, have undergone a period of accelerated change, particularly in the last 5–10 years. With the increased emphasis on local assessment, planning, provisional and evaluation of services, there is a wide variety of methods of assessing, quantifying and recording health and social need around the UK, and each locality plans and delivers its services according to its own priorities. The priority given to older people in the planning and delivery of services similarly varies considerably around the UK.

It has been suggested that something like 60% of NHS, and 50% of social services, budgets are for services for older people (McGlone, 1992), but estimating the use of services by older people is not straightforward. As the Medical Research Council (1994) highlights, health care utilisation depends not only on levels of ill health, but also on levels of provision of services, advances in treatment and care, expectations of individuals for their own health, individual's thresholds for self-referral, and professionals' thresholds for referral and use of specialist services. Thus a rise in health care utilisation does not necessarily reflect increased disease and disability, and self-reported illness, as in the general household surveys, may not accurately reflect absolute levels of morbidity, but rather individuals' expectations about their health and the services available. Therefore, from morbidity statistics based solely on health care utilisation, it is difficult to interpret trends in utilisation over time as a reflection of trends in levels of morbidity (Medical Research Council, 1994).

Reflection Point

When you prioritise your work, are your priorities in any way dictated by the value you place on individual patients as people? In other words, are your decisions influenced by a view that some individuals have intrinsically higher value than others?

Key Points

- Older people today are widely diverse individuals deriving from all social groups, backgrounds, social classes, income levels, and ranging in age from 50 to over 100.
- The living circumstances of older people vary but many live alone, commonly in poorer housing than younger people, and receive much lower incomes. These factors can adversely affect their health and ability to remain independent.
- The older population from minority ethnic groups is small at present but will increase within the next 10–20 years. These people are often particularly disadvantaged in income, housing and health.
- Many of the negative Western perceptions of older people derive not from factors intrinsic to them as a group, but rather from the way in which society disadvantages and marginalises them.
- There is a degree of scaremongering about increasing numbers of older people. More older people does not necessaraly mean a greater burden of dependency, and there is a 'breathing space' with respect to increasing age dependency until around 2020.
- Because of the dearth of research including older people, and the multiplicity of factors which influence statistics on health, illness and service utilisation in older age, these should be interpreted with caution.

THE HISTORY AND DEVELOPMENT OF NURSING OLDER PEOPLE

The roots of nursing older people lie in the workhouse infirmaries of the early twentieth century, and the specialty has struggled to free itself from such images. Research has consistently highlighted the pervading influence of the medical model and a warehousing approach to care.

The inherent 'cure' orientation of the medical model has hampered the development of nursing practice based on holism and caring. Isaacs (1981) highlights the inappropriateness of the standard medical paradigm for older sick people in that a single diagnosis is not always possible, as their disease manifestations may be multiple, and complicated by the effects of the ageing processes. Isaacs suggests that it is from the achievement of cure that the doctor derives his professional fulfilment and that the standard medical encounter is therefore geared towards this end. Older people, he says, with their 'poorly verbalised complaints and the limitless signs of past disease' may 'seem to offer little scope for therapeutic intervention'. This causes feelings of frustration and failure and, when this occurs, there may be a tendency to 'blame the victims, or to abrogate responsibility for them by labelling them for removal and storage'.

Research into the nursing of older people, including Norton *et al.* (1975), Baker (1978), Wells (1980), Evers (1981, 1984), Fielding (1986) and Reed (1989), has consistently revealed what Baker terms 'routine geriatric style', with its emphasis on meeting physical needs and 'getting through the work'.

Heath (1993) suggests that negative perceptions of nursing older people have been tainted by factors which do not derive from older people themselves and are not intrinsic to nursing them. When nurses feel negatively about working with older people, Heath argues, their perceptions have commonly been influenced by inferior care environments, inadequate equipment, low staffing levels, the lack of educational preparation and updating, the low priority given to the service by others, and the general perceptions of older patients as inferior in some way. Additional factors compounding this negative view can also derive from dealing with chronic illness, disability, dependency and death.

Nursing older people has faced many challenges in its development as a specialty. These include:

- Removing the 'stigma of the workhouse'
- Removing the label of older people as 'irremedial' and 'chronic' with no acute health care needs, and needing purely custodial care
- Shifting the focus from institutional care to rehabilitative care
- Overcoming inadequate facilities and chronic underfunding
- Challenging the view of nursing older people as 'just basic care'
- Dealing with staff who were 'relegated' to elderly care because they were considered unsuitable for 'more important' areas
- Developing and promoting suitable education, training and updating programmes
- Developing a positive research base.

Although the specialty has a history of disadvantage, the future is potentially brighter. Arguably some of the most visionary, articulate and pioneering nurses of recent decades have chosen to work with older people. Indeed, research demonstrates that more graduate nurses choose the specialty than any other. Some of the most fundamental changes in practice, such as primary nursing and therapeutic nursing, have developed through 'older people' nursing. There is currently a growing number of nurses and academics who are uniting the nursing of older people with the steadily burgeoning wealth of gerontology research. In terms of articulating and demonstrating the value of nursing, these people, and the body of knowledge they are creating, could be a formidable force in the future.

Reflection Point

When you formulate views about older people, or about working with them, are they factors that derive from the older people themselves, or peripheral issues such as funding, the environment, or other people's/nurses' perceptions?

WORKING WITH OLDER PEOPLE – FUNDAMENTAL VALUES AND PRINCIPLES

NURSES' ATTITUDES TOWARDS OLDER PEOPLE

How nurses view older people strongly influences how they work with them. A great deal of research has sought to analyse nurses' attitudes towards older people, and this has been periodically reviewed (Ingham and Fielding, 1985; Thomson, 1991; Pursey and Luker, 1995). However, the research into attitudes has been hampered by methodological difficulties deriving in part from a lack of conceptual clarity about, for example, the distinction between attitudes to older individuals, to older age, and to the process of ageing. In addition, the nature of the link between nurses' attitudes and how they behave towards older people has been difficult to define. Pursey and Luker (1995) also highlight the distinction between nurses' attitudes to older patients, and to the structural context of their work. For example, nurses may not feel positively about work with older people, but tend not to show this to the older patients themselves, with whom they often form close relationships.

In practice, staff attitudes communicate to older people in many, often subtle, ways. In Koch *et al.*'s study (1995), the older patients experienced 'being talked down to', 'spoken to as if one was a child or an imbecile', and not having their words taken seriously. This made them feel depersonalised. They attributed this behaviour to the staff categorising them in negative ways because they were old. The patients themselves resisted 'old' as a negative label.

In fact, there is a great deal to value about older people, both as individuals and in terms of their biographies.

VALUING BIOGRAPHIES AND LIFE EXPERIENCE

As discussed at the beginning of this chapter, older people have witnessed some of the most profound changes of any group at any time in history. They have overcome many social and personal challenges and have survived when their contemporaries have not.

Life experience has enriched the characters of older individuals in various ways. Contrary to the expectations of the stereotypes, expressed self-esteem remains high in later life (Baltes and Baltes, 1990; Coleman, 1993) and, in surveys, older people have expressed much higher rates of satisfaction with life than younger people. In Hunt's (1978) research into older people at home, the respondents expressed a greater degree of life satisfaction in all aspects of life, apart from health, than any other age group.

Research suggests that older people have learned self-reliance. For example, in Guttman's (1980) study psychiatrists observed that older patients could be maintained in the community with less frequent contact with therapists than younger people.

It is suggested that there are psychological characteristics which may have helped older individuals to surmount the various challenges of life (Hughes and Mtezuka, 1992). These include strength of character, a positive outlook and a desire to make life better for others (Grundy, 1994). Grimley Evans (1994) suggests that 'those people who insist on staying in control of their own lives, the wilful and cantankerous, live longer than the more compliant "sweet old folk" who make the "good patients" favoured by doctors and nurses'.

VALUING PERSONHOOD

Personhood is about valuing someone as 'worthy of being alive and having lived' (Hughes, 1995). Kitwood's (1993) concept of 'personhood' derives from his work with people with dementia but it is applicable to older people generally. Kitwood describes each person, whether old or young, ill or well, patient or nurse, as having accumulated resources (ways of being and doing learned from experience) and 'hang-ups' (defences, inadequacies, avoidances learned as a result of fear or hurt). He suggests that, rather than viewing patients as a set of symptoms or as a medical diagnosis, we should try to remove the 'them and us' barriers which result in, for example, nurses not wishing to use crockery used by patients/residents. Kitwood suggests that, in discovering the personhood of the older individuals with whom we work, we also discover something of ourselves.

VALUING RIGHTS, RESPONSIBILITIES, CHOICES AND RISK-TAKING

As citizens of society, older people have rights and responsibilities. Civil rights should not be eroded or disregarded when they enter a care environment, such as happens when older people living in nursing homes are not offered the right to vote.

Older people should also be offered choice in how they live their lives and the care they receive. Promoting and facilitating real choice for older people not only prevents the erosion of their rights, but also helps them to have control over their lives. It is important in these situations that nurses do not remove power and control from older people, but work to maintain this for as long, and in as many ways, as possible. It is also important that older people are encouraged and supported in making decisions, and that the choices they make are respected and acted upon. There may be cases where an older person is unable to make or express choices, and it is equally important that nurses facilitate that person's control as much as possible. This can be achieved by helping the older person to make choices in whatever ways they can (for example what to wear or what to do), and that they use their skills to help the older person succeed in whatever ways are possible, and always to maintain dignity (British Medical Association and Royal College of Nursing, 1995).

Research has demonstrated that choice and control contribute to positive health outcomes, and enhance both quality and quantity of life (Schultz, 1976; Rodin and Langer, 1977; Aasen, 1982; Ryden, 1984; Rodin, 1989). Loss of control is associated with ill health, psychological distress and increased mortality (Robertson, 1986).

The views of older people should also be respected when they wish to take risks. To facilitate the rights, responsibilities, choices and risk-taking, particularly when they are vulnerable, requires knowledge, understanding, sensitivity, skill and professionalism.

THE CARE ENVIRONMENT

Older people may have special needs with regard to the environment and nurses have a key role in manipulating the environment to enhance the functioning and quality of life. This can be assisted by:

- Facilitating individuality, e.g. by personal effects and photographs
- Facilitating personal space
- Facilitating freedom of movement, not arranging furniture so that it restricts moving around
- Facilitating privacy, not invading personal contemplation by intrusive noise or music
- Facilitating preferred lifestyle
- Helping the older person have choice in visitors
- Facilitating physical functioning by using appropriate furniture and equipment
- Helping to compensate for sensory loss or physical disabilities
- Facilitating social engagement, e.g. by the arrangement of furniture.

Social engagement, stimulating and meaningful activity are important. As Rabbitt (1988) describes:

'In the static environment, rehearsal of everyday minutiae makes poor conversation. When the theatre of the mind becomes the only show in town, archival memories begin to be actively explored for scripts.'

BUILDING RELATIONSHIPS WITH OLDER PEOPLE

UNDERSTANDING THE INDIVIDUAL WITHIN HIS/HER BIOGRAPHY

When nurses first encounter an older person in a care situation, that person may have experienced multiple changes and losses to which they are adjusting. These changes can be fundamental and can severely affect not only the older person's health but his/her self-perception, self-esteem and confidence. They could have a number of concerns:

- Is their health, vigour and ability to function independently declining?
- Are their symptoms due to a really serious illness? Could this be the end of life?
- Are their symptoms due to ageing? Should they 'bother' the doctor or nurse, and could anything be done?
- What will happen if their health continues to become worse, for example to their home, family, pets, treasured possessions?

For older people who are acutely ill and admitted to hospital, there may be overwhelming concerns about whether they will be able to remain independent and to return home.

For older people moving into a nursing or residential care home, there may be an overwhelming sense of loss as they, often against their will, give up their home, familiar surroundings, lifestyle and treasured possessions. For some, this experience can be devastating:

'For elderly people, moving into a nursing home meant the end of the line. It was as if they were crossing an invisible line; on the one hand they were people who had lives, possessions, identities and futures, and on the other they had none of these and would just live day by day. When people feel they have lost everything that they have spent their life building, and they know that they have neither the time nor the capacity to "start again", how can they perceive a future?'
(Nay, 1995)

Using a biographical approach to care can considerably enhance a nurse's understanding of an older person. Seeing an older person in the context of his/her biography, rather than detaching that person from his/her life experiences, can considerably enhance a nurse's understanding of that individual (Schofield, 1994):

> 'It is in the very process of unfolding a biography that relationships can be more fruitfully observed. It is the history which gives meaning to the major events which may not otherwise come to notice. In the setting of later life, such histories are vitally important. They provide the explanations which are needed when crises occur and professionals are deciding the future.'
>
> (Johnson, 1986)

COMMUNICATING WITH OLDER PEOPLE

There is potentially a great deal that nurses can learn from the ways in which older people communicate. As Nussbaum *et al.* (1989) state:

> 'Older people have participated in more relationships and in longer lasting relationships. They have had to adapt to more communicative situations than any other group of individuals. They have a wealth of communicative information to impart, and we simply have to listen!'

Communicating with older people can present challenges to nurses, particularly if the effects of psychological ageing have taken their toll on the older person's sight, hearing or movement. In addition, illness such as stroke, Parkinson's disease or dementia can drastically alter the way a person communicates.

Age-related changes affecting communication

Many age-related changes, including the speed of information processing and movement can affect communication, and the loss of abilities or opportunities to communicate can be very isolating.

Specific age-related changes in hearing (presbycusis) may result in:

- Impaired sensitivity to sound (the ability to hear high frequencies is usually lost first)
- Distorted loudness perception (causing distortion and pain)
- Impaired sound localisation
- Decreased ability to discriminate sound, especially speech.

Difficulties are exacerbated by background noise.

Age-related sight changes (presbyopia) may result in:

- Decreased visual accommodation (leading to difficulty focusing)
- Decreased tolerance of glare
- Decreased ability to adapt to dark and light
- Decreased peripheral vision (Pearce, 1981).

Difficulties are exacerbated by inadequate light.

Age-related changes in speaking can affect:

- Vocal production
- Speed of speech, which can become slower.

In addition, many older people wear dentures. This is not due to ageing as such, but to wear and tear, and inadequate nutrition or dental care in earlier years.

Non-verbal communication

Research suggests that older adults generally rely more on non-verbal than verbal cues, but that hearing and visual loss may reduce an older person's abilities to derive meaning from gestures such as a smile or nod. Touch can be particularly important for older people. Moore and Gilbert (1995) found that, at a time when their need for touch was greatest, older people had begun to think of themselves as untouchable. Touch raised their self-esteem by reassuring them that they are still loveable (Moore and Gilbert, 1995).

Verbal communication

Language is important both in terms of what is said, and how it is said. The words selected should acknowledge the language register of the individual and also any potential language difficulties. The pace at which speech is delivered should also acknowledge deficits such as hearing loss.

Intonation in the voice can convey power, authority and superiority, which reinforce powerlessness or dependence (Lanceley, 1985; Hewison, 1995a, b). Some speakers also modify the amount of feeling and nurture in their voices when talking to older people (Nussbaum *et al.*, 1989), but older people should not be patronised or infantilised.

Research in nurses' communication with older people

Research into how nurses communicate with older people has highlighted three areas of concern (Heath, 1997a):

- Staff attitudes (discussed above)
- Comparatively low priority given to communication
- Restricted communication styles.

THE PRIORITY GIVEN TO COMMUNICATION

Successive studies have demonstrated that nurses tend to focus on the completion of physical tasks of care. With physical priorities, talking to patients can become 'something to do after the "real" work has been completed' (Smith, 1992). An older woman in Koch *et al.*'s (1995) study highlighted this:

> 'they haven't got time to talk . . . wash, make you comfortable and that's it . . . they don't help how you *feel* . . . and I'd rather have that than the wash.'

RESTRICTED COMMUNICATION STYLES

Types of miscommunication identified by VanCott (1993), result from nurses:

- Using jargon or professional terms
- Using vague, ambiguous or unclear questions or statements
- Not explaining the purpose behind actions
- Ignoring, or failing to verify their own perception of the older person's statements.

An older person's hearing deficit and noise in the environment was also a factor.

Building therapeutic relationships can bring positive benefits to both the older person and the nurse:

> 'If younger individuals do not wish to become part of the relational world of [older people] who suffers? It can be argued that in the short run older people suffer. In the long run, however, it is the youth who will suffer, for one day they too will be old.'
>
> (Nussbaum *et al.*, 1989)

Reflection Point

When there are challenges or frustrations in your work with older people, for example extra time needed to communicate, from where do these originate? Could additional knowledge, experience or skills enhance your practice and potentially overcome the challenges?

Key Points

- Nursing older people has faced many changes in its development but, with its visionary, articulate and pioneering advocates and the growing alliances between nursing and gerontology, the future for gerontological nursing could be bright.
- The volumes of research into nurses' attitudes towards older people have been hampered by a lack of conceptual clarity (for example, in the distinction between attitudes to older individuals, older age, and the process of ageing), and by methodological difficulties.
- Key principles underpinning nursing practice with older people include valuing biographies, personhood, rights, responsibilities, choices and risk-taking.
- Nurses have a key role in creating a therapeutic environment, both in physical and psychosocial terms.
- In order to build relationships with older people, it can be helpful to acknowledge the individual's biography, and specifically the multiple changes and losses to which he/she may be adjusting on entering the care situation.
- Communicating with older people can be both rewarding and challenging. Nurses with sound skills based on a thorough understanding of communication processes in older age are more likely to reap the rewards.

ASSESSING OLDER PEOPLE

As has been highlighted throughout this chapter, each older person has individual needs, but older people as a group have distinct needs that require additional consideration. These derive from:

- The ageing processes, both physical and psychosocial, the effects of which are totally individual. In each person, systems of the body age at different rates and in individual ways, and the physical processes interact with the life experiences.
- Multiple pathology – the older an individual is, the more disease processes he/she is likely to experience. It is not uncommon for 80- and 90-year-olds to have upwards of four medical diagnoses. Partly because of the interaction between individual ageing processes and mul-

tiple pathology, diseases may be difficult to recognise and diagnose.

- Altered presentation of illness. Disease can present differently in older age. This altered presentation most often takes the form of some kind of physical or mental instability, immobility or incontinence. These manifestations have become known as 'the four Is', and were previously termed 'the giants of geriatrics'. An example of this would be that a chest infection would probably cause a raised temperature in a younger adult whereas, in an older adult, the first sign of an infection might be acute mental confusion.
- Polypharmacy and adverse drug reactions. When drugs are prescribed, particularly for multiple pathology, they tend to cause more adverse drug reactions, and these may be difficult to identify in the context of all the relevant factors.

When assessing an older person, therefore, a nurse is trying to unpick the complexities of individual ageing (both physical and psychosocial), multiple pathology, altered presentation of illness and drug reactions. Assessing an older person is therefore a complex activity, requiring high levels of skill and knowledge (see Box 26.1).

Box 26.1: Considerations when assessing older people

Old age is neither a disease nor a diagnosis and ageing is not synonymous with disease or disability. By itself, ageing does not cause aches, pains, depression, constipation, incontinence or forgetfulness. It is true that some functions, like sight or hearing, may become worse with ageing, and it may take longer to recover from illness or operations. But ageing, or old age, is never the sole reason for physical or mental illness. Remember – there is no disease which only affects people over the age of 65!

Older people are highly individual. With ageing, variations between individuals become more pronounced. Many variables influence the ageing process, genetic composition, lifestyle, the environment, education and socio-economic resources.

Health and social needs in older age are complex. Physical and psychosocial aspects interrelate, and the assessment of an older person is complex and challenging, for example:

- The older people become, the more problems they generally experience. A very old person can have upwards of four medical diagnoses (multiple pathology).
- Ill health can present differently in older age (altered presentation). Four common altered presentations are physical instability, mental instability, immobility and incontinence (the four 'Is'). Atypical or vague symptoms, such as lethargy, incontinence, increased mental confusion or agitation, reduced appetite, weight loss, sleeping disorders and falls, can indicate problems such as infection (particularly chest or urine), metabolic disorder (such as hypothyroidism), organ failure (such as cardiac), or mental change (such as depression).
- The consequences of deterioration in one function (e.g. hearing loss) may be most evident in the emergence of another problem (e.g. paraphemia).
- The prognosis of one problem (e.g. depression) may be dependent on the progress of another (e.g. physical illness).
- Judgements about action to be taken may be a matter of balancing priorities, as that which improves one aspect of health may aggravate another, particularly during drug treatment.
- Because older people have fewer adaptive mechanisms, one problem tends to exacerbate another. Health or social breakdown can start a 'domino effect', leading to decline or even death. Once breakdown has occurred health can deteriorate quickly.

There is a lack of generally agreed health and illness norms for older people, e.g. optimum blood glucose levels, or when to treat high blood pressure. Despite this, goals for care should be realistic and within the broad 'normal' age parameters.

Abilities and strengths, as well as disabilities and needs, should be acknowledged. Factors that have helped to maintain the older person's abilities and coping should be maximised, and threats to these, along with other stressors, identified. The person's goals for quality of life should be kept in focus.

Health promotion is effective into very old age in increasing well-being and delaying disability and premature death. Positive health practices should be recognised.

Despite time pressures, assessment should proceed at the older person's pace, allowing time for her/him to collect thoughts, formulate answers and

> verbalise concerns. Expressing interest and allowing for some degree of life review can elicit valuable information about long-term patterns of functioning, coping, preferred lifestyle and social support.
>
> If appropriate, information can be validated by family members/significant others. However, the views/needs of an older person and carer may differ, and seeing the older person and carer individually is recommended. Remember that one individual cannot give consent on behalf of another.

ASSESSING FUNCTION

To an older person, how they are functioning within their chosen lifestyle priorities and towards the achievement of life goals will generally be more important than a specific medical diagnosis. Areas of functioning include social (activities outside the home), domestic (activities within the home), and personal (self care). Loss of function tends to occur first in social activities, followed by domestic, and then personal (Williams and Wallace, 1993).

When assessing an older person, it is important to remember that he/she may function differently according to the environment, time of day, people around, physiological state or medication reactions. Functional impairment can indicate that there is an underlying health problem.

Social functioning

In later life, social functioning can be affected by many factors. These include change of role (from worker to retired person, wife to widow, parent to dependent), and altered self-image caused by changes in physical appearance and health. Opportunities for social functioning may be curtailed by loss of friends, loss of confidence or fear of crime. Accessibility to local services (e.g. laundry, pharmacy, bank, religious centre, library) can be affected by finance or the ability to use the telephone. Changes in local provision, such as the closure of small local shops in favour of large out-of-town supermarkets, coupled with the discontinuation of less economic transport services, can mean that older people are no longer independently able to access the services they need.

Social contact and networks have implications not only for how individuals experience older age, but also for their ability to continue living at home if they become ill or disabled. Wenger (1995, 1996) identified various types of support networks in older people:

- Family dependent network, which relies primarily on local kin
- Integrated network (in which the support derives from family, friends and neighbours)
- Private restricted networks, where there is no local kin and minimal contact with the local community.

Wenger found that approximately 50% of older people in the general population have social networks in the first two categories, and that these help them to remain in the community when they need help. Only a minority of older people have networks in the third category, but this type of network is most common on community care caseloads.

Family relationships are a central aspect of social functioning, but families function in very individual ways, and the roles assumed within each family vary greatly. It is important for nurses to be sensitive to these variations.

Some older people live with carers and, in fact, approximately 80% of community-based long-term care comes from informal networks of family and friends. There are about 6.8 million carers in Great Britain (OPCS, 1990); 13% of carers are 65 and over, and most are women. Around one million of these carers provide care for at least 35 hours a week and, in addition to their caring role, many have dependent children (Warner, 1994).

Caring can lead to profound changes in family and social life, as well as loss of income and additional expenditure. It can also be very detrimental to the carers themselves, and about two-thirds of carers say that their own health has suffered as a result of their caring responsibilities (Carers National Association, 1992). In the 1990 OPCS report, approximately 50% of carers said they had been caring for their dependent relative for at least 5 years, and 13% had not had a break from caring for 15 years or more. This signifies a heavy demand upon these individuals.

It is also important to recognise strains with a family, and particularly any family dysfunction, which may precede inadequate care or abuse, and there are indicators of these. Bennett (1990) suggests that the most common presentation usually involves combinations of poor hygiene, poor nutrition, frequent falls, confusion and poorly managed medical problems. When nurses go into a caring situation, it is important to appreciate that the needs of carers may be different from those of the older person. Carers should be seen alone so that they can raise any problematic issues (Warner, 1994).

Psychological and emotional functioning

There are many myths about how ageing affects mental functioning, and particularly memory. In fact, although there may be some slowing of thought and memory processes, Butler (1984) concluded that 75% of people can expect to retain sharp mental functioning, even if they live to a great old age, another 10–15% will experience mild to moderate memory loss, and only 5% will experience dementia. On other measures of intellectual functioning, such as the ability to organise and process visual materials, people have been shown to maintain high levels of performance into very old age, and studies have suggested that there is no strong age-related change in cognitive flexibility (Baltes and Shaie, 1982). The cumulative learning from life experiences can also enhance the ability of older people to solve problems, particularly when they practise generating their own solutions. In fact this ability can enhance over time (Blackburn et al., 1988).

Mental health in older age is difficult to define because the culmination of life experiences can accentuate some aspects of individual personalities and suppress others. Factors that can affect mental functioning include general health, fatigue or stress, and the manner in which information is presented.

Physical functioning

Physical functioning is affected by the multiple processes of ageing in the various systems of the body.

BREATHING
Age-related changes may cause shortness of breath, particularly in situations which increase the body's demand for oxygen. An individual's lifestyle will affect respiratory health in terms of occupation, exposure to environmental pollutants, and smoking habits. Pulmonary functioning may be compromised by lung tissue changes, decreased cardiac output, diminished immune system response, and a less efficient self-cleansing action of the respiratory cilia. Common problems experienced by older people include a reduced capacity for physical exertion, shortness of breath, dizziness, coughing, wheezing or recurrent chest infections (Ebersole and Hess, 1994).

MAINTAINING BODY TEMPERATURE
Due to deterioration of thermoregulation, reduced amounts of subcutaneous tissue, reduced sweat gland activity, and reduced metabolism or mobility, older people are sensitive to temperature extremes. They are at risk for hypothermia when environmental temperatures fall or they are not able to be active, such as after surgery.

HYDRATION AND NUTRITION
The thirst mechanism may become less efficient, and older people may not perceive a stimulus to take in fluid when they are at risk of dehydration. They are also at risk of undernutrition for reasons that may be physiological, psychological or social. Age-related changes which may compromise the ability to maintain nutritional status include diminished senses of smell, taste, touch and sight, plus reduced secretion of saliva, which may make chewing and swallowing more difficult and food less enjoyable. Poor dentition is also a factor. There are gastrointestinal changes, such as decreased hydrochloric acid secretion, with resultant reduction in the absorption of calcium and iron, or oesophageal changes resulting in dysphagia, heartburn and epigastric discomfort (Holmes, 1994). In older age there are lower energy requirements, due to a reduction in lean body mass, and older people may be more easily satiated, although the requirements for protein, minerals and vitamins are at least as great. In addition, lack of social stimulation can reduce the appetite, and mobility or joint problems can make shopping and preparing food more difficult for older people.

URINATION
Age-related changes can reduce the kidney's abilities to concentrate urine and cause reduced bladder elasticity, resulting in nocturia. Older men with prostatic hypertrophy commonly experience urinary retention. Some older adults experience

urinary tract infections, because the bladder may not contract effectively and urine may remain after voiding. This can increase the risk of bacterial growth. Urgency may occur because, unlike in younger people where the sensation of bladder fullness is felt when the bladder is about half full, in older people this urge may not be felt until the bladder is nearly full, therefore requiring an immediate response. Some older people experience continence problems, but incontinence is NOT an inevitable consequence of ageing. The condition may result from difficulties in walking to the lavatory, in retaining the urine for the necessary time, or in manipulating clothing.

BOWEL ELIMINATION

Constipation is not uncommon in older age. This may result from reduced mobility in the gastrointestinal tract, changes in the absorptive properties of the intestinal mucosa, slowing of nerve impulses, loss of muscle tone in the perineal floor and anal sphincter, and a history of using laxatives, which were believed to be valuable when the person was young. Older people who are immobile, particularly in hospital, are at high risk of constipation.

SEXUAL FUNCTIONING

Reduced opportunities to socialise, changes in self-image and body image, and self-confidence, can affect relationships and the expression of sexuality in older age. Physical age-related changes in sexual function may result in vaginal dryness in women, and a prolonged time taken to achieve erection, orgasm and recovery in men. However, sexual activity in later life is:

> 'the opportunity for the expression of passion, affection and loyalty: it affirms the value of one's body and its functions, it is a means of self-assertion and affirmation of life, it involves the pleasure of being touched and caressed; it defies the stereotype of ageing as the sexless older years, and it allows a continuing search for sexual growth and experience.'
>
> (Butler and Lewis, 1982)

MOVEMENT AND MOBILITY

Many of the major changes in functioning commonly seen in older people are associated with age-related changes in the muscles, joints and bones. Specific changes include decreased general strength and flexibility, limited range of motion in joints, mild reduction in physical endurance, gait changes (narrower standing base, wider sway when walking, shorter steps) leading to greater instability, decline in postural control, which affects balance, postural instability which is affected by medications, decreased visual and hearing acuity, and a decrease in handgrip strength. If older people become inactive, their muscle strength can decrease markedly, and they can experience a whole range of direct complications of not moving around.

Reflection Point

Have you every felt that it's not worth putting in such an amount of effort with older people because they cannot respond as well as younger people to treatment or therapeutic intervention?

PROMOTING HEALTH IN OLDER AGE

DEFINITIONS OF HEALTH

In older age, health can be viewed as the potential to achieve quality of life. Seedhouse (1986) suggests that a person's optimum state of health is equivalent to the state of the set of conditions which fulfil or enable a person to work to fulfil his or her realistic chosen and biological potentials. Some of these conditions are of the highest importance for all people. Others, Seedhouse suggests, are variable, dependent upon individual abilities and circumstances. The emphasis on potential is helpful in the context of nurses working with older people, in that their work can help maintain, reacquire or create the conditions which enable the older person to achieve these potentials, particularly in terms, not only of individual health status and health choices, but also potential lifestyle, and subjective perception of quality of life.

Studies have shown that the majority of older people can feel positively about their health, even if they have an illness or disability. Older people with physical problems may enjoy fulfilling mental activity, and vice versa. In one survey of older people, only 15% of respondents said they had no disease or disability, yet 75% of all respondents rated their health as good or excellent (Wade, 1993).

KEY AREAS FOR HEALTH PROMOTION

Nurses and health visitors have a key role in promoting health for older people, at all levels. Health promotion in a wide context could include social and political action as well as advocating for lifestyle changes. Measures to deal with poverty and cold-related illness, to reduce pollution, to improve housing and transport, and to combat ageism can make positive contributions to the health of older people. Health promotion in occupational settings can also contribute to a healthier older age through screening and health care for older workers, the maintenance of healthy work environments, and pre-retirement planning. There is also increasing emphasis on increasing the self-responsibility of older people in maintaining their health, such as in the UK Ageing Well initiative. The campaign 'aims to improve and maintain the health of older people recognising that they can be an important resource to themselves and others' (Ageing Well, 1996).

Lifestyle change

Much research demonstrates that the extent to which older people make positive lifestyle changes is dependent on their self-efficacy, the level of support they receive and the quality of health teaching (Allen, 1986; Brown and McCreedy, 1986; Shafer, 1989; Ebrahim and Williams, 1992; Gillis, 1993).

EXERCISE
Awareness is gradually growing of the significant role of exercise in the maintenance of physical and mental health, and functional ability at all ages (Edwards and Larson, 1992). There are also strong correlations between physical fitness and the retardation of cognitive change in old age (Rabbitt, 1988). Despite this, the participation of older people in exercise, and their physical fitness to do so, is below that required to ensure good functioning in daily life (National Fitness Survey, 1992). In fact 70% of men and 83% of women aged 50 and over do not participate in enough exercise to benefit their health (Health Education Authority, 1997).

NUTRITION
The principles of sound nutrition, such as eating a variety of foods from all sources, are consistent for older and younger people. However, because older people may eat less, it is important that their foods are rich in nutrients, or 'nutrient-dense'. Particular care is needed to ensure an adequate supply of calcium, iron, vitamins C and D, and fibre. Natural sources of fibre, such as fruit, vegetables and wholegrain cereals are preferable to raw bran which, in older people, can cause abdominal pain, and can also reduce the absorption of minerals such as iron and calcium (Holmes, 1994).

SENSORY FUNCTIONING
Nurses can help to promote sensory health by assisting an older person to arrange his/her living environment to maximum effect, with adequate levels of non-glare lighting, and appropriate positioning of objects, particularly for close work. Nurses can also check the older person's glasses or hearing aid, and should be able to give the address and telephone number of local opticians or hearing aid centres.

URINARY ELIMINATION
Nurses can promote health by recognising underlying problems (such as an infection), requesting appropriate diagnostic tests, rearranging the environment so that the older person can reach the lavatory quickly, advising on clothing that can be easily removed, offering health teaching (such as pelvic floor exercises), or referring for specialist advice and equipment.

BOWEL ELIMINATION
An adequate intake of natural dietary fibre can help to regulate bowel function. Exercise can help to strengthen muscles and stimulate peristalsis. Adequate fluid intake is also important, and the Nutrition Advisory Group for the Elderly (1992) advises at least eight full cups of liquid per day.

BREATHING
Upright posture and deep breathing can help to maintain respiratory functioning. Other measures include the avoiding of pulmonary irritants (such as cigarette smoke), exercising to maximum capacity, adequate fluid intake, influenza vaccinations and seeking medical advice for chest infections.

Health promotion in government target areas

Older people are explicitly excluded from many of the health gain targets of the four UK countries, due to the dearth of research on which targets could be formulated. However, the target areas are highly relevant to older people, as the following examples illustrate.

CORONARY HEART DISEASE AND STROKE

National health gain targets stress that adopting a healthy lifestyle, even in later life, is an important contributor towards the prevention of CHD and stroke. It emphasises that effective treatment and rehabilitation services are also vital for the health of older people. Studies have shown the benefits of controlling blood pressure at ages up to 80 years (Farnsworth and Heseltine, 1993). The link between cholesterol levels and CHD in older age is less clear (Manolio *et al.*, 1992) but the Medical Research Council (1994) suggests that, on current knowledge, 'a larger benefit from control of cholesterol might be expected in older compared with younger age groups'. Other factors which significantly link with CHD in people aged over 65 include male sex, diabetes, cigarette smoking, hypertension and left ventricular hypertrophy (Applegate *et al.*, 1991). Older people with CHD who abstain from smoking have improved outcomes, compared with those who do not (Hermanson, 1988). A reduction in smoking could also reduce morbidity from other diseases, such as respiratory disorders, for which it is a risk factor.

CANCER

Evidence suggests that screening women over 65 for breast and cervical cancer would improve survival rates and quality of life by the detection of invasive disease at an earlier stage when the prognosis following treatment is almost as good as at younger ages (Meanwell *et al.*, 1988). The efficacy of screening men for prostate cancer is currently the subject of debate.

SEXUAL HEALTH

The principles of safe sex are relevant for all age groups. Later life problems in sexual functioning may arise as a direct consequence of drug treatments. For example, some analgesics or antidepressants may reduce physiological arousal, whereas other drugs, such as levodopa, may increase arousal. Some anticholinergics, betablockers or diuretics can cause erectile dysfunction. Other drugs which cause problems include antihypertensives, sedatives, tranquillisers, sexual hormone preparations (such as stilboestrol), anticonvulsants and alcohol. Surgery, such as prostatectomy, radical pelvic surgery, aortoiliac surgery or sympathectomy, can also cause problems. If a person is sexually active, catheters or incontinence pads should be avoided, and specific treatments, such as lubricant gels, can help to alleviate vaginal dryness.

Nurses should try to be open-minded, nonjudgemental and sensitive in their approach to the whole area of sexuality and sexual health. Generational characteristics should be borne in mind, for example that sex was not generally discussed when older people were young. It may also be uncomfortable for an older person to seek advice, for example on safe sex, from a younger person.

ACCIDENTS

Improving environments and reducing hazards play a key role in reducing accidents. Most falls result from a combination of environmental hazards, physical disability, or risk-taking (Graham and Firth, 1992), but many falls could be prevented if contributory factors were removed. Assessment can identify environmental hazards (such as rugs, loose wiring or slippery surfaces), and physiological precursors (such as giddiness, 'legs giving way', stumbling or postural hypotension) (Downton, 1994). Reducing the risk of fractures by the preventing of osteoporosis could play a role. Chiropody and help/advice about suitable footwear can assist mobility.

Older people can and do want to learn more about their health (Pascucci, 1992), and health promotion can be effective even into advanced old age (Grimley Evans, 1994).

DYING AND BEREAVEMENT

Multiple loss is a prevalent theme in later life. Although retirement from paid employment may bring many benefits, it commonly results in reduced income, a change in identity, loss of the daily structure and reduced contact with people outside the home. If health deteriorates, this can lead to loss of independence and even loss of home and treasured possessions. Approximately 70% of deaths occur in the over 65 age group and, particularly if they had large families, older people can experience gradually diminishing social networks as they lose family members and contemporaries. The loss of a pet can also be significant (Lee, 1992). Multiple losses can cause 'bereavement overload' and this overwhelming grief can lead to a pervasive sense of helplessness, loneliness, disorientation and the risk of suicide.

The majority of research into grieving has taken place with younger people and Parkes (1988, page 46) suggests that 'there is reason to regard grief in old age as a rather different phenomenon from grief in young people'. Studies of older people experiencing bereavement have tended to concentrate on older women following the death of a spouse. Bowling and Cartwright (1982) found that the most frequent practical problems included adapting to living alone, coping with new household tasks and adjusting to lower income. Health problems were accentuated by loneliness and difficulties adjusting to altered status. There was reduced appetite, and increased anxiety, depression and sleeplessness. The risks of physical and emotional deterioration are high, particularly during the first year of bereavement, and especially for bereaved men (Herth, 1990). Although studies have focused on the first year after bereavement, there is strong indication that the bereavement period for older people often extends over several years (Herth, 1990).

Supportive networks, such as family, friends, clubs, or organisations such as CRUSE, are key in helping bereaved individuals to maintain self-esteem and a sense of hope for the future (Johnson *et al.*, 1986; Herth, 1990). Practical support to help the person adjust to new circumstances (such as handling money, using the telephone or using public transport) is important, as is health support provided by community nurses and general practitioners (Bowling and Cartwright, 1982).

Older people may also need special consideration as they approach death. The impact of advanced or terminal disease on an older person may be exacerbated by concurrent debilitating diseases, and the effects of bereavement exacerbated by other losses. There may be difficult ethical issues about active treatment in advanced disease in older people. Disease processes may not be as aggressive in older people, and palliative care or hospice services may not be geared to long-

term input. In addition, when there is pressure on these services, preference may be given to younger people, and it is not unknown for hospices to operate age-related admissions policies (Royal College of Nursing, 1994).

Nurses and health visitors have a key role in providing on-going support to older people who are bereaved or dying, and advocating for them to receive the services they need.

Key Points

- Older people are highly individual, but there are distinct and additional considerations when making a nursing assessment of an older person.
- To older people, how they function within their chosen lifestyles and towards the achievement of life goals will generally be more important than a specific medical diagnosis.
- Functional assessment should encompass not only physical, but social, psychological and emotional aspects.
- In older age, health goals may be related more to the quality of life than its prolongation.
- Nurses and health visitors have a key role in promoting health in older age. Health can be promoted at varying levels from public policy to individual lifestyle changes, and in various ways.
- Multiple loss is a prevalent theme in later life and older people need special consideration in terms of dying and bereavement support.

CONCLUSION

Older persons are highly individual and the only characteristic common to all older people is that they have lived for longer than younger people. Ageing is a continuous process and, because there are no particular points at which older age begins, terms such as 'the elderly' are unclear and unhelpful.

Current generations of older people have a diversity of life experience which encompasses some of the most profound social changes within any lifetime. Their lives and achievements are a cause for celebration. Their experiences have given them a richness of perspective on life, and sets of values, without which society would be impoverished. Their biographies can be used to enhance the nursing care offered, but to work effectively with older people requires not only a positive and caring attitude, but a sound knowledge of gerontological nursing, and high levels of skill. It requires that nurses be open, interested, flexible and creative. Nursing older people can be a fulfilling and life-enriching experience. The relationships formed can be rewarding, educational, and enjoyable for both the older person and the nurse. Older people constitute the majority of patients/clients in health and social care. It behoves us all to seek ways in which we can optimise the ways in which we work with them.

Reflection Point

If an understanding of older age or older people seems illusive, do not despair. We will learn best about older age when we become old ourselves. As Kierkegaard (1967) said 'life can only be understood backwards, but it must be lived forwards'.

Summary

This chapter has described various perspectives on ageing and older people, specifically how life experiences build into personal biographies, which act as 'filters' through which individuals view others. Some demographic characteristics of current older generations, including gender balance, ethnic mix, living conditions and economic circumstances, are offered, alongside a critique of common Western societal assumptions about health, ill health and dependency in older age. Key developments which influence nursing practice with older people and perceptions of the speciality are highlighted. The chapter discusses fundamental values and principles which can guide nurses working with older people and describes important principles for communicating and building relationships with them. It details the distinct and additional considerations for nurses when assessing older people, particularly when assessing an older person's functioning. It offers perspectives on the meaning of health in older age and describes the potential for nurses in key health promotion areas. Throughout, it emphasises the potential for the nursing of older people to be an enjoyable, enriching and life-enhancing experience.

REFERENCES

Aasen, N. (1982). Interventions to facilitate personal control. *Journal of Gerontological Nursing*, 13(6), 21–8.

Adams, J. (1991a). Human biography. Part (i): a personal approach. *Nursing Times*, 87(25), i–viii.

Adams, J. (1991b). Human biography. Part (ii): different lives, different perspectives. *Nursing Times*, 87(26), i–viii.

Ageing Well (1996). *The Ageing Well UK Programme: Guidelines for Partnership*. Age Concern England and the Health Education Authority, London.

Allen, J. (1986). New lives for old: lifestyle change initiatives among older adults. *Health Values*, 10(6), 8–18.

Applegate, W.B., Hughes, J.P. and Zwagg, R.V. (1991). Case-control study of coronary heart disease risk factors in the elderly. *Journal of Clinical Epidemiology*, 44, 409–15.

Baker, D. (1978). *Attitudes to Nurses to the Care of the Elderly*. Unpublished PhD Thesis, University of Manchester, Manchester.

Baltes, P.B. and Baltes, M.M. (1990). Psychological perspectives on successful ageing. In *Successful Ageing: Perspectives from the Behavioural Sciences*, Baltes, P.B. and Baltes, M.M. (eds). Cambridge University Press, New York.

Baltes, P.B. and Shaie, K.W. (1982). Ageing and IQ: the myth of the twilight years. In *Readings in Adult Psychology*, Allman, R.L. and Jaffe, D.T. (eds). Harper and Row, New York.

Barron, C.R., Foxall, M.J., Von Dolen, K. *et al.* (1994). Marital status, social support and loneliness in visually impaired elderly people. *Journal of Advanced Nursing*, 19, 272–80.

Bennett, G. (1990). Assessing abuse in the elderly. *Geriatric Medicine*, July, 49–51.

Berg, S., Mellstrom, D., Persson, G. and Swanorg, A. (1981). Loneliness in the Swedish aged. *Journal of Gerontology*, 36, 341–9.

Berger, K.S. (1994). *The Developing Person through the Lifespan*, 3rd edn. Worth Publishers, New York.

Bernard, M. and Meade, K. (eds) (1993). *Women Come of Age: Understanding the Lives of Older Women*. Edward Arnold, London.

Blackburn, J.A., Palalia-Finlay, D., Foye, B.F. and Serlin, R.C. (1988). Modifiaility of figural relations performance among elderly adults. *Journal of Gerontology*, 43, 87–9.

Bowling, A. and Cartwright, A. (1982). *Life After a Death: a Study of Elderly Widows*. Tavistock, London.

British Medical Association and Royal College of Nursing (1995). *The Older Person: Consent and Care*. British Medical Association, London.

Brouwer, A. (1990). The nature of ageing. In *Gerontology: Approaches to Biomedical and Clinical Research*, Horan, M.A. and Brouwer, A. (eds). Edward Arnold, London.

Brown, J.S. and McCreedy, M. (1986). The hale elderly: health and its correlates. *Research in Nursing and Health*, 9, 317–29.

Butler, R.A. (1963). The life review: an interpretation of reminiscence in the aged. *Psychiatry*, 26, 65–75.

Butler, R.A. (1984). Senile dementia: reversible and irreversible. *Counselling Psychologist*, 12(2), 75–9.

Butler, R.A. and Lewis, M.I. (1982). Cited in O'Leary, E. (1996). *Counselling Older Adults: Perspectives, Approaches and Research*. Chapman & Hall, London.

Bury, M. and Holme, A. (1991). *Life after Ninety*. Routledge, London.

Cameron, E., Badger, F. and Evers, H. (1989). District nursing, the disabled and the elderly: who are the black patients. *Journal of Advanced Nursing*, 14, 376–82.

Carer's National Association (1992). *Speak Up, Speak Out*. Carers National Association, London.

Central Statistical Office (1991). *Social Trends 21*. HMSO, London.

Coleman, P. (1993). Adjustment in later life. In *Ageing in Society: an Introduction to Social Gerontology*, 2nd edn, Bond, J., Coleman, P. and Pearce, S. (eds). Sage Publications, London.

Cumming, E. and Henry, W. (1961). *Growing Old: the Process of Disengagement*. Basic Books, New York.

Department of the Environment (1988). *English House Condition Survey 1986*. HMSO, London.

Department of Health (1992). The health of elderly people: an epidemiological overview. Central Health Monitoring Unit. *Epidemiological Overview Series*, Volume 1, HMSO, London.

Downton, J. (1994). Prevention of falls. *Care of the Elderly*, 6, 1.

Ebersole, P. and Hess, P. (1994). *Toward Healthy Ageing, Human Needs and Nursing Response*. Mosby, St Louis.

Ebrahim, S. and Williams, J. (1992). Assessing the effects of a health promotion programme for elderly people. *Journal of Public Health Medicine*, 14, 199–205.

Edwards, K.E. and Larson, E.B. (1992). Benefits of exercise for older adults. *Clinics in Geriatric Medicine*, 8, 35–50.

Erikson, E. (1950). *Childhood and Society*. Norton, New York.

Erikson, E.H., Erikson, J.M. and Knivick, H.Q. (1986). *Vital Involvement in Old Age*. Norton, New York.

Evandrou, M. and Falkingham, J. (1989). Benefit discrimination, *Community Care Supplement*, May 25, iii–iv.

Evers, H.K. (1981). Tender loving care? Patients and nurses in geriatric wards. In *Care of the Elderly*, Copp, L.A. (ed.) Churchill Livingstone, Edinburgh.

Evers, H.K. (1984). *Patients' Experiences and Social Relations in Geriatric Wards*. PhD thesis, University of Warwick, Warwick.

Falkingham, J. (1986). Dependency and ageing in Britain: a re-examination of the evidence. *Journal of Social Policy*, 18(2), 211–33.

Farnsworth, T. and Heseltine, D. (1993). Treatment of elderly hypertensives: some questions remain unanswered. *Age and Ageing*, 22, 1–4.

Fennell, G., Phillipson, C. and Evers, H. (1988). *The Sociology of Old Age*. Open University Press, Buckingham.

Fielding, P. (1986). *Attitudes Revisited*. Royal College of Nursing, London.

Garrett, G. (1983). *Health Needs of the Elderly*. The Macmillan Press Ltd, London.

Gillis, A.J. (1993). Determinants of a health promotion lifestyle: an integrative review. *Journal of Advanced Nursing*, 18(3), 345–53.

Graham, H.J. and Firth, J. (1992). Home accidents in older people: the role of the primary health care team. *British Medical Journal*, 305(30), 2.

Grimley Evans, J. (1994). Can we live to be a healthy hundred? *MRC Newsletter 64*, August. Medical Research Council, London.

Grimley, Evans, J., Goldacre, M.J., Jodkinson, M., Lamb, S. and Savory, M. (1992). *Health: Abilities and Wellbeing in the Third Age. The Carnegie Inquiry into the Third Age: Results Paper No. 9*. The Carnegie United Kingdom Trust, Dumfermline.

Grundy, E. (1994). Live old, live well. *MRC Newsletter 64*, August. Medical Research Council, London.

Gutemann, D.L. (1980). Psychoanalysis and ageing: a developmental view. In *The Course of Life: Psychoanalytic Contributions towards Understanding Personality*

Development. Vol III: Adulthood and the Ageing Process, Greenspan, S.I. and Pollock, G.H. (eds). US Department of Health and Human Science, Washington, DC.

Hasky, J. (1989). Families and households of the ethnic minority and white populations of Great Britain. *Population Trends*, 57, 8–19.

Hasky, J. (1995). The ethnic minority population of Great Britain: estimates by ethnic group and country of birth. *Population Trends*, 60, 35–8.

Havinghurst, R.J. (1952). *Developmental Tasks and Education*, 2nd edn. David McKay Co., New York.

Health Education Authority (1997). *Physical Activity in Later Life*. Health Education Authority, London.

Heath, H. (1993). *Solidarity between Generations: Older People and Young Nursing Students*. Paper presented at the Royal College of Nursing's 2nd Joint European Conference on Nursing Older People 'Positively Ageing: Reflections and Directions', Harrogate, Yorkshire, 5th November 1993.

Heath, H. (1997). Communicating with older people. *Nursing Standard*, 11(16), 48–56.

Help the Aged (1995). *Living Alone – Sharing Responsibility*. Help the Aged, London.

Hermanson, B. (1988). Benefit six year outcome of smoking cessation in older men and women with coronary heart disease. Results from the CASS Registry. *New England Journal of Medicine*, 9, 469–83.

Herth, K. (1990). Relationship of hope, coping styles, concurrent losses, and setting to grief resolution in the elderly widow(er). *Research in Nursing and Health*, 13, 109–17.

Hewison, A. (1995a). Power of language in a ward for the care of older people. *Nursing Times*, 91(21), 32–3.

Hewison, A. (1995b). Nurses' power in interactions with patients. *Journal of Advanced Nursing*, 21, 75–82.

Holmen, K., Ericsson, K., Andersson, L. and Winblad, B. (1992). Loneliness among elderly people living in Stockholm: a population study. *Journal of Advanced Nursing*, 17, 43–51.

Holmes, S. (1994). Nutrition and older people: a matter of concern. *Nursing Times*, 90(42), 31–3.

Hughes, B. (1995). *Older People and Community Care: Critical Theory and Practice*. Open University Press, Milton Keynes.

Hughes, B. and Mtezuka, E.M. (1992). Social work and older women. In *Women: Oppression and Social Work*, Langan, M. and Day, L. (eds). Routledge and Kegal Paul, London.

Hunt, A. (1978). *The Elderly at Home: a Study of People aged Sixty-five and Over Living in the Community in England*. Office of Population Censuses and Surveys, London.

Ingham, R. and Fielding, P. (1985). A review of nursing literature on attitudes towards old people. *International Journal of Nursing Studies*, 22(3), 171–81.

Institute of Actuaries (1993). *Financial Long-term Care in Great Britain*. Institute of Actuaries, Oxford.

Isaacs, B. (1981). Is geriatrics a speciality? In *Health Care of the Elderly*, Arie, T. (ed.). Croom Helm, London.

Johnson, M. (1985). That was your life: a biographical approach to later life. In *An Ageing Population*, Carver, V. and Liddiard, P. (eds). Open University, Milton Keynes.

Johnson, M.J. (1986). The meaning of old age. In *Nursing Elderly People*, Redfern, S. (ed.). Churchill Livingstone, Edinburgh.

Johnson, R.J., Lund, D.A. and Dimond, M.F. (1986). Stress, self-esteem and coping during bereavement among the elderly. *Social Psychology Quarterly*, 49(3), 273–9.

Jones, T. (1993). *Britain's Ethnic Minorities*, PSI Publishing, London.

Kane, R.L., Ouslander, J.G. and Abrass, I.B. (1994). *Essentials of Clinical Geriatrics*, 3rd edn. McGraw Hill, New York.

Kierkegaard (1967). Cited in Barber, P. (1993). Communicating for health. In *Nursing Practice and Health Care*, 2nd edn, Hinchliff, S.M., Norman, S.E. and Schober, J.E. (eds). Edward Arnold, London.

Kirkwood, T. (1994). The biological basis of ageing. *MRC Newsletter 64*, August. Medical Research Council, London.

Kitwood, T. (1993). Discover the person, not the disease. *Journal of Dementia Care*, 1(1), 16–7.

Koch, T., Webb, C. and Williams, A.M. (1995). Listening to the voices of older patients: an existential-phenomenological approach to quality assurance. *Journal of Clinical Nursing*, 4, 185–93.

Kuypers, J.A. and Bengston, V.L. (1984). Perspectives on the older family. In *Independent Ageing*, Quinn, W.H. and Hughston, G.A. (eds). Aspen Publications, Rockville, M.D.

Laing, W. and Hall, M. (1991). *The Challenges of Ageing: a Review of the Economic, Social and Medical Implications of an Ageing Population*. The Association of the British Pharmaceutical Industry, London.

Lanceley, A. (1985). Use of controlling language in the rehabilitation of the elderly. *Journal of Advanced Nursing*, 10, 125–35.

Lee, L. and Lee, M. (1992). *Absent Friend: Coping with the Loss of a Treasured Pet*. Heston Press.

McGlone, F. (1992). *Disability and Dependency in Old Age: a Demographic and Social Audit*. Family Policy Studies Centre, London.

Manolio, T.A., Pearson, T.A., Wenger, N.K. *et al.* (1992). Cholesterol and heart disease in older persons and women. Review of an NHLBI Workshop. *Annals of Epidemiology*, 2, 161–76.

Meanwell, C.A., Kelly, K.A., Wilson, S. *et al.* (1988). Young age as a prognostic factor in cervical cancer: analysis of population based data from 10,022 cases. *British Medical Journal*, 296, 386–91.

Medical Research Council (1994). *The Health of the UK's Elderly People*. Medical Research Council, London.

Moore, J.R. and Gilbert, D.A. (1995). Elderly residents: perceptions of nurses' comforting touch. *Journal of Gerontological Nursing*, 21(1), 6–13.

National Fitness Survey (1992). *The Allied Dunbar National Fitness Survey: a Report on Activity Patterns and Fitness Levels*. The Sports Council and Health Education Authority, London.

Nay, R. (1995). Nursing home residents' perceptions of relocation. *Journal of Clinical Nursing*, 4, 319–25.

Nolan, M. (1996). Developing a knowledge base in gerontological nursing: a critical appraisal. In *A Textbook of Gerontological Nursing: Perspectives on Practice*, Wade, L. and Walters, K. (eds). Baillière Tindall, London.

Norman, A. (1985). *Triple Jeopardy: Growing Old in a Second Homeland*. Centre for Policy on Ageing, London.

Norton, D., McLaren, R. and Exton-Smith, A.N. (1975). *An Investigation of Geriatric Nursing Problems in Hospital*, 2nd edn. Churchill Livingstone, London.

Nussbaum, J.F., Thompson, T. and Robinson, J.D. (1989). *Communication and Aging*. Harper and Row, New York.

Nutrition Advisory Group for the Elderly (1992). *Eating through the 90s*. NAGE, London.

OPCS (1980). *General Household Survey*. HMSO, London.

OPCS (1990). *General Household Survey*. HMSO, London.

OPCS (1993). *1991 Census: Persons aged 60 and over in Great Britain*. HMSO, London.

Parkes, C.M. (1986). *Bereavement: Studies of Grief in Adult Life*. Penguin Books, London.

Pascucci, M.A. (1992). Measuring incentives to health promotion in older adults. *Journal of Gerontological Nursing*, 18(2), 16–23.

Pearce, V. (1981). Sensory changes in old age. *Nursing*, 25, 1111–2.

Perks, D. (1984). Cited in Adams, J. (1991). Human biography II: different lives, different perspectives. *Nursing Times*, 87(26), i–viii.

Phillips, J. (1992). *Private Residential Care: the Admission Process and Reactions of the Public Sector*. Avebury Press, Aldershot, Hants.

Pursey, A. and Luker, K. (1995). Attitudes and stereotypes: nurses' work with older people. *Journal of Advanced Nursing*, 22, 547–55.

Rabbitt, P.M.A. (1984). Cited in Coleman, P. (1993). Adjustment in later life. In *Ageing in Society: an Introduction to Social Gerontology*, 2nd edn, Bond, J., Coleman, P. and Peace, S. (eds). Sage Publications, London.

Rabbitt, P.M.A. (1988). Social psychology, neuroscience and cognitive psychology need each other (and gerontology needs all three of them). *The Psychologist: Bulletin of the British Psychological Society*, 12, 500–6.

Reed, J. (1989). *All Dressed Up and Nowhere to Go: Nursing Assessment in Geriatric Care*. Unpublished PhD thesis, Newcastle Polytechnic, Newcastle upon Tyne.

Robertson, I. (1986). Learned helplessness. *Nursing Times*, 82(51), 28–30.

Rodin, J. (1989). Sense of control: potentials for intervention. *Annals of the American Academy of Political and Social Sciences*, (503), 29–42.

Rodin, J. and Langer, E.G. (1977). Longterm effects of a control-relevant intervention with the institutionalised aged. *Journal of Personality and Social Psychology*, 35(12), 897–902.

Royal College of Nursing (1994). *Older People and Nursing: Report of the RCN Task Force*. Royal College of Nursing, London.

Ryden, M.B. (1984). Morale and perceived control in institutionalised elderly. *Nursing Research*, 33(3), 130–6.

Schafer, S.L. (1989). An aggressive approach to health responsibility. *Journal of Gerontological Nursing*, 15(4), 22–7.

Schofield, I. (1994). A historical approach to care. *Elderly Care*, 6(6), 14–5.

Schultz, N.R. and Moore, D. (1984). Loneliness: correlates, attributions and coping among older adults. *Personality and Social Psychology Bulletin*, 10, 67–77.

Schultz, R. (1976). The effect of control and predictability on the psychological and physical wellbeing of the institutionalised aged. *Journal of Personality and Social Psychology*, 33, 563–73.

Seabrook, J. (1980). *The Way We Are*. Age Concern England, Hitcham, Surrey.

Seedhouse, D. (1986). *Health: the Foundations of Achievement*. John Wiley & Sons, Chichester.

Smith, P.A. (1992). *The Emotional Labour of Nursing*. Macmillan Education, Basingstoke.

Smythe, M. and Browne, F. (1992). *General Household Survey 1990*. HMSO, London.

Thomson, H. (1991). Attitudes to old people: a review. *Nursing Standard*, 5(30), 33–36, and 5(31), 33–5.

VanCott, M.L. (1993). Communicative competence during nursing admission interviews of elderly patients in acute care settings. *Qualitative Health Research*, 3(2), 184–208.

Victor, C.R. (1991). *Health and Health Care in Later Life*. Open University Press, Milton Keynes.

Wade, B. (1993). *The Changing Face of Community Care for Older People: Year 1: Setting the Scene*. Daphne Heale Research Unit, Royal College of Nursing, London.

Walker, A. (1981). Towards a political economy of old age. *Ageing in Society*, 1, 73–94.

Walker, A. (1990). Poverty and inequality in old age. In *Ageing in Society*, Bond, J. and Coleman, P. (eds). Sage Publications Ltd, London.

Warner, N. (1994). *Community Care: Just a Fairy Tale?* Carers National Association, London.

Warnes, A. and Law, C. (1985). Elderly population distributions and housing prospects in Britain. *Town Planning Review*, 56, 292–313.

Wells, T. (1980). Nurse/patient verbal communication in a geriatric ward. In *Problems in Geriatric Nursing Care*, Churchill Livingstone, Edinburgh.

Wenger, G.C. (1995). A comparison of urban with rural support networks; Liverpool and North Wales, *Ageing and Society* 15, 1.

Wenger, G.C. (1996). *Support Networks of Older People and the Demand for Community Care Services*. Centre for Social Policy Research and Development, University of Wales, Bangor.

Williams, E.I. and Wallace, P. (1993). Health checks for people aged 75 and over. *Occasional Paper 59*. Royal College of Practitioners, London.

Zusmann, J. (1966). Cited in Victor, C.R. (1989). *Old Age in Modern Society: a textbook of Social Gerontology*. Chapman & Hall, London.

FURTHER READING

Ebersole, P. and Hess, P. (1994). *Toward Healthy Ageing, Human Needs and Nursing Responses*, Mosby, St Louis.

A comprehensive text combining gerontological and nursing literature and dealing with some aspects not generally covered in nursing texts. Some information not relevant to the UK but the book is currently being revised for the UK market.

Ford, P. and Heath, H. (eds) (1996). *Older People and Nursing: Issues of Living in a Care Home*. Butterworth-Heinemann, Oxford.

Written specifically for nurses working in care homes but many aspects are more broadly relevant to the care of older people. Includes national frameworks and values, quality of life matters and selected clinical issues.

Phair, L. and Good, V. (1995). *Dementia: a Positive Approach*. Whurr, London.

A thought-provoking, practical and easy-to-use guide to working with people with dementia writtenb by a nurse and a social worker.

Redfern, S. (ed.) (1991). *Nursing Elderly People*. Churchill Livingstone, Edinburgh.

A comprehensive UK text covering aspects of ageing, health and social policy, and a broad range of clinical topics. Currently being revised.

Royal College of Nursing Booklets:

The Value and Skills of Nurses Working with Older People. 1993.
Guidelines for Assessing Mental Health Needs in Old Age. 1993.
Nursing Homes, Nursing Values. 1996.
How Nurses Can Help You: an RCN Guide for Older People and their Families. 1997.
What a Difference a Nurse Makes: Outcome Indicators for Nursing in the Continuing Care of Older People, 1998 (in press).

These succinct booklets are particularly useful in setting out the value of what nurses offer to older people. They are free of charge and available from the RCN in London (0171 409 3333).

Wade, L. and Walters, K. (eds) (1996). *A Textbook of Gerontological Nursing: Perspectives on Practice*. Baillière Tindall, London.

The first UK text heralding the progress and predicting the future of gerontological nursing. Selected aspects rather than a comprehensive text but important reading for gerontological nurses and students.

CHAPTER TWENTY-SEVEN

CARING FOR *the* DYING PATIENT – PRINCIPLES *of* PALLIATIVE CARE

Penny Smith

- Structure of services
- The team approach
- Philosophy of total pain
- The role of the nurse
- Nursing intervention in common symptoms
- Emotional care
- Spiritual care
- Cultural diversity
- Social needs
- Complementary therapies
- The last days of life
- Bereavement and the role of the nurse
- Evaluating care
- The cost of caring to the nurse
- Ethical issues
- Conclusion

This chapter aims to:

- Define the palliative care approach
- Discuss the structure of services within a rapidly changing health service
- Describe a philosophy of care, including the role of the nurse in physical, emotional and spiritual care.

Nursing the dying patient and his/her family will challenge the nurse at both a professional and personal level. The sure fact of life is our own death, which for most of us is a fearful prospect. As Woody Allen so famously said, 'I'm not afraid of death, I just don't want to be there when it happens'. Issues of death and dying are often not discussed with ease. It is therefore important that health professionals develop skills and strategies for caring for the dying patient and his/her family.

Palliative care is a recognised specialty and grew out of the modern hospice movement of the

1960s. The principles of the palliative care approach will be explained in this chapter. Although palliative care originally focused on patients with advanced cancer, the scope has now broadened. Palliative care is now offered to patients suffering from a wide range of life-threatening illnesses. Although much of the research conducted in palliative care relates to patients with cancer, the principles of patient-centred and family-centred care can be applied to people dying of non-malignant conditions. It is important the health professionals manage the care of the dying patient well. Giving appropriate care at this critical time will help the emotional health of the family, carers and friends.

Cancer remains a disease which causes death. It will account for the death of one in three people in the UK. Despite medical research only the haematological and childhood cancers have a significantly better outlook than 50 years ago.

The World Health Organization (WHO) has set out guiding principles. It states that palliative care:

- Affirms life and regards death as a normal process
- Neither hastens nor postpones death
- Provides relief from pain and other distressing symptoms
- Integrates the psychological and spiritual aspects of patient care
- Offers a support system to help patients live as actively as possible until death.

(WHO, 1990)

This palliative care approach described above offers a guiding principle for health professionals. Specialist palliative care will be needed by a proportion of those who are dying and is best provided by an expert multi-professional team. In the UK there are 223 hospice inpatient units (Hospice and Palliative Care Services, 1997) (Table 27.1).

Table 27.1: Inpatient care

Inpatient units	Units	Beds
Voluntary hospice units	147	2206
NHS managed units	50	557
Marie Curie Hospice Centres	11	291
Sue Ryder Homes	9	161
Total	217	3215

Source: Hospice Directory, 1997.

The WHO (1990) has defined palliative care as:

'The active, total care of patients whose disease no longer responds to curative treatment and for whom the goal must be the best quality of life for them and their families and carers. It focuses on controlling pain and other symptoms, easing suffering and enhancing the life that remains. It integrates the psychological and spiritual aspects of care, to enable patients to live out their lives with dignity as well as offering support to families both during the patient's illness and into bereavement.'

STRUCTURE OF SERVICES

INPATIENT CARE

Dame Cicely Saunders founded the first of the modern hospices at St Christopher's Hospice in Sydenham in 1967. It started as an inpatient unit but a home care service began some 2 years later. What differentiated this modern hospice from homes for people who were dying that had been in operation since the Middle Ages was that she aimed to 'combine scientific rigour with skilled compassionate care and education'.

COMMUNITY PALLIATIVE CARE TEAMS

Home care services began in the late 1960s and proliferated during the 1980s. There are around 400 teams in existence today. These teams are specially trained in advising on pain and symptom control and in giving emotional support to patients and their carers. They work with the primary health care teams and exist to augment care given and not to replace it.

MACMILLAN NURSES

Macmillan nurses account for a large part of the provision of palliative care at home. Introduced in 1976 by the charity Macmillan Cancer Relief they have funded over 1400 nursing posts. The funding for these posts is pump primed by the charity and at the end of 3 years becomes the responsibility of the health authority. Increasingly today, Macmillan nurses work in teams and are an important part of community palliative care.

MARIE CURIE NURSES

Marie Curie nurses are a practical nursing service founded in the 1950s. They also have charitable status and can provide 24-hour care for people dying at home.

DAY HOSPICES

Day hospices are currently a fast-growing part of palliative care provision. There are over 230 in operation, over two-thirds of which are attached to hospice inpatient units. Some are set up as socially led centres, bringing the patients away from the loneliness of their homes, giving them companionship and a programme of diversional activities. Other centres provide a directly therapeutic service following a medical model where all physical, emotional, social and spiritual needs are addressed within one environment.

HOSPITAL SUPPORT TEAMS

The other important area where palliative care teams exist is within the hospital setting. The majority of deaths from cancer and other non-malignant disease still occur in hospital. There are now about 275 such teams within the general hospital setting. They are usually small teams of nurses, a doctor and social worker who assess people with palliative care needs and give advice to the health professionals who have direct responsibility for their care.

STRATEGIC PLANNING ISSUES

Hospice and palliative care teams have mostly originated from the voluntary and charitable sectors. Until relatively recently, little thought has gone into strategic planning and communication and consultation with health authorities. The Community Care Act (Department of Health, 1990) which came into being in 1993 is doing much to change this. The English regional health

authorities now number only eight and decision making and resources lie with the local health authorities. The purchase of health care is now separated from the providers of health care, thus making the planning, evaluation and monitoring of services more effective.

The most recent reorganisation of cancer services in the Calman–Hine Report (Calman and Hine, 1996) is an attempt to provide services of equal quality nationwide. Cancer care will also be provided in cancer units where some district general hospitals will be designated to offer a wider range of services to people with cancer, such as day surgery, chemotherapy and outpatient services. There will also be large regional centres with surgical and radiotherapy facilities. The provision of palliative care will be an integral part of these units and centres. The report recommends that specialist palliative care teams should be multi-professional and pay particular attention to the psychosocial needs of the patient. It also identifies that palliative care needs to be offered at an earlier stage of a person's illness.

Care of people with advanced disease is now shifting to a community focus. General practitioners have greater purchasing power to support people and provide their care at home. Most patients' last year of life is spent at home although their death may occur in an inpatient setting.

The current changes in the health care system in the UK are an opportunity for palliative care services to be even more closely integrated with mainstream nursing and medical practice.

> **Key Points**
>
> - Palliative care and the modern hospice movement grew out of the voluntary sector.
> - Care of people with advanced disease is now shifting to a community focus.
> - Current changes in health care provide an opportunity for palliative care to be more closely integrated into main stream nursing.

THE TEAM APPROACH

Caring for people who are dying calls for far more skillls than one individual can command. The multi-professional team approach has already been developed in disciplines such as mental health and paediatrics. Nowhere is this approach more needed than in response to the expressed and perceived needs of dying people and their families. The team will involve the patient and family. Professionals who make up the teams will often consist of nurses, doctors, social workers, physiotherapists, occupational therapists, pharmacists and clergy.

If the patient is at home, the team is likely to consist of the district nurse, general practitioner, carers from the social services and the specialist palliative care team. Effective coordination of care is therefore crucial. Time spent in liaising with other professionals, agreeing a management plan and reviewing care is essential to coordinate activities to achieve good quality care. Teams that communicate well make better clinical decisions. In a multi-professional case discussion it can be the physiotherapist who only sees the patient weekly who is able to supply the missing information that is needed to inform a crucial clinical decision that is beneficial to the patient.

The need for multi-professional working in health care has been recognised at a high level. The National Association of Health Authority Trusts (1991) suggested that collaboration between professionals involved in health care provision is necessary in order to deliver a quality service.

Collaborative teamworking offers a safer approach to patients and families. For the individual professional it provides an opportunity for learning and self-appraisal. A team that works well provides a supportive environment for the professional and lessens stress. However, dysfunctional teams can be the most major source of stress (Vachon, 1995). It is important, therefore, to try to get it right. Teams that work well do not just happen. They are a result of good selection, leadership, agreed objectives for both the team and individual with the opportunity for regular review.

Taking the analogy of a football team who spend about 40 hours a week practising their teamwork for a 2-hour match, teams in organisations rarely spend 2 hours a year practising, when their ability to function as a team matters for 40 hours a week.

In order to function well, individuals need to be secure in their professional role. Stereotyping of other professionals is all too common. All team members need to feel they have the opportunity to influence a decision but different professionals have discrete areas of decision making and responsibility which must be respected. The process of consultation in decision making is time-consuming, but timely discussion and debate can avoid future conflict. As well as agreed leadership, key workers, structures and policies, teams have 'intangibles'. They demand trust, respect, honesty and occasional vulnerability from members.

Effective working in multi-professional teams is encouraging health care workers to move away from the paternalistic, autocratic medical approach. It is giving way to the right of the patient and family to make their own informed choices. Of course in an ideal world everyone ought to have the freedom to make their own decisions. This process can be reasonably straightforward to achieve for an articulate and well-informed patient and family, but more complex when caring for a confused, frail, inarticulate patient. Dying people are a vulnerable group and true autonomy must also imply a freedom not to be autonomous. A frail, dying patient may want the professional to make decisions regarding his/her care. The skill of the professional is to work sensitively, allowing the patient and family to participate as much or as little as they choose in decisions regarding care. In caring for dying people, health professionals must negotiate the difficult path of decision making, listening to the verbal and non-verbal communication of patients and families. Effective teamwork involves an equal partnership between professional carer, patients and their families.

> **Key Points**
> - Teams that work well are a result of careful selection, good leadership and agreed objectives.
> - Team members must respect the roles of others.
> - Teams need to share vulnerabilities as well as strengths.

PHILOSOPHY OF TOTAL PAIN

Teamwork is extremely important when trying to care for a family in pain. What follows has been built on Dame Cicely Saunders' model of 'Total Pain' (Saunders and Baines, 1995). The division of pain into three broad areas, physical, psychosocial and spiritual, may seem simplistic and artificial but it can be a useful way of attempting to analyse the different components in a patient and family who present with overwhelming distress. The pain the patient may describe may be the tip of the iceberg. Beneath the pain may be a range of factors and issues, physical, emotional, social and spiritual, all contributing to and entwined in the experience of pain. It is important, therefore, not to focus just on relieving physical pain.

PHYSICAL PAIN

The assessment and treatment of pain is covered in Chapter 15. It is important to remember the importance of assessment and evaluation of pain, looking for causal factors. Physical pain is present in 70% of people with advanced malignant disease (Twycross and Lack, 1990). The vast majority of pains can be controlled with analgesic drugs. The WHO (1996) has promoted the concept of an analgesic ladder for the management of cancer pain (Figure 27.1). Using this principle, non-opioids such as aspirin and paracetamol are used for mild pain.

If these are not adequate to control pain, then a drug of more potency in the form of a weak opioid, such as codeine, is used. If this is not strong enough, then a strong opioid such as morphine should be used. It is well recognised that at each stage it may be necessary to add in adjuvant medication. These are agents other than those classed as pure analgesics and when used appropriately will have useful analgesic effect.

Sadly, the reason why pain, even today, is not controlled is due to lack of understanding about the principles of pain relief. The appropriate strength analgesic should be used and given regularly before the pain returns. There remains unfounded fear about addiction. In cancer pain, morphine levels do not have a 'ceiling' but must be titrated against the level of pain the patient is experiencing. Addiction, an overpowering drive to take a drug for its psychological effects, does not appear to occur in patients taking opoids for cancer pain. Tolerance, the need to take a larger dose of the drug to achieve the same pharmacological effect, is also feared. In cancer pain an increase in dose may well be necessary, reflecting an increase in pain due to the the disease. This is not tolerance. Physical dependence may develop, but if pain control improves then it is possible to reduce the dose of morphine slowly without producing withdrawal symptoms.

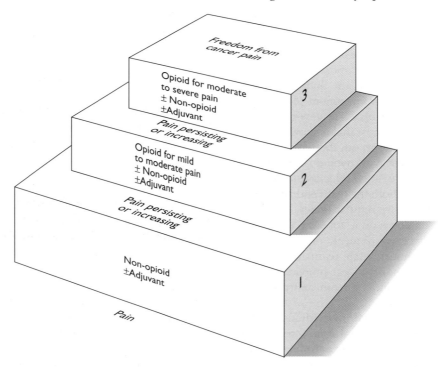

Figure 27.1: The WHO three-step analgesic ladder (reproduced with permission from WHO, 1996)

Morphine can cause constipation and so a laxative may be indicated. It can also cause nausea in about one-third of people and so initially an antiemetic may be needed. Other side-effects can be drowsiness and confusion. This usually lessens in a few days. Some patients complain of sweating and a dry mouth. Despite what may seem a disturbing list of possible side-effects, for the vast majority of patients the 'right' dose of morphine leaves them pain free, alert and comfortable.

Key Points: Pain control

- Establish the cause.
- Give appropriate treatment.
- Review.

THE ROLE OF THE NURSE

The role of the nurse is said to be central to the care of the dying patient and family, but it can be difficult to describe. Williams (1982) expounded the view that 'as the patient shifts from sick to dying role it is the nurse who assumes the dominant complementary role'. Williams differentiated between supportive and therapeutic roles. The therapeutic role is associated with active medical treatment and aimed at restoration of the patient to health, whereas the supportive role is that set of behaviours aimed at caring for the patient, supporting independent functioning and easing pain and discomfort. The supportive role prevails in the care of those who are dying and is primarily nursing's responsibility. A study by Davies and Oberle (1990) describes the clinical component of a supportive care nurse's role. A model of the supportive role was developed by them comprising six discrete but interwoven dimensions: valuing, connecting, empowering, doing for, finding meaning and preserving own dignity.

Practical nursing care is a skill delivered by the nurse alone amongst the professional carers. It requires attention to detail and the utmost sensitivity. Many dying people wish to remain independent for as long as possible. The nurse must judge carefully when more care is required and what aids to daily living are needed. The suggestion of a commode too soon, despite the patient's increasing weakness and frailty, can cause offence. Offering help at a time when the family carers are exhausted also requires sensitivity. Some family carers can feel usurped by a 'take-over bid by professionals', or can feel guilty if they have not followed through a promise to 'care until the end'. The nurse is in a key position to offer skilled supportive care to family carers. However, working in palliative care presents many complex situations and the nurse will need to be both flexible and creative in his/her approach.

It is important to have a knowledge of common symptoms, to understand the use of drugs to relieve these, and to know the side-effects of treatment. Such knowledge will help the nurse identify need and know when to call in medical help. The art of a skilled palliative care nurse is to know when to elicit the help of other professionals. Finlay (1991) described the symptoms that are commonly troublesome to the dying. Symptoms such as anorexia, sore and dry mouth and insomnia came top of the patient's list of concerns, most of which could be partially alleviated by nursing care outlined in a further section. The supportive role of the nurse will be more fully explained in the section on emotional and spiritual care.

Key Points

The nurse is in a key position to offer:

- Skilled supportive care to patients and families
- Sensitive nursing care enabling the patient to remain independent for as long as possible
- Reporting of presenting symptoms and monitoring of symptom control
- Coordination of care between the multi-professional team.

NURSING INTERVENTION IN COMMON SYMPTOMS

Understanding why a symptom has occurred is important, as it will guide the overall management. Cancers cause symptoms by direct or indirect pressure. The tumour mass can also cause metabolic effects, e.g. uraemia. Tumours themselves are sometimes metabolically active, secreting hormone-like substances such as parathormone, causing hypercalcaemia and cachexia, resulting in severe weight loss.

Symptoms can therefore be caused by the cancer itself, treatments both past and present and other concurrent illnesses. Achieving good symptom control requires a team approach. Discovering the cause of each symptom requires the best medical diagnostic skills and the most accurate nursing observations. The patient's experience of a symptom will be made worse by fear, worries and depression. The severity of the symptom is what the patient reports and not what the professional perceives. Some symptoms seem not to be taken seriously by professionals, e.g. itching, sweating, insomnia and dry mouth, when they may be more troublesome to the patient than pain or dyspnoea. If the professional continues to work with the patient with a positive attitude, attempting to alleviate the symptom, the patient will feel a greater degree of care and support.

In order for the nurse to manage the presenting symptoms, a detailed assessment will need to be made. This will include a detailed history of the symptom, finding out when it first occurred, how long it lasts, and whether anything makes it better or worse. The more information the nurse can obtain the easier it will be to find and treat the cause. There are some aspects of symptom control that will be directly helped by skilled nursing.

ANOREXIA

This is a common occurrence in people with advanced cancer. It is particularly distressing for carers who will have invested time and care into the preparation of food. Eating is one of the fundamental needs of the body associated with survival, well-being and even 'getting better'. An anorexic patient can cause a sense of helplessness in the carer. These feelings can be made worse by the emaciated appearance of some patients with advanced cancer, suggesting they are dying of starvation, a sign of extreme neglect. Metabolic studies have shown that there are several important differences between starvation and the cachexia of cancer (Giacosa et al., 1996). The changes that occur are not the result of the cancers using so much energy that the body starves; somehow they cause the metabolic systems to waste energy. There is no evidence that providing extra nutrition prolongs life. This is important information for the carer to understand as he/she is helped to adjust to the anorexic patient. The nurse

has a role in helping this adjustment process. Suggesting small, easy-to-swallow meals, served on a smaller plate, and attending to mouth care may be helpful. Sometimes a small amount of alcohol before meals may help to stimulate an appetite.

Many patients cannot tolerate feeling anorexic. They should be offered a trial of symptomatic treatments such as corticosteroids or progestogens to help increase their appetite. Many patients will tolerate nutrition in the form of food replacement drinks. It is possible to make some tempting cocktails out of these. The nurse would do well to liaise with a dietitian for ideas on the presentation of food supplements.

MOUTH CARE

Oral problems in advanced cancer can be divided into three categories: the disease process, treatments or medications and inadequate oral hygiene. The principal oral problems encountered in patients with advanced cancer are:

- Dirty mouth/coated tongue
- Dryness
- Infection
- Pain
- Halitosis
- Altered taste.

The nurse should assess the oral cavity. Loose-fitting dentures are a common problem. Regular oral hygiene twice a day should prevent most problems. A dirty mouth may need one of the following to help dissolve the coating:

- Sodium bicarbonate 2%, as a mouthwash
- Vitamin C, one-quarter of a gram of an effervescent tablet dissolved on the tongue four times a day.

The distress of a dry mouth can be helped with the stimulation of saliva flow by ice cubes, boiled lemon sweets or fresh pineapple chunks. Saliva-replacing sprays can be helpful.

Oral candida is a frequent problem for those with advanced cancer and should be treated with topical antifungals such as Nystan (nystatin) suspension 100 000 units/ml, 1–2 ml four times a day. This also comes in pastille form. Systemic antifungal medication may be necessary for some patients.

CONSTIPATION

Around 50% of people admitted to a hospice complain of constipation (Saunders and Sykes, 1993). Principal causes are the side-effect of medication such as morphine, decreased food intake and immobility. Advising a high fibre diet is usually inappropriate in palliative care. The nurse should foresee the need for laxatives and use them appropriately, provide privacy for defaecation and avoid, if possible, the use of bedpans. The patient should be encouraged to remain mobile for as long as possible.

Rectal measures, such as suppositories, only clear a few inches of bowel and should be used in conjunction with laxatives. Micralax enemas or glycerine and bisocodyl suppositories can help defaecation as can a phosphate enema. An arachis oil retention enema will help lubricate hard stools but the patient may well need a phosphate enema 12 hours later. Manual removal of faeces should be a last resort as it is extremely distressing. The patient should be offered analgesia and a muscle relaxant.

DYSPNOEA

The management of dyspnoea by non-pharmacological interventions has been researched by Corner *et al.* (1996) and shows a major role for nursing intervention. It is a symptom experienced by 30% of patients with cancer and 65% of patients with lung cancer. Their research is based on an intervention strategy. It includes counselling, breathing retraining, relaxation and the teaching of coping and adaptation strategies. It shows that this rehabilitative approach helps patients to increase their ability to function and to perform activities of daily living. These patients also experience significant reductions in the feeling of breathlessness. There are a range of pharmacological interventions that can also help to relieve breathlessness.

FUNGATING WOUNDS

A tumour fungating through the skin is a stark and visible sign of the presence of disease. The sight and smell of such lesions can have a deeply adverse psychological effect on patients and they require sensitive and skilled nursing care. The goals in nursing care differ from the goals in other wound care, as fungating lesions will not heal but will get progressively bigger as the tumour grows. The treatment aim is to contain the exudate, eradicate smell and achieve a dressing regimen that is cosmetically acceptable to the patient. Some dressings are not available in the community. This can be problematic for the patient being discharged from a hospital/hospic setting. Palliative radiotherapy may be effective in the management of fungating wounds as it can shrink the tumour and decrease the exudate.

Key Points

- Skilled nursing care can help to achieve better symtom control.
- Good symptom control requires accurate nursing observation combined with medical diagnostic skill.

EMOTIONAL CARE

'Cancer may not be catching but emotional pain is.'

(St Christopher's Hospice, 1992)

Terminal illness brings with it an enormous amount of loss. Some of the losses may include:

- Independence (holidays, trips out)
- Self-esteem (body image, appetite)
- Status and job
- Role and relationships
- Income
- A future.

These are enormous issues to adjust to. People with life-threatening disease may experience a variety of feelings and emotions that are in need of expression. Vachon (1988) identified considerable suffering directly resulting from poor communication and information from professional carers. A host of literature continues to show that professionals frequently communicate in an inadequate or misleading way. Health professionals working with those who are facing death have to confront their own personal fears and anxieties. They may worry about making the already bad situation worse, or precipitating an outburst of emotion, tears or anger by the patient and/or the family. They may have anxieties about not having the answers or about themselves identifying with the patient.

However, for those professionals working with dying people, these are anxieties that have to be faced. The nurse is not expected to be a professional counsellor but should be equipped with communication skills such as listening skills, and an ability to open up a conversation, helping the patient and family to express their feelings. The nurse should also be providing the patient and family with as much information as they request. The nurse should also recognise the limitations of his/her role and know when to seek more specialised help in the form of a counsellor or social worker, psychologist, psychotherapist or psychiatrist.

With regard to patients' insight into their illness, it is helpful for the nurse to ascertain the following:

- What does the patient understand about the illness?
- What else, if anything, does the patient want to know?

The medical profession are poor predictors of a patient's level of knowledge about a life-threatening illness. They often do not take into account the initial reaction of denial. This can be a healthy coping mechanism, enabling the patient to process information at his/her own rate. The important factor is that the patient is not left in isolation and further opportunities are given for information about the illness to be communicated. Some ways of beginning a conversation might be:

- What have the doctors told you about your illness? . . . What do you understand by that?
- How does that information make you feel?
- What do other family members know about your illness?
- What is the worst thing for you at the moment?
- What is worrying you most about your illness?
- Who is giving you most support?
- Who seems most affected by your illness?

It is appropriate to ask direct questions. They will not raise issues that the patient has not already thought of. Patients will soon make it clear if they do not want to take the question any further. They may do this by avoiding answering questions or by their body language. Such messages should be respected.

The impact of the news about a terminal illness will bring with it a host of strong and possibly unfamiliar emotions. The patient can feel out of control with a frightening mixture of confused emotions, including shock, denial, anxiety, anger, guilt and a deep sadness. The nurse needs to help the patient to understand that these feelings are normal, that talking through the worst fears will help regain some control and that living with uncertainty is always painful. A terminally ill patient will have a network of other relationships and it is important to see the patient within the context of these relationships. We will call them the family whether or not they are relatives. The impact of a terminal illness in a family can cause members to retreat into a conspiracy of fear and silence. Frightened people distance themselves from each other and become emotionally isolated just when they need most support and intimacy. Children in the family are often excluded from information in an effort to protect them, although they will sense something is seriously wrong and will often fantasise about their fears (Monroe, 1993). Ultimately, children cannot be protected from the truth; they have similar emotions and needs as adults and including them in the family's experience will help them to grieve and prepare them better for the death.

Meeting family members together with the patient can be enormously helpful. It is the task of the multi-professional team to determine which professionals should be present. For a family seeing professionals working together in this way models openness and gives the possibility for the truth about the illness to be shared. Gently breaking down the walls of isolation can help the family members find their own strengths and resources.

Key Points

- People with advanced disease will have strong and conflicting emotions.
- Encouraging expression of these emotions will help patients and families adjust to their situation.
- Meeting family members together can help to break down walls of isolation and help the family find their own strengths and resources.

SPIRITUAL CARE

Spirituality is addressed comprehensively in a Chapter 12. Spiritual care is much broader than religious issues. It is about our ultimate concerns, our search for meaning and values. It is often experienced in terms of relationships, possibly with God, but almost certainly with others and self. Religion, on the other hand, is the outward expression of a belief system. It is important to explore with the patient beyond the formal religious aspects. In a recent survey by the BBC (Coombe, 1996) it was shown that 70% of the population believed in a God concept, although only 12% practised organised religion.

Spiritual pain will not be a comfortable area for most health professionals to address as it usually means not having answers and challenges the professional's own belief system. The patient and family need the opportunity to examine the impact of the illness on their belief systems and they should be given the opportunity to ask the Why questions – Why me? Why now? What have I done to deserve this? Staying with this sort of spiritual pain and not being afraid of the questions is a helpful response from a nurse. Offering the support of the clergy or a relevant religious figure may be appropriate for some but not others. These deep questions should never be met with a trite response. Listening and being present is more appropriate and powerful in the face of the professional's powerlessness to understand and change the situation:

'Suffering is not so much a problem requiring an explanation as a mystery demanding a presence.'
(Unknown source)

Key Points
- Religion is the outward expression of a belief system.
- Spirituality is about ultimate concerns, a search for meaning and value.

CULTURAL DIVERSITY

We live in a rich multi-cultural society. Research has shown that there is unequal access to health services by black and ethnic minority groups (Hill,

1995) together with a lack of knowledge of services available. There is no evidence to suggest any difference in pattern for access to palliative care services. Culture is about our heritage, our inherited values and beliefs; it is about the way we live with our priorities and rituals. Religion and culture are often inextricably linked.

'One of the challenges of working with people from various cultural backgrounds is assessing where people are in their culture, i.e. which aspects of and to what extent their cultural background is important to them. Migration to a new country may have strengthened or diluted cultural practices and beliefs.'
(Olivier, 1993, page 204)

For health professionals working with those who are dying this represents a major challenge. Consider some of the areas of culture to which health professionals need to give thought.

Health professionals can be bound into practicalities, like issues of care and diet. These are important but if deeper issues are not further explored the service offered may fall short of meeting the needs of the patient and family.

An important question to be asked is 'How do I know that my practice is anti-discriminatory?' Making nursing practice relevant to people of many cultures is a constant challenge to the nurse. Reflection and review of care in these areas can be helpful in developing relevant nursing practice.

Key Points
Cultural diversity may relate to:
- The meaning of the illness
- Attitude to pain and symptoms and to medication
- Ways of coping with the illness
- Attitude to place of care, physical and emotional care
- Roles in the family
- Rituals around death, the funeral and bereavement.

SOCIAL NEEDS

The nurse is in a position to ensure that patients and families have adequate information regarding the benefits to which they may be entitled.

Disability living allowance (DLA)

If the patient is under 65 and needs help with personal care (i.e. help with washing, dressing, etc.) or getting around, he/she could be entitled to DLA, a tax free benefit.

To get DLA the patient must normally have needed help for 3 months and must be likely to need help for a further 6 months or more. But there are special rules for people who have an uncertain future because of their illness. These people do not have to wait to claim. Most people newly referred for hospice care, whether as an outpatient or an inpatient, will normally have an automatic right to claim DLA.

Attendance allowance

If the patient is over 65 and has an expected prognosis of less than 6 months, he/she will normally have an automatic right to claim the attendance allowance even if at the time of the claim he/she does not need nursing-type help from another person. Attendance allowance is tax free and does not affect any other income.

Both the disability living allowance and the attendance allowance can be claimed for the patient with his/her permission. The patient's doctor will need to complete one part of the form (DS1500) and the nurse can complete the rest.

Free prescriptions

If the patient is already claiming income support or family credit, or if he/she is aged over 60, he/she can get free prescriptions by ticking the appropriate box on the back of the prescription form. Alternatively, the patient can buy a pre-payment certificate which would save money. Pre-payment forms (FP95) are available from post offices, health authorities, benefit agencies and most pharmacists. However, there is also a further category whereby if a patient is unable to leave home without the assistance of another person, then he/she may also obtain free prescriptions. Form FP92a, together with booklet HC11 'Are you entitled to help with health costs?', which gives details of other exemptions, is available to the public through the same outlets as the pre-payment forms.

The following are other benefits to which patients may be entitled.

Housing benefit

If the patient is finding it hard to pay the rent, then he/she may apply for housing benefit. The housing officer or local council offices will be able to send the relevant application form. People can apply for housing benefit if they are working, if they are on benefit, or if they are in receipt of a pension.

Income support

If the patient has a low income, then it is always worth checking to see if he/she might qualify for income support. It is paid to top-up other benefits, or earnings from part-time work. It is not dependent on National Insurance contributions. Getting income support may also entitle the patient to other types of help, such as free prescriptions and dental treatment, housing renovation grants and help from the social fund.

Other payments

There are other payments from the Department of Social Security to which people may be entitled, i.e. community care grants/budgeting loans/crisis loans. Further information may be obtained from the local DSS office.

Council tax

If the patient is living permanently in a hospital/hospice/nursing home/residential home/ private hospital or hostel and receiving care/ treatment there, and has no other home, the he/she does not have to pay council tax. 100% Council tax benefit will be payable to people on income support, or those whose incomes are below income support level.

Who else can help?

If the patient is on a low income, some charities can help with the extra expenses in the household.

However, this will depend on how much money the patient has. Macmillan Cancer Relief gives grants to patients on low incomes who are terminally ill. Application for these grants can only be made through a health care professional and has to be supported by a medical certificate from the patient's GP or hospital doctor. These grants are available for many purposes, including clothing, furnishing, heating, holidays, nursing, telephones and travel expenses.

Finally, when people are terminally ill they may not have anyone who can collect their benefits, pay their bills and so on, and this can be a great worry to them. A relative, friend or solicitor can be given their Power of Attorney (the legal right to act on someone's behalf) or someone can become their 'appointee' in order that he/she can do these things for the patient. The patient may also find that he/she has wishes that can only be carried out properly if a Will has been drawn up. If the patient wishes to discuss these matters further, he/she should make contact with a local solicitor, or contact the social work department based at their hospital.

Key Points

The current key benefits available to people who are terminally ill are:

- Disability living allowance
- Attendance allowance
- Free prescriptions
- Crisis loans
- Grants for people on low incomes.

COMPLEMENTARY THERAPIES

Therapies complementary to orthodox medicine are becoming increasingly popular for people with cancer and therapies such as acupuncture, aromatherapy and reflexology have in some places been incorporated within National Health Service care. Perhaps their popularity is in part due to the failure of orthodox medicine to cure disease and to the increased time spent on a one-to-one basis with the therapist.

Research into the effect of many of the therapies is limited, although there is the Research Council for Complementary Medicine, which is a central body for registering research and which

has a database of current and completed studies. There are, however, some demonstrable advantages to some complementary therapies, such as helping patients take some positive control back when the situation feels out of control and chaotic. The patient will receive time, attention and skilled listening from the therapist. When orthodox medicine has reached its limits in terms of a possible cure, complementary therapies can have positive psychological effects. They are generally safe, and free from the side-effects of orthodox anti-cancer treatments.

Nurses who wish to practise complementary therapies as part of their professional role need to have done a recognised course or a period of study, and practise in full recognition of the United Kingdom Central Council's code of conduct (UKCC, 1992, Clause four). This states that the trained nurse must 'acknowledge her limitations in her knowledge and competence and decline any duties or responsibilities unless able to perform them in a safe and skilled manner'.

Key Points

Therapies most widely used in palliative care are:

- Aromatherapy
- Massage
- Reflexology
- Acupuncture.

THE LAST DAYS OF LIFE

Given the choice, most people would prefer to die at home (Townsend, 1990). However, only about 25% of people in the UK do so. As the illness progresses and families become more exhausted, another 30% change their minds, as shown in the study by Hinton (1994). He showed that for those patients who changed their minds their families made the same decision a week earlier. There is no 'right' place to die: it is where the patient and family choose. It is the nurse's responsibility to plan care effectively, whatever the setting. If it is in the community, then the resources required will need to be mobilised quickly and efficiently. A package of care is often needed involving:

- The district nurse
- The GP

- Social services
- The specialist palliative care team
- The Marie Curie nursing service.

As the patient becomes gradually weaker he/she will become more dependent on those around him/her to meet his/her physical needs. Maintaining comfort is paramount. As the weakness progresses, the last few days of life are likely to be spent in bed. Some patients remain mentally alert throughout whilst others may become confused. This can be due to biochemical changes or toxicity from infection. Anxieties and fear may need to be expressed and the nurse must listen actively to these. Some people fear terrible pain or dying in a dramatic fashion and the nurse can do much to reassure and comfort the patient on these issues. A few patients find the last days intolerable and it is compassionate for the medical and nursing team to offer medication that will sedate the patient. This decision is always a difficult one and if sedation is needed, it is usually for severe emotional anguish in the last days or hours of life. If this situation arises, it is important to discuss the issues fully with the family. The more normal process of death from advanced cancer is for the patient to become increasingly sleepy and to begin to lose interest in his/her surroundings. This sleepiness merges into drowsiness and unconsciousness. During this time the patient may develop noisy breathing due to increased secretions in the lungs and larynx. Suction is mostly inappropriate at this time and medication in the form of hyoscine hydrobromide or hyoscine butylbromide (the former also has sedative properties) may be needed in an attempt to dry up the secretions. 'Cheyne–Stokes' breathing may occur. These are respirations that involve a period of apnoea followed by more respirations which are repeated in a cycle until breathing ceases, the heart stops and death has occurred. The nurse has an important role in caring for both the patient and family around the last days and hours.

Questions commonly asked by families of dying patients and suggestions for responding

(For the purpose of this section, the male gender is being used as an example.)

He can no longer move himself. Will he get a pressure sore?

It is important that we change his position regularly from side to side. This is the best way of relieving pressure. Sometimes though, the skin is so fragile that it is not possible to prevent a pressure sore. If the skin begins to look red we will put a protective dressing on his hips and bony points. We will also gently exercise and massage his limbs when we turn him.

Will he need to eat now he is unconscious?

No. The body does not need food now. It will not prolong his life or make him any stronger.

What about drinking – does he need a drip?

No. There is no evidence that this prolongs life either. In fact, it could make him more uncomfortable as it can lead to increased urine output and increased secretions from his lungs. We will keep his mouth comfortable with mouth care.

Will he still need to go to the toilet?

He will probably not need to have his bowels open. He will continue to pass some urine. We will ensure his skin and bedclothes are protected. If this becomes a problem we would suggest using a catheter or a conveen. A conveen is a small tube with a rubber sheath that sits over the penis. A catheter is a small tube that is inserted into the bladder and collects the urine in a bag. Neither of these will be painful to him.

Will he need his tablets?

Most of his medicine can be stopped, but we will continue with his pain relief and his anti-sickness medicine. He may also need another medicine to dry up the secretions in his chest. We will need to give the medicine another way now. We will either give it via the 'back passage' (rectally) in the form of a suppository, or under the skin (subcutaneously) using a syringe driver. This is a syringe with a tube and small needle that is attached to a battery pump. It can deliver medicine over a 24-hour period. It does not hurt.

Will he get more pain?

No, he should not get more pain. If he does seem uncomfortable there is more analgesic medicine he can have. If he becomes restless he may need a small amount of a sedative medicine to keep him comfortable.

Can he hear me?

Hearing is thought to be one of the last senses to disappear. It is important that you continue to talk to him. There may be some important things you need to say. He still needs contact with you. Do you feel able to hold his hand and cuddle him?

Why is his breathing noisy?

It is due to the secretions in the back of his throat and lungs. He is unconscious and it will not be troubling him. It is much more traumatic for you to listen to. We will change his position to see if that helps. Suction does not usually help at this time. We can also give him some medicine called hyoscine to help dry up the secretions.

Will I know when he is dead?

Yes. His colour may change. His skin may look very pale or slightly tinged with blue on his face and hands. He will stop breathing and will not have a pulse. His eyes may be open and look glazed. His jaw may drop open. As the muscles relax at the point of death he may be incontinent of urine and faeces. Shortly after death his body will start to become cold.

I want to be with him, is that possible?

You should spend as much time with him as you want. No-one can predict the exact moment of death. Sometimes there is a little bit of warning. His breathing may change and he may have a long gap between breaths. At some point his breathing will stop. It usually happens so quietly that you will almost not have noticed it has happened. Be prepared, though, for the fact that he may die just when you have gone to the bathroom. It is not possible to predict the exact moment of death. If that happens it is important that you are gentle with yourself, and do not blame yourself.

WHAT TO DO AFTER THE PATIENT DIES

As soon as the patient has died the family should be able to spend as much time with the dead person as they want. There is no hurry. The hospital doctor or GP will need to be called to certify the death. It is helpful if the nurse shuts the patient's eyes and straightens his limbs. People will say their farewell in their own way. There is no need for children to be excluded from this time. If the patient dies at home the undertaker cannot remove the body until the death has been certified. Most undertakers operate a 24-hour service. However, there is no need to call them imme-

diately if the family are comfortable to keep the body in their home until the morning. In a hospital, hospice or nursing home the nurse will need to inform surrounding patients/residents of the death. If the patient has not been seen by a doctor within 14 days of the death, a post-mortem examination will be needed.

The final washing of the body (known as last offices) is usually performed by the nurse after the death. It is important for the nurse to know in advance the cultural values and religious beliefs of the family as it may not be acceptable for the nurse to carry out this task. Sometimes a relative will want to help. The body is washed and dressed in nightwear, a shroud or some other garments selected by the family. Catheters and other appliances should be removed and any dentures replaced. Orifices that are leaking fluid should be packed with gauze. The nurse should ask relatives whether jewellery should be left on or taken off the body. If the death has occurred in an institution, the body will need to be labelled and the property identified and stored.

The police will need to be informed only if the death was violent, accidental or suspicious. The coroner will arrange for a post-mortem examination to establish the cause of death. The coroner's inquest is an inquiry into the medical cause of death.

REGISTRATION OF DEATH

Once the death certificate has been issued the death must be registered within 5 days at the registrar's office in the district in which the death took place. It must be registered by the next of kin, a relative or the executor of the dead person's estate. It may also be registered by anyone who was present at the death or who is arranging the funeral. The person registering the death will be issued with a certificate of disposal to be given to the funeral director and a certificate of registration of death for social security purposes only. Extra copies of the death certificate can be issued at a small cost and may be needed for insurance purposes.

ORGAN DONATION

In many cases it is possible to transplant some organs of the dead person for the benefit of another person, provided there is no objection by the relative or next of kin. In patients with terminal cancer the corneas may be used. In patients under the age of 5 with a primary brain tumour the kidneys and heart valves may be used. Transplant coordinators are available to give nurses and relatives information, advice and support on these issues. Relatives often find comfort in the knowledge that someone else is benefiting from the death of their loved one. Nurses should not be afraid to ask as the relatives will make it immediately clear if they are not comfortable with this procedure.

FUNERAL ARRANGEMENTS

There is a national association of funeral directors who work to an agreed code of practice and it is advisable that people choose a funeral director who is registered. The relative has the choice of burial or cremation. Cremation forms need to be completed by two doctors. The will, where there is one, may contain instructions regarding the funeral although these are not binding. Families will need guiding through what to do after a death. For patients who die in a hospital, hospice or nursing home setting it is helpful for the nurse to invite the family to meet together with the nurse the following day. The family then have an opportunity to reflect on the illness and death, to ask questions and to receive practical instructions on what to do next. If the deceased person is still in the institution, they can be given the opportunity to view the body. It can be helpful for the community nurse to visit the following day, if the patient has died at home, for the same process to occur. It also gives the nurse a chance to say goodbye to the family. Families will also be able to view the body at the funeral directors.

Key Points

- The right place to die is where the patient and family choose.
- Clear explanations on the process of dying will support the family and help enable them to cope.

BEREAVEMENT AND THE ROLE OF THE NURSE

A nurse working with those who are dying needs to have an understanding of bereavement and how to recognise abnormal grief and to refer for more specialist help. Most of the country is now served by local bereavement services or national ones such as Cruse (see Useful Addresses at end of chapter).

Grief is not an illness. It is a recognised pattern of reactions that take place while the person adjusts to the death of their loved one. As Judy Tatelbaum (1980, page 7) says:

> 'The loss of a loved one throws every aspect of our lives out of balance. . . . It takes courage to grieve, to feel our pain and to face the unfamiliar. Grief experienced does dissolve. Unexpressed grief is like a powder keg waiting to be ignited.'

A helpful model for grief has been developed by William Worden (1991). He talks of four tasks of mourning which must be completed before equilibrium can be re-established. There is no linear pattern to grief and no defined time period for it to occur. Few are prepared for how long it goes on and how draining and exhausting it is. It begins at the moment that the relative knows his or her loved one is unlikely to recover, known as anticipatory grief.

In Worden's model the person first has to accept the reality of the loss. Then they need to experience all the painful feelings and emotion. This could involve despair, sadness, helplessness, loneliness, confusion, restlessness, depression, pining, denial, anger and guilt. Physical manifestations could include crying, sleep and appetite disturbance, pain, dreams, hallucinations, searching and calling out for the dead person. Some people feel they are going mad, and experience a frightening loss of control.

Next they must adjust to an environment in which the deceased is missing. This will involve taking on new roles and learning new skills. Finally, they must reinvest their emotional energy. This will involve re-establishing relationships and investing their emotion in living. Sometimes people need permisson for this as they can feel guilty and disloyal to the dead person.

THE ROLE OF THE NURSE IN BEREAVEMENT

The nurse is not expected to be a bereavement counsellor. The role of the nurse working in an institutional setting will primarily be before the patient has died. The nurse working in the community setting will care for people who are dying and also have the opportunity to offer support to relatives in bereavement. Research has shown that a well-managed death will help with the emotional health of a family. For the nurse in the community a single visit some weeks after death can be very helpful. It is difficult to asses how well the bereaved person will recover initially; this may depend on the support available at this time from family and friends. People who are bereaved need to be heard and understood. The presence of a nurse on a single visit implies concern and care. The acknowledgement of their pain and sorrow may help them move forwards.

The nurse needs a clear structure for the visit. This will help him/her be more focused, as the visit is not primarily social. In the visit the nurse can:

- Encourage and answer questions about the illness and death
- Encourage the expression of feelings through the telling of their story
- Assess the risk of abnormal grief and refer on
- Say goodbye.

The visit should not last more than about an hour. Making good eye contact and asking a series of direct questions is important. The following are guidelines for the visit:

- How are you yourself?
- How has it been since . . . ?
- Talk about the dead person in the past tense.
- What is the worst thing for you at the moment?
- Begin the flow of memories by sharing a personal memory of the dead person.
- How are you sleeping, eating?
- Where is your support coming from?
- Emphasise that grief is different for everyone.
- Recognise the family's role and achievements in the dead person's care.
- Acknowledge past losses and their re-awakened power to hurt.
- Help him/her consider the impact of the loss on important others especially children.

- Provide an opportunity for the relatives to say thank you and goodbye.
- Do not leave people with false hopes about seeing you again by saying, 'I'll pop in if I'm passing'. Make an ending.
- Leave written literature where appropriate about grief and information about further help.

RECOGNISING ABNORMAL GRIEF

- Are grief reactions prolonged, excessive and seeming incapable of resolution?
- Are grief reactions absent?
- Has grief been displaced or masked, e.g. by illness, drugs, alcohol or overwork?
- Was the relationship with the deceased person particularly ambivalent or dependent? Were the circumstances of the death unexpected or violent?

BEREAVED CHILDREN

Parents need to know that children grieve in similar ways to adults and need help and opportunities to express their feelings. They may, however, express their grief through their behaviour, e.g. sleep disturbance, clinging or bed wetting. Ideally, they need preparation before death and the opportunities to ask questions. Children do not need protecting from their sadness but need supporting in it. The nurse has a role in talking with parents about the grief their children will be facing. Parents need support in helping their children, as it is a difficult task and they may meet opposition from other friends and family.

Key Points

- The emotional health of the family will be helped by a well-managed death.
- A community nurse making a single structured bereavement visit can have a positive impact on the loss.
- A nurse needs to recognise abnormal grief and refer on.
- Children also need bereavement care.

EVALUATING CARE

Improving the quality of care is an objective of most palliative care professionals. Evidence suggests that palliative care practice varies between professionals. There is a need to know which models of care are most effective and which interventions work best. Audit of palliative care enables practitioners to identify problems in practice and set action plans to improve specific palliative care.

There are a number of tools and standards that practitioners can use to review and refresh their practice. For example:

- Symptom assessment schedule (Higginson, 1993)
- Edmonton symptom assessment schedule (Bruera *et al.*, 1991)
- Standards of palliative nursing (RCN, 1993).

Audit can also be useful for education and training as structured review allows analysis, comparison and evaluation of performance.

Key Point

- The multi-professional team need to agree a set of standards and choose the most appropriate tool for their organisation and practice.

THE COST OF CARING TO THE NURSE

Working closely with people who are dying can make the nurse aware of her own losses. Connecting with people in emotional distress can be painful. Nurses need adequate support systems in both their profesional and personal lives (see Chapter 14).

All professionals have different strategies for looking after themselves. The individual nurse should be familiar with signs of personal stress. The spacing of holidays and time off is important as is training and education. This can be stimulating and recharge lost energy. If an interaction with a patient and family has been stressful, it will be helpful to take time to debrief with a colleague. If a situation is likely to be difficult and stressful, it may be helpful to rehearse it with a colleague first.

It is helpful to take a few moments after a stressful situation to organise in your mind what rightly belongs to you and what rightly should be left to the patient and family. Thorough, concise written recording can be therapeutic and help the 'letting go' of the situation.

It is important to remember that nurses are professional health care workers offering skilled compassionate care. They are not family friends and should not behave as such. It is realistic that at times the nurse may connect closely with a patient or family. If this is the case, it is important that the nurse feels safe within the team to share feelings and gain support from colleagues.

The team can provide the most supportive environment, but it can also lead to stress. If any team member attempts to become heroic, it will be harmful to teamworking. Being honest and sharing vulnerabilities will help a team relate and work well together. If difficult conversations are anticipated, they are best conducted face to face. Some differences of opinion will need to be addressed and others relinquished. It is sometimes necessary to lose the battle in order to win the war.

Key Point

- The nurse needs to recognise internal signs of stress and develop strategies for coping.

ETHICAL ISSUES

In palliative care there are a number of difficult ethical dilemmas to be faced. Of course, respect for the choice of the individual should be paramount but this is not always straightforward as those who are dying are often frail and vulnerable. A sense of justice, fairness and kindness should be the guiding principles in difficult decisions.

Euthanasia, the active intentional killing of another, is illegal in the UK. The patient does not have the ultimate authority in this matter except in suicide, which was decriminalised in 1961. The patient who asks to be killed needs to be listened to and understood. As well as inadequately controlled symptoms there can often be deep emotional anguish behind such a request. The professional team need to be consistent and persistent in their attempts to relieve the patient's suffering. It is often difficult for families and carers to cope with the complex feelings aroused in them when a relative requests to be killed. Fortunately, patients dying of advanced cancer rarely continue to request euthanasia once adequate physical and psychological care is given. However, a few people persist in a rational request to die with help from the medical team. In such circumstances adequate time for debriefing and personal support is vital. This process will help professionals stay with the patient and family in their distress.

The ethical issues in palliative care are often based around selective non-treatment decisions. An example of this would be the decision not to give antibiotics to a terminally ill patient with pneumonia or a blood transfusion to a dying person who is bleeding. A patient has the right to refuse treatment as long as he/she is lucid and capable of understanding the decision (see Chapter 13 for further discussion on ethics, morality and nursing).

ADVANCE DIRECTIVES/LIVING WILLS

These are not legal documents. They are a set of directives that inform the medical profession of the health care a person would like to receive should he/she become incompetent and unable to make the decision. These directives usually contain an explanation of the circumstances in which the individual would like treatment withheld and desire not to be resuscitated.

> **Key Points**
> - Palliative care will involve difficult ethical issues. Euthanasia, the active intentional killing of a patient, is not legal in the UK.
> - Advance directives are written to inform the medical profession of the wishes of a patient should he/she become incompetent.

CONCLUSION

Care of the dying patient and family has been revolutionised in Britain in the last 30 years. As this specialist field of health care moves towards the twenty-first century, there remain many more challenges for health professionals. Research is needed into a variety of physical, psychosocial and spiritual issues. The services developed must be culturally sensitive and accessible to prospective users. The philosophy of the palliative care approach is transferable to patients dying of conditions other than cancer. Services must continue to be developed in the home setting in line with the choices of patients and families. Teaching and education to all levels of health professionals must continue to expand. Nurses are now able to undertake study in palliative care at diploma and degree level and multi-professional Masters programmes are being developed. Most important is a continuing dialogue between specialist palliative care services and commissioning authorities in order to ensure further integration of palliative care into mainstream health care.

The role of the nurse is central to the care of the dying patient. Helping a patient and family at this critical time in their lives can be very rewarding. The nurse often plays a key part in coordinating care and it is vital that the nurse develops palliative nursing skills in order to carry out this role effectively and enable the patient and family to find their own strengths and resources.

ACKNOWLEDGEMENT

The author would like to thank Barbara Monroe, Director of Social Work, St Christopher Hospice, for her material incorporated into the section on psychosocial and bereavement care.

USEFUL ADDRESSES

ACET (AIDS Education and Training)
PO Box 3693
London SW15 2BQ
Tel. 0181 780 0400

Age Concern
Astral House
1268 London Road
London SW16 4ER
Tel. 0181 679 8000

Breast Care and Mastectomy Association of Great Britain
26a Harrison Street
Kings Cross
London WC1H 8JG
Tel. 0171 837 0908

British Association for Counselling
1 Regent Place
Rugby
Warwickshire CV21 2PJ
Tel. 01788 578328

British Colostomy Association
38–39 Eccleston Square
London SW1V 1PB
Tel. 0171 828 5175

CancerBACUP
3 Bath Place
Rivington Street
London EC2A 3JR
Tel. 0171 608 1661
Tel. 0800 181199 (outside London)

CancerLink
17 Britannia Street
London WC1X 9JN
Tel. 0171 351 7811

Cruse Bereavement Care
Cruse House
126 Sheen Road
Richmond
Surrey TW9 1LF
Tel. 0181 940 4818

Hospice Information Service
St Christopher's Hospice
51–59 Lawrie Park Road
Sydenham SE26 6DZ
Tel. 0181 778 9252

Leukaemia Care Society
PO Box 82
Exeter
Devon EX2 5DP
Tel. 01392 218514

Macmillan Cancer Relief
Anchor House
15/19 Britten Street
London SW3 3TZ
Tel. 0171 351 7811

Marie Curie Cancer Care
28 Belgrave Square
London SW1X 8QG
Tel. 0171 235 3325

Sue Ryder Foundation
Cavendish
Sudbury
Suffolk CO10 8AY
Tel. 01787 280252

The Terrence Higgins Trust
52–54 Grays Inn Road
London WC1X 8JU
Tel. 0171 831 0330 (Administration)
Tel. 0171 242 1010 (Helpline)

REFERENCES

Bruera, E., Kuehn, N., Miller, M.J., Selmser, P. and Macmillan, K. (1991). The Edmonton symptoms assessment system; a simple method for the assessment of palliative care patients. *Journal of Palliative Care*, 7(2), 6–9.

Calman, K. and Hine, D. (1996). *A Policy Framework for Commissioning Cancer Service*. A report by the Expert Advisory Group on cancer to the chief medical officers Department of Health. DoH, London.

Coombe, V. (1996). Clairvoyancy and star signs 'are new religion'. *Daily Telegraph*, 12 November, page 6.

Corner, J., Plant, H., A'Hern, R. and Bailey, C. (1996). Non-pharmacological intervention in lung cancer. *Palliative Medicine*, 10(4), 299–305.

Davies, B. and Oberle, K. (1990). Dimensions of the supportive role of the nurse in palliative care. *Oncology Nursing Forum*, 17(1), 87–94.

Department of Health (1990). *National Health Service and Community Care Act, a Brief Guide*. Department of Health, London.

Finlay, I. (1991). *Results of Survey of 200 Consecutive Admissions to Holme Tower, Marie Curie Home, Penarth, Wales. Cancer Patients and Their Families at Home*. Interactive video disc, Marie Curie Education Department, London.

Giacosa, A., Frascio, F., Sukkar, S.G. and Roncella, S. (1996). Food intake and body composition in cancer cachexia. *Nutrition*, 12(1 Suppl), S20–S23.

Higginson, I. (1993). *Clinical Audit in Palliative Care*. Radcliffe Medical Press Ltd, Oxford.

Hill, D. (1995). *Opening Doors: Improving Access to Hospice and Specialist Palliative Care Services by Members of the Black and Ethnic Community*. National Hospice Council, London.

Hinton, J. (1994). Can home care maintain an acceptable quality of life for patients with terminal cancer and their relatives? *Palliative Medicine*, 8(3), 183–6.

Hospice Information Service (1997). *Directory of Hospice and Specialist Palliative Care Services*. St Christopher's Hospice, London.

Monroe, B. (1993). *Psycho-social Dimensions in Management of Terminal Malignant Disease*, 3rd edn, Saunders, C. and Sykes, N. (eds). Edward Arnold, London.

National Association of Health Authority Trusts (1991). *Care of People with Terminal Illness*. NAHAT, Birmingham.

Olivier, D. (1993). *Cross-cultural Principles of Care in Managment of Terminal Malignant Disease*, 3rd edn, Saunderss, C. and Sykes, N. (eds). Edward Arnold, London.

RCN (1993). *Standards of Palliative Nursing*. Scutari Press, London.

St Christopher's Hospice (1992). *A Team in Pain* (Video). St Christopher's Hospice, London.

Saunders, C. and Baines, M. (1995). *Living with Dying: a Guide to Palliative Care*, 3rd edn. Oxford University Press, Oxford.

Saunders, C. and Sykes, N. (eds) (1993). *Management of Terminal Malignant Disease*, 3rd edn. Edward Arnold, London.

Tatelbaum, J. (1980). *The Courage to Grieve*. Cedar Books, London.

Townsend, J. (1990). Patients' preference for place of death. *British Medical Journal*, 301, 415–17.

Twycross, R. and Lack, S. (1990). *Therapeutics in Terminal Cancer*. Churchill Livingstone, Edinburgh.

UKCC (1992). *Code of Professional Conduct*. UKCC, London.

Vachon, M. (1988). Counselling and psychotherapy in palliative care: a review. *Palliative Medicine*, 2(1), 36–50.

Vachon, M. (1995). Staff stress in hospice/palliative care; a review. *Palliative Medicine*, 9(2), 91–122.

WHO (1990). *Cancer Pain Relief and Palliative Care*. World Health Organization, Geneva.

WHO (1996). *Cancer Pain Relief*, 2nd edn. WHO, Geneva.

Williams, C.A. (1982). Role considerations in care of the dying patient. *Image*, XIV(1), 8–11.

Worden, W. (1991). *Grief Counselling and Grief Therapy*, 2nd edn. Routledge, London.

FURTHER READING

Kaye, P. (1994). *A–Z of Hospice and Palliative Medicine*. ELP Publications, Northampton.

Penson, J. and Fisher, R. (eds) (1995). *Palliative Care for People with Cancer*, 2nd edn. Arnold, London.

Saunders, C. and Sykes, N. (1993). *The Managment of Malignant Disease*, 3rd edn. Arnold, London.

Sims, R. and Moss, V. (1995). *Palliative Care for People with AIDS*, 2nd edn. Arnold, London.

Twycross, R. (1995). *Symptom Management in Advanced Cancer*. Radcliffe Medical Press Ltd, Oxford.

Worden, J.W. (1991). *Grief Counselling and Grief Therapy*, 2nd edn. Routledge, London.

GLOSSARY

Acidosis: a condition in which the blood pH is below 7.35.

Acupressure: the application of pressure to acupuncture sites (called Shiatsu in Japan).

Acupuncture: based on ancient Chinese medicine of needling the skin related to meridians, through which the life force flows (chi).

Addiction: a state of psychic or physical dependence (or both) on a drug, arising in a person following administration of that drug on a periodic or continuous basis. The characteristics of such a state will vary with the agents involved. Cardinal features are compulsive use, loss of control, and persistent use despite harm from the drug. It is rarely caused by the administration of opioids for pain relief.

Adult: ego state of transactional analysis concerned with testing reality and computing outcomes. Correlates with 'life as found to be'.

Advocacy: speaking on behalf of someone else, in support or defence of that person.

Agar: a polysaccharide made from seaweed and used to solidify bacteriological media.

Age-adjusted and standardised overall mortality: describes mortality rate when age and sex distributions have been taken into account.

Agoraphobia: morbid fear of open spaces, often associated with panic attacks. Such fears may be severe enough to limit social function.

Alarm reaction: this is the body's immediate reaction to a stressor.

Angina pectoris: thoracic pain originating from the heart, usually caused by a temporary lack of oxygen in a part of heart muscle as a consequence of insufficient blood supply (see **ischaemic heart disease**). Attacks are usually related to emotions, exertion or exposure to cold.

Anthropometric measurements: those measurements which incorporate weight/height ratios, e.g. body mass index (BMI) and skinfold thickness measurements - used to determine a more detailed nutritional assessment.

Antibody: a protein which is able specifically to combine with foreign molecules which are encountered in the body.

Antigen: any substance, usually proteins, which the body regards as foreign and produces antibodies against.

Anti-racism: an approach to race relations which stresses the role of institutional racism in structuring the experiences of black people in Britain. Anti-racists are politically committed to challenging racism in all the institutions of British society.

Aromatherapy: a specific form of therapy in which disorders are treated by body massage using aromatic oils; sometimes described as a 'complementary therapy'; any treatment which uses aromatic oils, obtained from a range of plants, for their medicinal purposes.

Arrhythmias: any deviation from the heart's normal rhythm.

Assessment: involves acquiring information about a person or situation that may include a description of the person's wants, needs wishes and ambitions. Part of a larger procedure and service to support planning towards goals which have been separately identified.

Asystole: absence of muscular contraction of the heart.

Atheroma: a deposit of lipid in the walls of a blood vessel.

Atherosclerosis: a narrowing and hardening of the arteries, typified by atheromatous or fatty plaques in the artery walls.

Atrial fibrillation: an atrial arrhythmia occurring at an extremely rapid atrial rate, lacking coordinated activity.

Authoritative: a style of responding characterised by prescriptive, confronting and informative interventions (see **Six Category Intervention Analysis**).

Autoclave: a machine in which materials can be exposed to steam under pressure and therefore to temperatures higher than boiling point; in order to sterilise them.

B-lymphocyte: one of the main cell types of the immune system responsible for the production of antibodies.

Bereweeke: a system of teaching skills which is accompanied by two checklists, one each for children and adults. It should be used as an integral component of the individual programme planning (IPP) process. Areas covered include language, self care, motor skills, social skills and cognitive skills. The main purpose is to develop individual teaching programmes.

Biofeedback: physiological responses associated with stress and tension are measured and displayed back to the patient, e.g. finger temperature, pulse or muscle electrical activity. It is often used with a relaxation technique so the patient has objective feedback from the impact of the relaxation.

Biographical approach: acknowledging a patient's/person's current point within his/her life and the influence of past experience and future life goals, and using this perspective as a basis for planning care.

Blastocyst: a hollow sphere of cells which develops from the morula stage of embryo development, prior to implantation into the endometrium of the uterus.

Capillary blood oxygenation: a pulse oximeter can be placed on a finger or an ear lobe (a non-invasive appliance). The electronic device measures the absorption of red and infrared light passing through living tissue. The reading closely responds to the arterial blood oxygen levels.

Capsule: a slimy substance, usually polysaccharides, which forms a protective layer around some bacterial cells.

Carbohydrate: a chemical compound consisting of carbon, hydrogen and oxygen which provides the most economical and the most readily digestible form of energy to the body. Carbohydrates can be monosaccharide (a single sugar, such as glucose), disaccharide (containing two sugars, such as sucrose) or polysaccharide (a complex compound containing many sugars, some of which may be digestible, such as starch, and others indigestible, such as cellulose).

Care management: a process introduced in the NHS and Community Care Act (1990) that provides a consistent approach for matching individual needs to services (rather than the other way around). The process depends upon the holistic assessment of individual needs and the appointment of a care manager who is responsible for the design and costing of a care package that will be systematically evaluated with respect to its effectiveness in meeting the identified needs of the client concerned.

Carotid sinus massage: massage to the area around the carotid artery, which contains specialised cells, which send sensory nerve stimulation to the brain stem to increase heart rate.

Categorisation: act of labelling people and events so as to confine them to a classification, rather than appreciate them for what they are.

Cerebral hypoxia: a reduced oxygen supply to brain tissue.

Cerebrovascular accident (CVA): destruction of brain tissue resulting from disorders of the blood vessels that supply the brain.

Child: ego state of transactional analysis concerned with feelings and expression, and addressing 'life as felt'.

Chlamydia: a bacterium recognised as a genital pathogen which is responsible for a variety of clinical syndromes, but may be asymptomatic in some cases. The genus *Chlamydia* comprises three species: *C. trachomatis*, *C. psittaci* and *C. pneumoniae*. Chlamydial infection not only undermines maternal health but also has implications for the fetus/neonate as it can be transmitted to the neonate during the birth process.

Cholesterol: a steroid found in mammalian tissue from which all other major steroids are synthesised, for example the hormone aldosterone. Cholesterol is synthesised mainly in the liver. A high plasma level of cholesterol is associated with atherosclerosis and coronary thrombosis.

Chromosome: this contains the genetic information of the cell. Chromosomes are composed of a long thread of DNA and associated proteins.

Circadian rhythms: changes in biochemical, physiological and psychological functions that exhibit 24-hour cycles, for example the cycle observed in body temperature which normally peaks during the day-time and reaches its lowest value during the night.

Classical conditioning: the construction of reflex responses by the presentation of paired stimuli. Theory devised by I.R. Pavlov in 1927.

Clinical waste: waste material from health care premises or veterinary practices which may be infectious, toxic or hazardous. This waste must usually be destroyed by incineration.

Cognitive-behavioural approach: focuses on the function and alteration in the quality of life caused by the pain, rather than the underlying disease. It aims to teach a person experiencing chronic pain how to cope with his/her pain and reduce the suffering.

Collusion: a conspiracy by some individuals – often people in controlling roles – to preserve their power covertly: i.e. the 'professional collusion' of a nurse and doctor to withhold information from a client, often justified on the grounds of confidentiality.

Colonisation: when a microbe establishes itself on or in part of the body without producing disease or symptoms.

Commensal: an organism which lives in association with another without either benefiting or harming it, e.g. normal flora of the gut.

Community learning disability teams: these teams have developed in the UK over the past two decades and are to be found in most areas in recognition of the fact that most people with a learning disability live in the community. Teams are based according to historical and geographical factors and generally include a community mental handicap nurse, a social worker, a clinical psychologist and other members of the health care team. The function of the team is to support people living in the community and their carers. This may be directly or by facilitation through generic health and community services.

Complement: a complex of proteins in the blood which promote the action of phagocytic cells and the killing of micro-organisms.

Compliance with treatment: an individual's acceptance and participation in treatment and his/her continued cooperation in carrying out prescribed treatment.

Conception: one of the various, debatable, meanings of a complex concept.

Congestive cardiac (heart) failure: a condition in which there is an excessive volume of blood within the chambers of the heart, with elevated intracardiac pressure. The right ventricle of the heart is not effective in pumping blood to the lungs. The consequences include: poor gaseous exchange in the lungs, congestion of blood in the venous circulation, which in turn increases congestion within the lungs, liver, kidneys and the peripheral circulation, leading to oedema.

Consumer: someone who uses goods or services which are designed to meet people's needs or desires.

Crackles: the sounds heard via a stethoscope when collapsed alveoli open explosively.

Crisis management: management that addresses change primarily in response to a crisis, rather than reflecting upon and planning for progress and the unexpected.

Culture: a way of life, including customs, values and beliefs, as well as family and other social arrangements. Culture can refer to the way of life of an entire society or to a particular group within a society, for example, a group based upon a shared ethnic identity.

Cyanosis: a bluish discoloration of the skin and mucous membranes due to reduced oxygenation of the blood. This can be caused by heart or respiratory failure.

Deamination: the removal of a group of atoms (NH_2; called an amino group) from an amino acid or similar. The amino group may be transferred to another molecule (ammonia, NH_3) which may be incorporated into urea for excretion.

Deep massage: the rubbing or kneading of different parts of the body, to aid circulation or to relax the muscles.

Defence mechanisms: strategies identified by psychoanalysts to reduce anxiety by distorting reality in some way and thereby deceive oneself about the presence of threat; examples include denial, repression, intellectualisation and projection.

Denial: the pushing from consciousness of unwanted awareness.

Depersonalisation: loss of a sense of oneself, along with feelings of non-being.

Depolarisation: cell membranes are electrically polarised by the uneven distribution of positive and negative ions, with the inside of the cell having excessive negative charge. Depolarisation is a reversal of the charge usually by the inward movement of positive ions. Observed when nerve cells or muscle cells are activated, and can be recorded (e.g. the electrocardiograph).

Deviance: types of action which are said to go against the socially acceptable ways of behaving, that is, the 'norms' or informal rules of society. Functionalism and symbolic interactionism regard illness as a form of deviance.

Disinfection: a process which reduces the number of micro-organisms to a level at which they are not harmful but which does not usually destroy spores. Disinfectant: chemicals which can be used to achieve disinfection.

Displacement: a subconscious defence mechanism where an individual receives feeling from one situation and expresses it in another where it does not belong: for example, you are reprimanded by your boss but express your frustrations upon your colleagues.

Distress: potentially harmful and occurs when increasing levels of stress become maladaptive because they exceed a person's adaptive ability to cope with the associated demands.

DNA: deoxyribonucleic acid, a large molecule composed of nucleotides which contain the sugar deoxyribose. It forms the genetic material of the organism.

Dominant gene: genes are normally found in cells in pairs. If each gene in the pair differs slightly, one will usually assume dominance and be expressed by the cell (the other member of the pair will be recessive and not be expressed).

DOMINO: domiciliary midwifery in and out; this is an option for delivery that may be offered to the pregnant woman.

Doula: a female companion who is not a midwife who, instead of the male partner, takes on a mothering role and provides social support for a woman during labour.

Dysmorphic: abnormality of shape or form, e.g. dysmorphic features.

Ecomap: a diagram portraying important connections between the family and others outside the family.

Effector organs or tissues: those that effect a homeostatic response, for example, the involvement of the peripheral circulation in the regulation of body temperature.

Elder abuse: a single or repeated act, or lack of appropriate action, occurring in any relationship where there is an expectation of trust, that causes harm or distress to an older person.

Electrocardiogram: a recording of the electrical currents within the myocardium. Heart rate, rhythm and electrical irregularities due to pathology or malformations can be recognised.

Emotion-focused coping: a means of reducing anxiety or stress that does not deal directly with the anxiety-provoking situation (e.g. defence mechanisms, use of alcohol or drugs).

Emphysema: pulmonary – a chronic disease where there is overdistension of fibrosed alveoli causing reduced surface area for gaseous exchange.

Empowerment: being enabled to take power or control over oneself.

Endogenous infection: caused by micro-organisms present on the body.

Endorphin: naturally occurring morphine-like substance produced by the body.

Enzyme: a protein which catalyses a biochemical reaction.

Epicanthic skin folds: a fold of the upper eyelid over the lower eyelid at the inner corner.

Epidemic: a definite increase in the incidence of a disease above its normal level; disease prevalent in a community for an isolated period.

Epidemiology: the study of the determinants and distribution of health and disease in populations.

Erythema: a flushing of the skin caused by dilation of capillary blood vessels, often a sign of inflammation or infection.

Eugenics: a theory or belief that 'survival of the fittest' can be applied to humans by encouraging the perceived fitter members of society to produce more children and discouraging, or coercing, the weaker not to have children.

Eukaryotic cell: a type of living cell found in higher animals and plants which is characterised by having a nucleus separated from the cytoplasm by a membrane.

Eustress: the term used to describe the positive form of stress that is needed for an active, healthy life.

Exhaustion: this is the final phase of the stress response and is generally due to persistent exposure to a stressor whereby the body is unable to maintain equilibrium, and death occurs.

Exogenous infection: micro-organisms causing the infection have been derived from another person or object, i.e. cross-infection.

Experiential: an approach – often linked with teaching – where the authority of individual experience is emphasised in the acquisition of knowledge. Emphasises the affective (feeling) rather than cognitive (intellectual) aspects of function.

Facilitation: the art of enabling others to explore and resolve their own problems rather than doing this for them and inducing independence (see **Facilitative; Six Category Intervention Analysis** for examples of facilitative interventions).

Facilitative: a style of responding characterised by cathartic, catalytic and supportive interventions (see **Six Category Intervention Analysis**).

False positives: the results of a screening test may wrongly identify people as having a disease when in fact they do not have the condition.

Family: a group of people who are bonded in some way and who share a number of beliefs and values.

Family-centred care: a systematic approach to meeting the needs of family members, either on an individual basis or collectively as a family unit.

Family psychotherapy: the application of psychotherapeutic techniques within a family context (see **Personal psychotherapy** below).

Fatty acid: a compound which contains oxygen and a chain of carbon atoms with attached hydrogen atoms. The degree to which the carbon atoms are loaded with hydrogen determines whether they are saturated or unsaturated. A saturated fatty acid has all its carbon atoms loaded with hydrogen and there are no double bonds. Unsaturated fatty acids have double bonds to which hydrogen can be added.

Fomites: inanimate objects which may have been contaminated with infectious pathogens and which could transmit infection to others.

Free radicals: chemical agents produced by metabolism which have oxidising properties that can damage membranes within cells. They are normally removed by 'scavengers' such as vitamin E.

Full employment: an economic term usually taken to be an unemployment rate of 3% or less. The unemployment rate is the percentage of the labour force that is unemployed at a particular point in time.

Fungus: a simple plant which lacks chlorophyll.

Gate control theory: proposed by Melzack and Wall (1965), this pain theory suggests that pain impulses can be regulated or even blocked by gating mechanisms along the central nervous system. Gating mechanisms can be altered by thoughts, feelings and memories.

Gene: a section of DNA which encodes the structure of a protein.

Genetic code: the information carried by DNA. It determines the sequence of amino acids in proteins and therefore governs the nature of all proteins in the cell.

Genetic deletion: the loss of sequences of bases within a section of DNA, leading to a change in gene structure.

Genogram: a diagram outlining a family's internal and external structure.

Gestalt: the perceptive pattern held by an individual as a product of his mental, emotional and environmental state at any one moment. Alludes to perception as being active and interpretive rather than a passive reception of external events.

Gillick competence: a principle set by law in 1985 indicating that a child below the age of 16 may give consent to treatment if she or he fully understands the nature and purpose of the proposed treatment and the likely consequences.

Glasgow coma scale: a tool designed to provide an objective method of assessing and recording conscious level; it focuses on the patient's eye opening ability, motor response and verbal response.

Gonadotropin: a hormone (e.g. follicle stimulating hormone) which stimulates the production of another hormone (e.g. oestrogen) from gonadal cells.

Gram stain: a method of colouring bacterial cells with dyes to distinguish the two main types of prokaryotic cell, Gram-negative and Gram-positive.

Growth: an individual's movement towards greater awareness, positive self-regard, enhanced personal and interpersonal skills and sensitivity.

Healthy alliances: describes projects and initiatives where there is collaborative action between statutory agencies including education, housing, health and social care as well as commerce, industry, voluntary agencies and the community itself.

High population mean: when the arithmetic average is calculated and it is found to be high in a particular population; e.g. the average number of people smoking or with a raised blood pressure is high.

Holistic care: an approach to health care which treats the individual as a whole person in relation to his or her environment.

Homeostasis: the maintenance of a constant internal environment (see Chapter 5).

Hospital-acquired infection: an infection acquired as a result of treatment in hospital or during a period of hospitalisation. Also called **nosocomial** infection.

Housing tenure: the legal basis in which houses are occupied, for example, rented or owned. There are four main housing tenures in Britain: owner-occupied, rented from local authorities, rented from housing associations, and rented from private landlords.

Hypovolaemic shock: a continued reduction in circulating volume of blood in the circulation, often followed by hypovolaemia.

Hypoxaemia: a term used to denote that the oxygen content of blood is below its homeostatic range (also **hypoxia**).

Idealisation: investing idealistic values in an object or person (for example, the projecting of 'parent-like' qualities on a teacher by a student who may then feel unrealistically safe and cared for).

Illness iceberg: that amount of illness which is socially 'invisible' because it is not reported to medical practitioners.

Immunisation: to confer immunity. Immunity is the natural reaction of the body to invading chemicals, known as antigens. The immune response to antigens results in the formation of antibodies which protect the body from future attacks. Immunity can be induced naturally (by contact with the disease itself) or artificially (by giving a vaccine). Artificial immunity can be active where the vaccine is a live or killed organism, or passive when an injection of prepared antibodies is given.

Immunodeficiency: impairment of the immune response rendering the host particularly susceptible to infection. May be caused by genetic disorder, underlying illness, chemotherapy or certain viral infections (= immunocompromised).

Incidence: the number of new cases occurring in a particular population over time.

Income support: a means-tested benefit for those aged over 18, who are either not in work or who work below a certain number of hours per week, and whose income falls below a minimum level set by Parliament. Income support replaced supplementary benefit in April 1988.

Individual programme planning (IPP): a system for making plans for one person based on the strengths and needs of that person as an individual with the assistance of people who are well known to him/her. A meeting is held to formulate the IPP at which objectives are set to be achieved within a specific time span. The person responsible for each of the needs is identified. Any service deficits which prevent the need from being met are also identified and managers are informed. In this way service provision can be based on the needs of clients.

Infection: entry of a micro-organism into tissues where it multiplies and causes damage.

Infectious disease: a disease which can be transmitted readily from one person to another.

Inflammation: response of tissue to infection or other injury characterised by swelling, heat, erythema and pain.

Intuition: those internal awarenesses and insights seemingly unconnected with external reality, but often appearing to have wisdoms of their own. May be linked with fantasy and creativity.

Invasive carcinoma (cervix): malignant changes affecting the tissues surrounding the cervical epithelium, including the vagina, uterine body and lymph nodes.

Involutional melancholia: an old term in psychiatry meaning mental illness involving depression and fears that are not always substantiated.

Ischaemic heart disease: inadequate blood supply to the muscle of the heart which causes temporary loss of function. If severe or sustained, the disorder can lead to cell death as in myocardial infarction.

Jaundice: a yellow discoloration of the skin and conjunctivae due to the presence of bile pigment in the blood. Can be caused by obstruction of the common bile duct, haemolysis or hepatitis.

Klinefelter's syndrome: a chromosomal disorder of males arising because of the inheritance of an extra X chromosome. Characteristics include underdeveloped testes, and poorly developed cognitive ability.

Labelling theory: this approach to deviance is associated with symbolic interactionism. It argues that instead of looking at deviance from the standpoint of who breaks society's rules and why they do so, one should instead focus on the issue of who makes and enforces the rules. Labelling theory is very much concerned with the effects of the application of the deviant 'label' on the rule-breaker.

Labour: the process which begins with the onset of regular, rhythmic and painful uterine contractions, and ends with the birth of the baby, placenta and membranes and control of bleeding from the placental site.

Lay referral: the interpretation of illness and the subsequent advice given to a sick individual by members of the family, friends or acquaintances.

Learned helplessness: a chronic form of dependence induced by authoritative methods of care which demotivate clients to care for themselves. A feeling of helplessness/apathy generated through subjecting organisms to trauma (such as electric shock, extremes of heat/cold) in a situation where they are unable to escape or avoid the aversive stimuli; this helplessness generalises to other situations.

Lipoprotein: a combination of a lipid and a protein. Lipoproteins may be structural components of cells, but also facilitate the transportation of lipid in blood by making it soluble in water.

Locus of control: refers to how much an individual believes the events in their lives are controlled.

Log-rolling: a method of turning patients whilst maintaining correct spinal alignment and protecting the cervical spine.

Luer lock: a screw-type connection fitted to intravenous administration sets and accessories to prevent accidental disconnection.

Lymphocyte: a type of white blood cell present in the blood, lymph system, gut wall and bone marrow. Lymphocytes are involved in the immune response and can be divided into B-lymphocytes, which produce antibodies, and T-lymphocytes, which are responsible for cell-mediated immunity.

Makaton: a manual signing or communication system designed for implementation with people with severe learning disabilities.

MEAC: minimum effective analgesic concentration. This can be different for individual patients.

Medical model: a model of health which suggests that health is the absence of disease in a person's body and that restoring a person to health is a matter of curing the disease. This model of health is associated with modern medicine and can be contrasted to the principles underlying holistic care.

Medicalisation: the process whereby natural and social phenomena are turned into 'diseases' or are treated as diseases by the medical profession.

Metabolism: the combined actions of biosynthesis (anabolism) and degradation (catabolism).

Mitochondria: organelles within a cell that are responsible for the production of energy, usually from glucose. Often referred to as the 'power houses' of the cell.

Mitochondrial DNA: small amounts of genetic material found in the walls of mitochondria of cells. Distinct from the DNA found in the nucleus of the cell.

Morbidity: relating to a disease or an abnormal or disordered condition.

Mortality: the ratio of the number of deaths to the total population.

Morula: this is the solid ball of cells formed following the fertilisation of the male and female gametes.

Multipara: a woman who has had two or more pregnancies that resulted in a viable offspring whether or not the offspring was alive at birth.

Myocardial infarction: the death of a part of heart muscle caused by obstruction in a coronary artery. Necrosis of tissue of the myocardium (the middle layer of the heart wall) due to an interrupted blood supply. Also known as 'heart attack'.

Needs: things that can be identified or assigned. They are presented as statements of fact which can be deduced by someone else.

Needs assessment: researching, describing and measuring the health care needs of a population in order to plan the provision of care.

Nerve blocks: injecting local anaesthetics blocks the function of sensory, motor and autonomic neurones supplying the affected area.

Neural tube defects: defects of the cerebrospinal system, usually relating to spina bifida.

Neurotransmitter: a chemical which facilitates the transmission of nerve impulses at junctions (synapses) between a nerve cell and another cell (nerve cell, muscle cell or gland cell). The transmitter that operates at junctions between nerve cells is considered to be excitatory if the impulse is passed on, and inhibitory if it is prevented. The nervous system contains a variety of neurotransmitters, such as the monoamines (e.g. noradrenaline, dopamine and serotonin).

New Right: a social theory which aims to explain social behaviour in terms of the actions of individuals. It is politically committed to the attempt to limit the role of the state in economic and social life in order for markets to operate in a manner free from state intervention.

Nociceptors: receptors in the skin and tissue which respond to stimuli from actual or potential tissue damage.

Non-essential amino acid: amino acids which can be synthesised in the liver from other amino acids (via transamination) and so need not be present in the diet. Essential amino acids cannot be synthesised and so must be present in the diet.

Normal flora: the community of micro-organisms which normally inhabits a surface of the body without causing any harm.

Nosocomial: see **hospital-acquired infection**.

NSAID: non-steroidal anti-inflammatory drugs; they exert their action by inhibiting the formation of prostaglandins. The latter sensitise nerve endings to pain.

Oedema: systemic – an effusion of fluid into the skin; pulmonary – an effusion of fluid into the tissue surrounding the lungs and into the alveoli. A serious cause of cyanosis.

Operant conditioning: the rewarding of desirable behaviours and the ignoring of undesirable ones. Often used with people experiencing chronic pain. A method used widely in behaviour modification, in which behaviours are altered by changing their consequences. It is a process of training operant behaviour using reinforcement techniques which involves four types of conditioning – positive reinforcement, negative reinforcement, punishment and extinction.

Operational definition: a stipulative definition which is formulated in such a precise way that it enables the scientific community to 'isolate' and measure the defined phenomenon. Note, once again, that this will not coincide with common usage; an operational definition of 'class', for example, will not measure all the things we associate with class.

Opiate: a compound specifically derived from the extract of the opium poppy (*Papaver somniferum*).

Opioid: a morphine-like drug whose action can be blocked by naloxone. This might be synthetic, naturally occurring or produced by the body (endogenous).

Opioid receptors: located in the brain and spinal cord. There are several types of receptor (e.g. mu, delta and kappa).

Opportunistic pathogen: a micro-organism which only causes infection in a host with an impaired immune system.

Organic: a compound that contains carbon.

Organogenesis: the formation of organs during the embryonic period.

Outbreak of infection: the occurrence of two or more related cases of the same infection or where the number of infections is more than would normally be expected.

Paraphemia: difficulty in finding the correct word in speech.

Parent: ego state of transactional analysis concerned with the, social world and 'life as taught'.

Pathogen: a micro-organism that is capable of causing disease.

Pathognomonic: a characteristic that positively identifies a condition, e.g. Koplik's spots on the buccal membrane in measles and the palm print of people with Down's syndrome.

Pectoralis muscles: broad, thick, triangular muscles, situated at the upper and fore part of the chest and in front of the axilla and extending from the clavicle to the seventh rib. They assist in the expansion of the rib cage during inspiration.

Perinatal mortality rate: the number of deaths per 1000 live births that occur between the 28th week of pregnancy and the 4th week after the birth.

Personal psychotherapy: treatment of emotional or psychosomatic disorders based on the application of psychological knowledge rather than on physical forms of treatment. Explores inner feelings and encourages the exploration of 'inner' coping strategies to deal with stress and life events.

Personality disorder: a cluster of disorders characterised by behaviours and inner experiences that are at variance with culturally accepted norms, which impair social, cultural or occupational functioning. The behaviour is largely not related to other mental health problems, organic damage or other physiological cause.

Phagocyte: a cell capable of ingesting material in a process called phagocytosis.

Phenylalanine: an amino acid which is needed for healthy brain growth and development. It is catalysed by the enzyme phenylalanine hydroxylase to tyrosine in the liver. The hereditary failure to produce this enzyme may lead to phenylketonuria if undetected and untreated.

Phenylketonuria: a condition caused by a deficiency of an enzyme (phenylalanine hydroxylase) in the body. Phenylalanine cannot be converted to tyrosine, an amino acid, and as a result phenylalanine builds up in the body, causing damage to the brain. Phenylpyruvic acid is excreted in the urine. The degree of learning disability may be severe unless detected and treated early in life. Untreated children have blue eyes, fair hair and dry (and sometimes eczematous) skin. This deficiency is routinely tested for in the UK and early treatment results in total recovery. The Guthrie test is generally used. Treatment is with a low phenylalanine diet. Blood screening for the measurement of phenylalanine is also necessary.

Placebo effect: the physical/emotional effects observed that reflect the expectation of an individual who believes that he/she has taken an active agent, but in fact has been given an inactive agent. Placebos are typically used in drug trials.

Plasmid: a circular strand of DNA found in some bacterial cells, which can carry genes for antibiotic resistance and can be copied and transferred to other cells.

Pneumothorax: air between the pleural layers of the lung resulting in abolition of the negative intrapleural pressure. A ruptured alveolus allows air into the pleural cavity, causing the associated lung to collapse which could be life-threatening. Can be spontaneous and is often found in fit young people.

Polyp: an overgrowth of tissue which extends from a mucous membrane into a cavity, but remains attached by means of a stalk.

Polypeptide: a molecule comprised of a chain of amino acids. Two or more polypeptides joined together comprise a protein.

Post-traumatic stress disorder (PTSD): an anxiety disorder caused by a stressful event such as a natural disaster which is outside the usual range of human experience; it includes a range of symptoms such as re-experiencing the trauma, feelings of detachment, avoiding thoughts and feelings associated with the traumatic event, and sleep disturbances.

Postural drainage: the patient/client is positioned in such a way as to allow the effects of gravity to aid the expulsion of fluid within the respiratory passages.

Pre-invasive carcinoma (cervix): epithelial changes in the cervix where cells are undifferentiated and immature, known as carcinoma in situ.

Primigravida: a woman who is pregnant for the first time.

Problem-focused coping: a direct means of reducing anxiety or stress by taking some conscious action to deal with the anxiety-provoking situation (e.g. provision of information or assertiveness training).

Projection: placing our own feelings on another and responding to these feelings as if they originated and belonged there. A subconscious mental defence mechanism.

Prokaryotic cell: one of the two main types of living cell which does not have a membrane around the nucleus and is simpler in structure than eukaryotic cells. All bacteria are prokaryotic cells.

Pro-life: this term is usually used to describe the anti-abortion lobby. They argue that the fetus has a right to be born.

Prostaglandins: generated from the breakdown of cell membranes. They are believed to increase sensitivity to pain.

Protozoa: single-celled, microscopic eukaryotic organisms. Can be either parasitic or free-living.

Psychoneuroimmunology: a new interdisciplinary field concerned with studying the link between psychological stress, immunological functioning and health. It enables us to investigate the psychophysiological associations between behaviour and disease.

Psychosis: a disordered mental reaction where there is loss of contact with conventional reality and withdrawal from usual social intercourse. A condition necessitating much psychiatric time and effort to address.

Psychotherapy: the helping of another by a practitioner trained in a specific counselling mode.

Psychotropic drugs: drugs which act upon the mind.

Pulmonary hypertension: higher than normal blood pressure within the lung circulation.

Quality of life measurement scale: a research instrument which employs a set of criteria to assess people's quality of life. These can be used for needs assessment or to measure, and compare, the effectiveness of therapies.

Reductionism: the process of 'reducing' a whole to some of its parts. In particular, it is the way in which humans can be regarded as bodies or objects of study. In itself, this is neither good nor bad, but it has the potential to cause problems.

Reflexology: reflexology is based on the principle that particular parts of the feet relate directly to various systems or organs of the body, and by gently stimulating specific areas, disorders can be alleviated or relieved.

Reliability: a key dimension of the usefulness of a measurement scale. A reliable measure will consistently give the same measure to the same phenomenon, and will thereby enable comparisons across time and space.

Repetitive strain injury: a term for a range of work-related disorders which affect the hand, arm and neck. They usually involve persistent pain and are often the result of rapid repetitive movements (e.g. typing).

Repression: the exile of unpleasant memories and material from consciousness, linked to mental defence mechanisms and cited to explain some of the content of the 'unconscious mind'.

Resistance or adaptation: the body attempts to control and adjust to a stressor to maintain normal bodily functions.

Ritual task performance: the reduction of behaviour to a right procedure. May be used defensively to limit personal involvement and disturbing feedback.

Role: the social expectations which are attached to a person's occupancy of a particular social position. These expectations are not necessarily realised in practice.

Saphrophytic bacteria: bacteria which live on dead organic material.

Sensory: refers to the qualities of the pain experience.

Sex selection: choosing the sex of the embryo for implantation following *in vitro* fertilisation.

Shaping: a behaviour modification teaching technique in which existing behaviours are built on and expanded. Initially, a response similar to the desired one is reinforced so that it occurs more frequently. The next stage is to reinforce it selectively when it is a nearer approximation to required response.

Shared action planning: a system based on the individual programme planning (IPP) approach which emphasises the importance of relationships and friendships as the core principle for the development of care plans. It ensures that service users share in all aspects of the process as joint decision makers. It involves goals, aims, assessment and provides strategies and actions to ensure that outcomes are evaluated in accordance with prescribed action plans.

Shock: a condition characterised by failure of the body to supply sufficient oxygen and nutrients to the cells to meet their metabolic needs.

Sickle cell anaemia: an inherited disease which affects the red blood cells and is found mainly amongst people of African or Caribbean descent.

Six Category Intervention Analysis: a model of intervention classification after Heron (1990; see references, Chapter 14) who distinguishes between authoritative and facilitative styles of responding.

Social defences: ways in which social systems are evolved to defend participants from disturbing features of their role – for example, the carer from the distress of the client.

Social mobility: the movement of individuals either up or down the class structure.

Spina bifida: a defect in the spinal column, in which the vetebral neural arches may be absent or fail to close. This may result in the protrusion of the spinal cord or its membranes, except in the case of spina bifida occulta.

Spore: a resistant casing which some bacteria use to enclose their cells when they encounter adverse environmental conditions. When conditions improve the spore germinates into a new cell.

Standardised mortality ratios: a measure of death rates.

Status: the respect and value the society invests in a role – for example, the bestowing of professional status on certain workers.

Sterilisation: a process which removes or destroys all micro-organisms, including spores.

Sternomastoid muscles: large thick muscles which pass obliquely across the side of the neck and extend to the upper border of the sternum. They assist in the expansion of the rib cage during inspiration.

Stipulative definition: a definition of a word which is decided by agreement, and set out systematically and explicitly. For these reasons it may not coincide with the normal usage of the word, which is likely to vary and have less clear boundaries.

Stress: a state that occurs when an individual encounters an event that (s)he perceives as potentially endangering his/her physical or psychological well-being.

Stress response: a reaction to an event perceived by an individual as potentially endangering his/her physical or psychological well-being. It may include physiological changes that prepare the individual to cope with an emergency (fight or flight response) and also psychological reactions such as anxiety, anger, aggression, apathy and depression.

Stressor: an event that is perceived by an individual potentially to endanger his/her physical or psychological well-being (i.e. stress as a stimulus). Anything that promotes a drain on body resources. Stressors may be aspects of social living (e.g. work activities, family relationships), environmental agents (e.g. drugs) or homeostatic disturbances in the body (e.g. cancer, HIV infection).

Stroke volume: the volume of blood ejected from each ventricle at each beat of the heart.

Syncope: temporary loss of consciousness caused by a reduction in cerebral blood flow.

Syndactyly: webbing of the fingers and toes.

T-lymphocyte: one of the two main cell types of the immune system, responsible for destroying intracellular parasites and coordinating the immune response.

Tachycardia: an abnormally rapid resting heart beat or pulse rate (over 100 beats per minute).

Tachypnoea: a respiratory rate greater than 20 breaths per minute.

Teratogens: drugs or other agents capable of disrupting normal growth and development, and which produce congenital malformations.

Thalassaemia: an inherited disease which affects the red blood cells and is found mainly amongst Cypriot, Greek, Turkish and Indian people.

Toxin: a poisonous substance produced by a living organism.

Tradition: that body of common practice which supports historically derived meanings and behaviours.

Transactional analysis: a model of ego structure and development suggested by Berne (1967; see references, Chapter 14), where personality is classified as consisting of parent, adult and child egos, the interplay of which produces characteristic behaviours and may be used to analyse interactions.

Transactional model of stress: assumes that stress reflects the relationship (transaction) between a person and his/her environment. Stress is not simply seen as either a stimulus or a response, but rather as the product of a person's interpretation of the significance of a potentially threatening event (the stimulus) and of their resources to cope with it (the response).

Transamination: the transfer of certain atoms (NH_2; called an amino group) from an amino acid to a keto acid, which results in the formation of a different amino acid.

Turner's syndrome: a chromosomal disorder in which the individual inherits a single X chromosome (the individual is always female). Characteristics include small stature, 'shield' chest, and poor development of gonads and secondary sexual characteristics.

Vaccination: a process of inducing immunity by administering a vaccine.

Vaccine: an agent inducing immunity. A vaccine can be live in that it infects, replicates and immunises in a similar way to the 'wild' strain but rarely causes the disease (for example, the measles vaccine). The vaccine may be inactivated, consisting of a suspension of the killed organisms (for example, the whooping cough vaccine).

Validity: the other key dimension of the usefulness of a measurement scale. A measure is valid if it gives a faithful and accurate picture of the phenomenon being measured.

Ventricular fibrillation: asynchronous ventricular contractions; will result in heart failure unless reversed by defibrillation.

Virulence: the ability of an organism to cause disease.

Virus: a micro-organism only capable of reproduction within living cells.

Well women clinics: clinics run for women with the aim of practising a holistic approach to women's health care needs. The emphasis is on allowing the female clients to determine their own health needs.

Wheezes: musical sounds heard from the airways either with or without a stethoscope.

Yeast: a unicellular fungus.

Young carers: children and young people whose lives are restricted by the responsibility of caring for a sick or disabled relative in the home.

INDEX

A&E department *see* first line care
ABCDE system, advanced trauma life
     support (ATLS) 586
abortion 405
   pro-life lobby 722
accident and emergency *see* first line
     care
accidents
   elderly people 684
   Health of the Nation targets 75
accountability 235–6, 306–7
Accountable Officers 235
acidosis, urine testing 639, 712
activities of daily living (ADLs) 671–2
Acts of Parliament
   Children Act (DoH, 1989) 215, 217,
      499, 504, 578
   Community Care Act (1990) 212, 550
   Community Care Act (1993) 473–4
   Control of Substances Hazardous to
      Health (COSHH) regulations 381
   Data Protection Act 303
   Environmental Protection Act
      (1990) 382
   Health and Safety at Work Act 45,
      380
   Mental Health (Patients in
      Community) Act (1995) 530, 531
acupressure, acupuncture 352, 712
acutely ill patients
   communication needs 646
   reducing sleep interruptions 651
   relatives' needs 649
adaptation, model 328
addiction 91, 94, 712
Addison's disease 188
addresses
   dying patient care and
      bereavement 709–10
   first line care 587
   maternity care 451–2
   patient communication 226
adolescence 405–9
adult, transactional analysis 712
advanced trauma life support
      (ATLS) 585–6
   A&E department 585
   ABCDE system 586
   definitive care phase 586
   Glasgow Coma Score 586
   mechanism of injury 585–6
   primary/secondary survey 586

   resuscitation phase 586
   trauma team 585–6
advocacy 304–5, 600-2, 712
   for children 491
   citizen 600
   collective or class 600
      SCOPE and MENCAP groups 600
   defined 305
   legal 600
   nurse assertiveness 603
   patient 224
   rights 555
   self 600
aerobic exercises 86
agar 712
Age Concern 219
age-adjusted mortality 712
ageing, cells 133
ageing *see* elderly people
aggression 583–4
   first line care 583–4
   indications of impending
      aggression 583
   self-defence 584
agoraphobia 712
AIDS *see* HIV/AIDS
airborne infections 369
alarm reaction 712
alcohol abusers, A&E department 581
alcohol consumption 407, 427–8
   background information 93–5
   coronary heart disease 93–5
   and fetal alcohol syndrome 427
   health inequalities 48–50
   legislative campaigns 96
   political actions 96
   social consequences 95
   standard units 427
allowances, attendance allowance 702
Alma-Ata Declaration 5, 74, 106–7
   WHO health targets 206
alternative medicine 208–9
Alzheimer's disease 533
ambulance personnel, first line
      care 569–70
analgesics, list 349, 696
angina pectoris 712
   pain perception 140
anorexia 406, 535–6
   dying patient care 698
antenatal care
   ethical aspects 439

   place of birth 436–8
   screening and diagnostic tests 438–40
anthropomorphic measurements 655,
      712
anti-racism 62–3, 712
antibiotics, sensitivity 366–7
antibody 712
antigen 712
anxiety 620
anxiety disorders, prevalence 532
Apgar score 445–6
Aristotle, on health 18
aromatherapy 209, 350, 712
arrhythmias 712
Art of Being Human 254
Asian Mother and Baby Campaign 58
assertiveness, nurses' rights and
      responsibilities 603
assessment *see* nursing practice,
      assessment of interventions
asystole 713
atheroma 138, 713
   genetic expression 138
atherosclerosis 83, 713
atrial fibrillation 626, 713
attendance allowance 702
attitudes and belief 292–301
audit, King's Fund Organisational
      Audit 240
Audit Commission, community health
      professionals identification 104
audit cycle, surveillance of HAI 377
authoritative vs facilitative
      nursing 330–2, 522
autoclave 713
autonomic nervous system
      (ANS) 617–22, 642
autonomy 598
awareness check list 320–3

B-lymphocytes 372–3, 713
bacteria 366, 367
   capsule 713
   microbiology laboratory 365–8
   plasmids 367, 721
   reservoirs of infection
      371
   resistant strains 367
   saprophytes 365, 723
   spores 723
   virulence factors 371

beliefs, attitudes and values 292–3
  five ethical principles 295–8
  rights and responsibilities 298–301
benefits
  attendance allowance 702
  disability living allowance (DLA) 702
bereavement 684–5
  children 707
  elderly people 684–5
  nurse's role 706–7
Bereweeke teaching system 560, 713
Bernard, Claude, homeostasis 125
bilirubin, urine testing 639
biofeedback 713
biographical approach 713
biographical model 665
biological determinants of
    health 124–34
biological theories of ageing 667–8
Black Report, health inequalities 40, 41,
    87
blastocyst 131–2, 713
blood
  analysis 638
  haematocrit levels 641
  haemoglobin levels 641
  plasma osmolality 641
blood pressure (BP) 629–31
  accurate measurement 633
  source of error 632
body mass index 426
Bordetella pertussis, whooping
    cough 78–9
bottle feeding 449–50
bowel elimination, elderly people 682,
    683
breast cancer 411
breast milk, species, comparisons 448
Breast Screening Programme, UK 21
breastfeeding 447–50 and
    substitutes 447
breathing
  elderly people 681, 683
  normal and abnormal 634–7
British Association of Cancer United
    Patients (CancerBACUP) 219
British Medical Association, alcohol
    consumption reduction
    targets 93–4
bronchitis 127
Bruhn, JJ, Art of Being Human 254
bulimia 536
Burford NDU model of hospital
    care 611–15
  documentation 656
  environment of care 614
  holism 612–13
  learning domains 614
  nurse-patient relationship 613–14
  nursing process 656
  recording and communicating
    nursing actions 614–15
  reflection 612
  situational meaning 612–13
  social viability 614

burnout syndrome 163, 329, 465

calcium, metabolism 407
cancer
  breast cancer 411
  British Association of Cancer United
    Patients (CancerBACUP) 219
  Calman–Hine Report 694
  cervical cancer 80–2, 409–10
  colorectal cancer 130–1
  elderly people 684
  fears and beliefs 81–2
  Health of the Nation targets 75
  and stress 195–6
candidiasis, oral 698
capillary blood oxygenation
    713
carbohydrates 85, 424, 713
cardiac failure 601, 714
care in the community 551–2
  learning disability 551-2
  risks and fears 554
care management 713
  interface with organisation
    management 244-6
Care Maps 241–2
care programme approach (CPA),
    mental health care 530
care-giving
  categories 208
    Committee of the Royal
      Commission on the National
      Health Service 208
  communication
    becoming a self-creating
      person 155–6
    supervision by example 160–4
  evidence-based 241
  family-centred care 457–77
  the five Cs 293, 295
  planning, effective practice 270–1
  requirements 463
  standards 240
  and women's health 416
  young carers 464–5
career matrix 545, 560
caring concepts 613
carotid sinus massage 626, 713
Casey's model of paediatric
    nursing 486–7
catalytic interventions 158
categorisation 713
catharsis 157
cell specialisation
  morula transition into blastocyst 131
  pre-implantation development 132
cellular ageing 133
central venous pressure (CVP) 631–4
  normal ranges 636
  water manometer measurement 635
cerebral hypoxia 713
cerebral palsy, learning disability 547–8
cerebrovascular accident 713
cervical cancer 409–10, 718
  pre-invasive carcinoma 722

screening programme 80–1
screening test objections and
    fears 81–2
change
  authoritative and healthy
    interactions 323–4
  avoidance by nurses 317–18
  awareness 320–3
  demands and outcomes 319
  learning to grow 318–20
Changing Childbirth 216
charities and further help, dying patient
    care 702–3
CHD see coronary heart disease
chemicals, decontamination
    381
child health care 215
  caring theory 487
  Casey's model 486–7
  developmental theory 486
  family-centred 505–6
  historical perspective 498–500
  interactional theory 487
  key principles and goals 483–4, 502–9
  legal issues 506
  Leininger's model 487–8
  mental health care 535
  nurses 483
  pain and pain assessment 339, 343–4
  parents' participation 503–4
  partnership model 504–5
  perceptions of illness 490
  stereotype 500
  systems theories 485–6
  see also children
Child Poverty Action Group 110
childbirth 441–4
  models 430–1
  National Childbirth Trust 219
  Winterton Report (DoH, 1992c) 431–2
children
  A&E department 577–8
  Action for Sick Children (1991) 577
  adolescence 405–9
  bereavement 707
  child abuse, A&E department 578
  confidentiality issues 506
  definitions 479–80
  development 496–8
  emotional–social competency 491–2
  empowerment 506–9
  Erikson's 8 stages 493
  Erikson's theory of psychosocial
    development 492
  intellectual competency 489–91
  physical competency 489
  sexual abuse 501–2
  smoking 50
  social constructions of
    childhood 498–502
  specific needs
    language 480–1
    love and security 480
    new experiences 480
    play 480, 482

praise and recognition 481
responsibility 482–4
understanding of health and
    illness 492–7
    8 stages 493
    age-related concepts 494–5
    comparing adult and child
        perceptions 496
    Piaget's theory 491, 493
    see also child health care
Children Act (DoH, 1989) 215, 217, 499,
    504, 505, 578
Children's Charter 215
Children's Rights Development Unit
    (UN, 1994) 505
Chlamydia 714
cholera 111
cholesterol 49, 714
    deposition in atheroma 138
    dietary control 84–5
chromosome 714
circadian rhythm 125, 714
    temperature measurement
        622
Citizen's Charter 220
class see social class
classical conditioning 714
clinical practice
    codes of practice 299–301
    effectiveness of health
        outcomes 239–40
    family-centred care 472–3
    management 244–5
clinical waste 714
codes of practice 299–301
cognitive behaviour therapy 533, 714
    investigation of effectiveness 196
College of Health 220
collusion 714
colonisation 714
colorectal cancer
    dominant gene 131
    genetic deletions 131
    occurrence 130–1
    polyps 131
    role of diet 131
coma, GCS 586, 617–20
commensals 365, 714
commissioning and purchasing
    agencies 112
Committee on Medical Aspects of Food
    Policy (COMA), diet
    recommendations 84–5
communicable disease see infections
communication 149–54
    assessment of interventions 644–7
    compulsive interventions 159
    core qualities 150–1
    cross-cultural 25
    degenerative interventions 158–60
    elderly people 677–8
    enhancement through developing the
        self 153–4
    factors affecting patients 647
    intervention analysis 156–8

key to personal service 255–7
listening skills 280–1
manipulative interventions 159
maternity care 434–5
mental defence mechanisms 161–2
pain assessment 644
patient, useful addresses 226
patient information 219–20
personal growth 152
relatives' dissatisfaction with
    information 467–8
role models 156
skills 280, 677
unskilled interventions 159–60
unsolicited interventions 158–9
Community Care Act (1990) see
    National Health Service and
    Community Care Act (1990)
Community Care Act (1993)
    family-centred care 473–4
    palliative care 694
community health care nursing 6
    areas of specialisms 116–17
    discipline 116
    profiling, caseload analyses 115–16
    see also care in the community
community health councils 214, 220
community health professionals 104
community learning disability
    team 561, 714
community psychiatric nurse
    (CPN) 516
competence 154
complaints, patient 220–2
complement 714
complementary medicine 208–9
    dying patient care 703
    holism 21–2, 123–4, 145, 606–8
compliance with treatment 714
conception of health 19–20, 28, 714
    caring concepts 613
confidentiality 224–5, 303–4
    children 506
    legal and ethical aspects 575
congestive cardiac failure 601, 714
constipation 699
Consultant in Communicable Disease
    Control 388–90
Consultant in Public Health
    Medicine 376
consumer 205, 218, 715
consumer surveys 223
consumerism, principles 217–18
contraception, pre-pregnancy 428
Control of Substances Hazardous to
    Health (COSHH) regulations 381
coping enhancement strategies (CES),
    mental health care 528
core and cue questions 616
coronary heart disease (CHD)
    alcohol's protective effect 93–5
    background information 83–6
    behaviour patterns 195
    cholesterol and dietary fat
        control 84–5

exercise, role of 85–6
Health of the Nation targets 75
high population mean 110
morbidity 84
older people 684
reduction targets 83
risk factors 84, 194–5
self-empowerment approach 83–9
self-empowerment and risk
    factors 86–9
smoking 90
and stress 194–5
type A/type B behaviour
    patterns 195
Western Collaborative Group
    Study 195
in women 49
coroner's court 576
cortisol
    anti-flammatory activity 185
    physiological effects 185
    secretion in acute and chronic
        stress 186–7, 189–90
council tax 702
counselling, in-hospital 192
crackles 715
crisis management 715
Cruse (bereavement) 706,
    710
cultural diversity 701
culture 715
Cumberlege Report 75
Cushing's syndrome 185
cyanosis 127, 715
cystic fibrosis, occurrence 130

daily hassles of life 177–8
data, Office for National Statistics 376
Data Protection Act 303
deamination process 130, 715
death see dying patient care
deep massage 715
defence mechanisms 715
dementia, mental health problems 533
denial 715
deontology 294–5
dependence cycle 671
depersonalisation 715
depolarisation 715
depression
    illness iceberg 48
    serotonin production 137
    social origins 97–8
    therapeutic approaches 135
    women 97
depressive disorders, mental health
    problems 532–3
deprivation index 43
deviance 715
diet
    Committee on Medical Aspects of
        Food Policy (COMA) 85
    decision-making 89
    fat control 84–5
    fatty acids 84–5

diet (*Cont.*)
  Finland 88
  health inequalities 48–50
disability 592–3, 671
  old age 671–2
  WHO definition 26
  see also learning disability
disability living allowance (DLA) 702
discrimination 246, 701
disease prevention, victim-blaming
      approach 74–5
disinfection 715
displacement 715
distress, defined 167, 715
district health authorities 232
district nurses, primary health care 105
DNA, defined 128, 715
DOMINO scheme 437, 715
donor cards, legal and ethical
      aspects 576–7
doula 445, 715
Down's syndrome
  features and characteristics
      547
  learning disability 546–7
drug abusers, A&E department 581
drug use/misuse 408, 581–2
  mental health problems 534
  women's health 402–3
dying patient care 692–709
  A&E department 580–1
  abnormal grief 707
  action at death 705
  advance directives/living wills 576,
      709
  anorexia 698
  attendance allowance 702
  bereavement
      children 707
      nurse's role 706–7
  charities and further help 702–3
  common symptoms 697–9
  community palliative care teams 693
  complementary therapies 703
  constipation 699
  council tax 702
  cultural diversity 701
  day hospices 694
  disability living allowance (DLA) 702
  DSS payments 702
  dyspnoea 699
  effects on nurses 708
  emotional care 699–700
  ethical issues 301–3, 708–9
  evaluation 708
  free prescriptions 702
  funeral arrangements 706
  fungating wounds 699
  hospices 693
  hospital support teams 694
  housing benefit 702
  income support 702
  informed consent 303
  inpatients 693
  last days 301–3, 703–6

MacMillan nurses 693–4
Marie Curie nurses 694
mouth care 698
multi-professional support
      team 694–5
nurse's role 697
organ donation 705–6
physical pain 696–7
registration of death 705
social needs 701–3
spiritual care 701
strategic planning issues 694
total pain philosophy 694–7
      Dame Cicely Saunders
      model 695–6
useful addresses 709–10
WHO three-step analgesic ladder 696
wills 709
Dynamic Standard Setting System,
      standards of care 240
dysfunction, model 327
dysmorphic 715
dyspnoea, dying patient care 699

eating disorders, mental health
      care 535–6
ecomap 716
economics 8–9
eczema care 503–4
effective assessment 263
effector organs or tissues 716
elder abuse 465, 716
elderly people 662–91
  A&E department 578–9
  abuse 579
  accidents 684
  ageing 591
      biographical theories 663–7
      perceptions and definitions 662–3,
      670
      perceptions of world events 664–5
      theoretical studies 666–8
  assessment 678–82
  building relationships 676–8
  cancer 684
  care patterns 680–1
  cellular and genetic aspects of
      ageing 133
  civil rights, responsibilities and
      choices 675–6
  communication 677–8
  dependence cycle 671
  disposable soma theory of ageing 667
  dying and bereavement 684–5
  economic circumstances 669
  environmental care 676
  equipment for A&E room 578
  error catastrophe theory of
      ageing 667
  ethnicity 669–70
  gene expression in ageing 133–4
  health 671–2, 682–4
      and social policy 672–3
  heart disease and stroke 684

history and development of
      nursing 673–4
housing and households 668–9
life experiences and satisfaction 675
lifestyle change 683
Marie Curie nurses 694
movement and mobility 682
nurses' attitudes and
      principles 674–5
pain 339
physical function 681–3
      body temperature
      maintenance 681
      breathing 681, 683
      elimination 681–2, 683
      hydration and nutrition 681, 683
      sexual health 682, 684
present day 668–70
psychological and emotional 681
social functioning 680–1
somatic mutation theory of
      ageing 667
stress theory 184
stroke 684
UK numbers 668
valuing 675
women's health 414–16
  see also palliative care
electrocardiogram (ECG) 628–30, 716
electroconvulsive therapy (ECT) 533
embryological development, tissue
      differentiation 128–9
emergency nurse practitioner
      (ENP) 572–4
emergency situations, A&E
      department 585–7
emotion-focused coping 716
emotional care, dying patient 699–700
emotional functioning, elderly
      people 681
emotional–social competency,
      children 491–2
emphysema 716
empowerment 211, 222, 716
  children 506–9
  defined 82, 222
  patients' control 604–5
  see also self-empowerment
endogenous infection 716
endorphins 141, 351, 716
enemas 699
environment
  genetic expression 137–8
  psychophysiological well-
      being 134–43
Environmental Protection Act
      (1990) 382
enzyme 716
enzyme synthesis 129–30
  gene expression 132
  intracellular metabolic
      homeostasis 131
epicanthic skin folds 716
epidemics 716
epidural analgesia 349–50

equipment
  prevention of infections 380–3, 387
  transmission of infections 369–70
Erikson's eight stages of man 493
Erikson's theory of psychosocial
    development 492
erythema 716
Escherichia coli 0157 infection, case
    study 388
essentially contestable definitions 18
ethical issues 295–8
  advocacy 304–5
  antenatal care 439
  decision-making 301–3
  dying patient care 708–9
  euthanasia 708
  goodness or rightness 296–7
  individual freedom 297–8
  innovative treatments 304
  justice or fairness 297
  models 294–8, 301–3
  morality and nursing 291–308
  natural law 295
  nurses 304–6
  patients 303–4
  response 295
  situation 295
  truth telling or honesty 297
  value of life 295–6, 301–2
  voicing concerns 305–6
ethnicity
  defined 53–4
  and health care 62–4
  and health inequalities 53–60
    artefact explanations 57
    cultural and behavioral
        explanations 57
    material and structural
        explanations 58
    natural selection 53
    racism 58
  and health service employment 63
  mental health care 536
  older people 669–70
  and perinatal mortality 56
  racism and mental health 59–60
  sensitivity 62–3
  SHARE project 64
  women's health 400–1
eugenics 716
eukaryotes 366, 716
Europe
  numbers and employment of
      nurses 8
  population 3, 234
  primary health care 5–6
  wider context 2–3
European Union 2–3
eustress 716
  defined 167
evidence-based care 241–3
evidence-based practice 9, 86, 433
  mental health care 519
executive and general
    managment 245–6

exercise
  elderly people 681
  lack of and health inequalities 48–50
  role in CHD reduction 85–6
exhaustion 716
exogenous infection 716
experiential 716
extra-contractual referrals (ECRs) 219

facilitative nursing
  vs authoritative 330–2, 522, 716
  relationship to functions and personal
      awareness 335
false positives 716
family 716
  cultural differences 465
  interventions, mental health care 529
  lay referral system 460
  and motherhood 403–5
  relatives' dissatisfaction with
      information 467–8
  as unit 457–8, 716
family-centred care 457–77, 505–6, 716
  compliance with treatment 460
  illness effects 461–9
  implications of practice 472–4
  involvement and needs of
      relatives 460–1, 465–7
  learned behaviour 459
  model 470–1
  in practice 469–71
  professional commitment 473
  reordered families 461
fat, CIMA recommendations 85
fat in diet 424
father, role 444–5
fatty acids 84–5, 717
feminism 36–7
fertility treatment 404–5
fetal development, tissue
    differentiation 128–9
fight or flight response 182–3, 190
Finland, diet study 88
first level assessment 616–17
first line care 565–89
  A&E organization 566, 568–70
  abuse
    children 578
    elderly patients 579
  addresses 587
  advanced trauma life support
      (ATLS) 585–6
  aggression and violence 583–4
    self-defence 584
  alcohol abusers 581
  ambulance personnel 569–70
  children's needs 577–8
  death of patient 580–1
  drug use/misuse 402–3, 408, 534,
      581–2
  elderly patients 578–9
  emergency nurse practitioner 572–4
  emergency situations 585–7
  hospital staff 569
  legal and ethical aspects 574–7

major incident preparation 586
minor injury units (MIU) 566–7
nursing scope 570–1
police force 570
pre-hospital care 567–8
primary health care team 570
problem patients 581–4
reception of patients 571–2
relatives and friends 579–81
resuscitation 585
  witnessed resuscitation 579–80
solvent abusers 581–2
staff stress 584–5
team working 569
trauma centres 567–8
triage and initial assessment 572–3
vagrants 582
folic acid 423–4
fomites 717
food
  consumption changes, government
      targets 85
  and exercise, attitudes 87–8
  nutritional groups 424
  transmission of infections
      370
  see also diet; nutrition
food manufacturers, advertising
    power 49
forensic mental nursing 534–5
formula feeding 449–50
free radicals 133, 717
full employment 717
functionalism 37
fundholding, primary health
    care 113–14
funding health care 233–4
  key points 234
funeral arrangements 706
fungi 366, 717

gastroenteritis, outbreak
    390
gate control theory of pain 141–2, 338,
    717
  higher centre descending
      control 141–2
  sensory neuron balance of
      activity 141
gender and health see women's health
gene expression 128–34
  ageing process 133–4
  dominant genes 715
  homeostasis and health link 129–31
  human development link 131–3
gene–environment (nature–nurture)
    interactions 134–9
  sensory perceptions 139–43
general adaptation syndrome (GAS)
  physiological responses 181, 189–90
  significance 181–2
general household survey (GHS) 671–2
general practice 233
  common goal 115
  nursing in primary health care 105–6

general practitioners
  contract 109
  fundholding 113–14
  primary health care 104–6
  trusts 233
genes 717
  the *Code of Life* 128–34
  dominant 715
  role 128–9
  synapse function 136
genetic code 717
genetic deletions 717
  colorectal cancer 131
genogram 649, 717
genotype 128
gestalt 717
Gillick competency ruling 506, 717
Glasgow Coma Scale 617–20, 717
  advanced trauma life support
    (ATLS) 586
  stimulation effects 618
global health status indices 115
glossary 712–25
glucocorticoid secretion
  control 185
  physiological effects 186
glucose, urine testing 639
glycogen 130
gonadotropin-releasing
    hormones 132–3, 717
goodness or rightness principle 296–7
Gram staining (bacteria) 366,
    717
grief, model 706–7
growth 717
growth-promoting aspects of
    function 326
*Guide to Consent for Examination or
    Treatment* 303
Guidelines for Professional Practice 300–1
  accountability 306

habituation/addiction 91, 94, 712
haematocrit 641
haemoglobin levels, blood 641
handicap, WHO definition 26
hands, transmission of infections 369
handwashing 378–9, 387
Harding Committee 114
Hassles Scale 177
health
  conceptions 19–20
  definition and measurement 18–19,
    27–9, 38–9, 151–2
  global health status indices 115
  and illness, concepts 205–6
  and individual responsibility,
    affecting factors 110–11
  philosophy 17–34
  WHO definition 22, 26, 206
  see also primary health care
Health Advisory Service (HAS) 535
Health Belief Model 87
health care assistants 12–13
health conceptions, WHO definition 22,

26, 28, 206
Health Divide 40, 110
  social class inequality
    explanations 47–52
health education, vs health
    promotion 72–3
health inequalities
  addressing 64–5
  artefact explanation 41–2, 57
  Black Report 40, 41
  cultural/behavioural
    explanations 42–3, 57–8
  explanations 41–6, 57–9
  health gap 3
  materialist/structuralist
    explanations 43–5, 58
  natural selection theories 57
  natural and social selection 42
  racism 58–9
  social support 45–6
  unemployment 43–4
  see also ethnicity; women's health
Health of the Nation 5, 232, 604–5
  nutrition recommendations 423
  poverty 110
  priority areas 111
  strategy 74–5
  targets 75, 206–7
    alcohol consumption reduction
      targets 93
    mental health care 75, 96–7
health needs assessment 116
  community health profiling 115–16
health promotion 71–102,
    206–7
  Alma-Ata Declaration 5, 74, 106–7
  challenges 75–82
  key points 75
  nursing 72–5
  perceptions 73
  preventive health care 108–10
  radical approach 92–8
  self-empowerment approach 82–92
  vs health education 72–3
  WHO principles 72
  WHO views 74
Health and Safety at Work Act 45, 380
health screening *see* screening
health services
  current shape 231–4
  leadership 234–44
  quality 239–43
  management 231–50
  reforms 212
    key points 212
health and social care
  elderly people 671–3, 682–4
  learning disability 543–6
  management 543–4
health status 645–6, 648
health visitors
  Nurses, Midwives and Health
    Visitors Rules Approval
    Order 270
  primary health care 105

health-damaging behaviours 80–1, 110
healthy alliances 717
heart disease and stroke, elderly
    people 684
heat treatment, decontamination 381
Heron's Six Category Intervention
    Analysis 522
high populaton mean 717
historical perspectives
  child health care 498–500
  development, nursing practice 673–4
  infections 364
  mental health 516–17
  nursing elderly people
    673–4
  women's health 399–400
HIV/AIDS, *Health of the Nation*
    targets 75, 76
holism 606–8, 612–13, 718
  complementary medicine 21–2,
    123–4, 145, 606–8
  conceptions 21–2, 124
  defined 123–4
  Florence Nightingale's concept 73,
    606
  interactional model 145
home care 118
homelessness
  health inequalites 44–5
  healthcare 61
homeopathic hospitals 209
homeostasis 122–48, 718
  assessment and nursing
    diagnosis 127–8
  control 126
  control theory 125–6
  defined 125
  enzyme production and
    inhibition 131
  gene expression link 129–31
  health and ill health link 125–8
  ill health 126–7
  nursing process 128
  principles in clinical practice: the
    nursing process 127–8
  process scheme 127
  systems theory, integration
    model 143–5
hormone replacement therapy 411, 412
hospices, dying patient care 693–4
hospital care 611–57
  assessment of interventions 615–56
  patient-focused hosptials 211
  see also Burford Nursing
    Development Unit (NDU) model;
    patients(s)
hospital closures 117–18
hospital stress rating scale 180
hospital-associated infections 373–6,
    718
  prevention 377–84
housing
  elderly people 668–9
  social class and health
    inequalities 44–5, 97

housing benefit 702
housing tenure 46, 718
human development, gene expression link 131–3
human papillomavirus 410
hydration, elderly people 681
hyperlipidaemia 138
hyperpyrexia 623–4
hypertension 630–1
  screening programme 80
hyperthermia 623–4
hypnosis 209
hypotension 629
hypothalamus, physiological stress responses 182
hypothermia 624
hypovolaemic shock 718
hypoxia, hypoxaemia 127, 638, 718

idealisation 718
ill health, assessment 29–32
illness iceberg 718
immune reponse 372, 374
  lymphocytes 372–3, 719
immune system, and stress 196–8
immunisation 718
  GP targets 79
  health inequalities 80
  informed decisions 79
  policies 78
  promotion 77–9
  schedule 385
immunodeficiency 718
impairment, WHO definition 26
incidence 718
income, social class and health inequalities 44, 92
income support 702, 718
  poverty indicator 39
incompetence 154
independent health sector 7
individual freedom principle 297–8
individual programme planning (IPP) 718
individualised patient care (IPC) 257–9
individuality, nature 257–9
Industrial Revolution 499
infants see children; neonates
infection control team 275–6
infections 363–95, 718
  defences 371–3
  endogenous 716
  exogenous 716
  history 364
  hospital-associated 373–6
  management 385–91
    isolation 385–8
  outbreaks 388–90
  prevention 377–84
    education and training 390–1
    equipment 380–3, 387
    handwashing 369, 378–9, 387
    protective clothing 379–80
    universal precautions 378
  reproductive tract 409–11

routes of transmission 367–71
susceptible patient 383–4
wounds 383–4
inflammatory reponse 372–3, 718
informatics 243–4
information
  patient 219–20
    useful addresses 226
  see also communication
informed consent 303
  legal and ethical aspects 574
innovative treatments, ethical issues 304
insects, transmission of infections 370
Integrated Care Management 242–3
integrated science
  clinical interventions and health education 125
  defined 123–4
  health and illness 124
internal market system, National Health Service 112–13
interpersonal relationships 264–6
  models 264–6
    aims 265
    definitions and meanings 265
    theories 266
interpretative skills 281–2
interventional analysis
  authoritative 156
    informative 157
  communication 156–8
  compulsive 159
  creating a workable synthesis 333–6
  facilitative, catalytic/cathartic 157–8
  Heron's six categories 331
  manipulative 159
  unnecessary 9
  unskilled 159–60
  unsolicited 158–9
  see also nursing practice
interviewing 521–2
intuition 718
involutional melancholia 718
iron, and metabolism 406, 407
ischaemic heart disease 719
isolation, management of infections 385–8

jaundice 719
justice of fairness principle 297

ketones, urine testing 639
key nurse theorists 264
King's Fund
  nursing records 270–1
  Organisational Audit 240
Klinefelter's syndrome, gene expression 132, 719
knowledge, defined 261
Korner Reports, informatics 243–4

labelling theory 719
labour and delivery 441–4, 719

Ladies' Sanitary Reform Association of Manchester and Salford 105
language development, children 480–1
LAS (local adaptation syndromes) 187
lay referral 719
LCU (life change units) 174
leadership components 235–9
  accountability 235–6
  authority 235
  interpersonal skills 236–7
  responsibility 236
  values clarification 237–9
learned helplessness, Seligman's theory 192, 719
learning cycle
  conscious competence/incompetence 154
  unconscious competence/incompetence 154–5
learning disability 540–64
  behavioural approaches 560–1
  behavioural shaping 560–1
  Bereweeke teaching system 560, 713
  biological causes 546–8
  care in the community 551–2
  care context 542–3
  definition 541–2
  generic health care services 562
  health and social care 543–6
  individual programme planning (IPP) 557–8
  instrumental nursing interventions 545
  interperonal nursing interventions 545
  interpersonal and scientific aspects 560
  intervention strategies 559
  maintenance of lifestyles 553–5
  multi-agency care 561–2
  nursing care 556–9
  nursing models 559
  nursing skills 544–6
  organisational nursing interventions 545–6
  philosophy of care 552–3
  prenatal and natal factors 549
  prevention and intervention 549–50
  responsibilities of NHS and social services 550–2
  rights
    advocacy and representation 555
    choice 554
    dignity and respect 554
    employment and leisure 554–5
    home ownership 554
    independence 555
    personal and sexual relationships 555
    to make mistakes 555
  risk taking 558–9
  social factors 549
  statement of principal entitlements and services 553
  views of service users 555–6

learning disability (*Cont.*)
  work practices and
    opportunities 554–5
legal and ethical aspects 217
  child health care 506
  confidentiality 575
  coroner 576
  donor cards 576–7
  first line care 574–7
  informed consent 574
  informing the police 575–6
  mental health care 530–1
  nursing notes 575
  patients' property 575
  refusal of treatment 574–5
  wills 576
Leininger's model of child
    nursing 487–8
life, value of life principle 295–6
life change units (LCU) 174
lifestyle change, elderly people 683
lifestyle diseases 110
lipoproteins 84, 138, 719
listening skills 280–1
living wills 576, 709
local adaptation syndromes (LAS) 181
local population, health needs
    assessment and sources of
    information 116
locus of control 719
log-rolling 719
London, mental health care 518
lone parent families 51
Luer lock 719
lung cancer
  death rates 90
  smoking relationship 90
lymphocytes 372–3, 713

MacMillan nurse 693–4
major incidents 586–7
makaton 719
Managed Care 242
management
  care management 713
  clinical practice 244–5
  executive and general
    management 245–6
  future 247–8
  health and social care 543–4
  Integrated Care Management 242–3
  interface with organisation
    management 244–6
  primary health care 230–50
Marie Curie nurse 694
Marxism 36
massage 209
materialism vs care skills 15
maternity care 403–5, 421–56
  antenatal care 436–41
    place of birth 436–8
    screening and diagnostic
      tests 438–40
  care of newborn 445–50
  communication 434–5

continuity of care 433–6
control 435–6
dissatisfaction 430
DOMINO scheme 437
empowerment 430
labour and delivery 441–4
models of childbirth 430–1
nutrition 422–5
postnatal care 444–5
pre-pregnancy care 421–9
requirements 433
rights of women 215–16
useful addresses 451–2
MEAC 719
medical model 719
medicalisation 719
Mencap 219
menopause 399, 412–14
menstruation 398–9, 406
mental defence mechanisms 161–2
mental health, definition 520
mental health care 216–17, 515–37
  anxiety 532
  care programme approach (CPA) 530
  case management 529–30
  child and adolescent 535
  collaboration with other professionals
    and agencies 519
  contemporary nursing values 518–20
  coping enhancement strategies
    (CES) 528
  dementia 533
  depressive disorders 532–3
  differentiation from psychiatric
    care 516
  eating disorders 535–6
  ethnicity 536
  ethnicity, racism and mental
    health 59–60
  evidence-based practice 519
  forensic nursing 534–5
  Health of the Nation targets 75, 96–7
  health promotion 96–8
  history and development 516–18
  incident and description 531–3
  interviewing 521–2
  legal issues 530–1
    care programme approach
      (CPA) 530
    Mental Health (Patients in the
      Community) Act (1995) 530–1
    supervision registers 530–1
  nature–nurture interactions 135–7
  nurse/client relationship 519
  nursing skills 520–3
  observation and data collection 521
  organization and delivery 529–30
  Patients' Charter 520
  privacy and dignity promotion
    520
  prodromal monitoring 528
  psychosocial interventions and
    support 527–9
  public attitudes 518
  research findings 56

risk assessment and
    management 522–3
schizophrenia 523–7
  symptoms 524
severe and enduring mental illness
    (SMI) 523–7
  clinical care 525–7
  collaborative assessment 525–7
  initial nursing goals 525, 527
social determinants 97–8
specific problem groups 534
Spectrum of Care 517
stress reduction 528
substance misuse 534
women's health issues 52–3, 399–400
mental health nurse 516
Mental Health Nursing Review Team
    (1994) 520–1
Mental Health (Patients in the
    Community) Act (1995) 530–1
mental hospitals 517
metabolism 719
microbiology *see* bacteria
midwifery care 215–16
  Nurses, Midwives and Health
    Visitors Rules Approval
    Order 270
  WHO on 3
Midwives' Information and Resource
    Service 432–3
millennium
  challenges and issues 117–19
  WHO health care goals 117
MIND 216, 219
mind–body interactions 144
minor injury units (MIU), first line
    care 566–7
mistakes, learning process 158–60
mitochondria 719
mitochondrial DNA 719
mobile team 568
mobility, elderly people 682
models of nursing 260–9
  see also Burford NDE model
Monitor, standards of care 240
morbidity rate measurement 38–9,
    719
mortality, age-adjusted and
    standardised overall health
    levels 106
mortality rate measurement 38, 719
  standardised mortality ratio 40
mortality ratios 40, 712, 723
morula 720
mosaicism 546
mouth care, dying patient 698
mRNA 130
MRSA (methicillin resistant
    Staphylococcus aureus) 367–8
multipara 720
Munchausen's syndrome 582
Myers Briggs Type Indicator
    (MBTI) 291
myocardial infarction 720
  pain perception 140